# DIAGNOSIS OF BONE AND JOINT DISORDERS

VOLUME 1

3rd
Edition

# DIAGNOSIS OF BONE AND JOINT DISORDERS

## Donald Resnick, M.D.

Professor of Radiology
University of California, San Diego
Chief of Osteoradiology Section
Veterans Administration Medical Center
San Diego, California

*With the Editorial Assistance of Catherine F. Fix*
*With the Technical Assistance of Debra J. Trudell*

## W.B. SAUNDERS COMPANY

*A Division of Harcourt Brace & Company*
Philadelphia    London    Toronto    Montreal    Sydney    Tokyo

**W.B. SAUNDERS COMPANY**
*A Division of*
*Harcourt Brace & Company*

The Curtis Center
Independence Square West
Philadelphia, Pennsylvania 19106

### Library of Congress Cataloging-in-Publication Data

Resnick, Donald

Diagnosis of bone and joint disorders / Donald Resnick.—3rd ed.

p.   cm.

Includes bibliographical references and indexes.

ISBN 0–7216–5066–X (set)

1. Musculoskeletal system—Diseases—Diagnosis.   2. Bones—Diseases—
Diagnosis.   3. Joints—Diseases—Diagnosis.   4. Diagnostic
imaging.   I. Title.

[DNLM: 1. Bone Diseases—diagnosis.   2. Joint Diseases—diagnosis.
3. Diagnosis Imaging.   WE 300 R434d 1995]

RC925.7.R47 1995

616.7′1075—dc20

DNLM/DLC                                                           93–48321

Diagnosis of Bone and Joint Disorders, 3rd edition

| | |
|---|---|
| Volume One | ISBN 0–7216–5067–8 |
| Volume Two | ISBN 0–7216–5068–6 |
| Volume Three | ISBN 0–7216–5069–4 |
| Volume Four | ISBN 0–7216–5070–8 |
| Volume Five | ISBN 0–7216–5071–6 |
| Volume Six | ISBN 0–7216–5072–4 |
| Six Volume Set | ISBN 0–7216–5066–X |

Printed in the United States of America.

Last digit is the print number:     9     8     7     6     5     4     3     2     1

## DEDICATION

*Once again, to my father who illuminated my first viewbox
and with it my mind, and to my mother, bless her, who
made certain the lights were off when we left the room.*

# CONTRIBUTORS

WAYNE H. AKESON, M.D.
Professor and Chairman, Department of Orthopaedics, University of California at San Diego, San Diego, California
*Articular Cartilage Physiology and Metabolism*

NAOMI ALAZRAKI, M.D.
Professor of Radiology, Co-Director, Division of Nuclear Medicine, Emory University and Affiliated Hospitals, Atlanta, Georgia
*Radionuclide Techniques*

DAVID AMIEL, Ph.D.
Professor of Orthopaedics, University of California at San Diego, San Diego, California
*Articular Cartilage Physiology and Metabolism*

MICHAEL ANDRÉ, Ph.D.
Associate Professor of Radiology and Chief, Physics and Engineering Division, University of California School of Medicine; Medical Physicist, Veterans Affairs Medical Center, San Diego, California
*Xeroradiography; Computed Tomography*

JOSEPH J. BOOKSTEIN, M.D.
Professor of Radiology, Emeritus, University of California at San Diego, San Diego, California
*Angiography*

RICHARD B. BUXTON, Ph.D.
Associate Professor of Radiology, University of California at San Diego; Director of Magnetic Resonance Research, UCSD Medical Center, San Diego, California
*Magnetic Resonance Imaging: Technical Considerations*

MURRAY K. DALINKA, M.D.
Professor of Radiology and Orthopedic Surgery, University of Pennsylvania Medical School; Chief, Musculoskeletal and Emergency Room Radiology, Hospital of the University of Pennsylvania, Philadelphia, Pennsylvania
*Radiation Changes*

MICHAEL D. FALLON, M.D.
Former Assistant Professor of Pathology, University of Pennsylvania School of Medicine, Philadelphia, Pennsylvania
*deceased
*Histogenesis, Anatomy, and Physiology of Bone*

FRIEDA FELDMAN, M.D.
Professor of Radiology and Orthopedic Surgery and Attending Radiologist, Columbia University College of Physicians and Surgeons, New York, New York
*Tuberous Sclerosis, Neurofibromatosis, and Fibrous Dysplasia*

ERICH FISCHER, M.D.
Professor of Radiology, University of Tübingen, Federal Republic of Germany; Robert Bosch Krankenhaus D 7000, Stuttgart, Federal Republic of Germany
*Low Kilovolt Radiography*

STEVEN R. GARFIN, M.D.
Professor of Orthopaedic Surgery, University of California at San Diego, UCSD Medical Center, San Diego, California
*Imaging After Spine Surgery*

HARRY K. GENANT, M.D.
Professor of Radiology, Medicine, and Orthopaedic Surgery; Chief, Musculoskeletal Section, and Director, Osteoporosis Research Group, Department of Radiology, School of Medicine, University of California, San Francisco, California
*Magnification Radiography; Xeroradiography; Quantitative Bone Mineral Analysis*

DAVID H. GERSHUNI, M.D., F.R.C.S.
Professor of Orthopaedic Surgery, University of California at San Diego, San Diego; Chief of Orthopaedic Surgery, Veterans Administration Medical Center, La Jolla, California
*Articular Cartilage Physiology and Metabolism*

THOMAS G. GOERGEN, M.D., F.A.C.R.
Associate Clinical Professor of Radiology, University of California at San Diego; Staff Radiologist, Palomar Medical Center, San Diego, California
*Physical Injury: Concepts and Terminology; Physical Injury: Extraspinal Sites*

AMY BETH GOLDMAN, M.D.
Professor of Radiology, Cornell University Medical College; Attending Radiologist, The Hospital for Special Surgery, New York, New York
*Heritable Diseases of Connective Tissue, Epiphyseal Dysplasias, and Related Conditions*

**GUERDON D. GREENWAY, M.D.**
Associate Clinical Professor, Department of Radiology, University of California at San Diego School of Medicine, San Diego, California; Clinical Associate Professor, Department of Orthopaedic Surgery, University of Texas Southwestern Medical Center at Dallas; Attending Radiologist, Baylor University Medical Center, Dallas, Texas
*Tumors and Tumor-Like Lesions of Bone: Imaging and Pathology of Specific Lesions*

**PARVIZ HAGHIGHI, M.D., F.R.C.P.A.**
Clinical Professor, Department of Pathology, University of California at San Diego; Staff Pathologist, Department of Veterans Affairs Medical Center, San Diego, California
*Myeloproliferative Disorders*

**VICTOR HAUGHTON, M.D.**
Professor of Radiology and Biophysics, Froedtert Memorial Lutheran Hospital and John L. Doyne Hospital, Milwaukee, Wisconsin
*Imaging Techniques in Intraspinal Diseases*

**TAMARA MINER HAYGOOD, Ph.D., M.D.**
Assistant Professor of Radiology, Department of Radiology, Bowman Gray School of Medicine; Staff Radiologist, North Carolina Baptist Hospital, Winston-Salem, North Carolina
*Radiation Changes*

**THOMAS E. HERMAN, M.D.**
Assistant Professor, Mallinckrodt Institute of Radiology, Washington University School of Medicine; Radiologist, St. Louis Children's Hospital, St. Louis, Missouri
*Osteochondrodysplasias, Dysostoses, Chromosomal Aberrations, Mucopolysaccharidoses, and Mucolipidoses*

**MICHAEL JERGAS, M.D.**
Visiting Researcher, Department of Radiology, Musculoskeletal Section, and Osteoporosis Research Group, University of California at San Francisco, San Francisco, California
*Quantitative Bone Mineral Analysis*

**PHOEBE A. KAPLAN, M.D.**
Professor of Radiology and Orthopedics and Co-Director, Musculoskeletal Imaging, University of Virginia Health Sciences Center, Charlottesville, Virginia
*Temporomandibular Joint*

**THEODORE E. KEATS**
Professor of Radiology and Orthopedics, University of Virginia School of Medicine; Radiologist, University of Virginia Health Sciences Center, Charlottesville, Virginia
*Plain Film Radiography: Sources of Diagnostic Errors*

**MICHAEL KYRIAKOS, M.D.**
Professor of Surgical Pathology, Washington University School of Medicine; Pathologist, Barnes Hospital, St. Louis, Missouri
*Tumors and Tumor-Like Lesions of Bone: Imaging and Pathology of Specific Lesions*

**LAURENCE A. MACK, M.D.**
Professor of Radiology, Adjunct Professor of Orthopedics, and Director of Ultrasound, University of Washington, Seattle, Washington
*Diagnostic Ultrasonography*

**JOHN E. MADEWELL, M.D.**
Professor and Chair, Department of Radiology, Penn State University, College of Medicine, The Milton S. Hershey Medical Center, Hershey, Pennsylvania
*Osteonecrosis: Pathogenesis; Tumors and Tumor-Like Lesions in or about Joints*

**STAVROS C. MANOLAGAS, M.D., Ph.D.**
Professor of Medicine and Director, Division of Endocrinology and Metabolism, University of Arkansas for Medical Sciences, Little Rock, Arkansas
*Histogenesis, Anatomy, and Physiology of Bone*

**WILLIAM H. McALISTER, M.D.**
Professor of Radiology and Pediatrics, Washington University School of Medicine and Mallinckrodt Institute of Radiology; Radiologist-in-Chief, Barnes, Jewish, and Shriners Hospitals, St. Louis, Missouri
*Osteochondrodysplasias, Dysostoses, Chromosomal Aberrations, Mucopolysaccharidoses, and Mucolipidoses*

**KEVIN W. McENERY, M.D.**
Assistant Professor of Radiology, Washington University School of Medicine and Mallinckrodt Institute of Radiology; Attending Radiologist, Barnes and Jewish Hospitals and Consulting Radiologist, St. Louis Children's Hospital, St. Louis, Missouri
*Magnetic Resonance Imaging: Practical Considerations*

**WILLIAM A. MURPHY, Jr., M.D.**
Professor and John S. Dunn, Sr., Chair and Head, Division of Diagnostic Imaging, University of Texas M.D. Anderson Cancer Center; Professor and Vice-Chairman, Department of Radiology, University of Texas School of Medicine, Houston, Texas
*Magnetic Resonance Imaging: Practical Considerations; Temporomandibular Joint*

**GEN NIWAYAMA, M.D., D.Med.Sc.***
Former Director, Autopsy Division, Department of Pathology, Brotman Medical Center, Culver City, California
**deceased*

**M. B. OZONOFF, M.D.**
Clinical Professor of Radiology, University of Connecticut School of Medicine; Senior Attending Radiologist, Newington Children's Hospital, Newington and Hartford Hospital, Hartford, Connecticut; Distinguished Scientist, Armed Forces Institute of Pathology, Washington, D.C.
*Spinal Anomalies and Curvatures*

**MINI N. PATHRIA, M.D., F.R.C.P.(C)**
Associate Professor of Radiology, University of California at San Diego, UCSD Medical Center, San Diego, California
*Imaging After Spine Surgery; Physical Injury: Spine*

**HELENE PAVLOV, M.D., F.A.C.R.**
Professor of Radiology, Cornell University Medical College; Attending Radiologist, Hospital for Special Surgery and New York Hospital, New York, New York
*Physical Injury: Sports Related Abnormalities*

**MICHAEL J. PITT, M.D.**
Professor of Radiology, University of Alabama at Birmingham; Staff, University Hospital, UAB Children's Hospital of Alabama, Birmingham, Alabama
*Rickets and Osteomalacia*

**DAVID J. SARTORIS, M.D.**
Professor of Radiology, University of California at San Diego; Chief, Quantitative Bone Densitometry, UCSD Medical Center; Professor of Radiology, VA Medical Center and Scripps Clinic, Green Hospital, La Jolla, California
*Plain Film Radiography: Routine and Specialized Techniques and Projections; Developmental Dysplasia of the Hip*

**WILLIAM SCHEIBLE, M.D.**
Radiologist, Portland Adventist Medical Center, Portland, Oregon
*Diagnostic Ultrasonography*

**DONALD E. SWEET, M.D.**
Chairman and Registrar, Department of Orthopedic Pathology, Armed Forces Institute of Pathology, Washington, D.C.
*Osteonecrosis: Pathogenesis; Tumors and Tumor-Like Lesions in or about Joints*

**ROBERT G. VOLZ, M.D.**
Lifetime Surgical Director, Arizona Arthritis Center, Arizona Health Sciences Center, Tucson, Arizona
*Basic Biomechanics*

**BARBARA N. WEISSMAN, M.D.**
Professor of Radiology, Harvard Medical School, Cambridge; Chief, Musculoskeletal Radiology Section and Assistant Chief for Ambulatory Services, Department of Radiology, Brigham and Women's Hospital, Boston, Massachusetts
*Imaging After Surgery in Extraspinal Sites; Imaging of Joint Replacement*

# PREFACE

▼

*Perceive the radiograph as but a mirror and its image a reflection of human anatomy and its modification by disease. Learn the anatomy and the reflection becomes that much clearer. Understand the disease and the perceived image takes on even deeper meaning.*

It has been said that an author's life might be better measured not in years but in editions, and now, as I write the Preface to this textbook, this saying takes on new meaning to me. As with the earlier edition, seven years have elapsed since the publication of the previous version, and as before, dramatic changes have occurred in the field of diagnostic radiology that make this new edition necessary. Foremost among these changes has been the further refinement of magnetic resonance (MR) imaging. This imaging method, above all others, displays human anatomy and its modification caused by disease. It does so through a series of sectional images, obtainable with countless variations in orientation and thickness. The images are made more vivid because of differences in contrast among the tissues that are governed by the choice of imaging parameters and pulse sequences and, in some cases, by the use of contrast media. To the observer, the MR imaging data at first may be perceived as overwhelming and impossible to master, but with time, patterns emerge that are recognized and interpreted correctly. Fundamental to accurate interpretation is knowledge of pertinent anatomy and of the pathology and pathophysiology of disease processes. Attempting to interpret MR images (or, for that matter, images derived from other techniques) without such knowledge leads to both missed diagnosis and misdiagnosis.

Owing to improvements in technology and changing concepts of disease, major modifications in organization, scope, and emphasis were required for this edition. Specifically, great emphasis is given to the expanded role of MR imaging in the assessment of musculoskeletal disorders. To this end, two chapters (Chapters 9 and 10) addressing the technical aspects of this imaging method are provided in Volume 1. Another chapter (Chapter 70, itself the size of a small book!) describes in detail the important applications of MR imaging to the evaluation of internal derangements of the major joints of the peripheral skeleton and, most importantly, places these applications into proper perspective by also including information on alternative techniques such as arthrography and computed tomography (CT). To further emphasize the important role played by MR imaging in the analysis of musculoskeletal trauma, individual chapters (Chapters 67, 68, 69, and 71) describe in great detail physical injuries of spinal and extraspinal sites as well as sports related injuries. Furthermore, throughout this textbook, in discussions of individual diseases, new emphasis is placed on the diagnostic value of MR imaging and CT scanning.

In no other specialty of medicine does the quality of the illustrated material have greater importance. Many of the less than optimal illustrations from the previous edition have been eliminated and the remaining ones often have been recropped and, in some instances, rephotographed. To these are added more than 3,000 new illustrations, the majority of them MR images. Each illustration has been carefully chosen, photographed, labeled, cropped, and oriented and each is accompanied by a detailed yet easy to read legend that, in the case of MR images, includes precise information on technical factors. The lists of references and the index are both complete and thorough. The references at the end of each chapter have been expanded by approximately 25 per cent, the vast majority of them being recent publications.

Once again, I have turned to authorities in the field of musculoskeletal imaging to provide valuable contributions to this textbook. Many have contributed to earlier editions of this work, whereas some present material for the first time. Their contributions speak to the expertise, energy, and enthusiasm that make them leaders in the field.

It is hoped that this textbook will serve as a reference for professionals involved in the interpretation of images of the musculoskeletal system. It is further hoped that the material contained herein will make the perceived images clearer and also easier to understand. Therein lies the real purpose of this work.

DONALD RESNICK, M.D.

# ACKNOWLEDGMENTS

▼

The success of any work, including this one, is related in large part to the contributions of others. Although my words may prove inadequate, I greatly appreciate the efforts of the many persons who have made this textbook possible. First, I wish to express my gratitude to the contributors of the various chapters who have given unselfishly of their time and energy, adhering to the strict deadlines that were imposed. Without their efforts, this textbook certainly would not have been possible.

A successful book requires close cooperation between the author (or editor) and the publisher. In this regard, I am fortunate to have chosen the W.B. Saunders Company and to have surrounded myself with a publishing team guided by high professional standards. Lisette Bralow, Vice President, Editor-in-Chief, Medical Books, who has been involved with this project for more than a decade (almost since its inception in 1978), served as my advisor and friend. The fact that she was only a phone call away gave me the fortitude that was needed on more than one occasion. Others, including Jacqui Brownstein, the Production Manager; Walt Verbitski, the Illustration Specialist; David Harvey, the Copy Editor; Joan Wendt, the Designer; and Susan Thomas, Roger Wall, and Mark Coyle, the Indexers, were of considerable help to me during the more than two years of preparation and production of this edition. To these persons, I offer my gratitude.

Throughout this work, within the legends of the illustrations, acknowledgment is given to the many physicians who shared their material with me. Their contributions were essential and I express my deep and sincere thanks. Among these persons, I would like to mention several whose contributions were extraordinary, well beyond the "call of duty." To Sevil Kursunoglu Brahme, Thomas Broderick, Anne Brower, Murray Dalinka, Steven Eilenberg, Arthur Newberg, Mini Pathria, and Mark Schweitzer, my thanks hardly seem sufficient. The contributions of Guerdon Greenway, a former colleague of mine, who has contributed scores of cases, must be singled out. Without his material, large gaps would have existed in this textbook. I deeply appreciate his energy and enthusiasm. Susan Brown was of great assistance in coordinating the illustrative material.

Finally, I must acknowledge the extraordinary efforts of three persons, two of whom have worked with me on previous editions of this textbook. To Michael Holbrook, my secretary, who was new to the task, I wish to express my deep appreciation for the dedication that he displayed. Debra Trudell, who has served as my laboratory assistant for more than twelve years, was instrumental in the preparation of most of the new illustrations that are contained in this edition; without her, this textbook would not have been possible. Finally, as before, I must acknowledge the assistance of Catherine Fix, an editor and a friend, who now has survived the preparation of three editions of this textbook. She has read and reread each sentence on each page, every table and legend, and she has done so without complaint and with patience, understanding, and incredible expertise. She has taught me more than anyone else the value of the written word, particularly when expressed in a clear (and grammatically correct) fashion.

# PREFACE TO THE SECOND EDITION

*It is often said or implied that, in our profession, a man cannot be both practical and scientific; science and practice seem to some people to be incompatible. Each man, they say, must devote himself to the one or the other. The like of this has long been said, and it is sheer nonsense.*

Sir James Paget, 1894

In the seven years that have elapsed since the publication of the first edition of this textbook, the specialties of diagnostic radiology and diagnostic osteoradiology have undergone dramatic change. In large part, such change has related to the introduction of new imaging methods, such as magnetic resonance, and the refinement of others, such as computed tomography. Indeed, the evaluation of many musculoskeletal disorders can now be likened to the construction of a building, with the conventional radiographic examination representing the cornerstone and other imaging methods representing the framework or scaffolding upon which the final edifice takes shape. To provide a solid foundation in diagnosis, however, the interpreter of the imaging studies must be cognizant of his or her responsibility to know or learn the pertinent anatomy and to understand fully the pathology and pathophysiology of the disease process. In this responsibility, the newer imaging methods afford both a unique challenge and a splendid opportunity. The transaxial display of computed tomography, for example, sorely tests the diagnostic acumen of the observer, requiring a thorough comprehension of cross-sectional anatomy so that the alterations produced by disease are recognized and interpreted correctly. Similarly, the signals derived from magnetic resonance imaging require knowledge of the biochemical composition and environment of normal and abnormal tissues for proper interpretation. Both techniques, however, disclose information that was previously difficult or impossible to obtain. As in the first edition, therefore, it is the purpose of this textbook to give new meaning to the perception of these diagnostic images by providing a comprehensive description of the anatomy and physiology of the musculoskeletal system and of the pathologic aberrations that accompany its disorders.

This second edition differs considerably in scope from its predecessor. The subtitle of the first edition, "With Emphasis on Articular Abnormalities," has been eliminated because equal attention is now given to osseous and soft tissue abnormalities as well. To accomplish this, it has been necessary to expand the size of the text significantly. By "tightening" the manner in which the information is displayed (publishing terminology that translates into an elimination of free or unused space), however, it was possible to add considerably more information without greatly exceeding the page count of the first edition. Many of the chapters have been revised completely, additional ones appear for the first time, and a few have been eliminated. Chapters concerned with computed tomography, physical trauma, bone dysplasias, and tumors and tumor-like lesions of bone have been expanded dramatically, and those dealing with magnetic resonance imaging, histomorphology of bone, spinal anomalies and curvatures, as well as other topics, are offered for the first time. As in the first edition, close radiographic-pathologic correlation represents the fundamental method by which each disease is examined, although throughout, the reflection of the pathology in the image displays derived from computed tomography, magnetic resonance, scintigraphy, and additional techniques is illustrated. As in the first edition, contributing authors, each known for his or her expertise in the field of musculoskeletal disease, provide the substance essential to a full understanding of the disease process.

Once again, great care has been exercised in the choice of the illustrations and, whenever possible, they are shown as if the same side of the body is affected, to facilitate comparison of one disease with another. Similarly, as before, a complete bibliography, with emphasis on recent publications, and an extensive index are included to provide the interested reader with easy access to information contained both in other sources and within this textbook.

Preparation of a second edition of a textbook is sometimes viewed as an opportunity to indicate superficially what has transpired since the first edition and to offer that information in a form that resembles an addendum. It should be emphasized, therefore, that this edition is the culmination of three years of research, organization, and writing. As before, the effort has been a labor of love, fueled by the inspiration derived from the inquisitive minds of residents and, especially, fellows who frequently have asked not what, when, or where, but why. It is offered as both a scientific and practical approach to the diagnosis of musculoskeletal disorders, and it should be viewed as an attempt by the authors to prove that scientific and practical matters are indeed compatible.

DONALD RESNICK, M.D.

# CONTENTS

▼

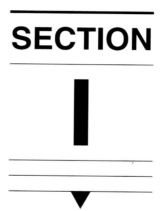
# Radiography and Related Diagnostic Techniques in the Evaluation of Bone, Joint, and Soft Tissue Diseases

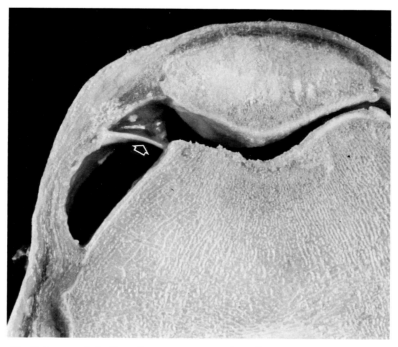

**Medial synovial plica:** A transverse section of the knee at the level of the patellofemoral space reveals this prominent synovial fold (arrow).

# 1

## Plain Film Radiography: Routine and Specialized Techniques and Projections

*David J. Sartoris, M.D., and Donald Resnick, M.D.*

The radiographic evaluation of osseous and articular disease begins in the x-ray room. Without high quality radiographs of properly positioned patients, the physician frequently is unable to detect significant abnormalities and thereby establish a correct diagnosis. Although there is no substitute for a well-trained radiologic technician who is aware of methods and techniques of skeletal radiography, both the referring physician and the radiologist must be familiar with these available techniques so that the proper radiographs are ordered and obtained. Ideally, neither too few nor too many images are acquired. Careful clinical evaluation of the patient prior to radiography, therefore, is of utmost importance. As an example of this, a patient selection protocol for posttraumatic radiographs has been described.[117] Strict adherence to this strategy for evaluation would have reduced usage by 12 per cent for the upper extremities and by 19 per cent for the lower extremities. Actual reductions noted in the investigation by Brand and coworkers were 5 per cent and 16 per cent, respectively.

This chapter summarizes various radiographic projections that are available for the evaluation of bones, joints, and soft tissues.[1-3, 118-121] Some are general projections that are used for the examination of patients with many types of disorders, including arthritis. Other projections have more limited indications. At the conclusion of the discussion of each region of the body, a recommended screening examination is included for the evaluation of a patient with symptoms or signs in that region. At the end of the entire chapter, a discussion of appropriate arthritic and osseous radiographic surveys is given. Specialized radiographic procedures and related examinations investigating patients with bone and joint diseases are discussed in some of the following chapters.

### FINGERS AND HAND

Adequate radiographic evaluation of the fingers requires posteroanterior and lateral projections (Fig. 1–1). The particular position employed for obtaining a lateral radiograph of one of the four ulnar (medial) digits will depend upon the specific digit being examined. Placing the hand on a step wedge permits separation of individual fingers in the lateral projection, allowing all digits to be examined on a single radiograph. Positioning of the thumb is unique because its axis differs from that of the other digits (Fig. 1–2). Stress views of the first metacarpophalangeal articulation may be required for evaluation of injuries of the ligaments of this joint.[4]

The radiographic examination of the hand uses posteroanterior, oblique, and lateral projections (Fig. 1–3). The posteroanterior projection is the best conventional view for demonstrating malalignment, joint space narrowing, and

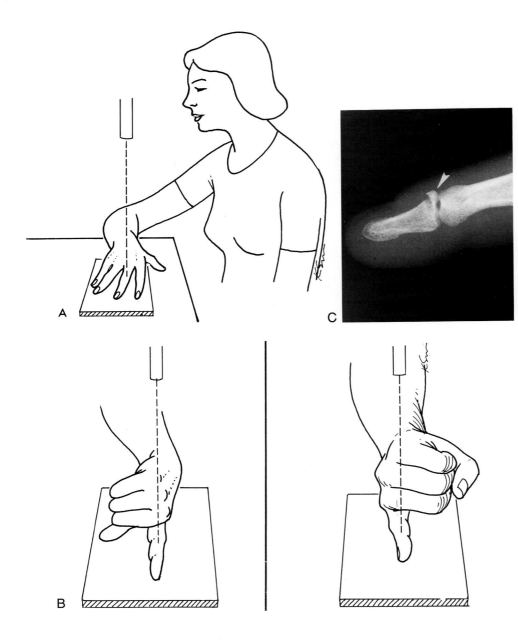

**FIGURE 1–1**. Fingers: Routine radiographs.

**A** Posteroanterior radiograph. The fingers should be separated slightly to provide better visualization of the osseous and articular structures.

**B** Lateral radiograph. Note that the position of the hand will vary depending on which digit is being examined. The involved finger is extended and the remaining digits are folded into a fist.

**C** Lateral radiograph: Dorsal fracture. The intra-articular fracture is well delineated (arrowhead).

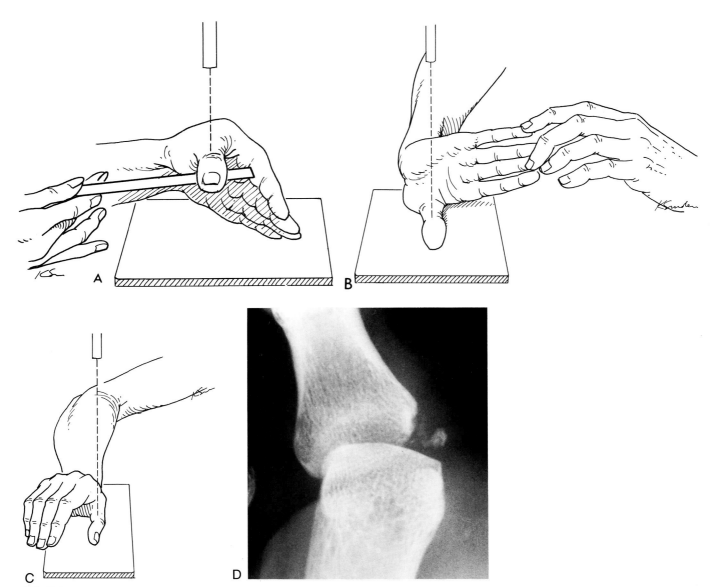

**FIGURE 1–2**. Thumb: Routine radiographs.
   **A, B** Posteroanterior **(A)** and anteroposterior **(B)** radiographs. Either view is satisfactory.
   **C** Lateral radiograph.
   **D** Stress radiograph of first metacarpophalangeal joint: Gamekeeper's thumb. With radial stress, laxity of the ulnar aspect of the joint and avulsion fractures are observed.

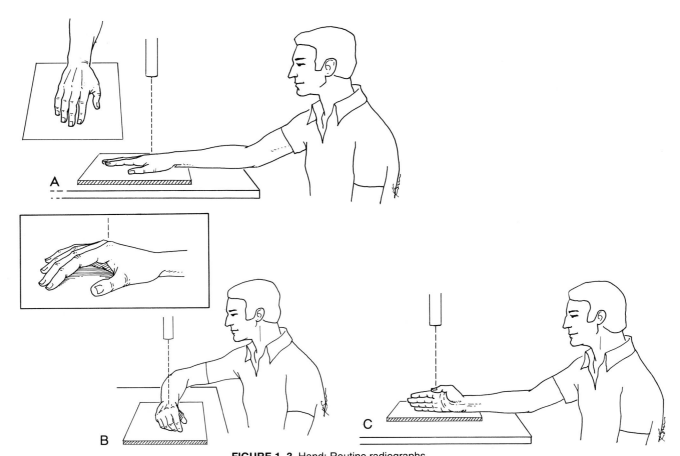

**FIGURE 1–3**. Hand: Routine radiographs.
**A** Posteroanterior radiograph.
**B, C** Oblique **(B)** and lateral **(C)** radiographs.

soft tissue abnormalities in early rheumatoid arthritis. Radiographic magnification is more sensitive than conventional radiography for evaluating erosive disease, but otherwise it is no better than the conventional posteroanterior view. [122] In fact, a prospective study to determine the optimum number of radiographic projections needed to assess applications for veteran's compensation for service-related hand disease or injury has indicated that a frontal view alone is sufficient.[123]

Occasionally anteroposterior and lateral flexion radiographs may be useful to further evaluate the dorsum of the hand and the metacarpophalangeal joints. The value of traction during radiography of the metacarpophalangeal joints (as well as the wrist) has been described.[105] During this procedure, the absence of release of intra-articular gas is indicative of an effusion. A similar technique has been used to evaluate the hip.

*Basic Examination: Hand*
Posteroanterior
Oblique
Lateral

## WRIST

Frontal and lateral radiographs of the wrist are routine (Fig. 1–4). The posteroanterior radiograph is best obtained with the arm abducted 90 degrees from the trunk and the forearm flexed at 90 degrees to the arm.[162] For the evaluation of arthritis, oblique projections also are necessary. These latter projections should include radiographs exposed with the wrist in both a semipronated oblique and a semisupinated oblique position. Of importance, an indistinct cortex on such views has been found not to be specific for early rheumatoid arthritis, having been identified in both inflammatory and noninflammatory arthritides and apparently representing variations in cortical morphology rather than true erosions.[124] On the semisupinated oblique projection, however, the pisiform-triquetral joint is well seen.[6]

Radiographs obtained during radial and ulnar deviation of the wrist are useful for visualizing the carpal bones, particularly the scaphoid (ulnar deviation), and for assessing carpal mobility (Fig. 1–5). Similarly, lateral radiographs may be obtained in palmar flexion and dorsiflexion. Furthermore, a tangential posteroanterior radiograph of the wrist with the ulnar border of the hand elevated 20 degrees from the top of the table has been described for the evaluation of scapholunate dissociation. A similar examination can be accomplished by leaving the hand in a flat position and angulating the x-ray beam accordingly. Both of these approaches are thought to be superior to others that have been suggested, including supination anteroposterior and clenched fist views, because they do not require patient movement that might cause pain.[125]

Specialized projections for the scaphoid may be required for detection of fractures.[7–9] The carpal tunnel view (Fig. 1–5) delineates the osseous structures and soft tissues of the carpal canal, including the hook of the hamate, pisiform, trapezium, trapezoid, and tuberosity of the scaphoid.[10–13] It should be noted that the carpal tunnel view obtained using the Gaynor-Hart method, an inferosuperior projection, may create a confusing ring artifact representing an end-on view of the fifth metacarpal superimposed on the carpal bones,

with the central radiolucent area corresponding to the medullary canal.[126] A carpal bridge view (Fig. 1–5) demonstrates the osseous and soft tissue structures on the dorsum of the wrist.[14] A lateral view using 30 degrees of supination and ulnar deviation of the wrist also has been recommended for optimal visualization of an os styloideum.[127, 128]

Radiographs obtained by angulating the beam along the axis of the radiocarpal joint allow better visualization of this articulation; a lateral radiograph from the radial side of the joint should be obtained with the beam angulated 15 degrees proximally, and a posteroanterior radiograph should be obtained with the beam angulated 10 degrees proximally.

A specialized anteroposterior projection with beam angulation has been used to define changes in the first carpometacarpal joint[15] (Fig. 1–5). Coned frontal and lateral views of the first carpometacarpal joint allow a more precise analysis of arthritis and traumatic lesions, such as Bennett's fractures. By taking these films in positions of maximal flexion and extension as well as anteposition and retroposition, it is possible to measure the range of motion of the articulation.[129] To measure the motions of this joint quantitatively, a radiographic method has been developed and tested using T-shaped metal markers, a special cassette-holder, and biplane radiographs.[130]

*Basic Examination: Wrist*
Posteroanterior
Lateral
Semisupinated Oblique
Semipronated Oblique

## RADIUS AND ULNA

Routine radiographic evaluation of the bones of the forearm consists of anteroposterior and lateral views, which should include both the elbow and the wrist. The lateral projection is obtained with the elbow joint flexed 60 to 90 degrees and the medial aspect of the elbow and fifth finger placed against the film. Oblique views may be necessary in specific situations, such as fracture assessment in the presence of an internal fixation plate.

*Basic Examination: Radius and Ulna*
Anteroposterior
Lateral

## ELBOW

Standard examination of the elbow includes anteroposterior and lateral radiographs and, in many cases, an oblique film (Fig. 1–6). The frontal radiographs should be obtained with supination of the hand so that rotation of radius and ulna does not occur. On the oblique radiograph, the coronoid process is well visualized, and the lateral projection, taken in elbow flexion, allows identification of the important fat pads about this joint. Additional radiographs that occasionally are used are frontal radiographs with acute flexion of the elbow to visualize the olecranon process[2] and angulated[16] and axial radiographs to better delineate the radial head[1, 2] and olecranon process[17, 18] (Fig. 1–7). A special radial head-capitulum view has proved useful in the evaluation of elbow trauma. Minimally displaced fractures of the radial head, capitulum, and coronoid process are

*Text continued on page 12*

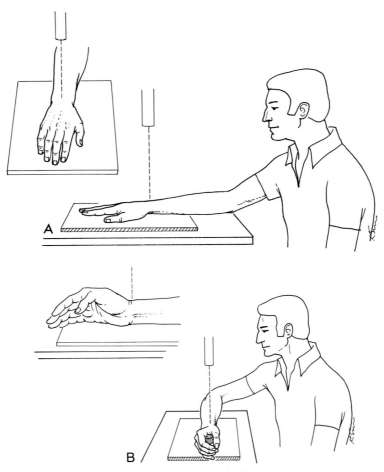

**FIGURE 1–4**. Wrist: Routine radiographs.
 **A** Posteroanterior radiograph.
 **B** Lateral radiograph.
 *Illustration continued on opposite page*

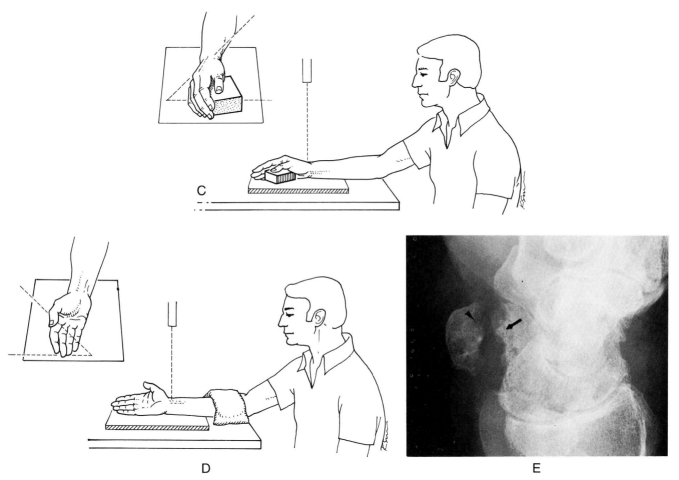

**FIGURE 1–4** *Continued*
  **C** Semipronated oblique radiograph. This view allows evaluation of the radial aspect of the wrist, particularly the scaphoid and radial styloid.
  **D** Semisupinated oblique radiograph.
  **E** Semisupinated oblique radiograph: Rheumatoid arthritis. Characteristic erosions occur in the dorsal surface of the pisiform (arrowhead) and the volar surface of the triquetrum (arrow) related to synovitis in the pisiform-triquetral compartment.

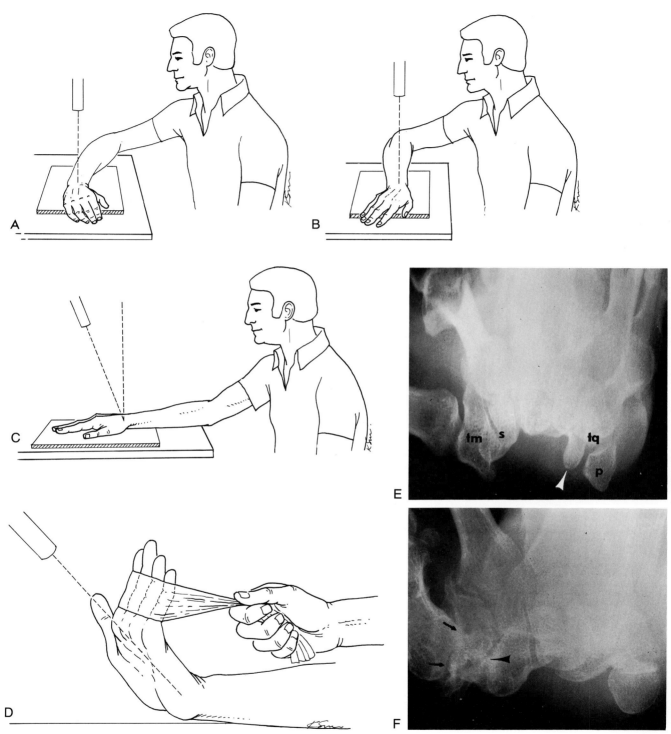

**FIGURE 1–5.** Wrist: Additional radiographs.

**A, B** Radial **(A)** and ulnar **(B)** deviation.

**C** Scaphoid: Specialized view. The hand and wrist are placed horizontally on the film and the central ray is directed 20 degrees toward the elbow. The scaphoid is projected free of adjacent osseous structures.

**D–F** Carpal tunnel view. The drawing **(D)** indicates that the long axis of the hand is placed in a vertical direction and the central ray is directed at an angle of 25 to 30 degrees to this long axis. In the normal situation **(E)**, the trapezium *(tm)*, scaphoid *(s)*, triquetrum *(tq)*, pisiform *(p)*, and hook of the hamate (arrowhead) can be delineated. In the abnormal situation **(F)**, observe considerable degenerative disease at the first carpometacarpal joint (arrows) and trapezioscaphoid area of the midcarpal joint (arrowhead).

*Illustration continued on opposite page*

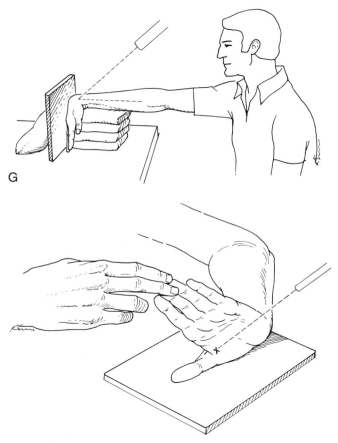

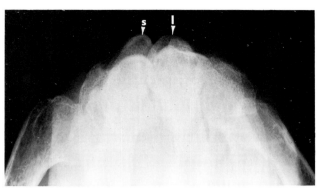

**FIGURE 1–5** *Continued*

   **G, H** Carpal bridge view. The drawing indicates that the wrist is flexed to approximately 90 degrees and the central ray is angled at 45 degrees in a superoinferior direction. This view demonstrates the scaphoid *(s)* and lunate *(l)* and is useful for diagnosing fractures, foreign bodies, and soft tissue swelling on the dorsal aspect of the wrist.

   **I** First carpometacarpal joint: Specialized view. The hand is hyperextended and the thumb is placed in a horizontal position. The central ray is angled approximately 45 degrees toward the elbow.

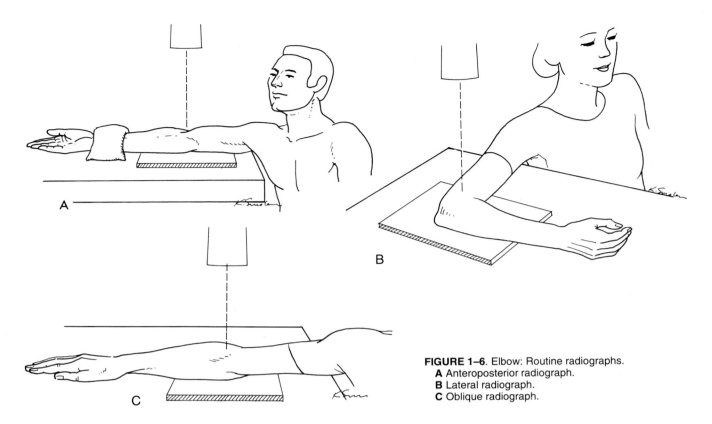

**FIGURE 1–6**. Elbow: Routine radiographs.
**A** Anteroposterior radiograph.
**B** Lateral radiograph.
**C** Oblique radiograph.

better demonstrated on this view than on traditional radiographs of the elbow. The radial head-capitulum view is particularly useful in the demonstration of fractures involving the posterior half of the radial head, which are difficult to diagnose on the traditional lateral projection[131–133] (see Chapter 68).

*Basic Examination: Elbow*
Anteroposterior
Lateral

## HUMERUS

Frontal and lateral radiographs of this bone constitute the basic examination. Both views should include the elbow and joints of the shoulder, with the elbow manifesting a true lateral configuration in the lateral projection. Under certain circumstances, oblique views may provide additional information.

*Basic Examination: Humerus*
Anteroposterior
Lateral

## GLENOHUMERAL JOINT

Anteroposterior radiographs are obtained in external and internal rotation of the arm (Fig. 1–8). The former reveals the greater tuberosity in profile and is useful in detecting calcification in the supraspinatus tendon. A radiolucent area in the greater tuberosity is a normal variation, termed the humeral pseudocyst; it is most prominent on radiographs obtained with external rotation of the humerus. As the arm

is rotated internally, the greater tuberosity is projected en face over the humerus, and the lesser tuberosity may overlie the glenohumeral joint. In this position, calcification in the infraspinatus and teres minor tendons is seen on the outer aspect of the humerus, and calcification in the subscapularis tendon is seen adjacent to the lesser tuberosity. These views may be obtained with 15 degrees of caudal angulation of the x-ray beam to better demonstrate the area of the subdeltoid bursa between the humeral head and acromion.[19] Additional projections for detecting calcification in the teres minor and subscapularis tendons have been described.[2]

It should be recognized that an anteroposterior radiograph of the shoulder is not a true anteroposterior radiograph of the scapula, nor does it allow adequate visualization of the glenohumeral joint space. A true anteroposterior radiograph of the scapula is obtained with the patient in a 40 degree posterior oblique position and is the most favorable projection for visualizing the joint, as this articulation is projected tangentially in this view.[20, 21]

In evaluating the shoulder after trauma, an additional radiograph at approximately right angles to the frontal radiographs is mandatory to determine the relative positions of the humeral head and glenoid. This can be accomplished in one of several ways. An axillary projection is particularly useful (Fig. 1–8),[113] and although it too can be obtained in several different ways,[2] it may be difficult to acquire in patients with fractures and dislocations about the shoulder. A transthoracic projection has been used in some patients,[1] but it may be difficult to interpret. The most favorable view makes use of a true lateral projection of the scapula (Fig. 1–8), which is acquired with the patient in a 60 degree anterior oblique position.[22–24, 112] It may be obtained in an

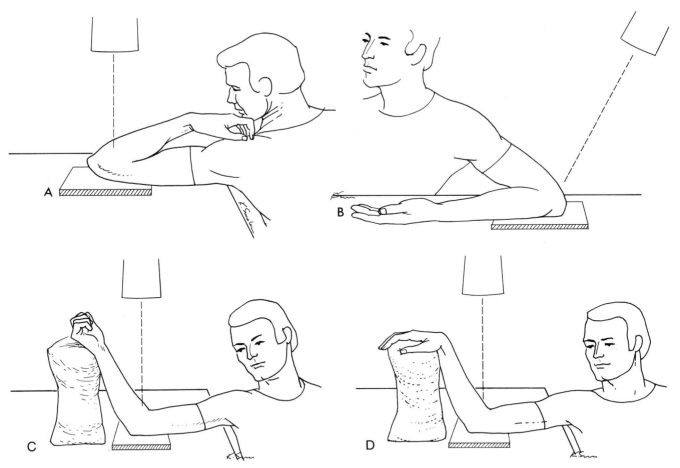

**FIGURE 1–7**. Elbow: Additional radiographs.
**A, B** Flexion views.
**C, D** Radial head: Supinated and pronated flexion views of the elbow.

upright or recumbent position, whichever is more comfortable for the patient. The projection is superior to a semiaxial anteroposterior projection, which has been recommended by some investigators for evaluation of the glenohumeral joint.[2] An apical oblique view (45 degree posterior oblique projection with 45 degree caudal angulation of the central ray) may be used as a supplementary projection in the analysis of shoulder trauma.[164]

Several different radiographic projections have been described to evaluate patients with previous anterior dislocations of the glenohumeral joint (Fig. 1–9). These radiographs are used to delineate a typical compression fracture of the posterolateral aspect of the humeral head, the Hill-Sachs lesion, which is associated with such dislocations,[25] and include an angulated internal rotation projection, [26–27] Hermodsson's tangential projection,[24] the "notch" view of Stryker,[28] and the Didiee view.[29] A West Point projection also is described. Multiple radiographs obtained in varying degrees of internal rotation also are helpful in delineating this fracture.

In the diagnosis of posterior dislocation of the glenohumeral joint, additional radiographic projections have been used, including modified axillary and angle-up views.[30] (Fig. 1–10). To visualize the bicipital groove, a radiograph

obtained in a superoinferior projection is recommended[31] (Fig. 1–11). A cephaloscapular radiographic projection has been advocated for diagnosing subluxation about the glenohumeral joint.[134] When the patient has been positioned properly for this view, the acromion, glenoid region, humeral head, and coracoid process can be seen in independent relief. The relatively radiolucent clavicle overlies the area of interest but does not obscure these landmarks.

An axial projection of the glenohumeral joint has been described that uses fluoroscopy and spot radiography to test the functional integrity of the joint capsule.[135] Such integrity also can be assessed with autotraction stress radiography.[163]

Because of the density differences of the structures about the shoulder, equalization filters may be helpful.[110] A silicone filter that overcomes peripheral overpenetration has been developed, which is said to facilitate better demonstration of the acromiohumeral window and adjacent structures.[136]

*Basic Examination: Glenohumeral Joint*
Anteroposterior (Internal Rotation)
Anteroposterior (External Rotation)
40 Degree Posterior Oblique

*Text continued on page 18*

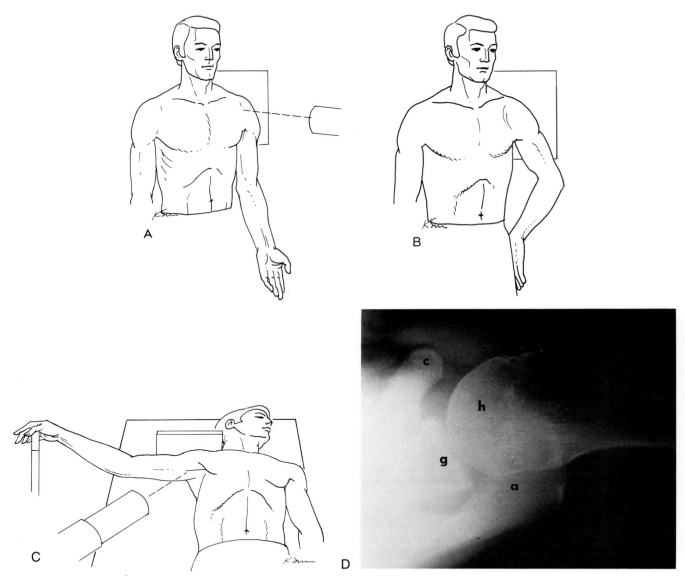

**FIGURE 1–8.** Glenohumeral joint: Routine radiographs.
  **A** External rotation.
  **B** Internal rotation.
  **C, D** Axillary view: Normal. Visualized structures are the glenoid cavity *(g)*, coracoid process *(c)*, acromion *(a)*, and humeral head *(h)*.

*Illustration continued on opposite page*

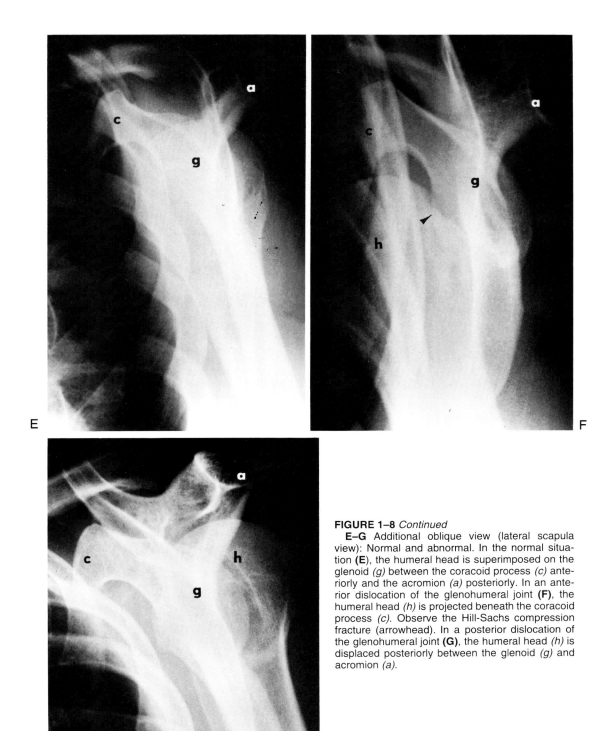

**FIGURE 1–8** *Continued*
**E–G** Additional oblique view (lateral scapula view): Normal and abnormal. In the normal situation **(E)**, the humeral head is superimposed on the glenoid *(g)* between the coracoid process *(c)* anteriorly and the acromion *(a)* posteriorly. In an anterior dislocation of the glenohumeral joint **(F)**, the humeral head *(h)* is projected beneath the coracoid process *(c)*. Observe the Hill-Sachs compression fracture (arrowhead). In a posterior dislocation of the glenohumeral joint **(G)**, the humeral head *(h)* is displaced posteriorly between the glenoid *(g)* and acromion *(a)*.

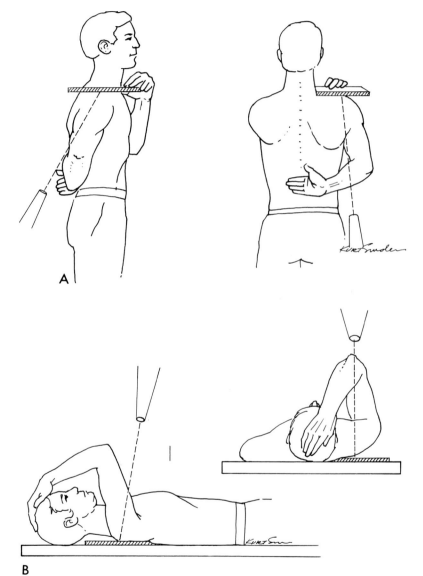

**FIGURE 1–9**. Glenohumeral joint: Evaluation of patients with previous anterior dislocation of glenohumeral joint.

**A** Hermodsson view. The dorsum of the hand is placed over the upper lumbar vertebrae with the thumb pointing upward. The central ray is directed at a 30 degree angle from the vertical, with the film held on the shoulder, parallel to the floor.

**B** "Notch" view. The palm is placed on top of the head. The central ray is directed 10 degrees cephalad.
*Illustration continued on opposite page*

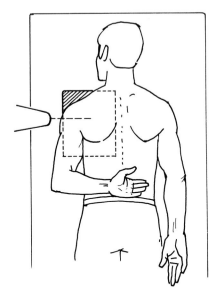

**FIGURE 1–9** *Continued*

**C** Modified Didiee view. The hand is placed on the iliac crest with the thumb directed upward. The central ray is angled 45 degrees in a lateral to medial direction.

**D** West Point view. In the prone position, the patient abducts the arm 90 degrees and the hand is placed over the end of the table. The central ray is angled 25 degrees in a cephalad direction and 25 degrees in a lateral to medial direction.

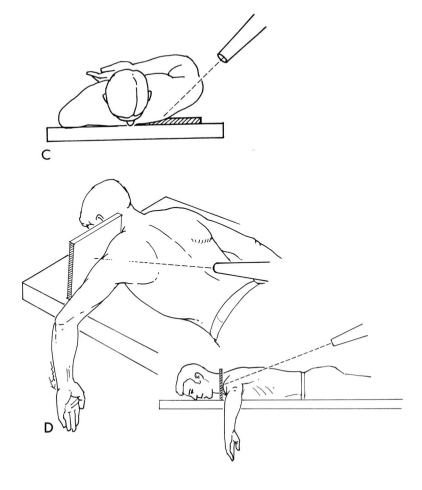

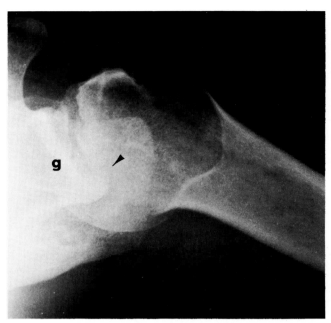

**FIGURE 1–10.** Glenohumeral joint: Evaluation of patients with posterior dislocation of the glenohumeral joint. In a modified axillary projection, observe the subluxed humeral head, which is displaced posteriorly with respect to the glenoid *(g)*. The latter structure is producing an impaction fracture of the humerus (arrowhead).

## ACROMIOCLAVICULAR JOINT

Although the acromioclavicular joint is visualized in routine views of the shoulder, it may be superimposed on other osseous structures. Radiographs obtained in the frontal projection with cephalad tilt of the incident beam of approximately 15 degrees are superior in delineating abnormalities of this articulation[32, 33] (Fig. 1–12). A lateral projection of this joint also has been described [2, 33] and an additional technique includes a frontal radiograph taken in a lordotic position.[2]

Stress radiographs frequently are necessary to diagnose

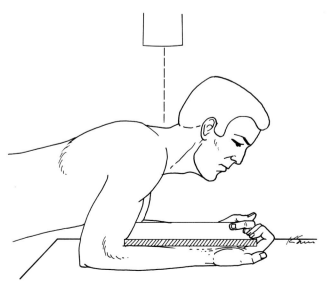

**FIGURE 1–11.** Glenohumeral joint: Bicipital groove view. The patient flexes the trunk across the table and holds the cassette on the forearms. The central ray is directed vertically.

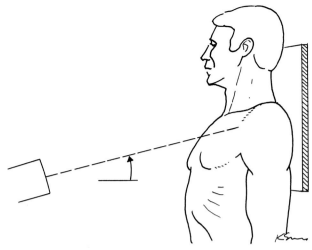

**FIGURE 1–12.** Acromioclavicular joint: Routine radiographs. Anteroposterior radiograph. The central ray is angled 15 degrees in a cephalad direction.

acromioclavicular joint subluxation and dislocation. These are obtained by having the patient hold a 2.3 to 7 kg (5 to 15 lb) mass (weight) in the hand or tying this weight to the wrist. If possible, it is beneficial to view both acromioclavicular joints on a single film. This allows comparison of the two joints, with the radiologist carefully observing the distance between the coracoid process and clavicle on both sides.[24, 34] A shoulder-forward projection and an axial projection have been recommended as additional methods in diagnosing abnormalities of the clavicle and acromioclavicular joint subluxation.[35–37] Furthermore, stress radiography accomplished with the patient's arm forcefully adducted across the body may be more sensitive than routine projections in the diagnosis of osteoarthritis of the acromioclavicular joint.[165]

*Basic Examination: Acromioclavicular Joint*
Anteroposterior with 15 Degrees of Cephalad
Angulation

## STERNUM AND STERNOCLAVICULAR JOINT

The radiographic evaluation of the sternum requires oblique and lateral projections. Long exposure times are useful, as the patient's breathing during several phases of respiration will produce blurring of overlying lung and rib shadows. The lateral projection can be obtained in an erect or a recumbent position.

Adequate radiographs of the sternoclavicular joints are difficult to obtain. Oblique and frontal radiographs of the sternum frequently do not provide optimal visualization of this articulation (Fig. 1–13). Many special views have been recommended.[38–40] The Hobbs view, a superoinferior projection of the sternoclavicular joint,[41] and lordotic projection[24] may both be helpful, particularly in evaluating a patient with a possible dislocation of the sternoclavicular joint (Fig. 1–14). One additional projection, the Heinig view, which is similar to Kurzbauer's lateral projection,[40] also can document dislocation of this joint.[42, 43] Using an ultrafine focal spot tube and a short focal spot–patient distance allows differential magnification with projection of the ster-

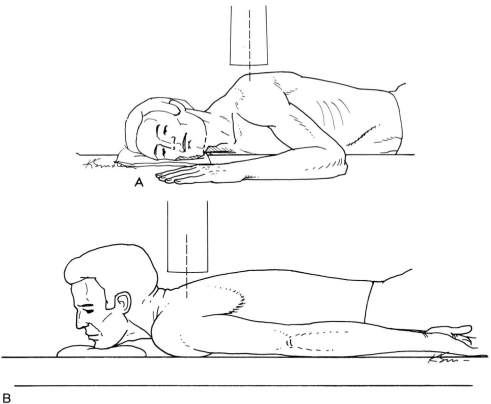

**FIGURE 1–13.** Sternoclavicular joint: Routine radiographs.
**A** Oblique radiograph.
**B** Posteroanterior radiograph.

noclavicular joints to either side of the thoracic spine on an anteroposterior projection.[106]

*Basic Examination: Sternum and*
*Sternoclavicular Joint*
Posteroanterior
Oblique
Lateral

## SPINE

The radiographic examination of the spine varies considerably, depending upon the vertebral segment being examined and the specific indication for the examination.

### Cervical Spine

Although a screening examination of the cervical spine in a patient with widespread articular disease may require only anteroposterior and lateral flexion radiographs, a more complete evaluation may be necessary in a patient with neck pain and is mandatory in a patient who has sustained neck trauma.[44–48]

The standard examination of the cervical spine consists of multiple views (Fig. 1–15). A frontal radiograph is obtained with the patient either recumbent or erect in an anteroposterior projection with approximately 15 degrees to 20 degrees of cephalad angulation of the tube. Mandibular motion during the exposure allows more favorable visualization of the upper cervical vertebrae in this projection.[49]

The lateral radiograph usually is obtained with the head in neutral position but may be supplemented with lateral radiographs obtained with head flexion and extension. Forty-five degree oblique projections are obtained with the patient sitting or standing. Although these projections are useful in the analysis of the intervertebral foramina, those in the lower cervical spine are better demonstrated on 55 degree oblique radiographs.[166] An anteroposterior open-mouth projection allows visualization of the atlas and axis.[50] A pillar view for demonstration of the vertebral arches is obtained in an anteroposterior or posteroanterior position with neck extension. In the former position, the central ray is angulated 25 to 30 degrees toward the feet[51]; in the latter position, the central ray is angulated 40 degrees cephalad. Certain modifications of the pillar view have been suggested.[48] One such technique employs turning the mandible to each side to eliminate overlying soft tissue and osseous structures that may obscure the cervical spine. The authors prefer to have the patient maintain a central position of the mandible, as this position facilitates comparison between the two sides.

After significant cervical spine trauma, initial radiographs should include cross-table lateral and anteroposterior views, which may be obtained without disturbing the patient. After this screening examination, further radiographs can be taken. The complete cervical spine examination in these patients should include those projections that have previously been noted: anteroposterior view with 20 degree cephalad angulation of the tube; open-mouth view; right and left 45 degree oblique views; lateral views in neutral

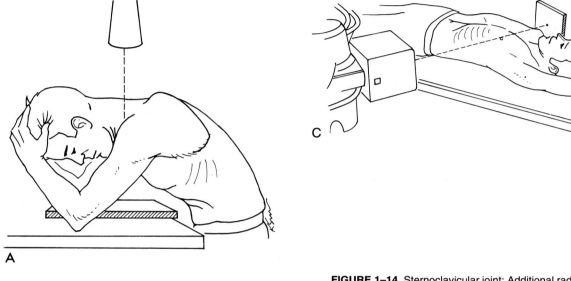

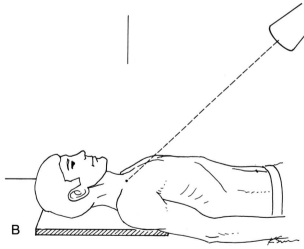

**FIGURE 1–14**. Sternoclavicular joint: Additional radiographs.

**A** Hobbs view. This radiograph is obtained with the patient bent over the table, hands placed on the head.

**B** Lordotic view. The central ray is directed with a 40 to 50 degree cephalad tilt.

**C** Heinig view. The patient is recumbent. The shoulder closest to the tube is abducted. The central ray is centered at the sternoclavicular joint and directed along the axis of the clavicle.

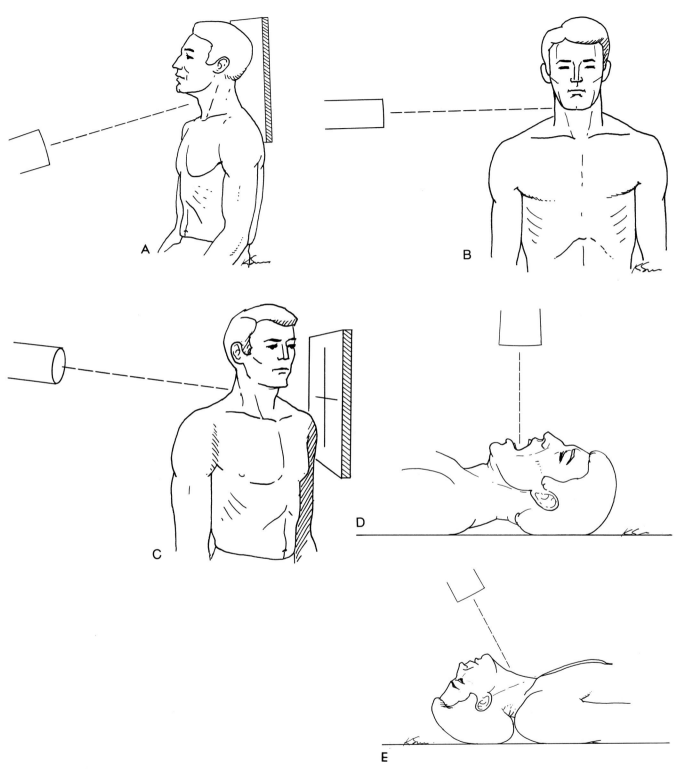

**FIGURE 1–15**. Cervical spine: Routine radiographs.
 **A** Anteroposterior radiograph.
 **B** Lateral radiograph.
 **C** Oblique radiograph.
 **D** Open-mouth radiograph.
 **E** Pillar radiograph. In an anteroposterior position, the central ray is angulated 25 to 30 degrees toward the feet.

position, flexion, and extension; and pillar view.[138] Additionally, shallow oblique radiographs (approximately 20 degrees of obliquity) may be needed. The 60 degree supine oblique view of the cervical spine also can be useful in delineating fractures of the articular processes or pedicles and constriction of the intervertebral foramina. The fact that the film is placed under the patient's shoulder, without disturbing the potentially fractured cervical spine, is its most attractive characteristic. This view separates the anterior and posterior structures in a side-to-side projection, allowing for an elongated but detailed view of the articular processes, pedicles, and intervertebral foramina.[137] Certain flexion injuries of the cervical spine may be evident radiologically only if radiographs are obtained in the erect position.[139]

For some portions of the cervical spine, additional radiographs are suggested (Fig. 1–16). Specific projections are designed for the cervicobasilar region.[2, 52] An abnormal relationship between the upper cervical spine and the base of

the skull that becomes evident on these projections is known as basilar impression or invagination and is defined radiographically by reference to several parameters (see Chapter 22).[140] For the cervicothoracic region, recommended views include the swimmer's projection,[2] a lateral view with the arms pulled down,[47] flying angel projection with traction on a single arm,[47] and a supine oblique projection.[53] A simple traction device has been developed to facilitate radiography of the lower cervical spine, which assumes particular importance in the setting of acute trauma.[141]

To better delineate alterations at the atlantoaxial joint, multiple open-mouth views may be necessary.[54] These are obtained with the patient in the frontal position, with rotation of the head of 10 to 15 degrees to either side and with lateral tilting of the head to either side. A modified basal projection for demonstration of fractures involving the anterior arch of the atlas has been described. The central ray is angled 10 degrees with respect to a line perpendicular to

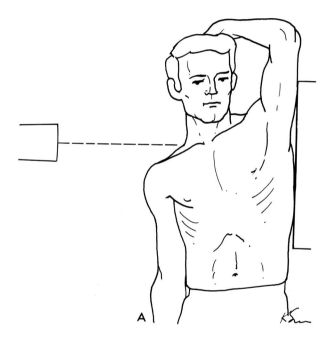

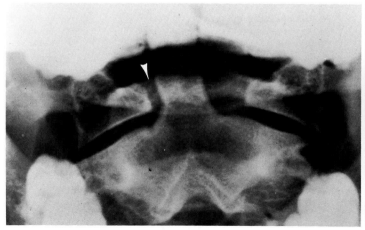

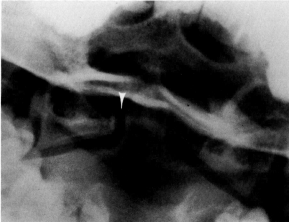

**FIGURE 1–16.** Cervical spine: Additional radiographs.

**A** Swimmer's position radiograph. The lateral radiograph is obtained with one arm elevated. This allows evaluation of the cervicothoracic junction.

**B, C** Open-mouth views: Rotary fixation of the atlas and axis. These two radiographs were taken with the patient tilting the head to either side. They demonstrate persistent asymmetry at the atlantoaxial junction, with the odontoid more closely associated with the right lateral mass (arrowheads). This indicates rotary fixation at the atlantoaxial junction.

A

B

C

the orbitomeatal line, with the head in neutral position and rotated 30 degrees to either side.[142]

*Basic Examination: Cervical Spine*
Anteroposterior
Pillar View
Lateral in Neutral Position and in Flexion
Open-mouth
Obliques

## Thoracic Spine

A radiographic series of the thoracic spine should include anteroposterior and lateral radiographs and a swimmer's view of the lower cervical and upper thoracic vertebrae (Fig. 1–17). The anteroposterior projection places the spine adjacent to the x-ray film. Because of the normal thoracic kyphosis, diverging incident rays are relatively parallel to the upper and lower aspects of the vertebrae in this position. Certain modifications in the technique may allow more uniform density throughout the entire radiograph.[55] On the lateral radiograph nonsuspended respiration may blur the overlying shadows of the thoracic cage. Radiographs exposed with the patient positioned in slight obliquity allow visualization of the apophyseal joints of the thoracic spine.[2, 56, 57]

In patients with scoliosis in the thoracic spine, a clinical study has indicated that measurements of the curve on paired posteroanterior and anteroposterior upright radiographs of the spine differ by a small but statistically signif-

icant amount. The posteroanterior scoliotic angles were larger than anteroposterior angles by a mean of 2.4 degrees for the thoracic curves and a mean of 1.71 degrees for the lumbar curves[143] (see Chapter 89). Additional methods allowing evaluation of vertebral rotation in patients with scoliosis have been described.[160]

*Basic Examination: Thoracic Spine*
Anteroposterior
Lateral

## Lumbar Spine

The frontal radiograph of the lumbar spine can be obtained in the posteroanterior or anteroposterior projection with the patient erect or recumbent (Fig. 1–18). The recumbent anteroposterior radiograph should be taken with the hips and knees flexed, which reduces the lumbar lordosis and better delineates the vertebral bodies and intervertebral discs. The lateral outlines of the pedicles and the lateral borders of the body of the fifth lumbar vertebra are not normally imaged on these conventional frontal radiographs, owing to the deviant morphology of this segment compared with the third and fourth lumbar vertebrae. This anatomic feature may be of assistance in identifying the specific vertebrae in transitional spines.[144]

The lateral radiograph also is exposed with slight flexion of the hips and knees. A coned-down lateral projection of the lumbosacral junction also is included. Oblique radiographs allow evaluation of the posterior elements of the

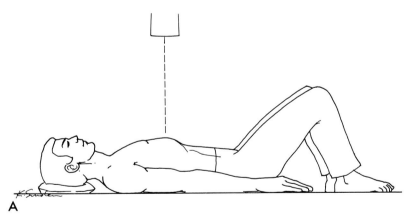

**FIGURE 1–17**. Thoracic spine: Routine radiographs.
**A** Anteroposterior radiograph. The flexed position of the knees produces some straightening of the normal thoracic kyphosis.
**B** Lateral radiograph.

A

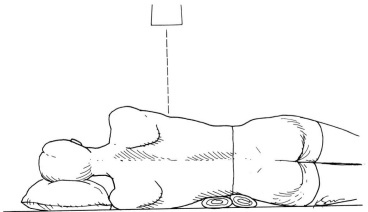

B

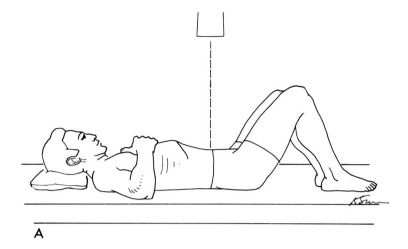

A

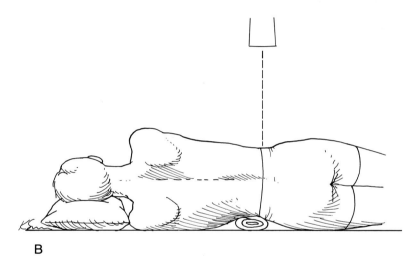

B

**FIGURE 1–18**. Lumbar spine: Routine radiographs.
   **A** Anteroposterior radiograph. The knees and hips are flexed to reduce the degree of lumbar lordosis.
   **B** Lateral radiograph. The knees and hips again are flexed.
   **C** Oblique radiograph.

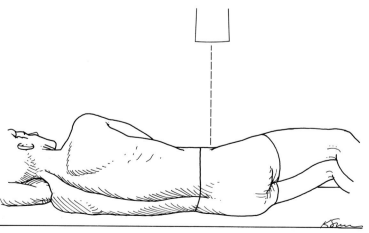

C

lumbar spine, although some regard the oblique projections as unnecessary.[111] These radiographs can be obtained in anteroposterior or posteroanterior positions by turning the patient 45 degrees. Unilateral spondylolysis may be extremely difficult to demonstrate even using such oblique radiographs; 20 degree cephalad angulation of the x-ray tube may allow more precise diagnosis.[146]

An anteroposterior view of the pelvis generally is included in the evaluation of the lumbosacral spine. To evaluate the laminae and articular processes in this region, an axial radiograph (in infants)[107] or an anteroposterior radiograph with 45 degrees of caudal angulation of the beam can be obtained.[58] The latter view is particularly helpful in delineating congenital, posttraumatic, and postsurgical changes, as well as capsular calcifications involving the articular facets and neural arch.[145]

An anteroposterior radiograph with the incident beam angled 15 to 30 degrees cephalad will allow visualization of tangential surfaces of the inferior aspect of the fifth lumbar vertebral body and the superior aspect of the first sacral segment.[2] An oblique semiaxial projection provides delineation of the inferior intervertebral foramina.[59]

Examination of motion of the lumbar spine may provide useful information.[60] To accomplish this, lateral radiographs may be obtained during flexion and extension, and frontal radiographs may be obtained during lateral bending of the spine.

*Basic Examination: Lumbar Spine*
Anteroposterior
Lateral
Lateral Coned to L5-S1
Obliques
Anteroposterior of Pelvis

## PELVIS

The standard radiographic view for the pelvis is obtained in an anteroposterior position with the patient supine (Fig. 1–19). The feet are placed in approximately 15 degrees of internal rotation. This is done to overcome the normal anteversion of the femoral necks and to place their longitudinal axes parallel to the film. To evaluate the pubis, a posteroanterior radiograph probably is superior to an anteroposterior radiograph and may be supplemented with axial projections obtained by angulating the beam or torso.

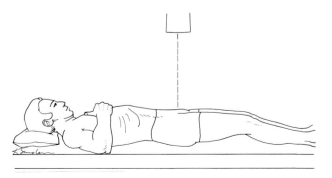

**FIGURE 1–19.** Pelvis: Routine radiographs. Anteroposterior radiograph. Internal rotation of the lower legs allows elongation of the femoral necks.

Various methods have been used to examine the sacroiliac joints (Fig. 1–20); none is ideal, as the normal undulating articular surfaces make evaluation of these joints extremely difficult. Oblique views of this joint can be obtained in either the supine or the prone position.[61, 62] In either instance, the side of the body is elevated approximately 25 degrees, and the beam can be directed perpendicular to the film or angulated to the feet or head. Radiographs of both right and left sacroiliac joints are obtained.

A better method for radiography of the sacroiliac joints uses the frontal projection (Fig. 1–20). An anteroposterior radiograph can be taken with the tube angulated 25 to 30 degrees in a cephalad direction or a posteroanterior radiograph can be taken with 25 to 30 degrees of caudal angulation of the tube. In either case, both sacroiliac joints are exposed on a single film, facilitating comparison of the two joints. Although the authors favor the anteroposterior projection, proponents of the posteroanterior projection claim its superiority because of the normal inclination of the joint.

A craniocaudal axial view of the sacroiliac joint may better delineate abnormalities along the anterior aspect of the joint[63] (Fig. 1–21). In this view, the patient sits on the x-ray table with slight forward flexion of the trunk. The tube is angled approximately 10 to 20 degrees along the craniocaudal axis of the articulation. This view may be modified by increasing or decreasing the degree of trunk flexion and by not angulating the x-ray tube.[2] Other modifications also have been suggested.[108]

Obtaining anteroposterior views with the patient erect, with the weight borne first on one leg and then on the other, may provide information about motion at the sacroiliac joint and symphysis pubis.[2, 64] This examination also can be accomplished under fluoroscopy[65] or with stereophotogrammetry.[109] The sacroiliac joints and symphysis pubis are part of a single functional unit. Any increase in mobility of the sacroiliac joint is transferred to the symphysis pubis and appears as abnormal motion at this latter site. A 1 mm displacement of the symphyseal part of the pubic bone probably is within normal limits,[64] and a permanent displacement of the symphysis pubis occasionally may be noted in certain patients, particularly multiparous women. True instability of the symphysis pubis and sacroiliac joint is indicated by abnormal widening of either articulation or rotation of one pubic bone in relation to the other on these specialized views.

*Basic Examination: Sacroiliac Joint*
Anteroposterior with 30 Degrees of Cephalad
Angulation

## SACRUM AND COCCYX

The radiographic examination of the sacrum and coccyx includes frontal and lateral projections (Fig. 1–22). To visualize the upper sacrum, an anteroposterior radiograph is obtained with 15 degrees of cephalad angulation of the tube. To visualize the lower sacrum, an anteroposterior radiograph without beam angulation is useful. To visualize the coccyx, an anteroposterior radiograph with 10 degrees of caudal angulation of the tube is required. All of these films can be done in a prone rather than supine position; in the prone position, the direction of beam angulation is re-

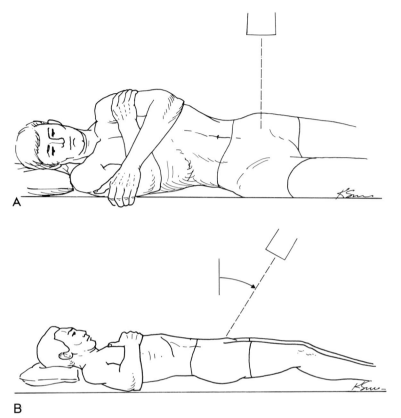

A

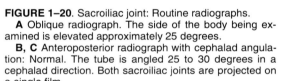

B

**FIGURE 1–20**. Sacroiliac joint: Routine radiographs.
   **A** Oblique radiograph. The side of the body being examined is elevated approximately 25 degrees.
   **B, C** Anteroposterior radiograph with cephalad angulation: Normal. The tube is angled 25 to 30 degrees in a cephalad direction. Both sacroiliac joints are projected on a single film.

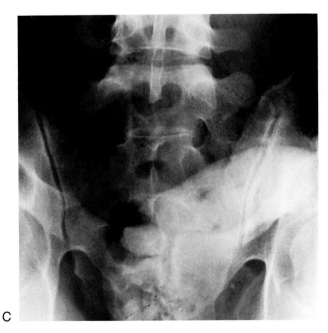

C

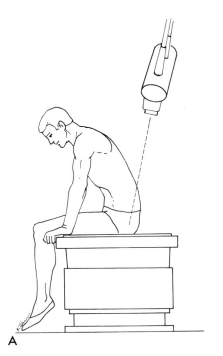

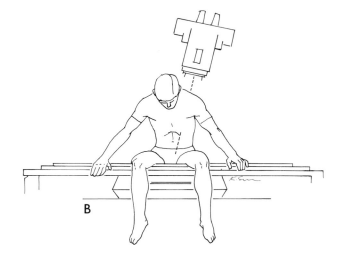

**FIGURE 1–21.** Sacroiliac joint: Additional radiographs. **A, B** A craniocaudal axial view is obtained with the patient sitting on the x-ray table. The tube is angled 10 to 20 degrees in a lateral to medial direction. Anterior angulation also may be utilized.

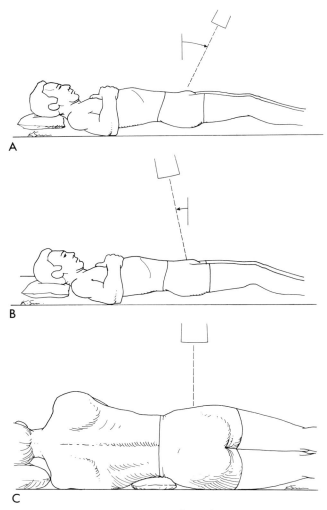

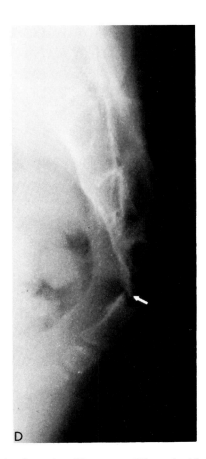

**FIGURE 1–22.** Sacrum and coccyx: Routine radiographs.
   **A–C** Frontal radiographs of sacrum **(A)** use 15 degrees of cephalad angulation; frontal radiographs of the coccyx **(B)** require 10 degrees of caudal angulation. The lateral radiograph **(C)** also is obtained.
   **D** Lateral radiograph of sacrum: Fracture. The displaced fracture can be observed (arrow).

versed. A lateral projection of the sacrum or coccyx is the second required view.

*Basic Examination: Sacrum, Coccyx*
Anteroposterior with 30 Degrees of
Cephalad Angulation (Sacrum) or 10
Degrees of Caudal Angulation (Coccyx)
Lateral

## HIP

The most common method of examining the hip joint includes an anteroposterior radiograph of the pelvis and a coned-down anteroposterior radiograph of the hip, both obtained with internal rotation of the foot to elongate the femoral neck, and a frog-leg view obtained with the hip abducted (Fig. 1–23). Supplementary views are suggested in certain clinical situations. These views include a semiaxial projection, the Chassard-Lapiné position, obtained with the patient sitting on the table and the central ray directed vertically through the lumbosacral region,[66, 67] an axial lateral projection, obtained in an inferosuperior direction, and an angulated lateral projection.[68]

In the evaluation of the hip joint and acetabulum following trauma, 45 degree anterior and posterior oblique projections have been recommended to visualize the anterior and posterior acetabular rims and important bony columns of the pelvis.[69] The authors' investigation has indicated that shallower oblique projections may be more useful[70] (Fig. 1–24). A lateral acetabular view also has been recommended.[71] A projection obtained with the patient supine and the central ray angled 40 degrees cephalad elongates the femoral neck and shows it to optimum advantage. This angled or "upshot" view allows detection of nondisplaced fractures of the femoral neck that are not apparent on standard views.[148] Furthermore, a technique for the early detection and classification of collapse of the femoral head after transcervical fracture on conventional frontal radiographs also has been described.[149]

Radiographs of the hip obtained during traction of 14 to 23 kg (30 to 50 lb) have been recommended as a useful technique in a variety of articular disorders.[72] This maneuver produces spontaneous intra-articular release of gas, the "vacuum" phenomenon. The pneumoarthrogram is not obtained if the patient has a hip effusion. Traction radiography thus affords an easy and noninvasive means for detecting fluid in the hip joint.[150] In the absence of an effusion, a vacuum arthrogram will show the shape, thickness, and extent of the cartilage. The degree of diastasis that can be achieved depends on muscular development, muscle tone, laxity of the joint capsule and ligaments, age, and sex. In children and adolescents, especially girls, it is easy to induce a vacuum phenomenon, whereas in advanced osteoarthritis, diastasis is limited by capsular thickening and muscular spasm. Demonstration of the limbus in developmental dysplasia of the hip generally has been unsuccessful using this technique.[151] In the presence of osteonecrosis, gas may be released into the separated fragment of subchondral bone, allowing earlier diagnosis of this condition.[73]

Radiographs of the hip obtained while the patient is bearing weight generally are not useful, although this technique may be applied to the evaluation of the postoperative hip.[161]

*Basic Examination: Hip*
Anteroposterior View of Pelvis
Anteroposterior View of Hip
Frog-leg View of Hip

## FEMUR

Lateral and anteroposterior radiographs are the components of a routine evaluation of the femur. Both are obtained with the leg rotated medially about 20 degrees. The hip and knee should be visualized on both views even if this requires two separate exposures with different centering in each projection. In the detection of occult fractures or the presence of orthopedic hardware, additional oblique views may be necessary.

*Basic Examination: Femur*
Anteroposterior
Lateral

## KNEE

An anteroposterior radiograph of the knee is obtained with the beam directed 5 to 7 degrees toward the head, and

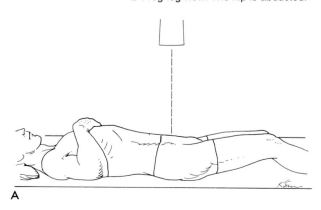

FIGURE 1–23. Hip: Routine radiographs.
**A** Anteroposterior radiograph.
**B** Frog-leg view. The hip is abducted.

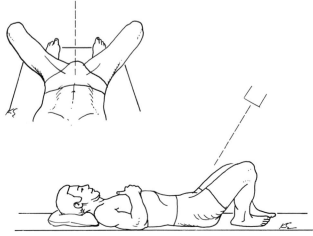

A                                                                                          B

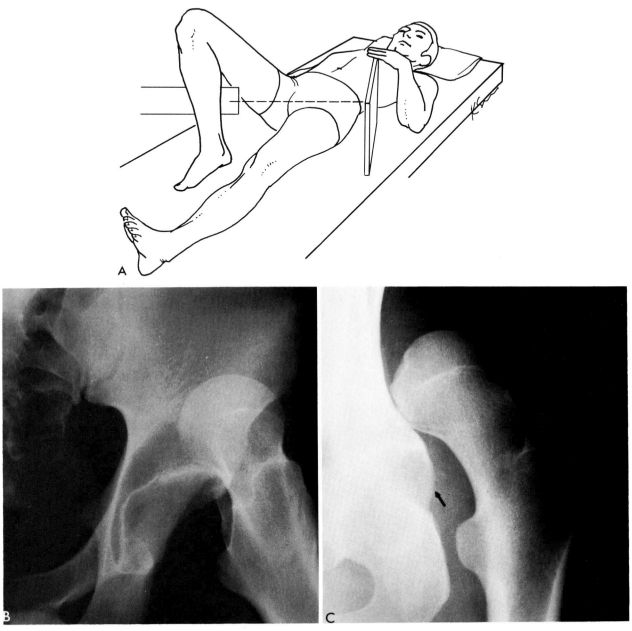

**FIGURE 1–24.** Hip: Additional radiographs.

  **A** Inferosuperior radiograph. This technique provides a lateral view of the hip. The tube is placed beneath the flexed knee and the central ray is angled in a superior direction.

  **B, C** Anteroposterior and oblique radiographs: Posterior dislocation of the hip. Although the frontal radiograph **(B)** demonstrates that the femoral head is displaced superiorly, the oblique radiograph **(C)** reveals its posterior displacement and provides information regarding the posterior acetabular rim (arrow).

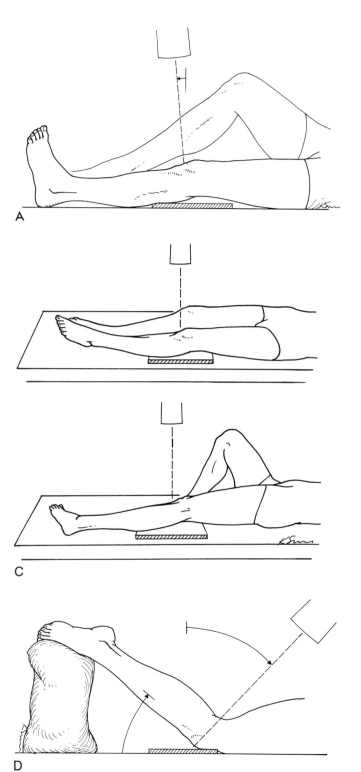
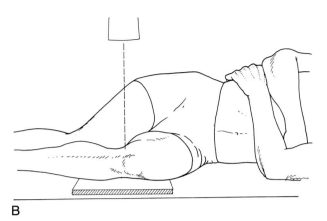

**FIGURE 1–25.** Knee: Routine radiographs.

**A** Anteroposterior radiograph. Observe that the central ray is directed in a cephalad direction with an angle of 5 to 7 degrees.

**B** Lateral radiograph. The knee is flexed 20 to 35 degrees.

**C** Oblique radiographs. These films are obtained with the patient turned 45 degrees in either direction.

**D** Tunnel view. The knee is flexed 40 to 50 degrees and rests on a sandbag. The central ray is angulated 40 to 50 degrees in a caudal direction.

a lateral radiograph is obtained with the knee flexed 20 to 35 degrees (Fig. 1–25). Although investigations have indicated that these two views (anteroposterior and lateral) are adequate in the assessment of most disorders of the knee,[123] complete evaluation of patients with knee effusions after acute trauma may require additional views to ensure that occult fractures are not overlooked.[155] Forty-five degree oblique projections usually are necessary in a patient who has experienced knee trauma and in a patient whose problems relate to the proximal tibiofibular articulation. An angulated frontal view with the knee flexed 40 to 50 degrees, the tunnel view, is used to visualize the intercondylar notch.[74] This can be obtained in an anteroposterior or posteroanterior projection. Some investigators have suggested that radiographs should be obtained in a greater degree of knee flexion to provide better visualization of the articular space and intercondylar area.[75] In patients with knee trauma, a cross-table lateral projection should be added to the examination, allowing demonstration of fat-fluid levels, indicative of fractures with release of medullary fat into the articular cavity (Fig. 1–26). The cross-table lateral view, however, has been found to be less sensitive than the routine overhead lateral view in the detection of knee joint effusions, owing to fluid shift into the lateral recesses of the suprapatellar bursa with the patient in the supine position.[152]

Various techniques have been described for adequate evaluation of the patellofemoral joint (Fig. 1–27). Original descriptions suggested using the prone position with acute knee flexion (the sunrise view).[76] This degree of knee flexion results in the patella's becoming deeply situated within the intercondylar fossa. As most cases of subluxation of the patella occur in lesser degrees of knee flexion, this view is not ideal. Furthermore, the sunrise view fails to demonstrate the articular surfaces of the patellofemoral joint and can be painful for the acutely traumatized patient.[153] Hughston[77] suggested that a view obtained with the patient prone and the knee flexed to 50 or 60 degrees was a more suitable technique for visualization of the patellofemoral joint, although in this view distortion is created by severe angulation of the incident beam. Subsequently, some investigators described techniques in which the patient was examined supine.[78–80] Merchant and coworkers[81] proposed a technique in which the patient is positioned supine on the table with the leg flexed 45 degrees over the end of the table. The tube is angulated 30 degrees toward the floor. Unfortunately, this method requires a special film-holding apparatus and patellar magnification is apparent. The direction of the beam can be reversed (i.e., from the ankle toward the knee) and radiographs can be obtained at various degrees of knee flexion, perhaps providing a more accurate appraisal of the patellofemoral area.[82, 83, 114] These radiographs with reversed angulation of the beam are well tolerated by the patient, require no special equipment, and provide a better view of the articulating surfaces of the patellofemoral compartment than the sunrise view; subluxation, fracture, and degenerative joint disease thus may be detected more easily.[153]

Weight-bearing radiography of the knee is particularly helpful in the evaluation of degenerative joint disease, providing a more accurate assessment of the articular space[84–86] (Fig. 1–28). In the authors' experience,[87] these views should be obtained on vertically oriented 7 × 17 inch films with the patient standing on the leg being examined. This allows better delineation of the degree of angulation and subluxation at the knee and is a more reliable indication of the extent of joint space loss. In addition, a preoperative radiographic analysis of the whole leg in the standing position has been described as a diagnostic aid prior to high tibial osteotomy for osteoarthritis of the knee. This analysis provides information about the mechanical condition of the knee, the extent of osseous deformity, and the exact size of the wedge of bone that needs to be excised surgically.[154] Similar weight-bearing radiographs are valuable in the preoperative assessment of patients who are to undergo total joint replacements.

Radiography performed during varus and valgus stress of the knee allows evaluation of ligament instability.[88] Stress radiography is especially useful in the assessment of the cruciate ligaments.[167]

*Basic Examination: Knee*
Anteroposterior
Lateral
Tunnel View
Merchant View

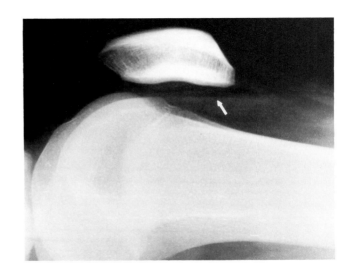

**FIGURE 1–26.** Knee: Additional radiograph. Cross-table lateral projection: Fat-fluid level in a patient with a tibial plateau fracture. Note the sharply delineated horizontal radiodense line representing the fat-fluid interface (arrow). The fat originated in the medullary cavity and was released into the joint following the fracture.

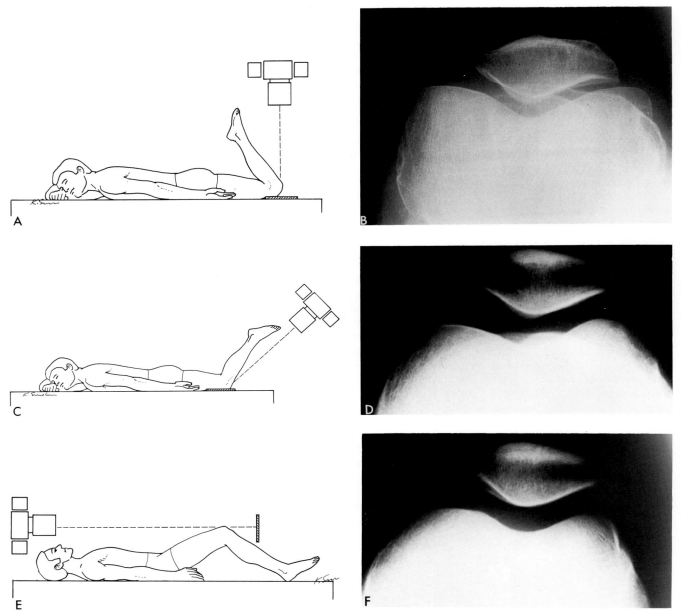

**FIGURE 1–27.** Patellofemoral joint: Routine and specialized radiographs.

**A, B** Sunrise view: Normal. This can be obtained with the knee flexed more than 90 degrees. The patella is situated deep within the intercondylar fossa.

**C, D** Hughston view: Normal. In this projection, the knee is flexed 50 to 60 degrees. The patella is not so closely applied to the femur.

**E, F** Knutsson view: Normal. The patient is supine and the slightly flexed knee rests on the table. A special film holder is necessary.

*Illustration continued on opposite page*

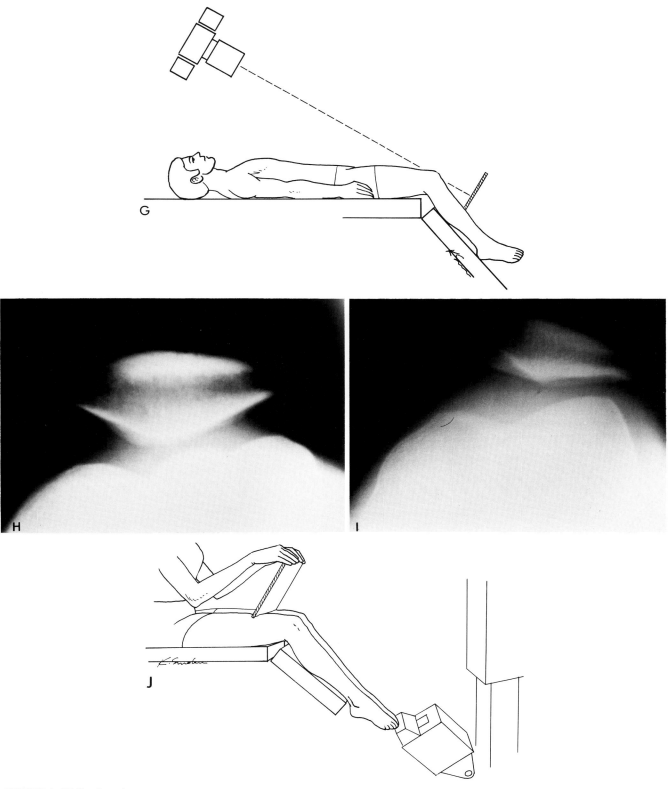

**FIGURE 1–27** *Continued*

    **G–I** Merchant view: Normal and abnormal. The patient is placed supine on the table and the knees are flexed 45 degrees over the end of the table **(G)**. The central ray is angled 30 degrees from the horizontal in a caudal direction. The normal **(H)** and abnormal **(I)** appearances are illustrated. In the latter situation, observe the lateral subluxation and tilting of the patella.

    **J** Inferosuperior view. Direction of the beam has been reversed. There is less distortion of the patella and the patient is able to hold the film.

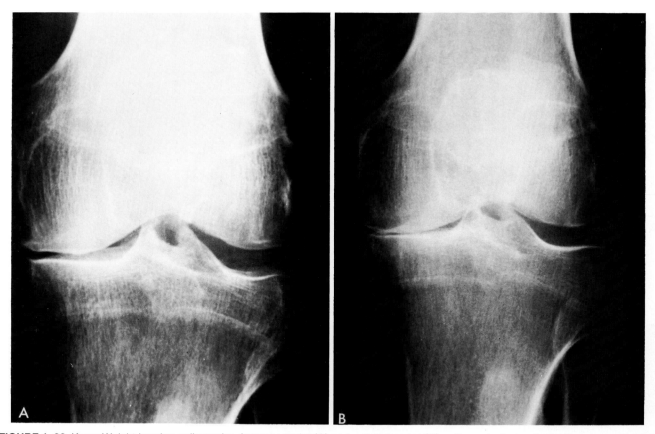

**FIGURE 1–28.** Knee: Weight-bearing radiography. Anteroposterior **(A)** and weight-bearing **(B)** radiographs in a patient with degenerative joint disease. With weight-bearing, there is further loss of joint space between the medial femoral condyle and tibia, allowing more accurate appraisal of the articular cartilage.

## TIBIA AND FIBULA

Standard radiographic assessment of the bones of the lower leg includes anteroposterior and lateral projections. In the frontal view, the center of the lateral malleolus should lie approximately 1 cm closer to the film than that of the medial malleolus, whereas for the lateral projection, the lateral malleolus should be positioned this same distance behind an imaginary line perpendicular to the film through the medial malleolus. Two radiographs with different centering in each projection may be required to visualize both the knee and the ankle joints. Supplementary oblique projections may be beneficial in occasional instances.

*Basic Examination: Tibia and Fibula*
Anteroposterior
Lateral

## ANKLE

Anteroposterior and lateral radiographs of the ankle are considered routine (Fig. 1–29). To better evaluate the medial articular space, an anteroposterior radiograph with 15 to 20 degrees of internal rotation of the foot—the mortise view—is optimal[89] to compensate for the fact that the ankle is oriented at approximately 15 to 20 degrees of external rotation in reference to the coronal plane of the knee.[90] Forty-five degree medial and lateral oblique radiographs

also are useful in the patient with a history of trauma to better evaluate the osseous structures, including the malleoli. In this clinical situation, anteroposterior radiographs obtained with varus and valgus stress and lateral radiographs accomplished during the application of anterior and posterior stress will document the presence of ligamentous damage.[156, 157] A "poor" (poorly positioned, steep oblique) lateral view obtained during slight external rotation of the foot will better delineate the posterior tibial lip.[91, 115, 116]

Weight-bearing radiographs of the ankle joint have not been found to provide additional information in the evaluation of arthritis at this site.[158]

*Basic Examination: Ankle*
Anteroposterior
Lateral
Mortise

## FOOT

Anteroposterior, medial oblique, and lateral projections are standard views for evaluation of the foot (Fig. 1–30). Of these, the single best view for evaluation of the joints of the midfoot and forefoot is the medial oblique projection. Similarly, for visualization of the toes, frontal, oblique, and lateral radiographs are necessary.

Adequate radiography of the sesamoid bones beneath the first metatarsal head requires an axial projection[92, 93] and,

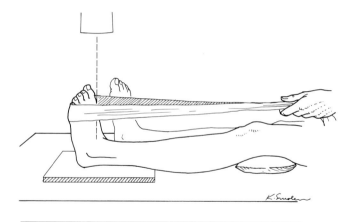

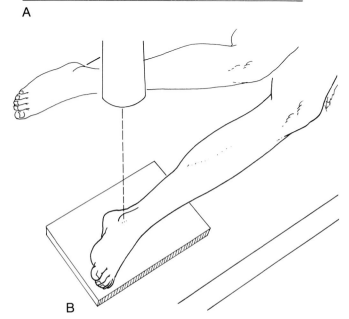

**FIGURE 1–29.** Ankle: Routine radiographs.
  **A** Anteroposterior radiograph. A sling may be used to provide mild dorsiflexion of the ankle.
  **B** Lateral radiograph.

views also are helpful in visualization of the subtalar and talocalcaneonavicular joints.[97, 98]

In children or adults with foot deformities, additional radiographs are suggested. In general, weight-bearing radiography is necessary using a lateral view of the foot in dorsiflexion and an anteroposterior view with the sagittal

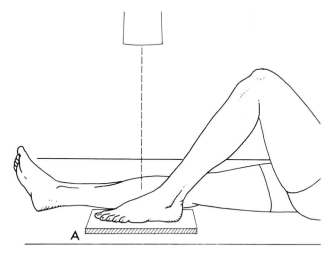

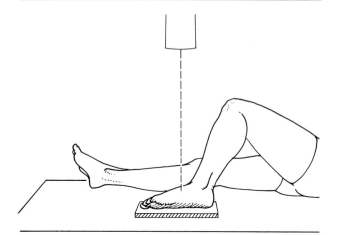

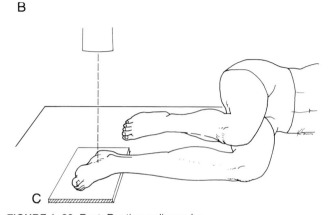

**FIGURE 1–30.** Foot: Routine radiographs.
  **A** Anteroposterior (dorsoplantar) radiograph.
  **B** Medial oblique radiograph.
  **C** Lateral radiograph.

rarely, an angulated lateral view[94] (Fig. 1–31). Axial radiographs of the forefoot are particularly helpful in evaluating patients with metatarsalgia.[159, 168]

Evaluation of the calcaneus can be accomplished by using a lateral projection, similar to that obtained for evaluation of the ankle, and an angulated frontal view, which can be obtained in an anteroposterior or posteroanterior direction (Fig. 1–32).

The tarsal joints require special radiographic projections (Fig. 1–33). A penetrated axial view, the Harris-Beath view, is utilized for demonstration of the subtalar joint and that portion of the talocalcaneonavicular joint about the middle facet of the calcaneus.[95] This view, which is similar to the angulated frontal view of the calcaneus, must be obtained with high kilovoltage technique so that the subtalar joints are identified. In addition, it is advantageous to obtain several axial radiographs with varying degrees of beam angulation, as some variation occurs in the configuration of these articulations.[96] Medial and lateral oblique

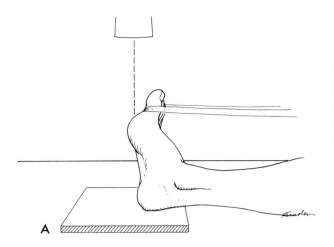

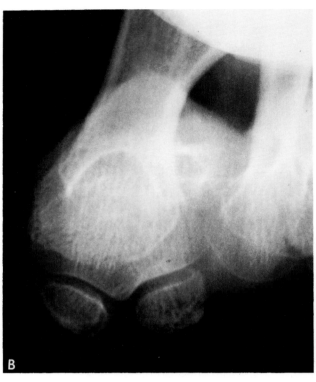

**FIGURE 1–31.** Sesamoid bones: Radiography—normal. The patient is supine. The toes are extended and a tangential radiograph demonstrates normal sesamoid bones beneath the first metatarsal head.

plane of the leg perpendicular to the film.[99, 100] Additional radiographs also are described.[101–103]

*Basic Examination: Foot*
Anteroposterior
Oblique
Lateral

## SURVEY RADIOGRAPHS

Survey radiographs are obtained in the initial evaluation of patients with polyarticular disorders and at various intervals during subsequent examinations. The type of radiographs required will depend in large part on the specific disorder that is suspected clinically and its distribution, as indicated by the patient's symptoms and signs. Thus, survey articular radiographs must be tailored to each patient and carefully monitored. In this fashion, abnormalities may

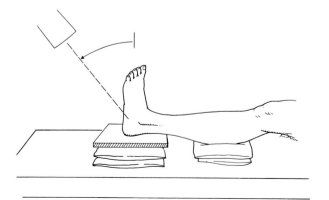

**FIGURE 1–32.** Calcaneus: Angulated frontal radiograph. With the patient supine, the central ray is angled at 40 degrees with the long axis of the foot.

be detected on initial films, and additional views may be obtained for better delineation of these alterations. Despite this necessity for individualizing the survey examination in articular disorders, certain general comments are appropriate.

Initial survey radiographs in a patient with polyarticular disease, particularly when the exact diagnosis has not yet been established clinically, must reveal enough information to delineate the type and extent of the disorder without representing an overuse either of the patient's, technician's, and physician's time or of radiation and expense. This can be accomplished by following a protocol that includes a minimal number of high-yielding radiographs.[104] The authors' experience has suggested that a protocol relying on the following projections is most useful in these patients:

| | |
|---|---|
| Hands: | Posteroanterior |
| | Semipronated oblique |
| Wrists: | Posteroanterior |
| | Lateral |
| | Semipronated oblique |
| | Semisupinated oblique |
| Shoulders: | 40 degree posterior oblique |
| Feet: | Medial oblique |
| Ankles: | Lateral, to include heel |
| Knees: | Anteroposterior |
| | Lateral |
| Pelvis: | Anteroposterior |
| Cervical Spine: | Lateral, with neck flexion |

It should be emphasized that these guidelines will require modifications depending upon the specific diagnosis that is to be established and the clinical questions that need to be answered. For example, in a patient with ankylosing spondylitis, emphasis must be placed on obtaining radiographs of the axial skeleton, including the sacroiliac joints,

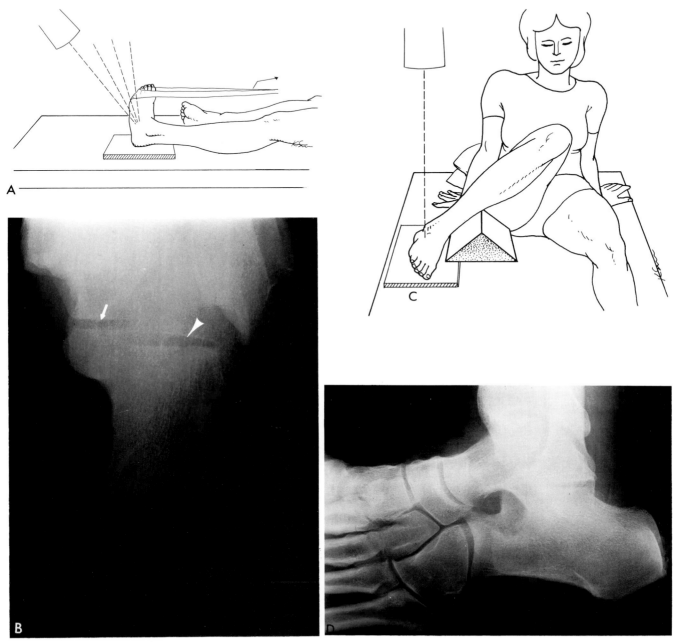

**FIGURE 1–33**. Tarsal joints: Normal radiography.

**A, B** Axial (Harris-Beath) view. The central ray can be directed at various angles. The posterior subtalar joint (arrowhead) and talocalcaneal portion of the anterior talocalcaneonavicular joint (arrow) are demonstrated.

**C, D** Oblique radiograph. The lateral aspect of the foot is elevated approximately 45 degrees. A vertical beam is used. The tarsal bones and joints are well seen.

whereas in a patient with calcium pyrophosphate dihydrate crystal deposition disease, a radiographic search for the presence or absence of cartilage calcification should include a coned-down view of the symphysis pubis, posteroanterior radiographs of the wrist, and anteroposterior radiographs of the knees. Furthermore, when a patient with polyarticular disease has more severe symptoms in one or two specific joints, a more detailed radiographic analysis of these joints must be obtained.

Follow-up radiographic examinations in patients with widespread articular disorders need not be as extensive as the initial survey. Attention should be paid to known target areas of the specific disorder and to additional areas that are symptomatic. In this way, radiographs can assess the distribution and extent of disease and its response to therapy.

Skeletal surveys in patients with neoplastic disease should not be performed prior to scintigraphic evaluation, owing to the greater sensitivity of the latter in the detection of metastatic foci. Radiographs of only those areas determined to be abnormal on the basis of bone scan findings then should be obtained. Exceptions to these rules occur in multiple myeloma, histiocytosis X, and neuroblastoma, in which a high percentage of lesions yield false-negative results on radionuclide studies. Skeletal surveys also are justified in the unconscious patient after major trauma to evaluate possible clinically occult injuries and in the diagnosis and follow-up of certain metabolic bone diseases, particularly renal osteodystrophy.

## References

1. Clark KC: Positioning in Radiography. 8th Ed. New York, Grune ) Stratton, 1964, p 1.
2. Merrill V: Atlas of Roentgenographic Positions. Vol 1. 3rd Ed. St Louis, CV Mosby Co, 1967, p 3.
3. Meschan I, Farrer-Meschan RMF: Radiographic Positioning and Related Anatomy. Philadelphia, WB Saunders Co, 1968, pp 29, 169.
4. Resnick D, Danzig LA: Arthrographic evaluation of injuries of the first metacarpophalangeal joint: Gamekeeper's thumb AJR 126:1046, 1976.
5. Norgaard F: Earliest roentgen changes in polyarthritis of the rheumatoid type. Continued investigations. Radiology 92:299, 1969.
6. Resnick D: Early abnormalities of pisiform and triquetrum in rheumatoid arthritis. Ann Rheum Dis 35:46, 1976.
7. Stecher WR: Roentgenography of the carpal navicular bone. AJR 37:704, 1937.
8. Bridgman CF: Radiography of the carpal navicular bone. Med Radiogr Photogr 25:104, 1949.
9. Ziter FMH Jr: A modified view of the carpal navicular. Radiology 108:706, 1973.
10. Templeton AW, Zim ID: The carpal tunnel view. Missouri Med 61:443, 1964.
11. Nisenfeld FG, Neviaser RJ: Fracture of the hook of the hamate: A diagnosis easily missed. J Trauma 14:612, 1974.
12. Carter PR, Eaton RG, Littler JR: Ununited fracture of the hook of the hamate. J Bone Joint Surg [Am] 59:583, 1977.
13. Stark HH, Jobe FW, Boyes JH, et al: Fracture of the hook of the hamate in athletes. J Bone Joint Surg [Am] 59:575, 1977.
14. Lentino W, Lubetsky HW, Jacobson HG, et al: The carpal bridge view. J Bone Joint Surg [Am] 39:88, 1957.
15. Burman M: Anteroposterior projection of the carpometacarpal joint of the thumb by radial shift of the carpal tunnel view. J Bone Joint Surg [Am] 40:1156, 1958.
16. Schmitt H: Die röntgenologische Darstellung des Radiusköpfchens. Roentgenpraxis 11:33, 1939.
17. Laquerrière A, Pierquin: De la nécessité d'employer une technique spéciale pour obtenir certains détails squelettiques. J Radiol Electrol Med Nucl 3:145, 1918.
18. Viehweger G: Zum Problem der Deutung der Knöchernen Gebilde distal des Epikondylus medialis humeri. ROFO 86:643, 1957.
19. Berens DL, Lockie LM: Ossification of the coraco-acromial ligament. Radiology 74:802, 1960.
20. Slivka J, Resnick D: An improved radiographic view of the glenohumeral joint. J Can Assoc Radiol 30:83, 1979.
21. Cleaves EN: A new film holder for roentgen examination of the shoulder. AJR 45:288, 1941.
22. Rubin SA, Gray, RL, Green WR: The scapular ''Y'': A diagnostic aid in shoulder trauma. Radiology 110:725, 1974.
23. Neer CS II: Displaced proximal humeral fractures. J Bone Joint Surg [Am] 52:1077, 1970.
24. Neer CS II, Rockwood CA Jr: Fractures and dislocations of the shoulder. In CA Rockwood Jr, DP Green (Eds): Fractures. Philadelphia, JB Lippincott, 1975, p 585.
25. Hill HA, Sachs MD: The grooved defect of the humeral head. A frequently unrecognized complication of dislocations of the shoulder joint. Radiology 35:690, 1940.
26. Hermodsson I.: Röntgenologische Studien über die traumatischen und habituellen Schultergelenkverrenkungen nach vorn und nach unten. Acta Radiol Suppl 20:1, 1934.
27. Adams JC: The humeral head defect in recurrent anterior dislocations of the shoulder. Br J Radiol 23:151, 1950.
28. Hall RH, Isaac F, Booth CR: Dislocation of the shoulder with special reference to accompanying small fractures. J Bone Joint Surg [Am] 41:489, 1959.
29. Didiee J: Le radiodiagnostic dans la luxation récidivante de l'épaule. J Radiol Electrol Med Nucl 14:209, 1930.
30. Bloom MH, Obata WG: Diagnosis of posterior dislocation of the shoulder with use of Velpeau axillary and angle-up roentgenographic views. J Bone Joint Surg [Am] 49:943, 1967.
31. Fisk C: Adaptation of the technique for radiography of the bicipital groove. Radiol Technol 37:47, 1965.
32. Zanca P: Shoulder pain: Involvement of the acromioclavicular joint. Analysis of 1000 cases. AJR 112:493, 1971.
33. Alexander OM: Radiography of the acromioclavicular articulation. Med Radiogr Photogr 30:34, 1954.
34. Bearden JM, Hughston JC, Whatley GS: Acromioclavicular dislocation: Method of treatment. J Sports Med 1:5, 1973.
35. Alexander OM: Dislocation of the acromio-clavicular joint. Radiography 15:260, 1949.
36. Tarrant RM: The axial view of the clavicle. X-ray Techn 21:358, 1950.
37. Quesada F: Technique for the roentgen diagnosis of fractures of the clavicle. Surg Gynecol Obstet 42:424, 1926.
38. Kattan KR: Modified view for use in roentgen examination of the sternoclavicular joints. Radiology 108:8, 1973.
39. Ritvo M, Ritvo M: Roentgen study of the sternoclavicular region. AJR 58:644, 1947.
40. Kurzbauer R: The lateral projection in roentgenography of the sternoclavicular articulation. AJR 56:104, 1946.
41. Hobbs DW: Sternoclavicular joint: A new axial radiographic view. Radiology 90:801, 1968.
42. Heinig CF: Retrosternal dislocation of the clavicle: Early recognition, x-ray diagnosis and management. J Bone Joint Surg [Am] 50:830, 1968.
43. Lee FA, Gwinn JL: Retrosternal dislocation of the clavicle. Radiology 110:631, 1974.
44. Christenson PC: The radiologic study of the normal spine. Cervical, thoracic, lumbar and sacral. Radiol Clin North Am 15:133, 1977.
45. Weir DC: Roentgenographic signs of cervical injury. Clin Orthop 109:9, 1975.
46. Miller MD, Gehweiler JA, Martinez S, et al: Significant new observations on cervical spine trauma. AJR 130:659, 1978.
47. Scher A, Vambeck V: An approach to the radiological examination of the cervicodorsal junction following injury. Clin Radiol 28:243, 1977.
48. Smith GR, Abel MS, Cone L: Visualization of the posterolateral elements of the upper cervical vertebrae in the anteroposterior projection. Radiology 115:219, 1975.
49. Jacobs LG: Roentgenography of the second cervical vertebra by Ottonello's method. Radiology 31:412, 1938.
50. George AW: Method for more accurate study of injuries to the atlas and axis. Boston Med Surg J 181:395, 1919.
51. Dorland P, Frémont J, Parer, et al: Techniques d'examen radiologique de l'arc postérieur des vertèbres cervicodorsales. J Radiol Electrol Med Nucl 39:509, 1958.
52. Buetti C: Zur Darstellung der Atlanto-epistropheal-gelenke. bzw. der Procc. transversi atlantis und epistrophei. Radiol Clin 20:168, 1951.
53. McCall I, Park W, McSweeney T: The radiological demonstration of acute lower cervical injury. Clin Radiol 24:235, 1973.
54. Wortzman G, Dewar FP: Rotary fixation of the atlantoaxial joint: Rotational atlantoaxial subluxation. Radiology 90:479, 1968.
55. Fuchs AW: Thoracic vertebrae. Radiogr Clin Photogr 17:2, 1941.
56. Oppenheimer A: The apophyseal intervertebral articulations roentgenologically considered. Radiology 30:724, 1938.
57. Fuchs AW: Thoracic vertebrae. II. Radiogr Clin Photogr 17:42, 1941.
58. Abel MS, Smith GR: Visualization of the posterolateral elements of the lumbar vertebrae in the anteroposterior projection. Radiology 122:824, 1977.
59. Kovacs A: X-ray examination of the exit of the lowermost lumbar root. Radiol Clin North Am 19:6, 1950.
60. Gianturco C: A roentgen analysis of the motion of the lower lumbar vertebrae in normal individuals and in patients with low back pain. AJR 52:261, 1944.
61. Resink JEJ: Zur Röntgenologie der sacroiliakalen Gelenke. Acta Radiol 38:313, 1952.
62. Jaeger E: Zur Aufnahmetechnik der Sacroiliocalgelenke. ROFO 71:630, 1949.
63. Dory MA, Francois RJ: Craniocaudal axial view of the sacroiliac joint. AJR 130:1125, 1978.

64. Chamberlain WE: The symphysis pubis in the roentgen examination of the sacroiliac joint. AJR *24*:621, 1930.

65. Kamieth H, Reinhardt K: Der ungleiche Symphysenstand, ein wichtiges Symptom der Beckenringlockerung. ROFO *83*:530, 1955.

66. Chassard, Lapine: Étude radiographique de l'arcade pubienne chez la femme enceinte: Une nouvelle méthode d'appréciation du diamètre biischiatique. J Radiol Electrol Med Nucl *7*:113, 1923.

67. Broderick TF: Complementary roentgenographic view of the hip. J Bone Joint Surg [Am] *37*:295, 1955.

68. Johnson CR: A new method for roentgenographic examination of the upper end of the femur. J Bone Joint Surg *14*:859, 1932.

69. Judet R, Judet J, Letournal E: Fractures of the acetabulum: Classification and surgical approaches for open reduction—preliminary report. J Bone Joint Surg [Am] *46*:1615, 1964.

70. Armbuster TG, Guerra J Jr, Resnick D, et al: The adult hip: An anatomic study. I. The bony landmarks. Radiology *128*:1, 1978.

71. Dunlap K, Swanson AB, Penner RS: Studies of the hip joint by means of lateral acetabular roentgenograms. J Bone Joint Surg [Am] *38*:1218, 1956.

72. Martel W, Poznanski AK: The value of traction during roentgenography of the hip. Radiology *94*:497, 1970.

73. Martel W, Poznanski AK: The effect of traction on the hip in osteonecrosis. A comment on the ''radiolucent crescent line.'' Radiology *94*:505, 1970.

74. Camp JD, Coventry MB: Use of special views in roentgenography of the knee joint. US Naval Med Bull *42*:56, 1944.

75. Holmblad EC: Postero-anterior x-ray view of the knee in flexion. JAMA *109*:1196, 1937.

76. Settegast: Typische Roentgenbilder von normalen Menschen. Lehmanns Med Atlanten *5*:211, 1921.

77. Hughston JC: Subluxation of the patella. J Bone Joint Surg [Am] *50*:1003, 1968.

78. Wiberg G: Roentgenographic and anatomic studies on the femoropatellar joint. Acta Orthop Scand *12*:319, 1941.

79. Knutsson F: Über die Röntgenologie des Femoropatellargelenks sowie eine gute Projektion für das Kniegelenk. Acta Radiol *22*:371, 1941.

80. Furmaier A, Breit A: Uber die Roentgenologie des Femoropatellargelenks. Arch Orthop Unfallchir *45*:126, 1952.

81. Merchant AC, Mercer RL, Jacobsen RH, et al: Roentgenographic analysis of patellofemoral congruence. J Bone Joint Surg [Am] *56*:1391, 1974.

82. Ficat P, Phillipe J, Bizour H: Le défilé fémoro-patellaire. Rev Méd Toulouse *6*:241, 1970.

83. Ficat RP, Hungerford DS: Disorders of the Patello-Femoral Joint. Baltimore, Williams & Wilkins Co, 1977, p 40.

84. Leach RE, Gregg T, Ferris JS: Weight-bearing radiography in osteoarthritis of the knee. Radiology *97*:265, 1970.

85. Arlbück S: Osteoarthrosis of the knee. A radiographic investigation. Acta Radiol Suppl *277*:7, 1968.

86. Leonard LM: The importance of weight-bearing x-rays in knee problems. J Maine Med Assoc *62*:101, 1971.

87. Thomas R, Resnick D, Alazraki N, et al: Compartmental evaluation of osteoarthritis of the knee: A comparative study of available diagnostic modalities. Radiology *116*:585, 1975.

88. Jacobsen K: Radiologic technique for measuring instability in the knee joint. Acta Radiol (Diagn) *18*:113, 1977.

89. Goergen TG, Danzig LA, Resnick D et al: Roentgenographic evaluation of the tibiotalar joint. J Bone Joint Surg [Am] *59*:874, 1977.

90. Hutter CG Jr, Scott W: Tibial torsion. J Bone Joint Surg [Am] *31*:511, 1949.

91. Mandell J: Isolated fracture of the posterior tibial lip at the ankle as demonstrated by an additional projection, the ''poor'' lateral view. Radiology *101*:319, 1971.

92. Holly EW: Radiography of the tarsal sesamoid bones. Med Radiogr Photogr *31*:73, 1955.

93. Lewis RW: Non-routine views in roentgen examination of the extremities. Surg Gynecol Obstet *67*:38, 1938.

94. Causton J: Projection of sesamoid bones in the region of the first metatarsophalangeal joint. Radiography *9*:39, 1943.

95. Harris RI, Beath T: Etiology of peroneal spastic flat foot. J Bone Joint Surg [Br] *30*:624, 1948.

96. Brodén B: Roentgen examination of the subtaloid joint in fractures of the calcaneus. Acta Radiol *31*:85, 1949.

97. Isherwood I: A radiological approach to the subtalar joint. J Bone Joint Surg [Br] *43*:566, 1961.

98. Feist JH, Mankin HJ: The tarsus: Basic relationships and motions in the adult and definition of optimal recumbent oblique projection. Radiology *79*:250, 1962.

99. Freiberger RH, Hersh A, Harrison MO: Roentgen examination of the deformed foot. Semin Roentgenol *5*:341, 1970.

100. Ritchie GW, Keim HA: A radiographic analysis of major foot deformities. Can Med Assoc J *91*:840, 1964.

101. Cobey JC: Posterior roentgenogram of the foot. Clin Orthop *118*:202, 1976.

102. Kandel B: Suroplantar projection in congenital club foot of the infant. Acta Orthop Scand *22*:161, 1952.

103. Gamble FO: A special approach to foot radiography. Radiogr Clin Photogr *19*:78, 1943.

104. Mink J, Gold R, Bluestone R: Radiographic arthritis survey. Arthritis Rheum *20*:1564, 1977.

105. Yousefzadeh DK: The value of traction during roentgenography of the wrist and metacarpophalangeal joints. Skel Radiol *4*:29, 1979.

106. Abel MS: Symmetrical anteroposterior projections of the sternoclavicular joints with motion studies. Radiology *132*:757, 1979.

107. Shackelford GD, McAlister WH: Axial radiography of the spine: A projection for evaluation of the neural arches in children. Radiology *130*:798, 1979.

108. Chevrot A: Incidence cranio-caudale oblique unilatérale de l'articulation sacro-iliaque. J Radiol *60*:143, 1979.

109. Egund N, Olsson TH, Schmid H, et al: Movements in the sacroiliac joints demonstrated with roentgen stereophotogrammetry. Acta Radiol (Diagn) *19*:833, 1978.

110. Sauser DD, Billimoria PE: Equalization filter for the shoulder. AJR *133*:952, 1979.

111. Rhea JT, DeLuca SA, Llewellyn HJ, et al: The oblique view: An unnecessary component of the initial adult lumbar spine examination. Radiology *134*:45, 1980.

112. DeSmet AA: Anterior oblique projection in radiography of the traumatized shoulder. AJR *134*:515, 1980.

113. DeSmet AA: Axillary projection in radiography of the nontraumatized shoulder. AJR *134*:511, 1980.

114. Laurin CA, Dussault R, Levesque HP: The tangential x-ray investigation of the patellofemoral joint: X-ray technique, diagnostic criteria and their interpretation. Clin Orthop *144*:16, 1979.

115. Van Moppes FI, Van Engelshoven JMA, Van de Hoogenband CR: Comparison between talar tilt, anterior drawer sign and ankle arthrography in ankle ligament lesions. J Belge Radiol *62*:441, 1979.

116. Seligson D, Gassman J, Pope M: Ankle instability: Evaluation of the lateral ligaments. Am J Sports Med *8*:39, 1980.

117. Brand DA, Frazier WH, Kohlhepp WC, et al: A protocol for selecting patients with injured extremities who need X-rays. N Engl J Med *306*:333, 1982.

118. Kreel L (Ed): Clark's Positioning in Radiography. Vol 2. 10th Ed. Chicago, Year Book Medical Publishers, 1981.

119. Balinger PW (Ed.): Merrill's Atlas of Radiographic Positions and Radiologic Procedures. 5th Ed. St Louis, CV Mosby Co, 1982.

120. Cullinan JE, Cullinan AM: Illustrated Guide to X-ray Technics. 2nd Ed. Philadelphia, JB Lippincott, 1980.

121. Bontrager KL, Anthony BT: Textbook of Radiographic Positioning and Related Anatomy. Denver, Multi-Media Publishing, 1982.

122. Hartley RM, Liang MH, Weissman BN, et al: The value of conventional views and radiographic magnification in evaluating early rheumatoid arthritis. Arthritis Rheum *27*:744, 1984.

123. Eisenberg RL, Hedgcock MW, Williams EA, et al: Optimum radiographic examination for consideration of compensation awards. III. Knee, hand, and foot. AJR *135*:1075, 1980.

124. DeSmet AA, Martin NL, Fritz SL, et al: Radiographic projections for the diagnosis of arthritis of the hands and wrists. Radiology *139*:577, 1981.

125. Moneim MS: The tangential posteroanterior radiograph to demonstrate scapholunate dissociation. J. Bone Joint Surg [Am] *63*:1324, 1981.

126. Fodor J III, Malott JC, Moulton J: Carpal tunnel ring artifact. AJR *144*:765, 1985.

127. Conway WF, Destouet JM, Gilula LA, et al: The carpal boss: An overview of radiographic evaluation. Radiology *156*:29, 1985.

128. Cuono CB, Watson HK: The carpal boss. Surgical treatment and etiological considerations. Plast Reconstr Surg *63*:88, 1979.

129. Kapandji A, Moatti E, Raab C: Specific radiography of trapezio-metacarpal joint and its technique. Ann Chir *34*:719, 1980.

130. Cooney WP III, Lucca MJ, Chao EYS, et al: The kinesiology of the thumb trapeziometacarpal joint. J Bone Joint Surg [Am] *63*:1371, 1981.

131. Greenspan A, Norman A: The radial head-capitellum view: Useful technique in elbow trauma. AJR *138*:1186, 1982.

132. Greenspan A, Norman A, Rosen H: Radial head-capitellum view in elbow trauma: Clinical application and radiographic-anatomic correlation. AJR *143*:355, 1984.

133. Hall-Craggs MA, Shorvon RJ, Chapman M: Assessment of the radial head-capitellum view and the dorsal fat-pad sign in acute elbow trauma. AJR *145*:607, 1985.

134. Oppenheim WL, Dawson EG, Quinlan C, et al: The cephaloscapular projection. A special diagnostic aid. Clin Orthop *195*:191, 1985.

135. Fagerlund M, Ahlgren O: Axial projection of the humeroscapular joint. Acta Radiol (Diagn) *22*:203, 1981.

136. Vezina JA: Compensation filter for shoulder radiography. Radiology *155*:823, 1985.

137. Abel MS: The exaggerated supine oblique view of the cervical spine. Skel Radiol *8*:213, 1982.

138. Pope TL Jr, Riddervold HO, Frankel CJ: Right or left intervertebral foramina? A simple method. J Can Assoc Radiol *32*:236, 1981.

139. Scher AT: The value of erect radiographs in cervical spine injury. S Afr Med J *58*:574, 1980.

140. Pozo JL, Crockard HA, Ransford AO: Basilar impression in osteogenesis imperfecta. A report of three cases in one family. J Bone Joint Surg [Br] *66*:233, 1984.

141. Boger D, Ralls PW: New traction device for radiography of the lower cervical spine. AJR *137*:1202, 1981.

142. England AC III, Shippel AH, Ray MJ: A simple view for demonstration of fractures of the anterior arch of C1. AJR *144*:763, 1985.

143. DeSmet AA, Goin JE, Asher MA, et al: A clinical study of the differences between the scoliotic angles measured on posteroanterior and anteroposterior radiographs. J Bone Joint Surg [Am] 64:489, 1982.

144. vanSchaik JJP, Verbiest H, vanSchaik FDJ: Morphometry of lower lumbar vertebrae as seen on CT scans: Newly recognized characteristics. AJR 145:327, 1985.

145. Abel MS, Smith GR, Allen TNK: Refinements of the anteroposterior angled caudad view of the lumbar spine. Skel Radiol 7:113, 1981.

146. Porter RW, Park W: Unilateral spondylolysis. J Bone Joint Surg [Br] 64:344, 1982.

147. Vanhoute JJ, Raeside DE: A generalization of Chevrot's method for determining the anteversion and cervico-diaphyseal angles. Radiology 128:251, 1978.

148. Eisenberg RL, Hedgcock MW, Akin JR: The 40 degree cephalad view of the hip. AJR 136:835, 1981.

149. Ru-Bin C, Qiang-de N: Early detection and classification of collapse of femoral head after transcervical fracture. Chin Med J 95:25, 1982.

150. van den Broek HAC, Vegter J: Traction radiography of the hip and fluid in the hip joint. Diagn Imaging 52:76, 1983.

151. Vegter J, van den Broek JAC: The diagnostic value of traction during radiography in diseases of the hip. A preliminary report. J Bone Joint Surg [Br] 65:428, 1983.

152. Singer AM, Naimark A, Felson D, et al: Comparison of overhead and cross-table lateral views for detection of knee-joint effusion. AJR 144:973, 1985.

153. Bradley WG, Ominsky SH: Mountain view of the patella. AJR 136:53, 1981.

154. Hagstedt B, Norman O, Olsson TH, et al: Technical accuracy in high tibial osteotomy for gonarthrosis. Acta Orthop Scand 51:963, 1980.

155. Cockshott WP, Racoveanu NT, Burrows DA, et al: Use of radiographic projections of knee. Skel Radiol 13:131, 1985.

156. Cox JS, Hewes TF: "Normal" talar tilt angle. Clin Orthop 140:37, 1979.

157. Cass JR, Morrey BF: Ankle instability: Current concepts, diagnosis and treatment. Mayo Clin Proc 59:165, 1984.

158. Bauer M, Bergstrom B, Hemborg A: Arthrosis of the ankle evaluated on films in weight-bearing position. Acta Radiol (Diagn) 20:88, 1979.

159. Pritsch M, Heim M, Horoszowski H, et al: The significance of the axial foot projection in the diagnosis of metatarsal pathology. Arch Orthop Trauma Surg 98:139, 1981.

160. Drerup B: Improvements in measuring vertebral rotation from the projections of the pedicles. J. Biomechanics 18:369, 1985.

161. Turula KB, Friberg O, Haajanen J, et al: Weight-bearing radiography in total hip replacement. Skel Radiol 14:200, 1985.

162. Hardy DC, Totty WC, Reinus WR, et al: Posteroanterior wrist radiography: Importance of arm positioning. J Hand Surg [Am] 12:504, 1987.

163. Jalovaara P, Myllylä V, Päivänsalo M: Autotraction stress roentgenography for demonstration of anterior and inferior instability of the shoulder joint. Clin Orthop 284:136, 1992.

164. Kornguth PJ, Salazar AM: The apical oblique view of the shoulder: Its usefulness in acute trauma. AJR 149:113, 1987.

165. Stenlund B, Goldie I, Marions O: Diminished space in the acromioclavicular joint in forced arm adduction as a radiographic sign of degeneration and osteoarthrosis. Skel Radiol 21:529, 1992.

166. Marcelis S, Seragani FC, Taylor JAM, et al: Reevaluation of oblique radiography of the cervical spine: Comparison of 45 degree and 55 degree anteroposterior oblique projections. Radiology 188:253, 1993.

167. Rijke AM, Tegtmeyer CJ, Weiland DJ, et al: Stress examination of the cruciate ligaments: A radiologic Lachman test. Radiology 165:867, 1987.

168. Dreeben S, Thomas PBM, Noble PC: A new method for radiography of weight-bearing metatarsal heads. Clin Orthop 224:260, 1987.

# 2

# Plain Film Radiography: Sources of Diagnostic Errors

*Theodore E. Keats, M.D.*

*The diagnostician must be familiar with normal variation if he is not to give his patients diseases which they do not have.*
JOHN CAFFEY

The routine radiographic examination represents a major contribution to the diagnosis and differential diagnosis of skeletal disorders. This is particularly true because the identification of the disease process and its differentiation from other disorders often is still a difficult process by clinical and laboratory examination. It therefore is of great importance that the physician be aware of the many anatomic variants and radiographic pitfalls that may mislead in the assessment of the patient with skeletal complaints.

Nature has supplied myriad anatomic variations that complicate the radiographic examination. Many of these are simply the changes of growth, others are variations in individual development, and still others are positional artifacts, but all of them potentially are misleading.

Because of space limitation, the author has chosen from a large amount of material a number of entities that often are confused with true disease or that have potential for harm if they are misinterpreted. This survey is by no means exhaustive, and the interested reader is urged to consult more comprehensive works on the subject of normal anatomic variation for help with problems that are not presented here.[1, 2]

## CERVICAL SPINE

Erosion and destruction of the odontoid process is a well-recognized characteristic of a number of inflammatory ar-
thritides, and minor variations of configuration should not be confused with manifestations of this inflammatory process (Figs. 2–1 and 2–2). Similarly, in the search for involvement of the apophyseal joints of the cervical spine, these joints in the midcervical spine may not be well seen and give the appearance of fusion, owing to positioning of the spine and the direction of the x-ray beam (Fig. 2–3). This matter is resolved easily by obtaining oblique projections that will show well-defined articular surfaces in the normal person.

Another apparent abnormality that may be produced by faulty positioning is factitial calcification of the posterior spinal ligament as a result of slight rotation of the spine at the time of filming, so that two posterior aspects of the vertebral bodies are seen (Fig. 2–4). This situation, too, will

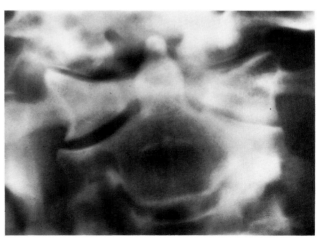

FIGURE 2–1. Normal pointed configuration of the odontoid tip.

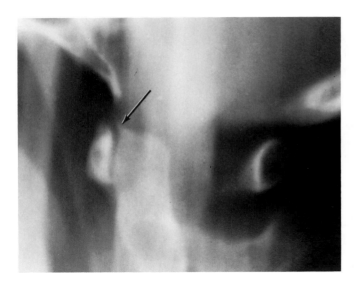

**FIGURE 2–2**. Pointed configuration of the superior aspect of the tip of the odontoid process (arrow), which should not be mistaken for an erosive alteration.

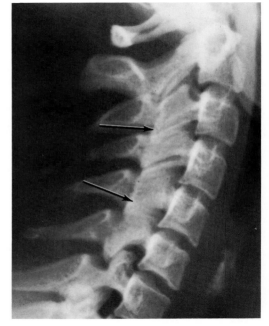

**FIGURE 2–3**. Simulated fusion of the posterior cervical elements produced by projection (arrows).

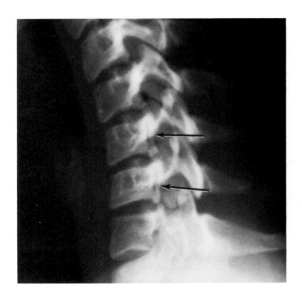

**FIGURE 2–4**. Simulated posterior spinal ligament calcification (arrows) produced by rotation of the neck at the time of filming.

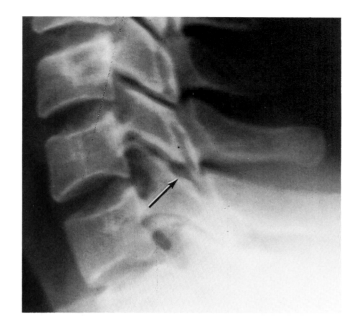

**FIGURE 2–5.** Normal notching of the apophyseal joint surface (arrow) of the lower cervical spine should not be mistaken for erosion or fracture.

be resolved by repetition of the examination with correct positioning of the spine.

The superior articular surfaces of the fifth to seventh cervical vertebrae in some normal persons may show a groove or depression, which should not be mistaken for an erosive process or traumatic alteration[3] (Fig. 2–5).

## CLAVICLE AND RIBS

The point of insertion of the rhomboid ligament at the inferior aspect of the medial portion of the clavicle in some persons is reflected as a deep and, at times, irregular fossa. These fossae are not always present bilaterally, nor are they symmetric if they occur bilaterally. At times, they are sufficiently striking to be confused with a destructive process.

A potential pitfall in the radiologic search for evidence of arthritis is the appearance of the medial ends of the clavicles in adolescence (Fig. 2–6). Before the secondary centers appear at approximately the age of 17 years, the medial ends of the clavicles appear cupped and irregular,

and this appearance might be mistaken for an inflammatory arthritis or as evidence of a metabolic bone disorder.

Loss of the cephalic margins of the posterior aspects of the upper ribs is a recognized phenomenon that occurs in a variety of diseases, including the collagen vascular disorders. It most commonly is seen in rheumatoid arthritis and in hyperparathyroidism. It also may be seen in the elderly, however, as a manifestation of the restrictive lung disease of the aged (Fig. 2–7). The common denominator in all the conditions in which it has been described probably is disuse.[4]

## UPPER EXTREMITY

Marginal irregularities of the edges of the glenoid fossa, a common finding in pubertal children, may simulate marginal joint destruction of arthritis (Fig. 2–8). Such irregularities are particularly marked at the superior margin. These irregularities disappear by the time the secondary centers of ossification become evident.

**FIGURE 2–6. A,** Plain film, and **B,** conventional tomogram, of normal irregularity of the medial ends of the clavicles of an adolescent before development of the secondary ossification centers.

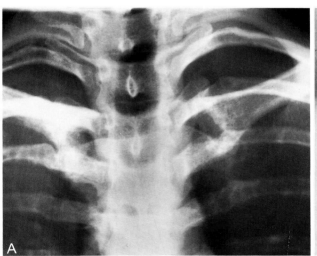
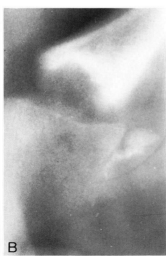

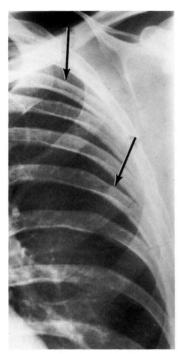

**FIGURE 2–7**. Loss of the cephalic margins of the posterior aspects of the ribs (arrows) may be seen in the elderly as a manifestation of restrictive lung disease.

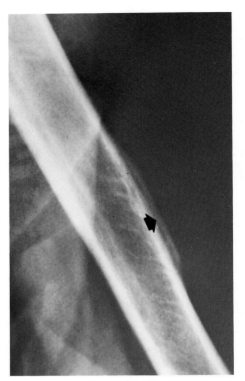

**FIGURE 2–9**. Changes at the insertion site of the deltoid muscle (arrow) may simulate those of neoplasm.

The insertion of the deltoid muscle may result in an area of bone sclerosis or an appearance simulating periostitis (Fig. 2–9).

Notches or shallow grooves in the medial cortex of the metaphysis of the proximal end of the humerus are seen as a normal variant in children between the ages of 10 and 16 years (Fig. 2–10). They are asymptomatic and apparently represent a transient event in the growth period. These cortical alterations may be unilateral or bilateral and are of concern only in that they may be mistaken for an inflammatory or neoplastic alteration.[5]

The greater tuberosity of the humerus in some persons contains a large amount of cancellous bone, which projects

on the radiograph as a circumscribed area of radiolucency (pseudocyst) that may simulate a destructive lesion (Fig. 2–11).

The thin flange of bone that constitutes the lateral cortical margin of the distal portion of the humerus often is projected in a fashion that simulates periosteal proliferation (Fig. 2–12). This is misinterpreted as evidence of reactive new bone formation. Similarly, the thin flanges of bone that serve as the attachment of the interosseous membrane in the forearm may be mistakenly thought to be abnormal periostitis (Fig. 2–13).

Patients in whom the ulna is relatively short in compari-

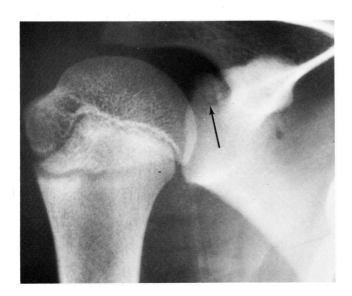

**FIGURE 2–8**. Normal developmental irregularity of the glenoid fossa in a 14 year old boy (arrow).

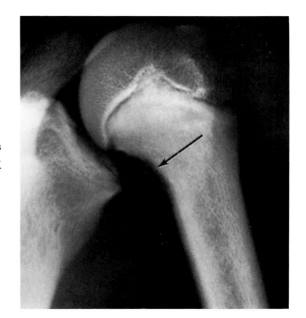

FIGURE 2–10. Upper humeral notch (arrow) in a 10 year old girl. These notches are seen between the ages of 10 and 16 years, and represent a phase of growth. They probably are similar to the cortical lesions seen in the metaphyses of other long bones in adolescence, particularly in the distal end of the femur.

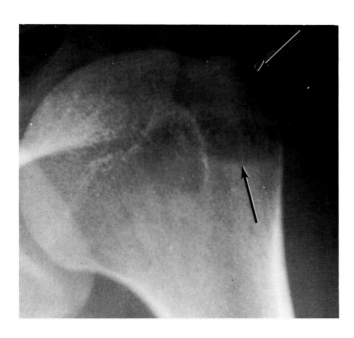

FIGURE 2–11. Simulated destruction of the greater tuberosity. This normal finding (arrows) appears to represent the fusion line of the lateral portion of the physis. Its position in relationship to the physeal line should help differentiate it from a true lesion.

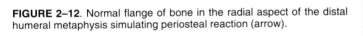

FIGURE 2–12. Normal flange of bone in the radial aspect of the distal humeral metaphysis simulating periosteal reaction (arrow).

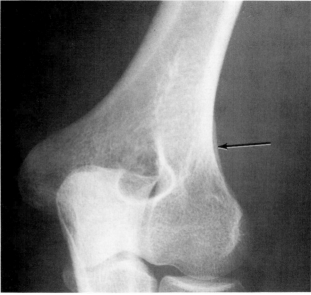

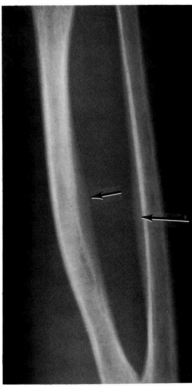

**FIGURE 2–13**. Normal bony flanges for the insertion of the interosseous membrane that may simulate new bone formation (arrows).

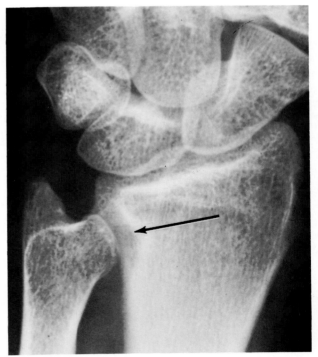

**FIGURE 2–14**. In patients who have a relatively short ulna, the fossa at the inferior radioulnar articulation should not be mistaken for a destructive or arthritic process (arrow).

son to the radius often show a relatively deep fossa at the site of the inferior radioulnar joint, which may simulate an inflammatory arthritic process (Fig. 2–14).

The triangular cartilage of the wrist just distal to the end of the ulna frequently is a site of abnormal calcification. It should be kept in mind that there is an accessory bone, the os triangulare, that may be found in this position as well (Fig. 2–15), and it often occurs bilaterally.

Congenital fusions of the carpal bones often are a famil-ial trait. These fusions most commonly involve the lunate and triquetral bones (Fig. 2–16) but may involve others, such as the scaphoid and trapezium (Fig. 2–17).

The pisiform is a sesamoid bone and ossifies in an irregular fashion, best seen in the lateral projection. Such irregularity should not be confused with a pathologic process in young children (Fig. 2–18).

Narrow medullary cavities of the metacarpal bones are normal variations in development and are without pathologic significance (Fig. 2–19).

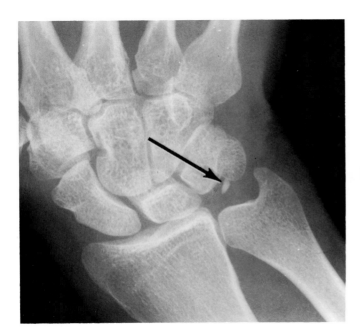

**FIGURE 2–15**. The os triangulare, an accessory ossicle (arrow).

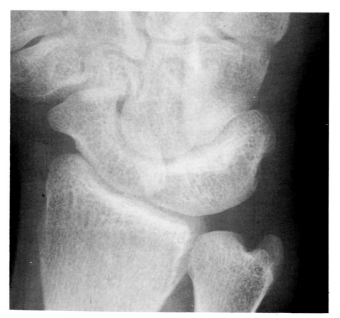

**FIGURE 2–16.** Congenital fusion of the lunate and triquetral bones.

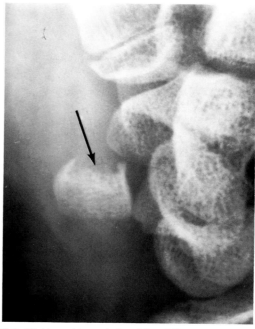

**FIGURE 2–18.** Normal irregularity of the pisiform bone in an 11 year old boy (arrow).

Spurlike extensions of the medial aspects of the epiphyses of the distal ends of the metacarpal bones represent a transient event in the ossification of this end of the bone (Fig. 2–20). In some persons, after completion of growth, a spurlike extension of the radial side of the metaphysis of the distal ends of the metacarpal bones may be seen in the oblique projection (Fig. 2–21).

Common sources of confusion in the early diagnosis of rheumatoid arthritis are apparent small defects in the bases of the proximal phalanges (Fig. 2–22). These can be disregarded if there are no associated erosions in the metacarpal heads or disturbances in joint architecture.[6]

The nutrient canals of the distal ends of the proximal phalanges may be quite prominent and cast shadows that simulate areas of intraosseous bony destruction (Fig. 2–23).

The bony ridges and projections seen in the proximal phalanges, which represent areas of insertion of muscles, should not be confused with reactive new bone formation (Fig. 2–24).

Ivory epiphyses in the hands of healthy children may be seen as an anatomic variant (Fig. 2–25). At times, there may be an associated delay in maturation of the hand, particularly the phalanges. There apparently is no associa-

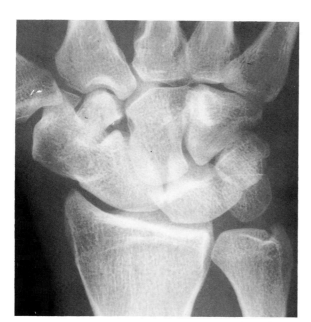

**FIGURE 2–17.** Congenital fusion of the scaphoid and trapezium.

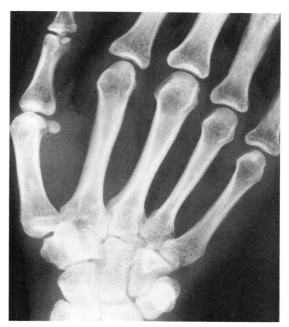

**FIGURE 2–19.** Narrowing of the medullary cavities of the metacarpal bones, a normal variant.

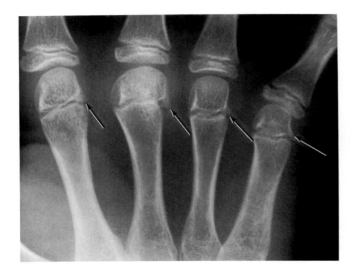

**FIGURE 2–20.** Developmental excrescences (arrows) of the metacarpal heads in a normal 13 year old boy.

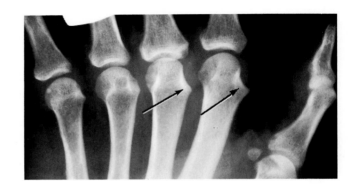

**FIGURE 2–21.** Normal osteophyte-like projections of the metacarpal heads (arrows).

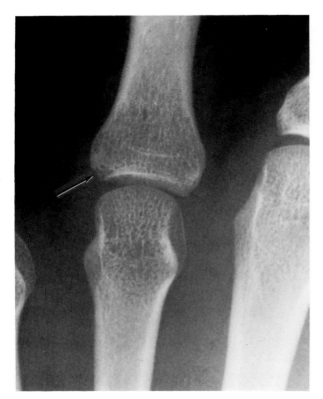

**FIGURE 2–22.** Small notches at the bases of the proximal phalanges (arrow) should not be mistaken for the erosions of inflammatory arthritis, which usually first involve the heads of the metacarpal bones.

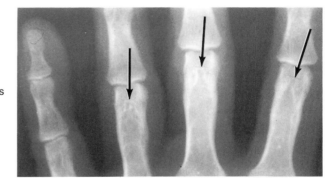

**FIGURE 2–23**. Nutrient canals in the heads of the proximal phalanges (arrows).

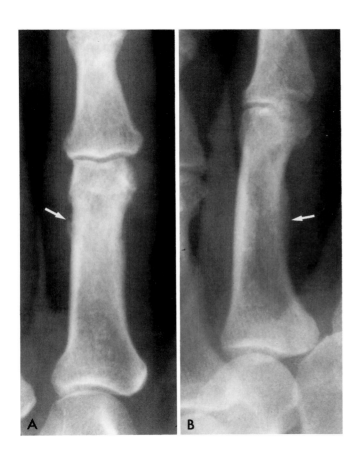

**FIGURE 2–24**. Normal ridges and projections on the phalanges associated with muscular insertions, not to be mistaken for periosteal new bone (arrows).

**FIGURE 2–25**. Ivory epiphyses of the bases of the distal phalanges of the second and fifth fingers in a normal 12 year old girl.

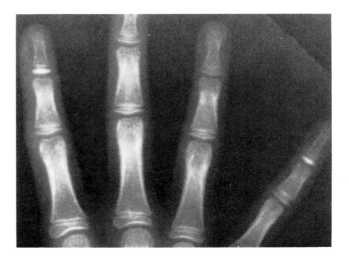

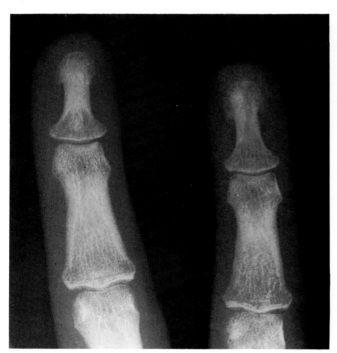

**FIGURE 2–26**. Sclerosis of the terminal phalanges in a patient with no associated disease.

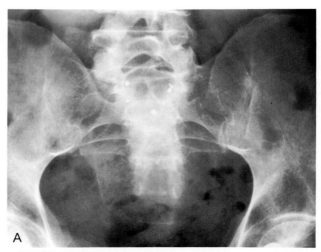

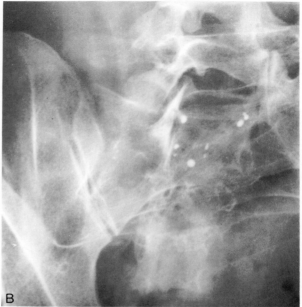

**FIGURE 2–28. A** Simulated obliteration of the right sacroiliac joint produced by rotation of the pelvis.
**B** Oblique sacroiliac view shows normal joint.

tion with ischemic necrosis of these ossification centers.[7] Similarly, sclerosis of the terminal phalanges may be seen in healthy adults, particularly in women over the age of 40 years[8] (Fig. 2–26).

### PELVIS

The appearance of the sacroiliac joints in adolescents bears a distinct resemblance to the changes of ankylosing spondylitis (Fig. 2–27). It is well to bear in mind that, in youngsters, the joint spaces are wide, with irregular and often dense joint margins.

Obliquity of the pelvis at the time of filming may simulate obliteration of one sacroiliac joint (Fig. 2–28A). Improved positioning or sacroiliac joint views will reveal the true state of affairs (Fig. 2–28B).

The preauricular sulci are anatomic variants evident as

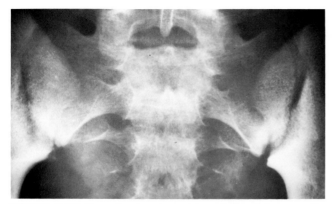

**FIGURE 2–27**. Normal sclerosis and irregularity of the sacroiliac joints in a 14 year old boy resemble the changes of ankylosing spondylitis.

fossae in the ilia adjacent to the inferior margins of the sacroiliac joint (Fig. 2–29). They are seen only in women and should not be confused with areas of bone destruction.

Cephalad angulation of the x-ray beam will produce a double contour of the superior margins of the pubic bones that simulates periosteal new bone formation (Fig. 2–30). This effect is not seen when the beam is directed perpendicularly to the film.

In the aged, the bone of the brim of the pelvis often appears laminated and thickened, an appearance that may be confused with Paget's disease (Fig. 2–31).

The normal pubertal symphysis pubis is wide, with irregular joint margins (Fig. 2–32). This appearance may mimic a destructive arthritis.

Alterations in the symphysis pubis occur after parturition (Fig. 2–33A). With passage of time, the density of the bone regresses and cystlike areas of radiolucency remain as permanent stigmata (Fig. 2–33B).

The normal ischiopubic synchondroses are a source of

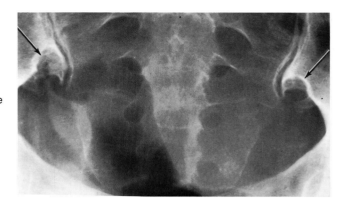

**FIGURE 2–29.** Preauricular sulci (arrows). This is a characteristic of the female pelvis and is not necessarily bilaterally symmetric.

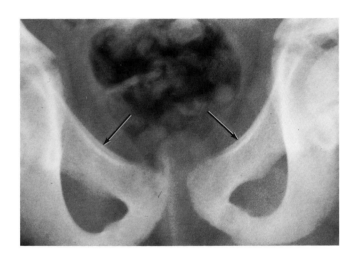

**FIGURE 2–30.** Simulated periosteal proliferation of bone of the superior margins of the pubic bones (arrows) due to cephalad angulation of the x-ray beam.

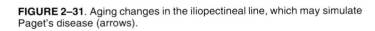

**FIGURE 2–31.** Aging changes in the iliopectineal line, which may simulate Paget's disease (arrows).

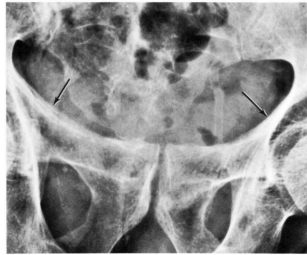

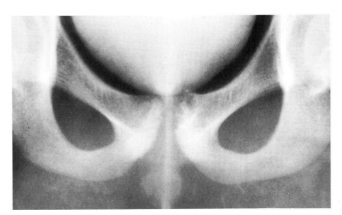

**FIGURE 2–32.** Normal developmental irregularity of the symphysis pubis in a 12 year old boy. Incidentally noted is contrast material in the bladder.

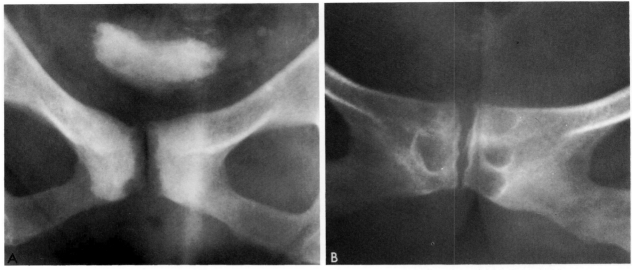

FIGURE 2–33. Postpartum changes in the symphysis pubis. **A**, Recent changes. **B**, Old changes.

confusion, as they often appear as swollen, radiolucent areas in young children (Fig. 2–34A). This is a normal phenomenon of growth and not evidence of disease. It is important to remember that these synchondroses do not always close synchronously (Fig. 2–34B) and, at times, may reappear after initial closure.

The inferior aspects of the ischia may be markedly irregular in adolescents. This phenomenon is thought to be the result of strong muscular pull at the sites of insertion and is self-limited (Fig. 2–35). These irregularities disappear with completion of growth and are not of clinical significance. A similar alteration also may be seen at the anteroinferior iliac spine at the point of insertion of the rectus femoris muscle[9] (Fig. 2–36).

## HIP

The capital femoral epiphysis may ossify from multiple centers rather than from a single center (Fig. 2–37). This appearance in an ossification center should not be taken as a manifestation of disease, such as ischemic necrosis. In like fashion, the roofs of the acetabula in young children often are grossly irregular, representing areas of ossification in the cartilaginous matrix (Fig. 2–38).

Protrusio acetabuli is a normal phenomenon in children from approximately 4 to 12 years of age and is not a reflection of acetabular abnormality (Fig. 2–39).[10]

The fossae for the nutrient vessels in the acetabulum may be mistaken for a destructive lesion in the femoral head if

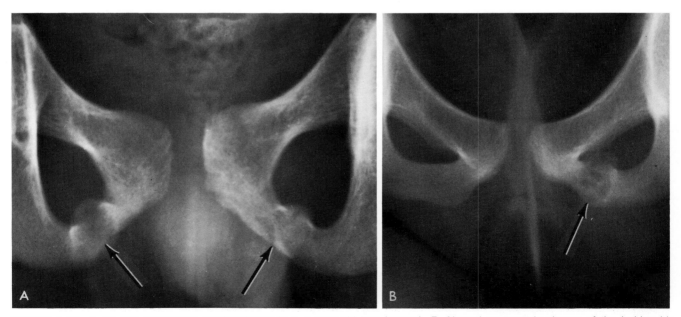

FIGURE 2–34. **A**, Normal ischiopubic synchondroses in a 4 year old boy (arrows). **B**, Normal asymmetric closure of the ischiopubic synchondroses in a 12 year old boy (arrow).

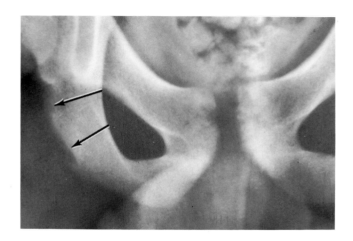

FIGURE 2–35. Normal irregularity of the ischium in a 16 year old boy (arrows). These changes usually are asymmetric and disappear with increasing age. They represent "tug" lesions due to the pull of the hamstring muscles.

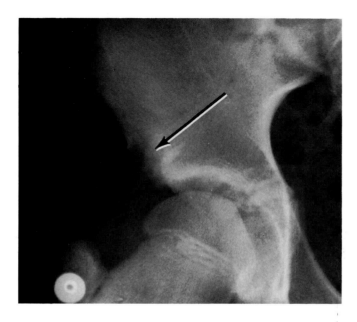

FIGURE 2–36. Irregularity of the anteroinferior iliac spine (arrow) in an adolescent boy. This represents a "tug" lesion at the insertion of the rectus femoris muscle and should not be mistaken for the changes caused by neoplasm.

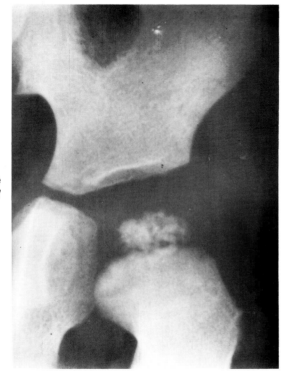

FIGURE 2–37. Normal irregular ossification of the capital femoral epiphysis of the left hip in a young child. This appearance in a single center does not necessarily indicate the presence of disease.

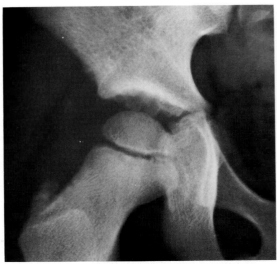

**FIGURE 2–38**. Normal irregularity of the acetabular roof in a 5½ year old child.

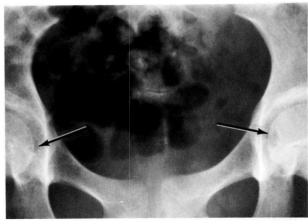

**FIGURE 2–40**. Fossa for nutrient vessel of the acetabulum (arrows) simulating a destructive lesion in the left femoral head owing to overlap of osseous structures.

they are fully superimposed on the head (Fig. 2–40). In addition, the fovea capitis of the femoral head should not be confused with an erosion of the articular surface (Fig. 2–41). Additional spurious shadows in the acetabulum may be produced by an undulation in the anterior margin of the acetabulum coupled with superimposition of the shadow of the ischium (Fig. 2–42) or by superimposition of bony shadows of the posterior wall of the acetabulum projected through the femoral head (Fig. 2–43). Similar overlapping shadows of the acetabulum may produce an area of double density that may be confused with ischemic necrosis of the femoral head (Fig. 2–44).

Brown[11] has shown that apparent bulging of the "capsular" shadow of the hip can be produced by filming the hip in abduction and external rotation, leading to an appearance suggesting fluid in the joint (Fig. 2–45). Comparison of the soft tissue shadows about the hip from side to side requires that both hips be in neutral position to obtain useful information.

The secondary ossification centers for the posterior margin of the acetabulum often are multiple and not necessarily symmetric bilaterally (Fig. 2–46). Remnants of these ossification centers may be confused with fractures.

## LOWER EXTREMITY

The superior margins of the femoral necks are poorly defined in young children and, at times, may have an appearance that suggests new bone formation. This is particularly prominent at about the age of 4 or 5 years (Fig. 2–47). In older children, similar growth irregularities may be seen in the greater trochanter (Fig. 2–48).

Several somewhat striking cortical irregularities are seen in the distal femoral metaphysis in adolescents, which may lead to needless concern and investigation. One of these is seen in the lateral projection in the anterior cortex[12] and the others in the posterior cortex on the medial side[13] (Fig. 2–49). The posterior irregularity is larger and, therefore, its cause has been the subject of considerable debate. It has been considered to be a fibrous cortical defect[14] as well as an avulsive lesion.[15] In any case, the irregularity commonly

*Text continued on page 59*

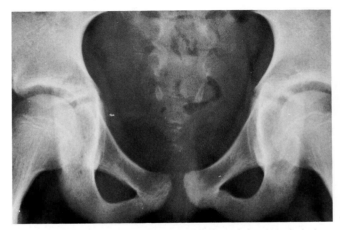

**FIGURE 2–39**. Normal intrapelvic protrusion of the acetabula in a 9½ year old girl.

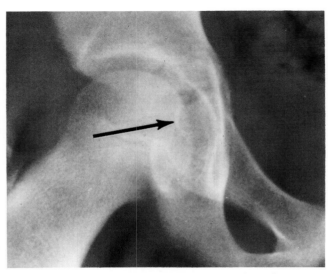

**FIGURE 2–41**. The normal fovea capitis (arrow).

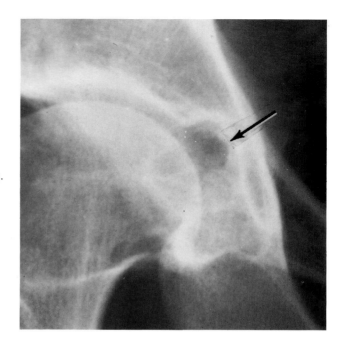

FIGURE 2–42. Pseudocyst of the acetabulum (arrow).

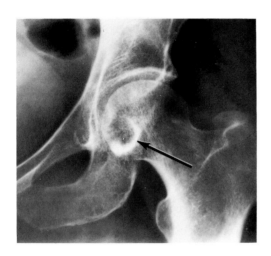

FIGURE 2–43. Simulated destructive lesion of the femoral head produced by a bony strut in the posterior wall of the acetabulum projected through the femoral head (arrow).

FIGURE 2–44. Overlapping shadows of the femoral head and acetabulum simulating ischemic necrosis (arrow).

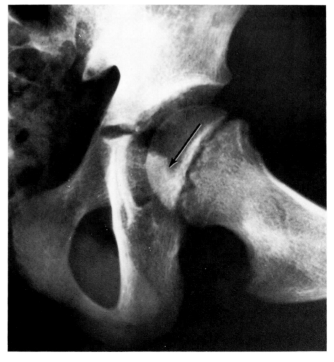

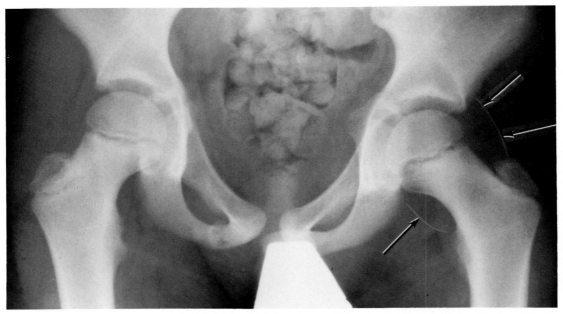

**FIGURE 2–45.** Apparent bulging of the "joint capsule" of the left hip in a 9 year old boy (arrows) due to malpositioning of the hip at the time of filming. Compare with shadows of the opposite side. (Illustration has been altered to accentuate the findings.)

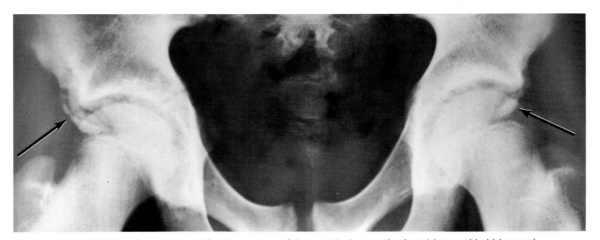

**FIGURE 2–46.** Secondary ossification centers of the acetabular margins in a 14 year old girl (arrows).

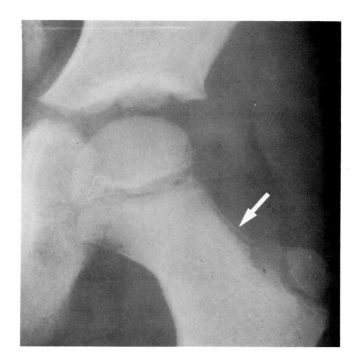

FIGURE 2–47. Normal irregularity of the superior margin of the femoral neck in a 4 year old child (arrow).

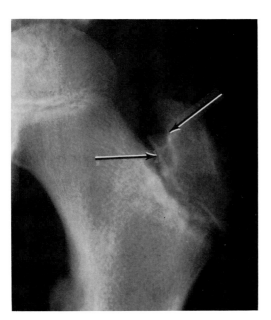

FIGURE 2–48. Normal irregularities of ossification of the greater trochanter in a 12 year old boy (arrows).

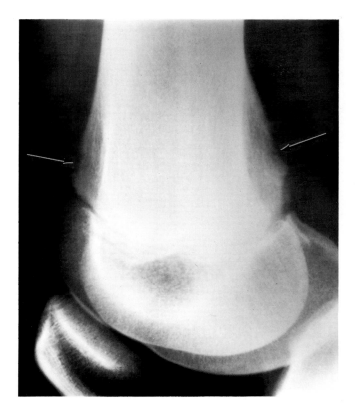

**FIGURE 2–49.** Normal cortical irregularities on the anterior and posterior aspects of the distal end of the femur in a 15 year old boy (arrows).

**FIGURE 2–50.** Irregularity of the cortex of the medial aspect of the distal femoral metaphysis (arrows) is a common finding between the ages of 12 and 16 years. This is a fibrous lesion, which often demonstrates fine perpendicular spiculation of bone and which may be mistaken for a malignant bone neoplasm.

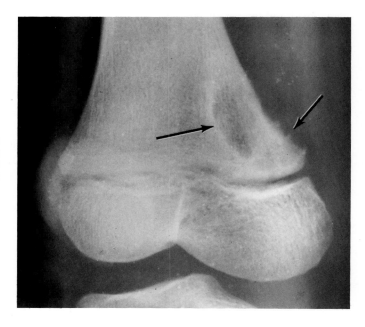

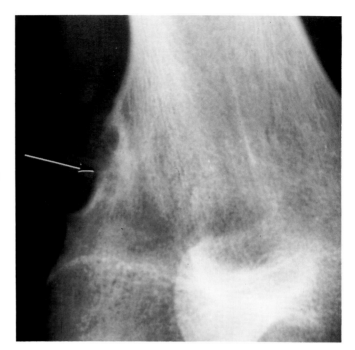

**FIGURE 2–51.** Remnants of the posterior femoral cortical irregularity in a 21 year old man (arrow).

is seen posteriorly as well as posteromedially (Fig. 2–50) and should not be mistaken for an inflammatory or neoplastic lesion. It is sufficiently characteristic radiographically. Evidence of this same process often can be found in the adult, manifested as a fossa in the cortex (Fig. 2–51).

The nutrient foramen at the distal end of the femur is intra-articular and is seen as one or several discrete areas of radiolucency, which may be mistaken for a destructive lesion in the intercondylar area (Fig. 2–52).

The patella may be partitioned into two or more segments, and the resulting appearance can be mistaken for fracture (Fig. 2–53). The segmentation usually occurs in the lateral aspect of the patella. Observation of the well-defined spaces between the segments and the sharp bone margins is

helpful in its differentiation from fracture. This can be demonstrated best in the tangential view of the patella.

The distal articular surface of the femur in young children radiologically is grossly irregular, representing islands of ossification in the cartilaginous epiphysis[16] (Fig. 2–54). These irregularities are best seen from the ages of 6 to 12 years and are confused with osteochondritis dissecans. They are well delineated in the tunnel projection (Fig. 2–54A) and are most evident in the posterior aspects of either or both condyles (Fig. 2–54B). They can be differentiated from osteochondritis dissecans by their occurrence in a younger age group and by their appearance in areas of the condyles that usually are not involved in osteochondritis dissecans.

In adults, grooves may be seen in the articular surface of the medial condyle in tangential patellar views and are a source of misinterpretation[17] (Fig. 2–55). These grooves may be evident in the lateral projection as well (Fig. 2–56).

The ossification of the distal femoral epiphysis may be quite irregular in children, particularly in its lateral aspect,

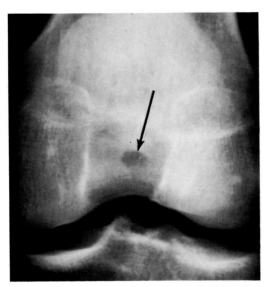

**FIGURE 2–52.** The nutrient foramen of the distal end of the femur (arrow).

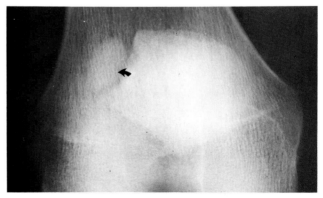

**FIGURE 2–53.** Bipartite patella. Note the irregular superolateral bone fragment (arrow).

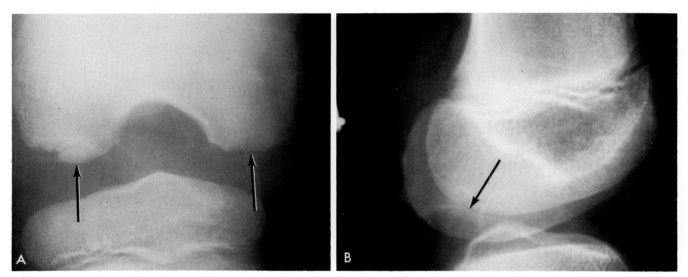

**FIGURE 2–54. A** Normal irregularity of ossification of the articular surfaces of the distal end of the femur in a 10 year old boy, simulating osteochondritis dissecans (arrows).
   **B** These irregularities are located posteriorly, as illustrated in a 12 year old boy (arrow).

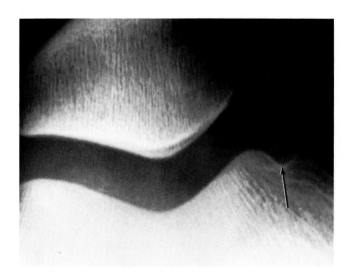

**FIGURE 2–55.** Normal groove in the articular surface of the medial condyle of the femur, seen in a tangential patellar view (arrow).

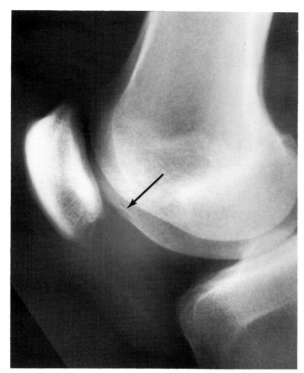

**FIGURE 2–56**. Normal depression of the articular surface of the medial condyle of the femur (arrow).

and this results in areas of relative radiolucency that may be quite alarming[18] (Fig. 2–57).

A circumscribed radiolucent defect may be seen in the dorsal aspect of the patella in young people, usually as an incidental finding (Fig. 2–58). The defect is self-limited and apparently represents a variant in ossification. It is not a manifestation of osteochondritis dissecans of the patella.[19]

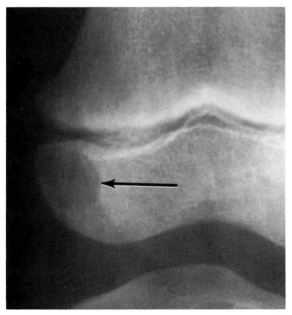

**FIGURE 2–57**. Normal developmental area of radiolucency in the lateral aspect of the distal femoral epiphysis in a 6 year old boy (arrow).

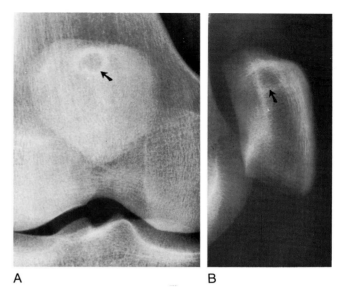

A                                                    B

**FIGURE 2–58**. Dorsal patellar defect. These radiolucent shadows (arrows) are of no clinical significance and should not be confused with osteochondritis dissecans of the patella.

The tibial tubercle is notoriously irregular in its ossification, and this irregularity in itself is not necessarily a reflection of traumatic avulsion or "osteochondrosis" (Fig. 2–59). Furthermore, the lateral aspect of the tibial tubercle in the adult may be seen in the frontal projection as a laminated-appearing mass on the lateral aspect of the tibia and may be confused with a lesion producing new bone (Fig. 2–60). Similar spurious thickening of the lateral cortex of the tibia and the medial cortex of the fibula may be produced by slight external rotation of the leg (Fig. 2–61).

Another reported source of misinterpretation is the soleal line of the tibia, which is a cause of tibial pseudoperiostitis. The origin of the soleus muscle may result in a prominent osseous crest, which mimics a large area of periostitis in the posterior aspect of the proximal portion of the shaft of the tibia (Fig. 2–62). It always is associated with normal, undisturbed architecture of the underlying bone.

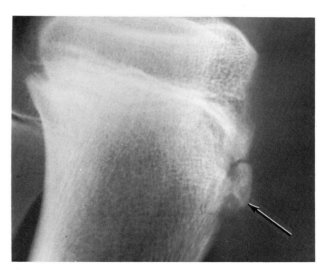

**FIGURE 2–59**. Normal variation in appearance of the ossification center of the tibial tubercle in an adolescent (arrow).

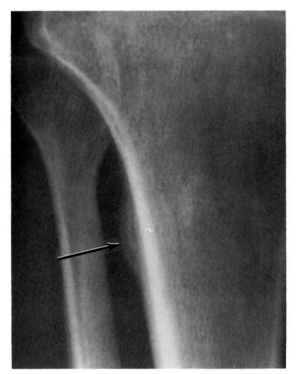

**FIGURE 2–60**. The tibial tubercle simulating laminated periostitis (arrow).

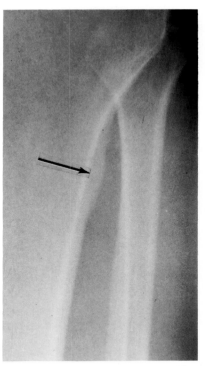

**FIGURE 2–61**. Pseudoperiostitis of the tibia, simulated by the tibial tuberosity (arrow). Note also the spurious thickening of the lateral cortex of the tibia and the medial cortex of the fibula due to slight external rotation of the leg.

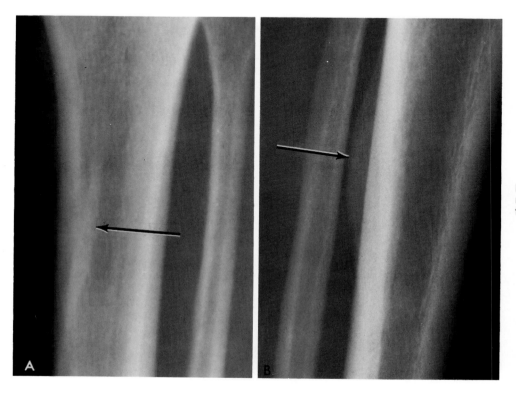

**FIGURE 2–62**. The soleal line (arrows) represents a "tug" lesion at the insertion of the soleus muscle.

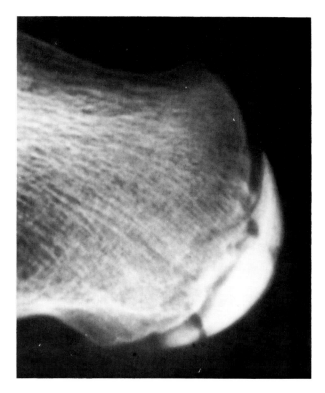

FIGURE 2–63. Normal density and "fragmentation" of the calcaneal apophysis.

The ossification of the calcaneal apophysis is associated with two troublesome radiologic aspects. It normally is dense in children who walk, and it also may develop from multiple centers (Fig. 2–63). Neither of these findings should be confused with ischemic necrosis or osteochondritis. Similar irregularities in ossification without increased density may be seen in the tarsal navicular bones (Fig. 2–64). Invariably these centers unite and form a single bone. In the stage of irregular ossification, the lack of sclerosis will differentiate this normal finding from osteochondritis (Köhler's disease).

In children with painful feet, the irregular ossification of

the developing sesamoid bones should not be mistaken for pathologic calcification in the plantar soft tissues (Fig. 2–65).

The os intermetatarseum is an accessory bone that arises from the base of the first or second metatarsal bone. It is variable in its size and shape and may be seen on the dorsum of the foot (Fig. 2–66). The apophysis of the base of the fifth metatarsal bone may not fuse and may remain as a separate bone throughout life. It should not be mistaken for a fracture (Fig. 2–67).

The ossification center of the base of the proximal phalanx of the great toe is similar to the calcaneal apophysis in

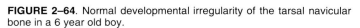

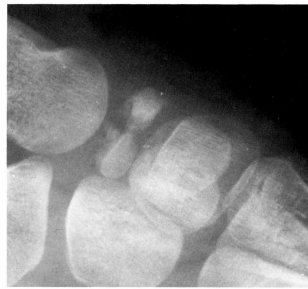

FIGURE 2–64. Normal developmental irregularity of the tarsal navicular bone in a 6 year old boy.

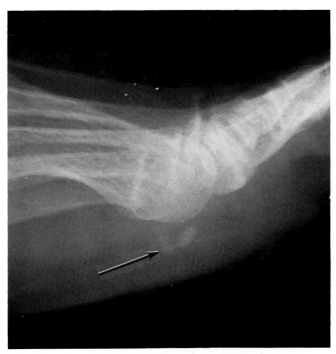

FIGURE 2–65. The normal irregular appearance of the ossifying sesamoid bones in the foot of a 12 year old boy (arrow).

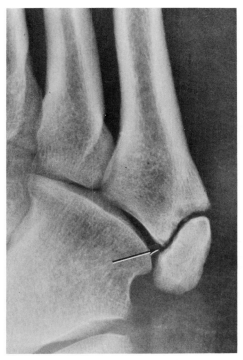

FIGURE 2–67. An ununited apophysis (arrow) of the base of the fifth metatarsal bone.

that it usually is dense and occasionally may be bifid. Both alterations are normal variants of growth (Fig. 2–68).

Cone-shaped epiphyses are seen in the proximal phalanges in many normal children and are not necessarily expressions of generalized or local disease (Fig. 2–69).

In the search for early periosteal bone formation in the phalanges as an expression of inflammatory arthritis, the normal osseous excrescences of the proximal phalanges should not be mistaken for periostitis (Fig. 2–70).

Many normal persons do not develop distal interphalangeal joints in their toes. This is seen most commonly in the fifth toe but also may occur in the third and fourth toes. This condition, therefore, is not a manifestation of acquired ankylosis (Fig. 2–71).

The ungual tufts of the toes may not be seen in children and some adults, resulting in a pointed configuration of the distal phalanx. This does not represent a resorptive phenomenon (Fig. 2–72).

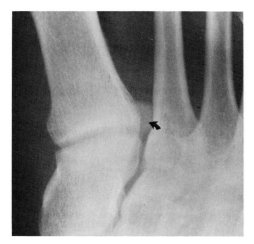

FIGURE 2–66. Os intermetatarseum. The accessory bone (arrow) is projected between the bases of the first and second metatarsal bones.

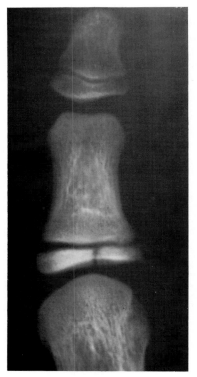

FIGURE 2–68. A dense ossification center at the base of the proximal phalanx of the great toe with or without a midline cleft is a normal variation of growth.

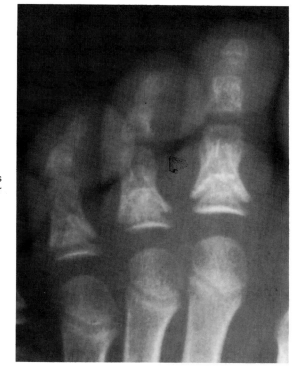

**FIGURE 2–69**. Cone-shaped epiphyses at the bases of the proximal phalanges may occur in normal children and are unrelated to any skeletal dysplasia or arthropathy.

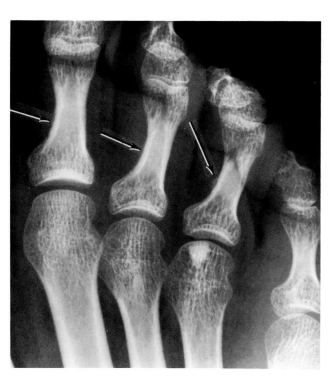

**FIGURE 2–70**. Normal bony excrescences in toes (arrows), not to be mistaken for periosteal proliferation.

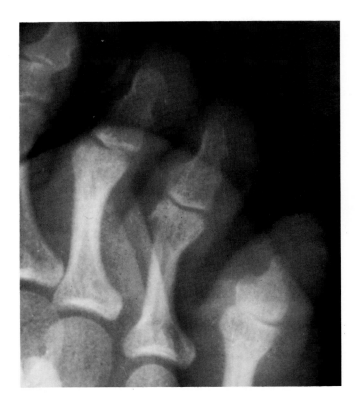

FIGURE 2–71. Nonsegmented middle and distal phalanges in the third, fourth, and fifth toes.

FIGURE 2–72. Pointed terminal phalanges without tufts may be seen as a normal variant in young children and are unrelated to disease. In this subject, note also the variations in growth of the middle phalanges.

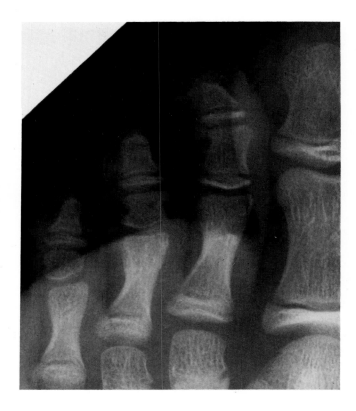

## SUMMARY

The examples of variation in development described in this chapter are only a few of the problems that beset any physician who uses routine radiography in the study of skeletal disease. It is obvious that a broad appreciation of the alterations that are part of the normal growth of the skeleton, as well as a knowledge of many of the normal variations of the adult skeleton that may mimic significant disease, is necessary to avoid errors of commission.

---

I wish to express my appreciation to the Year Book Medical Publishers for permission to reproduce material from my book, Atlas of Normal Roentgen Variants That May Simulate Disease. Copyright © 1973, 1979, 1984, 1988, and 1992 by Mosby–Year Book, Inc., Chicago.

## References

1. Keats TE: Atlas of Normal Roentgen Variants That May Simulate Disease. 5th Ed. St. Louis, Mosby–Year Book, 1992.
2. Köhler A, Zimmer EA: Borderlands of Normal and Early Pathologic Findings in Skeletal Radiography. 4th Ed. New York, Thieme Medical Publishers, 1993.
3. Keats TE, Johnstone WH: Notching of the lamina of C7: A proposed mechanism. Skel Radiol 7:233, 1982.
4. Keats TE: Superior marginal rib defects in restrictive lung disease. AJR 124:449, 1975.
5. Ozonoff MB, Ziter FMH Jr: The upper humeral notch. Radiology 113:699, 1974.
6. Stelling CB, Keats MM, Keats TE: Irregularities at the bases of the proximal phalanges. AJR 138:695, 1982.
7. Kuhns LR, Poznanski AK, Harper HAS, et al: Ivory epiphyses of the hands. Radiology 109:643, 1973.
8. Goodman N: The significance of terminal phalangeal osteosclerosis. Radiology 89:709, 1967.
9. Murray RO, Jacobson HG: The Radiology of Skeletal Disorders. 2nd Ed. New York, Churchill Livingstone, 1977.
10. Alexander C: The aetiology of primary protrusio acetabuli. Br J Radiol 38:567, 1965.
11. Brown I: A study of the "capsular" shadow in disorders of the hip in children. J Bone Joint Surg [Br] 57:175, 1975.
12. Keats TE: The distal anterior femoral metaphyseal defect: An anatomic variant that may simulate disease. AJR 121:101, 1974.
13. Barnes GR, Gwin JL: Distal irregularities of the femur simulating malignancy. AJR 122:180, 1974.
14. Brower A, Culver JE Jr, Keats TE: Histological nature of the cortical irregularity of the medial posterior distal femoral metaphysis in children. Radiology 99:389, 1971.
15. Bufkin WJ: The avulsive cortical irregularity. AJR 112:487, 1971.
16. Dunham WK, Marcus NW, Enneking WF, et al: Developmental defects of the distal femoral metaphysis. J Bone Joint Surg [Am] 62:801, 1980.
17. Harrison RB, Wood MB, Keats TE: The grooves of the distal articular surface of the femur—a normal variant. AJR 126:751, 1976.
18. Caffey J: Pediatric X-Ray Diagnosis. 8th Ed. Chicago, Year Book Medical Publishers, 1985.
19. Haswell DM, Berne AS, Graham CB: The dorsal defect of the patella. Pediatr Radiol 4:238, 1976.
20. Levine AH, Pais J, Berinson H, et al: The soleal line: A cause of tibial pseudoperiostitis. Radiology 119:79, 1976.

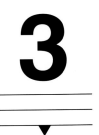

# Fluoroscopy

*Donald Resnick, M.D.*

Fluoroscopy is a diagnostic tool that is a fundamental part of many radiologic procedures, including barium studies of the gastrointestinal tract and angiography. Its application to the evaluation of musculoskeletal disorders is readily apparent when considering that fluoroscopic guidance is a prerequisite for arthrography, tenography, bursography, sinography, myelography, and biopsy procedures (Chapters 12, 13, and 16). With regard to arthrographic examinations, earlier methods using overhead radiographic filming to delineate meniscal or ligament abnormalities after contrast opacification of the knee have been entirely replaced with fluoroscopic monitoring and recording of such abnormalities, and fluoroscopic techniques can be used as an adjunct to routine radiography in defining arthrographic alterations in the glenohumeral joint, hip, ankle, wrist, and other locations. In fact, the experienced arthrographer knows full well that fluoroscopic monitoring immediately after the introduction of small amounts of contrast material or air will document that the needle has been placed properly in the joint (as the contrast agent will flow freely from the tip of the needle), lessening the possibility of technical failure of the examination. During biopsy of the bones or soft tissues, the position of the advancing needle or guide often is defined by single plane or biplane fluoroscopy, and fluoroscopic spot films document the precise location from which the tissue sample is removed. Although computed tomography (CT) also can be used to monitor biopsy procedures, fluoroscopy is the preferred technique primarily because of its convenience.

Fluoroscopic assistance in a number of orthopedic and neurosurgical procedures also is well recognized.[1, 2] Insertion of dynamic hip screws, Kuntscher rods, and Ender nails is best accomplished with fluoroscopic guidance in the operating room.[3] Fluoroscopy also defines the precise vertebral level prior to spinal surgery.

Additional applications of fluoroscopy to the assessment of musculoskeletal disease are less well known. Many of these are described in appropriate sections of this book, but a few of particular importance are summarized here.

## NORMAL AND ABNORMAL JOINT MOTION

Fluoroscopy with videotaping (or cineradiography) is useful in the evaluation of articular movement. Careful monitoring of vertebral position during flexion, extension, and lateral bending provides information defining the presence and level of spinal instability; abnormal findings include abrupt or jerky movement of one vertebra with respect to its neighbors and asymmetric widening of apophyseal joints, and the instability is confirmed by the identification of secondary signs such as narrowing of the intervertebral disc space, vacuum phenomena, and traction enthesophytes at the discovertebral junction.

The kinematics of the wrist are complex, yet when alterations occur in the normal integrated function of the carpal bones, significant symptoms and signs arise. Conventional plain radiographs, even when obtained as static images in positions of flexion, extension, and radial and ulnar deviation, may not indicate the source of the clinical manifestations. The analysis of wrist motion is better accomplished using either (1) fluoroscopy with spot filming or videotaping, or (2) cineradiography,[4-9] sometimes in combination with arthrography.[8] Such motion also can be evaluated with dynamic studies using magnetic resonance (MR) imaging. During fluoroscopy, the positions of the carpal bones as the patient reproduces the painful wrist motion and their movements during radial and ulnar deviation with an open and clenched hand in both the frontal and the lateral projections are observed and recorded with an attempt to identify irregular movement and abnormal widening of the intercarpal spaces.[9] The application of external stress to the wrist during the fluoroscopic examination also is helpful in delineating subtle and transient subluxations of the carpal bones.[10]

Fluoroscopic monitoring and spot filming while stress is applied by the examiner may provide important diagnostic information in cases of posttraumatic instability in many additional sites. Examples of this include injuries of the cruciate ligaments of the knee, medial and lateral ligaments of the ankle, and acromioclavicular and coracoclavicular ligaments. Although routine radiography during the application of stress will allow identification of some or all of these injuries, the diagnosis is provided more easily by carefully monitored studies accomplished with fluoroscopy.

## FRACTURES

The most important method allowing the initial identification of fractures after acute trauma remains the conventional radiograph. Most physicians suggest that, when the initial radiographs are equivocal, additional radiographic projections be used. This approach is time-consuming and commonly is unsatisfactory. Fluoroscopy with spot filming represents a more successful alternative approach to this diagnostic problem. The patient can be evaluated in multiple positions until the optimal projection is identified and the findings are recorded on the film.[11] The procedure is quick and direct and avoids the excessive radiation dose and the frustration on the part of the x-ray technician that accompany multiple overhead projections.

The extent of the fracture and its relationship to adjacent articulations also are well defined by fluoroscopy. The fluoroscopic examination, when combined with the application of external stress, is useful in demonstrating a fracture nonunion by profiling the involved osseous surfaces and documenting movement among the fracture fragments. It often is essential in the diagnosis of the Hill-Sachs lesion of the humeral head.

## OSTEOCHONDRITIS DISSECANS

The adequate evaluation of curved and angular bone contours is especially difficult with routine radiography. As these sites not uncommonly are involved in osteochondritis dissecans, it is not surprising that fluoroscopy aids in the assessment of this injury.[11] Five minutes spent in the fluoroscopic suite as the examiner views the injured area from different perspectives commonly is sufficient to establish a diagnosis of osteochondritis dissecans. This technique particularly is important in evaluating osteochondral fractures of the talar dome, as they may not be projected in a tangential fashion on the conventional radiographs. Fluoroscopic spot filming in various degrees of plantar flexion and dorsiflexion of the foot usually is successful in defining the location and the extent of the fracture (Fig. 3–1).

## INTRA-ARTICULAR OSTEOCHONDRAL BODIES

Fluoroscopy with or without the instillation of contrast material or air into the joint represents an important procedure in identifying intra-articular osteochondral fragments or bodies (Fig. 3–2). The precise position of the radiodense fragment with respect to the articular cavity is evident during the procedure, and additional bodies not seen on the conventional radiographs may be detected. A typical tumbling or rolling motion of the osseous body generally confirms an intra-articular or intrabursal location and that the body is loose or unattached to the synovial lining.[12] Less freely movable radiodense shadows that do not tumble or roll may indicate bodies attached to the synovial membrane or capsule or lying outside the joint.

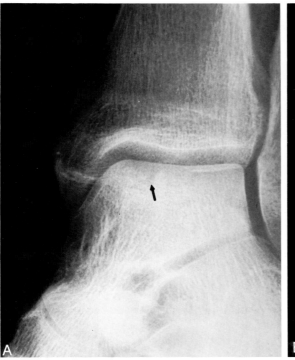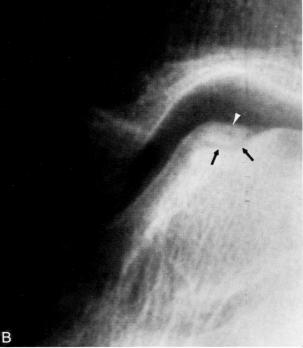

**FIGURE 3–1.** Fluoroscopy: Osteochondritis dissecans of the talus.
   **A** The initial radiograph shows an area of radiolucency in the superomedial portion of the talus (arrow).
   **B** A fluoroscopic spot film, accomplished with the patient in an oblique position and with plantar flexion of the foot, reveals a depression of the articular surface (arrows) containing an osseous body (arrowhead).

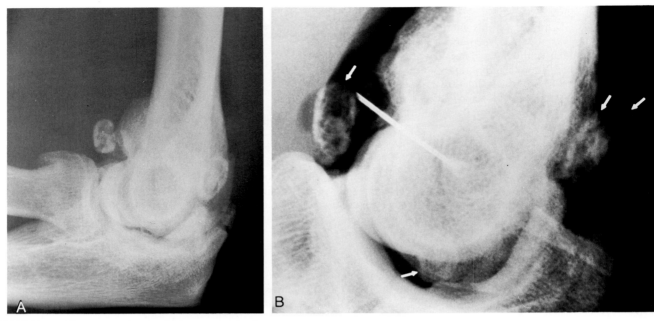

**FIGURE 3–2.** Fluoroscopy: Intra-articular osseous bodies.

**A** A lateral radiograph of the elbow reveals multiple osseous radiodense areas of various sizes in front of and behind the distal portion of the humerus.

**B** A fluoroscopic spot film obtained during the introduction of intra-articular air confirms that the osseous bodies (arrows) are within the joint.

## SHOULDER IMPINGEMENT SYNDROME

The shoulder impingement syndrome is an important source of shoulder pain that occurs when the bone and soft tissue structures of the superior aspect of the shoulder encroach on the coracoacromial ligamentous arch during abduction of the arm[13] (see Chapters 13, 39, and 70). Subacromial bursitis, bicipital tendinitis, and rotator cuff disruption are common sequelae of this abnormality. Although the clinical examination commonly is diagnostic, evidence supporting the shoulder impingement syndrome is provided by routine radiography that indicates osseous excrescences (subacromial enthesophytes) arising from the anteroinferior aspect of the acromion and flattening and sclerosis of the greater tuberosity of the humerus. Fluoroscopic examination (with or without subacromial bursography) reveals bone contact between the greater tuberosity and the subacromial enthesophyte during abduction of the arm (Fig. 3–3) or close approximation of this tuberosity and the acromion during abduction at a time when the patient experi-

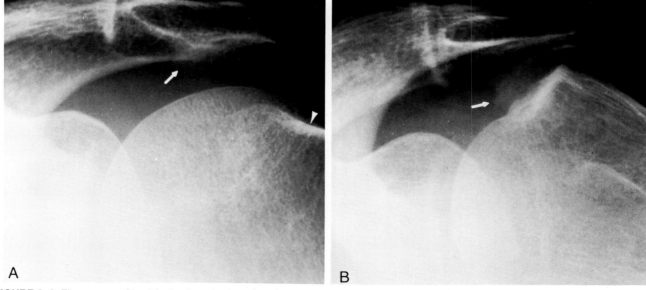

**FIGURE 3–3.** Fluoroscopy: Shoulder impingement syndrome.

**A** An initial radiograph shows a subacromial enthesophyte (arrow) and sclerosis of the greater tuberosity (arrowhead).

**B** With fluoroscopy, the abnormal contact of the enthesophyte (arrow) and the sclerotic and flattened greater tuberosity as the patient abducts his arm are apparent.

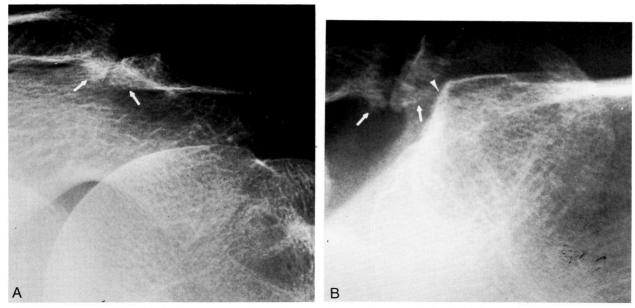

**FIGURE 3–4**. Fluoroscopy: Shoulder impingement syndrome. Fluoroscopic spot films are obtained with the arm in a neutral position **(A)** and abducted **(B)**. Osteophytes arising from the inferior margin of the acromioclavicular joint (arrows) approximate the greater tuberosity (arrowhead) in the abducted position.

ences typical pain and restriction of motion. Less commonly, shoulder impingement may result from osteophytes at the inferior margin of the acromioclavicular joint (Fig. 3–4).

## ORTHOPEDIC APPLIANCES

Metal contained in orthopedic appliances creates diagnostic problems during conventional radiography by obscuring adjacent osseous and soft tissue structures. Fluoroscopy allows the examiner to choose an appropriate patient position carefully in which obscurity is less prominent.[11] It also promotes the examination of the orthopedic device itself, defining its relationship to the adjacent bone and joint. This is of particular importance in the assessment of patients who have had pins or screws placed within the bone. Establishing that the orthopedic device has been inserted improperly and has penetrated the cortical surface or joint cavity can be difficult using routine radiography.[14]

## FOREIGN BODIES

The detection and the localization of foreign bodies in the soft tissues with conventional radiography can be extremely difficult. Clarifying their presence and location is better accomplished with ultrasonography and fluoroscopy,[11] and the latter technique can be of great help both before and during surgical removal of the foreign body.[15]

## SUMMARY

An overview is provided of the usefulness of fluoroscopy in the evaluation of a number of musculoskeletal problems.

Although the technique commonly is combined with other diagnostic methods, such as arthrography, myelography, and angiography, it also represents an important independent means of supplementing nondiagnostic or equivocal routine radiographs, saving considerable time and effort, and lessening the radiation dose to the patient. At times, fluoroscopy serves as an inexpensive alternative to CT scanning or MR imaging.

### References

1. Giachino AA, Cheng M: Irradiation of the surgeon during pinning of femoral fractures. J Bone Joint Surg [Br] 62:227, 1980.
2. Miller ME, Davis ML, MacClean CR, et al: Radiation exposure and associated risks to operating-room personnel during use of fluoroscopic guidance for selected orthopaedic surgical procedures. J Bone Joint Surg [Am] 65:1, 1983.
3. Bohler J: Closed intramedullary nailing of the femur. Clin Orthop 60:51, 1968.
4. Arkless R: Cineradiography in normal and abnormal wrists. AJR 96:837, 1966.
5. Arkless R: Rheumatoid wrists: Cineradiography. Radiology 88:543, 1967.
6. Youm Y, McMurtry RY, Flatt AE, et al: Kinematics of the wrist. I. An experimental study of radial-ulnar deviation and flexion-extension. J Bone Joint Surg [Am] 60:423, 1978.
7. Protas JM, Jackson WT: Evaluating carpal instabilities with fluoroscopy AJR 135:137, 1980.
8. Braunstein EM, Louis DS, Greene TL, et al: Fluoroscopic and arthrographic evaluation of carpal instability. AJR 144:1259, 1985.
9. Gilula LA, Destouet JM, Weeks PM, et al: Roentgenographic diagnosis of the painful wrist. Clin Orthop 187:52, 1984.
10. White SJ, Louis DS, Braunstein EM, et al: Capitate-lunate instability: Recognition by manipulation under fluoroscopy. AJR 143:361, 1984.
11. Choplin RH, Gilula LA, Murphy WA: Fluoroscopic evaluation of skeletal problems. Skel Radiol 7:191, 1981.
12. Hudson TM: Joint fluoroscopy before arthrography: Detection and evaluation of loose bodies. Skel Radiol 12:199, 1984.
13. Cone RO III, Resnick D, Danzig L: Shoulder impingement syndrome: Radiographic evaluation. Radiology 150:29, 1984.
14. Turner A, Taylor JF, Carty H, et al: The radiological evaluation of multiple pin fixation of the femoral head. Br J Radiol 57:887, 1984.
15. Puhl RW, Altman MI, Seto JE, et al: The use of fluoroscopy in the detection and excision of foreign bodies in the foot. J Am Podiatry Assoc 73:514, 1983.

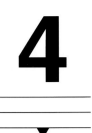

# Magnification Radiography

*Harry K. Genant, M.D., and Donald Resnick, M.D.*

The quality of a radiographic image is important for accurate and detailed assessment of subtle skeletal abnormalities. To maximize diagnostic information, high-resolution radiographic techniques have been developed. The purpose of this chapter is to examine quantitatively the fundamental imaging properties and qualitatively the clinical applications of conventional and high-resolution magnification techniques.

Magnification techniques have received increased attention for skeletal radiography and in recent years have been applied widely.[1-22] The expanded application of magnification has resulted from three factors: (1) advances in radiologic sciences; (2) optimization of physical parameters and exposing factors; and (3) delineation of the meaningful areas for clinical use. High-resolution magnification is achieved by two different techniques.[2,3,6] The first is optical magnification of fine-grain films, and the second is direct radiographic magnification (Fig. 4–1).

The *optical magnification* technique consists of contact exposures obtained with conventional radiographic equipment and fine-grain industrial films, such as Kodak Type M. The resultant image is viewed with optical enlargement. Clinical studies with this technique are not new. In the early

1950s, Fletcher and Rowley[23] reported their experience with fine-grain films and photographic enlargement in the study of peripheral skeletal abnormalities. In a monograph published in 1969, Berens and Lin[24] reported their observations in rheumatoid arthritis with the use of industrial films and optical magnification. Subsequently, Meema and associates,[10,25] Weiss,[13] Genant and coworkers,[3,4,26,27] Mall and coworkers,[9,28] and Jensen and Kliger[29] have reported extensive experience with this technique in various metabolic and arthritic skeletal disorders. Thus, the clinical importance of the optical magnification technique appears established for selected skeletal examinations.

*Direct radiographic magnification* for skeletal radiography[3,5-8,11,12,30-32] has received less attention than has optical magnification. Only with the development of x-ray tubes having small focal spots (100 to 150 μm) and adequate output for clinical examination has this technique become available. Limited clinical experience with direct radiographic magnification of the skeleton has been reported by Gordon and associates,[7] Sundaram and coworkers,[31] Ishigaki,[8] Doi and colleagues,[2] Genant and coworkers,[3,5,6] and Buckland-Wright and associates.[17,19-21] The results have been promising, and applications for both thin and thick body parts have been established.

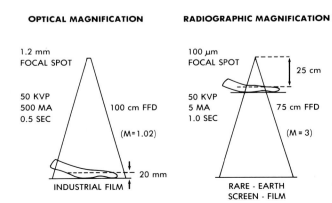

**FIGURE 4–1**. Comparison of optical and radiographic magnification.

## RADIOGRAPHIC TECHNIQUES

### Optical Magnification

The standard technique[3] for optical magnification employs Kodak industrial Type M film, (Fig. 4–1). A conventional x-ray tube with a 1.2 mm focal spot is used for these contact exposures, and the inherent magnification for thin parts is low (approximately 1.01 to 1.04 times).[2, 33] Thus, for the peripheral skeleton, exposure times are kept relatively short, and geometric unsharpness is minimal because of the low degree of inherent magnification. The industrial film must be developed manually or by means of an industrial processor. A rapid-process fine-grain film such as Kodak RP/M may be substituted for ease of X-omat processing at a modest loss of image quality. The completed industrial radiograph is surveyed without magnification initially, then viewed with a hand lens or a projector for optical magnification (Fig. 4–2).[3, 10, 28]

Inherent in the optical magnification technique is obtaining a contact radiograph of high quality. A comparison[4] of the imaging properties of the Type M film technique and two widely used conventional techniques for peripheral skeletal radiography is given in Figure 4–3. The small wire structures are best imaged with the Type M technique because of its higher resolution, lower noise, and greater contrast.

The modulation transfer function (MTF) is a measure of sharpness and describes the signal-transmitting capability of the imaging system in the spatial frequency domain, which may be compared to the frequency response of a "hi-fi" system.[34, 35] The MTF is defined as the ratio of the amplitude of the image to the amplitude of the sinusoidal object, expressed as a function of the spatial frequency. The higher the MTF value, the better the imaging system (i.e., the more closely the image obtained resembles the object). An ideal imaging system with regard to resolution is one that contains a flat MTF curve such as that derived for Type M film (Fig. 4–4). The MTF for imaging components may be measured by a number of methods[36, 37]—for example, the Fourier transformation of slit images was used for these experimental data.[4]

The Wiener spectral value of noise is plotted against the spatial frequency in Figure 4–5. For Wiener spectra of similar shape, the higher the spectral value, the greater the noise level. The noise at high frequencies corresponds to the fine noise pattern, whereas the low frequency component corresponds to the coarse pattern. The Wiener spectra are determined by an electronic Fourier analysis method,[36] in which the film is scanned circularly by a light spot and the fluctuating noise signal in a photomultiplier that corresponds to the radiographic noise is analyzed by an electronic wave analyzer.

The characteristic or "H&D" curve of a screen-film system may be derived by several methods[38] and reflects the relative speed, latitude, and contrast of the recording system. The gradient curve is a plot of gradient or contrast as a function of film density. The H&D and gradient curves for the three comparison techniques are shown in Figure 4–6.

Of the two conventional techniques displayed in Figure 4–3 and quantified in Figures 4–4 to 4–6, the cardboard technique has higher resolution and lower contrast than the detail screen-film system, and the noise is comparable. The overall image quality for the cardboard and detail screen-film techniques is comparable and is far inferior to that obtained with the Type M technique. Thus, the superior imaging properties of the Type M technique permit optical magnification of up to 10 times for improved detection of subtle abnormalities. Radiation exposure is high,[4] however, resulting in approximately 1 centigray (rad) to the hand or foot, three times the dose given with the cardboard technique, and 70 times the dose for detail screens. For this

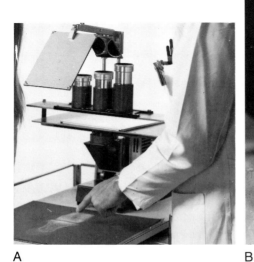
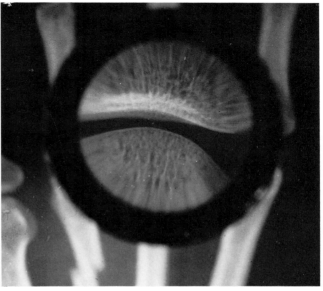

A                B

**FIGURE 4–2.** Optical magnification achieved by two methods.
  **A** For group viewing, a projector, such as the Leitz Macro Promar, is used.
  **B** For individual viewing, a loupe or hand lens is placed in direct contact with the fine-grain industrial film and the image is viewed at close range.

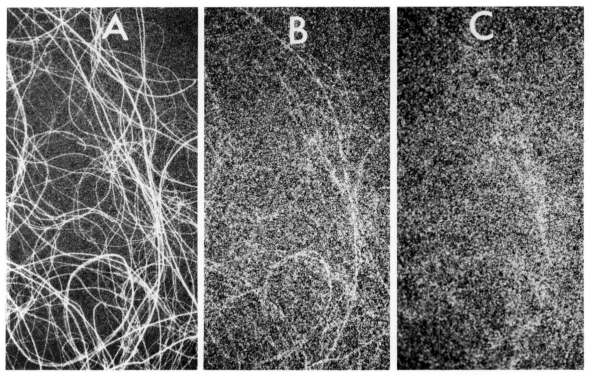

**FIGURE 4–3**. For qualitative comparison, fine steel wool has been radiographed with Type M technique **(A)**, nonscreen cardboard technique with medical RP film **(B)**, and fine screen-film system, RP-Detail **(C)**. Type M technique affords higher resolution, greater contrast, and lower noise compared with the other two standard techniques. Images in **B** and **C** are fairly comparable. (From Genant HK, et al: Invest Radiol *11*:486, 1976.)

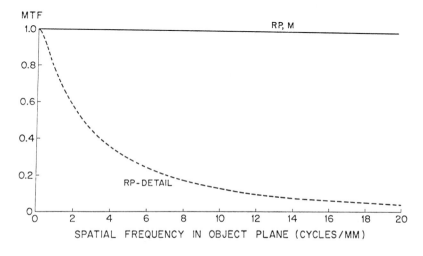

**FIGURE 4–4**. The modular transfer functions (MTFs) of recording systems. The MTFs for direct exposure of RP and Type M film show only 1 per cent decline in the demonstrated range of spatial frequency. The MTF for RP-Detail is quite poor by comparison. (From Genant HK, et al: Invest Radiol *11*:486, 1976.)

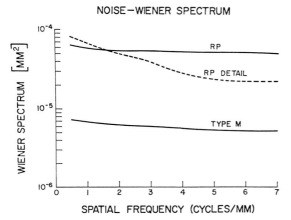

NOISE—WIENER SPECTRUM

**FIGURE 4–5**. The Wiener spectrum values for Type M, medical RP, and RP-Detail techniques are shown. The noise with Type M is appreciably lower than with either of the other two techniques. (From Genant HK, et al: Invest Radiol *11*:486, 1976.)

reason, the industrial film with optical magnification should be used selectively in those instances in which delineation of subtle abnormalities in the peripheral skeleton is important.

## Radiographic Magnification

More proximal to the peripheral skeleton, where body parts become thicker, the optical magnification technique with Type M film becomes less feasible. The limitations are attributed to the high radiation exposure that is required and the degradation of image quality related to increased geometric unsharpness, blurring by motion, and scattered radiation. Direct radiographic magnification with a microfocus x-ray tube provides a reasonable alternative.

In radiographic magnification, a screen-film system and geometric enlargement of two to four times are employed in conjunction with a microfocus x-ray tube having a nominal focal spot size of 100 μm. This technique may overcome some of the limitations of optical magnification, including the high radiation dose to the patient and the special viewing procedure required.[6]

The magnification technique affects the quality of the radiographic image in a complex way.[6] The technical *ad-*

*vantages* of radiographic magnification are based on the following: (1) the sharpness effect, (2) the noise effect, (3) the air-gap effect, and (4) the visual effect.[2, 5, 12, 39–42] The potential *disadvantages* of radiographic magnification result from the following: (1) the size of the body part examined is limited to small areas compared to those able to be examined with contact exposure; (2) the proper positioning of the area with the lesion may be difficult; and (3) the skin dose is high compared to that with the conventional screen-film technique, although it is low compared to that with Type M film and optical magnification.[3]

**Sharpness Effect.** The most widely recognized advantage of the magnification technique may be called the sharpness effect. When the x-ray pattern is enlarged, the relative or effective unsharpness of the recording system, which is the unsharpness relative to the input x-ray pattern, is reduced. Therefore, the resolution of the recording system can be improved linearly by the magnification factor. Thus, at 4× magnification, the resolution at the recording system is better by a factor of 4. Similarly, the transfer characteristic of the imaging system—namely, the MTF of the recording system—at 4× magnification is derived from the conventional MTF at contact exposure by shifting of the spatial frequency by a factor of 4.

**Noise Effect.** The reason for the noise effect in magnification radiography is similar to that for the sharpness effect. The inherent noise of the recording system does not change, regardless of the magnification. When the x-ray pattern is enlarged, however, the "effective noise," which is the noise relative to the magnified object, is reduced by the square of the magnification factor.[40]

Theoretical study[40] indicates that the effect of radiographic magnification on the Wiener spectrum of the effective noise in the recording system is twofold: (1) the Wiener spectral value decreases by a factor equal to the square of the magnification and (2) the spatial frequency increases by a factor equal to the magnification. Thus, the general result is that the higher the magnification, the more drastic the reduction of effective noise by the radiographic magnification technique.

**Air-Gap Effect.** The air-gap effect has been known for many years to be a technical advantage of magnification radiography.[12, 42, 43] The air gap usually reduces the scattered radiation relative to contact exposure and thus enhances the contrast of the x-ray pattern used as input to the recording

**FIGURE 4–6**. The characteristic and gradient curves for Type M and RP medical film techniques, as well as RP-Detail screen-film technique, are shown. The contrast or gradient with RP medical film technique is quite low compared with that of the other two techniques. (From Genant HK, et al: Invest Radiol *11*:486, 1976.)

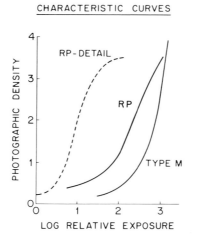

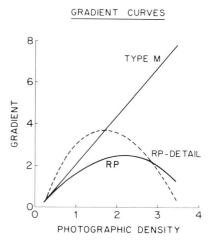

system. The contrast gained, however, may not be as high as that obtained by contact exposure using a grid technique.

**Visual Effect.** The advantage of magnified radiographs to the observer is called the visual effect. Enlargement of the image usually is helpful for either visual detection or recognition of fine details in the radiograph. It is not helpful, however, for large, low-contrast images because the MTF of the visual system decreases at low spatial frequencies. In practice, therefore, large, low-contrast images are viewed at a greater distance from the radiographs or by a minification lens. These viewing methods are advantageous because noise is suppressed as well. The MTF of the human visual system has been measured,[44, 45] and numerous reported experimental results now are available. These results vary considerably; one common point, however, is that the MTF of the visual system peaks at an intermediate spatial frequency and drops on both the high and low frequency sides. The approximate peak position is near the spatial frequency of 1 cycle per mm (an object 1 mm in diameter) at the normal viewing distance of 30 cm but varies with the brightness of the scene. Enlargement of the image detail is equivalent to shifting the frequency of this detail to the lower side (to the left) in the MTF curve. Therefore, when the image is very large, the enlargement may cause a decrease in the MTF of the visual system unless optical minification is employed.

**Effect of Focal Spot Size on Magnification.** The selection of the size of the focal spot in magnification radiography affects the resolution of the imaging system but does not affect contrast or noise. Inherent in achieving the sharpness effect in the direct geometric magnification technique is minimizing the adverse effect of focal spot unsharpness. The potential effect of geometric unsharpness is shown dramatically in Figure 4–7, where fine steel wire has been radiographed at contact as well as elevated 4 cm and 8 cm from a fine-grain film.[27] A standard 1.2 mm focal spot was used at 100 cm focus-film distance. It can be seen that with such a large focal spot, even small degrees of magnification introduce considerable geometric unsharpness due to the focal spot penumbra.

**Image Comparison and Dosimetry.** Despite its excellent imaging characteristics, direct radiographic magnification, like optical magnification, should be used selectively because of its potentially high radiation exposure. Magnification results in an approximately fourfold increase in exposure per surface area (skin dose) compared with conventional techniques when recording-system speeds, air gap, and grid are considered.[46] The size of the field with magnification is significantly reduced, however, which helps lower the total body radiation to a level nearly equivalent to that of conventional techniques.

A variety of experimental and, now, commercially available screen-film systems have been used for direct magnification to help reduce radiation exposure. Most of these consist of rare-earth screen-film systems that have high photon-absorption efficiency and high light-conversion efficiency, thus providing an approximately 50 per cent reduction in exposure compared with conventional calcium-tungstate screens.[47] For thin anatomic parts, single-emulsion, single-screen systems often are used, whereas for thicker anatomic parts, double-screen, double-emulsion systems are used.

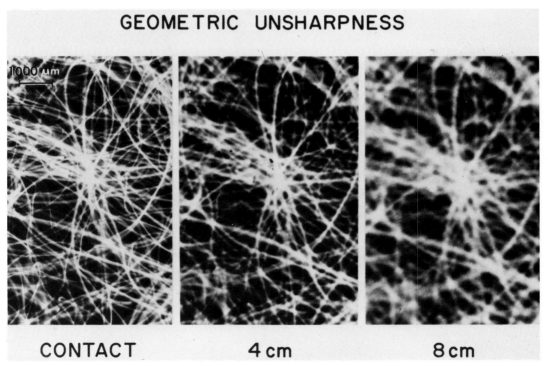

**FIGURE 4–7.** Fine steel wire radiographed at contact and elevated 4 cm and 8 cm from a fine-grain film using a standard 1.2 mm focal spot at 100 cm focus-film distance (FFD).

## CLINICAL APPLICATIONS OF MAGNIFICATION RADIOGRAPHY

The clinical applications of magnification radiography will be considered. There also is considerable application of magnification radiography to the evaluation of a variety of other skeletal disorders as illustrated in appropriate sections throughout the textbook.

### Articular Disorders

**Rheumatoid Arthritis.** The largest area of clinical application for high-resolution skeletal radiography has been the assessment of rheumatoid arthritis. High-resolution radiography using industrial film and *photographic* enlargement first was used in investigations by Fletcher and Rowley[23] in rheumatoid arthritis patients in the 1950s. Berens and Lin[24] later employed fine-detail radiography routinely in the clinical evaluation of patients with various arthritides, including rheumatoid arthritis. Mall and collaborators[9] studied the hands in 25 patients with proved but early rheumatoid arthritis[48] and 20 controls who were normal or had osteoarthritis. Their results demonstrated conclusively that fine-detail radiography was more sensitive than conventional radiography for the detection and evaluation of erosive disease in early rheumatoid arthritis. Further analysis indicated that severe erosions were observed in about the same number of patients with each technique, but minimal erosions usually were detectable only with fine-detail radiography because of its increased sensitivity. These subtle erosive changes were identified most easily as a sawtooth or a "dot-dash" appearance in the metacarpal head (Fig. 4–8) or ulnar styloid (Fig. 4–9) but also were noted in other locations, described by Martel as "bare areas."[49] The detection of soft tissue swelling also was improved by the high contrast of fine-detail radiography.

Hartley and coworkers[18] evaluated various conventional radiographic projections and radiographic magnification techniques in 54 patients with suspected early rheumatoid arthritis. These investigators confirmed the sensitivity of magnification radiography in detecting osseous erosions, a finding that is in agreement with the results of other studies.[15] Joint space narrowing was detected equally well by both routine and magnification radiography.[18]

**Other Arthritides.** Magnification radiography may be helpful not only in detecting erosive disease but also in characterizing and differentiating the appearances of various joint afflictions. For example, the erosions seen in psoriatic arthritis, Reiter's syndrome, and the other HLA B-27—associated arthritides are characterized by bony proliferation producing a fluffy appearance in juxta-articular regions as well as a linear periosteal new bone response in the adjacent shafts of bones (Fig. 4–10). Another form of arthritis, calcium pyrophosphate dihydrate crystal deposition disease, is characterized radiographically by chondrocalcinosis. When subtle, the fine linear and punctate calci-

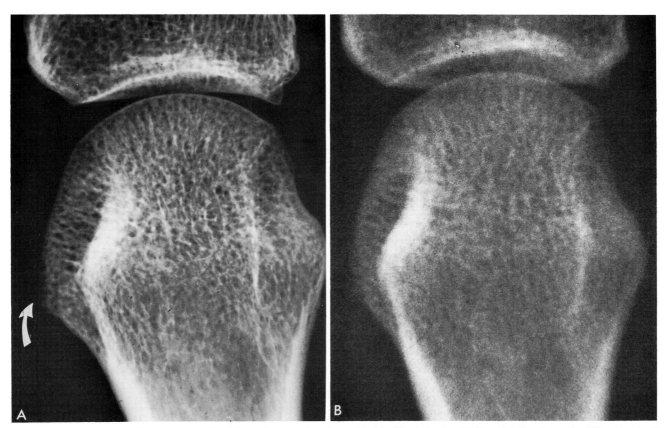

**FIGURE 4–8.** The "dot-dash" appearance of subtle surface erosion (arrow) is identified clearly with fine-detail radiography **(A)**, but not with conventional radiography **(B)**.

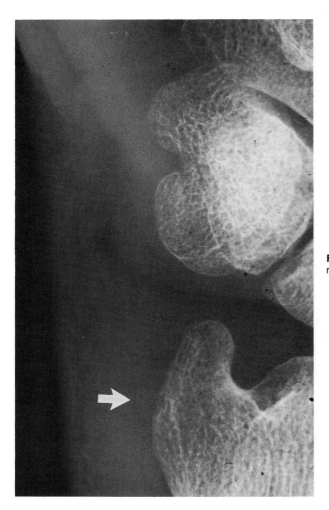

**FIGURE 4–9.** Subtle surface erosion (arrow) of ulnar styloid illustrated by magnification radiography.

fications in the hyaline cartilage and fibrocartilage may be detected only with high resolution magnification techniques (Fig. 4–11). Advanced articular calcification is recognized easily with conventional radiographic techniques.

### Metabolic Disorders

**Hyperparathyroidism.** The radiographic assessment of osseous changes in hyperparathyroidism has undergone substantial modification in recent years. The classic findings of advanced hyperparathyroid skeletal disease, with striking cortical erosions and cystic brown tumors, rarely are seen today.[11, 26, 50] This change probably reflects the earlier stage of detection[46] and the greater preponderance of benign chemical hyperparathyroidism.[51, 52] In a large study[26] of primary hyperparathyroidism, subperiosteal bone resorption limited to the phalanges was revealed by conventional radiography in only 7 of 87 patients (8 per cent). This experience contrasts with the prevalence (and severity) of bony abnormalities in hyperparathyroid patients cited in the earlier classic radiologic reviews of Pugh,[53] who reported a 33 per cent prevalence in 1951, and of Steinbach and coworkers,[54] who reported a prevalence of 23 per cent in 1961. For this reason, high resolution radiographic techniques were introduced to detect subtle resorptive changes in the peripheral skeleton.[10, 13, 25–27, 51] Fine-detail radiography will dem-

onstrate clearly the irregular resorption of the outer cortical margins that is pathognomonic of hyperparathyroidism (Figs. 4–12 and 4–13).[53–55] When subperiosteal bone resorption becomes advanced, high-resolution radiographic techniques are not necessary for detection. However, for monitoring the course of the disease or the response to therapy, magnification may be helpful (Fig. 4–14).

The second, more sensitive but less specific, finding in hyperparathyroidism is *cortical striation* or *tunneling* (Fig. 4–15). It corresponds histologically to widened haversian systems and resorptive spaces that result from excessive bone resorption in the hyperparathyroid state,[25, 26, 56] and it is detected only on fine-detail radiographs unless extremely advanced.[10, 25, 51] It is not a specific change, however, because it occurs in a variety of conditions with high bone turnover, such as renal osteodystrophy, thyrotoxicosis, immobilization, reflex sympathetic dystrophy, osteomalacia, and rheumatoid arthritis.[57] The changes of increased intracortical tunneling are not limited to the small tubular bones of the hands but may be seen in the long bones as well (Fig. 4–16).[55, 56, 58]

### Infectious Disorders

The diagnosis of osteomyelitis or septic arthritis generally is made on the basis of clinical symptoms and findings

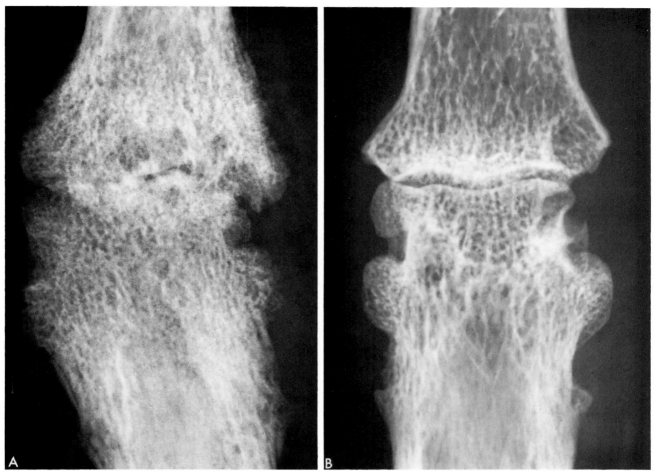

**FIGURE 4–10.** Proliferative erosions and periostitis of psoriatic arthritis **(A)** differ in appearance from the well-defined erosions and reactive bone formation of gouty arthritis **(B)**.

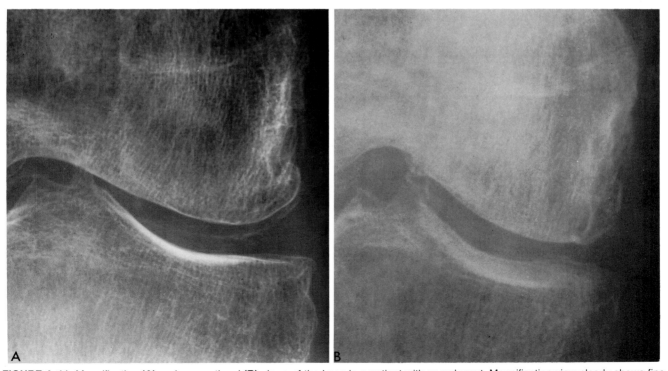

**FIGURE 4–11.** Magnification **(A)** and conventional **(B)** views of the knee in a patient with pseudogout. Magnification view clearly shows fine linear calcification of the hyaline cartilage and fibrocartilage, diagnostic of calcium pyrophosphate dihydrate crystal deposition disease. The conventional radiograph fails to reveal definite chondrocalcinosis.

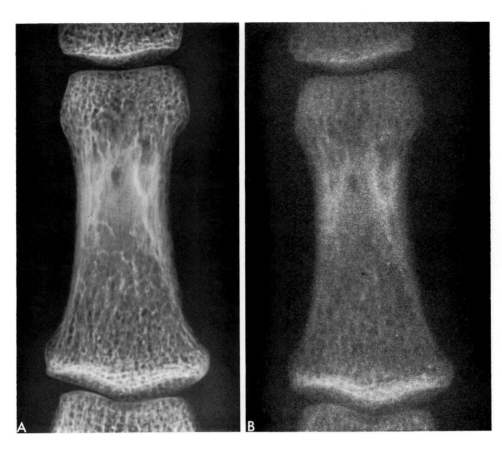

FIGURE 4–12. Radiograph of a phalanx of a hyperparathyroid patient. Type M film **(A)** shows the irregular resorption of the outer cortical margin not detected in the detail screen-film system **(B)**. (From Genant HK, et al: Radiology *109*:513, 1973.)

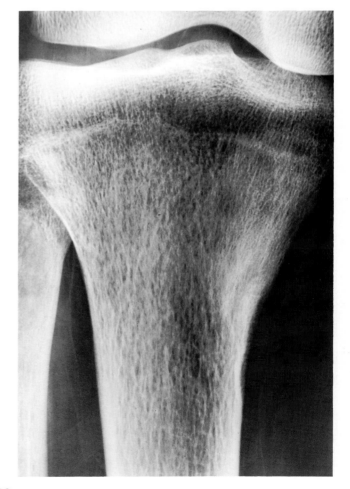

FIGURE 4–13. Magnification radiograph of a knee of a child with chronic renal disease demonstrates definite subperiosteal resorption of the proximal medial metaphysis of the tibia, as well as mild osteosclerosis of trabecular bone, nearly pathognomonic of renal osteodystrophy.

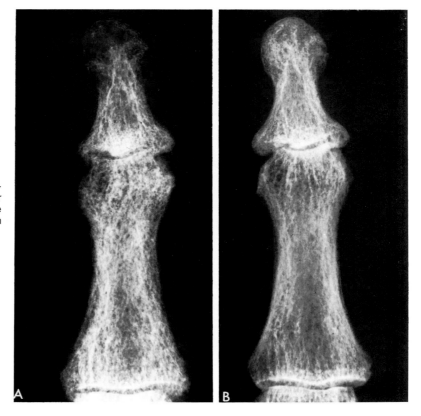

FIGURE 4–14. Advanced subperiosteal bone resorption accompanying chronic renal disease **(A)**. After parathyroidectomy, remarkable reconstitution of the cortex and healing of the subperiosteal bone resorption occurred **(B)**.

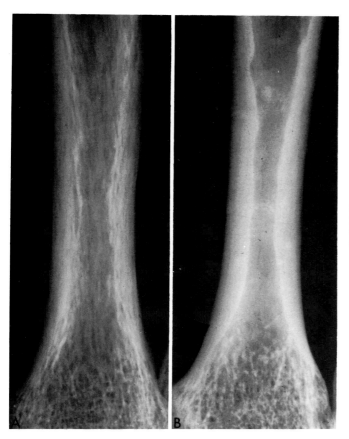

FIGURE 4–15. Radiographs of metacarpal bones of a hyperparathyroid patient **(A)** and of a normal patient **(B)**. Intracortical striation is excessive in **A**, compared with solid cortex in **B**. (From Genant HK, et al: Radiology *109*:513, 1973.)

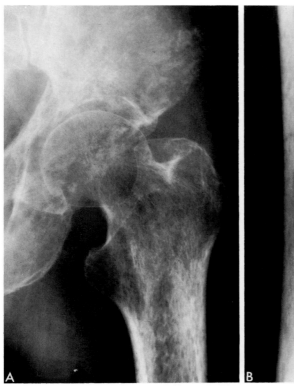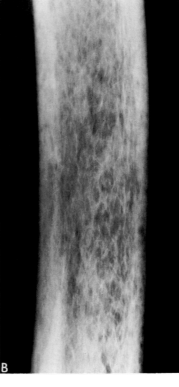

**FIGURE 4–16.** Radiograph of the left hip and femoral shaft **(A)** in a patient who had sustained a pathologic fracture of the acetabulum 3 months earlier. The magnification view **(B)** of the femur demonstrates the increased intracortical tunneling as well as the extensive resorption of the endosteal surface, all indicative of an aggressive disuse osteoporosis.

because conventional radiography demonstrates characteristic features only later in the course. Occasionally, however, magnification radiography may be helpful in delineating subtle cortical destruction or periosteal new bone prior to its demonstration on conventional films. For example, a problem frequently is encountered in an elderly, osteoporotic patient who has ulceration of the soft tissues of the foot related to diabetes mellitus or arterial insufficiency (Fig. 4–17). The diagnostic problem is to determine whether or not there is underlying osteomyelitis.[22] In this setting, conventional radiography often fails to visualize the bone margins adequately because of the low inherent subject contrast of osteopenic bone. Magnification radiography, however, may clearly delineate the cortical margins and reveal irregular destruction of the outer cortical surfaces, thus permitting a specific diagnosis. Similar diagnostic advantages are encountered in the analysis of other skeletal sites as well (Figs. 4–18 and 4–19).

### Neoplastic Disorders

Both primary and metastatic neoplasms of bone have been examined with magnification techniques.[30] These examinations are largely of the thick skeletal parts, such as the ribs, pelvis, hips, spine, and femora, and, therefore, direct radiographic magnification is employed. In some applications, conventional radiographs appear normal or equivocal, and magnification serves to delineate permeative, lytic destruction or subtle periosteal reaction. In other instances, conventional radiography readily demonstrates the presence of the lesion; however, the character or pattern of host response or aggressiveness is best determined by

magnification (Fig. 4–20). Frequently, direct magnification is initiated after a positive bone scan and conventional radiographs provide inconclusive results. Serial assessment of the progression of the neoplasm or the response to therapy also is improved by magnification.

The largest application of magnification for assessing metastatic disease has been in imaging the ribs (Fig. 4–21). Although it aids in demonstrating the presence and extent of metastatic involvement at this site as well as other sites, magnification radiography usually does not supply new information that is critical for the management of the patient.

### Traumatic Disorders

Magnification radiography has had more limited application in the evaluation of trauma because the detection of fractures by conventional radiography generally is adequate (Fig. 4–22). Occasionally, however, magnification radiography may be helpful in delineating and defining subtle fractures, especially in the ribs, carpal scaphoid, and femoral neck.

### SUMMARY

For most skeletal areas in which magnification (optical or geometric) proves useful, subtle abnormalities of clinical importance are present at bone surfaces or at host-lesion interfaces. This is particularly true for arthritis and metabolic and infectious disorders of bone. In additional instances, serial assessment of the progression of disease or its response to therapy is enhanced by magnification. When gross abnormalities are present, however, the findings are

*Text continued on page 87*

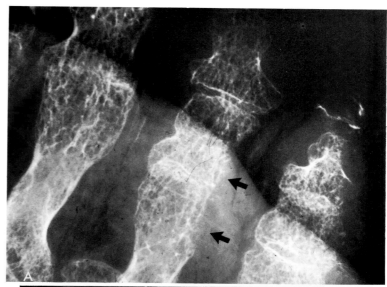

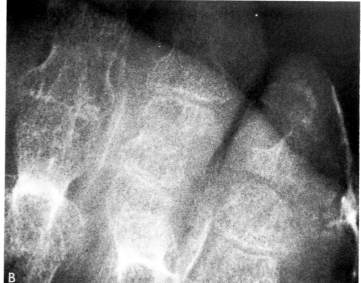

**FIGURE 4–17**. Distal aspect of the foot of a diabetic patient with suspected osteomyelitis.

**A** Cortical destruction of the lateral aspects of the middle and proximal phalanges of the fourth digit (arrows) readily is detected with the Type M technique.

**B** The cortical outlines are delineated inadequately for accurate interpretation with the cardboard technique.

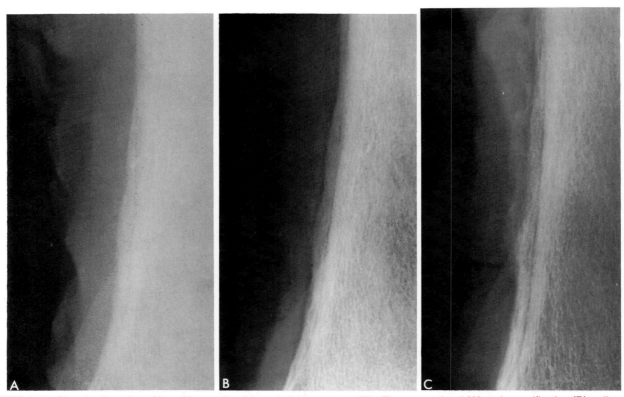

**FIGURE 4–18.** Chronic ulceration of leg with questionable underlying osteomyelitis. The conventional **(A)** and magnification **(B)** radiographs both demonstrate thick periosteal new bone along the shaft of the distal portion of the tibia, with overlying soft tissue ulceration. Additionally, the fine, spiculated periosteal new bone seen to extend into the adjacent soft tissues in the magnification film indicates an evolving process and supports a diagnosis of active osteomyelitis. Serial magnification view **(C)** 1 month later shows further progression of periosteal new bone, confirming the dynamic nature of the process. Such serial assessment is enhanced by magnification. (From Genant HK, et al: Radiology *123*:47, 1977.)

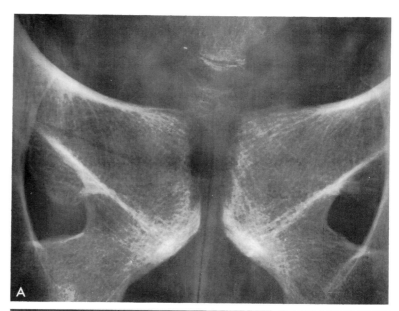

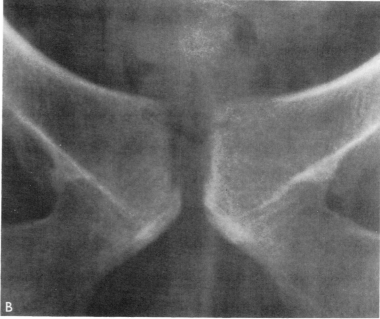

**FIGURE 4–19**. Magnification **(A)** and conventional radiographs **(B)** demonstrate widening of the symphysis pubis. The magnification study, in addition, shows irregular destruction of the subchondral cortical line, producing a ragged, lacelike appearance. These features indicate an aggressive, evolving process and support the diagnosis of infectious osteitis pubis. (From Genant HK, et al: Radiology *123*:47, 1977.)

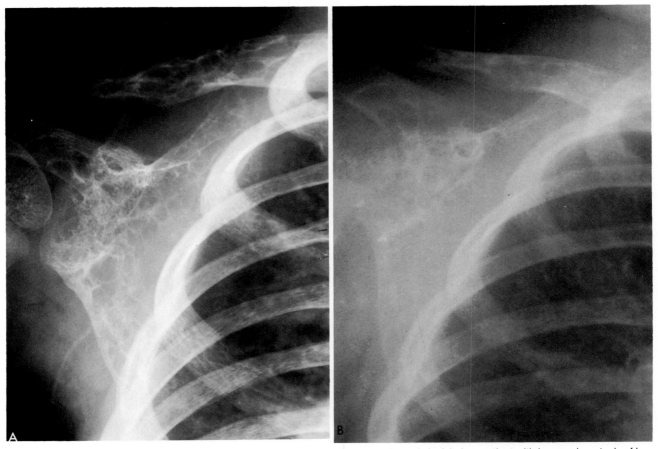

**FIGURE 4–20.** Multiple well-defined cystic and lytic destructive lesions in the scapula and clavicle in a patient with hemangiomatosis of bone. Although large lesions are seen with both magnification and conventional techniques, evaluation of extent of involvement is far superior in the magnification view **(A)**.

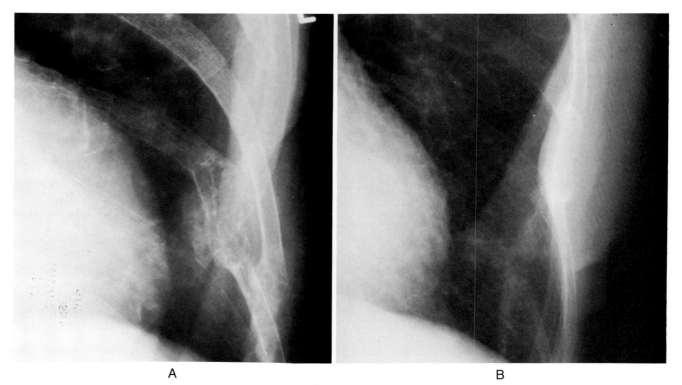

A                                                                          B

**FIGURE 4–21.** Metastatic carcinoma of breast producing mixed lytic and sclerotic osseous destruction, as well as expansion of bone. Direct magnification technique **(A)** is used frequently when rib lesions are suspected on conventional radiography of the chest. Conventional radiograph of the chest **(B)** shows lateral soft tissue mass and rib destruction; however, the extent of involvement is not well defined.

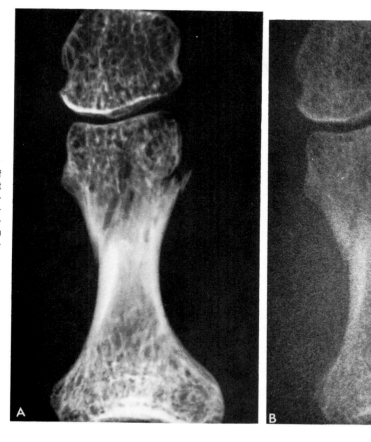

**FIGURE 4–22.** Oblique fracture of the proximal phalanx of the left foot. Although the Type M technique **(A)** demonstrates the fracture more clearly, it does not provide additional useful information over that of the cardboard technique **(B)**.

obvious on conventional radiography, and magnification is not necessary. Thus, the magnification techniques appear to provide important diagnostic information, depending on the anatomic part that is studied and the clinical question that is posed. From dosimetry measurements, it is apparent that relatively high radiation doses result from magnification techniques. For this reason and because of the somewhat greater technical difficulty of performing the examination, magnification is recommended only as a selective procedure. Such selection may be based on analysis of the clinical history and suspected diagnosis or may be in response to the inadequacies of conventional radiography. When employed in this manner, magnification radiography may be an important tool in the diagnostic study of skeletal diseases.

### References

1. Chinn D, Genant HK, Quivey J, et al: Heterotopic bone formation in metastatic tumor from transitional cell carcinoma of the urinary bladder: A case report. J Bone Joint Surg [Am] 58:881, 1976.
2. Doi K, Genant HK, Rossmann K: Comparison of image quality obtained with optical and radiographic magnification techniques in fine-detail skeletal radiography: Effect of object thickness. Radiology 118:189, 1976.
3. Genant HK, Doi K, Mall JC: Optical versus radiographic magnification for fine-detail skeletal radiography. Invest Radiol 10:160, 1975.
4. Genant HK, Doi K, Mall JC: Comparison of non-screen techniques (medical vs. industrial film) for fine-detail skeletal radiography. Invest Radiol 11:486, 1976.
5. Genant HK, Doi K, Mall JC, et al: Direct radiographic magnification for skeletal radiology. An assessment of image quality and clinical application. Radiology 123:47, 1977.
6. Genant HK, Doi K: High-resolution skeletal radiography: Image quality and clinical applications. Curr Probl Diagn Radiol 7:3, 1978.
7. Gordon SI, Greer RB, Weidner WA: Magnification roentgenographic technic in orthopedics. Clin Orthop 91:169, 1973.
8. Ishigaki T: First metatarsal-phalangeal joint of gout—macroroentgenographic examination in 6 times magnification. Nippon Acta Radiol 33:839, 1973.
9. Mall JC, Genant HK, Silcox DC, et al: The efficacy of fine-detail radiography in the evaluation of patients with rheumatoid arthritis. Radiology 112:37, 1974.
10. Meema HE, Schatz DL: Simple radiologic demonstration of cortical bone loss in thyrotoxicosis. Radiology 97:9, 1970.
11. Sakuma S, Ayakawa Y, Fujita T: Macroroentgenography in twenty-fold magnification taken by means of 50μ focal spot x-ray tube and evaluation of its reduced image. Nippon Acta Radiol 30:205, 1971.
12. Takahashi S, Sakuma S: Magnification Radiography. New York, Springer-Verlag, 1975.
13. Weiss A: A technique for demonstrating fine detail in bones of the hands. Clin Radiol 23:185, 1972.
14. Guilford WB: Enhanced skeletal radiography using microfocus x-ray tubes. Revista Interam Radiol 8:59, 1983.
15. Buckland-Wright JC: Microfocal radiographic examination of erosions in the wrist and hand of patients with rheumatoid arthritis. Ann Rheum Dis 43:160, 1984.
16. De Smet AA, Goin JE, Martin R: A radiographic model for simulating rheumatoid erosions. Invest Radiol 18:353, 1983.
17. Buckland-Wright JC: Advances in the radiological assessment of rheumatoid arthritis. Br J Rheum 22(Suppl):34, 1983.
18. Hartley RM, Liang MH, Weissman BN, et al: The value of conventional views and radiographic magnification in evaluating early rheumatoid arthritis. Arthritis Rheum 27:744, 1984.
19. Buckland-Wright JC, Carmichael I, Walker SR: Quantitative microfocal radiography accurately detects joint changes in rheumatoid arthritis. Ann Rheum Dis 45:379, 1986.
20. Buckland-Wright JC: A new high-definition microfocal x-ray unit. Br J Radiol 62:201, 1989.
21. Buckland-Wright JC, Bradshaw CR: Clinical applications of high-definition microfocal radiography. Br J Radiol 62:209, 1989.
22. Lee SM, Lee RCL, Wilinsky J, et al: Magnification radiography in osteomyelitis. Skel Radiol 15:625, 1986.
23. Fletcher DE, Rowley KA: Radiographic enlargements in diagnostic radiology. Br J Radiol 24:598, 1951.
24. Berens DL, Lin RK: Roentgen Diagnosis of Rheumatoid Arthritis. Springfield, Ill, Charles C. Thomas, 1969.
25. Meema HE, Meema S: Comparison of microradioscopic and morphometric findings in the hand bones with densitometric findings in the proximal radius in thyrotoxicosis and in renal osteodystrophy. Invest Radiol 7:88, 1972.
26. Genant HK, Heck LL, Lanzl LH, et al: Primary hyperparathyroidism: Comprehensive study of clinical, biochemical and radiographic manifestations. Radiology 109:513, 1973.
27. Genant HK, Doi K, Rossmann K, et al: Fine-detail radiography—theoretical and

practical considerations. *In* Z Jaworski (Ed): Proceedings of the First International Workshop on Bone Morphometry. Ottawa, Ontario, University of Ottawa Press, 1976, p 63.

28. Mall JC, Genant HK, Rossmann K: Improved optical magnification for fine-detail radiography. Radiology *108*:707, 1973.
29. Jensen PS, Kliger AS: Early radiographic manifestations of secondary hyperparathyroidism associated with chronic renal disease. Radiology *125*:645, 1977.
30. Genant HK, Doi K: High-resolution radiographic techniques for the detection and study of skeletal neoplasms. *In* Encyclopedia of Medical Radiology. Vol 6, Bone Tumors. New York, Springer-Verlag, 1977, p 677.
31. Sundaram MB, Brodeur AE, Burdge RE, et al: The clinical value of direct magnification radiography in orthopedics. Skel Radiol *3*:85, 1978.
32. De Smet AA, Templeton AW: Direct magnification radiography using conventional radiographic equipment. AJR *135*:858, 1980.
33. Doi K, Genant HK, Rossmann K: Effect of film graininess and geometric unsharpness on image quality in fine-detail skeletal radiography. Invest Radiol *10*:35, 1975.
34. Rossmann K: Point spread function, line spread function and modulation transfer function. Radiology *93*:257, 1969.
35. Rossmann K: Image quality and patient exposure. Curr Probl Diagn Radiol *2*(2):3, 1972.
36. Doi K, Rossmann K: Measurements of optical and noise properties of screen-film systems in radiography. *In* Proceedings of the Symposium on Application of Optical Instrumentation in Medicine. Vol 56. Bellingham, Washington, Society of Photo-Optical Instrumentation Engineers, 1975, p 45.
37. Doi K, Fromes B, Rossmann K: A new device for accurate measurement of the x-ray intensity distribution of x-ray tube focal spots. Med Phys *2*:268, 1975.
38. Haus AG, Rossmann K: X-ray sensitometer for screen-film combinations used in medical radiology. Radiology *94*:673, 1970.
39. Ayakawa Y: Optimal magnification ratio of direct macroradiography in high magnification. Modulation transfer function study on system combined with intensifying screen-film and object. Nagoya J Med Sci *34*:227, 1972.
40. Doi K, Imhof H: Noise reduction by radiographic magnification. Radiology *122*:479, 1977.
41. Greenspan RH, Simon AL, Ricketts HJ, et al: In vivo magnification angiography. Invest Radiol *2*:419, 1967.
42. Moore R, Krause D, Amplatz K: A flexible grid-air gap magnification technique. Radiology *104*:403, 1972.
43. Bookstein JJ, Powell TJ: Short-target-film rotating-grid magnification. Comparison with air-gap magnification. Radiology *104*:399, 1972.
44. Campbell FW, Kulikowski JJ, Levinson J: The effect of orientation on the visual resolution of gratings. J Physiol (Lond) *187*:427, 1966.
45. Lowry EM, DePalma JJ: Sine-wave response of the visual system. The Mach phenomenon. J Opt Soc Am *51*:740, 1961.
46. Boonstra CE, Jackson CE: Hyperparathyroidism detected by routine serum calcium analysis: Prevalence in a clinic population. Ann Intern Med *63*:468, 1964.
47. Buchanan RA, Finkelstein SI, Wickersheim KA: X-ray exposure reduction using rare-earth oxysulfide intensifying screens. Radiology *105*:185, 1972.
48. Ropes MW, Bennett GA, Cobb S, et al: 1958 revision of diagnostic criteria for rheumatoid arthritis. Bull Rheum Dis *9*:175, 1958.
49. Martel W: The pattern of rheumatoid arthritis in the hand and wrist. Radiol Clin North Am *2*:221, 1964.
50. Forland M, Strandjord NM, Paloyan E, et al: Bone density studies in primary hyperparathyroidism. Arch Intern Med *122*:236, 1968.
51. Genant HK, Vander Horst J, Lanzl LH, et al: Skeletal demineralization in primary hyperparathyroidism. *In* RB Mazess (Ed): Proceedings of the International Conference on Bone Mineral Measurement. Washington, D.C., National Institute of Arthritis, Metabolism, and Digestive Diseases, 1973, p 177.
52. Purnell DC, Smith LH, Scholz DA, et al: Primary hyperparathyroidism: A prospective clinical study. Am J Med *50*:670, 1971.
53. Pugh DG: Subperiosteal resorption of bone: Roentgenologic manifestation of primary hyperparathyroidism and renal osteodystrophy. AJR *66*:577, 1951.
54. Steinbach HL, Gordan GS, Eisenberg E, et al: Primary hyperparathyroidism: A correlation of roentgen, clinical and pathologic features. AJR *86*:329, 1961.
55. Genant HK, Kozin F, Bekerman C, et al: Reflex sympathetic dystrophy syndrome: A comprehensive analysis using fine-detail radiography, photon absorptiometry, and bone and joint scintigraphy. Radiology *117*:21, 1975.
56. Duncan H: Cortical porosis: A morphological evaluation. *In* Z Jaworski (Ed): Proceedings of the First Workshop on Bone Morphometry. Ottawa, Ontario, University of Ottawa Press, 1976, p 78.
57. Wilson JS, Genant HK: In vivo assessment of bone metabolism using the cortical striation index. Invest Radiol *14*:131, 1979.
58. Herrmann LG, Reineke HG, Caldwell JA: Post-traumatic painful osteoporosis: Clinical and roentgenological entity. AJR *47*:353, 1942.

# 5

# Low Kilovolt Radiography

*Erich Fischer, M.D.*

The mammography technique, which uses a molybdenum target and filter and a voltage range between 28 and 35 kilovolts (KV), also is well suited to the extensive diagnostic evaluation of the extremities. The reduced penetration of this low energy x-ray spectrum and the increased radiation exposure restrict the applicability of the technique to thinner body parts, mainly the hands and feet. Low KV radiography results in greater contrast between fat and water-equivalent tissues and between water-equivalent tissues and bone (calcium)[1] and allows more specific soft tissue diagnosis and more precise analysis of the margins and thinner portions of the bone. Although delineating the soft tissues to some extent, conventional radiography lacks sensitivity in this regard.[2-12] This lack of sensitivity for soft tissues especially is evident in rheumatoid arthritis, which begins with soft tissue changes and throughout its course is accompanied by soft tissue abnormalities. The importance of such changes was recognized in 1936 by Ferguson.[13]

Low KV radiography of the extremities is a specialized procedure that requires meticulous technique that differs from conventional radiographic methods. For example, as the hand consists of two main parts, the fingers and the wrist, that vary considerably in thickness, delineation of both regions with low KV radiography requires precise radiation exposures as well as comprehensive radiographic projections.

## METHODS AND TECHNIQUES

Low KV radiography, at least of the hands, can be performed with routine mammography equipment. An immersion technique for the fingers, accomplished by immersing the hand and forearm (or the forefoot) in 70 per cent ethanol solution,[14-16] improves the resolution of skin and subcutaneous structures over that possible with nonimmersion low KV radiography, because the uniformly deep liquid layer equalizes the differences in thickness of the fingers. One of the disadvantages of this technique is that it is possible to obtain only posteroanterior (PA) views of the fingers and the forefoot. Lateral views of the second, third, fourth, and fifth fingers also are possible if these fingers can be extended and spread sufficiently, although overlapping of the proximal portions of the phalanges is inevitable. This becomes important in rheumatoid arthritis, in which the tendon sheaths of the fingers are not always dilated over their whole lengths by tenosynovitis but sometimes are dilated only in this overlapped region.[17]

An advantage of xeroradiography over low KV radiography lies in its broad latitude in recording different densities and thicknesses. Important disadvantages of xeroradiography are edge enhancement (which may falsely provide sharp contours to contours that are not sharp) and a halo effect (in which small soft tissue shadows adjacent to bone may disappear). MR imaging and, to a lesser extent, CT scanning are effective for the analysis of soft tissue structures, but both techniques are expensive in comparison to low KV radiography.

Nonimmersion ("dry") low KV radiography of the hands and feet using three views offers comprehensive visualization of the changes in the soft tissues[18-21] as well as in the bones.[17, 22-28] The "double film technique" of the fingers in the true PA projection is a modification of dry low KV radiography that is used to evaluate diseases associated with increased bone turnover. Two single packed fine-grain films with different exposure factors are placed one over the other and exposed with a radiation dose that is sufficient for the low sensitivity film. Thin bones, the margins of thicker bones, the soft tissues, and small calcifications are well shown on the low sensitivity film, and thicker osseous parts are well penetrated on the more sensitive film. Single packed industrial fine-grain films provide the utmost resolution and have the best type of gradation for both bones and soft tissues but require higher radiation exposure. All rare-earth screen-film combinations result in perceptibly reduced sharpness and resolution.

### Three-View Examination of the Hand, Wrist, and Forefoot

Because the radiation tube and film support assembly are rigidly interconnected by a C-arm in low KV machines, a firm wedge is needed to bring the hand or the foot into the desired oblique position. The film lies on the wedge and remains in direct contact with the object. The C-arm then is rotated so that a comfortable position is achieved for the patient.[29]

#### Fingers

The fingers are spread moderately. Three views are required: a true PA view and two oblique views in a PA projection with the radial or ulnar aspect of the fingers elevated 25 degrees relative to the direction of the central beam of the x-ray. The abducted thumb is included to the extent permitted by the film size.

#### Wrist

The three required views are a true PA projection with the hand in slight ulnar deviation so that the radius and the second metacarpal bone are aligned, an anteroposterior (AP) projection with the radial aspect of the hand elevated 25 degrees and with abduction of the thumb, and a true lateral radioulnar projection. In each view, the metacarpophalangeal joints and the soft tissues of the metacarpal region are projected somewhat differently, which often is useful for precise analysis.[19]

#### Forefoot

The forefoot radiographs are taken in three views, corresponding to those of the fingers.

### Horizontal Beam Lateral View of the Ankle

For the tibiofibular view, the foot is in midposition and rotated slightly inward so that the fibula is projected on the middle third of the tibia. This inward rotation compensates for lateral tibial torsion and is necessary to see the anterior surface of the Achilles tendon exactly in profile. Radiographs obtained with the extremity not positioned precisely will lead to an unsharpness of the Achilles tendon that mimics a pathologic finding and prohibits measuring the thickness of the tendon. In addition, the horizontal beam lateral view shows the soft tissues around the tibiotalar joint. The retrocalcaneal bursa lies in the fatty wedge between the Achilles tendon and the calcaneal surface and is seen only if it is enlarged.[30]

## SYNOPSIS OF SOFT TISSUE CHANGES

In the range of 28 to 35 KV, the following tissues are of "water density": skin, tendons, ligaments, tendon sheaths, joint capsules, muscles, blood vessels, and cartilage. Fatty tissue is interspersed with blood vessels and fine strands of connective tissue.

### Thickened Soft Tissues

The thickness of the skin shows individual variation and is influenced by occupational stress and abnormal conditions, such as scars, edema, scleroderma, acromegaly, myxedema, Down's syndrome, pachydermoperiostosis, pachydermodactyly,[31] and Fabry's disease. Thickening of tendons and ligaments occurs in rheumatoid arthritis, the seronegative spondyloarthropathies, stress related conditions, lipid storage diseases, gout, hydroxyapatite crystal deposition disease, and amyloidosis.

Dilation of joint capsules may relate to the patient's age and gender, manual work,[20, 32] rheumatoid arthritis, the seronegative spondyloarthropathies, osteoarthritis, gout, amyloidosis, Fabry's disease, multicentric reticulohistiocytosis, and other conditions, such as multiple epiphyseal dysplasia.

### Thinned Soft Tissues

Thinning related to atrophy can be demonstrated in the skin and muscles. In some cases, the reduced volume of an entire muscle or a portion of it will be partially compensated for by its replacement with fatty tissue. In the metacarpal region, atrophy of muscle indicates long-standing reduced physical activity.[19, 21]

### Hazy Soft Tissue Margins

Normally, most soft tissues of water density have distinct contours if they are located adjacent to a fatty layer of adequate thickness. A normal hazy margin results when the fatty layer is too thin or when the skin and the underlying synovial compartments are connected by localized increased strands of connective tissues.[18, 20] A pathologic hazy margin is caused by irritation of a synovial compartment or within the enveloping tissue of a tendon.

### Increased Number and Thickness of Vessels

The vessels that are recognizable in areolar tissue, for the most part, are veins. Normally, there is marked symmetry in both the width and the number of subcutaneous veins. Inflammation leads to an increased localized circulation,[33] and resulting venous alterations can be detected with low KV radiography. During acute phases of rheumatoid arthritis and related diseases, the veins about the wrist may become greatly dilated and tortuous.[20] Reversal of these abnormal vascular patterns indicates a decrease in the extent of local inflammation.

### Changes in Structure of Fine Connective Tissue

Normal fat contains a fine pattern of connective tissue variously formed in terms of length, width, direction, and quantity.[18–20, 34, 35] Edema leads to widening and an increase in the number of thin strands of connective tissue. Furthermore, structures not normally seen will become visible when enlarged owing to edema or bleeding. Edematous fatty tissue increases the distance between the fascial layers and the muscles or skin, and such tissue becomes water-equivalent in density.

In scleroderma, the strands of the subcutaneous tissue, especially in the fingers, may be pathologically broadened and augmented.[36]

### Soft Tissue Masses

Gouty tophi, rheumatoid nodules,[19, 37] and localized sacculations of synovial compartments (analogous to synovial cyst formation) are causes of such masses.

### Calcifications and Opaque Foreign Bodies

As a consequence of the technical improvements in low KV radiography, minimal calcifications and opaque foreign bodies easily are recognizable. Beginning in the third decade of life, soft tissue calcifications may be seen; they are frequent, diverse in shape and size, and, in many cases, may resolve spontaneously. Most often they occur in the ungual tufts, adjacent to joints (especially those of the fingers), and at the volar side of the pisiform bone. Their importance as a sign of a generalized disturbance of mineral metabolism or connective tissue disease should not be overestimated.

Vascular calcifications also are common. As a rule, arterial calcifications occur at an earlier time in the feet than in the hands. When they occur in the metacarpal region they usually are a sign of severe generalized atherosclerosis.

Because of their contact with fatty tissue, embedded foreign bodies, such as glass, wood chips, thorns, and plastic particles, easily are recognizable with low KV radiography.[38–42]

### CLINICAL EXAMPLES OF LOW KV RADIOGRAPHY

#### Fingers

Two kinds of soft tissue calcifications are observed in the distal portions of the fingers or toes, or both. Subungual calcifications in the normal nail bed of the fingers[43] (Fig. 5–1) are seen in elderly adults, especially women. In elderly women, their frequency is 7 per cent.[44] Similar calcifica-

tions in the toes appear in women during the third decade of life, and are frequent (47 per cent) in elderly women; in men, they generally appear two decades later and are less common (14 per cent) in the elderly.[45] These calcifications occur independently of diseases associated with soft tissue calcifications.[43]

A second pattern of soft tissue calcification occurs in close proximity to the ungual tuft.[46] These asymptomatic calcifications appear in the second decade of life and often disappear within a few months (Fig. 5–2). The mean frequency of such calcifications in a normal adult population is 7 per cent with a maximum frequency of 14 per cent in the fifth decade of life. In patients with rheumatoid arthritis and in those undergoing chronic hemodialysis, these calcifications are not more frequent but, in progressive systemic sclerosis without tuftal resorption, their frequency is about 50 per cent. Long-term corticosteroid therapy increases the frequency of such calcifications[47] (Fig. 5–2).

Calcifications are seen also in the periarticular regions. Small calcifications occur near the insertions of the fibrous capsule of the joints and other entheses. These have been detected in 2 per cent of patients with rheumatoid arthritis (Fig. 5–3) and in 5 per cent of those with secondary hyperparathyroidism undergoing hemodialysis[48, 49] (Figs. 5–4 and 5–5). No constant relationship has been found between these calcifications and osseous erosions; one finding typically occurs independently of the other.

The thin cancellous bones (ungual tufts) are early target sites in disorders of increased bone turnover. Bone remodeling, consisting of both bone formation and resorption, is a normal finding but one that increases in frequency in rheumatoid arthritis.[23, 24, 27] In secondary hyperparathyroidism, this remodeling is very common, occurring simultaneously in several areas of the fingers. One important site of involvement is the proximal corner on each side of the ungual tuft (Figs. 5–5 and 5–6). A second site of involvement is the entheses in the fingers (Fig. 5–7).

Osteoarthritic changes in the fingers[22] are better evaluated with oblique projections. Initially, osteophytes in the phalangeal bases are oriented predominantly in a dorsolateral direction, appearing as early as the third decade of life. The changes in the phalangeal heads begin at the medial or lateral volar margin with localized thickening of the subchondral bone plate (Fig. 5–8) accompanied by degenerative erosions of varying size (Fig. 5–9) or laterally located cystlike changes.[22]

The normal radiographic anatomy of the water-equivalent tissues of the fingers is shown in Figure 5–10 in a PA view. The periarticular soft tissues of the fingers are com-

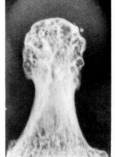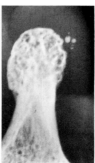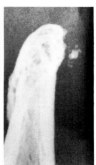

**FIGURE 5–1.** Subungual calcifications in the right second finger. The calcifications are better seen in the oblique view (radiograph in the center) and the lateral view (right), because in the posteroanterior (PA) view (left), the calcifications are covered by the ungual tufts. These subungual calcifications, which also were evident in other fingers, diminished during the following 7 months in this 58 year old woman whose nails were clinically normal. (From Fischer E: ROFO *137*:580, 1982.)

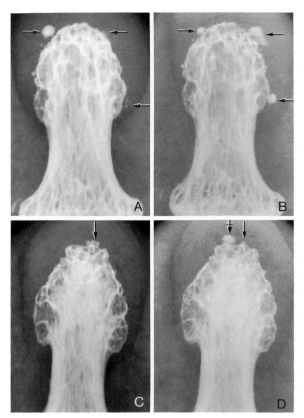

FIGURE 5–2. Calcifications in close proximity to the ungual tufts. The patient is a 34 year old man with bronchial asthma for 20 years who had been treated with corticosteroids for 9 years, and who also had steroid-induced diabetes mellitus and adrenal hypofunction.

**A** In the left second finger, approximately 10 calcifications of different sizes are present (arrows). The stripelike calcification at the base of the phalanx is not related to the ungual calcifications.

**B** Four months after **A,** there is a decrease as well as an increase in size of some of the calcifications (arrows). The stripelike calcification at the base of the phalanx has decreased in size.

**C** In the left fourth finger, three closely spaced calcifications are evident (arrow).

**D** Four months after **C,** two calcifications have disappeared (arrow) and a new large calcification has developed (arrow with cross). Similar calcifications were present in three other fingers. Note the bone loss in some portions of the ungual tufts and in some submarginal trabeculae in **B** and **D.**

(From Fischer E: Radiologe *25*:93, 1985.)

posed of joint capsules and their contents and collateral ligaments in the interphalangeal joints, with the addition of interosseous and lumbrical muscles about the metacarpophalangeal joints. In oblique views, the mass of the tendon sheaths contributes to the volar prominence of the periarticular soft tissues. The thickness of these tissues is determined by measuring the maximal transverse diameter of the periarticular soft tissues and subtracting the maximum transverse diameter of the base of the corresponding phalanx (Fig. 5–10); this measurement is called the "relative width of the periarticular soft tissues" and is relatively

independent of the different diameters of the bones and any osteophytes. The width of the periarticular soft tissues changes from the second through the fifth fingers in both the true PA and the oblique views, is larger in the oblique than in the true PA projection, and increases from a distal to a proximal direction in a digit.[18] As the normal periarticular soft tissues vary considerably in width, caution should be exercised in diagnosing abnormality, and the opposite side and neighboring joints should be compared meticulously. Pathologic enlargement of the soft tissues first is

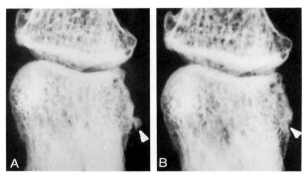

FIGURE 5–3. Disappearance of periosseous calcification with development of adjacent erosion. Right fifth distal interphalangeal joint in an 81 year old woman who had had rheumatoid arthritis for 4 years.

**A** Calcification at the dorsoulnar margin of the phalangeal head (arrowhead).

**B** One year after **A,** the calcification has resolved with the development of an adjacent erosion (arrowhead).

(From Fischer E: ROFO *141*:87, 1984.)

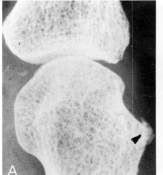
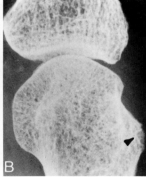

FIGURE 5–4. Calcification and bone erosion. Right fifth metacarpophalangeal joint in a 64 year old woman who for 5 years had been on hemodialysis.

**A** Eighteen months after the beginning of hemodialysis, a calcification appears at the metacarpal tubercle (arrowhead).

**B** Thirty months after **A,** the calcification has disappeared with resorption of the corner of the tubercle (arrowhead). Similar changes occurred at other periarticular sites in additional fingers.

(From Fischer E: ROFO *141*:87, 1984.)

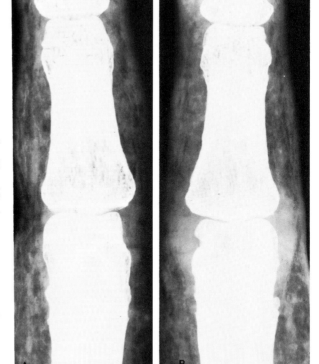

**FIGURE 5–12.** Rheumatoid arthritis with subcutaneous edema and moderate thickening of the veins.

**A** The left index finger possesses a normal but slightly accentuated subcutaneous venous texture.

**B** In the right index finger, moderate thickening of the veins, edema-induced unsharpness of soft tissue contours, and an augmented width of the areolar tissue related to an inflamed and dilated proximal interphalangeal joint capsule are seen.

(From Fischer E: Radiologe *19*:119, 1979.)

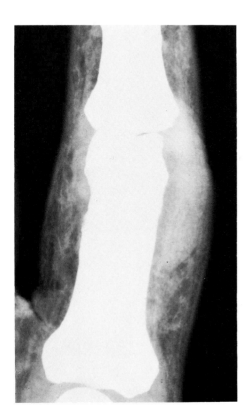

**FIGURE 5–13.** Left index finger, 25 degree PA oblique view with ulnar elevation. Enormous engorgement of the capsule of the proximal interphalangeal (PIP) joint is present at the radial aspect only. (From Fischer E: Radiologe *19*:119, 1979.)

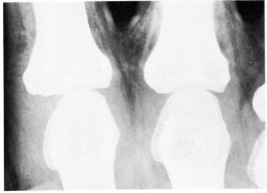

A

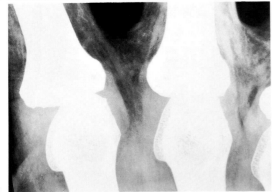

B

**FIGURE 5–14.** Second and third right metacarpophalangeal joints, true PA views, in a 28 year old woman with early and acute rheumatoid arthritis.

**A** Minor thickening of the periarticular soft tissues with narrowing of the interdigital fatty wedge is visible.

**B** Eighteen months after **A,** normalization of the interdigital fatty wedge following reversal of enlargement and edema of adjacent joint capsules is seen.

(From Fischer E: Radiologe *19*:119, 1979.)

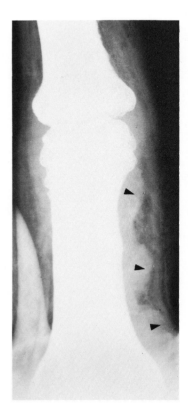

**FIGURE 5–15.** Left third finger, 25 degree PA oblique view with radial elevation. Threefold herniation of the tendon sheaths at the MCP joint with only minor engorgement of the sheaths (arrowheads). The herniations were not palpable.

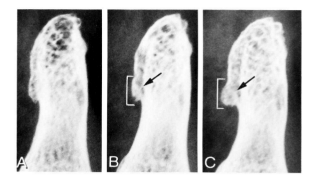

**FIGURE 5–16.** Rheumatoid arthritis with development of extrasynovial osseous changes. Right fifth distal phalanx, 25 degree oblique view with radial elevation.

**A** Five months after the onset of the disease that led to rapidly severe joint destruction in the hand, there are no local osseous abnormalities.

**B** Five months after **A,** a small entheseal erosion with an adjacent sclerotic reaction is seen at the proximal corner of the ungual tuft (arrow).

**C** Fifteen months after **B,** considerable new bone has formed at the proximal corner of the ungual tuft (arrow).

(From Fischer E: Akt Rheumatol *9*:135, 1984.)

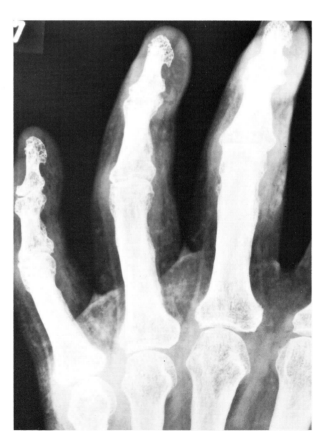

**FIGURE 5–17.** Reflex sympathetic dystrophy (Sudeck's atrophy). The syndrome developed 4 months after a fracture of the distal portion of the radius in a 63 year old woman. Uniform enlargement of all of the joint capsules and the tendon sheaths of the left third, fourth, and fifth fingers is seen. Note the erosion at the medial side of the head of the fourth proximal phalanx.

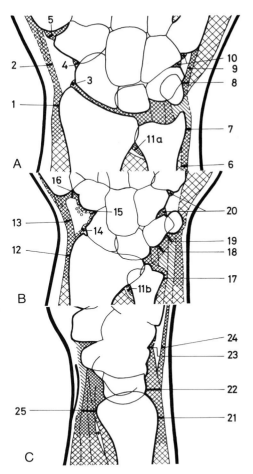

**FIGURE 5–18.** Schematic outline of the soft tissues and bones of the wrist in three views. Joint capsules, tendon sheaths, and tendons: fine crosshatched area; variants of size of tendon sheaths: obliquely lined area; muscles: coarse crosshatched area; constantly sharp borders of the soft tissues: uninterrupted lines; intertenosynovial thin fatty stripes: interrupted lines within the tendon sheaths distal to the ulna in **A** and **B** and at the volar side in **C**; thick line within the soft tissues: suitable position and direction to record soft tissue changes.

**A** Posteroanterior view. 1, 2, Tendon sheath of abductor pollicis longus and extensor brevis muscles of the thumb. 3, 4, 5, Joint capsules of the radiocarpal, trapezioscaphoid, and trapezium–first metacarpal joint. 6, 7, Proximal portion of the tendon sheath of the extensor carpi ulnaris muscle. 8, Overlap of the joint capsule of the pisiform–triquetral joint with the tendon sheath of the extensor carpi ulnaris muscle. 9, Pisometacarpal ligament as a continuation of the tendon sheath of the extensor carpi ulnaris muscle. 10, Joint capsules of the triquetrum–hamate and hamate–fifth metacarpal joints (these soft tissue masses may merge into each other in abduction or by synovial dilation). 11a, Saccular recess of the inferior radioulnar joint.

**B** Twenty-five degree anteroposterior (AP) oblique view, radial elevation. 12, 13, Tendon sheath of the extensor and abductor pollicis longus muscles of the thumb, which may be separated distally by a thin fatty stripe. 14, 15, 16, The same joint capsules as 3, 4, and 5 in **A**. 17, Joint capsule of the inferior radioulnar joint (in normal condition, sometimes overlapped with the tendon sheath of the extensor carpi ulnaris; with synovitis of both compartments the dilation of the joint capsule dominates). 18, Radiocarpal joint capsule at the proximal prominence of the triquetrum, sometimes overlapped by the ulnar bursa. 19, Pisiform–triquetral joint capsule (which normally may be prominent). 20, The same as 10 in **A**. 11b, The same as 11a in **A** (normally sized saccular recess is seldom seen in this view; with synovial dilation and surrounding edema, the saccular recess is better outlined in the AP oblique than in the true PA projection). The small circles in the fatty triangle between 15 and 16 represent veins.

**C** Lateral view. 21, Extensor tendon sheaths at the metaepiphyseal junction (sometimes overlapped by intertendineal bony ridges). 22, Combined width of the radiocarpal joint and extensor tendon sheaths at the proximal corner of the lunate bone. 23, Joint capsule of the triquetrum–hamate joint. 24, Tendon sheaths of the extensor digitorum muscle. 25, Tendon sheaths of the flexor digitorum profundus and superficialis muscles. +, Fatty plane between the pronator quadratus muscle and the tendon sheaths of the flexors (reduced from the front by tenosynovitis and extended dorsally by atrophy of the pronator quadratus).

(From Fischer E: Radiologe 25:562, 1985.)

## Wrist

The normal anatomy of the soft tissues in this location is shown for each of the three views in Figure 5–18.

In the early stages of rheumatoid arthritis, the frequency of enlarged joint capsules decreases in a proximal to distal direction.[20] In reference to Figure 5–18, the most common enlargements of the joint capsule occur at points 14, 11a, 4, 15, 17, 18, 22, and 23, in order of decreasing frequency (Figs. 5–19 and 5–20). In the true PA view, a mass adjacent to the ulnar styloid process can be caused by tenosynovitis of the extensor carpi ulnaris tendon sheath, by dilation of the joint capsule around the ulnar head, and by marked dilation of the prestyloid recess of the radiocarpal joint (Fig.

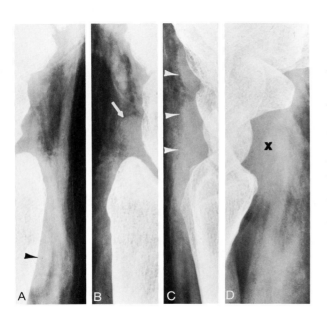

**FIGURE 5–19.** Soft tissue changes in rheumatoid arthritis. Three views of the left wrist in a 54 year old woman who had had rheumatoid arthritis for 6 months.

**A** True PA view, radial aspect. Note joint capsule dilations between trapezioscaphoid joint and trapezium–first metacarpal joint, with only borderline width of the radiocarpal joint capsule. The tendon sheath of the abductor pollicis longus and extensor brevis muscles of the thumb is shifted by a synovial outpouching from an adjacent tendon sheath (arrowhead).

**B** Anteroposterior oblique view, 25 degree radial elevation, radial aspect. The considerable dilation of the radiocarpal joint capsule is seen only in this view (arrow). Compare with **A**.

**C** Lateral view, dorsal side. All of the joint capsules from the radius through the capitate are enlarged (arrowheads). The dorsal edema of the inflamed joint capsules makes the contours of the extensor tendon indistinct.

**D** Lateral view, palmar side. The dilated joint capsules between the radius and the scaphoid shift the flexor tendon sheaths and blend with them, producing a uniform mass (X).

(From Fischer E: Radiologe 25:562, 1985.)

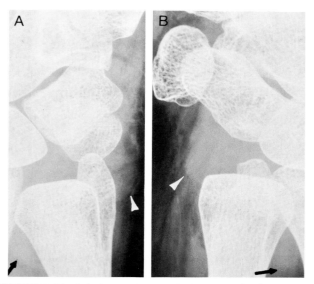

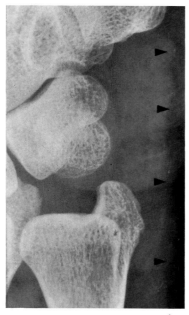

**FIGURE 5–20.** Soft tissue changes in rheumatoid arthritis. Ulnar aspect of the right wrist in a 58 year old woman who had had rheumatoid arthritis for 2 years.

**A** True PA view. Observe the bulging mass at the lateral side of the ulnar styloid (arrowhead) without dilation of the tendon sheath of the extensor carpi ulnaris muscle. The mass is caused by a pathologic enlargement of the prestyloid recess, as seen in **B.** Further joint capsule enlargements are the saccular recess (arrow) and the capsules of the triquetrum–hamate and the hamate–fifth metacarpal joints.

**B** Anteroposterior oblique view, 25 degree radial elevation. The prestyloid recess (arrowhead) of the radiocarpal joint is enlarged. Note the considerable dilation of the saccular recess (arrow) without dilation of the capsule of the radioulnar joint.

(From Fischer E: Radiologe 25:562, 1985.)

5–20). The dilated saccular recess of the inferior radioulnar joint can be recognized (Fig. 5–20).

The frequency of tenosynovitis in rheumatoid arthritis is less than that of dilation of the joint capsules.[20] This is most commonly apparent in the extensor carpi ulnaris tendon sheath (point 7 in Fig. 5–18). The distal part of this tendon sheath (point 9 in Fig. 5–18) is affected less frequently (Fig. 5–21). The first changes in rheumatoid arthritis related to osteopenia and bone erosions in the wrist appear at the proximal midportion of the triquetrum (Fig. 5–22).

De Quervain's disease, caused by stress damage of the tendon sheaths at the radial and dorsoradial aspects of the wrist, is seen as individual enlargements of the tendon sheaths at points 1, 2, 12, and 13 in Figure 5–18.[55] Storage diseases may enlarge the synovial compartments or tendons in the hand and wrist. They do not produce surrounding edema, dilated vessels, localized periarticular osteopenia, or bone erosions. Examples of such diseases are Fabry's disease, amyloidosis,[56, 57] and xanthomatosis.

### Forefoot

Normal as well as slightly enlarged periosseous soft tissues of the toes are more difficult to recognize radiographically than those of the fingers. Apparently the thick pads on the undersurface of the toes, which contain substantial fatty tissue, may abolish many soft tissue contours. If perceptible, normal periarticular soft tissues of the second through fourth metatarsophalangeal joints are not wider

**FIGURE 5–21.** Ulnar aspect of the right wrist. Substantial thickening of the entire tendon sheath of the extensor carpi ulnaris muscle with globular distention of its distal portion (arrowheads).

than the transverse diameter of the adjacent bases of the respective phalanges.

The essential soft tissue signs of rheumatoid arthritis and the seronegative spondyloarthropathies are thickening of periarticular soft tissues and, more importantly, periarticular edema (Fig. 5–23).

An acute attack of gout causes moderate inflammatory distention of the capsule of the involved joint, as well as

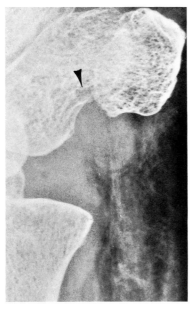

**FIGURE 5–22.** Typical site of early erosion in rheumatoid arthritis in the ulnar aspect of the wrist. Anteroposterior oblique view, 25 degree radial elevation. Note the erosion in the palmar midportion of the triquetrum at the proximal border of the pisiform–triquetral joint (arrowhead). Multiple small erosions are seen in the pisiform bone. Moderate dilation of the joint capsule around the ulnar head also is present. (From Fischer E: Radiologe 25:562, 1985.)

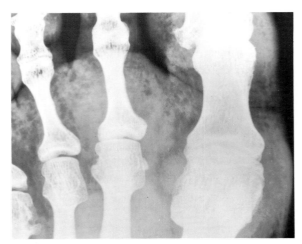

**FIGURE 5–23.** Rheumatoid arthritis. Left first through third toes. Note distention of the capsules of the first and second metatarsophalangeal (MTP) joints and of the first interphalangeal (IP) joint. Substantial capsular edema is visible only in the vicinity of the second proximal phalanx. Periarticular soft tissues of the third and fourth MTP joints are normal.

periarticular edema and an augmentation of surrounding veins.

### Ankle Region

The Achilles tendon normally is between 4 and 9 mm thick. The tendon is thinnest in its distal third and commonly increases in thickness proximally. Its junction with the triceps surae muscle is somewhat extended; terminal fascicles of the muscle sometimes insert asymmetrically into the distalmost portion of the tendon. With proper radiographic positioning, the Achilles tendon has well-defined margins anteriorly, and, if there is sufficient fatty tissue between it and the skin, posteriorly as well. Nevertheless, there are thin opaque areas accompanying the anterior margin produced by slender lateral extensions of the tendon. These opaque regions may be caused by the plantaris tendon as well, which frequently courses alongside the medial aspect of the Achilles tendon.[58]

In normal posture, the slightly curved contour of the skin posterior to the Achilles tendon forms an obtuse angle of at least 150 degrees, opening posteriorly (Toygar's angle).[6] Because the skin and tendon are closely parallel, the contour formed by the margin of the skin reflects the tension of the Achilles tendon.

Lesions related to overstrain of the Achilles tendon range from irritation of the paratenon to complete rupture, usually secondary to degenerative changes that reduce the strength of the tendon. The signs of paratenonitis (crepitans) achillea are increased thickness and unsharpness of the anterior margin as a result of edema (Fig. 5–24), which may extend considerably into the preachilles fatty tissue.

The signs of incomplete rupture of the Achilles tendon depend on the time interval between the causative event and the low KV radiographic examination. A few hours after the event, the tendon frequently is thickened owing to intratendinous edema and bleeding with localized thickening at the site of incomplete rupture. The normal gently curved course of the tendon is straightened by the presence of marked edema in the preachilles fatty tissue (Fig. 5–25).

Perifocal edema and bleeding as well as shredding of the severed ends of the Achilles tendon are likely to abolish its outline at the site of complete rupture. However, even when its contours are well outlined and its thickness is normal, an increase in the anterior curvature of the tendon reducing Toygar's angle to less than 150 degrees indicates complete rupture.

Spontaneous healing of an incomplete rupture usually is manifested initially as localized thickening, whereas surgically treated ruptures commonly lead to shortening and considerable thickening.

The entire Achilles tendon may be involved in rheumatoid arthritis and its variants. The edematous paratenon causes the outlines of the tendon to broaden, with possible blurring of its contours and with edema in the preachilles fatty tissue.[57] The thickness of the tendon may be nearly twice normal.

The retrocalcaneal bursa frequently is involved in rheumatoid arthritis and the seronegative spondyloarthropathies. The radiographic sign is an opaque area of water density of varying size situated between the Achilles tendon and the superoposterior limit of the calcaneal tubercle (Fig. 5–26). Mechanical factors aggravate the irritation of an already inflamed bursa, as has been shown in Haglund's disease.[57] Retrocalcaneal bursitis frequently causes thickening of the adjacent Achilles tendon as evidence of secondary localized rheumatoid paratenonitis.

The Achilles tendon may be thickened diffusely or focally by deposition of cholesterol in hyperlipoproteinemia,[58] and by gout. Soft tissue prominence in the vicinity of the Achilles tendon may be caused by cutaneous or subcuta-

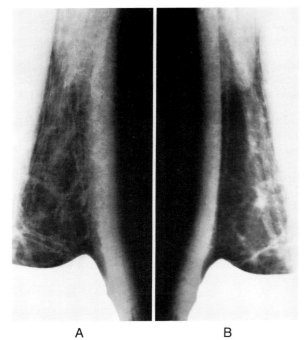

A                                   B

**FIGURE 5–24.** Ankle joint of 31 year old woman with painful right ankle after 4 weeks of strenuous gymnastic exercise.

**A** Right ankle: Paratenonitis achillea due to overstrain. Note moderate thickening and hazy and irregular anterior margin of the Achilles tendon with increased opacity of the preachilles fat pad due to edema.

**B** Normal left ankle of same patient for comparison. (From Fischer E: Radiologe *14*:457, 1974.)

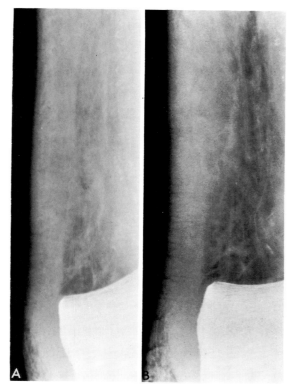

**FIGURE 5–25.** Paratenonitis achillea with subsequent incomplete rupture.

**A** Left Achilles tendon. Note substantial thickening of the tendon with slight bulging in its middle part. Observe its straight course as a result of edematous stiffness within the tendon and edema in the preachilles fat pad. The tendon damage was caused by 2 weeks of strenuous digging by this 70 year old man.

**B** Two weeks after **A,** while descending from a ladder, the patient experienced sudden, excruciating pain in the Achilles tendon with a clearly audible "pop." Note incomplete rupture with unsharpness of the anterior tendinous contour due to bleeding or localized augmented edema. This was treated with conservative management. After 3 years, the Achilles tendon almost was normal in thickness and shape.

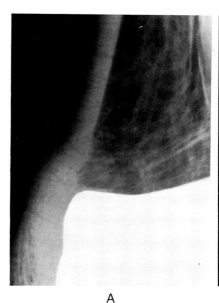

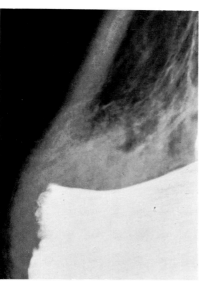

A B

**FIGURE 5–26.** Retrocalcaneal bursitis in ankylosing spondylitis; 22 year old woman.

**A** Note edema in the vicinity of the bursa as the only radiologic sign of bursitis. A moderate degree of thickening of the adjacent distal Achilles tendon is observed.

**B** Two years after **A.** Substantial destruction has taken place at the posterior margins of the calcaneal tubercle, and there is marked distention of the bursa proximally and substantial streaky edema proximal to the bursa.

neous rheumatoid nodules, gouty tophi, or cutaneous thickening or chronic irritation by the hard edge of a boot.

## SUMMARY

Because of the increase in contrast and resolution obtainable with low KV radiography, many minute details of bones and soft tissues clearly are perceptible that would otherwise not be visible. Similar and, sometimes, superior information, however, is provided by other methods, particularly MR imaging, but such methods often are more costly.

The investigations on low KV radiography of the extremities were supported by the Robert-Bosch Foundation.

## References

1. Ter-Pogossian MM: The Physical Aspects of Diagnostic Radiology. New York, Hoeber Medical Division, Harper and Row, 1969, p 173.
2. Révész V: Röntgenbilder normaler peripherischer Blutgefässe. ROFO 20:39, 1913.
3. Bonola A: Sulla interpretazione radiografica delle ombre normali e pathologiche delle parti molli del ginocchio senza mezzi di contrasto. Chir Organi Mov 23:39, 1936.
4. Carty JR: Soft tissue roentgenography. Anatomical, technical and pathological considerations. AJR 35:474, 1936.
5. Frantzell A: Röntgenologische Weichteilsstudien von Cutis and Subcutis. Ein Beitrag zur röntgenologischen Oedemdiagnostik. Acta Radiol (Stockh) 25:460, 1944.
6. Toygar O: Subkutane Ruptur der Achillessehne (Diagnostik und Behandlungsergebnisse). Helv Chir Acta 14:209, 1947.
7. Bonse G: Anwendungsmöglichkeiten röntgenologischer Weichteildiagnostik ohne Kontrastmittel. ROFO 74:450, 1951.
8. Chiappa S: Stuido radiologico sulle parti molli articolari e periarticolari. Le parti molli dell'articolazione tibiotarsica nel quadro normale e nelle lesioni da trauma. Radiol Med (Torino) 38:621, 1952.
9. Norell HG: Roentgenologic visualization of the extra-capsular fat: Its importance in the diagnosis of traumatic injuries to the elbow. Acta Radiol (Stockh) 42:205, 1954.
10. MacEwan W: Changes due to trauma in the fat-plane overlying the pronator quadratus muscle: A radiologic sign. Radiology 82:879, 1964.
11. Weston WJ: The soft tissue signs of the enlarged ulnar bursa in rheumatoid arthritis. J Can Assoc Radiol 24:282, 1973.
12. Curtis DJ, Downey EF, Brower AC, et al: Importance of soft-tissue evaluation in hand and wrist trauma: Statistical evaluation. AJR 142:781, 1984.
13. Ferguson AB: Roentgenographic features of rheumatoid arthritis. J Bone Joint Surg 18:297, 1936.
14. Tabár L, Dean PB: Magnification immersion radiography: Better soft tissue visualisation in the hands. ROFO 136:444, 1982.
15. Tabár L, Dean PB, Mäkelä P, et al: Magnification immersion radiography of the distal extremities. Appl Radiol, 1984, p 99.
16. Mäkelä P, Haaslahti JO: Immersion technique in soft tissue radiography. Acta Radiol (Diagn) 19:89, 1977.
17. Fischer E: Die Leistungsfähigkeit der Drei-Ebenen-Weichstrahl-radiographie an den Fingern bei der chronischen Polyarthritis. Akt Rheumatol 8:200, 1983.
18. Fischer E: Die Weichteilveränderungen der Finger bei der rheumatischen Polyarthritis. Ergebnisse nach Weichstrahlaufnahmen in drei Ebenen. Radiologe 19:119, 1979.
19. Fischer E: Weichteilveränderungen an der Mittelhand bei der chronischen Polyarthritis. ROFO 141:561, 1984.
20. Fischer E: Weichteilveränderungen am Handgelenk bei der chronischen Polyarthritis. Ergebnisse nach Weichstrahlaufnahmen in drei Ebenen. Radiologe 25:562, 1985.
21. Fischer E: Synovitische und enthesitische Veränderungen an der Hand bei der Reflexdystrophie. Radiologe 25:554, 1985.
22. Fischer E: Frührthrose der Fingergelenke. Ergebnisse nach Weichstrahlaufnahmen in drei Ebenen. ROFO 140:566, 1984.
23. Fischer E: Die quantitative Entwicklung von fibroostitischen im Vergleich zu synovitischen Reaktionen am Fingerskelett bei chronischer Polyarthritis. Akt Rheumatol 9:92, 1984.
24. Fischer E: Fibroostitische Erosionen am Fingerskelett bei der chronischen Polyarthritis. Akt Rheumatol 9:135, 1984.
25. Fischer E: Subligamentäre Resorptionen am Finger als Frühzeichen eines Hyperparathyreoidismus. ROFO 140:704, 1984.
26. Fischer E: Die Entstehung von Erosionen am Fingerskelett bei der Auflösung periossärer Verkalkungen. ROFO 141:87, 1984.
27. Fischer E: Ossäre Tenosynovitisfolgen an Fingern und Zehen bei der chronischen Polyarthritis. Radiologe 24:573, 1984.
28. Fischer E: Exo- und endomarginale Reaktionen an der Hand bei der diffusen idiopathischen Skeletthyperostose, ihre Quantifizierung und Altersabhängigkeit. ROFO 142:85, 1985.
29. Fischer E: Weichstrahlradiographie an Händen und Füssen. Aufnahme-material, Einstelltechnik, Ausstattung des Weichstrahlgerätes, Zubehör, Röntgenmorphologie, Indikationen. MTA Praxis 28:290, 1982.
30. Fischer E: Weichteildiagnostik an den peripheren Extremitäten mittels Weichstrahltechnik. Teil III. Der Nachweis diskreter Reizzustände der Bursa subachillea. Radiologe 14:468, 1974.
31. Fleeter TB, Myrie C, Adams JP: Pachydermodactyly: A case report and discussion of the pathologic entity. J Hand Surg [Am] 9:764, 1984.
32. Mäkelä P, Virtama P, Dean PB: Finger joint swelling: Correlation with age, gender, and manual labor. AJR 132:939, 1979.
33. Wegelius U: Angiography of the hand. Acta Radiol (Suppl) 315:86, 1972.
34. Bohndorf W: Uber die Röntgendiagnostik der Hautkrankheiten. Radiologe 5:39, 1965.
35. Schraub S: Radiographie de la peau. In T Trial, M Laval-Jeantet, M-C Plainfossé (Eds): Traité de radiodiagnostic. Rhumatologie, articulations, parties molles. Paris, Masson, 1976, p 423.
36. Fischer E: Die progressive Sklerodermie der Finger im Weichstrahlbid. ROFO 119:372, 1973.
37. Brower AC, NaPombejara C, Stechschulte DJ, et al: Rheumatoid nodulosis: Another cause of juxtaarticular nodules. Radiology 125:669, 1977.
38. Fischer E: Der Nachweis von Holz- und kleinen Glassplittern durch die Weichstrahlaufnahme. ROFO 118:309, 1973.
39. Lewis RW: A roentgenographic study of glass and its visibility as a foreign body. AJR 27:853, 1932.
40. Goldhahn WE, Buttenberg H: Zur röntgenologischen Darstellung inkorporierter Glassplitter bei Handverletzungen. Dtsch Gesundh 20:517, 1965.
41. Felman AH, Fisher MS: The radiographic detection of glass in soft tissue. Radiology 92:1529, 1969.
42. Woesner ME, Sanders I: Xeroradiography: A significant modality in the detection of nonmetallic foreign bodies in soft tissues. AJR 115:636, 1972.
43. Fischer E: Subunguale Verkalkungen. ROFO 137:580, 1982.
44. Fischer E: Subunguale Verkalkungen im normalen Nagelbett der Finger. Hautarzt 34:625, 1983.
45. Fischer E: Subunguale Verkalkungen im normalen Nagelbett der Zehen. Radiologe 24:31, 1984.
46. Fischer E: Weichteilverkalkungen am Rande der Tuberositas phalangis distalis der Finger. ROFO 139:150, 1983.
47. Fischer E: Steroideinfluss auf die Entstehung von Weichteilverkalkungen am Rand der Tuberositas phalangis distalis der Finger. Radiologe 25:93, 1985.
48. Meneghello A, Bertoli M, Romagnoli GF: Unusual complication of soft tissue calcification in chronic renal disease: The articular erosions. Skel Radiol 5:251, 1980.
49. Andresen J, Nielsen HE: Juxta-articular erosions and calcifications in patients with chronic renal failure. Acta Radiol (Diagn) 22:709, 1981.
50. Fischer E: Die normale Sehnenscheidenbreite des 2.—5. Fingers auf Schrägaufnahmen. ROFO 140:75, 1984.
51. Kalliomäki JL, Vastamäki M: Chronic diffuse oedema of the rheumatoid hand. A sign of local lymphatic involvement. Ann Rheum Dis 27:167, 1968.
52. Weston WJ, Palmer DG: Soft Tissues of the Extremities. A Radiologic Study of Rheumatic Disease. Berlin, Springer Verlag, 1978, pp 13, 14.
53. Jacobs JH, Hess EV, Beswick IP: Rheumatoid arthritis presenting as tenosynovitis. J Bone Joint Surg [Br] 39:288, 1957.
54. Genant HK, Kozin F, Bekerman C, et al: The reflex sympathetic dystrophy syndrome. Radiology 117:21, 1975.
55. Weston WJ: De Quervain's disease. Br J Radiol 40:446, 1967.
56. Gordon DA, Pruzanski W, Ogryzlo MA, et al: Amyloid arthritis simulating rheumatoid disease in five patients with multiple myeloma. Am J Med 55:142, 1973.
57. Fischer E: Weichteildiagnostik an den peripheren Extremitäten mittels Weichstrahltechnik. Teil II. Erkrankungen der Achilles-sehne und ihrer angrenzenden Gewebe. Radiologe 14:457, 1974.
58. Gatterau A, Davignon J, Langelier M, Levesque HP: An improved radiological method for the evaluation of achilles tendon xanthomatosis. Can Med Assoc J 108:39, 1973.

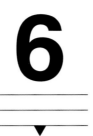

# 6

# Xeroradiography

*Harry K. Genant, M.D., and Michael André, Ph.D.*

Xeroradiography is an electrostatic imaging system that uses selenium as a photoconductor. It is a radiographic application of the xerographic process first discovered by Carlson in 1937. This methodology initially was applied in the field of graphic arts, where the process was used as a photographic recording medium. McMaster and Schaffert[1] first used the selenium plate with x-rays for the nondestructive testing of metal castings. The initial medical adaptation of xeroradiography was undertaken in the early 1950s by Roach and Hilleboe,[2–4] who explored the system as a means of providing diagnostic x-ray facilities during civilian disasters. Subsequent investigations were limited, despite some very good results, because these early units were unreliable and required higher radiation doses.

The pioneering effort in the medical use of xeroradiography as it is used today was directed by Wolfe.[5–8] His perseverance and collaboration with the Xerox Corporation led to the development of the first production units in 1971. Wolfe and others have written extensively on xeroradiography as an imaging technique for mammography[9, 10] and also have supported its use in other areas of radiography. These applications include skeletal trauma, metabolic bone disease, musculoskeletal neoplasms, arthritis, and radiation therapy beam verification.

The image produced by xeroradiography is very different from that obtained by conventional film radiography. It is a completely dry process, requires no darkroom, and records the final image on paper. Additionally, the exposure latitude is very wide compared to that for film, soft tissues and bone may be recorded with the same emphasis, the enhancement of edges gives the appearance of improved resolution, and either a positive or a negative recording mode may be selected.

## TECHNICAL CONSIDERATIONS

The physical qualities of semiconductors form the basis for the xeroradiographic imaging process.[4, 8, 11] The ability of a semiconductor to change from a material of high electrical resistance in the resting state to one of relatively low resistance when activated by radiant energy is the fundamental principle of formation of the latent image in xeroradiography. The xeroradiographic plate on which the latent image is formed has an aluminum base that is coated with a thin photoconductive layer of vitreous selenium. Selenium is a photoconductor that behaves as an insulator until it is exposed to a source of photons (light or x-ray). Although a number of semiconductors are available, selenium has been used most extensively.

### Image Production

Briefly, the steps in image production are as follows[4, 8, 11]: The metal plate is charged to a high positive potential by coronal discharge; then it is placed in a light-tight cassette and used as an image receptor similar to a conventional screen-film system; when the x-rays strike the selenium plate, photoconduction occurs, reducing the electrical charge locally, and resulting in a latent charge image of the object; the latent image is made visible by the use of charged developer particles or toner particles, which are brought into close proximity to the plate; finally, the resultant powder image is transferred to a paper and fused thermally, providing a permanent opaque image.

The operator controls three steps in producing a xeroradiograph: (1) charging of the selenium plate, (2) amount of x-ray exposure, and (3) development of the image. The quality of the final image may be changed considerably by a variation in any of these steps.[12]

### Edge Enhancement

One of the unique features of the xeroradiographic imaging process is the phenomenon of edge enhancement. To understand this process, it is necessary to examine closely

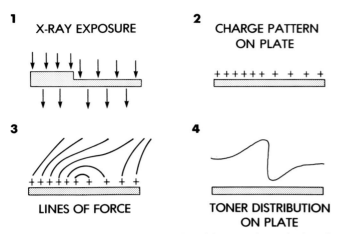

**1** X-RAY EXPOSURE

**2** CHARGE PATTERN ON PLATE

**3** LINES OF FORCE

**4** TONER DISTRIBUTION ON PLATE

**FIGURE 6–1.** Schematic representation of the steps in production of the xeroradiographic image. (From Xerox Corporation: Technical Application Bulletin 3, November 1975.)

the mechanism of image production in xeroradiography[8, 11, 13] (Fig. 6–1).

Prior to x-ray exposure, the xeroradiographic plate undergoes *relaxation,* a process of heating that removes any residual charge pattern on the plate.[11, 14] This relaxation prevents ghosting or the faint persistence of information from the previous image on the new image. After relaxation, the plate can be charged to a uniform level of surface potential.

For the image to be captured, the plate must be charged by submitting the plate to a uniform surface charge, thus sensitizing it for x-ray exposure. The surface charge is applied by a series of coronal discharge wires that are electromechanically passed close to the selenium plate, depositing a positive electrostatic charge on the surface of the selenium.

During radiographic exposure, x-rays are transmitted through the object and are absorbed by the selenium plate, causing a selective *discharge.* The amount of discharge is proportional to the radiation striking the selenium plate. The information in the transmitted x-ray beam is converted to a residual charge pattern on the plate, a *latent image.* Although the latent image is not edge enhanced, charge differences in the latent image and the resulting electric fields do cause edge enhancement during later steps in development. To make the latent image visible, the selenium plate is processed, during which a cloud of negatively charged fine powder, called toner, is attracted to the charge pattern on the plate. This attraction is related to the amount of residual charge and is controlled by the *electrical fields* occurring during development.

Electric fields exist during development as a result of two phenomena. First, a voltage is applied to the back of the plate and the development chamber. This provides a uniform contribution to the electric field and aids in delivering toner near the plate. Second, charge differences in the latent image cause *fringe fields.* These are strong near the plate surface and contribute to the electric field nonuniformly. Fringe fields are strongest at the boundary between areas of different charge and are weakest in areas of uniform charge. The latter phenomenon results in broad area contrast suppression. Wherever there is an abrupt change in charge, as shown for the step edge exposure (Fig. 6–1), the fringe

field directs more toner to the high charge side of the step edge and less toner to the lower charge side, producing the edge effect.

Thus, following the distribution of the lines of electric force, an edge or boundary is developed with increased toner on one side producing a darker band juxtaposed to a lighter band with less toner deposition. This accentuated toner distribution at contrast interfaces then produces the *edge enhancement* characteristic of xeroradiography.[8, 11]

## IMAGE QUALITY AND DOSIMETRY

The recording characteristics of *edge enhancement* and *broad latitude* found with the xeroradiographic system can be appreciated from Figure 6–2, which demonstrates the density tracings of a step-wedge exposure using xeroradiography, a screen-film system, and a nonscreen system.[11, 15] The exaggerated edge effect and the suppressed broad area contrast of the xeroradiographic system can be appreciated from the tracing and are the result of the electric lines of force discussed previously. With the screen-film system, a blurred edge effect can be seen, which represents unsharpness resulting from light diffusion in the phosphor screen. This blurring is characteristic of screen-film systems. The nonscreen-film technique demonstrates a sharp edge interface but no edge enhancement, as with xeroradiography. Additionally, the nonscreen technique has lower contrast than the screen-film system but does not show the broad area contrast suppression of the xeroradiographic system.

It is of importance to note that the amount of edge enhancement and the degree of broad area contrast suppression can be manipulated by appropriate selection of the kilovoltage for exposure, the amount of charge potential initially placed on the plate, and the level of back voltage applied during developing.[11] The last two steps provide added recording flexibility, which is not achievable with conventional radiography. Generally, a relatively high kilo-

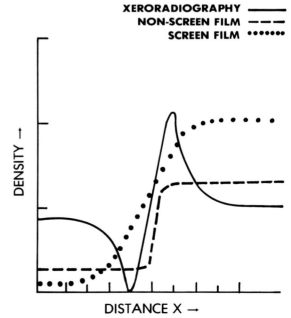

XERORADIOGRAPHY ——————
NON-SCREEN FILM — — —
SCREEN FILM ••••••

DENSITY →

DISTANCE X →

**FIGURE 6–2.** Schematic representation of density tracings of a step wedge for three recording systems (adapted from Fender[15]).

voltage exposure (~ 120 kVp) is selected for musculoskeletal applications[16] to increase the recording latitude and to diminish the excessive edge enhancement, which can produce a halo effect or toner deletion at the high contrast interfaces between bone and soft tissue. It can be inferred from Figure 6–2 that the sharpness or *spatial resolution* of the xeroradiographic system is high relative to conventional screen-film radiography but is less than that of nonscreen techniques using medical or industrial film.[17] The mottle or *noise* of the xeroradiograph similarly falls between that of a conventional screen-film system and that of a nonscreen-film technique. As a result of these inherent image characteristics, a xeroradiograph may be magnified optically 1.5 to 2 times using a hand lens, and additional useful information occasionally may be derived. The use of higher degrees of optical magnification, as commonly are employed for industrial film radiography, however, does not provide additional diagnostic information for xeroradiography. Here, the four- to eightfold enlargement simply produces a greater visual awareness of the inherent unsharpness and mottle of the xeroradiographic image.

The *radiation exposure* required for xeroradiography is relatively high compared to that needed for conventional screen-film radiography, but it is lower than that for nonscreen industrial film.[6, 7, 18, 19] Typically skin doses of 0.3 to 2.0 centigrays (cGy)(rad) are needed for musculoskeletal applications, which generally limits the use of xeroradiography to the thinner body parts.

## CLINICAL APPLICATIONS

By far the largest clinical application for xeroradiography has been in the area of *mammography*.[5, 7, 20, 21] In this field the broad latitude of the recording system and the edge enhancement have proved valuable in assessing the breast for benign and malignant neoplasms. In comparison with the nonscreen industrial film technique used earlier by Egan,[22] xeroradiography provides lower radiation exposure and possibly greater ease of interpretation. These factors have contributed to the widespread use of xeroradiography as a mammographic recording system. With the advent of the low-dose, high-resolution screen-film systems for mammography,[23–26] however, the continued use of the higher dose xeromammography is in question.

Owing to the availability of other techniques, such as CT, MR imaging, and ultrasonography, that can be used effectively to study the soft tissues, xeroradiography has not been widely employed as a recording medium for anatomic parts other than the breast. Although studies have been reported outlining its value in selected applications, a widespread use of xeroradiography in routine clinical practice has not been observed. It appears to have greatest potential in the depiction of *soft tissue masses*[6, 27, 28] in an extremity or limb girdle, in which situations the broad recording latitude and the edge enhancement show the subtle density interfaces of the soft tissue lesions to advantage (Fig. 6–3). Differentiation between benign and malignant soft tissue neoplasms has been observed in some cases. This application, however, has rapidly been supplanted by CT and MR imaging (see Chapters 8 to 10), which have far superior density resolution and the advantage of providing cross-sectional display.

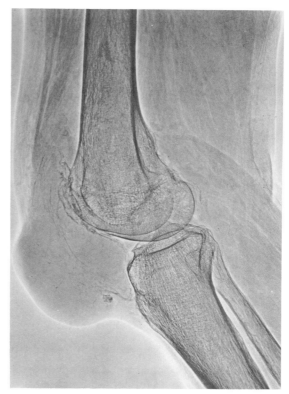

**FIGURE 6–3.** Xeroradiograph of the knee, which demonstrates an osteolytic process with a large soft tissue component that has replaced the patella. The edge enhancement and broad latitude of the xeroradiographic system can be appreciated.

Another area in which xeroradiography has found some success is in the depiction of subtle skeletal abnormalities in patients with early *arthritis* or *metabolic bone disease*.[6, 16, 29] In the former situation the ability to show with a single radiographic exposure the osseous structures of the joint as well as the periarticular soft tissues is a potential advantage (Figs. 6–4 and 6–5). It appears, however, that for this application, the use of magnification techniques, either optical or radiographic, are accepted more widely, because they provide superior images.[26, 30–35] Similarly, in the assessment of subtle structural changes in the hands or feet in metabolic bone disease, xeroradiography, although superior to conventional screen-film radiography, is inferior to the alternative high-resolution magnification techniques.[32, 33, 36–40]

In selected cases, xeroradiography has been shown to provide high-quality images for viewing the *cervical spine* and *ribs*.[6, 28] In these cases xeroradiography can record many tissues of different density and thickness; for example, bone, fat, air, and muscle readily are delineated on a single image. On a lateral view of the cervical spine, the primary areas of interest (the vertebrae) can be seen easily, as can the thinner, less dense parts such as the trachea, epiglottis, and valleculae (Fig. 6–6). Thus, when the soft tissues of the neck are of particular importance, xeroradiography may be used.[41] Similarly, the detection of subtle abnormalities in the rib cage may be difficult with conventional radiography owing to the broad latitude required, and xeroradiography may be used.

Xeroradiography has had some success in imaging the

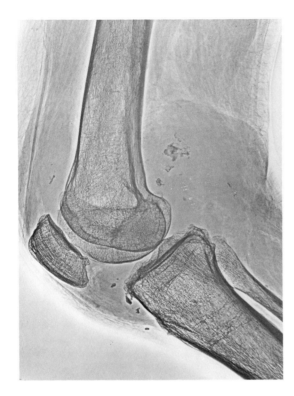

**FIGURE 6–4.** Xeroradiograph of the knee demonstrating moderately advanced osteoarthritis complicated by a large joint effusion and a popliteal cyst. The soft tissue planes are well demonstrated by xeroradiography.

**FIGURE 6–5.** Xeroradiograph of the distal portion of the hand of a patient with primary generalized osteoarthritis. Articular and periarticular structures are well shown with the xeroradiographic technique.

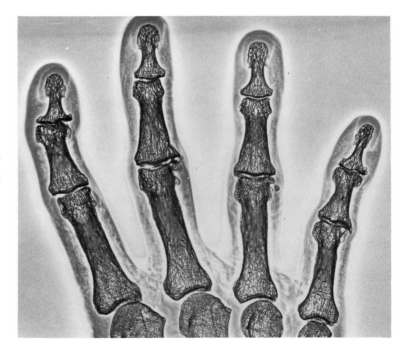

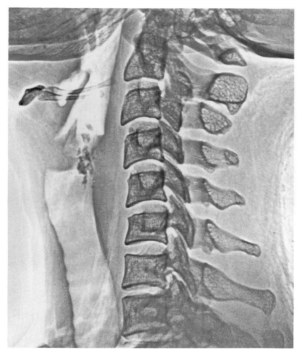

**FIGURE 6–6.** Xeroradiograph of the neck demonstrates the osseous as well as the soft tissue structures to advantage.

skeletal structures of an extremity that has been immobilized in a *plaster cast.*[42] In this situation, the superimposition of structures and the broad range of subject density make visualization by conventional radiography difficult. The xeroradiographic process, with the high kilovoltage generally applied, permits the cast to be penetrated readily, whereas the edge enhancement and wide recording latitude permit the edges of bones and fractures to be detected easily. Likewise, xeroradiography has proved excellent for evaluating the fit of the prosthetic socket for the stump after below-the-knee amputation.[43, 44]

## SUMMARY

The xeroradiographic imaging process differs considerably from conventional screen-film or nonscreen radiography, having unique imaging characteristics of edge enhancement, subdued broad area response, and large object latitude. These imaging characteristics make this technique useful in selected cases for imaging low-contrast objects that are defined by sharp edges. Nevertheless, widespread acceptance and usage of xeroradiography for routine musculoskeletal examinations appear unlikely owing to the relatively high radiation exposure required, the comparatively limited availability of the system, and the presence of alternative methods, such as CT, MR imaging, ultrasonography, and magnification radiography.

## References

1. McMaster RC, Schaffert RM: Xeroradiography—a basic development in x-ray. Nondestructive Testing 9:11, 1950.
2. Roach JF, Hilleboe HE: Xeroradiography. Arch Surg 69:594, 1954.
3. Roach JF, Hilleboe HE: Xeroradiography. AJR 73:5, 1955.
4. Roach JF: Xeroradiography. Radiol Clin North Am 8:271, 1970.
5. Wolfe JN: Xerography of the breast. Radiology 91:231, 1968.
6. Wolfe JN: Xeroradiography of the bones, joints and soft tissues. Radiology 93:583, 1969.
7. Wolfe JN, Dooley R, Harkins LE: Xeroradiography of the breast: A comparative study with conventional film mammography. Cancer 28:1569, 1971.
8. Wolfe JN: Xeroradiography: Image content and comparison with film roentgenograms. AJR 117:690, 1973.
9. Wolfe JN: Xeroradiography of the Breast. Springfield, III, Charles C Thomas, 1972.
10. Egan RL: Mammography and breast diseases. In LL Robbins (Ed): Golden's Diagnostic Radiology. Baltimore, Williams & Wilkins, 1970, p 240.
11. Kearns WJ: Xeroradiography—Principles and Practice. In Quantitative Imagery in the Biomedical Sciences. Proceedings of the Society of Photo-Optical Instrumentation Engineers, Bellingham, Washington, Vol 26, 1971.
12. Paulus DD: Xeroradiography: An in-depth review. CRC Crit Rev Diagn Imaging 3:309, 1980.
13. Xerox Corporation: What is edge enhancement and how does it affect the mammographic image? Pasadena, California, Technical Application Bulletin 1, November 1974.
14. Xerox Corporation: What are the most common xeroradiographic terms and what do they mean? Pasadena, California, Technical Application Bulletin 3, November 1975.
15. Fender WD: Radiographic image analysis through application of the radiographic modulation transfer function and system phase response. In Quantitative Imagery in the Biomedical Sciences. Proceedings of the Society of Photo-Optical Instrumentation Engineers, Bellingham, Washington, Vol 26, 1971.
16. Xerox Corporation: Xeroradiography for extremities. Pasadena, California, Xerox Medical Application Bulletin 117, December 1973.
17. Xerox Corporation: How does the resolution capability of xeroradiography compare with that of films used in mammography? Pasadena, California, Technical Application Bulletin 2, 1974.
18. Jaeger SS, Cacak RK, Barnes JE, et al: Optimization of xeroradiographic exposures. Radiology 128:217, 1978.
19. Lester RG: Risk versus benefit in mammography. Radiology 124:1, 1977.
20. Martin JE: Xeromammography—an improved diagnostic method. A review of 250 biopsied cases. AJR 117:90, 1973.
21. Rothenberg LN, Kirch RLA, Snyder RE: Patient exposure from film and xeroradiographic mammographic techniques. Radiology 117:701, 1975.
22. Egan RL: Mammography, xerography, and thermography of the breast. J Med Assoc Ga 61:151, 1970.
23. Chang CHJ, Sibala JL, Martin NL, et al: Film mammography: New low radiation technology. Radiology 121:215, 1976.
24. Ostrum BJ, Becker W, Isard HJ: Low-dose mammography. Radiology 109:323, 1973.
25. Sickles EA, Doi K, Genant HK: Magnification film mammography: Image quality and clinical studies. Radiology 125:69, 1977.
26. Sickles EA, Genant HK: Controlled single-blind clinical evaluation of low-dose mammographic screen-film systems. Radiology 130:347, 1979.
27. Jing BS: Xeroradiography of the soft tissues. Cancer Bull 26:31, 1974.
28. Otto RC, Pouliadis GP, Kumpe DA: The evaluation of pathologic alterations of juxtaosseous soft tissue by xeroradiography. Radiology 120:297, 1976.
29. Xerox Corporation: Xeroradiography for detection of hyperparathyroidism. Pasadena, California, Xerox Medical Application Bulletin 108, June 1973.
30. Berens DL, Lin RK: Roentgen Diagnosis of Rheumatoid Arthritis. Springfield, III, Charles C Thomas, 1969.
31. Doi K, Genant HK, Rossmann K: Comparison of image quality obtained with optical and radiographic magnification techniques in fine-detail skeletal radiography: Effect of object thickness. Radiology 118:189, 1976.
32. Genant HK, Doi K, Mall JC: Optical versus radiographic magnification for fine-detail skeletal radiography. Invest Radiol 10:160, 1975.
33. Genant HK, Doi K, Mall JC, et al: Direct radiographic magnification for skeletal radiology: An assessment of image quality and clinical application. Radiology 123:47, 1977.
34. Genant HK, Doi K: High-resolution skeletal radiography: Image quality and clinical applications. Curr Probl Radiol 7:3, 1978.
35. Mall JC, Genant HK, Silcox DC, et al: The efficacy of fine-detail radiography in the evaluation of patients with rheumatoid arthritis. Radiology 112:37, 1974.
36. Doyle FH: Radiological patterns of bone disease associated with renal glomerular failure in adults. Br Med Bull 28:220, 1972.
37. Genant HK, Heck LL, Lanzl LH, et al: Primary hyperparathyroidism. A comprehensive study of clinical, biochemical and radiographic manifestations. Radiology 109:513, 1973.
38. Meema HE, Schatz DL: Simple radiologic demonstration of cortical bone loss in thyrotoxicosis. Radiology 97:9, 1970.
39. Meema HE, Meema S: Comparison of microradioscopic and morphometric findings in the hand bones with densitometric findings in the proximal radius in thyrotoxicosis and in renal osteodystrophy. Invest Radiol 7:88, 1972.
40. Weiss A: A technique for demonstrating fine detail in bones of the hands. Clin Radiol 23:185, 1972.
41. Doust BD, Ting YM: Xeroradiography of the larynx. Radiology 110:727, 1974.
42. Xerox Corporation: Xeroradiography for casted extremities. Pasadena, California, Xerox Medical Application Bulletin 105, June 1973.
43. Jing BS, Villanueva R, Dodd, GD: A new radiological technique in evaluation of prosthetic fitting. Radiology 122:534, 1977.
44. Irwin GAL, Friedman L, Shapiro D: Use of xeroradiography in evaluating the adequacy of prosthetic socket fit. Radiology 157(P):177, 1985.

# 7

# Conventional Tomography

## Donald Resnick, M.D.

The role of conventional tomography in the evaluation of musculoskeletal disorders has diminished significantly since the introduction and refinement of alternative (and commonly superior) techniques, especially CT and MR imaging. In fact, in many radiology departments, conventional tomographic equipment has been sacrificed in an attempt to create needed space for newer CT equipment. Nonetheless, as there remain important applications of conventional tomography to the assessment of disease of the bones, joints, and soft tissues, a brief summary of these applications is included here. A comprehensive discussion of the physics and techniques of conventional tomography is beyond the scope of this book, and the interested reader should consult other available sources.[1–3]

## BASIC CONCEPTS AND TERMINOLOGY

The particular aim of conventional tomography is the imaging of structures lying in a predetermined plane of tissue while eliminating or at least blurring those structures located in other planes. All conventional tomographic techniques involve motion of two of three objects: the x-ray tube, the patient, or the film. Most systems move the x-ray tube and the film while the patient remains stationary. The basic mechanism is designed so that structures in the focal plane always are imaged at the same relative location on the film, whereas structures above or below the focal plane are imaged in various locations on the film, thereby effectively eliminating them from the image by motion blurring.

The precise pattern of motion used in conventional tomography can be classified as either unidirectional or pluridirectional. The unidirectional motion most often is termed linear tomography. The pluridirectional motion can be further described as circular, elliptical, spiral, pseudosinusoidal, or hypocycloidal. The amplitude of motion is specified by the angle through which the tube moves (tomographic angle) or the angle through the particular ex-

posure (exposure angle). Nonsymmetric pluridirectional motions, including elliptical, hypocycloidal, and spiral motions, require two angles for their specification; these most often are the minimum and maximum angles achieved in the course of the complex motion. Each type of tube-film motion has a characteristic blur pattern. The most basic principle of any tomographic system is that all parts of the objects to be blurred that are perpendicular to the direction of the tube motion are maximally blurred, whereas those parts that are parallel to the direction of motion are not blurred but merely elongated.

The thickness of the focal plane is inversely proportional to the exposure angle. The optimal thickness used in conventional tomography as well as the spacing of the tomographic sections will vary according to the body part that is being examined and the clinical questions that need to be answered. Hypocycloidal tube motion is able to provide extremely thin tomographic sections and can be very helpful in evaluating structures with complex anatomy, such as the vertebral column and inner ear. Narrow angle conventional tomography, also termed zonography, produces relatively thick sections, a technique that has been applied successfully to the evaluation of the sacroiliac and sternoclavicular joints. The author most commonly employs hypocycloidal motion with thin sections, usually spaced at 5 mm intervals, although the examination is carefully monitored and additional tomograms may be obtained at selected intervals (or in another projection) to supplement the initial tomographic images.

Specialized tomographic techniques that have been developed include axial transverse tomography (which has been completely eliminated owing to the widespread availability and superiority of CT scanning) and panoramic radiography, which is used predominantly to evaluate the curved osseous surfaces of the mandible and maxilla.[4]

One of the disadvantages of conventional tomography is the length of the examination, which, when images are obtained one section at a time, can be quite long (30 to 60 min). A method of obtaining several cuts simultaneously is provided by the use of a book cassette in which several film-screen layers are separated by spaces (with the spacing equal to the desired section spacing) and exposed simulta-

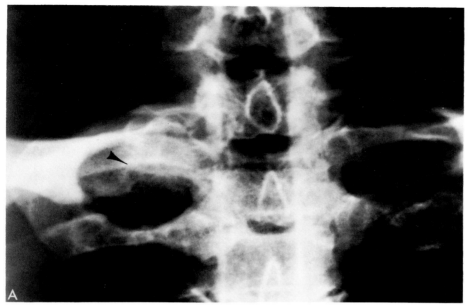

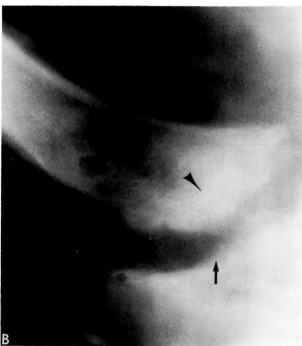

**FIGURE 7-1.** Sternoclavicular joint: Osteomyelitis and septic arthritis.

**A** The initial radiograph outlines erosion and eburnation (arrowhead) of the medial aspect of the right clavicle. Sternal alterations are not well delineated.

**B** Hypocycloidal tomography reveals considerable osseous erosion of both clavicle (arrowhead) and sternum (arrow). The extensive bony sclerosis, loss of articular space, and superior subluxation of the clavicle are readily apparent.

neously. A second disadvantage of conventional tomography is the radiation exposure to the patient, which obviously increases with the number of "cuts" that are obtained and is particularly high for the skin.

## CLINICAL APPLICATIONS

Many skeletal structures can be evaluated readily with routine radiographs. Specialized views, coned-down projections, and fluoroscopic monitoring are additional methods that may supplement initial films, providing adequate visualization of most skeletal sites. Certain structures, such as the vertebral column, sternum, ribs, and sella turcica, are more difficult to evaluate because of their size, particular orientation in the body, or surrounding tissues. Likewise,

certain joints may not be visualized adequately during initial radiography, necessitating application of conventional tomography. This is particularly true for the sternoclavicular (Fig. 7–1), temporomandibular (Fig. 7–2), sacroiliac, costovertebral, apophyseal, atlanto-occipital, atlantoaxial, subtalar (Fig. 7–3), and intertarsal joints[5–10] (Fig. 7–4).

Conventional tomographic evaluation of musculoskeletal disorders can be accomplished in several ways. Preliminary films must be studied prior to tomography and should be available during the procedure. These radiographs also must be available when the tomograms are being interpreted. The optimal patient position during tomography generally can be ascertained from the plain films; the patient should be placed in an attitude that best demonstrates the part to be examined. In general, conventional tomograms in a frontal

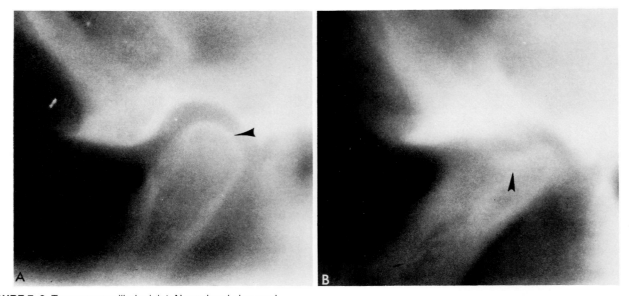

**FIGURE 7–2.** Temporomandibular joint: Normal and abnormal.

**A** Normal situation. Conventional tomogram reveals a smooth condylar head (arrowhead) and temporal fossa and normal joint space.

**B** Posttraumatic degenerative joint disease. Conventional tomography delineates flattening of the condylar head with bony eburnation (arrowhead) and loss of articular space.

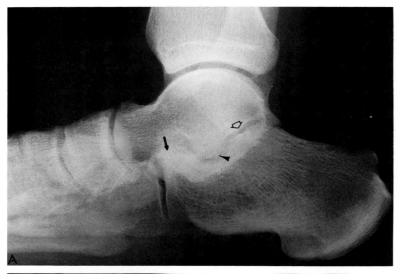

**FIGURE 7–3.** Talocalcaneal joints: Tarsal coalition.

**A** An initial lateral radiograph of the ankle and foot reveals narrowing of the posterior subtalar joint (open arrow), enlargement of the lateral process of the talus (arrowhead), and poor definition of the anterosuperior aspect of the calcaneus (arrow).

**B** Conventional tomography in the lateral projection confirms the osseous coalition (arrowheads) between the sustentaculum tali and inferior surface of the talus.

110

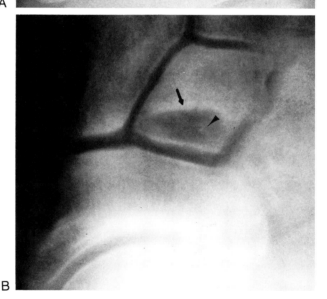

**FIGURE 7–4.** Cuneonavicular joint: Posttraumatic osteonecrosis.

**A** Frontal radiograph demonstrates soft tissue swelling, bony fragmentation, and a radiolucent lesion of the intermediate cuneiform bone (arrow).

**B** Frontal conventional tomogram better delineates the size of the lesion (arrow), a central sequestrum (arrowhead), surrounding bony eburnation, and normal articular space. A subsequent biopsy documented posttraumatic osteonecrosis of this bone.

projection are most helpful in visualizing the sacrum and sacroiliac and sternoclavicular joints; those in an oblique projection may be beneficial in evaluating the costovertebral and apophyseal joints; and conventional tomograms obtained in both the frontal and the lateral projections may be required to delineate the temporomandibular, atlanto-occipital, atlantoaxial, and subtalar joints, as well as the vertebrae and sternum.

Although there is a general tendency to use CT scanning rather than conventional tomography in many patients with musculoskeletal problems, the amount of time available in the CT suite often is limited owing to the clinical demand. Furthermore, certain problems are equally well or better evaluated with conventional tomography. Depending on the body part being examined, the way in which the patient can be placed in the CT scanner may be somewhat limited, resulting in primary CT scans that also are limited in terms of the imaging plane. As an example, CT of the vertebral column uses transaxial or transverse sections, an imaging strategy that is not ideal for delineating alterations (such as pseudarthrosis after spinal fusion) that also lie in the transverse plane. Although reformation of the CT image data in a coronal or sagittal plane is possible, information is lost with such image reconstruction. In these cases, conventional tomography represents an important alternative diagnostic method.[11, 12] Similarly, when it is necessary to image a long segment of a bone or bones owing to the presence of an extensive lesion or multiple lesions, conventional tomography rather than CT might be preferred.

The clinical situations that may be evaluated with conventional tomography are many. Only a few will be mentioned here; others are indicated elsewhere in the book. Conventional tomography can be applied in cases of skeletal trauma to detect and delineate vertebral column (Fig. 7–5), tibial plateau (Fig. 7–6), and carpal (Figs. 7–7 and 7–8) and femoral fractures; to identify osteochondral defects

*Text continued on page 117*

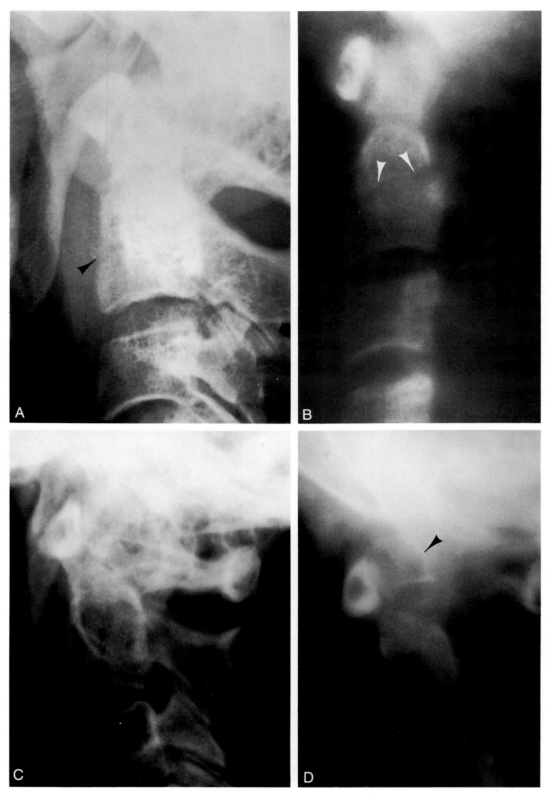

**FIGURE 7–5.** Spinal fractures.

**A, B** Fracture of the axis. An initial lateral radiograph **(A)** reveals probable disruption (arrowhead) of the anterior surface of the vertebral body, but the fracture (arrowheads) is much better delineated with conventional tomography **(B)**.

**C, D** Fracture of the odontoid process (os odontoideum). Although the odontoid process appears abnormal in the routine radiograph **(C)**, the characteristics of a separated tip of the odontoid process (arrowhead) and its relationship to the anterior arch of the atlas are better shown with conventional tomography **(D)**. This condition results from a previous fracture rather than a congenital abnormality.

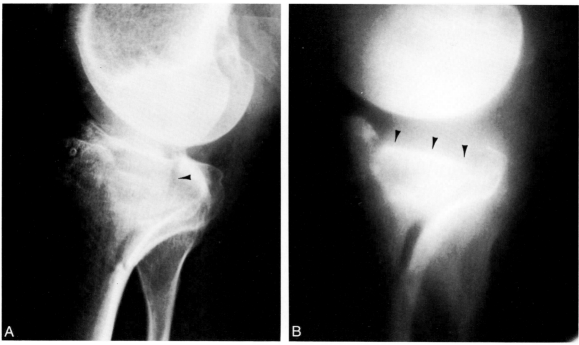

**FIGURE 7–6.** Fracture of the tibial plateau. In this patient, the fracture (arrowhead) is evident in the lateral radiograph **(A),** but the degree of depression of the articular surface (arrowheads) is better revealed with conventional tomography **(B).**

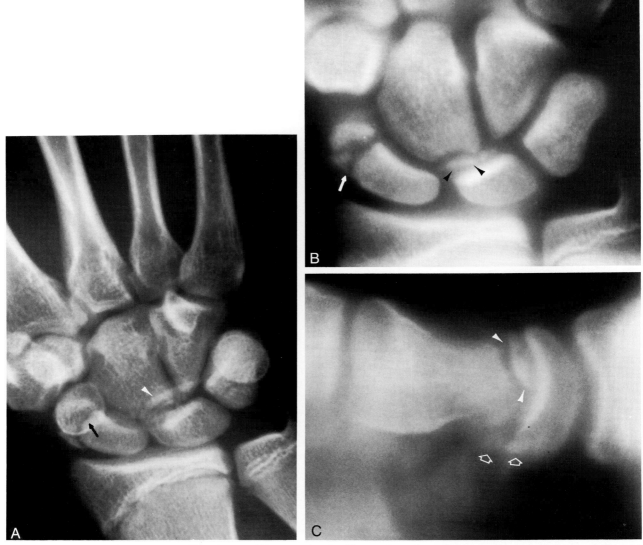

**FIGURE 7–7.** Scaphocapitate syndrome. This 16 year old boy was involved in a motorcycle accident, resulting in hyperflexion of the wrist. A closed reduction of a "perilunate" dislocation was attempted, and the patient subsequently was evaluated with additional radiographs.

**A** A posteroanterior radiograph shows a scaphoid fracture (solid arrow) and irregular osseous contours at the junction of the capitate and lunate (arrowhead).

**B, C** Frontal **(B)** and lateral **(C)** conventional tomograms reveal the scaphoid fracture (solid arrow), a fracture of the proximal portion of the capitate with 180 degrees of rotation of the bone fragment (arrowheads), and a fracture of the lower portion of the lunate (open arrows).

(Courtesy of G. Greenway, M.D., Dallas, Texas.)

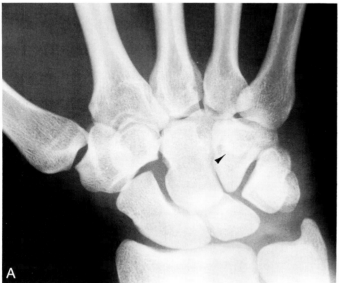

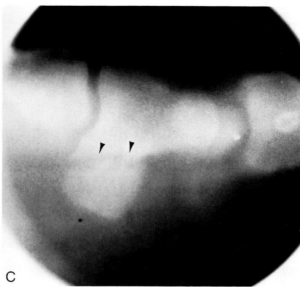

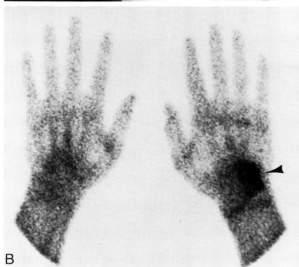

**FIGURE 7–8.** Fracture of the hook of the hamate.

**A** The initial radiograph is essentially unremarkable. The hook of the hamate can be identified (arrowhead).

**B** The bone scan reveals abnormal accumulation of the radionuclide in the region of the hamate (arrowhead).

**C** A conventional lateral tomogram reveals the fracture site at the base of the hook of the hamate (arrowheads). CT scanning also is well suited to the diagnosis of this injury.

(Courtesy of V. Vint, M.D., San Diego, California.)

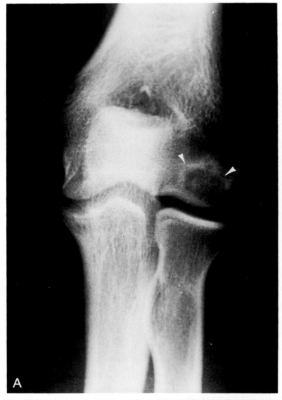

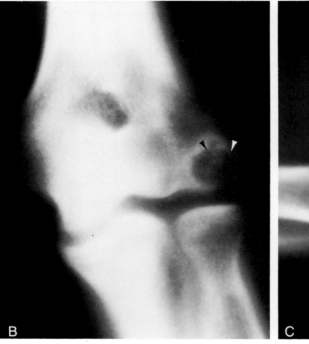

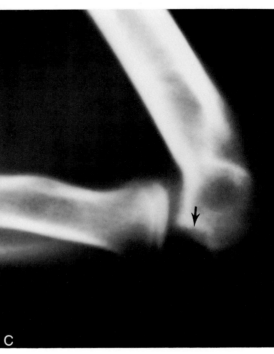

**FIGURE 7–9.** Osteochondral fracture: Capitulum.

**A** In a 15 year old boy, the initial radiograph shows an osteolytic lesion with a sclerotic margin in the capitulum (arrowheads).

**B, C** Frontal and lateral conventional tomograms demonstrate the area of abnormality (arrowheads) and reveal the deformity of the articular surface (arrow).

(Courtesy of L. Danzig, M.D., Santa Ana, California.)

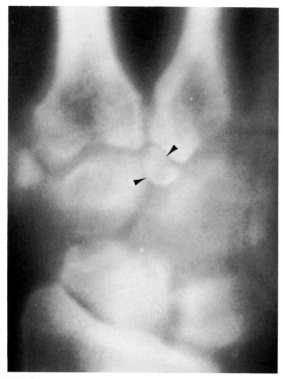

**FIGURE 7–10.** Carpe bossu (carpal boss). Conventional tomography shows a separate os styloideum (arrowheads) at the bases of the second and third metacarpal bones. This bone or an osteophyte in this region usually is asymptomatic, although ganglia or tendon abnormalities may accompany it. (Courtesy of J. Mink, M.D., Los Angeles, California.)

(Fig. 7–9); and to evaluate fracture healing. Intra-articular or periarticular osseous bodies (Fig. 7–10) can be outlined with conventional tomography; intra-articular cartilaginous bodies may require arthrotomography. Correct differentiation between severe osteoporosis and infection necessitates scrutiny of subchondral bone to detect early osseous destruction. In this situation, conventional tomography allows evaluation of the articular bone. Conventional tomography

also can be beneficial in evaluating patients with chronic osteomyelitis by identifying areas of cortical disruption and sequestra, findings that imply active disease. Conventional tomographic evaluation of bone neoplasms may identify a nidus of an osteoid osteoma, matrix calcification in cartilaginous tumors, and soft tissue extension of malignant disease.

## SUMMARY

It is apparent that conventional tomography is a useful adjunct to plain film radiography, may be competitive with CT in the evaluation of certain musculoskeletal problems, and should be used when standard and specialized views fail to provide needed information for correct diagnosis and adequate treatment. Its role, however, has diminished in recent years owing to the introduction and refinement of CT and MR imaging techniques.

## References

1. Christensen EE, Curry TS, Nunnally J: Introduction of Physics of Diagnostic Radiology. Philadelphia, Lea & Febiger, 1972.
2. Andrews JR: Planigraphy. I. Introduction and history. AJR 36:575, 1936.
3. Littleton JT, Crosby EH, Durizch ML: Adjustable versus fixed fulcrum tomographic systems. A microdensitometric examination of two tomographic systems. AJR 117:910, 1973.
4. Langland OE, Langlais RP, Morris CR: Principles and Practices of Panoramic Radiology Including Intraoral Radiographic Interpretation. Philadelphia, WB Saunders, 1982.
5. Wilkinson M, Meikle JAK: Tomography of the sacro-iliac joint. Ann Rheum Dis 25:433, 1966.
6. Morag B, Shahin N: The value of tomography of the sterno-clavicular region. Clin Radiol 26:57, 1975.
7. Hazan H, Labrune M, Massias P, et al: Etude tomographique de la charnière cervico-occipitale au cours des polyarthrites rheumatoides. A propos de 50 observations. Ann Radiol 19:743, 1976.
8. Reichmann S: Tomography of the lumbar intervertebral joints. Acta Radiol 12:641, 1972.
9. Elhabali M, Scherak O, Seidl G, et al: Tomographic examinations of sacroiliac joints in adult patients with rheumatoid arthritis. J Rheumatol 6:417, 1970.
10. Hermann G, Rothenberg RR, Spiera H: The value of tomography in diagnosing infection of the sternoclavicular joint. Mt Sinai J Med 50:52, 1983.
11. Clader TJ, Dawson EG, Bassett LW: The role of tomography in the evaluation of the postoperative spinal fusion. Spine 9:686, 1984.
12. Dawson EG, Clader TJ, Bassett LW: A comparison of different methods used to diagnose pseudarthrosis following posterior spinal fusion for scoliosis. J Bone Joint Surg [Am] 67:1153, 1985.

# 8

# Computed Tomography

*Michael André, Ph.D., and Donald Resnick, M.D.*

CT has matured into a reliable and prominent tool for study of the musculoskeletal system. When it was introduced in 1973,[1] it was unique in many ways and posed a challenge to interpretation. It is in these unique features, however, that its advantages lie in comparison with conventional techniques. These advantages will be described as they relate to a spectrum of important applications in orthopedics and rheumatology.

Like conventional tomography, CT is planar but CT images are transaxial and unhindered by overlying tissue. This technique has superior contrast resolution with a capacity to provide quantitative measures of the skeleton. In a dramatic departure from film methods, the CT image is produced in a computer that allows manipulation of the display. These powerful features may be used improperly, however, causing distortion or masking of structures; for this reason, it is important to understand the limitations of CT scans.[2, 3] Careful attention to the technical details also will improve interpretation of CT scans and enhance their diagnostic and therapeutic utility. To this end, the operational features of the CT scanner are presented.

The principles of image reconstruction from projections were described as early as 1917 by Radon,[4] and the technologic tools to build a CT scanner were available 20 years before Hounsfield developed a working prototype in 1970. The transfer of this method to medicine may appear to have been slow in coming, but its dissemination was not. CT rapidly revolutionized neurologic diagnosis and has been so widespread and important to health care that it is difficult to imagine its absence.[5]

## CT SCANNER

The essential components of a CT system consist of a scanning gantry with patient couch, x-ray generator, and computer processing and display system. The total cost for such a system, depending on performance requirements, ranges from a few hundred thousand dollars to more than $1.5 million.

CT scanning involves passing a thin beam of x-rays through the patient and measuring with a detector the number that are transmitted to the other side (Fig. 8–1). The amount of x-ray transmission is determined by the combined attenuating properties of tissues through which the rays pass.[6]

In the simplified scheme of Figure 8–2, a narrow x-ray beam passes through an object containing a lesion. Sequential transmission measurements are made by translating (moving) the x-ray tube (Fig. 8–2 A), producing a scan projection.[7] By measuring many additional projections at different angles, enough information is obtained for the

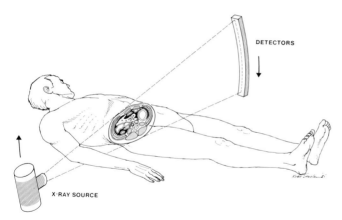

**FIGURE 8–1.** A CT scanner produces a cross-sectional image of the patient by confining its beam to a thin transaxial slice.

computer to produce an image by a method called filtered backprojection, as shown in Figure 8–2.[8, 9]

The so-called first generation scanners, which no longer are produced, used the method illustrated in Figures 8–2 and 8–3A to scan the patient.[1] These first generation scanners used inefficient translate-rotate geometry, and data acquisition was slow. Scan times therefore were long, typically 3 to 5 min. These early units served to demonstrate the potential of CT but rapidly became obsolete.

The second generation CT scanners greatly decreased scan times by increasing the number of detectors and using a fan-shaped beam (Fig. 8–3B). By using up to 30 detectors, many more measurements are made during translation, so fewer rotational increments are needed. With a rotation of 10 degrees, only 18 translations are required for a 180 degree scan, which makes possible scan times as short as 20 sec. This dramatic improvement in speed made body scanning possible.

It was a logical extension from the second generation scanners to increase the size of the fan beam and the number of detectors still further to encompass the entire body cross section. One x-ray pulse provides a complete view or projection, and linear translation is not needed. The pure rotational motion of the tube and detector array is diagrammed for this third generation design in Figure 8–3C. Xenon gas–filled detectors and scintillators are used in

these units because they have excellent stability during the rapid rotation and may be made very densely packed, with more than 700 elements in the array. A major advantage of third generation systems is the incorporation of a predetector collimator, which functions much like a radiographic grid to reduce x-ray scatter and improve contrast resolution. These systems put considerable heat stress on the x-ray tubes and are sensitive to detector artifacts. Scan times as short as 1 sec are common.

An alternative to rotating the detector array is to place the x-ray tube inside a stationary 360 degree ring of detectors (Fig. 8–3D). From the point of view of the computer reconstruction, this approach is analogous to the third generation design, although, owing partly to marketing considerations, the scanners usually are referred to as the fourth generation. These systems have between 720 and 4000 solid state detectors, which provide a very high absorption efficiency of nearly 100 per cent. Detector size and spacing reduce the total detection efficiency, however, such that third and fourth generation scanners are approximately equal. Like second generation units, each detector is calibrated during the scan to minimize detector artifacts.

Third and fourth generation scanners offer similar features and performance at comparable scan times, and they dominate the market. Detector and computer designs are nearly optimal, so that big improvements in image quality without significant increase in patient radiation doses are not anticipated. However, substantial improvement in data acquisition was accomplished with the introduction of "slip ring" technology (Fig. 8–4). This approach, which is applicable to both third and fourth generation designs, allows the x-ray tube to rotate continuously on a slip ring within the gantry. Electrical connections are made by sliding contacts from the stationary gantry to the rotating ring. These systems also have large data acquisition memories so that many scans may be performed in rapid succession, which permits the study of some dynamic processes. Scan times of 0.6 to 0.75 sec are possible.

Very short scan times are possible with a scanner design that utilizes no mechanical motion. The "ultrafast" CT scanner does not use a conventional x-ray tube at all; instead, a scanning electron beam is swept along a curved tungsten target ring that wraps around the patient (Fig. 8–5). A detector ring wraps around the opposite side. Scan

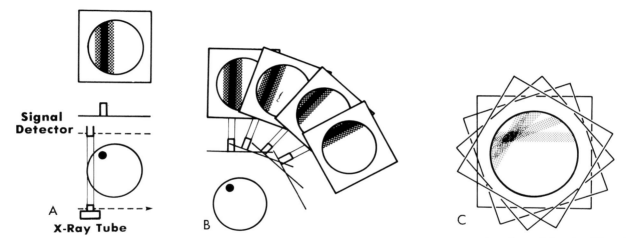

**FIGURE 8–2.** Reconstruction of an image from scan projections is shown schematically.[3] By translating the tube and detector (**A**), a single ray may produce a view. Multiple views are taken (**B**) and combined by the backprojection process (**C**) to form an image.

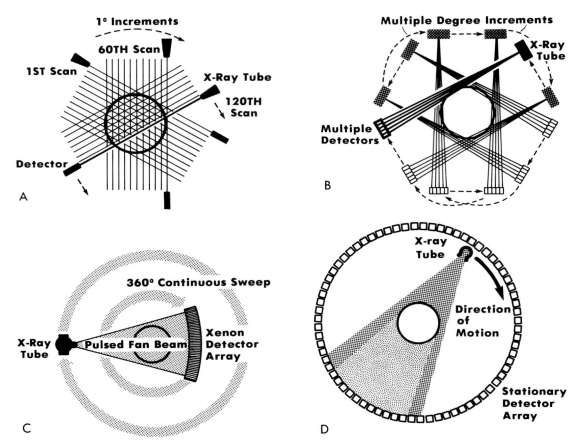

**FIGURE 8–3.** Schematic representation of first generation (**A**), second generation (**B**), third generation (**C**), and fourth generation (**D**) CT scanners.

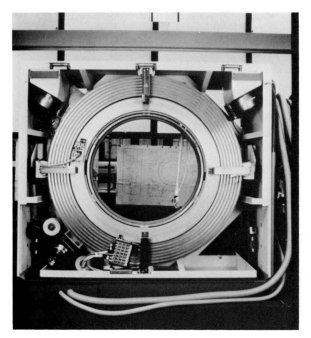

**FIGURE 8–4.** The slip ring components are visible when the covers are removed from the gantry. The x-ray tube is mounted on the inside ring and is able to rotate continuously.

times were designed to freeze 50 msec with only 8 msec between scans.[308] This excellent dynamic scanning capability holds promise for joint motion studies.

CT image quality for all scanner designs depends to a great extent on the computer algorithms used for reconstruction, in which area development and progress continue. Several operational features common to all scanners affect the image display and are surveyed in the next section.

### DISPLAY CHARACTERISTICS

The manner of image computation and presentation by CT scanners is shown schematically in Figure 8–6. The cross-sectional plane of the patient is divided into a rectangular matrix of usually 512 elements on a side called *pixels*. Each pixel corresponds to a region in the patient and is assigned a numerical value according to its relative attenuation. The pixel in the two-dimensional image actually represents a volume of tissue—a *voxel*—in which the depth of the element equals the slice thickness.

The attenuation values are expressed as a standardized unit, the Hounsfield unit (HU), which is normalized to water according to the following relation:

$$HU = \frac{\mu_t - \mu_w}{\mu_w} 1000$$

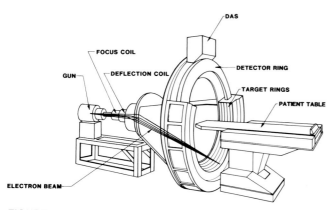

**FIGURE 8–5.** With no moving parts, a scanning electron beam system is capable of very short (50 msec) scans and rapid dynamic scanning.

**TABLE 8–1. Sample CT Numbers for Various Tissues**

| Tissue | CT Number (HU) |
| --- | --- |
| Bone | 1000 |
| Liver | 40 to 60 |
| White matter (brain) | 46 |
| Gray matter (brain) | 43 |
| Blood | 40 |
| Muscle | 10 to 40 |
| Kidney | 30 |
| Cerebrospinal fluid | 15 |
| Water | 0 |
| Fat | −50 to −100 |
| Air | −1000 |

in which $\mu_t$ is the attenuation value for the tissue of interest and $\mu_w$ is the known value for water. By definition, the CT number for water is 0 HU. Air is the least attenuating material encountered and has a value of −1000 HU, whereas dense bone is +1000 HU. This represents a very large dynamic range of data—significantly greater than that for radiography—and is the principal reason for the success of CT; much finer distinction between tissues is possible despite poorer spatial resolution. Representative values of CT numbers are given in Table 8–1.

It is the task of the display computer to convert this matrix of numbers into a recognizable anatomic form. The CT numbers are assigned to a range of gray shades, varying from black for air to white for bone, and these are displayed on a monitor. Unfortunately, monitors have a very limited gray scale and are unable to portray all of the available CT numbers. Displays, therefore, have ''windowing'' capabilities, which allow the available shades of gray to be assigned to a selectable range of CT numbers, as shown in Figure 8–7. In this example, the window center is set to a level of 200 HU and the window width is 400 HU. For a display that has 32 gray shades, CT numbers from 0 to 400 HU will be displayed, with each gray shade representing 12.5 HU. CT numbers greater than and equal to 400 HU (mostly bone) will be white, and those less than and equal to 0 HU will be black. To detect more subtle tissue differences than 12 HU, the viewer must use a narrower window, if image noise permits. A wider window is used to display a greater range of tissues but there is a resulting loss of fine discrimination.

The effect of adjusting the level of the window is shown for a CT scan of the chest in Figure 8–8. All three images are from the same scan and are displayed with a window width of 200 HU. Figure 8–8A shows a low window level, the center being set to −400 HU, in which all soft tissues and bone appear white (CT number greater than −200 HU). Raising the window level to 0 HU distributes the gray shades to soft tissues; bone appears white and lung appears black (Fig. 8–8B). Note that the lesion apparent in the left lung of Figure 8–8A is not seen in Figure 8–8B. A window

## CT BODY SECTION

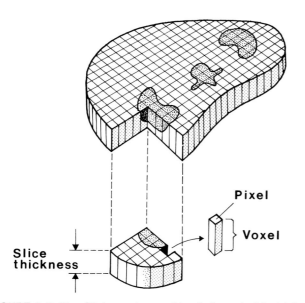

**FIGURE 8–6.** The CT image is a matrix of elements (pixels) that correspond to a volume of tissue (voxel).

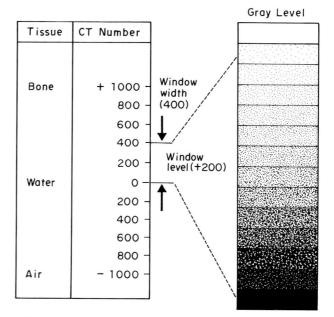

**FIGURE 8–7.** CT numbers are assigned a shade of gray for display using windowing to select the range of tissues viewed.

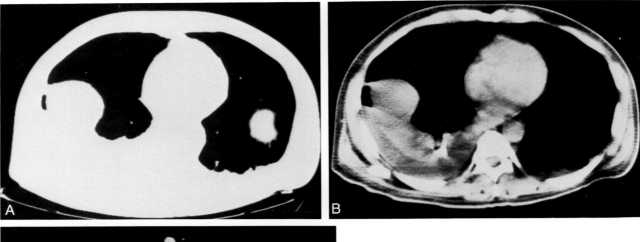

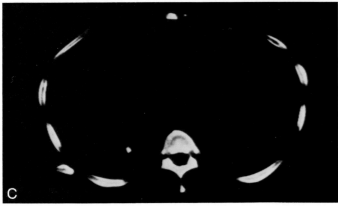

**FIGURE 8–8.** Adjusting the level of the window center determines the tissues that are displayed. A level of −400 HU **(A)** excludes bone and soft tissues in favor of lung. A window of 0 HU **(B)** displays soft tissues, and raising the center to 200 HU **(C)** displays only bone.

center of 200 HU displays nearly all soft tissues and air as black (Fig. 8–8*C*) but provides contrast discrimination in bone.

The data processing systems in CT scanners are electronic marvels close to the present state of the art, which perform thousands of computations in seconds and handle enormous quantities of data. A 512 × 512 image matrix requires attenuation values to be computed for 262,144 pixels from as many as 2.5 million detector measurements. Radon's equations of 1917 could not be applied practically until the advent of such digital computers. All CT scanners achieve fast image reconstruction, as little as 1 sec, through the use of special computing machines called array processors. These dedicated processors are distinguished by very high speeds but limited flexibility. The data storage requirements of CT are large because a single image may occupy 0.5 million bytes.

Multiformatting film cameras are used to record monitor displays. Variations in film characteristics and processing may make the film copy appear different from that of the monitor. The greatest amount of information is available by viewing the monitor directly and making use of the window controls.

## CT IMAGE QUALITY

A number of parameters under the control of the operator affect the quality of the CT scan as well as the radiation dose to the patient. The effects of these parameters are considered in two categories: (1) spatial resolution factors, and (2) contrast resolution or noise factors.

### Spatial Resolution

When two objects that are close together can be distinguished as separate entities they are said to be resolved. The spatial resolution or sharpness produced by a scanner is determined primarily by its design. The number, size, and spacing of detectors, the number of measurements made by each detector, and the characteristics of the patient all affect image resolution but normally are not modifiable by the operator. The operator, however, can select the matrix size for display, the reconstruction algorithm, the size of the scan field, and the thickness of the slice.

Increasing the number of elements in the image matrix—for example, from 20 × 20 to 40 × 40 (Fig. 8–9)—decreases the size of the pixel. Four pixels are needed in Figure 8–9*B* to represent the area of one pixel in Figure 8–9*A*. Decreasing pixel size does not by itself increase resolution, however. It also is necessary to increase the number of transmission measurements to have enough information to compute attenuation values for the greater number of pixels. Patient dose also increases. Figure 8–9*C* shows a resolution pattern scanned on a fourth generation unit for a 256 × 256 reconstruction matrix, and Figure 8–9*D* shows the same pattern scanned on a 512 × 512 matrix. The largest holes (2.5 mm) are not resolved in the former image, whereas the latter image clearly resolves the 1.25 mm holes.

An in-depth treatment of the principles of image reconstruction is beyond the scope of this chapter, but the choice of algorithm available on most machines can have considerable effect on image resolution.[10] A CT scan of a spine,

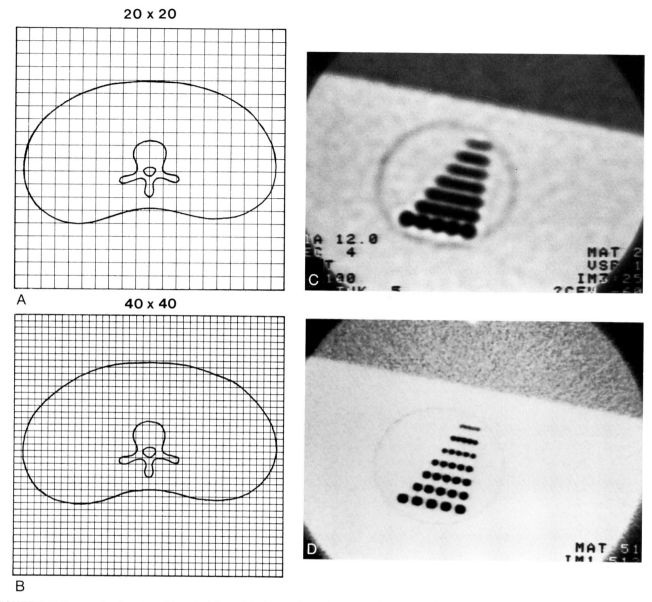

**FIGURE 8–9.** Decreasing the size of the pixel, from **A** to **B**, requires a larger matrix to cover the same cross-sectional area. Better resolution is seen in **D**, a 512 × 512 matrix, than in **C**, a 256 × 256 matrix.

reconstructed with two different algorithms, is shown in Figure 8–10. The image in Figure 8–10*B* is sharper, with better resolution of the apophyseal joints. Figure 8–10*B* also is more grainy and mottled, however, which can sometimes obscure low contrast detail.

Better resolution is achieved with a small scan field of view, such as the 12.5 cm diameter field of Figure 8–10, than with a large body-sized field of 40 cm or more. Each pixel in the image from a small scan field corresponds to a smaller region of the patient. The radiologist does not always know in advance where an abnormality will be, so the more limited field of view may be inappropriate. An alternative possibility is to use the projection data from a larger field, select only those rays that pass through the smaller desired region, and reconstruct an image with smaller pixels at potentially higher resolution. This process, called enlarged reconstruction or target scanning, can ob-

viate having to rescan an anatomic region. The resolution of this enlarged reconstruction is not quite as good as that obtained by scanning directly with a smaller field.

The concept of enlarged reconstruction often is confused with simple display magnification, which does not involve projection data or reconstruction at all. To magnify the displayed image, the operator simply instructs the computer to rewrite the image such that the information in one pixel is distributed over four pixels, as diagrammed in Figure 8–11*A*. Figure 8–11*B* is a magnified display of a scan acquired with a 40 cm field of view and does not show an increase in resolution.

Slice thickness in modern CT scanners ranges between 1 and 10 mm and determines the axial component of resolution. It is rare that a boundary between tissues, such as the surface of a bone or a fracture, is exactly perpendicular to the slice. As a result, a number of voxels contain both types

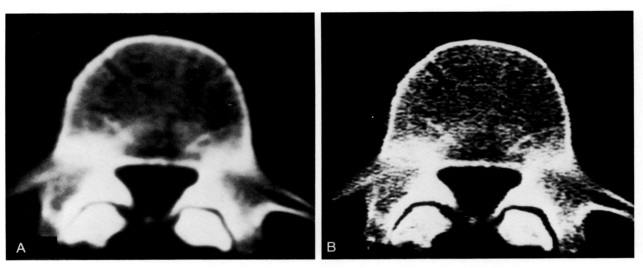

**FIGURE 8–10.** CT scan of the spine reconstructed with a smooth **(A)** and a sharp **(B)** algorithm.

of tissue. Partial volume averaging[11] reduces both the tissue contrast and the apparent sharpness of the boundary, and can obscure a fracture. When an object is smaller than the slice thickness or projects only partially into the slice, this partial volume effect may cause streaks or bridging to occur, as in the petrous pyramids of the temporal bone. Thinner slices reduce this effect.

Modern CT scanners can resolve high contrast objects as

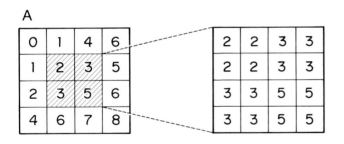

A

ORIGINAL ENLARGED

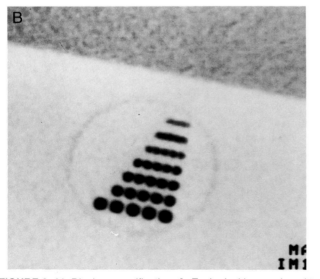

**FIGURE 8–11.** Display magnification. **A,** Each pixel is reassigned to a larger area in the display. **B,** Resultant image is magnified.

small as 0.25 to 0.5 mm, which corresponds to a maximum resolving power of 0.5 to 0.75 line pair/mm. Image intensifiers in fluoroscopy provide a somewhat better resolution of 1 to 2 line pairs/mm, whereas screen-film systems under normal circumstances resolve 2.5 to 4 line pairs/mm.

### Contrast Resolution

It would be expected that, if a scan were made of a uniform region of the patient, such as muscle or liver, all of the pixels in that tissue would have the same CT number. This is never the case and, in fact, for even a pure substance, such as water in a calibration phantom, CT numbers vary from pixel to pixel. This statistical fluctuation limits the ability to image low contrast objects and is called noise. The ability to detect a small difference in pixel values (attenuation) is known as contrast resolution.

The contrast resolution of CT scanners (0.3 per cent) is much better than that of conventional radiography. It is this fact that has made CT so prominent despite its lower spatial resolution. Contrast resolution is determined by the size and composition of the tissue of interest but also is affected by radiation dose, scan time, pixel size, slice thickness, and reconstruction algorithm.

Figure 8–10 demonstrated that the reconstruction algorithm could improve resolution. The price paid for a sharper algorithm is increased noise and a corresponding loss of contrast resolution. Scans of a water-filled phantom that have been reconstructed with smooth and sharp algorithms are shown in Figure 8–12A and 8–12B, respectively. Although noise is present in both images, the sharp filter greatly enhances the random fluctuations of the uniform regions. The choice of algorithm is a balance between sharpness and noise.

Radiation dose is controlled most readily by the x-ray tube's current setting in milliamperes (mA) and the scan time in seconds (sec). Increasing either factor will increase dose proportionally but will decrease the noise in the image and possibly improve contrast resolution. The scan in Figure 8–12C was obtained at 50 mAs and exhibits greater noise than that in Figure 8–12A, which was scanned at 400

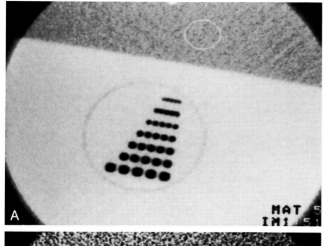
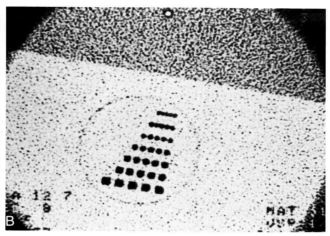
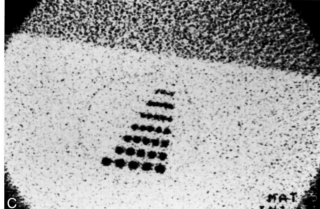

**FIGURE 8–12.** Effect of reconstruction algorithm and mAs on image noise. Scans obtained at 400 mAs with smooth algorithm **(A)**, 400 mAs with sharp algorithm **(B)**, and 50 mAs with smooth algorithm **(C)**.

mAs. To double contrast resolution by reducing noise, a fourfold increase in patient dose is required.[12]

Increasing either the pixel size or the slice thickness (larger voxel) will increase the number of counts detected per pixel and will decrease the statistical noise. Contrast resolution of large objects will increase.

The ultimate challenge for any imaging system is to provide high spatial resolution and contrast resolution in the same scan. An example of such a challenge occurs in the evaluation of the lumbar spine, in which it is necessary to detect small soft tissue structures such as nerve roots and epidural veins and, at the same time, to delineate bone morphology and discal herniations. This task may require a higher patient dose.

Sample performance characteristics of CT scanners are given in Table 8–2.

## SPECIAL FEATURES

A number of special developments have appeared in CT that greatly enhance its utility.

### Scan Projection Images

The CT scanner may be used to make a digital radiograph of the patient, which is very useful for identifying the exact region of interest for scanning. Scan projection images are produced by fixing the x-ray tube at one position in the gantry, turning on the beam, and passing the patient through it as the table is advanced. Images from any desired projection may be made and are displayed with the same windowing functions as used in the CT scan.

### Image Plane Reformation

CT scans are acquired normally in the transverse or transaxial plane (Fig. 8–13). Limitations in positioning of the patient in the gantry prevent the direct scanning of certain anatomic regions in another plane, such as sagittal or coronal, even though this sometimes is desirable. When a set of contiguous transaxial scans is acquired, it still is possible to produce an image by pixel rearrangement in essentially any desired plane.[52] Scans with thinner or overlapping sections produce a better reformatted image because the voxel is nearly cubic, but patient dose may be increased substantially by this technique.

It sometimes is possible to improve the appearance of reformations, particularly for oblique and "curved"[51]

**TABLE 8–2. CT Scanner Performance Characteristics**

| | |
|---|---|
| Spatial resolution | 0.3 mm |
| Contrast resolution | 0.3 per cent |
| Scan time | 0.7–10 sec |
| Total imaging time | 20–40 min |
| Slice thickness | 1.0–10 mm |
| Pixel size | 0.1–1.9 mm |
| Patient dose | 1–4 cGy (rad) or higher |

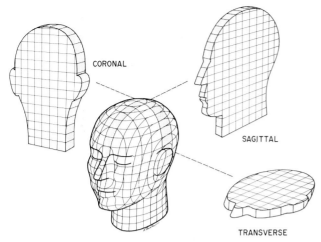

**FIGURE 8–13.** Scans acquired in a transaxial (transverse) plane may be rearranged to produce images in other planes.

planes, by interpolating between slices to produce very thin sections prior to rearranging the pixels.[13]

## Volume Scanning

The advent of slip ring and electron beam scanners provides a new procedure variously called volume, spiral, or helical scanning. The x-ray source is continuously energized and rotated while the patient table is continuously moved through the beam (Fig. 8–14).[305] Cross-sectional images may be reconstructed from this large volumetric set of data at any desired point along the patient axis. Volume scanning permits an entire organ such as the liver or lung to be scanned in a single breath-hold, greatly reducing motion artifacts. The resultant stack of images facilitates multiplanar reformation and three-dimensional renderings.

## Three-Dimensional Image Display

A set of adjacent transaxial scans (Fig. 8–13) contains information about all three dimensions of the patient. With the development of sophisticated computer-aided design systems in industry capable of pseudo–three-dimensional displays, musculoskeletal applications using CT data have appeared.[14, 55, 56, 275–281]

The quality and accuracy of the three-dimensional image are improved with thin adjacent slices. The additional step of interpolation and smoothing between scans, permits each

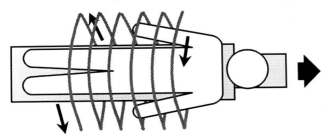

**FIGURE 8–14.** Volume scanning is accomplished with slip ring or electron beam scanners by moving the patient through the continuously rotating x-ray beam.

voxel to be reduced to a symmetric cube. Resampling the voxel in this way provides a uniform spatial interval in all three dimensions.

The technical features related to three-dimensional imaging have been summarized by Fishman and coworkers[282] in a review of the subject. Although three-dimensional displays derived from CT (or MR) imaging data can be accomplished with hardware or software designed specifically for this purpose, many of the currently available display systems are based mostly on software. The rendering techniques that transform conventional serial transaxial CT (or MR) data into simulated three-dimensional images can be divided into two types: thresholding, or surface-based (binary), techniques and percentage, or semitransparent (continuum) volume-based, techniques. Either technique consists of three steps: volume formation, classification, and image projection. Volume formation consists of the actual acquisition of the imaging data, the combining or stacking of the resultant data to form a volume, and some form of preprocessing. The classification step involves the determination of the types of tissue that are present in each voxel (i.e., fat, soft tissue, or bone). The image projection step relates to the manner in which the classified volume data is projected.

The thresholding-based imaging techniques were the first to be explored. The tissue to be imaged (e.g., bone) is assigned two numbers, or thresholds, on the basis of its attenuation values (Hounsfield units). The low threshold value (for bone, a value of about 100 Hounsfield units) serves to indicate an attenuation value below which this tissue type will not possess, and the high threshold value (for bone, a value of 3000 Hounsfield units or more) similarly indicates the uppermost attenuation value that will be exhibited by this tissue type. With thresholding classification, each voxel is assumed to contain only one type of tissue, and if the attenuation value of that voxel falls between the two threshold values, that voxel is considered to contain 100 per cent of the tissue of interest. Each voxel is analyzed, and a volume can be classified. As the thresholding technique of classification assumes the existence of only one type of tissue in each voxel, significant errors are introduced by volume averaging, in which a voxel containing more than one type of tissue (e.g., bone and muscle) is incorrectly analyzed. Volume averaging artifacts affect tissue surface interfaces most dramatically and lead to imaging irregularities of these interfaces, characterized as spaces or holes or as erroneous accessory fragments (or tags) of tissue.

Percentage-based imaging represents a more recently developed departure from thresholding-based imaging and, as summarized by Fishman and colleagues,[282] has definite advantages over the latter technique. By assuming that any individual voxel may contain more than one type of tissue, percentage classification allows more accurate analysis of the content of each of the voxels by the determination of the amounts, or percentages, of each type of tissue. Although requiring more computer power than threshold classification, percentage classification leads to fewer and less pronounced computer-generated artifacts.

Our experience has been mainly with thresholding-based imaging techniques. With this method, the edge or surface of the desired structure is viewed as though all surrounding tissue were removed. To accomplish this, as indicated ear-

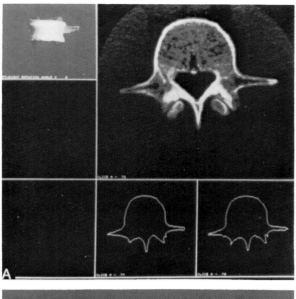

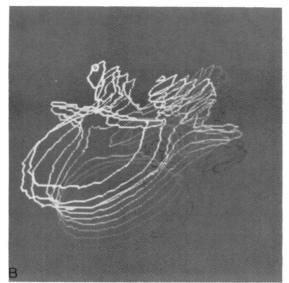

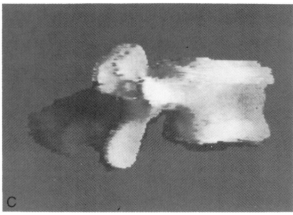

**FIGURE 8–15.** Generation of a three-dimensional CT display. A surface contour is produced for each CT slice **(A)**, contours are stacked according to slice separation **(B)**, and shading is used to give perspective **(C)**.

lier, the surface, generally the outer edge of skeletal bone, is defined in each interpolated slice by selecting the appropriate CT number value. Several refinements of this threshold method exist, but the end result is a contour for each section that outlines the bone (Fig. 8–15A). The contours are stacked according to the separation between slices and may be displayed in this form for a crude appreciation of shape (Fig. 8–15B).

A variety of graphic display schemes may be used to "fill in" the contours and produce a solid surface display. Figure 8–15C presents a light reflectance technique that computes the angle and distance of a point on the surface from a simulated light source and assigns a gray shade accordingly. This is not a true three-dimensional display but rather one that gives the impression of perspective and depth by shading.

Surface contours may be edited or moved in three dimensions to separate joint surfaces or remove overlying structures, as was done in Figure 8–15. The resultant three-dimensional data are quantitative and can be used to operate a numerically controlled milling machine for the production of life-sized models of the bone or custom-fit prostheses. Detailed surgical planning also may be done.

True three-dimensional images of CT, MR, and sonographic data have been produced on film using hologra-

phy.[309] This method allows viewing of volumetric data on a simple light box and does not require elaborate operator effort, as do the computer-based displays. This method has shown promise for visualization of complex fractures of the face, pelvis, and hip and for MR angiograms and fetal sonograms.

## ARTIFACTS

The quality of the CT image may be degraded by the presence of artifacts, which can be thought of as errors induced by the scanner or the patient.[25] The nature of artifacts produced and the machine's sensitivity to artifacts are unique to a particular scanner model and are a primary difference between products.

Artifacts originating within the patient are due mainly to motion, both voluntary and involuntary, and high density foreign objects. Barium contrast material and surgical clips or prostheses are common causes of streaking.

A rapid change in attenuation, such as at the boundary between gas and barium, may cause a ringing artifact, which results from the reconstruction algorithm. The image reconstruction programs assume that a monoenergetic x-ray beam is used for the transmission measurements, which can lead to an error in pixel value owing to the beam-hardening

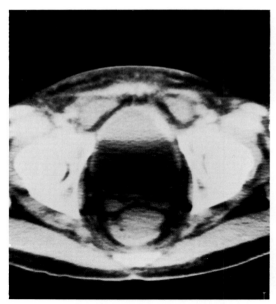

**FIGURE 8–16.** Beam-hardening effect visible in the bladder.

effect.[15] This effect commonly is seen in the bladder (Fig. 8–16), where a portion of the beam passes through dense bone in the pelvis and is filtered.

Detector errors are a main cause of machine-induced artifacts. Detector failures in third generation scanners produce dark concentric rings or circles. Fourth generation scanners may be less affected by a faulty detector because the computer may be instructed to ignore the data without significant loss of image quality. Variations in x-ray tube output produce gross divergent streaks emanating from outside the patient. Some calibration errors produce more subtle effects, such as nonuniformity, which may be mistaken for lesions. It may be difficult to determine from a scan if an apparent lesion is related to the pathologic condition of the patient or is a scanner artifact. Artifacts may be important in the determining of machine malfunction.

## SAFETY CONSIDERATIONS

CT scanning is a procedure that produces patient radiation doses intermediate between those from conventional film radiography at the lower end and interventional procedures, which use fluoroscopy extensively, at the higher end. The operator controls several factors that can alter dose by a factor of 10 or more. In general, patient dose increases with scan parameters that improve image quality such as thinner or overlapping slices, higher mA, and smaller fields of view. It is prudent to optimize scan parameters for the diagnostic task and to limit the number of slices. For example, during CT-guided biopsy, in which the same region of the patient is scanned repeatedly, it is possible to greatly reduce mA with no significant impact on needle visualization.

Occasionally, with trauma patients or during a difficult biopsy, it is necessary for a staff member to remain in the scan room. Although this is not routine practice, it is possible with modern CT scanners to avoid the majority of scattered radiation emanating from the patient. Figure 8–17

shows typical exposures around a scanner, and it is clear that the best place to stand is on either side of the gantry.

## TECHNICAL CONSIDERATIONS

Although general guidelines applicable to CT evaluation of the musculoskeletal system can be provided, the ideal examination is one tailored to the diagnostic requirements of the individual patient. As such, CT is best planned after a review of the clinical records and results of other imaging studies, which allows the examiner to comprehend the specific indications for the examination and the clinical questions that require answers. The development of general CT protocols is a natural consequence of two decades of clinical investigation and experimentation, and the guidelines certainly are useful in the setting of a busy radiology department, in which CT is performed from the early morning hours to late at night. These protocols also are useful at times when a radiologist may not be able to monitor the study closely. Nevertheless, unmonitored examinations using standard protocols are those most likely to be inadequate technically.

### Availability of Conventional Radiographs and Scan Projection View

As a general rule, it is unwise to perform CT in the absence of preliminary radiographs of the area of the body to be examined. Such radiographs commonly will provide information that will influence the strategy to be employed even in those cases in which the abnormality itself is not visible. The presence and location of metallic prostheses or foreign bodies, objects which lead to scanning artifacts, may require modifications in the examination or abandonment of CT altogether. The existence of abnormal or accentuated spinal curvatures may indicate that a particular patient position or angulation of the gantry is advisable.

A scan projection view is fundamental to the success of most CT examinations, allowing localization of the region of interest and display of the planned imaging strategy, but it is not a substitute for the conventional radiographs. External radiopaque markers facilitate the localization of the

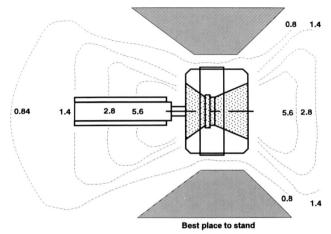

**FIGURE 8–17.** Top view of a typical CT scanner. Dotted lines represent the distribution of scattered radiation in milliroentgens (mR) per scan.

area of interest in the projection view and are especially important in patients with palpable but small soft tissue masses that would otherwise be difficult to locate. Scan projection views also ensure that the position chosen for the patient maintains anatomic symmetry of the skeleton, a measure that aids in the detection of subtle differences in the osseous or soft tissues on the two sides of the body.

### Scanning Strategy

Theoretically, it is best to obtain initial CT scans in the plane of interest (transaxial, coronal, or sagittal) rather than depend on reformation of image data that initially were acquired in another plane, which would result in the deterioration of image resolution. Practically, the choice of a scanning plane often is severely restricted as a result of human anatomy. Transverse, or transaxial, scans of the central skeleton (vertebral column and pelvis) in the supine or prone adult patient are mandated by the size and location of the area of interest, although direct sagittal CT in the adult has been employed in the evaluation of the head.[16-19] In addition, in the child, direct sagittal or coronal CT of centrally located structures such as the chest, pelvis, or spine is more feasible.[20] In some cases, acquisition of image data in these latter planes requires modification of the table and a large gantry aperture. Direct sagittal image acquisition can be used to evaluate the temporomandibular joint[21, 22, 241, 242] (Fig. 8–18), although again accessory or modified equipment and awkward patient position are required. In more peripherally located regions, the choice of image orientation is more flexible. Direct sagittal or coronal imaging of the forearms, elbows, hands (Fig. 8–19), wrists, and feet is possible[23, 24] and, in some cases, indispensable for accurate diagnosis, whereas that of the knee, shoulder, and hip is more difficult.

The choice of a prone or supine position of the subject during CT commonly is based on patient comfort and convenience, although it becomes more significant in certain

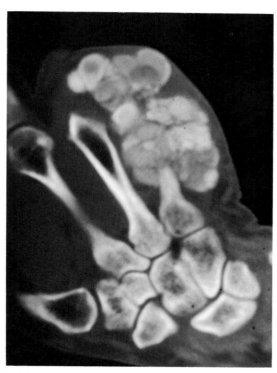

**FIGURE 8–19.** Scanning strategy: Direct coronal image acquisition—hand and wrist. In this patient with chronic renal disease and calcium hydroxyapatite crystal deposition in the soft tissues of the hand, direct coronal CT imaging is useful in demonstrating the relationship of the calcification to the fourth metacarpal bone and osseous erosion. (Courtesy of G. Bock, M.D., Winnipeg, Manitoba, Canada.)

situations, including examinations of the lower spine (in which a supine position and knee flexion produce flattening of the normal lumbar lordosis); examinations of joints by computed arthrotomography (in which the distribution of air or radiopaque contrast material is influenced by the precise patient position); and examinations of acutely injured patients (in whom certain positions may be contraindicated owing to respiratory problems or fracture location). CT monitoring of biopsy or aspiration procedures requires precise patient positioning that allows proper placement and advancement of the needle. The position selected for any CT study and the use of stabilizing or restraining belts or weights ideally should guarantee the absence of patient movement, which is detrimental to routine CT scanning and disastrous when reformation and three-dimensional display are being considered.

Symmetric placement of the patient in the gantry is employed during most CT examinations, although exceptions to this rule occasionally are required to allow the use of a small scan field diameter in the examination of laterally located areas such as the shoulder and to avoid artifacts created by contralateral metallic implants, as in the hip. In the latter situation, an oblique position of the patient may be necessary.

Since most current CT scanners allow as much as 20 degrees of angulation of the gantry in either direction, one further technical consideration is whether or not gantry angulation is necessary in the examination of a specific patient. Certain structures, such as the sacrum, are oriented

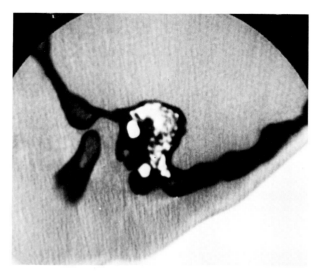

**FIGURE 8–18.** Scanning strategy: Direct sagittal image acquisition—temporomandibular joint. This technique can be useful in the evaluation of the temporomandibular joint, although modification of the table or the application of a special apparatus to hold the patient's head, or both, may be required. (Courtesy of T. Armbuster, M.D., Fort Wayne, Indiana.)

in the body in such a fashion that true transaxial sections are not possible without gantry angulation. In other locations, such as the hindfoot, limitations in positioning the body part imposed by the gantry itself can be overcome by such angulation, allowing direct coronal scans, which would otherwise be difficult or impossible to obtain. The evaluation with CT of the lower lumbar intervertebral discs is limited by normal or accentuated lordosis in this region, which prevents an ideal image display without angulation of the gantry. Direct sagittal image acquisition in the knee or temporomandibular joint also is enhanced by this technique.

The choice of slice thickness and table incrementation between slices (overlapping versus contiguous scans) is based on considerations of radiation dosage and examination time; the type, size, and location of the abnormality; the need for image data reformation; and, in many cases, the personal preference of the individual examiner. A commonly employed imaging strategy for soft tissue neoplasms consists of contiguous 1.0 cm-thick slices, whereas for bone lesions contiguous or overlapping 0.3 to 0.5 cm slices frequently are used. In the cervical spine, hands, wrists, and feet, thinner scan slices may be required.[270]

### Measurement of Attenuation Coefficient

The use of CT numbers (in the form of Hounsfield units) as absolute values allowing characterization of the tissue within a lesion assumes that the value of a given pixel depends only on the average attenuation coefficient of that voxel and disregards other variables, such as beam hardening, reconstruction artifacts, scanner variability, and departure from standard scan geometry.[25] As it has been shown experimentally that there are significant differences in absolute CT numbers between most scanners, even those of the same manufacturer, and that these numbers are influenced significantly by the location of the body in the scanner and by technical factors (such as kilovoltage) used to obtain the scans,[25] the strict application of CT numbers in a clinical setting will result in diagnostic errors. The inclusion of a calibration phantom in the field with the patient could minimize some of these errors, effectively teaching the scanners to speak the same language and to remember that language from day to day.[26] Short of that, a less rigid reliance by the examiner on the ability of attenuation coefficients to predict minor histologic variations in a lesion would suffice.

The expectation that lesions composed solely or predominantly of fat will produce negative CT numbers is justified,[27, 28] usually, but not invariably, allowing a diagnosis of a lipoma (Fig. 8–20). Modifications of these numbers by sarcomatous foci in a lipoma also are expected and useful diagnostically in some cases, although extensive fibrotic components and calcification may alter the attenuation coefficient to such an extent that a specific fatty component of the lesion can no longer be identified.[29] Furthermore, some types of liposarcoma contain great amounts of fat and some forms of lipoma reveal abundant nonfatty tissue, leading to diagnostic difficulty in the CT assessment of these tumors. A lesion whose attenuation value is close to that of water is consistent with, but not specific for, a cyst, whereas hematomas characteristically demonstrate inhomogeneous areas with both high attenua-

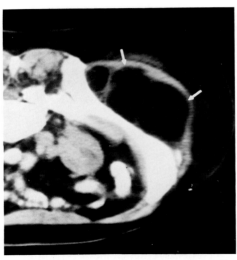

**FIGURE 8–20.** Measurement of attenuation values: Negative CT numbers—fat in lipoma. Smooth, homogeneous soft tissue lesions with negative CT numbers generally represent lipomas. In this case, with the patient in the prone position, a large lipoma in the gluteal region is evident (arrows). Note its internal septation and composition, the latter being identical to that of the subcutaneous fat. (Courtesy of T. Broderick, M.D., Orange, California.)

tion (approximately 50 HU) and low attenuation (approximately 10 HU) regions in their subacute stage and homogeneous areas with low attenuation (1 to 20 HU) in their chronic stage.[27]

The measurement of attenuation values of intraosseous lesions may be more difficult, especially in narrow bones in which the contribution of the cortex may prohibit accurate assessment. The expected replacement of fatty marrow (with its negative CT numbers) with inflammatory or tumorous tissue possessing higher attenuation values has been used to judge the extent of infective or neoplastic processes. This technique is more reliable when care is exercised in the choice of a region of interest, when irregularities of the endosteal surface of the cortex are recognized as potential causes for error in the measurements, and when the opposite (uninvolved) side is used for comparison purposes.

The limitation of absolute CT numbers as a means of distinguishing among lesions with similar histologic composition perhaps is best exemplified by the problems that arise in the evaluation of patients with significant symptoms after low back surgery. The two leading causes of such symptoms are a hypertrophic extradural scar and a recurrent herniated intervertebral disc. Although the attenuation value of a scar (50 to 75 HU) typically is slightly less than that of a discal herniation (90 to 120 HU),[30] relatively common exceptions to this rule limit its applicability and have led to interest in other differentiating features, including the change in attenuation value that accompanies intravenous administration of contrast material (see later discussion),[31] as well as to interest in other imaging methods, such as MR imaging (see Chapter 12).

The identification of gas in soft tissue or bone by CT is possible owing to its very low attenuation. This assumes clinical importance in cases in which a gas-containing discal fragment is present in the spinal canal,[32–34] although such vacuum phenomena can be identified in the canal or even in the retroperitoneal tissues in the absence of discal

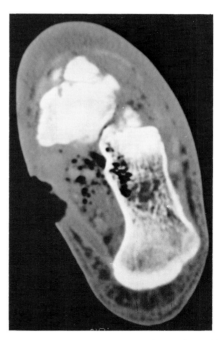

**FIGURE 8–21.** Measurement of attenuation values: Negative CT numbers—gas in osteomyelitis. A transverse CT scan of the foot reveals soft tissue ulceration and gas in both the soft tissues and the calcaneus. (Courtesy of A. Deutsch, M.D., Los Angeles, California.)

herniation.[35] Similarly, gas within a vertebral body documented by CT (or even by routine radiography) is an important sign of ischemic necrosis of bone.[36] Intraosseous gas also is identified in some cases of osteomyelitis (Fig. 8–21) and in subchondral cysts (''pneumatocysts'') (Fig. 8–22), particularly in the ilium and vertebral bodies.

Finally, in an age in which close imaging-pathologic correlation is being used increasingly to provide further understanding of disease processes, alterations in attenuation values (as well as tissue volumes) that accompany specimen freezing must be recognized.[271]

## Administration of Contrast Material

The intravenous, intraspinal, or intradiscal administration of radiopaque contrast material or the intra-articular administration of radiopaque contrast material or air can be a useful adjunct to CT of the musculoskeletal system.

Potential applications of intravenous contrast material include the identification of a suspected soft tissue mass when initial CT scans are unremarkable; the assessment of the vascularity of a soft tissue or osseous lesion when this feature is of diagnositc or therapeutic significance; and the delineation of the relationship of a tumor and adjacent vascular structures. Certain limitations exist in these applications. Hypervascularity is not synonymous with malignancy so that this feature cannot be used as a reliable means of differentiating between benign and malignant lesions. Furthermore, distinguishing displacement from actual invasion of vessels is difficult by CT, a problem that assumes major importance in patients with soft tissue neoplasms.

It has been suggested that enhancement of a soft tissue mass in the spinal canal after the intravenous administration of contrast material is a reliable means of differentiating by CT between a postoperative hypertrophic scar (which is associated with marked contrast enhancement) and a recurrent herniated intervertebral disc (which is associated with only a thin rim of enhanced tissue)[31, 37, 38, 272] (Fig. 8–23). The value of this sign remains controversial,[39] and, in fact, delayed contrast enhancement of an extradural mass is regarded by some investigators as an important means of

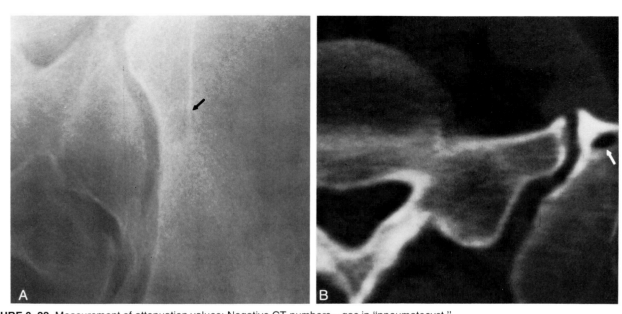

**FIGURE 8–22.** Measurement of attenuation values: Negative CT numbers—gas in "pneumatocyst."
  **A** The initial radiograph reveals a well-defined subchondral radiolucent lesion in the ilium (arrow).
  **B** A transaxial CT scan documents that gas, with its large negative CT number, is present in the lesion (arrow). This gas, presumably representing nitrogen, is derived from the nearby joint. In fact, a vacuum phenomenon was evident in the sacroiliac joint with CT, although it is not well demonstrated in this reproduction.

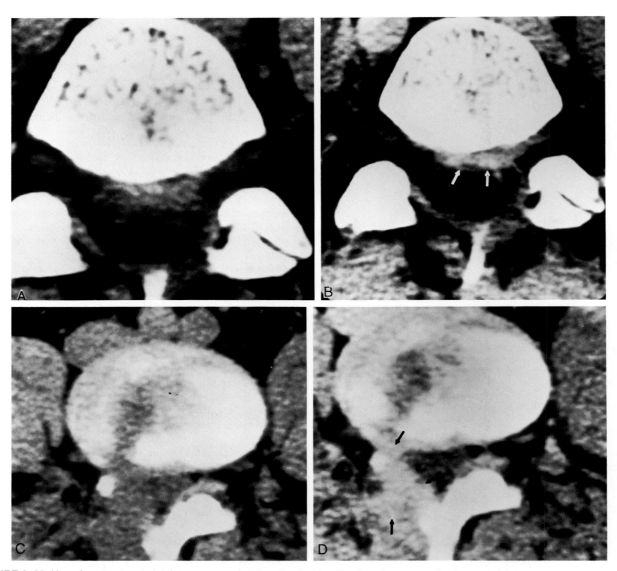

**FIGURE 8–23.** Use of contrast material: Intravenous administration for identification of postoperative hypertrophic scar.

**A, B** Preinjection **(A)** and postinjection **(B)** transaxial CT scans reveal contrast enhancement of a soft tissue mass (arrows) behind the vertebral body, consistent with postoperative hypertrophic scar formation. Note strandlike radiodense regions extending from the mass. (Courtesy of J. Mink, M.D., Los Angeles, California.)

**C, D** Preinjection **(C)** and postinjection **(D)** transaxial CT scans in a different patient again reveal contrast enhancement (arrows) compatible with the diagnosis of postoperative fibrosis. (Courtesy of A. Polansky, M.D., San Diego, California.)

identifying sites of discal herniation.[40] Furthermore, intraspinal tumors also may reveal enhancement after the introduction of intravenous contrast material.[251]

The precise indications for CT combined with metrizamide myelography as opposed to myelography or CT alone also are a matter of controversy and heated debate (see Chapter 12). The combined examination is recommended frequently for the evaluation of the postoperative spine[41] and modifications in technique, including the placement of the patient in a prone position,[42, 43] have been employed. CT after discography represents an additional method that has been used to define sites of discal herniation. Despite these many potential modifications of CT technique that improve its diagnostic accuracy when applied to the assessment of pathology of the intervertebral disc, the increasing use of

MR imaging for this purpose indicates that none of these modifications is ideal (see Chapter 12).

CT after the injection of air or radiopaque contrast material into a joint is useful in defining a periarticular soft tissue mass when one of the diagnostic considerations is a synovial cyst (Fig. 8–24A). This technique has been recommended for the identification of intra-articular osteocartilaginous bodies, especially in the knee[44] but also in the hip, ankle, and elbow (Fig. 8–24B). Computed arthrotomography is advantageous in evaluating the glenoid labrum,[45, 46] patellar cartilage,[47, 48] synovial plicae[49] and cruciate ligaments of the knee,[50] and osteochondritis dissecans of the talus, although in some instances, the benefits of this technique over those of CT or arthrography alone or conventional tomography are questioned (Fig. 8–24C, D). Fur-

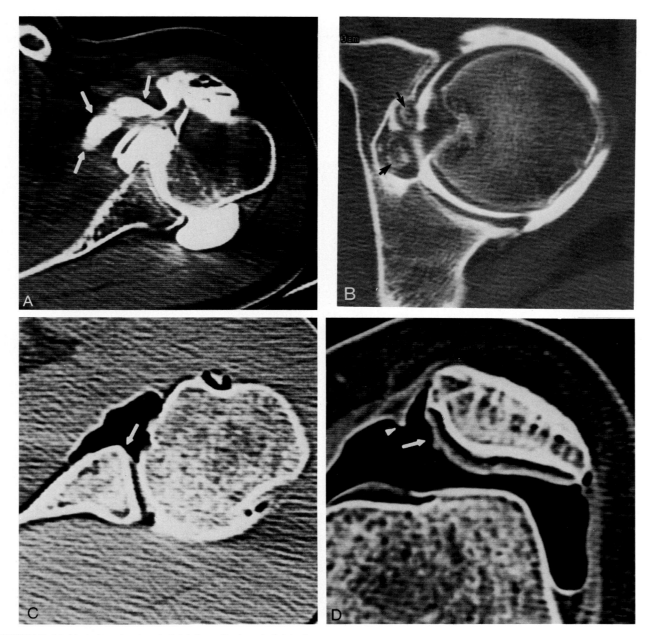

**FIGURE 8–24.** Use of contrast material: Intra-articular administration.

**A** Synovial cyst. In this elderly man with rheumatoid arthritis, CT after the introduction of radiopaque contrast material into the glenohumeral joint reveals an anterior synovial cyst (arrows) communicating with the bicipital tendon sheath.

**B** Computed arthrotomography using radiopaque contrast material demonstrates intra-articular osseous bodies (arrows) in the acetabular fossa in a patient with idiopathic synovial (osteo)chondromatosis. (Courtesy of P. Kindynis, M.D., Geneva, Switzerland.)

**C** Bankart lesion of the glenoid labrum. After the introduction of both air and radiopaque contrast material into the glenohumeral joint, a transaxial CT scan documents the absence of the anterior portion of the glenoid labrum (arrow), consistent with a Bankart lesion resulting from a previous anterior dislocation of this articulation. A Hill-Sachs humeral fracture also was present but is not well seen at this level.

**D** Chondromalacia and medial synovial plica. Transaxial computed arthrotomography, using both air and radiopaque contrast material, allows identification of chondromalacia of the patella, characterized by cartilage irregularity and imbibition of contrast material (arrow) and a medial plica or synovial fold (arrowhead).

thermore, MR imaging provides superior information in most of these situations.

### Image Display and Reformation

Although the choice of window width and level is best accomplished at the video console on the basis of diagnostic information that is required in any individual case, a near-maximum window width (1000 to 2000 HU) and a relatively high window level (200 to 250 HU) allow good visualization of musculoskeletal structures and commonly are used for hard copy images in which bone detail is required. For soft tissue detail, a window width of 400 to 600 HU and a window level of 0 to 100 HU generally are acceptable.

It is difficult to generalize about the need for reformation of image data in a plane or planes different from that in which such data were acquired (Fig. 8–25). Any decision in this regard is based on, among other factors, the anatomic area and type of abnormality being studied, the plane of the original CT scans, and the personal bias of the examiner. Many authorities believe that the vast majority of CT examinations can be interpreted without reformatted images. As such images do not provide new data (only presenting the information in another fashion), possess less resolution than the original CT images, and require a commitment in

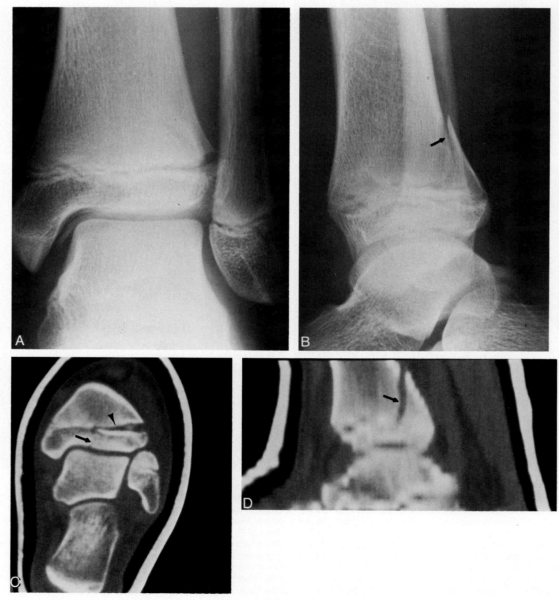

**FIGURE 8–25.** Use of reformatted image data: Triplane fracture of the tibia.

**A, B** In the frontal and lateral radiographs of the ankle, the epiphyseal extension of the fracture is not readily apparent. The metaphyseal component (arrow) is seen, suggesting a type II physeal injury.

**C** A direct coronal CT scan shows the extent of the physeal widening (arrowhead) and the epiphyseal fracture line (arrow).

**D** A sagittal reformatted image reveals the metaphyseal fracture (arrow) and posterior displacement of the epiphysis. Note that the presence of a cast has not interfered significantly with the CT image displays.

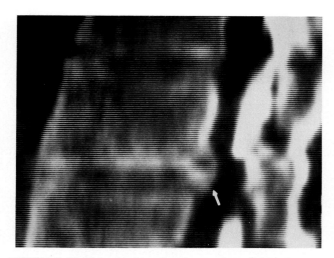

**FIGURE 8–26.** Use of reformatted image data: Spinal disorders. Acquired spinal stenosis. A sagittal reformatted CT image shows an osteophyte (arrow) arising from the posterior aspect of the vertebral body, leading to narrowing of the spinal canal.

time and effort from the technician and physician, this opinion is understandable. When a particular plane of image display is preferable but unobtainable initially owing to the restrictions in patient positioning imposed by the gantry of the CT scanner, reformatted images become more important. In response to this clinical need, manufacturers of CT equipment have continued to provide software capabilities that allow the generation of secondary images oriented differently from standard reformatted views as well as of those that follow the shape of a particular anatomic structure ("curved" reformations).[51] Software programs have been developed that allow real-time display of high resolution CT reformations in all three standard planes as well as oblique planes, with large image display format, reconstruction of entire data set, and interactive techniques.[273] Improvement in image detail through the use of edge-enhancement postprocessing filters has been accomplished.[274]

Disagreement certainly exists regarding the need for reformatted CT images in the evaluation of spinal disorders (Fig. 8–26). Imaging protocols vary from those containing a standard set of transaxial views alone to those that employ sagittal, coronal, or oblique reformatted images routinely.[52, 53] A compromise position suggests that reformatted image displays are required only when diagnostic uncertainty exists at the time of review of the transaxial CT scans.[54]

### Three-Dimensional Image Display

As indicated previously, three-dimensional display represents a further modification of image data provided by various graphic options contained in newer computer systems. The clinical applications of this technique are expanding rapidly. With regard to the musculoskeletal system, applications include the analysis of regions of complex anatomy, such as the face, pelvis, spine, shoulder, wrist, knee, midfoot, and hindfoot[55–59, 243, 244, 252–254, 262–265, 275–284] (Figs. 8–27 and 8–28). The preoperative assessment of articular disorders of the hip and traumatic abnormalities of the spine and shoulder has represented a major indication for three-dimensional image display from which solid plas-

tic models may be created. Three-dimensional imaging techniques may define better the extent of osseous stenosis of the central canal, lateral recesses, and neural foramina in the spine, although the three-dimensional delineation of soft tissue structures, such as the intervertebral disc and ligamenta flava, may be more difficult. In all instances, high quality three-dimensional images derived from CT data require closely spaced initial scans (leading to an increase in examination time and radiation exposure) and absence of patient movement. As is the case with two-dimensional reformatted images, in actuality no new information is provided by three-dimensional image displays; rather, the standard CT data are displayed in a format that may be more familiar to many physicians. In this fashion, the amount of information comprehended by the observer may be increased.

The ability to provide plastic models of a diseased area is an important extension of three-dimensional imaging, which facilitates operative planning and even allows rehearsal surgery of complex osteotomies or other reconstructive procedures (Fig. 8–29). These models, derived from the interfacing of the three-dimensional image data with a computer numerically controlled milling machine, are highly accurate with regard to size and configuration. A further extension of this process is the design and manufacture of customized replacements, as in articular surgery, which can shorten the time of surgery.[281]

### Spiral, or Helical, Scanning

Spiral, or helical, CT scanning recently has been developed in which image data are acquired rapidly from a volume of tissue.[305] The advantages of this method when applied to the musculoskeletal (or any) system are many, including decreased patient motion; and thin collimation with a resultant increase in sectional data ensures high quality two-dimensional and three-dimensional images.[306, 307] Spiral CT also allows scanning to be accomplished during the time of maximum tissue enhancement provided by the intravenous injection of contrast material.[307]

### CLINICAL APPLICATIONS

It is not the authors' intent in this chapter to discuss the myriad musculoskeletal applications of CT. The diagnostic value of CT is discussed and illustrated throughout this textbook and, where possible, scans are compared with images derived from other techniques, such as scintigraphy and MR imaging, to provide appropriate perspective. What follows here is an overview of some of the more important indications for CT of the musculoskeletal system, to serve as a guide to the interested reader, who should then consult other chapters for more detailed information.

### Anatomic Regions

As a generalization, with regard to bones and joints, the more complex the anatomy of a specific region of the body or the more difficult the task of obtaining adequate conventional radiographs, the greater the likelihood that CT will provide additional diagnostic information (Fig. 8–30). CT is a well-established technique in the evaluation of abnormalities of the bony pelvis,[60–62] hip,[63–67, 285, 286] sacrum and

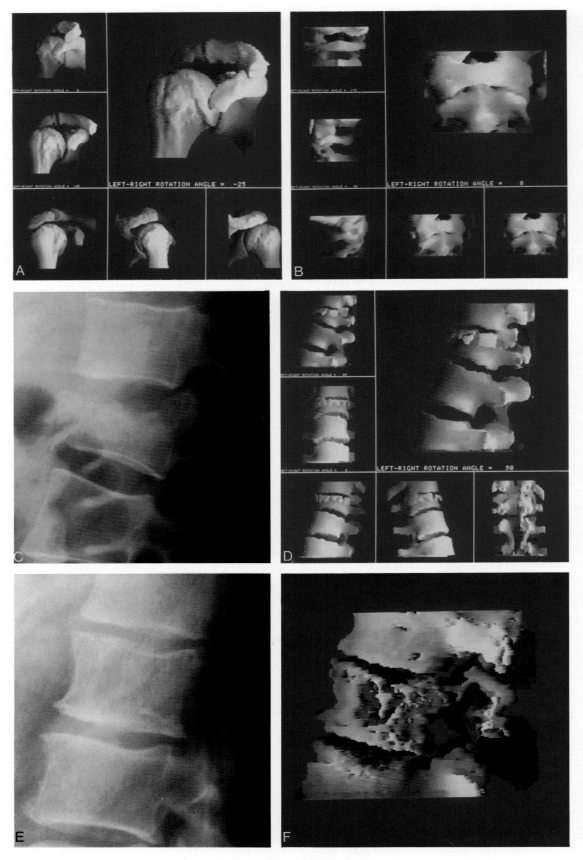

**FIGURE 8–27** *See legend on opposite page*

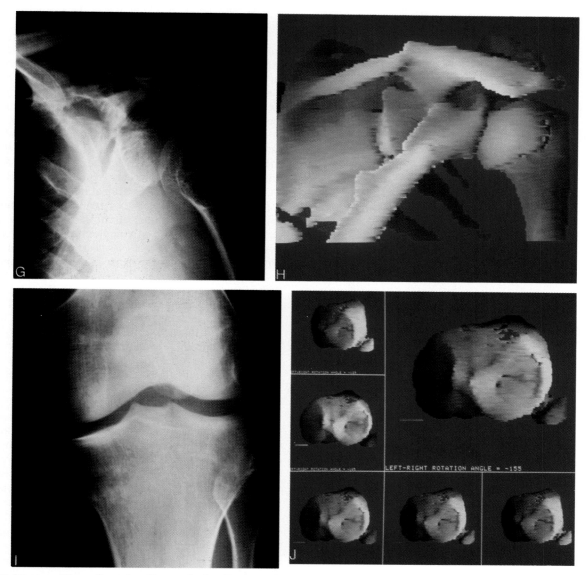

**FIGURE 8–27.** Use of three-dimensional image display: Regions of complex anatomy. Note that in some of the displays, the area of interest has been rotated with the rotated images placed about the primary image.

**A** Shoulder: Normal situation.

**B** Cervical spine: Atlantoaxial rotary fixation. The lateral mass of the atlas that is located on the viewer's left has moved forward with respect to the axis, and the opposite mass has moved backward to an equal extent. The odontoid process is located closer to the anteriorly positioned lateral mass of the atlas.

**C, D** Thoracolumbar spine: Complex fracture.

**E, F** Lumbar spine: Plasma cell myeloma.

**G, H** Shoulder: Scapular fracture in osteogenesis imperfecta.

**I, J** Knee: Depressed fracture of the lateral tibial plateau. The degree of osseous depression is well seen on the three-dimensional image, which shows the appearance of the tibial plateau as viewed from above.

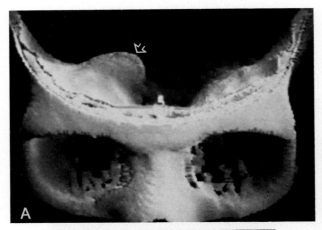

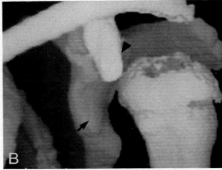

**FIGURE 8–28.** Use of three-dimensional image display: Regions of complex anatomy.

 **A** Skull and facial bones: Ossifying fibroma (arrow).

 **B** Shoulder: Hypoplasia (dysplasia) of the glenoid neck. Note the malformed scapular neck (arrow) and coracoid process (arrowhead).

 (**B**, Courtesy of A. Deutsch, M.D., Los Angeles, California.)

sacroiliac joint,[68–72] glenohumeral and sternoclavicular joints,[46, 73] sternum,[73–75, 287] spine (including the occipitoatlantoaxial region),[76, 77, 288, 289] midfoot and hindfoot,[78, 255, 256, 266, 267, 290] temporomandibular joint,[291] and wrist.[79, 270, 292, 293] With regard to soft tissues, the potential applications for CT are even greater owing to its superior contrast resolution over that of conventional radiography. This ability to distinguish between tissues differing only slightly in contrast characteristics explains the benefits of CT in defining the presence, location, and, in some cases, nature of soft tissue masses, which produce nonspecific findings or escape detection altogether on routine radiographs. Such soft tissue masses include hematomas, abscesses, tumors, and cysts. Among the many areas of the body in which the soft tissue applications of CT to musculoskeletal problems are most beneficial, the spinal canal, pelvis, wrist, knee, and other regions of the extremities should be emphasized. Although the superiority of CT over conventional radiography in imaging the soft tissues in these sites and others is not debated, it is fairer to compare this technique to xeroradiography and MR imaging. In particular, in the delineation of the soft tissues, MR imaging possesses definite advantages over CT, not the least of which is the absence of radiation exposure, and this technique has influenced dramatically the manner in which CT is used.

## Specific Disorders

In the two decades that have passed since the introduction and refinement of CT, the number of its clinical applications with respect to the musculoskeletal system has increased exponentially, as documented in countless scientific articles and numerous textbooks. These applications are best considered according to specific categories of disease.

**Trauma.** The general benefits of CT in the area of skeletal trauma include its ability to define the presence and extent of a fracture or dislocation, to delineate intra-articular abnormalities, including cartilage damage and osteocartilaginous bodies, and to assess the adjacent soft tissues (see Chapters 67 and 68). The CT examination of the injured patient usually is accomplished with a greater degree of patient comfort than routine radiography as the patient can be placed in a single position. Furthermore, the presence of casts does not cause significant deterioration of CT images, whereas their presence represents a considerable barrier to high-quality conventional radiographs.[65]

In the spine, CT largely has replaced conventional tomography as the technique of choice after routine radiography in the evaluation of complex fractures and dislocations (see Chapter 69). It is best employed not as a screening examination but rather as a directed examination through a specific area of known or suspected injury.[80] Although disagreement exists regarding the precise technique of the CT examination, including the need for intraspinal contrast material, there is little debate about the ability of CT to display osseous, cartilaginous, and soft tissue abnormalities in the traumatized spine. Although considerable information is provided by transaxial CT images, many examiners also emphasize the benefits of coronal or sagittal reformations, or both, in this clinical setting, especially if the fractures are oriented horizontally.

The presence of bone fragments in the spinal canal after fractures of the vertebral column easily is overlooked on conventional radiographs but is well shown with CT[81–88] (Fig. 8–31). In the thoracolumbar region, such fragments generally arise from the superior aspect of the vertebral body and they frequently migrate and rotate craniocaudally.[84] Although the degree of spinal canal narrowing as depicted by CT in these cases reflects the final resting position of the fragments and is not equivalent to that which may have occurred during the traumatic incident, and does not correlate with the degree of neurologic impairment,[85] the data provided by the CT examination are still regarded as important in the assessment of patients with spinal fractures. Furthermore, CT can be employed following the treatment of such fractures with Harrington or other instruments, displaying significant information despite some imaging degradation owing to the presence of the metallic rods.[89–91]

With regard to the posterior osseous elements, CT is superior to conventional radiography in defining the extent of injury at any level of the spine.[80, 92, 93] Pediculate or laminar fractures and disruption of the capsule about the apophyseal joints are examples of abnormalities that are well shown with CT. Injuries of the cervical spine that are optimally delineated with this technique include Jefferson or burst fractures of the atlas and atlantoaxial rotational fixation.[80, 94] More complex cervical injuries arising from

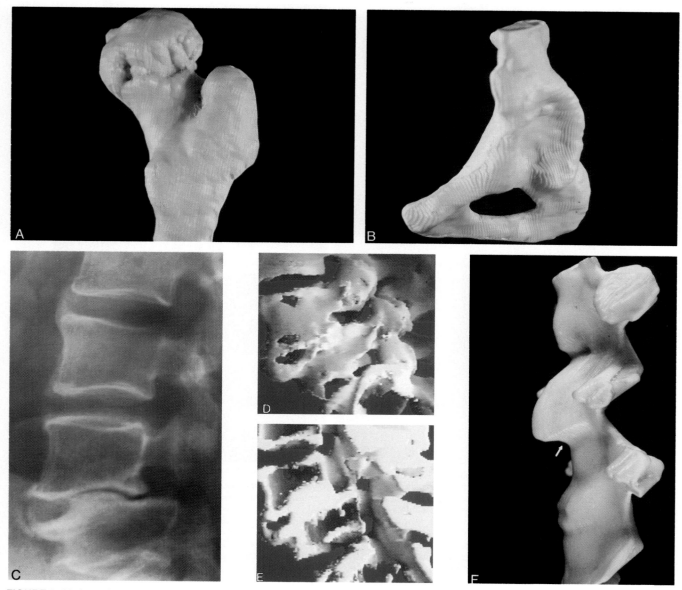

**FIGURE 8–29.** Use of plastic models created from three-dimensional CT data: Various applications.

**A, B** Hip. Corresponding models of the femoral head and acetabulum can be viewed together or separately.

**C-F** Lumbar spine. This patient developed symptoms and signs suggesting central spinal stenosis. The lateral radiograph **(C)** shows bilateral spondylolysis and spondylolisthesis of L4 and discal narrowing and osteophytosis at the L4-L5 spinal level. Three-dimensional images of the involved area **(D)** and of a sagittal section of this area **(E)** reveal the extent of vertebral slippage and narrowing of the central spinal canal. A plastic model of the interosseous canal **(F)** shows the degree of deformity of the anterior surface of the canal (arrow) at the L4-L5 spinal level. The neural foramina are of normal size.

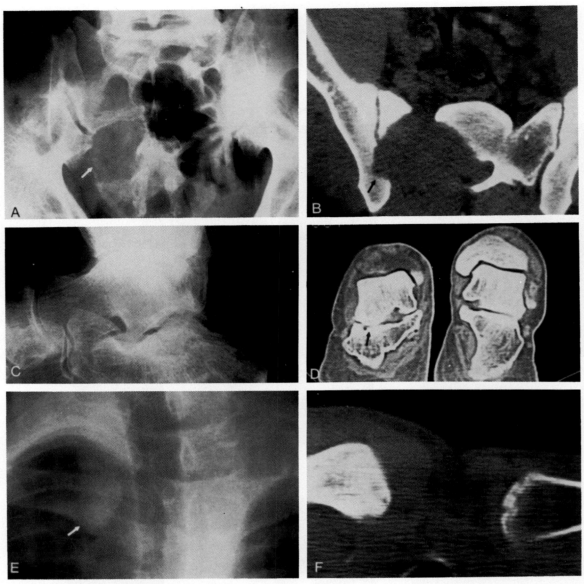

**FIGURE 8–30.** Use of CT: Regions of complex anatomy.
   **A, B** Osseous pelvis: Skeletal metastasis from renal carcinoma. An osteolytic lesion in the sacrum (arrow) is evident in the frontal radiograph **(A)**. Its transarticular extension (arrow) is shown with transaxial CT **(B)**. (Courtesy of G. Greenway, M.D., Dallas, Texas.)
   **C, D** Hindfoot: Posttraumatic osteoarthritis of the subtalar joint. The lateral radiograph **(C)** reveals an old calcaneal fracture with flattening of Bohler's angle. **D,** The degree of deformity and narrowing of the posterior subtalar joint (arrow) is demonstrated with direct coronal CT imaging. Compare to the opposite (normal) side.
   **E, F** Sternoclavicular joint: Stress changes. In this amateur right-handed tennis player, sclerosis of the medial end of the right clavicle (arrow) is evident on the routine radiograph **(E)** but is better demonstrated on the transaxial CT scan **(F)**. The clavicular head also is subluxated anteriorly. The findings resemble those of condensing osteitis of the clavicle.

compression, hyperflexion, or hyperextension can be evaluated with CT (with some limitations),[245] although conventional tomography also is used commonly in such cases.

In the bony pelvis, CT is best used for the evaluation of acute or stress fractures of the sacrum, complex fractures of the pelvic ring, and those fractures that extend into the acetabulum.[66, 95] With regard to the first application, the configuration and the anatomic orientation of the sacrum are factors that explain, in part, the diagnostic difficulties that arise when conventional radiographs alone are used to identify sacral fractures (or other lesions). Obscuration of bone by overlying gas and soft tissues further compli-

cates this analysis. The transaxial images of the sacrum provided by CT are more optimal than those in the sagittal or coronal plane derived from conventional tomography, and angulation of the CT gantry represents an additional technical modification that may further enhance the CT display.[97]

Although complex fractures of the bony pelvis are detected with routine radiographs, the extent of injury is better defined with CT.[60, 66, 95] A 10 section CT protocol has been recommended as a diagnostic approach that allows visualization of important anatomic landmarks in the pelvis[62]; however, the CT examination is better accomplished on the

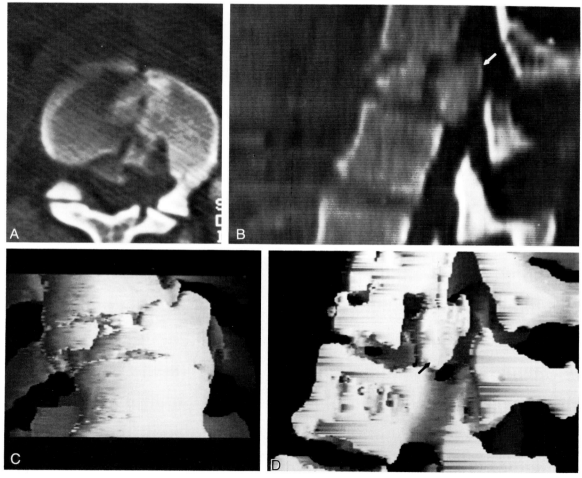

**FIGURE 8–31.** Trauma: Spinal fracture. The transaxial CT scan **(A)** shows a comminuted fracture of the twelfth thoracic vertebral body with intraspinal fragments and a fracture of the lamina with subluxation of the ipsilateral apophyseal joint. A sagittal reformatted image **(B)** delineates the complexity of the fracture of the vertebral body and the presence of a large fragment, arising from the posterior surface of the vertebral body, displaced into the spinal canal (arrow). A three-dimensional surface display **(C)**, viewed from the front, shows the extent of vertebral collapse. A three-dimensional sagittal sectional display **(D)** again documents the presence of an intraspinal fragment (arrow).

basis of specific characteristics of the injury in a particular patient. In such cases, CT represents an excellent method for demonstrating fracture extent as well as soft tissue injury and has particular merit in patients with double vertical fractures or subluxations of the hemipelvis or an iliac fracture with extension into the acetabulum, or in patients with major injuries of the hemipelvis that are to be treated with open reduction and internal fixation of the posterior part of the pelvic ring.[95]

It is in the area of acetabular and hip fractures that CT has had an even greater clinical impact.[57, 98–105, 275, 294] The pioneering work of Judet and his collaborators[108] simplified the complexities of such fractures by defining a logical classification system based on mechanistic and therapeutic considerations; their work also established the need for a thorough radiographic examination of the pelvis, including oblique projections. The subsequent application of CT to the evaluation of the injured acetabulum and hip, although not detracting in any way from the value of Judet and colleagues' investigations, has represented a major clinical advancement, providing imaging data in an anatomically complex area of compound curves.[109] CT identifies occult acetabular fractures that are difficult to visualize with con-

ventional techniques, disruptions of the posterior and anterior acetabular margins that accompany dislocations of the hip, subtle injuries of the femoral head, and intra-articular osteocartilaginous bodies (Fig. 8–32). It provides information about the integrity of the acetabular dome, quadrilateral surface, and iliopubic and ilioischial bone columns.[257] CT also can be used after surgical reduction of pelvic fractures or hip dislocations, delineating the adequacy of the reduction, the position of metallic fixation devices, the presence of intra-articular fragments, and, later, the degree of healing and the amount of heterotopic bone formation[66] (Fig. 8–33).

Dislocations of the sternoclavicular joint are extremely difficult to diagnose by conventional imaging techniques, requiring specialized projections that test the experience of the x-ray technician and the patience and expertise of the examiner. Although anterior dislocations of this joint are more frequent than posterior dislocations, the latter represent a more challenging diagnostic problem to the clinician and potentially are a more serious event owing to the proximity of the displaced clavicle to the trachea, esophagus, and great vessels. The transaxial plane provided by CT allows immediate documentation of the malpositioned clav-

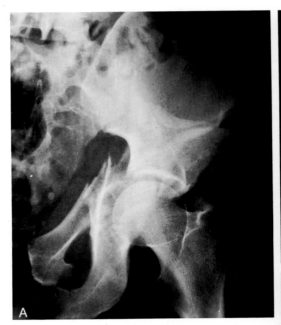

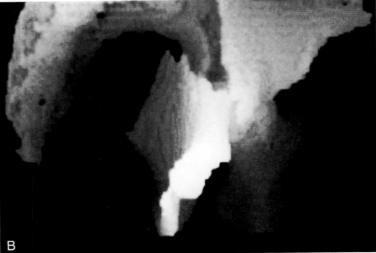

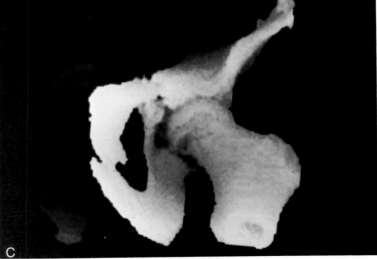

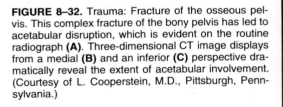

**FIGURE 8–32.** Trauma: Fracture of the osseous pelvis. This complex fracture of the bony pelvis has led to acetabular disruption, which is evident on the routine radiograph **(A)**. Three-dimensional CT image displays from a medial **(B)** and an inferior **(C)** perspective dramatically reveal the extent of acetabular involvement. (Courtesy of L. Cooperstein, M.D., Pittsburgh, Pennsylvania.)

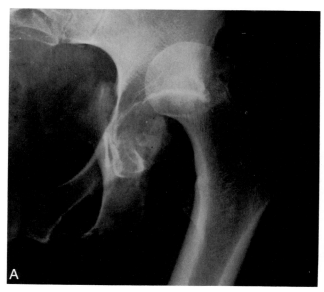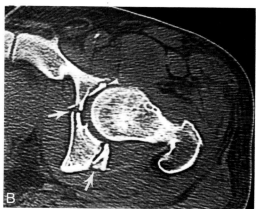

**FIGURE 8–33.** Trauma: Fracture-dislocation of the hip.
 **A** The initial radiograph reveals a posterior dislocation of the hip with fractures of the medial wall and posterior rim of the acetabulum.
 **B** After reduction of the dislocation, a transaxial CT scan shows the fractures of the acetabulum (arrows) and an intra-articular fragment (arrowhead) with persistent widening of the joint space.

icle, whether it be located anteriorly or posteriorly with respect to the adjacent sternum, as well as evaluation of any soft tissue injury [46, 110] (Fig. 8–34).

Dislocations of the glenohumeral joint are common, occur in an anterior, posterior, inferior, or superior direction in order of decreasing frequency, and are associated with bony or cartilaginous injuries, or both. The accurate diagnosis of dislocation is not difficult if the humeral head remains in an abnormal position with respect to the glenoid cavity of the scapula, but in cases in which spontaneous relocation occurs prior to the patient's being seen by a physician, the nature of the injury as well as its propensity to recur may be unclear. Routine radiographs supplemented with special projections have been advocated in the latter instances to document the presence of osseous and cartilaginous residua of the dislocation, including the Hill-Sachs lesion of the humeral head and the Bankart lesion of the glenoid cavity, which indicate previous anterior dislocation. When large and bony, one or both of these lesions will be detected by the conventional studies but when the osseous

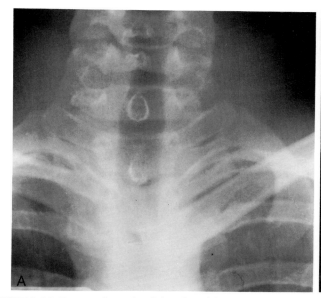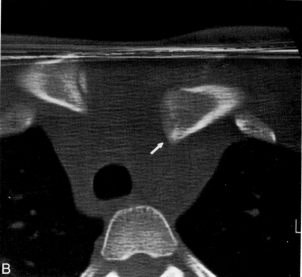

**FIGURE 8–34.** Trauma: Posterior dislocation of the sternoclavicular joint.
 **A** In the frontal radiograph, asymmetry in the position of the medial ends of the clavicles, with the left one being lower than that on the right, is evident.
 **B** Transaxial CT shows posterior displacement of the left clavicular head (arrow). Note that the adjacent clavicular epiphysis, which normally is seen (as evident on the opposite side), is not identifiable.

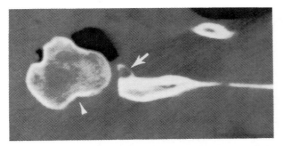

**FIGURE 8–35.** Trauma: Anterior dislocation of the glenohumeral joint. In this patient, transaxial CT following the introduction of air into the glenohumeral joint shows an osseous Bankart lesion (arrow). Note the Hill-Sachs lesion as well (arrowhead).

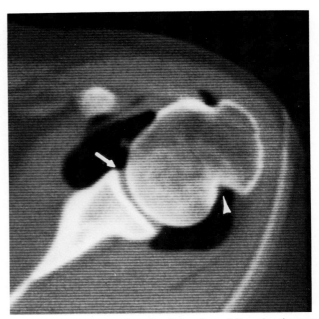

**FIGURE 8–36.** Trauma: Anterior dislocation of the glenohumeral joint. Transaxial computed arthrotomography shows loss of the normal anterior portion of the glenoid labrum (arrow), redundancy of the anterior capsule, intra-articular cartilaginous debris, and a Hill-Sachs lesion (arrowhead).

defect in the humeral head or scapula is small, CT may be required (Fig. 8–35). In addition, CT allows the identification of intra-articular osseous bodies.[46, 111–113] When the Bankart lesion primarily is cartilaginous, computed arthrotomography, using air alone (Fig. 8–36) or air combined with a small amount of radiopaque contrast material, is one method of choice.[46] Capsular abnormalities may be detected in this manner.[260] CT also may be used to investigate posterior dislocations of the glenohumeral joint (Figs. 8–37 and 8–38). Competing techniques in the assessment of glenohumeral joint instability include standard MR imaging and MR arthrography, all of which present diagnostic difficulties in some cases owing to normal variations in glenoid labral morphology (see Chapter 70).

Although conventional radiography provides useful information in cases of fractures of the proximal portion of the humerus, the precise position of fracture fragments, which influences the Neer classification of the injury, sometimes is better defined with CT. Displaced fractures of the greater and lesser tuberosities of the humerus and impaction fractures of the humeral head may require CT assessment.[295]

CT occasionally is required in the analysis of fractures or dislocations about the knee, ankle, elbow, and wrist (Figs. 8–39 and 8–40). Examples of specific applications of this technique are subluxations or dislocations of the pa-

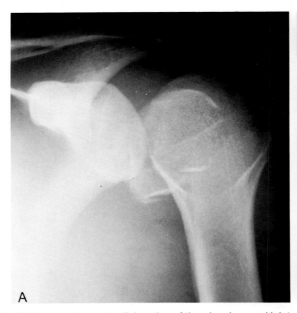
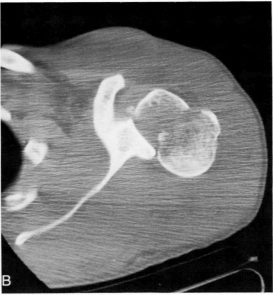

**FIGURE 8–37.** Trauma: Posterior dislocation of the glenohumeral joint.

**A** Findings on the frontal radiograph include a humerus held in internal rotation, widening of the glenohumeral joint with an "empty glenoid" sign, and fragmentation of the lesser tuberosity of the humerus.

**B** Transaxial CT documents the posterior position of the humeral head and a fracture of the lesser tuberosity. (Courtesy of A. Deutsch, M.D., Los Angeles, California.)

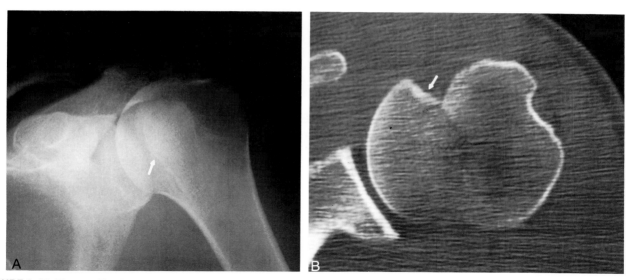

**FIGURE 8–38.** Trauma: Previous posterior dislocation of the glenohumeral joint.

**A** With routine radiography, the humeral head is documented to be situated normally with respect to the glenoid cavity. A radiodense area overlies the head of the humerus (arrow).

**B** A transaxial CT scan confirms a normal relationship of the humeral head and the glenoid cavity, as well as a trough fracture in the anterior surface of the humeral head (arrow), consistent with a previous posterior glenohumeral joint dislocation.

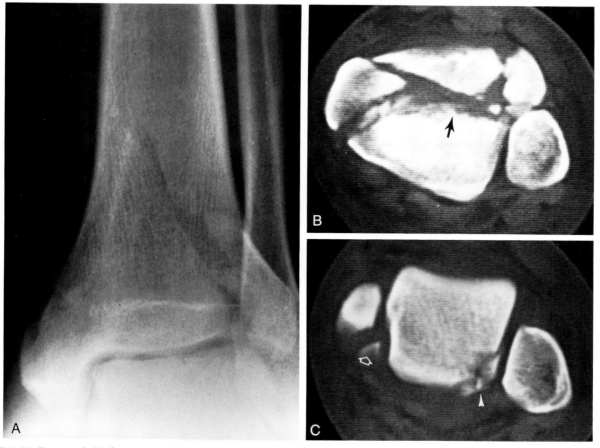

**FIGURE 8–39.** Trauma: Ankle fracture.

**A** An anteroposterior radiograph of the ankle reveals a fracture of the distal portion of the tibia.

**B, C** The comminuted nature of the tibial fracture (solid arrow) with involvement of the medial malleolus (open arrow) and the talus (arrowhead) is well shown in two transaxial CT scans. **B** is located at a level slightly above that in **C**.

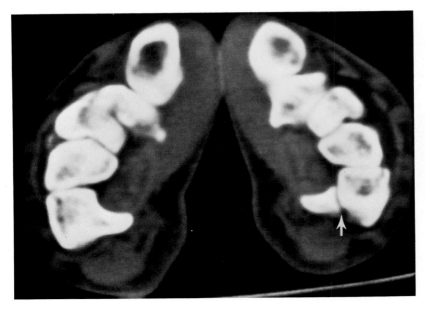

**FIGURE 8–40.** Trauma: Fracture of the hook of the hamate bone. CT represents an important technique for the identification of such fractures (arrow). This scan was obtained with the ulnar aspect of the hands in a dependent position. The opposite side is normal and can be used for comparison purposes. (Courtesy of G. Greenway, M.D., Dallas, Texas.)

tella,[114] fractures of the tibial plateau,[115] dislocations of the proximal tibiofibular joint, complex fractures of the distal portions of the tibia and fibula,[116, 117] triplane fractures of the distal portion of the tibia,[118, 119] disruptions of the inferior radioulnar joint,[120–122] and fractures of the hook of the hamate.[123] When CT is used to provide further information in cases of acute scaphoid fracture or chronic fracture malunion, thin (1.5 mm) sections oriented parallel to the long axis of the body of the scaphoid bone may be required.[270] In the midfoot and hindfoot, CT is best used to analyze extensive fractures of the calcaneus (Fig. 8–41) and talus and fractures and dislocations about the tarsometatarsal joints.[78, 124, 125] The assessment of patellar subluxations and other causes of patellofemoral pain with CT may be improved when a series of static transaxial images are obtained with varying degrees of knee flexion or when ultrafast techniques including cine-CT[304] are employed. In any articular location, CT (often combined with arthrography) can further delineate osteochondral fractures and intra-articular osteocartilaginous bodies.[44, 126, 127] In the long tubular bones of the extremities, especially the tibia and the femur, this technique is best applied to complex or spiral fractures in which the degree of separation of the osseous fragments governs subsequent surgical planning and patient prognosis.[258]

The role of CT in the diagnosis of certain intra-articular cartilaginous and ligamentous injuries, especially in the knee and temporomandibular joint, is limited and, in situations in which MR imaging is available, may be nonexistent. The advantages of CT in such diagnosis over arthrography are not clear. Injuries of the menisci and, to a lesser extent, the collateral and cruciate ligaments in the knee have long been considered an indication for arthrography, although the deficiencies of this technique, especially in the diagnosis of cruciate ligament disruption, also have been recognized. The increasing popularity of MR imaging and arthroscopy has lessened dramatically the role of arthrography in detecting internal derangements of the knee (and other joints). Potential applications of CT in defining cartilaginous and ligamentous integrity[128, 129, 246, 247, 259] (Fig. 8–

42) have been indicated. The advisability of first injecting radiopaque contrast material or air into the knee prior to the CT examination of the ligaments and cartilage has been emphasized in some reports.[44, 130] The province of arthrography or CT alone or CT arthrography has been compromised by the application of MR imaging (as well as ultra-

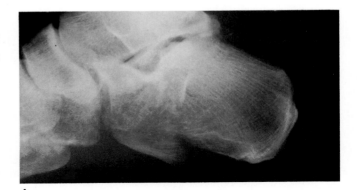

A

B

**FIGURE 8–41.** Trauma: Calcaneal fracture. Routine radiography **(A)** and three-dimensional CT display **(B)** are used to illustrate the features of this complex fracture of the calcaneus. In **B**, a perspective of the fracture from the lateral side of the foot is shown. (Courtesy of L. Cooperstein, M.D., Pittsburgh, Pennsylvania.)

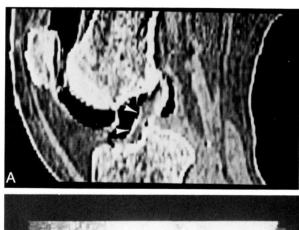
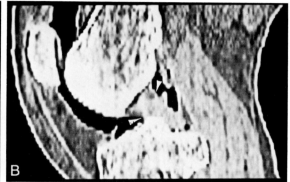
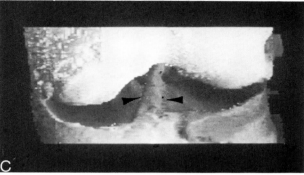

**FIGURE 8–42.** Trauma: Normal cruciate ligaments in the knee. The identification of these ligaments with CT can be accomplished either after the intra-articular injection of air (as in this case) or after the injection of both air and radiopaque contrast material or without such injection.

 **A** Normal anterior cruciate ligament (arrowheads) on sagittal CT scan.

 **B** Normal posterior cruciate ligament (arrowheads) on sagittal CT scan.

 **C** Normal anterior cruciate ligament (arrowheads) on frontal three-dimensional CT display.

sonography) to the analysis of the rotator cuff musculature of the shoulder.

CT has been offered as an attractive alternative choice to arthrography in evaluating the meniscus of the temporomandibular joint.[21, 22, 131–133, 291] Direct transaxial or sagittal CT images of this articulation allow identification of discal displacement or dislocation, but more detailed information about this meniscus, including its perforation, still may require arthrography.[134] MR imaging, however, has unique advantages in the evaluation of the temporomandibular joint and now is considered by many to be the imaging method of choice (see Chapter 49).[135, 136]

**Infection.** The indications for CT in cases of bone, joint, or soft tissue infection are less numerous than those in traumatic disorders. The early diagnosis of osteomyelitis is best left to scintigraphy or MR imaging, but defining the intraosseous extent of disease can be accomplished with CT. As noted previously, the negative CT numbers (Hounsfield units) of fat-containing marrow are altered in the presence of osteomyelitis owing to the accumulation of infected tissue.[137] This finding is not specific, being observed in any process that involves the intramedullary portion of the bone, such as tumor, trauma, certain types of anemia, storage diseases, and primary bone marrow disorders.[65] It is a more sensitive indicator of abnormality in bones that contain large amounts of fatty marrow and is less useful in small bones whose dimensions complicate accurate CT measurement. In rare instances, the identification of intraosseous gas allows a more specific diagnosis of infection,[138] as does gas in the soft tissues and fat-fluid levels in osseous or soft tissues.[139]

In cases of chronic osteomyelitis, CT has been used to identify single or multiple sequestra (Fig. 8–43), bone ab-

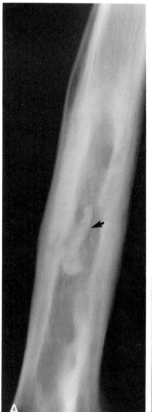
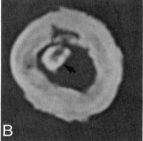

**FIGURE 8–43.** Infection: Chronic osteomyelitis with sequestration. Conventional tomography **(A)** and CT **(B)** are competing techniques for the investigation of sequestered bone (arrows) in osteomyelitis.

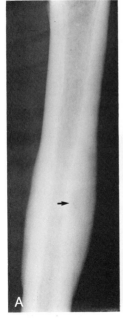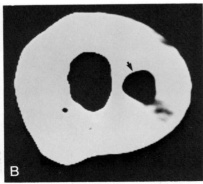

**FIGURE 8–44.** Infection: Chronic osteomyelitis with cortical abscess. Although the cortical abscess (arrow) and periosteal bone formation in the femoral diaphysis are seen with routine radiography **(A)**, the abscess (arrow) is better demonstrated with transaxial CT **(B)**. The appearance simulates that of an osteoid osteoma. (Courtesy of A. G. Bergman, M.D., Stanford, California.)

scesses (Fig. 8–44), and soft tissue abscesses and sinus tracts,[140, 141] and in both chronic and acute osteomyelitis, this technique may guide aspiration or biopsy attempts when the diagnosis is not clear or when causative organisms are sought.

Although the ability of CT to document the extent of soft tissue involvement in instances of infection (as well as tumor) affecting the axial skeleton, such as the spine and pelvis, has had major therapeutic impact,[261] use of CT in judging the extent of primary soft tissue infections in the appendicular skeleton has received less attention. CT can

be used to define the proximal limit of soft tissue abnormality in the infected foot of a diabetic patient when such information will influence directly the amputation level chosen by the surgeon; it also is used for the infected finger or hand[142] when a choice of conservative versus operative intervention is required.

The major indication for CT in patients with septic arthritis relates to the analysis of the adjacent soft tissues. Extension of infection in deep joints such as the hip and sacroiliac, glenohumeral, and sternoclavicular joints to the surrounding soft tissues is well delineated by this method.[69, 310] Defining similar extension of vertebral infection to intraspinal or paraspinal tissues represents another important indication for CT (Fig. 8–45). The early diagnosis of septic arthritis in spinal or extraspinal sites is better accomplished by other techniques, such as MR imaging or scintigraphy.

**Neoplasm.** In assessing the role of CT in the evaluation of neoplasms of the musculoskeletal system, it is necessary to consider this role independently of that of MR imaging, which generally is regarded as a superior diagnostic method in the assessment of most musculoskeletal tumors, particularly those arising in soft tissues. The value of CT in such assessment is increased when MR imaging capabilities are not available. Furthermore, in addressing the role of CT in the evaluation of musculoskeletal neoplasms, it is best to consider separately those arising in bone and those originating in soft tissue. Although the identification of the relative clinical contributions of routine radiography and CT in patients with bone neoplasms is complicated because the latter technique almost always is undertaken in conjunction with the former, conventional radiography represents the superior technique in establishing a specific diagnosis and defining the tumor position, pattern of bone destruction, presence of visible tumor matrix, and presence and type of periosteal reaction, characteristics that provide important clues to the nature of the lesion. Clearly, then, CT has not replaced conventional radiographic techniques in the diagnosis of primary and secondary bone tumors; however, CT is better able to judge the osseous and soft tissue extent of the process. Intraosseous extension of the neoplasm leads to the conversion of fatty marrow, with its negative CT

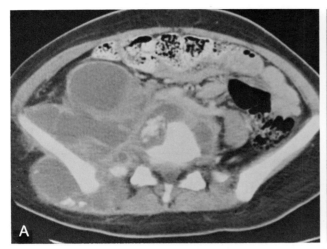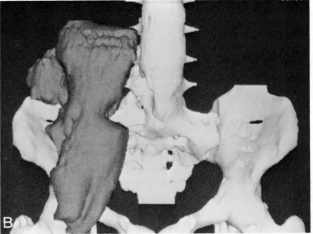

**FIGURE 8–45.** Infection: Tuberculous spondylitis with paraspinal and psoas extension. Transaxial CT scan at a low lumbar level **(A)** and three-dimensional reconstruction of CT data **(B)** show the full extent of bone and soft tissue involvement. (Courtesy of B. Howard, M.D., Charlotte, North Carolina.)

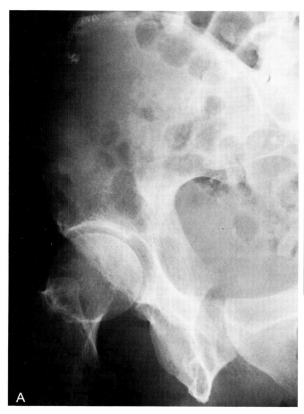

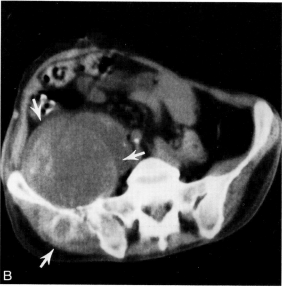

**FIGURE 8–46.** Neoplasm: Skeletal metastasis from carcinoma of the colon. Compared with routine radiography **(A)**, CT **(B)** is superior in the delineation of the soft tissue extent of the metastatic lesion (arrows).

numbers, to marrow containing tumorous tissue, with higher CT numbers. The assessment of marrow attenuation coefficients with CT, however, requires careful positioning of the patient, the evaluation of a bone that normally would contain fatty marrow, and the knowledge that tumor necrosis after radiotherapy or chemotherapy produces similar modification of CT numbers.[143] Intracortical extension of a medullary lesion can be judged better by CT than by routine radiography, an attribute that assumes clinical importance in instances of skeletal metastasis in a long tubular bone, particularly the femur, when prophylactic internal fixation is being considered.[302, 303] The ability of CT to delineate the soft tissue extent of a bone neoplasm (as well as of a primary soft tissue neoplasm) is a consequence of its excellent contrast resolution (Fig. 8–46) and allows this technique to compare favorably with others, such as arteriography.[144] The relationship between the tumor and major neurovascular bundles can be demonstrated effectively by CT,[145] especially if intravenous contrast material is administered,[146] although the differentiation of neurovascular invasion and displacement remains difficult.

These comments indicate that CT is more important in the surgical planning than in the actual diagnosis of primary bone neoplasms; however, there are specific instances in which this technique has definite diagnostic value. In anatomically complex areas, such as the spine and pelvis, or in areas with curved or angulated bones, such as the cranial vault, cross-sectional display obtained by CT may allow identification of lesions that are obscured on the conventional radiographs (Fig. 8–47). By defining the absorption coefficient of the intraosseous process, CT allows differentiation of a cystic and fibrous lesion[147] and the documentation of fat within it (as in an intraosseous lipoma) (Fig. 8–48). As none of these findings is entirely specific, the application of rigid criteria will lead to diagnostic error. Similarly, although the demonstration with CT of a radiolucent region with surrounding bone sclerosis strongly supports the diagnosis of an osteoid osteoma[148] (Fig. 8–49), and a gas-fluid or fluid-fluid level generally indicates a solitary or aneurysmal bone cyst[149, 150] (Fig. 8–50), exceptions to these rules, too, will be encountered.[248] Intraosseous calcification, indicative of a cartilaginous tumor, occasionally is better delineated by CT than by conventional radiography or tomography, and CT has been used with variable success to

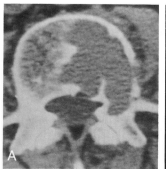
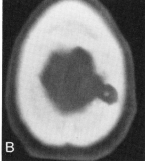

**FIGURE 8–47.** Neoplasm: Tumors or tumor-like lesions.

**A** Plasmacytoma of a vertebra. The osteolytic lesion involving the vertebral body and left pedicle is well shown with transaxial CT.

**B** Eosinophilic granuloma of the cranial vault. In this transaxial CT display, the osteolytic lesion containing a button sequestrum is seen easily.

(**B**, Courtesy of S. K. Brahme, M.D., La Jolla, California.)

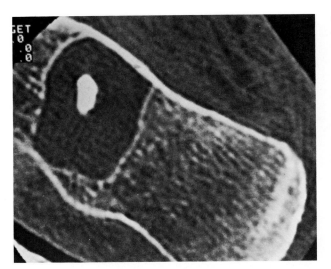

**FIGURE 8–48.** Neoplasm: Intraosseous lipoma. This CT scan of the calcaneus shows a well-defined lesion containing fat and an osseous spicule, findings characteristic of a lipoma.

define the thickness of a cartilaginous cap of an osteochondroma,[151] a finding that assumes clinical importance, owing to the thicker cartilage that characterizes a chondrosarcoma. Although other CT features allowing differentiation of an osteochondroma and chondrosarcoma also have been formulated,[152] biopsy of the lesion commonly is required.

The diagnostic value of CT is more established in patients with primary soft tissue tumors in which conventional radiography provides little specific information. Low attenuation numbers are characteristic of a lipoma, forming the basis for the CT diagnosis of this soft tissue neoplasm. Although many such lipomas readily are apparent on routine radiographs, CT is particularly useful in evaluating those that behave unexpectedly[153] or are located in parts of the body that are less accessible to conventional radiographic techniques.[146] Liposarcomas may possess areas of both low and high attenuation, whereas discrete zones of high density indicative of lesions of mixed cellularity occur in some cases of angiolipomas and fibrolipomas.[146] Cyst formation, cystic necrosis, and cartilage or bone formation are additional CT characteristics of a soft tissue lesion, which, when combined with information regarding location, size, and type of interface with surrounding structures, are invaluable in defining the nature of a soft tissue process.

With regard to both primary and secondary soft tissue and osseous neoplasms, CT often is fundamental to successful aspiration or biopsy procedures. The likelihood of obtaining diagnostic tissue from a scintigraphically positive bone lesion is increased if that lesion is visible with CT alone or with both CT and conventional radiography. In the spine and pelvis, the ability to monitor the initial placement and advancement of the needle or trephine represents an important advantage of the cross-sectional display provided by CT. Similarly, the chances of successful biopsy of a soft tissue tumor increase dramatically when such a lesion,

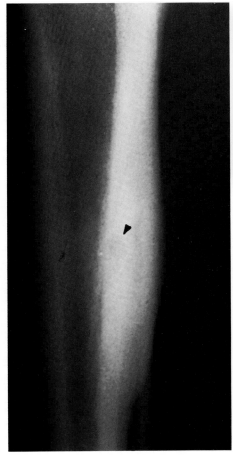

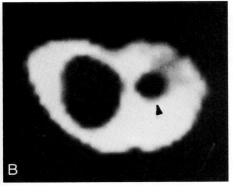

**FIGURE 8–49.** Neoplasm: Osteoid osteoma.

**A** The lateral tomogram of the lower leg reveals cortical thickening involving the posterior portion of the tibia. A radiolucent nidus (arrowhead) also is seen.

**B** Transaxial CT at the level of the lesion confirms the presence of a nidus (arrowhead) in the thickened tibial cortex.

(Courtesy of Mallinckrodt Institute of Radiology, St. Louis, Missouri.)

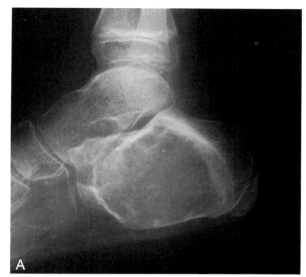

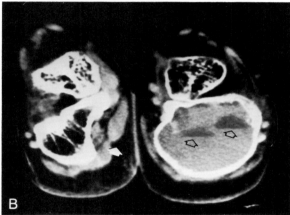

**FIGURE 8–50.** Neoplasm: Aneurysmal bone cyst.
**A** A large, expansile lesion of the calcaneus in this child has a well-defined, partially sclerotic margin and a hazy interior.
**B** A coronal CT scan through the lesion documents osseous expansion of the calcaneus and fluid-fluid levels (arrows).
(Courtesy of T. Broderick, M.D., Orange, California.)

which may be invisible on routine radiographs, is detected with CT.

CT represents an excellent technique for monitoring the effects of radiation therapy or chemotherapy on soft tissue and bone neoplasms. Tumor regression, growth, or recurrence can be defined in this fashion.

In summary, the major indications for CT in patients with primary or secondary bone or soft tissue neoplasms are detecting the extent of the process, aiding in surgical planning, judging the effects of therapy, and providing diagnostic information related to either the CT characteristics of the lesion or the ability of CT to monitor biopsy or aspiration procedures.[65, 146, 154–157] Early reports dealing with MR imaging assessment of such neoplasms, however, clearly indicated the relative benefits of this technique,[158, 159, 268] and subsequent reports certainly have confirmed this (see Chapters 83, 84, 85, and 95). Imaging protocols in institutions in which both CT and MR imaging are available frequently emphasize the latter technique, diminishing the importance of CT in the assessment of musculoskeletal neoplasms.

**Articular Disease.** CT generally is not required in the diagnosis of articular disorders, particularly those that are polyarticular in distribution. Monoarticular processes, including pigmented villonodular synovitis and idiopathic synovial (osteo)chondromatosis, also are associated with characteristic radiographic and arthrographic findings, severely restricting the diagnostic usefulness of CT. Occasionally, CT will better define the extent of osseous involvement in such disorders, especially in the hip[160] and knee[161] (Fig. 8–51); and in pigmented villonodular synovitis as well as in hemophilia, CT has a theoretical value in delineating the increased attenuation values attributable to an elevated iron content in the synovial membrane. Hemosiderin deposition, however, also is clearly defined with MR imaging.

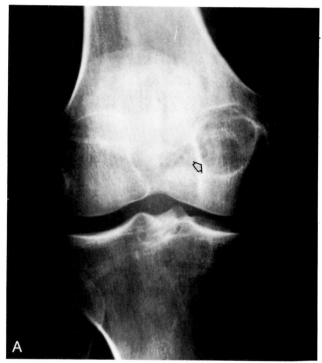

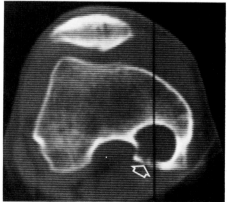

**FIGURE 8–51.** Articular disease: Pigmented villonodular synovitis in the knee.
**A,** A frontal radiograph of the knee reveals well-defined cystic lesions, especially in the femur (open arrow). The findings are compatible with the diagnosis of pigmented villonodular synovitis.
**B** A transaxial CT scan documents the size of the femoral cystic lesion (open arrow).

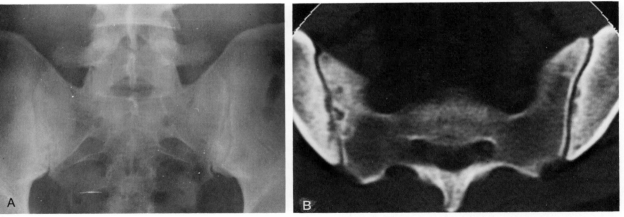

**FIGURE 8–52.** Articular disease: Sacroiliitis. In this patient with Reiter's syndrome and bilateral, asymmetric sacroiliitis, the extent of the joint abnormalities is not so well shown with routine radiography **(A)** as with CT **(B)**.

The identification of the presence and extent of disease by CT becomes more important in those joints that are difficult to visualize with usual imaging techniques. Such sites include the apophyseal, costovertebral, sternoclavicular, and temporomandibular joints,[299] although in these locations, examination with CT frequently requires meticulous positioning of the patient and the use of reformatted images.

The contribution of CT to the diagnosis of sacroiliitis (Fig. 8–52) is a subject on which there is no uniform agreement. Although initial studies indicated that CT was more sensitive and specific than other radiographic techniques in allowing detection of sacroiliitis,[70, 71] subsequent investigations have cast doubt on the accuracy of some of the reported abnormalities. The presence of nonuniform and poorly defined iliac sclerosis and focal joint space narrowing in asymptomatic (and commonly older) persons makes these findings less valuable in confirming sacroiliitis[296]; more helpful in establishing this diagnosis are increased sacral subchondral sclerosis, bone erosions, and intra-articular osseous fusion.[72] Furthermore, there is no single opinion regarding the optimal CT technique for evaluating the sacroiliac joints; rather, opinions vary as to whether the patient should be prone or supine and whether or not angulation of the gantry is required. It is the authors' belief that high-quality radiographs of the sacroiliac joints, including specialized views, generally eliminate the need for CT in most patients with sacroiliitis. CT occasionally is useful in the evaluation of patients with septic arthritis or osteoarthritis (Fig. 8–53) in the sacroiliac articulation.

A more fundamental role for CT exists in those patients with septic arthritis, especially in deep articulations, such as the hip, sacroiliac and glenohumeral joints, and joints of the spine. In these instances, the cross-sectional display provided by CT is better able to allow detection of cartilaginous and osseous destruction and, more importantly, to allow identification of extra-articular spread of infection in the form of abscesses, fistulae, and sinus tracts (Fig. 8–54). CT also can be used to monitor joint aspiration.

The propensity for rheumatoid arthritis to affect the cervical spine has led to considerable interest in evaluating the extent of such disease with CT.[162–166] Most attention has been directed toward the occipitoatlantoaxial level owing to

its anatomic complexity and the many serious complications of rheumatoid arthritis that occur in this region. The transaxial CT display facilitates evaluation of soft tissue, ligament, and spinal cord involvement,[163] and the use of reformatted coronal or sagittal images and of intraspinal contrast material may enhance this diagnostic information[165] (Fig. 8–55). Most investigators would agree, however, that CT is not a routine requirement for adequate visualization of cervical spine involvement in rheumatoid arthritis and should be reserved for diagnostically or therapeutically difficult cases; they also would agree that MR imaging with its excellent contrast resolution and sagittal imaging capability provides superior information regarding compromise of the spinal cord.

The use of CT in further defining the nature of a subchondral radiolucent lesion often is better accomplished if air or radiopaque contrast material, or both, is first injected into the joint. The subsequent CT detection of the contrast agent or air in the lesion documents intra-articular extension and, in most cases, provides strong evidence that the process represents a cyst or has arisen as a result of abnormalities in the joint itself. Intraosseous ganglia may lead to similar abnormalities, although articular communication is less likely, and accompanying soft tissue masses, sometimes containing radiolucent areas themselves, are characteristic.[167]

With regard to joint disease, CT perhaps is best suited to the evaluation of para-articular soft tissue masses. Synovial cysts (Fig. 8–56) arising adjacent to the glenohumeral joint, hip, knee, and apophyseal joint are well visualized in this fashion,[168, 169] although the simultaneous administration of an arthrographic contrast agent may be required. Isolated iliopsoas bursitis or that associated with hip disease leads to a mass that is well characterized by CT.[170, 171, 310] In hemophilia, hemorrhagic collections in periarticular soft tissues as well as in muscles and bones are identified with this technique.[172–174]

In recent years, three-dimensional analysis of CT data with the subsequent creation of plastic models of diseased areas has provided the orthopedic surgeon with diagnostic information displayed in a new and exciting fashion, which can have profound impact on the preoperative assessment of patients with joint disease. This technique is best applied

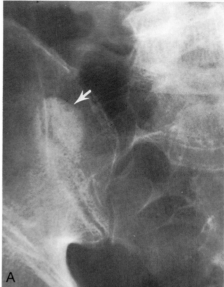

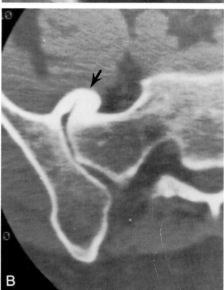

**FIGURE 8–53.** Articular disease: Osteoarthritis in the sacroiliac joint.
**A** Note a radiodense area (arrow) overlying the superior region of the right sacroiliac articulation.
**B** Transaxial CT shows that the cause of the abnormality is a large, bridging, anteriorly located osteophyte (arrow).

to a hip or glenohumeral joint involved with osteoarthritis, rheumatoid arthritis, calcium pyrophosphate dihydrate crystal deposition disease, and ischemic necrosis of bone (see later discussion).

**Neuromuscular Disease.** Even a glance at a typical transaxial CT scan through virtually any portion of the body would indicate the advantages of this technique over routine radiography for allowing identification of individual muscles and muscle bundles. Yet, few of the initial reports dealing with CT of the musculoskeletal system indicated its potential to provide information regarding the size and density of the skeletal muscle, information that would be vital in assessments of the extent and severity of neuromuscular diseases. Although this capability now is well recognized, MR imaging will play a more essential role than CT in the

future design of imaging strategies devoted to neuromuscular diseases (see Chapter 77).

After the establishment of some normal and reproducible values for size and density of individual muscles,[175, 176] standard CT protocols were developed that included scans of the body, neck, shoulder girdle, pelvic girdle, thigh, and lower leg.[65] Many of the types of neuromuscular disease are characterized by specific distributions of abnormalities affecting proximal or distal muscles or those of the neck, body, or extremities.[65] Furthermore, primary neural disorders generally first appear as muscle atrophy, with decreased density in the muscles occurring later in the course of the disease; primary muscle diseases show an early decrease in density in the muscles, with atrophy occurring later.[177] These CT abnormalities indicative of neuromuscular processes must be distinguished from normal age-progressive phenomena that include fatty replacement of paraspinal muscles, especially in the lumbosacral spine and in women,[178] as well as CT findings related to the muscles in immobilized patients and in those with such diseases as ankylosing spondylitis (which is associated with paraspinal muscle atrophy).

In the paralyzed patient, decubitus ulcerations produce soft tissue infections that subsequently may affect nearby bones and joints. CT has been used to evaluate this complication.[179, 180]

Additional applications of CT to diseases of nerves include the detection of neurofibromas, schwannomas,[181] and compressive neuropathies,[182–184] especially those of the sciatic and median nerves[185, 186]; other CT applications to diseases of muscles include the evaluation of abscesses, hematomas, tumors, and "myositis ossificans." The last-mentioned disorder does not necessarily affect the muscles but leads to a characteristic CT pattern in which a peripheral rim of ossification surrounds a more radiolucent soft tissue area[27] (Fig. 8–57).

**Vascular Disease.** As with other soft tissue abnormali-

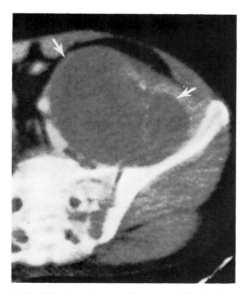

**FIGURE 8–54.** Articular disease: Septic arthritis in the sacroiliac joint. A major advantage of transaxial CT is the delineation of the extent of a soft tissue abscess (arrows) in patients with septic arthritis of this articulation. Note the osseous destruction in the ilium and sacrum.

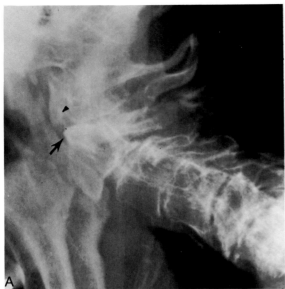

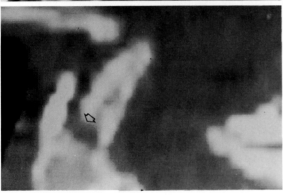

**FIGURE 8–55.** Articular disease: Rheumatoid arthritis in the cervical spine.

**A** Findings on this lateral radiograph include diffuse narrowing of multiple intervertebral discs with irregularity of the discovertebral junctions, apophyseal joint bone erosions and sclerosis, and malalignment at multiple levels including the atlantoaxial region. With regard to the last, note that the anterior arch of the atlas (arrowhead) is located slightly posterior to the anterosuperior surface of the axis (solid arrow), indicating a probable fracture of the odontoid process.

**B** Sagittal CT reformation documents the fracture of the base of the odontoid process (open arrow).

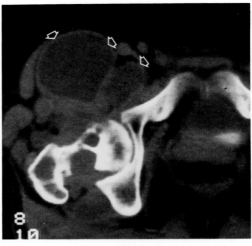

**FIGURE 8–56.** Articular disease: Synovial cyst of the hip in rheumatoid arthritis. In this region, a synovial cyst (open arrows) may create a mass that leads to an erroneous diagnosis of an inguinal hernia. Note the destruction of the ipsilateral femoral neck and joint space narrowing.

disease compared with those seen when bone-seeking radiopharmaceutical agents and MR imaging are used. More importantly, cross-sectional CT displays of the femoral head, when combined with sagittal, coronal, and three-dimensional reconstruction of the image data, provide important information in the later stages of ischemic necrosis, when verification of collapse of subchondral bone affects operative planning directly[191, 249] (Fig. 8–58). Furthermore, in these cases, as well as in related conditions, such as Legg-Calvé-Perthes disease and spontaneous osteonecrosis about the knee, CT can delineate intra-articular osseous fragments.[67]

**Congenital Disease.** Among the many applications of CT to congenital disorders of the musculoskeletal system, several deserve emphasis. The technique can be used to evaluate the degree of osseous deformity, position of the iliopsoas tendon and acetabular labrum, and concentricity of closed reduction in children with developmental dyspla-

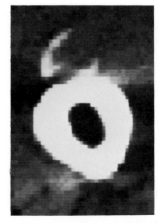

**FIGURE 8–57.** Neuromuscular disease: "Myositis ossificans." A transaxial CT scan through the diaphysis of the femur reveals a partial peripheral rim of calcification, which suggests the diagnosis of posttraumatic heterotopic ossification.

ties, CT provides diagnostic information in patients with masses related to aneurysms and pseudoaneurysms and arterial entrapment syndromes.[187] CT characteristics of an aneurysm are peripheral curvilinear or punctate calcifications on noncontrast scans and partial opacification of its lumen and contrast enhancement of its wall on postcontrast scans; similar enhancement of the rim of a mass may be seen on the CT scans of pseudoaneurysms.[27]

With regard to ischemic necrosis of bone, the early diagnosis is best accomplished with other techniques, such as scintigraphy and MR imaging. Although reports have documented the presence of subtle alterations in the trabecular pattern within the necrotic femoral head using CT[189, 190] (including modification of the normal asterisk sign that is created by the thick, crossed weight-bearing trabeculae), such findings occur relatively late in the course of the

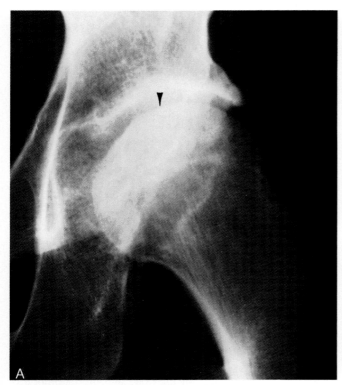

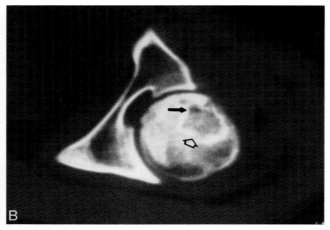

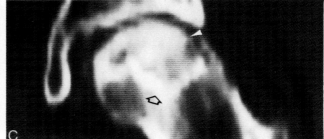

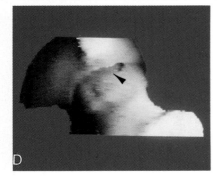

**FIGURE 8–58.** Vascular disease: Ischemic necrosis of the femoral head.

**A** An initial radiograph reveals patchy lucent and sclerotic regions in the femoral head and subtle flattening of the subchondral bone (arrowhead).

**B, C** Tranaxial **(B)** and coronal reformatted **(C)** CT scans obtained somewhat later document fissures in the femoral head (solid arrow), curvilinear osteosclerosis (open arrows), and articular collapse (arrowhead).

**D** A three-dimensional display, viewed from the front, of the CT data confirms the presence of osseous collapse (arrowhead).

sia of the hip[67, 192–194] (Fig. 8–59). CT provides an easy, accurate, and reproducible method to measure femoral anteversion and tibial torsion.[65, 67, 193, 197–200] The degree of rotation of vertebrae in scoliosis can be calculated using transaxial CT scans,[195] and the amount of leg length discrepancy can be measured by CT digital radiography.[196, 297] Congenital tarsal coalition, especially that between the talus and the calcaneus, is well shown by direct coronal CT imaging[78, 201, 202] (Fig. 8–60). Although CT can be used for other types of coalition as well,[203] some of these are visualized adequately with more conventional techniques.

In the spine, diastematomyelia,[204, 205] the tethered conus syndrome,[206] anomalies of the posterior osseous structures of the vertebrae, including absent or hypoplastic pedicles and laminae,[207–210, 298] dorsal dysraphism with or without lipomas,[211] and meningoceles[212, 213] can be identified with CT, which, in some cases, should be combined with myelography.

**Metabolic Disease.** In view of the prevalence of osteoporosis, especially in an elderly population, and its propen— ————— ignificant morbidity, mortality, and public ————— is not surprising that considerable

time and effort have been devoted to the development of quantitative techniques that allow sensitive and reproducible assessment of bone mineral content. Although all would agree that routine radiographs are remarkably inaccurate in

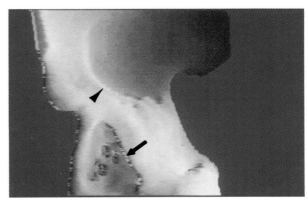

**FIGURE 8–59.** Congenital disease: Developmental dysplasia of the hip. Three-dimensional CT display of a type 3 dysplasia shows the hypoplastic true acetabulum (arrow) and the pseudoacetabulum (arrowhead).

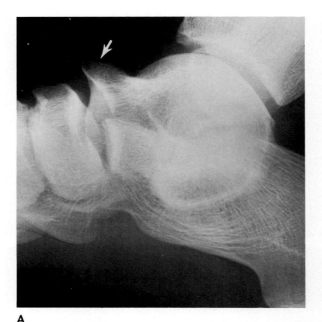

**FIGURE 8–60.** Congenital disease: Tarsal coalition.

**A** Findings on a lateral radiograph that suggest the correct diagnosis include the inability to visualize the talocalcaneal joints and a large talar excrescence, the talar beak (arrow).

**B** A direct coronal CT scan shows a solid bone fusion (arrowhead) between the talus and the calcaneus in the region of the sustentaculum tali. Compare with the opposite (normal) side.

this assessment, the choice of an alternative method has met with less uniformity of opinion. Photon absorptiometry and neutron activation are among the proposed techniques for measuring bone mineral content, and in the last decade, quantitative CT (as well as dual energy x-ray absorptiometry) has become an additional established method in this analysis (see Chapter 52).

With the application of different methods to bone mineral measurements, it has become increasingly apparent that not only do cortical and trabecular bone show different responses to physiologic and abnormal stimuli but also variations in bone mineral may be found in individual bones or parts of a bone.[214] Thus, the selection of a specific anatomic osseous site for such analysis becomes important. The interest in finding one particular area of the skeleton that was sensitive to changes in bone mineral content stimulated a search for appropriate regions that were amenable even to conventional radiography and led to the identification of trabecular modifications in the femoral neck (Singh index) and calcaneus as well as of changes in vertebral shape in patients with osteoporosis. Site selection for CT analysis of bone mineral likewise is not uniformly agreed on, with some investigators favoring locations in the appendicular skeleton (femur, tibia, and radius)[215, 216] and others favoring the spine.[217] This choice is of more than academic interest as information derived from one site does not necessarily correspond to that obtained from a different site and, ideally, the chosen location would be one most sensitive to fluctuations in bone mineral content produced by metabolic disorders. In recent years, vertebral spongiosa has gained widespread support as an appropriate target area for analysis of bone mineral content (whether accomplished with CT, with x-ray absorptiometry, or with radionuclide techniques), because it contains cancellous bone, highly responsive to metabolic stimuli, that can be separated spatially from less responsive cortical bone.[218]

The analysis of bone mineral content by CT does not distinguish reliably between osteoporotic persons who are likely to develop fractures and those who are not. This lack of discrimination relates to wide biologic variation in the normal population and a limited correlation between absolute bone mass or bone strength and fracture.[219] Bone mass represents only one of the determinants of fracture risk, others being the quality of the bone and the likelihood of any person's suffering a traumatic injury.[219] Despite this, CT of the spine remains a useful, noninvasive means of determining quantitative bone mineral, and serial values in any one person are of particular value.[220] Although the technique possesses high precision and sensitivity in this regard, a major stumbling block to reproducibility of results is the difficulty in repositioning exactly the same section of bone in the scan plane, which may be combined with additional, less significant errors related to intrinsic drift and beam-hardening effects.[221]

The application of CT to the evaluation of other metabolic diseases is more limited. Although quantitative analysis of bone mineral content has definite importance in patients with osteomalacia and primary or secondary hyperparathyroidism, limited data are available in this area. Various complications of renal osteodystrophy and transplantation, including ischemic necrosis of bone, and complications of Paget's disease (not truly a metabolic disorder), including articular abnormalities,[222] spinal stenosis,[223, 224] and sarcomatous degeneration, also may require CT analysis.

**Low Back Pain.** Although a full discussion of the manner in which CT is used to evaluate patients with low back pain and other spinal problems is beyond the scope of this chapter (see Chapters 12 and 40 for further information), a few comments are appropriate here. Without question, CT has profoundly influenced imaging protocols designed for vertebral disorders, owing to both its superior contrast resolution (compared with routine radiography) and its cross-sectional display. The diagnostic advantages provided by sectional images of the osseous, cartilaginous, and soft tissue elements of the spine that are not obscured by the overlying shadows that plague the conventional radiographs were obvious even during the early years when first generation CT scanners were the rule, and such advantages have become more obvious with each technical advance in the field.[225–227] Currently, despite occasi

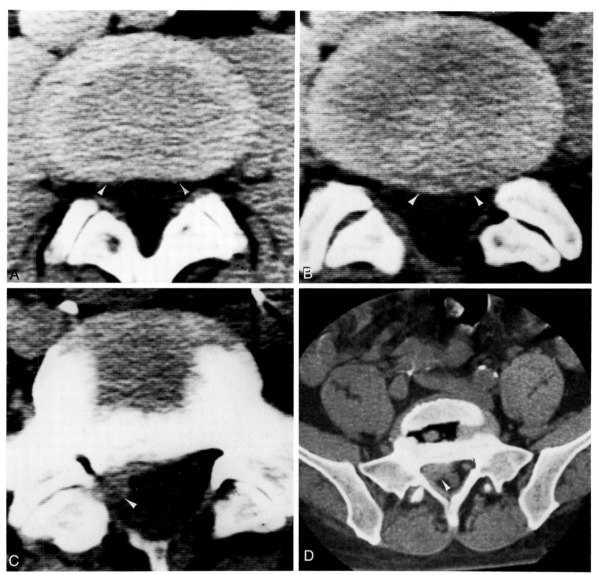

**FIGURE 8–61.** Low back pain: Bulging anulus fibrosus versus discal herniation.

  **A** Normal situation. The posterior margin of the lumbar intervertebral discs (with the exception of that at L5-S1) usually is concave (arrowheads).

  **B** Bulging anulus fibrosus. A general extension of the posterior discal margin is seen (arrowheads).

  **C** Herniated intervertebral disc. Observe focal extension of discal material (arrowhead) with obliteration of the adjacent nerve root.

  **D** Herniated intervertebral disc. A situation similar to that in **C** is evident (arrowhead).

the idea, CT (and MR imaging) has become the imaging method of choice in the evaluation of patients with low back pain. Those who doggedly maintain that myelography alone is diagnostically superior to CT in this clinical setting are becoming fewer, although there is continued support for the combination of both CT and myelography in the delineation of spinal disease, especially at the cervical level. CT and myelography produce different images of the spine, the former providing a cross-sectional direct display of the bony canal, the intervertebral discs, the thecal sac and segmental nerves, and the dural and epidural spaces and the latter displaying the subarachnoid space and its contents alone.[228] The two techniques are not incompatible, however, and the sequential use of myelography followed by CT with myelography has definite advantages, even when applied to problems of the lower lumbar spine. Although the results of comparison studies of myelography, CT, and CT combined with myelography have not been uniform,[228–230] it must be remembered that in those clinical situations in which CT and myelography compare favorably with each other, the former technique, because it is a noninvasive technique with a lower rate of patient complications and morbidity, should be preferred. Furthermore, in certain situations, such as extreme lateral discal herniation,[231, 233] CT possesses definite superiority over myelography. In other situations, such as in the evaluation of recurring symptoms and signs after back surgery, a strong argument can be made for using CT and myelography together. Finally, MR imaging with its remarkable soft tissue contrast resolution and its ability to allow imaging of the spine directly in the sagittal and coronal planes as well as the transaxial plane, and to allow differentiation between the anulus fibrosus and the nucleus pulposus of the intervertebral disc, has had a major clinical impact in the last few years.[232]

There is no uniform agreement regarding the technical aspects of the CT examination of the lumbosacral spine. In addition to differing philosophies regarding the need for intraspinal contrast material, the position of the patient (prone versus supine), the use of contiguous transaxial sections at every lower lumbar level versus sections at preselected levels alone, and the requirement for gantry angulation are decisions about which opinions vary. Reformation of transaxial image data in the coronal or sagittal plane is an additional technical modification that many investigators regard as superfluous in most cases and a few investigators regard as indispensable.

The CT characteristics of a herniated intervertebral disc need not be discussed in detail here other than to note the diagnostic difficulty that occasionally may arise in differentiating a bulging anulus fibrosus and a true discal herniation. With a bulging anulus fibrosus, a general extension of the discal margin beyond that of the vertebral body is seen, whereas with true discal herniation, a focal extension of the intervertebral disc is evident[234] (Fig. 8–61). These diagnostic features are not uniformly reliable, however, especially in patients with significant alignment abnormalities of the spine. Reformatted images may provide supplementary evidence favoring one diagnosis over the other,[235] although generally they are not necessary.

The extruded (sequestered) intervertebral disc, characterized by discal penetration of the posterior longitudinal ligament, appears on CT as an epidural mass that may either be contiguous with the remaining portions of the intervertebral disc or be separated from them by epidural fat.[236, 238] These discal fragments commonly migrate caudally or rostrally and may extend into the neural foramen.

The herniated intervertebral disc must be distinguished from other causes of extradural masses, including a dilated nerve root sheath (Fig. 8–62), conjoined nerve roots (Fig. 8–63), and benign and malignant neoplasms[236] (Fig. 8–64). The enlarged nerve root sheath typically produces a rounded mass in the region of the intervertebral foramen that is isodense with the cerebrospinal fluid in the subarachnoid space and that may be accompanied by enlargement of the foramen itself owing to scalloped erosion of the posterolateral aspect of the vertebral body.[237] The intrathecal presence of metrizamide will confirm this diagnosis.[236] Conjoined, or composite, nerve roots represent uncommon congenital anomalies in which two nerve roots arise from the thecal sac together.[239] They are identified most commonly at the lumbosacral level in a unilateral distribution. The division of the soft tissue mass into its separate nerve root components allows accurate CT diagnosis in most cases. Benign epidural tumors usually are smoother than discal fragments and may lead to pressure erosion of adjacent bone; malignant epidural tumors may be irregular or smooth, and they too produce bone abnormalities consisting of sclerosis or destruction.[236] Bone erosion is an infrequent finding in disc herniations.[300]

Failure of spinal surgery to alleviate symptoms and signs and to permit the patient to return to a normal level of physical activity postoperatively is not rare, appearing in as

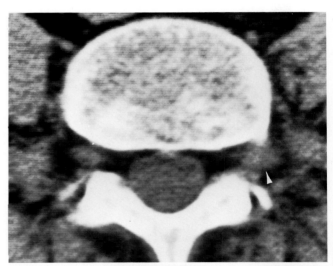

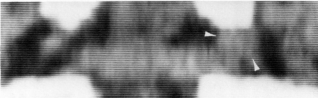

**FIGURE 8–62.** Low back pain: Cystic dilatation of nerve root sheath. The apparent enlargement of the left nerve root (arrowheads) seen in transaxial and coronal reformatted CT images was proved to relate to a dilated sheath, although conjoined nerve roots were considered a second diagnostic possibility on the basis of CT images.

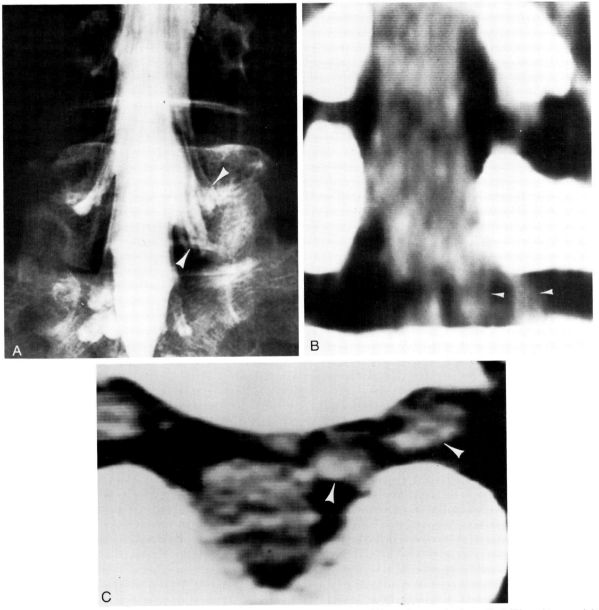

**FIGURE 8–63.** Low back pain: Conjoined nerve roots. On the basis of myelography **(A)**, and coronal reformatted **(B)** and transaxial **(C)** CT scans, conjoined nerve roots (arrowheads) are identified at the L5-S1 spinal level. (Courtesy of A. Stauffer, M.D., San Diego, California.)

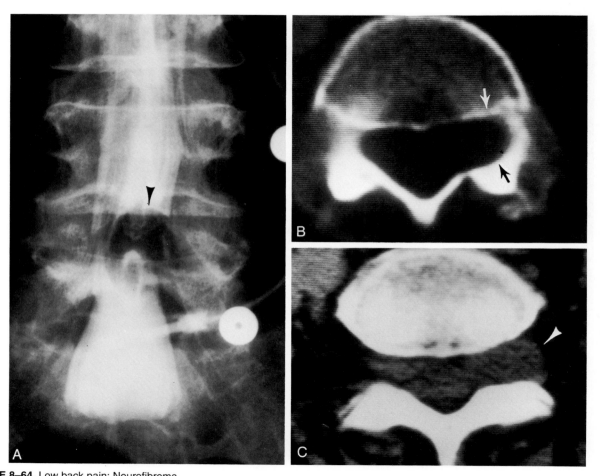

**FIGURE 8–64.** Low back pain: Neurofibroma.

**A** A mass at the L4-L5 spinal level has led to a well-defined defect (arrowhead) in the contrast material during myelography.

**B, C** Two transaxial CT scans (at different levels and window settings) show the smooth mass (arrowhead) and pressure erosion of neighboring bone (arrows).

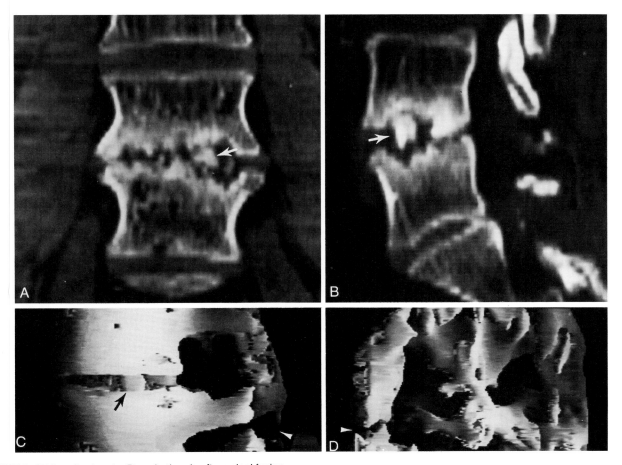

**FIGURE 8–65.** Low back pain: Pseudarthrosis after spinal fusion.

**A, B** Coronal **(A)** and sagittal **(B)** reformatted CT scans in a patient who had had a previous attempted anterior and posterior fusion at the L4 to S1 spinal levels show that the osseous graft (arrows) in the L4-L5 intervertebral disc is not incorporated into the vertebral bodies.

**C, D** Three-dimensional CT displays viewed from the anterolateral **(C)** and posterior **(D)** aspects of the spine document the unfused bone graft in the L4-L5 disc (arrow) and a pseudarthrosis (arrowheads) in the posterior fusion mass.

many as 30 per cent of patients after surgery. The CT evaluation of such patients is more difficult than that of persons who have not undergone surgery, and the diagnostic success of the study depends more on the experience and expertise of the examiner. Modifications in CT technique commonly are advised for the ''failed back surgery syndrome'' and include prone positioning of the patient, intravenous injection of contrast material, and use of intraspinal metrizamide.[31, 41, 250, 269, 272, 301]

Causes of this syndrome include inappropriate or inadequate surgery, recurrent discal herniation at the same vertebral level or another level, bone proliferation with spinal stenosis, arachnoiditis, subluxation of the facet joints, infection, and hypertrophic scars.[30, 31, 34, 240] When fusion also has been employed, pseudarthrosis represents an additional cause of new or persistent clinical manifestations (Fig. 8–65).

The extradural scar appears as a soft tissue dense shadow within the spinal canal, usually possessing a higher CT number than the thecal sac and a lower CT number than the intervertebral disc. It occurs on the side of operation, generally in one or more of three specific sites: in the posterior part of the canal at the site of the laminectomy and ligamentum flavum excision; in the anterior part of the

canal at the site of a diskectomy; and in the lateral wall of the canal at the site of a facetectomy.[30] CT characteristics of the postdiskectomy scar simulate those of a recurrent discal herniation with some minor differences: retraction of the thecal sac toward the soft tissue lesion; mass formation that contours itself around the thecal sac; linear strandlike radiodense shadows; a location that often is above or below the intervertebral disc space; a mass that is not continuous with the intervertebral disc itself; and a CT number of approximately 75 HU, which may increase following the intravenous administration of a contrast material.[30]

Spinal stenosis is discussed elsewhere (see Chapters 12 and 40). The cross-sectional display afforded by CT is well suited to the identification of stenosis of the central canal, lateral recesses, and neural foramina in the lumbar region. In addition to congenital and developmental causes of such stenosis (Fig. 8–66), acquired causes include intervertebral (osteo)chondrosis, bulging of the anulus fibrosus, hypertrophy of the ligamenta flava, and osteoarthritis of the apophyseal joints.

The excellent demonstration of the apophyseal joints provided by CT has been welcomed by those caring for patients with low back pain, a reaction that is not surprising on considering the mounting evidence that supports a rela-

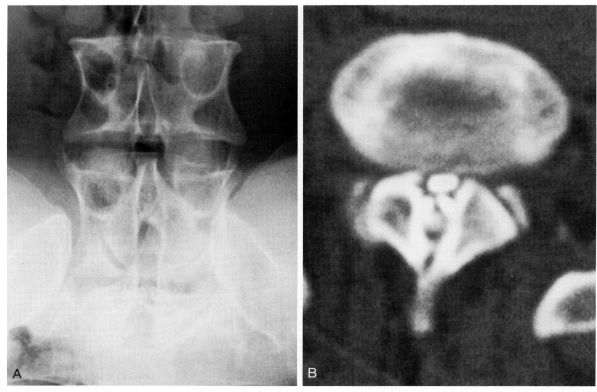

**FIGURE 8–66.** Low back pain: Spinal stenosis in achondroplasia. Routine radiography **(A)** demonstrates progressive narrowing of the interpediculate distance on proceeding caudad. After metrizamide myelography, a transaxial CT scan **(B)** documents extreme spinal stenosis.

tionship between modifications in the apophyseal joints, and significant clinical manifestations, as well as the inability of conventional techniques to image these areas in a satisfactory manner.[299] Intra-articular entrapment of meniscus-like structures, synovial cyst formation, and a variety of joint disorders, including osteoarthritis and ankylosing spondylitis (Fig. 8–67), are among the potential diseases or

occurrences that localize in or near the apophyseal joints. CT may provide direct diagnostic information by demonstrating the osteophytes, bone fragmentation, and spinal stenosis that accompany osteoarthritis (Fig. 8–68); the in-

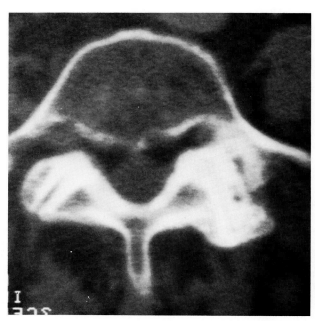

**FIGURE 8–68.** Low back pain: Osteoarthritis of the apophyseal joint. Transaxial CT ideally can reveal osteophytosis and bone sclerosis of the apophyseal joints, changes that are indicative of osteoarthritis. In this case, the left apophyseal joint at the L5-S1 spinal level is affected, and involvement has led to distortion of the spinal canal and neural foramen.

**FIGURE 8–67.** Low back pain: Arachnoid diverticula in ankylosing spondylitis. Scalloping of the laminae in the lumbar spine is characteristic of this complication.

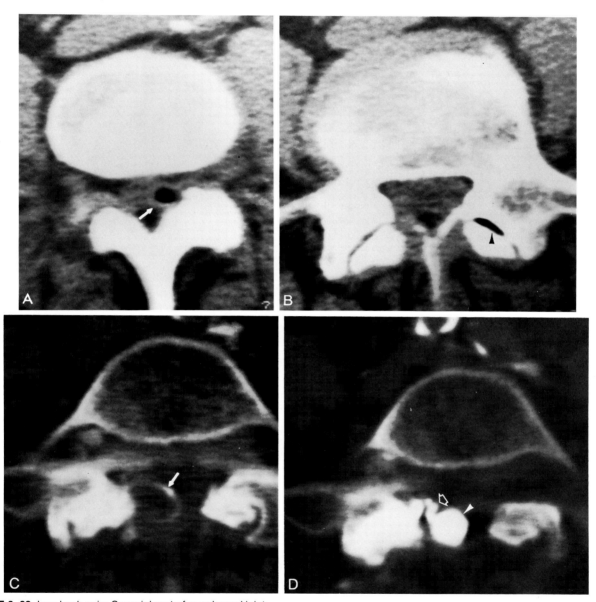

**FIGURE 8–69.** Low back pain: Synovial cyst of apophyseal joint.

   **A, B** In this example, a mass containing a vacuum phenomenon (arrow) at the level of the left L4-L5 apophyseal joint is evident **(A)**. The gas arose from the joint itself (arrowhead) **(B)**, indicating that the synovial cyst communicated with the joint.

   **C, D** In a second patient, the synovial cyst possesses a calcific rim (solid arrow) and is adjacent to a degenerative right apophyseal joint at the L5-S1 spinal level **(C)**. A similar transaxial CT scan **(D)** obtained after the introduction of corticosteroid preparations and radiopaque contrast material into the joint shows that the cyst has opacified (arrowhead), indicating its articular communication. Note the presence of a channel between the cyst and the joint (open arrow). The patient's symptoms and signs decreased dramatically after this injection.

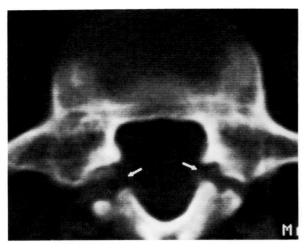

**FIGURE 8–70.** Low back pain: Spondylolysis. Bilateral defects in the pars interarticularis are evident (arrows).

tra-articular bone fusion that appears in ankylosing spondylitis; and the extradural mass containing a peripheral rim of calcification or gas that characterizes a synovial cyst (Fig. 8–69). Furthermore, this technique can be used to monitor the injection of corticosteroid preparations, lidocaine, and radiopaque contrast material into these joints (see Chapter 13).

Spondylolysis (Fig. 8–70), spondylolisthesis, ossification of paraspinal and intraspinal ligaments (Figs. 8–71 and 8–72), cartilaginous (Schmorl's) nodes (Fig. 8–73), arachnoid cysts, infections, tumors, fractures, and dislocations are among the many additional spinal disorders that can be evaluated with CT.

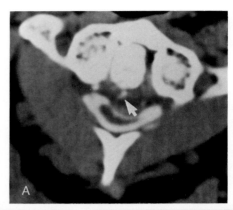

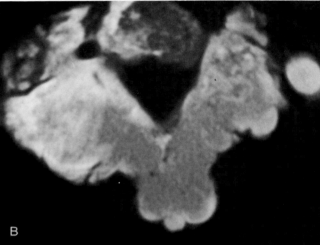

**FIGURE 8–72.** Cervical spine pain: Calcification of intraspinal and paraspinal tissues.

**A** Calcium pyrophosphate dihydrate crystal deposition disease. Calcification in the transverse ligament (arrow) is seen. (Courtesy of P. Kaplan, M.D., Charlottesville, Virginia.)

**B** Calcium hydroxyapatite crystal deposition disease. Massive intraspinal and paraspinal calcification and bone destruction are seen. The patient had no underlying systemic disease. (Courtesy of D. Witte, M.D., Memphis, Tennessee.)

## SUMMARY

An overview is provided of the prominent role played by CT in the analysis of musculoskeletal diseases. Cross-sectional display, excellent contrast resolution, and the ability to allow the measurement of specific attenuation values are important characteristics of CT that underscore its potential to delineate and define soft tissue and bone alterations that may be undetectable with conventional radiography. Reformation of transaxial images in the coronal or sagittal plane and three-dimensional analysis of image data represent significant additional advantages of CT. The prominent place of this technique as a diagnostic tool available to clinicians of many different specialties cannot be questioned, although the introduction and refinement of MR imaging already have required and will continue to require adjustments in imaging protocols applied to the evaluation of musculoskeletal disorders.

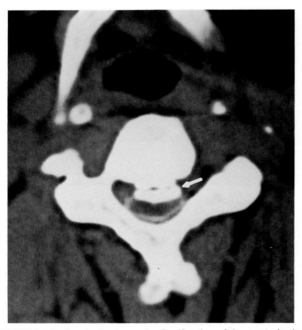

**FIGURE 8–71.** Cervical spine pain: Ossification of the posterior longitudinal ligament. The ossified ligament (arrow) is well shown with transaxial CT, accomplished after myelography.

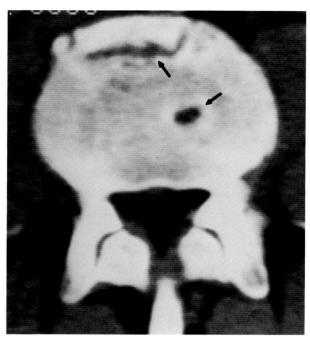

**FIGURE 8–73.** Low back pain: Cartilaginous (Schmorl's) nodes. Two sites of intraosseous discal displacement (arrows) are apparent.

## References

1. Hounsfield GN: Computerized transverse axial scanning (tomography). I. Description of a system. Br J Radiol 46:1016, 1973.
2. McCullough EC: Factors affecting the use of quantitative information from a CT scanner. Radiology 124:99, 1977.
3. Baxter BS, Sorenson JA: Factors affecting the measurement of size and CT number in computed tomography. Invest Radiol 16:337, 1981.
4. Radon J: On the determination of functions from their integrals along certain manifolds. Ber Saech Akad Wiss Leipzig Math Phys Kl 69:262, 1917.
5. Baker HL: The impact of computed tomography on neuroradiologic practice. Radiology 116:637, 1975.
6. McCullough EC: Photon attenuation in computed tomography. Med Physics 2:307, 1975.
7. Introduction to Computed Tomography. Milwaukee, Wisconsin, General Electric Company, Medical Systems Division, 1976.
8. Brooks RA, DiChiro G: Theory of image reconstruction in computed tomography. Radiology 117:561, 1975.
9. Gordon R, Herman GT, Johnson SA: Image reconstruction from projections. Sci Am 233:56, 1975.
10. Blumenfeld SM, Glover G: Spatial resolution in computed tomography. In TH Newton, DG Potts (Eds): Radiology of the Skull and Brain. Technical Aspects of Computed Tomography. St Louis, CV Mosby Co, 1981, p 3918.
11. Glover GH, Pelc NJ: Nonlinear partial volume artifacts in x-ray computed tomography. Med Physics 7:238, 1980.
12. Brooks RA, DiChiro G: Statistical limitations in x-ray reconstructive tomography. Med Physics 3:237, 1976.
13. Glenn WV, Johnston RJ, Morton PE, et al: Image generation and display techniques for CT scan data. Thin transverse and reconstructed coronal and sagittal planes. Invest Radiol 10:403, 1975.
14. Herman GT, Liu HK: Display of three-dimensional information in computed tomography. J Comput Assist Tomogr 1:155, 1977.
15. Joseph PM, Spital RD: A method for correcting bone induced artifacts in computed tomography scanners. J Comput Assist Tomogr 2:209, 1978.
16. Bluemm R: Direct sagittal (positional) computed tomography of the head. Neuroradiology 22:199, 1982.
17. Haverling M, Johanson H, Ahren L: Approximate sagittal computer tomography of the sellar and suprasellar region. Acta Radiol Diagn 19:918, 1978.
18. Osborn AG, Anderson RE: Direct sagittal computed tomographic scans of the face and paranasal sinuses. Radiology 129:81, 1978.
19. Mondello E, Savin A: Direct sagittal computed tomography of the brain. J Comput Assist Tomogr 3:706, 1979.
20. Altman N, Harwood-Nash DC, Fitz CR, et al: Evaluation of the infant spine by direct sagittal computed tomography. Am J Neuroradiol 6:65, 1985.
21. Sartoris DJ, Neumann CH, Riley RW: The temporomandibular joint: True sagittal computed tomography with meniscus visualization. Radiology 150:250, 1984.
22. Manzione JV, Katzberg RW, Brodsky GL, et al: Internal derangements of the temporomandibular joint: Diagnosis by direct sagittal computed tomography. Radiology 150:111, 1984.
23. Nesbit D, Levine E, Neff JR: Direct longitudinal computed tomography of the forearm. J Comput Assist Tomogr 5:144, 1981.
24. Azouz EM: Longitudinal CT of the forearm in children. J Can Assoc Radiol 35:388, 1984.
25. Levi C, Gray JE, McCullough EC, et al: The unreliability of CT numbers as absolute values. AJR 139:443, 1982.
26. Mull RT: Mass estimates by computed tomography: Physical density from CT numbers. AJR 143:1101, 1984.
27. Heiken JP, Lee JKT, Smathers RL, et al: CT of benign soft-tissue masses of the extremities. AJR 142:575, 1984.
28. Hermann G, Yeh H-C, Schwartz I: Computed tomography of soft-tissue lesions of the extremities, pelvic and shoulder girdles: Sonographic and pathological correlations. Clin Radiol 35:193, 1984.
29. DeSantos LA, Ginaldi S, Wallace S: Computed tomography in liposarcoma. Cancer 47:46, 1981.
30. Teplick JG, Haskin ME: Computed tomography of the postoperative lumbar spine. AJR 141:865, 1983.
31. Teplick JG, Haskin ME: Intravenous contrast enhanced CT of the postoperative lumbar spine: Improved identification of recurrent disk herniation, scar, arachnoiditis, and diskitis. AJR 143:845, 1984.
32. Orrison WW, Lilleas FG: CT demonstration of gas in a herniated nucleus pulposus. J Comput Assist Tomogr 6:807, 1982.
33. Gulati AN, Weinstein ZR: Gas in the spinal canal in association with lumbosacral vacuum phenomenon: CT findings. Neuroradiology 20:191, 1980.
34. Teplick GH, Teplick SK, Goodman L, et al: Pitfalls and unusual findings in computed tomography of the lumbar spine. J Comput Assist Tomogr 6:888, 1982.
35. Beers AJ, Carter AP, Leiter B, et al: CT detection of retroperitoneal gas associated with gas in intervertebral disks. J Comput Assist Tomogr 8:232, 1984.
36. Resnick D, Niwayama G, Guerra J, et al: Spinal vacuum phenomena: Anatomical study and review. Radiology 139:341, 1981.
37. Schubiger O, Valavanis A: CT differentiation between recurrent disc herniation and postoperative scar formation: The value of contrast enhancement. Neuroradiology 22:251, 1982.
38. Raininko R, Torma T: Contrast enhancement around a prolapsed disk. Neuroradiology 24:49, 1982.
39. Braun IF, Lin JP, Benjamin MV, et al: Computed tomography of the asymptomatic postsurgical lumbar spine: Analysis of the physiologic scar. AJR 142:149, 1984.
40. De Santis M, Crisi G, Vici FF: Late contrast enhancement in the CT diagnosis of herniated lumbar disk. Neuroradiology 26:303, 1984.
41. Meyer JD, Latchaw RE, Roppolo HM, et al: Computed tomography and myelography of the postoperative lumbar spine. Am J Neuroradiol 3:223, 1982.
42. Tehranzadeh J, Gabriele OF: The prone position for CT of the lumbar spine. Radiology 152:817, 1984.
43. Barmeir E, Blinder GE, Sasson AA, et al: Prone computed tomography metrizamide myelography: A technique for improved diagnosis of lumbar disc herniation. Clin Radiol 35:479, 1984.
44. Sartoris DJ, Kursunoglu S, Pineda C, et al: Detection of intra-articular osteochondral bodies in the knee using computed arthrotomography. Radiology 155:447, 1985.
45. Deutsch AL, Resnick D, Berman JL, et al: Computerized and conventional arthrotomography of the glenohumeral joint: Normal anatomy and clinical experience. Radiology 153:603, 1984.
46. Deutsch AL, Resnick D, Mink HH: Computed tomography of the glenohumeral and sternoclavicular joints. Orthop Clin North Am 16:497, 1985.
47. Reiser M, Karpf P-M, Bernett P: Diagnosis of chondromalacia patellae using CT arthrography. Eur J Radiol 2:181, 1982.
48. Boven F, Bellemans M-A, Geurts J, et al: The value of computed tomography scanning in chondromalacia patellae. Skel Radiol 8:183, 1982.
49. Boven F, De Boeck M, Potvliege R: Synovial plicae of the knee on computed tomography. Radiology 147:805, 1983.
50. Reiser M, Rupp N, Karpf PM, et al: Erfahrunger mit der CT-Arthrographie der Kreuzbänder des Kniegelenkes. ROFO 137:372, 1982.
51. Rothman SLG, Dobben GD, Rhodes ML, et al: Computed tomography of the spine: Curved coronal reformations from serial images. Radiology 150:185, 1984.
52. Rhodes ML, Glenn WV, Azzawi YM: Extracting oblique planes from serial CT sections. J Comput Assist Tomgr 4:649, 1980.
53. Glenn WV, Rhodes ML, Altschuler EM, et al: Multiplanar display computerized body tomography application in the lumbar spine. Spine 4:282, 1979.
54. Rosenthal DI, Stauffer AE, Davis KR, et al: Evaluation of multiplanar reconstruction in CT recognition of lumbar disk disease. Am J Neuroradiol 5:307, 1984.
55. Totty WG, Vannier MW: Complex musculoskeletal anatomy: Analysis using three dimensional surface reconstruction. Radiology 150:173, 1984.
56. Vannier MW, Marsh JL, Warren JO: Three dimensional CT reconstruction images for craniofacial surgical planning and evaluation. Radiology 150:179, 1983.
57. Burk DL Jr, Mears DC, Kennedy WH, et al: Three-dimensional computed tomography of acetabular fractures. Radiology 155:183, 1985.
58. Weeks PM, Vannier MW, Stevens WG, et al: Three-dimensional imaging of the wrist. J Hand Surg [Am] 10:32, 1985.

59. Armstrong EA, Smith TH, Salyer KE: Three dimensional image reconstruction of computed tomograms of the head and neck in the pediatric age group. Ann Radiol 28:241, 1985.
60. Gilula LA, Murphy WA, Tailor CC, et al: Computed tomography of the osseous pelvis. Radiology 132:107, 1979.
61. Naidich DP, Freedman MT, Bowerman JW, et al: Computed tomography in the evaluation of the soft tissue component of bony lesions of the pelvis. Skel Radiol 3:144, 1978.
62. Naidich DP, Freedman MT, Bowerman JW, et al: Ten section approach to computed tomography of the pelvis. Skel Radiol 5:213, 1980.
63. Rubenstein J, Kellam J, McGonigal D: Cross-sectional anatomy of the adult bony acetabulum. J Can Assoc Radiol 33:137, 1982.
64. Dihlmann W, Nebel G: Computed tomography of the hip joint capsule. J Comput Assist Tomgr 7:278, 1983.
65. Riddlesberger MM Jr: Computed tomography of the musculoskeletal system. Radiol Clin North Am 19:463, 1981.
66. Dalinka MK, Arger P, Coleman V: CT in pelvic trauma. Orthop Clin North Am 16:471, 1985.
67. Hernandez RJ, Poznanski AK: CT evaluation of pediatric hip disorders. Orthop Clin North Am 16:513, 1985.
68. Shirkhoda A, Brashear HR, Zelenek ME, et al: Sacral abnormalities—computed tomography versus conventional radiography. J Comput Tomogr 8:41, 1984.
69. Bankoff MS, Sarno RC, Carter BL: CT scanning in septic sacroiliac arthritis or periarticular osteomyelitis. Comput Radiol 8:165, 1984.
70. Kozin F, Carrera GF, Ryan LM, et al: Computed tomography in the diagnosis of sacroiliitis. Arthritis Rheum 24:1479, 1981.
71. Carrera GF, Foley WD, Kozin F, et al: CT of sacroiliitis. AJR 136:41, 1981.
72. Vogler JB III, Brown WH, Helms CA, et al: The normal sacroiliac joint: A CT study of asymptomatic patients. Radiology 151:433, 1984.
73. Destouet JM, Gilula LA, Murphy WA, et al: Computed tomography of the sternoclavicular joint and sternum. Radiology 138:123, 1981.
74. Hatfield MK, Gross BH, Glazer GM, et al: Computed tomography of the sternum and its articulations. Skel Radiol 11:197, 1984.
75. Goodman LR, Teplick SK, Kay H: Computed tomography of the normal sternum. AJR 141:219, 1984.
76. Roach JW, Duncan D, Wenger DR, et al: Atlanto-axial instability and spinal cord compression in children—diagnosis by computerized tomography. J Bone Joint Surg [Am] 66:708, 1984.
77. Daniels DL, Williams AL, Haughton VM: Computed tomography of the articulations and ligaments at the occipito-atlantoaxial region. Radiology 146:709, 1983.
78. Martinez S, Herzenberg JE, Apple JS: Computed tomography of the hindfoot. Orthop Clin North Am 16:481, 1985.
79. Patel RB: Evaluation of complex carpal trauma: Thin-section direct longitudinal computed tomography scanning through a plaster cast. J Comput Tomogr 9:107, 1985.
80. Handel SF, Lee Y-Y: Computed tomography of spinal fractures. Radiol Clin North Am 19:69, 1981.
81. Lindahl S, Willen J, Irstam L: Computed tomography of bone fragments in the spinal canal. An experimental study. Spine 8:181, 1983.
82. Brant-Zawadski M, Jeffrey RB Jr, Minagi H, et al: High resolution CT of thoracolumbar fractures. AJR 138:699, 1982.
83. Colley DP, Dunsker SB: Traumatic narrowing of the dorsolumbar spinal canal demonstrated by computed tomography. Radiology 129:95, 1978.
84. Guerra J Jr, Garfin Sr, Resnick D: Vertebral burst fractures: CT analysis of the retropulsed fragment. Radiology 153:769, 1984.
85. Shuman WP, Rogers JV, Sickler ME, et al: Thoracolumbar burst fractures: CT dimensions of the spinal canal relative to postsurgical improvement. AJR 145:337, 1985.
86. Brown BM, Brant-Zawadzki M, Cann CE: Dynamic CT scanning of spinal column trauma. AJR 139:1177, 1982.
87. McAfee PC, Huan HA, Fredrickson BE, et al: The value of computed tomography in thoracolumbar fractures. J Bone Joint Surg [Am] 65:461, 1983.
88. Kilcoyne RF, Mack LA, King HA, et al: Thoracolumbar spine injuries associated with vertical plunges: Reappraisal with computed tomography. Radiology 146:137, 1983.
89. Golimbu C, Firooznia H, Rafii M, et al: Computed tomography of thoracic and lumbar spine fractures that have been treated with Harrington instrumentation. Radiology 151:731, 1984.
90. Willen J, Lindahl S, Irstam L, et al: Unstable thoracolumbar fractures. A study by CT and conventional roentgenology of the reduction effect of Harrington instrumentation. Spine 9:213, 1984.
91. White RR, Newberg A, Seligson D: Computed tomographic assessment of the traumatized spine before and after Harrington instrumentation. Clin Orthop 146:150, 1980.
92. Faerver EN, Wolpert SM, Scott M, et al: Computed tomography of spinal fractures. J Comput Assist Tomogr 3:657, 1979.
93. O'Callaghan JP, Ullrich OG, Yuan HA, et al: CT of facet distraction in flexion injuries of the thoracolumbar spine: The ''naked'' facet. AJR 134:563, 1980.
94. Steppe R, Bellemans M, Boven F, et al: The value of computed tomography scanning in elusive fractures of the cervical spine. Skel Radiol 6:175, 1981.
95. Gill K, Bucholz RW: The role of computerized tomographic scanning in the evaluation of major pelvic fractures. J Bone Joint Surg [Am] 66:34, 1984.
96. Rubenstein JD: Radiographic assessment of pelvic trauma. J Can Assoc Radiol 34:228, 1983.
97. Burk DL Jr, Mears DC, Herbert DL, et al: Pelvic and acetabular fractures: Examination by angled CT scanning. Radiology 153:548, 1984.
98. Mack LA, Duesdieker GA, Harley JD, et al: CT of acetabular fractures: Postoperative appearances. AJR 141:891, 1983.
99. Rafii M, Firooznia H, Golimbu C, et al: The impact of CT on clinical management of pelvic and acetabular fractures. Clin Orthop 178:228, 1983.
100. Rubenstein J, Kellam J, McGonigal D: Acetabular fracture assessment with computerized tomography. J Can Assoc Radiol 34:19, 1983.
101. Walker RH, Burton DS: Computerized tomography in assessment of acetabular fractures. J Trauma 22:227, 1982.
102. Mack JA, Harley JD, Winquist RA: CT of acetabular fractures: Analysis of fracture patterns. AJR 138:407, 1982.
103. Blumberg ML: Computed tomography and acetabular trauma. Comput Tomogr 4:47, 1980.
104. Shirkhoda A, Brashear HR, Staab EV: Computed tomography of acetabular fractures. Radiology 134:683, 1980.
105. Griffiths HJ, Standertskjold-Nordenstam OG, Burke J, et al: Computed tomography in the management of acetabular fractures. Skel Radiol 11:22, 1984.
106. Sauser DD, Billimoria PE, Rouse GA, et al: CT evaluation of hip trauma. AJR 135:269, 1980.
107. Adam P, Labbe JL, Alberge Y, et al: The role of computed tomography in the assessment and treatment of acetabular fractures. Clin Radiol 36:13, 1985.
108. Judet R, Judet J, Letournel E: Fractures of the acetabulum: Classification and surgical approaches for open reduction. Preliminary report. J Bone Joint Surg [Am] 46:1615, 1964.
109. Hansen ST Jr: CT for pelvic fractures. AJR 138:592, 1982.
110. Levinsohn EM, Bunnell WP, Yuan HA: Computed tomography in the diagnosis of dislocations of the sternoclavicular joint. Clin Orthop 140:12, 1979.
111. Danzig L, Resnick D, Greenway G: Evaluation of unstable shoulders by computed tomography. A preliminary study. Am J Sports Med 10:138, 1982.
112. Seltzer SE, Weissman BN: CT finding in normal and dislocating shoulders. J Can Assoc Radiol 36:41, 1985.
113. Gould R, Rosenfield AT, Friedlaender GE: Loose body within the glenohumeral joint in recurrent anterior dislocation: CT demonstration. J Comput Assist Tomgr 9:404, 1985.
114. Martinez S, Korobkin M, Fondren FB, et al: Computed tomography of the normal patellofemoral joint. Invest Radiol 18:249, 1983.
115. Rafii M, Firooznia H, Golimbu C, et al: Computed tomography of tibial plateau fractures. AJR 142:1181, 1984.
116. Karrholm J, Hansson LI, Laurin S: Computed tomography of intraarticular supination-eversion fractures of the ankle in adolescents. J Pediatr Orthop 1:181, 1981.
117. Friedburg H, Hendrich V, Wimmer B, et al: Computertomographie bei komplexen sprunggelenksfrakturen. Radiologe 23:421, 1983.
118. Spiegel PG, Mast JW, Cooperman DR, et al: Triplane fractures of the distal tibial epiphysis. Clin Orthop 188:74, 1984.
119. Cone RO III, Nguyen V, Flournoy JG, et al: Triplane fracture of the distal tibial epiphysis: Radiographic and CT studies. Radiology 153:763, 1984.
120. Mino DE, Palmer AK, Levinsohn EM: The role of radiography and computed tomography in the diagnosis of subluxation and dislocation of the distal radioulnar joint. J Hand Surg 8:23, 1983.
121. Scheffler R, Armstrong D, Hutton L: Computed tomographic diagnosis of distal radio-ulnar joint disruption. J Can Assoc Radiol 35:212, 1984.
122. Mino DE, Palmer AK, Levinsohn EM: Radiography and computerized tomography in the diagnosis of incongruity of the distal radio-ulnar joint. A prospective study. J Bone Joint Surg [Am] 67:247, 1985.
123. Norman A, Nelson J, Green S: Fractures of the hook of hamate: Radiographic signs. Radiology 154:49, 1985.
124. Goiney RC, Connell DG, Nichols DM: CT evaluation of tarsometatarsal fracture-dislocation injuries. AJR 14:985, 1985.
125. Heger L, Wulff K, Seddigi MSA: Computed tomography of calcaneal fractures. AJR 145:131, 1985.
126. Patel RB, Barton P, Green L: CT of isolated elbow in evaluation of trauma: A modified technique. Comput Radiol 8:1, 1984.
127. Zinman C, Reis ND: Osteochondritis dissecans of the talus: Use of the high resolution computed tomography scanner. Acta Orthop Scand 53:697, 1982.
128. Passariello R, Trecco F, Depaulis F, et al: Computed tomography of the knee joint: Technique of study and normal anatomy. J Comput Assist Tomogr 7:1035, 1983.
129. Passariello R, Trecco F, DePaulis F, et al: Computed tomography of the knee joint: Clinical results. J Comput Assist Tomogr 7:1043, 1983.
130. Pavlov H, Freiberger RH, Deck MF, et al: Computer-assisted tomography of the knee. Invest Radiol 13:57, 1978.
131. Thompson JR, Christiansen EL, Hasso AN, et al: Dislocation of the temporomandibular joint disk demonstrated by CT. Am J Neuroradiol 5:115, 1984.
132. Helms CA, Vogler JB III, Morrish RB Jr, et al: Temporomandibular joint internal derangements: CT diagnosis. Radiology 152:459, 1984.
133. Roberts D, Pettigrew J, Udupa J, et al: Three-dimensional imaging and display of the temporomandibular joint. Oral Surg 58:461, 1984.
134. Thompson JR, Christiansen E, Sauser et al: Dislocation of the temporomandibular joint meniscus: Contrast arthrography vs. computed tomography. AJR 144:171, 1985.
135. Katzberg RW, Schenck J, Roberts D, et al: Magnetic resonance imaging of the temporomandibular joint meniscus. Oral Surg 59:332, 1985.
136. Roberts D, Schenck J, Joseph P, et al: Temporomandibular joint: Magnetic resonance imaging. Radiology 155:829, 1985.

137. Kuhn JP, Berger PE: Computed tomographic diagnosis of osteomyelitis. Radiology 130:503, 1979.
138. Ram PC, Martinez S, Korobkin M, et al: CT detection of intraosseous gas: A new sign of osteomyelitis. AJR 137:721, 1981.
139. Rafii M, Firooznia H, Golimbu C, et al: Hematogenous osteomyelitis with fat-fluid level shown by CT. Radiology 153:493, 1984.
140. Wing VW, Jeffrey RB Jr, Federle MP, et al: Chronic osteomyelitis examined by CT. Radiology 154:171, 1985.
141. Seltzer SE: Value of computed tomography in planning medical and surgical treatment of chronic osteomyelitis. J Comput Assist Tomogr 8:482, 1984.
142. Hauser H, Rheiner P: Computed tomography of the hand. Part II. Pathological conditions. Medicamundi 28:129, 1983.
143. Hermann G, Rose JS, Strauss L: Tumor infiltration of the bone marrow: Comparative study using computed tomography. Skel Radiol 11:17, 1984.
144. Berger PE, Kuhn JP: Computed tomography of tumors of the musculoskeletal system in children: Clinical applications. Radiology 127:171, 1978.
145. Heelan RT, Watson RC, Smith J: Computed tomography of lower extremity tumors. AJR 132:933, 1979.
146. Rosenthal DI: Computed tomography of orthopedic neoplasms. Orthop Clin North Am 16:461, 1985.
147. de Santos LA: The radiology of bone tumors: Old and new modalities. CA 30:66, 1980.
148. Gamba JL, Martinez S, Apple J, et al: Computed tomography of axial skeletal osteoid osteoma. AJR 142:769, 1984.
149. Hahn PF, Rosenthal DI, Ehrlich MG: Case report 286. Skel Radiol 12:214, 1984.
150. Hertzana Y, Mendelsohn DB, Gottschalk F: Aneurysmal bone cyst of the calcaneus. Radiology 151:51, 1984.
151. Hudson TM, Springfield DS, Spanier SS, et al: Benign exostoses and exostotic chondrosarcomas: Evaluation of cartilage thickness by CT. Radiology 152:595, 1984.
152. Kenney PJ, Gilula LA, Murphy WA: The use of computed tomography to distinguish osteochondroma and chondrosarcoma. Radiology 139:129, 1981.
153. Lloyd TU, Paul D: Erosion of the scapula by a benign lipoma: Computed tomography diagnosis. J Comput Assist Tomogr 3:679, 1979.
154. de Santos LA, Goldstein HM, Murray JA, et al: Computed tomography in the evaluation of musculoskeletal neoplasms. Radiology 128:89, 1978.
155. Lukens JA, McLeod RA, Sim FH: Computed tomographic evaluation of primary osseous malignant neoplasms. AJR 139:45, 1982.
156. Jones ET, Kuhns LR: Pitfalls in the use of computed tomography for musculoskeletal tumors in children. J Bone Joint Surg [Am] 63:1297, 1981.
157. Levine E, Lee KR, Neff JR, et al: Comparison of computed tomography and other imaging modalities in the evaluation of musculoskeletal tumors. Radiology 131:431, 1979.
158. Zimmer WD, Berquist TH, McLeod RA, et al: Bone tumors: Magnetic resonance imaging versus computed tomography. Radiology 155:709, 1985.
159. Hudson TM, Hamlin DJ, Enneking WF, et al: Magnetic resonance imaging of bone and soft tissue tumors: Early experience in 31 patients compared with computed tomography. Skel Radiol 13:134, 1985.
160. Goldberg RP, Weissman BN, Naimark A, et al: Femoral neck erosions: Signs of hip joint synovial disease. AJR 141:107, 1983.
161. Ginaldi S: Computed tomography feature of synovial osteochondromatosis. Skel Radiol 5:219, 1980.
162. Castor WR, Miller JDR, Russell AS, et al: Computed tomography of the craniocervical junction in rheumatoid arthritis. J Comput Assist Tomogr 7:31, 1983.
163. Braunstein EM, Weissman BN, Seltzer SE, et al: Computed tomography and conventional radiographs of the craniocervical region in rheumatoid arthritis. A comparison. Arthritis Rheum 27:26, 1984.
164. Raskin RJ, Schnapf DJ, Wolf CR, et al: Computerized tomography in evaluation of atlantoaxial subluxation in rheumatoid arthritis. J Rheumatol 10:33, 1983.
165. Kaufman RL, Glenn WV Jr: Rheumatoid cervical myelopathy: Evaluation by computerized tomography with multiplanar reconstruction. J Rheumatol 10:42, 1983.
166. Kaiser MC, Veiga-Pires JA, Capesius P: Atlanto-axial impaction and compression of the medulla oblongata and proximal spinal cord in rheumatoid arthritis evaluated by CT scanning. Br J Radiol 56:764, 1983.
167. McBeath AA, Neidhart DA: Acetabular cyst with communicating ganglion. A case report. J Bone Joint Surg [Am] 58:267, 1976.
168. Lee KR, Tines SC, Price HI, et al: The computed tomographic findings of popliteal cysts. Skel Radiol 10:26, 1983.
169. Schwimmer M, Edelstein G, Heiken JP, et al: Synovial cysts of the knee. CT evaluation. Radiology 154:175, 1985.
170. Sartoris DJ, Danzig L, Gilula L, et al: Synovial cysts of the hip joint and iliopsoas bursitis: A spectrum of imaging abnormalities. Skel Radiol 14:85, 1985.
171. Penkava RR: Iliopsoas bursitis demonstrated by computed tomography. AJR 135:175, 1980.
172. Shirkhoda A, Mauro MA, Staab EV, et al: Soft-tissue hemorrhage in hemophiliac patients. Computed tomography and ultrasound study. Radiology 147:811, 1983.
173. Guilford WB, Mintz PD, Blatt PM, et al: CT of hemophilic pseudotumors of the pelvis. AJR 135:167, 1980.
174. Pettersson H, Ahlberg A: Computed tomography in hemophilic pseudotumor. Acta Radiol Diagn 23:453, 1982.
175. Haggmark T, Jansson E, Saune B: Cross-sectional area of the thigh muscle in man measured by CT. Scand J Clin Lab Invest 38:355, 1978.
176. Termote J-L, Baert A, Crolla D, et al: Computed tomography of the normal and pathologic muscular system. Radiology 137:439, 1980.
177. Hawley RJ Jr, Schellinger D, O'Doherty DS: Computed tomographic patterns of muscles in neuromuscular diseases. Arch Neurol 41:383, 1984.
178. Hadar H, Gadoth N, Heifetz M: Fatty replacement of lower paraspinal muscles: normal and neuromuscular disorders. AJR 141:895, 1983.
179. Firooznia H, Rafii M, Golimbu C, et al: Computerized tomography in diagnosis of pelvic abscess in spinal-cord-injured patients. Comput Radiol 7:335, 1983.
180. Firooznia H, Rafii M, Golimbu C, et al: Computerized tomography of pelvic osteomyelitis in patients with spinal cord injuries. Clin Orthop 181:126, 1983.
181. Powers SK, Norman D, Edwards MSB: Computerized tomography of peripheral nerve lesions. J Neurosurg 59:131, 1983.
182. Tysvaer AT: Computerized tomography and surgical treatment of femoral compression neuropathy. Report of two cases. J Neurosurg 57:137, 1982.
183. Firooznia H, Golimbu C, Rafii M, et al: Computerized tomography in diagnosis of compression of the common peroneal nerve by ganglion cysts. Comput Radiol 7:343, 1983.
184. Stewart JD, Schmidt B, Wee R: Computed tomography in the evaluation of plexopathies and proximal neuropathies. Can J Neurol Sci 10:244, 1983.
185. Pech P, Haughton V: A correlative CT and anatomic study of the sciatic nerve. AJR 144:1037, 1985.
186. Cone RO, Szabo R, Resnick D, et al: Computed tomography of the normal soft tissues of the wrist. Invest Radiol 18:546, 1983.
187. Heiken JP, Lee JKT, Smathers RL, et al: CT of benign soft-tissue masses of the extremities. AJR 142:575, 1984.
188. Muller N, Norris ED, Nichols DM: Popliteal artery entrapment demonstrated by CT. Radiology 151:157, 1984.
189. Dihlmann W: CT analysis of the upper end of the femur: The asterisk sign and ischaemic bone necrosis of the femoral head. Skel Radiol 8:251, 1982.
190. Dihlmann W: Computed tomography of the hip joint. Medicamundi 28:29, 1983.
191. Casteleyn PP, DeBoeck H, Handelberg F, et al: Computed axial tomography and disulphine blue in the evaluation of osteonecrosis of the femoral head. Int Orthop (SICOT) 7:149, 1983.
192. Hernandez RJ: Concentric reduction of the dislocated hip: Computed tomographic evaluation. Radiology 150:266, 1984.
193. Hernandez RJ: Evaluation of congenital hip dysplasia and tibial torsion by computed tomography. J Comput Tomogr 7:101, 1983.
194. Hernandez RJ, Tachdjian MO, Dias LS: Hip CT in congenital dislocations: Appearance of tight iliopsoas tendon and pulvinar hypertrophy. AJR 139:335, 1982.
195. Aaro S, Dahlborn M, Svensson L: Estimation of vertebral rotation in structural scoliosis by computed tomography. Acta Radiol Diagn 19:990, 1978.
196. Aitken AGF, Flodmark O, Newman DE, et al: Leg length determination by CT digital radiography. AJR 144:613, 1985.
197. Hernandez RJ, Tachdjian MO, Poznanski AK, et al: CT determination of femoral torsion. AJR 137:97, 1981.
198. Jend H-H, Heller M, Dallek M, et al: Measurement of tibial torsion by computed tomography. Acta Radiol Diagn 22:271, 1981.
199. Laasonen EM, Jokie P, Lindholm TS: Tibial torsion measured by computed tomography. Acta Radiol Diagn 25:325, 1984.
200. Weiner DS, Cook AJ, Hoyt WA Jr, et al: Computed tomography in the measurement of femoral anteversion. Orthopedics 1:299, 1978.
201. Deutsch AL, Resnick D, Campbell G: Computed tomography and bone scintigraphy in the evaluation of tarsal coalition. Radiology 144:137, 1982.
202. Azouz EM: Tarsal pseudo-coalition. J Can Assoc Radiol 33:105, 1982.
203. Sarno RC, Carter BL, Bankoff MS, et al: Computed tomography in tarsal coalition. J Comput Assist Tomogr 8:1155, 1984.
204. Weinstein MA, Rothner AD, Duchesneau P, et al: Computed tomography in diastematomyelia. Radiology 118:609, 1975.
205. Arredondo F, Haughton VM, Hemmy DC, et al: The computed tomographic appearance of the spinal cord in diastematomyelia. Radiology 118:609, 1975.
206. Kaplan JO, Quencer RM: The occult tethered conus syndrome in the adult. Radiology 137:387, 1980.
207. De Boeck M, De Smedt E, Potvliege R: Computed tomography in the evaluation of a congenital absent lumbar pedicle. Skel Radiol 8:197, 1982.
208. Wortzman G, Steinhardt MI: Congenitally absent lumbar pedicle: A reappraisal. Radiology 152:713, 1984.
209. Tatler G, Kendall B, Saunders A: Case report 206. Skel Radiol 8:311, 1982.
210. Cox HE, Bennett WF: Computed tomography of absent cervical pedicle. J Comput Assist Tomogr 8:537, 1984.
211. Naidich TP, McLone DG, Mutluer S: A new understanding of dorsal dysraphism with lipoma (lipomyeloschisis): Radiologic evaluation and surgical correction AJR 140:1065, 1983.
212. Modesto MA, Servadei F, Greitz T, et al: Computed tomography for anterior sacral and intracorporal meningoceles. Neuroradiology 21:155, 1981.
213. Grivegnee A, Delince P, Ectors P: Comparative aspects of occult intrasacral meningocele with conventional x-ray, myelography and CT. Neuroradiology 22:33, 1981.
214. Wahner HW, Dunn WL, Riggs BL: Assessment of bone mineral. Part I. J Nucl Med 25:1134, 1984.

215. Jensen PS, Orphanoudakis SC, Rauschkolb EN, et al: Assessment of bone mass in the radius by computed tomography. AJR *134*:285, 1980.

216. Revak CS: Mineral content of cortical bone measured by computed tomography. J Comput Assist Tomogr *4*:342, 1980.

217. Cann CE, Genant HK: Precise measurement of vertebral mineral content using computed tomography. J Comput Assist Tomogr *4*:493, 1980.

218. Genant HK, Ettinger B, Cann CE, et al: Osteoporosis: Assessment by quantitative computed tomography. Orthop Clin North Am *16*:557, 1985.

219. Cann CE, Genant HK, Kolb FO, et al: Quantitative computed tomography for prediction of vertebral fracture risk. Bone *6*:1, 1985.

220. Genant HK, Cann CE, Ettinger B, et al: Quantitative computed tomography of vertebral spongiosa: A sensitive method for detecting early bone loss after oophorectomy. Ann Intern Med *97*:699, 1982.

221. Breatnach E, Robinson PJ: Repositioning errors in measurement of vertebral attenuation values by computed tomography. Br J Radiol *56*:299, 1983.

222. Heller M, Dihlmann W: Computertomographie der Paget-koxopathie. ROFO *138*:427, 1983.

223. Newmark H III: Paget's disease of a vertebral body seen on computerized tomography. Comput Radiol *6*:7, 1982.

224. Helms CA, Vogler JB III, Genant HK: Characteristic CT manifestations of uncommon spinal disorders. Orthop Clin North Am *16*:445, 1985.

225. Williams AL, Haughton VM, Syvertsen A: Computed tomography in the diagnosis of herniated nucleus pulposus. Radiology *135*:95, 1980.

226. Carrera GF, Williams AL, Haughton VM: Computed tomography in sciatica. Radiology *137*:433, 1980.

227. Meyer GA, Haughton VM, Williams AL: Diagnosis of herniated lumbar disk with computed tomography. N Engl J Med *301*:1166, 1979.

228. Raskin SP, Keating JW: Recognition of lumbar disk disease: Comparison of myelography and computed tomography. Am J Neuroradial *3*:215, 1982.

229. Haughton VM, Eldevik OP, Magnaes B, et al: A prospective comparison of computed tomography and myelography in the diagnosis of herniated lumbar disks. Radiology *142*:103, 1982.

230. Anand AK, Lee BCP: Plain film and metrizamide CT of lumbar disk disease: Comparison with myelography. Am J Neuroradiol *3*:567, 1982.

231. Godersky JC, Erickson DL, Seljeskog EL: Extreme lateral disk herniation: Diagnosis by computed tomography scanning. Neurosurgery *14*:549, 1984.

232. Richardson ML, Genant HK, Helms CA, et al: Magnetic resonance imaging of the musculoskeletal system. Orthop Clin North Am *16*:569, 1985.

233. Williams AL, Haughton VM, Daniels DL, et al: CT recognition of lateral lumbar disk herniation. Am J Neuroradiol *3*:211, 1982.

234. Williams AL, Haughton VM, Meyer GH, et al: Computed tomographic appearance of the bulging annulus fibrosus. Radiology *142*:403, 1982.

235. Williams JP, Joslyn JN, Butler TW: Differentiation of herniated lumbar disc from bulging annulus fibrosus. Use of reformatted images. J Comput Tomogr *6*:89, 1982.

236. Williams AL, Haughton VM, Daniels DL, et al: Differential CT diagnosis of extruded nucleus pulposus. Radiology *148*:141, 1983.

237. Neave VCD, Wycoff RR: Computed tomography of cystic nerve root sleeve dilatation. J Comput Assist Tomogr *7*:881, 1983.

238. Dillon WP, Kaseff LG, Knackstedt VE, et al: Computed tomography and differential diagnosis of the extruded lumbar disc. J Comput Assist Tomogr *7*:969, 1983.

239. Helms CA, Dorwart RH, Gray M: The CT appearance of conjoined nerve roots and differentiation from a herniated nucleus pulposus. Radiology *144*:803, 1982.

240. Heithoff KB, Burton CV: CT evaluation of the failed back surgery syndrome. Orthop Clin North Am *16*:417, 1985.

241. Simon DC, Hess ML, Smilak MS, et al: Direct sagittal CT of the temporomandibular joint. Radiology *157*:545, 1985.

242. Manco LG, Messing SG, Busino LJ, et al: Internal derangements of the temporomandibular joint evaluated with direct sagittal CT: A prospective study. Radiology *157*:407, 1985.

243. Hemmy DC, Tessier PL: CT of dry skulls with craniofacial deformities: Accuracy of three-dimensional reconstruction. Radiology *157*:113, 1985.

244. Woolson ST, Dev P, Fellingham LL, et al: Three-dimensional imaging of the ankle joint from computerized tomography. Foot Ankle *6*:2, 1985.

245. Pech P, Kilgore DP, Pojunas KW, et al: Cervical spinal fractures: CT detection. Radiology *157*:117, 1985.

246. Passariello R, Trecco F, de Paulis F, et al: Meniscal lesions of the knee joint: CT diagnosis. Radiology *157*:29, 1985.

247. Ghelman B: Meniscal tears of the knee: Evaluation by high-resolution CT combined with arthrography. Radiology *157*:23, 1985.

248. Kahmann R, Gold RH, Eckardt JJ, et al: Case report 337. Skel Radiol *14*:301, 1985.

249. Magid D, Fishman EK, Scott WW Jr, et al: Femoral head avascular necrosis: CT assessment with multiplanar reconstruction. Radiology *157*:751, 1985.

250. Braun IF, Hoffman JC Jr, Davis PC, et al: Contrast enhancement in CT differentiation between recurrent disk herniation and postoperative scar: Prospective study. AJR *145*:785, 1985.

251. Lapointe JS, Graeb DA, Nugent RA, et al: Value of intravenous contrast enhancement in the CT evaluation of intraspinal tumors. AJR *146*:103, 1986.

252. Woolson ST, Fellingham LL, Dev P, et al: Three dimensional imaging of bone from analysis of computed tomography data. Orthopedics *8*:1269, 1985.

253. Woolson ST, Dev P, Fellingham LL, et al: Three-dimensional imaging of bone from computerized tomography. Clin Orthop *202*:239, 1986.

254. Gillespie JE, Isherwood I: Three-dimensional anatomical images from computed tomographic scans. Br J Radiol *59*:289, 1986.

255. Sartoris DJ, Feingold ML, Resnick D: Axial computed tomographic anatomy of the foot. Part I: Hindfoot. J Foot Surg *24*:392, 1985.

256. Sartoris DJ, Feingold ML, Resnick D: Axial computed tomographic anatomy of the foot. Part II: Midfoot. J Foot Surg *24*:413, 1985.

257. Saks BJ: Normal acetabular anatomy for acetabular fracture assessment: CT and plain film correlation. Radiology *159*:139, 1986.

258. Gershuni DH, Skyhar MJ, Thompson B, et al: A comparison of conventional radiography and computed tomography in the evaluation of spiral fractures of the tibia. J Bone Joint Surg [Am] *67*:1388, 1985.

259. Manco LG, Kavanaugh JH, Fay JJ, et al: Meniscal tears of the knee: Prospective evaluation with CT. Radiology *159*:147, 1986.

260. Rafii M, Firooznia H, Golimbu C, et al: CT arthrography of capsular structures of the shoulder. AJR *146*:361, 1986.

261. Raininko RK, Aho AJ, Laine MO: Computed tomography in spondylitis. CT versus other radiograhic methods. Acta Orthop Scand *56*:372, 1985.

262. Altman NR, Altman DH, Wolfe SA, et al: Three-dimensional CT reformation in children. AJR *146*:1261, 1986.

263. Kursunoglu S, Kaplan P, Resnick D, et al: Three-dimensional computed tomographic analysis of the normal temporomandibular joint. J Oral Maxillofac Surg *44*:257, 1986.

264. Armstrong EA, Smith TH, Oshman DG, et al: Clinical applications of three-dimensional reconstruction of computed tomograms. IM *7*:209, 1986.

265. Woolson ST: Three-dimensional bone imaging and preoperative planning of reconstructive hip surgery. Contemp Orthop *12*:1, 1986.

266. Solomon MA, Gilula LA, Oloff LM, et al: CT scanning of the foot and ankle. 1. Normal anatomy. AJR *146*:1192, 1986.

267. Solomon MA, Gilula LA, Oloff LM, et al: CT scanning of the foot and ankle. 2. Clinical applications and review of the literature. AJR *146*:1204, 1986.

268. Aisen AM, Martel W, Braunstein EM, et al: MRI and CT evaluation of primary bone and soft-tissue tumors. AJR *146*:749, 1986.

269. Weisz GM: The value of CT in diagnosing postoperative lumbar conditions. Spine *11*:164, 1986.

270. Bush CH, Gillespy T III, Dell PC: High-resolution CT of the wrist: Initial experience with scaphoid disorders and surgical fusions. AJR *149*:757, 1987.

271. Pech P, Bergström K, Rauschning W, et al: Attenuation values, volume changes and artifacts in tissue due to freezing. Acta Radiol Diagn *28*:779, 1987.

272. Firooznia H, Kricheff II, Rafii M, et al: Lumbar spine after surgery: Examination with intravenous contrast-enhanced CT. Radiology *163*:221, 1987.

273. Ney DR, Fishman EK, Magid D, et al: Interactive real-time multiplanar CT imaging. Radiology *170*:275, 1989.

274. Fishman EK, Ney DR, Kawashima A, et al: Effect of image display on the quality of multiplanar reconstruction of computed tomography data. Invest Radiol *28*:146, 1993.

275. Fishman EK, Drebin B, Magid D, et al: Volumetric rendering techniques: Applications for three-dimensional imaging of the hip. Radiology *163*:737, 1987.

276. Lobregt S, Schaars HWGK: Three-dimensional imaging and manipulation of CT data. Part I. General principles. Medicamundi *32*:92, 1987.

277. Zonneveld FW, van der Meulen JC, van Akkerveeken PF, et al: Three-dimensional imaging and manipulation of CT data. Part II. Clinical applications in orthopaedic and craniofacial surgery. Medicamundi *32*:99, 1987.

278. Hoehne KH, Delapaz RL, Bernstein R, et al: Combined surface display and reformatting for the three-dimensional analysis of tomographic data. Invest Radiol *22*:658, 1987.

279. Herman GT: Three-dimensional imaging on a CT or MR scanner. J Comput Assist Tomogr *12*:450, 1988.

280. Lang P, Hedtmann A, Steiger P, et al: Dreidimensionale Computertomographie bei Erkrankungen der Knochen und Gelenke. Z Orthop *125*:418, 1987.

281. Robertson DD, Walker PS, Granholm JW, et al: Design of custom hip stem prosthesis using three-dimensional CT modeling. J Comput Assist Tomogr *11*:804, 1987.

282. Fishman EK, Magid D, Ney DR, et al: Three-dimensional imaging. Radiology *181*:321, 1991.

283. Gillespie JE, Isherwood I, Barker GR, et al: Three-dimensional reformations of computed tomography in the assessment of facial trauma. Clin Radiol *38*:523, 1987.

284. Rothman SLG, Chaftez N, Rhodes ML, et al: CT in the preoperative assessment of the mandible and maxilla for endosseous implant surgery. Work in progress. Radiology *168*:171, 1988.

285. Resnick CS, Kerr R, Sartoris DJ, et al: The architecture of the proximal femur: An imaging analysis. CRC Crit Rev Diagn Imaging *27*:49, 1987.

286. O'Sullivan GS, Goodman SB, Jones HH: Computerized tomographic evaluation of acetabular anatomy. Clin Orthop *277*:175, 1992.

287. Stark P: Computed tomography of the sternum. CRC Crit Rev Diagn Imaging *27*:321, 1987.

288. Wojcik WG, Edeiken-Monroe BS, Harris JH Jr: Three-dimensional computed tomography in acute cervical spine trauma: a preliminary report. Skel Radiol *16*:261, 1987.

289. Raila FA, Aitken AT, Vickers GN: Computed tomography and three-dimensional reconstruction in the evaluation of occipital condyle fracture. Skel Radiol *22*:269, 1993.

290. Adler SJ, Vannier MW, Gilula LA, et al: Three-dimensional computed tomography of the foot: Optimizing the image. Comput Med Imaging Graphics *12*:59, 1988.

291. Christiansen EL, Thompson JR, Hasso AN, et al: CT number characteristics of malpositioned TMJ menisci. Diagnosis with CT number highlighting (blink-mode). Invest Radiol 22:315, 1987.
292. Belsole RJ, Hilbelink D, Llewellyn JA, et al: Scaphoid orientation and location from computed, three-dimensional carpal models. Orthop Clin North Am 17:505, 1986.
293. Biondetti PR, Vannier MW, Gilula LA, et al: Wrist: Coronal and transaxial CT scanning. Radiology 163:149, 1987.
294. Magid D, Fishman EK: Computed tomography of pelvic trauma. In JL Bloem, DJ Sartoris (Eds): MRI and CT of the Musculoskeletal System. A Text-Atlas. Baltimore, Williams & Wilkins, 1992, p 337.
295. Kilcoyne RF: Computed tomography of shoulder trauma. In JL Bloem, DJ Sartoris (Eds): MRI and CT of the Musculoskeletal System. A Text-Atlas. Baltimore, Williams & Wilkins, 1992, p 285.
296. Jeandel P, Chouc PY, Briant JF, et al: Valeur et limites de la tomodensitométrie appliquée au diagnostic des sacro-iliites chez l'adulte jeune: Etude de 200 dossiers. Rev Rhum Mal Ostéoartic 59:413, 1992.
297. Kogutt MS: Computed radiographic imaging: Use in low-dose leg length radiography. AJR 148:1205, 1987.
298. Helms CA, Vogler JB III, Hardy DC: CT of the lumbar spine: Normal variants and pitfalls. RadioGraphics 7:447, 1987.
299. Pathria MN, Sartoris DJ, Resnick D: Osteoarthritis of the facet joints: Accuracy of oblique radiographic assessment. Radiology 164:227, 1987.
300. Vadalà G, Dore R, Garbagna P: Unusual osseous changes in lumbar herniated disks: CT features. J Comput Assist Tomogr 9:1045, 1985.
301. Yang PJ, Seeger JF, Dzioba RB, et al: High-dose IV contrast in CT scanning of the postoperative lumbar spine. AJNR 7:703, 1986.
302. Leggon RE, Lindsey RW, Panjabi MM: Strength reduction and the effects of treatment of long bones with diaphyseal defects involving 50% of the cortex. J Orthop Res 6:540, 1988.
303. McBroom RJ, Cheal EJ, Hayes WC: Strength reductions from metastatic cortical defects in long bones. J Orthop Res 6:369, 1988.
304. Shapeero LG, Dye SF, Lipton MJ, et al: Functional dynamics of the knee joint by ultrafast, cine-CT. Invest Radiol 23:118, 1988.
305. Kalender WA, Seissler W, Klotz E, et al: Spiral volumetric CT with single-breath-hold technique, continuous transport, and continuous scanner rotation. Radiology 176:181, 1990.
306. Ney DR, Fishman EK, Kawashima A, et al: Comparison of helical and serial CT with regard to three-dimensional imaging of musculoskeletal anatomy. Radiology 185:865, 1992.
307. Fishman EK, Wyatt SH, Bluemke DA, et al: Spiral CT of musculoskeletal pathology: preliminary observations. Skel Radiol 22:253, 1993.
308. Peschmann KR, Napel S, Couch J, et al: High-speed computed tomography: Systems and performance. Appl Optics 24:4052, 1985.
309. Bosch E, André MP, Hart SJ, et al: Multiplexed transmission holograms: A novel technique for three-dimensional display of CT and MR images. Radiology 185(P):339, 1992.
310. Lenchik L, Dovgan DJ, Kier R: CT of the iliopsoas compartment: Value in differentiating tumor, abscess, and hematoma. AJR 162:83, 1994.

# 9

# Magnetic Resonance Imaging: Technical Considerations

*Richard B. Buxton, PhD*

The phenomenon of nuclear magnetic resonance (NMR) was first investigated nearly 50 years ago.[1, 2] Since then it has become a standard tool in chemistry,[3] and in the last two decades has served as the basis for a remarkably powerful and flexible medical imaging technique.[4] This chapter explains the basic physics that underlies the phenomenon of NMR and describes how a measurable signal is produced and used to form an image. The local NMR signal determines the intensity at each point in a magnetic resonance (MR) image, so that the contrast characteristics of MR images all follow from the physics of NMR. (In current usage the less specific term MR is used to refer to imaging applications, rather than NMR. Another related phenomenon, electron spin resonance [ESR], also falls in the category of MR, although there are not yet any medical imaging applications of ESR.)

A number of methods have been developed for creating an image of the NMR signal, and each has advantages and disadvantages in terms of imaging time and image contrast. In addition to providing anatomic images with good soft tissue contrast, MR imaging also is uniquely sensitive to blood flow, and noninvasive MR angiography techniques now are used widely.

## OVERVIEW OF NMR

### The NMR Experiment

The simplest form of the pulsed NMR experiment requires just two components: a magnet and a coil. The magnet produces a uniform magnetic field with magnitude $B_0$. The coil is arranged so that its axis is perpendicular to the magnetic field direction (Fig. 9–1). The coil can be as simple as a loop of copper and is connected to two devices: a power circuit, which can drive an oscillating electrical current through the coil; and a sensitive detector circuit, which measures small currents in the coil. For typical MR imagers, the currents oscillate at frequencies in the range of 20 to 80 MHz, producing fields in the radio frequency (RF) region of the electromagnetic spectrum. A sample, such as a human body, is placed in the magnet near the coil. The experiment has two parts: a transmit period and a receive period.

1. Transmit: The detector is turned off and an oscillating voltage is applied to the coil, creating in the sample an additional oscillating magnetic field $B_1$, referred to as the *RF magnetic field*. After a few milliseconds, $B_1$ is turned off.

2. Receive: The detector circuit is turned on to measure any signal returned from the sample.

**TABLE 9–1. Some Nuclei that Exhibit NMR**

| Nucleus | Gyromagnetic Ratio (MHz/T) |
|---------|----------------------------|
| $^1$H | 42.6 |
| $^{19}$F | 40.1 |
| $^{31}$P | 17.2 |
| $^{23}$Na | 11.3 |
| $^{13}$C | 10.7 |
| $^{17}$O | 5.8 |

### The NMR Phenomenon

If this experiment were performed on the human body, varying the oscillation frequency of $B_1$ and the magnitude of $B_0$, the following phenomena would be noted:

1. Resonance: For a few specific frequencies a weak, transient signal is produced and detected with the coil. Each of these frequencies constitutes the *resonant frequency* (or *Larmor frequency*) of a particular nucleus (Table 9–1). At these frequencies the nuclei absorb energy from the RF magnetic field and then return some of that energy to the coil during the receive part of the experiment.

2. Field Dependence: The resonant frequency is directly proportional to the magnetic field: $f_0 = \gamma B_0$, where $f_0$ is the resonant frequency and $\gamma$ is the *gyromagnetic ratio*, which

## Transmit

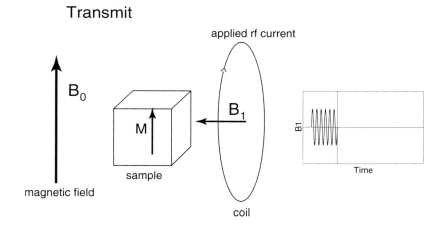

## Receive

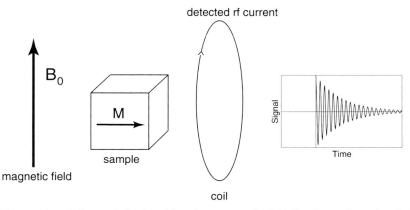

**FIGURE 9–1.** The basic NMR experiment. A sample is placed in a large magnetic field $B_0$ with a coil nearby. During the transmit part of the experiment an oscillating current in the coil creates an oscillating magnetic field $B_1$ in the sample. During the receive part of the experiment the coil acts as a detector to measure the precessing magnetization $M$ in the sample.

is a different constant for each nucleus. In standard MR imaging the nucleus of interest is hydrogen (H), which has a resonant frequency of 63 MHz in a magnetic field of 1.5 Tesla (T). The linear relationship between resonant frequency and magnetic field is the physical basis for MR imaging.

3. Chemical Shift: For a particular nucleus, the resonant frequency varies by a few parts per million (ppm) depending on the chemical form of the nucleus (e.g., for H in water and lipids the difference is 3.5 ppm). This chemical shift is the basis for the use of NMR as an analytical tool in chemistry. The effect occurs because molecular electronic orbitals create additional magnetic fields that combine with $B_0$ to shift the magnetic field at the location of the nucleus and thus shift the resonant frequency.

### Origin of the NMR Signal

In brief the physical picture of NMR is illustrated in Figure 9–2. Certain nuclei (such as hydrogen) have an intrinsic magnetic moment, so that they behave like small magnets when placed in a magnetic field. The nuclear magnetic moments tend to align with $B_0$, creating a magnetization $(M)$ in the sample. $M$ essentially is a weak magnetic field parallel to $B_0$. The oscillating field $(B_1)$ at the resonant

frequency $f_0$ tips $M$ away from $B_0$. At this point $M$ can be viewed as consisting of two parts: a *longitudinal* component $(M_L)$ parallel to $B_0$, and a *transverse* component $(M_T)$ perpendicular to $B_0$. The transverse magnetization $(M_T)$ rotates around $B_0$ *(precession)* with frequency $f_0$, generating a signal in the detector coil which is proportional to the magnitude of $M_T$. Over time $M$ gradually realigns with $B_0$ *(relaxation)* and the signal decays as $M_T$ decays.

The precessing magnetization $M_T$ is the source of the signal measured in all NMR experiments, from spectrometer studies in analytical chemistry to MR imaging. In MR imaging the local image intensity is proportional to the local magnitude of $M_T$. To understand why NMR happens, and in particular to understand the phenomena of precession and relaxation, the physics of a nucleus in a magnetic field must be considered.

### PRINCIPLES OF NUCLEAR MAGNETIC RESONANCE

#### Physics of NMR

##### Coils: Electric Currents and Magnetic Fields

Two basic principles of the physics of electricity and magnetism are involved in the generation and detection of

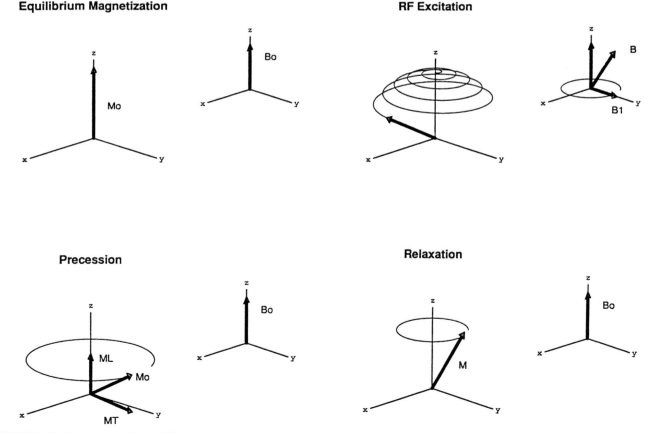

**Equilibrium Magnetization**

Mo     Bo

**RF Excitation**

B     B1

**Precession**

ML    Mo    MT     Bo

**Relaxation**

M     Bo

**FIGURE 9–2.** The physics of the NMR phenomenon. Hydrogen nuclei possess a magnetic dipole moment, and when placed in a constant magnetic field $B_0$ they tend to align with the field creating a local magnetization $M$. When a radio frequency (RF) magnetic field $B_1$ oscillating at the resonant frequency is applied, the magnetization tips away from the main field direction, creating a transverse component $M_T$ and a longitudinal component $M_L$. The magnetization precesses around $B_0$ and generates a signal proportional to $M_T$. Over time $M$ relaxes back toward the equilibrium alignment with $B_0$.

**Magnetic Field of a Circular Coil**

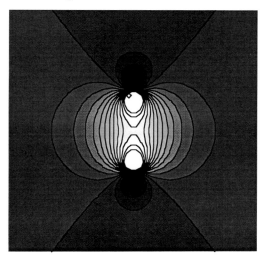

**FIGURE 9–3.** The magnetic field pattern produced by a simple circular coil. The magnetic field at each point is a vector, and only the component in the horizontal direction is shown. The contour map shows the magnitude of this component of the field in a plane perpendicular to the plane of the coil. The coil intersects the plane at the two bright spots.

the NMR signal:[3] Electric currents produce magnetic fields; and changing magnetic fields produce electric currents. Electric currents in a coil (either constant or changing) produce magnetic fields in the vicinity of the coil, and these fields are strongest close to the coil. The magnetic field produced by a simple circular coil is illustrated in Figure 9–3. Changing magnetic fields in the vicinity of a coil produce currents in the coil *(induction),* but constant magnetic fields do not. The current in the coil is strongest when the coil is near the source of the changing magnetic field.

These principles come into play in several ways in the NMR experiment. The main magnetic field $B_0$ is generated by a large cylindrical coil carrying a constant current. High field (greater than 0.3 T) imagers use superconducting magnets in which the coil carrying the current is cooled to the temperature of liquid helium. At this low temperature, the electrical resistance of the conductor is zero, so the high current can be maintained without supplying any additional power to the system.

The two principles also apply to the two parts of the NMR experiment. During the transmit portion, the oscillating current in the RF coil produces an oscillating magnetic field $(B_1)$ in the vicinity of the coil. During the receive portion, the precessing transverse magnetization $(M_T)$ in the sample (a changing magnetic field) generates a detectable current in the coil. Often in MR imaging two separate coils are used for the transmit and receive parts of the measurement, to optimize the coils for each role. For the transmit coil the $B_1$ field should be as uniform as possible over the body, so that all areas are equally excited. For signal detection, however, the signal to noise ratio can be significantly improved by using a smaller receive coil. By placing the small coil closer to the location of the oscillating magnetization, the current produced in the coil is larger. In addition, because the noise in an MR imaging system arises primarily

from the body itself, a small coil that is sensitive only to a small part of the body receives less noise as well.

## Nuclear Spin and Magnetic Dipole Moment

Protons and neutrons possess an intrinsic angular momentum called *spin.* Like mass and charge, spin is a fundamental characteristic of subatomic particles. The concept of an intrinsic angular momentum comes from the quantum mechanical description of nature and has no analogue in the macroscopic world of everyday experience. Although we are familiar with many spinning objects, from tops to entire planets, the "spin" is not an inseparable feature of these bodies: we can stop a spinning top and we can at least imagine stopping a spinning planet. In other words, these objects could exist with zero angular momentum. But a proton always has angular momentum, and the only aspect that can be changed is the direction of the spin axis. Protons and neutrons combine to form a nucleus such that their spins mutually cancel (opposite spin axes), so that the nucleus has no net spin unless there are an odd number of protons or neutrons. Thus the nuclei of $^1$H (one proton) and $^{13}$C (six protons and seven neutrons) have a net spin, whereas $^{12}$C does not.

Nuclei with a net spin also possess another important physical property: a magnetic dipole moment. Each proton behaves like a magnet with the north-south axis aligned with the spin axis. The association of a magnetic moment with angular momentum of the nucleus can be understood from a simple (and naive) picture of the nucleus as a spinning charged ball. The rotational motion of the charges constitutes a current, which in turn creates a magnetic field. It is the magnetic moment of the nucleus that leads to the phenomenon of NMR, so only nuclei with a net spin exhibit NMR.

## Precession in a Magnetic Field

A magnetic dipole moment has two key properties: a magnitude ($\mu$) and a directional axis. When a magnetic dipole is placed in a uniform magnetic field it has an energy that is proportional to $\mu$ but also depends on its orientation. Aligned with the field is the lowest energy state, and opposite to the field is the highest energy state. A compass needle thus aligns with the earth's magnetic field because it is seeking its lowest energy state. However, when a nucleus is placed in a magnetic field, its intrinsic angular momentum prevents it from immediately aligning with the field. The field exerts a torque on the dipole, which, by itself, would rotate the dipole into alignment with the field. However, when this change in angular momentum is added to the existing angular momentum of the dipole, the net change is a *precession* of the dipole axis around the field. That is, the dipole axis rotates while keeping the same angle with the magnetic field.

This is an example of the peculiar nature of angular momentum, and is exactly analogous to the behavior of a spinning top or bicycle wheel. A spinning top tipped at an angle to the vertical would be in a lower energy state if it simply fell over; instead, the rotation axis precesses around a vertical line. For a nucleus in a magnetic field the frequency of precession is directly proportional to the product $\mu B_0$; the stronger the field, the stronger the torque on the dipole and the faster the precession. The precession frequency ($f_0$) is the resonant frequency of NMR.

## Relaxation

The foregoing considerations apply to a single nucleus in a magnetic field, and from the precession arguments it might be concluded that a proton would never align with the main field. But in a real sample, $B_0$ is not the only source of magnetic field. The magnetic moments of other nuclei produce additional magnetic fields. For example, in a water molecule, an H nucleus feels the field produced by the other H in the molecule. Because the molecules are rapidly tumbling owing to their thermal motions, the total field felt by a particular nucleus fluctuates around the mean field $B_0$. These fluctuations alter both the total magnetic field magnitude and the direction. As a result, the proton's precession is more irregular, and the axis of precession fluctuates. Over time, the protons gradually tend to align more with $B_0$, a process called *relaxation.*

Because the energy associated with the orientation of the magnetic dipole moment of a hydrogen nucleus in a magnetic field is small compared with the thermal energy of a water molecule, the average degree of alignment with the field is small, corresponding to a difference of only about one part in $10^5$ between those nuclei aligned with the field and those opposite. However, this is sufficient to produce a slight net magnetization ($M$) of the water. The creation of $M$ can be understood as a relaxation toward thermal equilibrium. When a sample is first placed in a magnetic field the magnetic dipoles are oriented randomly, so that the net magnetization is zero. This means that the dipoles possess a higher energy owing to their orientation than they would if they were partly aligned with the field. (The lowest possible energy would correspond to complete alignment.) As the system relaxes, this excess energy is dissipated as heat, the dipoles align more with the field, and $M$ grows toward its equilibrium value, $M_0$.

The time constant for relaxation is called T1 and varies from about 0.2 to 4.0 sec in the body.[5] In a pure water sample the main source of a fluctuating magnetic field is the field produced by the other H nucleus in the same water molecule. But the presence of other molecules in the liquid (such as protein) can alter the relaxation rate by changing either the magnitude or the frequency of the fluctuating fields. A large molecule will tumble more slowly than a water molecule, so that a water molecule that transiently binds to the large molecule will experience more slowly fluctuating fields. The magnitude of the fluctuating fields can be increased significantly in the presence of paramagnetic compounds. Paramagnetic compounds have unpaired electrons, and electrons have magnetic moments more than a thousand times larger than a proton. This is the basis for the use of paramagnetic contrast agents, such as gadopentetate dimeglumine, as a way of reducing the local relaxation time.

The fact that T1 varies by an order of magnitude between different tissues is important because this is the source of most of the contrast differences between tissues in MR images. The differences are attributable to differences in the local environment (e.g., chemical composition, biologic structures). In general, the higher the water content of a tissue, the longer the T1. The strong dependence of the relaxation time on the local environment is exactly analogous to everyday experiences of relaxation phenomena. A cup of hot coffee sitting in a cool room is not in thermal equilibrium. Over time, the coffee will cool to room temperature (thermal equilibrium), but the time constant for this relaxation depends strongly on the local environment. If the coffee is in a thin-walled open cup, it may cool in a few minutes, whereas if it is in a covered, insulated vessel, cooling may take hours. Regardless of how long it takes, however, the final equilibrium state is the same.

## Generating the NMR Signal

### Radio Frequency Pulse

The fact that the protons tend to align with the field, producing a net magnetization ($M$), does not lead to any measurable signal (a constant magnetic field produces no currents). However, if $M$ is tipped away from the direction of $B_0$, it will precess; all of the nuclear dipoles will precess together if they are tipped over, so the net magnetization $M$ also will precess at the same frequency. The transverse component of $M$ then is a changing magnetic field and will generate a signal in a nearby detector coil.

The tipping is accomplished during the RF pulse of our basic NMR experiment by applying an oscillating magnetic field ($B_1$) perpendicular to $B_0$ and oscillating at the proton precession frequency. $M$ then begins to precess around the net time-varying magnetic field. To see why this tips $M$ away from $B_0$, imagine viewing $M$ in a reference frame that rotates at the precession frequency $f_0$.[6] If $M$ is tipped away from $B_0$, it will precess in the laboratory frame, but in the rotating frame it will be stationary, so that in this frame it appears as if the magnetic field is zero (Fig. 9–4). Similarly, the magnetic field $B_1$, which is oscillating in the laboratory frame with frequency $f_0$, appears to be a stationary field in the rotating frame. The complex picture of precession around a time varying net magnetization in the laboratory frame then reduces to a simple precession around $B_1$ in the rotating frame.

After $B_1$ is turned off, $M$ continues to precess around $B_0$ and generates a signal in the detector coil. Over time, $M$ will relax until it is again aligned with $B_0$. Because the action of an RF pulse is to tip $M$ away from $B_0$, such pulses usually are described by the *flip angle* (or *tip angle*) they produce (e.g., a 90 degree RF pulse or a 180 degree RF pulse). The flip angle is adjusted by changing either the duration or the amplitude of the RF pulse.

From the thermodynamic point of view, the process of tipping $M$ can be interpreted as the system of magnetic dipoles absorbing energy from the RF field, because the alignment of $M$ is changing, and then dissipating this energy over time as heat as the system relaxes back to equilibrium. For this reason, the RF pulse sometimes is described as an *excitation pulse* because it raises the system to an excited (higher energy) state.

### Free Induction Decay

After an RF excitation pulse (e.g., a 90 degree pulse) occurs the signal generated in the detector coil is called a *free induction decay.* "Free" relates to free precession, "induction" is the physical process in which a varying magnetic field (the precessing magnetization $M$) produces a current in a coil, and "decay" indicates that the signal dies out over time. It might be expected that the time constant for this decay would be T1, the time constant for relaxation

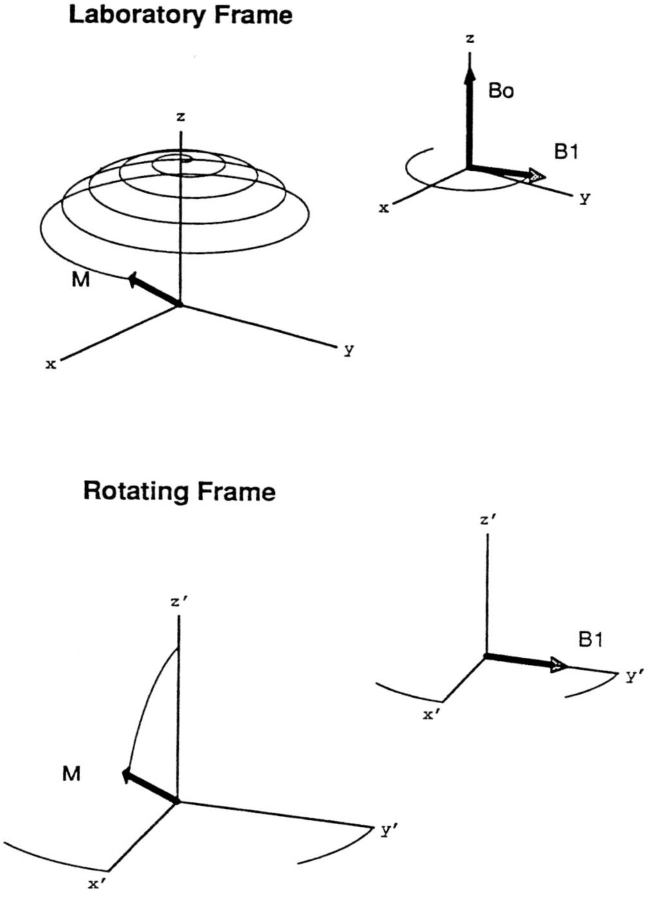

## Laboratory Frame

## Rotating Frame

**FIGURE 9–4.** The rotating reference frame. The process of RF excitation is understood most easily by viewing the magnetization from a frame of reference that rotates at the same rate as the magnetization $M$ precesses. In the rotating frame $M$ appears to be stationary, and so it appears that $B_0$ is zero. The field $B_1$, which also is rotating with the same frequency in the laboratory frame, appears to be a constant field in the rotating frame. The motion of $M$ then is a simple precession around $B_1$ in the rotating frame, and appears as a widening spiral when viewed in the laboratory frame.

to equilibrium. However, the decay of the signal usually is much faster than would be expected from T1. For this reason it is necessary to introduce a second time constant, T2, to describe the signal decay.

### Relaxation Times: T1, T2, and T2*

The two relaxation times T1 and T2 apply to the longitudinal and the transverse components of the magnetization, respectively. At equilibrium, $M$ is purely longitudinal (aligned with $B_0$), and after a 90 degree RF pulse it is purely transverse (perpendicular to $B_0$). Because the measured signal is proportional to the transverse component of $M$, the time constant governing the decay of the signal is T2, and this process often is termed *transverse relaxation.* On the other hand, the relaxation back to thermal equilibrium is related to changes in the longitudinal component, the growth of the net magnetization. T1 thus is the time constant for *longitudinal relaxation.* In the human body at field strengths typical of MR imagers, T1 is about eight to ten times larger than T2.

In practice, experimentally the free induction decay often

is found to decay much more quickly than would be expected for the T2 of the sample. This frequently is described qualitatively by saying that the decay time is T2*, with T2* less than T2. The reason for this is simply inhomogeneity of the magnetic field. If two regions of the sample feel different magnetic fields, the precession rates will differ, the local transverse magnetization vectors will quickly get out of phase with each other, and the net magnetization will decrease owing to *phase dispersion.* However, this signal decay is due to constant field offsets within the sample and not to the fluctuating fields that produce T2 decay. Because of this, the additional decay due to inhomogeneity is reversible.

### Spin Echoes

Signal loss due to inhomogeneity can be reversed by applying a second RF pulse that causes the magnetization vectors to come back into phase and create an echo of the original free induction decay signal (a *spin echo*) at a time TE (the *echo time*) after the original excitation pulse.[7] To see how this remarkable effect comes about, imagine two small magnetized regions in slightly different magnetic fields. After a 90 degree excitation pulse, the magnetization vectors are tipped into the transverse plane (Fig. 9–5). As they begin to precess at slightly different frequencies, the phase difference between them grows larger. After waiting a time TE/2, a 180 degree RF pulse is applied. The action of the 180 degree pulse is to flip the transverse plane like a pancake, reversing the *sign* of the phase of each magnetization vector. In other words, the phase $\phi_1$ of the first magnetization is changed to $-\phi_1$, and the phase $\phi_2$ of the second group is changed to $-\phi_2$. After the RF pulse the phase of each magnetization continues to evolve, just as before, so that after another time delay TE/2 the first group again acquires an additional phase $\phi_1$, and the second group again acquires an additional phase $\phi_2$. But the net phase of each group then is zero, meaning they are back in phase and add coherently to form a strong net signal (the echo) at time TE. In fact, the echoing process is quite general, and any RF pulse will create an echo, although with flip angles other than 180 degrees the refocusing is not complete.

Note that although an 180 degree pulse will correct for field inhomogeneities, it will *not* refocus T2 decay (Fig. 9–6). An echo forms because the phase acquired during the interval before the 180 degree pulse is exactly the same as the phase acquired during the interval after the pulse, so that by reversing the sign of the phase at the halfway point the net phase will be zero. But the phase variations associated with T2 decay are due to *fluctuating* fields, and the pattern of fluctuations is not repeated before and after the RF pulse. In short, a spin echo reverses the dephasing effects of static fields but not fluctuating fields. As a result, the echo signal intensity is weaker than the initial free induction decay signal owing to T2 decay during the interval TE. After the echo the signal again decays because of T2* effects, but another 180 degree RF pulse will create another echo. This can be continued indefinitely, but each echo will be weaker than the last because of T2 decay.

### Spin Echo Pulse Sequence

The basic spin echo pulse sequence can be summarized as follows:

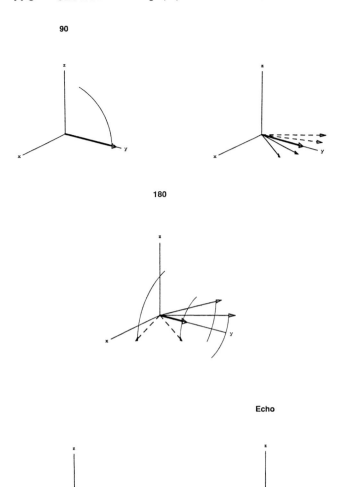

**FIGURE 9–5.** The formation of spin echoes. A 90 degree RF pulse tips over all spins to create a coherent transverse magnetization. Owing to magnetic field inhomogeneity, spins in different locations precess at different rates, leading to a spread of phase angles and a reduction in the net transverse magnetization. After a time TE/2, a 180 degree RF pulse flips the plane of magnetization vectors, reversing the phase that each spin has acquired. Continued precession for another interval TE/2 brings the spins back in phase to create an echo of the original magnetization at the echo time TE.

90 degree RF pulse—wait TE/2—180 degree RF pulse—wait TE/2—echo

Typically, this pulse sequence is repeated at a regular interval, called the *repetition time* (TR). In a normal MR imaging setting it is necessary to repeat the pulse sequence many times to collect all of the data needed to reconstruct the image. The contrast between one tissue and another in the image will depend on the magnitude of the spin echo signal generated at each location.

### Spin Echo Signal Intensity

Two pulse sequence parameters are operator controlled: the repetition time (TR) and the echo time (TE). The measured signal intensity depends strongly on both of these parameters (Fig. 9–7). The effect of TE has already been

discussed. By lengthening TE (i.e., waiting a longer time after the excitation pulse before looking at the signal), more time is allowed for transverse (T2) decay. TR, on the other hand, controls how much longitudinal relaxation is allowed to happen before the magnetization is tipped over again. During the period TR, a sample with T1 much shorter than TR will relax nearly completely, so that the longitudinal magnetization just before the next 90 degree pulse is large, but a sample with T1 longer than TR will be relaxed only partly and the longitudinal magnetization will be smaller. After the next 90 degree pulse, this longitudinal magnetization becomes the transverse magnetization and generates a signal, so the short T1 sample will produce a stronger signal.

In addition to T1 and T2, the signal intensity also is proportional to the local density of nuclei. In MR imaging this ususally is called the *hydrogen density* or *proton density*. These relationships can be summarized by the following approximate equation:[8, 9]

$$S \cong S_0 \, e^{-TE/T2} \, (1 - e^{-TR/T1})$$

where $S$ is the measured signal (e.g., the brightness of a particular pixel in an image), $S_0$ is proportional to the local proton density, the first exponential term describes T2 decay, and the second exponential term describes T1 relaxation. The signal thus depends on three properties of the tissue ($S_0$, T1, and T2) and two operator-controlled parameters (TR and TE).

### Spin Echo Tissue Contrast

The proton density is always a determining factor in the signal, but *in vivo* the water content does not vary over as great a range as do T1 and T2. Good contrast therefore is produced by making the measured signal sensitive to the relaxation times, and the relative importance of T1 and T2 can be adjusted by changing TR and TE (Fig. 9–7). With a short TR, tissues with short T1 will relax much more than tissues with a long T1, and thus T1 will affect the signal strongly. The signal then is said to be T1-weighted. How-

### Spin Echoes

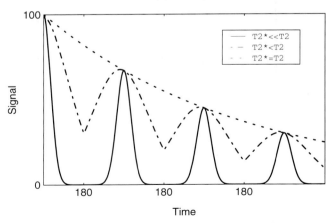

**FIGURE 9–6.** Spin echo signal decay. After an RF pulse creates a transverse magnetization, the rate of signal decay depends on T2* and T2. T2* is the apparent decay time, which includes the effects of field inhomogeneity as well as transverse relaxation (T2 decay). A series of 180 degree RF pulses will create echoes in which the inhomogeneity effects are reversed, but each echo peak still is reduced by T2 decay.

**T1-Weighted SE Contrast**

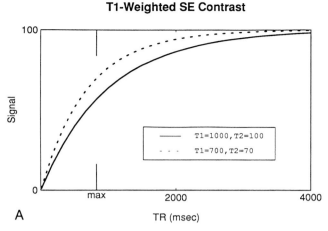

A

**T2-Weighted SE Contrast**

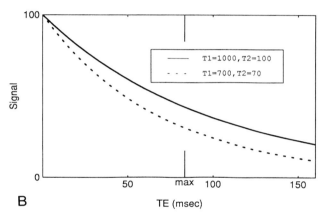

B

**SE Contrast**

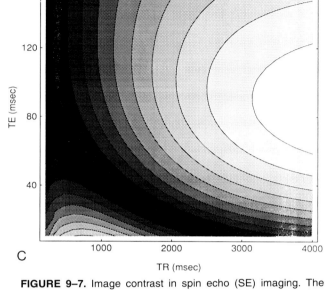

C

**FIGURE 9–7.** Image contrast in spin echo (SE) imaging. The plots show the effect on signal and contrast of the two operator-adjustable parameters, TR (the repetition time) and TE (the echo time). Signal curves are plotted for two hypothetical tissues with different relaxation times, and the contrast between the tissues is the difference between the two curves. **A,** TR dependence of the signal, assuming TE is short. **B,** TE dependence of the signal, assuming TR is long. **C,** Contour plot showing contrast for different choices of TR and TE. Note that many choices of TR and TE produce poor contrast. The two islands of high contrast are at TR≈4000 and TE≈90 (T2 weighted) and at TR≈600 with TE at the minimum possible value (T1 weighted).

ever, with long TR (several times the longest T1) all tissues will relax nearly completely and T1 will have little effect on the signal. With a long TE, differences in T2 will affect the signal strongly (T2 weighting), but with a short TE there is little time for decay and T2 will not have an effect. These arguments lead to the following loose characterization of contrast in SE pulse sequences:

> short TR: T1-weighted, short T1 tissues are bright
> long TE: T2-weighted, long T2 tissues are bright

A central problem with tissue contrast in MR imaging is that the relaxation times are positively correlated: tissues with a long T1 also are likely to have a long T2. For this reason it is rarely desirable to have both substantial T1 weighting and T2 weighting in the same image. With T1 weighting a tissue with short relaxation times will tend to be bright, but with T2 weighting it will tend to be dark. As a result of this conflict, tissue contrast can be destroyed. For this reason, TR and TE should be chosen not only to emphasize sensitivity to one of the relaxation times but also to *suppress* sensitivity to the other:

> "T1-weighted": short TR, short TE
> "T2-weighted": long TR, long TE
> "proton density weighted": long TR, short TE

The terminology here is necessarily loose, and the quotation marks are meant to indicate that these terms should be used with caution. The third pulse sequence is proton density weighted, but in fact all three are proton density weighted; it is just that in the third one the additional sensitivity to T1 and T2 has been suppressed. Note also that "short" and "long" in this context are relative to T1 and T2, and these vary substantially in the body. For example, a spin echo image obtained with a TR of 2000 msec and a TE of 20 msec would be proton density weighted for white matter in the brain (T1 ≅ 700 msec) but T1-weighted for cerebrospinal fluid (T1 ≅ 3000 msec).

## Inversion Recovery Pulse Sequence

The *inversion recovery* (IR) pulse sequence typically requires three RF pulses. It begins with an 180 degree inversion pulse, and after a time delay TI (the *inversion time*) a spin echo pulse sequence is started:

> 180 degree RF—wait TI—90 degree RF—wait TE/2—180 degree RF—wait TE/2—echo

The effect of the inversion pulse is to flip the longitudinal magnetization from the positive *z*-axis to the negative *z*-axis. This does not produce any signal because there is still no transverse magnetization. After the inversion pulse the magnetization begins to relax back toward equilibrium (alignment with the positive *z*-axis). But after a time TI, before complete relaxation can occur, the 90 degree pulse

**Inversion Recovery**

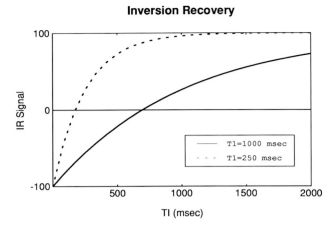

**FIGURE 9–8.** The inversion recovery (IR) signal as a function of the inversion time (TI). The initial 180 degree inversion pulse flips the longitudinal magnetization from the positive $z$-axis to the negative $z$-axis. The magnetization is allowed to relax for a time TI and then is tipped over with a 90 degree RF pulse to create a strongly T1-weighted signal. The time TI when the longitudinal magnetization passes through zero is called the null point, and no signal is generated. By using a short TI, the signal from tissues with a short T1 (such as fat) can be suppressed substantially.

tips over the longitudinal magnetization to create a transverse magnetization. The final 180 degree pulse then creates an echo of the transverse magnetization for measurement. The signal received depends on how much relaxation occurred during the interval TI, and so is strongly T1-weighted (Fig. 9–8).

Note that as the magnetization relaxes it passes through a *null point* at which the longitudinal magnetization is zero. If the 90 degree pulse is applied at this time, no signal will be generated. This effect is exploited with a short TI inversion recovery (STIR) pulse sequence to suppress the fat signal by choosing the TI to be at the null point of fat.

## PRINCIPLES OF MAGNETIC RESONANCE IMAGING

### Basic Imaging Techniques

#### Field Gradients

MR imaging exploits the physical fact that the resonant frequency $f_0$ is directly proportional to the magnetic field. By altering the magnetic field in a controlled way, so that it varies linearly along a particular axis, the resonant frequency also will vary linearly with position along that axis. Such a linearly varying field is called a *gradient field* and is produced by additional coils in the scanner. An MR imager is equipped with three orthogonal sets of gradient coils, allowing a field gradient to be produced along any axis. Because these gradient fields usually are turned on for only a few milliseconds at a time, they are referred to as *pulsed gradients.*

Compared to the main magnetic field ($B_0$), the field variations produced by the gradients are small. Typical gradient strengths used for imaging are a few milliTesla per meter (mT/m), and conventional MR imagers usually have maximum strengths of 10 mT/m. At maximum strength the magnetic field variation across a 30 cm object is 3 mT, only 0.2 per cent of a typical $B_0$ of 1.5 T. For the discussion of

spatial encoding on the following pages it is convenient to express field gradients in units of the resonant frequency change they produce per centimeter (Hz/cm): 10 mT/m = 4258 Hz/cm for protons.

Field gradients are used in three ways to encode the spatial location of a signal: (1) *slice selection,* (2) *frequency encoding,* and (3) *phase encoding.* These three methods are used for the three spatial axes; in the following sections slice selection is used on the $z$-axis, frequency encoding on the $x$-axis, and phase encoding on the $y$-axis. This is an image-based coordinate system, with the image in the $x$-$y$ plane, and should not be confused with the magnet-based coordinate system in which $B_0$ is considered as being in the ''$z$'' direction and ''$x$-$y$'' is in the transverse plane. These two coordinate systems have no fixed relationship with each other; an image may be made in any orientation with respect to the main field.

Figure 9–9 is a diagram of how these methods are implemented in a spin echo imaging pulse sequence. Time is plotted along the horizontal axis and the rows show when different gradients or RF pulses are turned on and off. The phase encoding gradient is diagrammed as a series of gradient steps, indicating that it is changed each time the pulse sequence is repeated.

### Slice Selection

The simplest application of a gradient field is to limit the excitation of the protons to just one desired slice. If the RF pulse with center frequency ($f_0$) has only a small bandwidth ($\Delta f$), then with a $z$-gradient ($G_z$) turned on, only a narrow band in $z$ with a width $\Delta z = \Delta f / G_z$ will be excited. That is, for spins above or below this slice, the resonant frequency is either too high or too low to be excited by the RF pulse, so that only the magnetization in the band $\Delta z$ is tipped over to produce a signal.

### Frequency Encoding

After the 90 degree excitation pulse, the $z$-gradient can be turned off, and only the selected slice will produce a

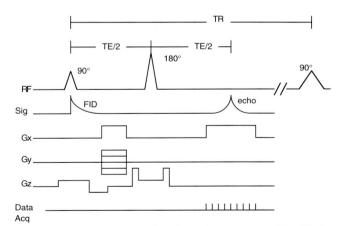

**FIGURE 9–9.** The spin echo imaging pulse sequence. The 90 degree RF pulse creates a free induction decay signal (which is not measured) and the 180 degree RF pulse creates an echo of that signal at time TE. Data acquisition is centered on the echo time. Field gradient pulses along different axes are used for slice selection in $z$, for frequency encoding in $x$, and for phase encoding in $y$. The entire pulse sequence is repeated after a repetition time TR, and with each repetition the phase encoding gradient is changed to a new value.

signal. The *x*-axis then is frequency encoded by turning on an *x*-gradient during data collection (sometimes called a *read-out gradient*). In this way, each spin will precess with a frequency (*f*) that is proportional to its position along *x*. The net signal therefore is a sum of many individual signals with different frequencies, and the amplitude of each frequency can be determined from the data by the mathematical operation of a Fourier transform (discussed in more detail later). The signal at each frequency is the total signal at the corresponding position *x* summed over (or projected along) *y*.

## Phase Encoding

Phase encoding is a more subtle technique. The procedure is to turn on a gradient field in *y* after the slice select gradient in *z* and before the frequency encoding gradient in *x*. The gradient is left on for a few milliseconds and then turned off. While the gradient is on, protons at a positive *y* position will precess faster than those at negative *y*, so a linear variation in phase along *y* will develop. Once the *y*-gradient is turned off, all spins again will precess at the same rate but the linear phase variation will be locked in. When the data are read out, with the *x*-gradient on, the total signal measured for each position *x* is a sum of all the signals on a line running in *y* at that value of *x*. Because of the locked-in phase variations, these signals will not add coherently; there can be some cancellation. Subsequently, the whole pulse sequence is repeated, but with a different *y*-gradient strength. Again the result of the frequency encoding will be to give a summation of all the signals along *y* at each *x* position, but because the phase variation along *y* is now different, in effect the signals are added with different weighting factors. By stepping through 128 different phase encoding gradient strengths, the signal along a *y*-projection can be separated into 128 distinct values.

In fact, the results of phase encoding and frequency encoding are mathematically identical (Fig. 9–10). With fre-

quency encoding, data collection consists of a series of measurements that sample the total signal with an interval Δ*t* between samples. With each successive sample the phase difference between signals from different locations increases because the gradient is on for a longer time. With phase encoding, the sampling can be thought of as occurring every TR (instead of Δ*t*) as the pulse sequence is repeated and the phase encoding gradient is increased to the next value. For each phase encoding sample the amplitude of the gradient pulse is increased but the duration is the same. However, increasing the amplitude with a constant duration has the same effect on the local phases as increasing the duration with constant amplitude (as in frequency encoding); the relative phase changes are determined just by the product of amplitude and duration. Thus, the samples measured every TR with different phase encode steps are exactly analogous to the samples measured every Δ*t* with frequency encoding. Just as frequency encoding yields data that are the Fourier transform of the signal distribution in *x*, phase encoding yields data that are the Fourier transform of the signal distribution in *y*.

## Spin Echo Imaging Pulse Sequence

The key features of the pulse sequence diagram in Figure 9–9 are the timings of the RF pulses and the gradient pulses used for slice selection, frequency encoding, and phase encoding. A few additional gradient pulses also are included in the diagram: (1) the *x*-gradient pulse between the 90 degree and 180 degree RF pulses, called the *x-compensation pulse,* (2) the negative *z*-gradient pulse immediately after the first slice selection gradient, called the *z-compensation pulse,* and (3) the large *z*-gradient pulses before and after the second slice selection pulse, sometimes called *crusher pulses.* These additional pulses are involved in producing *gradient recalled echoes* (GRE) and in *gradient spoiling.*

### Gradient Spoiling and Gradient Echoes

If a gradient pulse is applied after an RF excitation pulse, spins at different positions along the gradient axis will precess at different rates. The net effect of the gradient pulse is thus to produce a large dispersion of phase angles, and the net signal is severely reduced *(spoiled)*. However, if an opposite gradient pulse is then applied for the same duration, each spin will acquire a phase angle opposite to the phase it acquired during the first pulse (Fig. 9–11). The phase dispersion therefore is removed, and all spins add coherently to produce a strong signal called a *gradient recalled echo.* If a 180 degree RF pulse is placed between the two gradient pulses, the two gradients must have the same sign for a gradient echo to occur. The 180 degree RF pulse will reverse the phase of each spin group, and the second gradient pulse will then bring them back into phase.

### x-Compensation Pulse

The *x*-compensation pulse is used to create a gradient echo at the center of data collection. At the middle of the read-out gradient the newly acquired phase of each group due to the read-out gradient just balances the phase acquired from the *x*-compensation pulse. All spins are back in phase, and the net signal again is large, creating the gradient echo. All this is done because the data samples

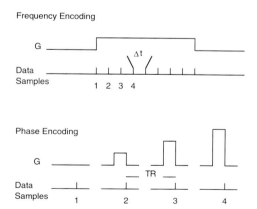

**FIGURE 9–10.** Comparison of frequency encoding and phase encoding, showing the essential similarity of the two encoding processes. In frequency encoding, successive data samples are separated by a time interval Δ*t*, and for each sample the phase effects of the gradient are increased because the gradient has been on for a longer time. In phase encoding, data samples are separated by a time TR, and for each successive sample the phase effects are increased because the amplitude of the gradient pulse is increased. Because the phase changes produced by a field gradient pulse are proportional to the product of the gradient amplitude and duration (the area in this diagram), the signal measured in corresponding samples is the same.

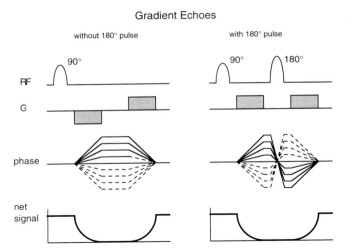

**FIGURE 9–11.** Gradient recalled echoes (GRE). A field gradient pulse creates phase changes proportional to the spin's position, and the resulting phase dispersion spoils the signal. A second opposite gradient pulse brings the spins back into phase and creates a gradient echo. If a 180° RF pulse occurs after the first gradient pulse, the phase of each spin is reversed, and a second gradient pulse with the same sign as the first then will create the gradient echo.

near the time when all of the spins are in-phase are critical for reconstructing the image. Without the $x$-compensation pulse these samples would occur at the beginning of the read-out gradient. In practice a gradient cannot be turned on instantly; some time is required for it to ramp up and stabilize. For this reason it is desirable that these samples occur in the center of the read-gradient window. By adjusting the strength (amplitude times duration) of the $x$-compensation pulse the time of the gradient echo can be shifted.

Note that there are thus two echoing processes involved in an imaging spin echo pulse sequence. The $x$-compensation gradient is adjusted so that the gradient echo occurs at the center of data collection, and the timing of the 180 degree pulse also is adjusted so that the RF echo occurs at the same time. If the time of the RF echo is deliberately shifted from the time of the gradient echo, the resulting pulse sequence is referred to as an *asymmetric spin echo*. Asymmetric spin echo pulse sequences can be useful for chemical shift imaging, such as fat-water separation. Because the fat and water magnetizations precess at slightly different frequencies, the relative phase difference between the fat signal and the water signal is proportional to the time shift between the RF echo and the gradient echo. By adjusting the time shift so that fat and water are 180 degrees out of phase, the signals will subtract, and tissues containing both fat and water (such as vertebral marrow) will be dark in the MR image.

### z-Compensation Pulse

The $z$-compensation pulse is necessary because spins at different $z$-positions within the slice are getting out of phase with each other as they precess during slice selection. Reversing the gradient and leaving it on for the right amount of time will bring all the spins back in phase; a spin that acquired a phase $\phi$ during the slice selection pulse will acquire an additional phase $-\phi$ during the compensation pulse. In other words, another gradient echo occurs. The

only difference between this gradient echo and the one formed by the $x$-gradient is that there is no 180 degree pulse between the two gradient pulses to reverse the first phase, so the sign of the gradient must be reversed. For the 180 degree slice selection gradient pulse there *is* a 180 degree pulse in the center, so this gradient is automatically compensated.

### Crushers

The crusher gradients are designed to eliminate problems associated with imperfect 180 degree RF pulses. If the refocusing pulse is not exactly 180 degrees, some new transverse magnetization will be generated, and the signal produced will create artifacts in the image. The large gradient pulse after the 180 degree RF pulse will produce a large phase dispersion in the unwanted magnetization and thus crush (or spoil) the net signal. In order not to crush the desired transverse magnetization generated by the 90 degree RF pulse, a second large gradient pulse must be put before the 180 degree RF pulse. Then these two crusher gradients create a gradient echo of the desired magnetization and thus have no effect on the desired signal.

## Fourier Transforms and *k*-Space

### *k*-Space

At the heart of the imaging process is the concept of the Fourier transform.[10] Any signal that is a function of time can be decomposed into a sum of contributions of simple sine waves with different frequencies and amplitudes (Fig. 9–12). The signal can be specified either as a series of amplitudes at different time points (referred to as the *time domain*) or as a series of amplitudes of different frequency components (the *frequency domain*). The Fourier transform (FT) is the mathematical procedure for calculating the amplitudes in one domain given the amplitudes in the other domain, and time and frequency are called an FT pair. Figure 9–12 shows how a time domain function can be approximated by adding up the contributions of a limited range of frequencies. With only a few of the low frequencies, the approximation is poor, large ripples are apparent, and small details cannot be seen. But as higher frequencies are included, the approximation improves and finer detail can be seen.

In a similar way we can consider the distribution of magnetization along a spatial direction $x$ as the sum of many sine waves with different amplitudes and spatial frequencies $(k_x)$, where $k_x$ is 1/wavelength. Spatial position $(x)$ and spatial frequency $(k_x)$ also form an FT pair. These one-dimensional arguments can be expanded to describe a two-dimensional FT between an image space with coordinates $(x,y)$ and a $k$-space with coordinates $(k_x,k_y)$, as illustrated in Figure 9–13. Because the measured local magnetization is a vector quantity it is described by two numbers: a magnitude and a phase. The image space thus consists of a magnitude image and a phase image, with the phase image reflecting the local precessional phase at the center of data collection. In conventional MR imaging, only the magnitude image is displayed, but with some pulse sequences the phase image can contain information on local velocity or field offsets.

Each point in $k$-space represents the amplitude of a par-

## Fourier Transforms

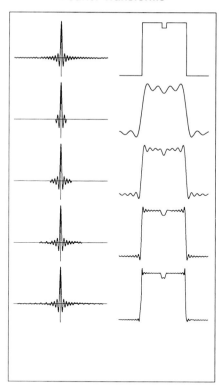

**FIGURE 9–12.** Fourier transforms. Each pair of curves is a Fourier transform pair. The curve in the top right could be a spatial distribution of signal intensity. The curve on the left then shows the contribution of different spatial frequencies. To represent the original spatial distribution curve completely, an infinite number of frequencies would be required. Successive plots show how increasing the number of spatial frequencies included provides a better approximation to the curve. Note in the bottom pair that even with a large number of frequencies a characteristic overshoot occurs at sharp edges (Gibbs phenomenon).

## Symmetry of k-Space: Partial Fourier Imaging

For an ideal situation in which all of the signals generated in the imaged volume are in phase, k-space is symmetric so that only the upper (positive $k_y$) or lower (negative $k_y$) halves need to be measured. This is the basis of the partial Fourier techniques, in which only 50 or 75 per cent of the $k_y$ values are measured and the imaging time is correspondingly reduced. Similarly, the partial echo techniques measure only a fraction of the $k_x$ values, and the others are calculated from the assumed symmetry of k-space. In practice the assumption of perfect symmetry usually is not true. However, by imaging somewhat more than half of the k-space plane (e.g., 75 per cent of the $k_y$ lines or 60 per cent of a full echo) corrections can be made for the imperfect symmetry.

## Fast Imaging: Fast Spin Echo and Echo Planar Imaging

It often is helpful in understanding novel schemes for faster imaging to examine how these methods sample (or measure) k-space. In conventional imaging one line in k-space is measured with each repetition of the pulse sequence (each phase encode step moves the sampling to a

ticular spatial pattern: the point at ($k_x, k_y$) corresponds to a spatial pattern in which intensity varies sinusoidally in the x direction with frequency $k_x$ and in the y direction with frequency $k_y$ across the entire image plane (Fig. 9–14). Thus, the amplitude of each point in k-space affects the intensity in all parts of the image.

**Measuring k-Space.** Consider now what happens during frequency encoding in MR imaging. When the frequency encoding gradient is on, the frequency of the MR signal generated at x is proportional to x, so that as the data are collected the net signal as a function of time is a sum of contributions from many frequencies. The FT of the net signal will give the distribution of amplitudes at different frequencies, and thus at different x positions. Therefore, the net signal measured as a function of time can be directly interpreted as the spatial FT of the image. Similarly, the FT of the phase encoded data gives the spatial distribution in y. Imaging consists of measuring a matrix of values in k-space, and this matrix is then Fourier transformed to produce the reconstructed image. With each phase encoding step a new line is measured in k-space. The matrix of measured k-space values (e.g., 128 × 256) will produce the same size matrix of image pixel values.

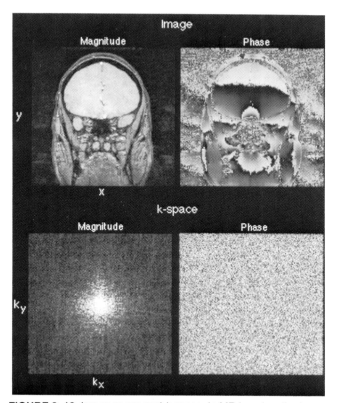

**FIGURE 9–13.** Image space and k-space. In MR imaging, the image domain consists of a magnitude and a phase at each point. The magnitude is proportional to the amplitude of the local transverse magnetization, and the phase is the precessional phase of the magnetization at the center of data acquisition. The two-dimensional Fourier transform of the image domain is called the k-space representation of the image, which consists of a magnitude and a phase for each spatial frequency. In standard MR imaging, one line in k-space is measured each time the pulse sequence is repeated, and the image is then calculated by computing the Fourier transform.

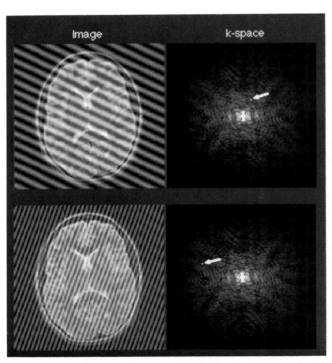

**FIGURE 9–14.** The contribution of a single point in *k*-space to the image. Examples illustrating how a single point in *k*-space represents the amplitude of a particular spatial frequency and produces a wave pattern that extends over the entire image. In each example the point marked with an arrow in the *k*-space representation was increased to create the artifactual images.

new *k*-space line). Full measurement of a *k*-space matrix with 128 $k_y$ values then requires 128 TR periods. With the *fast spin echo* technique, several lines in *k*-space are measured in each TR interval by creating multiple echoes with 180 degree pulses and applying a different phase encoding pulse to each echo.[11] For example, if an echo train of eight echoes is used, the required imaging time is reduced by a factor of eight. In *echo planar* imaging the gradients are switched so rapidly that the entire *k*-space is sampled with the signal generated by just one RF pulse, leading to the acquisition of the full image in a few tens of milliseconds.[12] Echo planar imaging requires special hardware.

## Image Properties

As described earlier, MR imaging can be viewed as measuring a matrix of values in the *k*-space (Fourier transform) of the image. This matrix usually is adjustable, but changes produce changes in resolution, field of view, and signal to noise ratio in the reconstructed image.

### Resolution

Image resolution is determined by the highest spatial frequencies that are measured and thus depends on how far out in *k*-space sampling is done (Fig. 9–15). The high spatial frequency samples are measured when the gradient effects are at their maximum: either the largest gradient amplitudes used in phase encoding or the last samples with the longest gradient duration in frequency encoding.

Resolution also can be understood by considering that if two regions that are very close together are to be distin-

guished, there must be some measured data sample in which the signals from the two points have a phase difference of at least 180 degrees. Otherwise the two signals always will add approximately coherently and there will be no detectable difference in their signals. For frequency encoding, the phase difference of the signals from two nearby points is greatest in the last data sample, when the gradient has been on for the longest time. The resolution ($\Delta x$) is then the distance between two points such that their phase difference in the last data sample is 180 degrees.

### Field of View

The field of view is determined by the spacing of the measurements in *k*-space (Fig. 9–15). Phase considerations also clarify this concept. Consider the data sampling that is done during frequency encoding, in which samples are separated by a short time interval $\Delta t$. For the first sample, all of the signals from different regions are in phase. For the second sample (after a delay $\Delta t$), however, phase differences will develop. If we compare the phase of the signal at a particular point with the phase at other points, the phase difference will be greater as the distance between the points increases. For a particular distance $L = 1/G_x\Delta t$ the phase difference acquired during $\Delta t$ is 360 degrees. This point therefore is back in phase with the first point, and for all subsequent samples it will just go through another complete rotation. As a result, these points are indistinguishable in our data; there is never a time when they are out of phase. The signals from these two points will thus be mapped to the same pixel in the image. This is the *wrap-around* artifact (or *aliasing*), and it appears as if the part of the image that continues beyond an edge were just cut off and pasted onto the other side.

### Signal to Noise Ratio

In MR imaging, noise enters the data uniformly at all frequencies (usually) and is unrelated to the signal itself. Provided that the RF filter is matched to the data sampling interval $\Delta t$, the following equation can be used to gauge the cost of different imaging choices on signal to noise ratio (SNR):

$$\text{SNR} \approx V \sqrt{n_s\Delta t}$$

where $V = \Delta z\Delta x\Delta y$ or the voxel volume (the product of the slice thickness and the resolutions in $x$ and $y$) and $n_s = n_x n_y n_{avg}$ or the total number of data samples (the product of the number of frequency encoding samples, the number of phase encoding steps, and the number of averages). For volume imaging (discussed later), $n_s$ also includes a factor $n_z$, the number of phase encoding steps in $z$.

Thus the reason for the extreme cost of high resolution imaging becomes obvious: cutting each of the voxel dimensions by a factor of two directly decreases the signal to noise by a factor of eight due to the factor $V$. To recover the original signal to noise ratio, the number of averages (and thus the imaging time) would have to be increased by a factor of 64.

Other changes in the acquisition parameters also affect the signal to noise ratio. Increasing the total data collection time ($T = n_x\Delta t$) increases signal to noise ratio. This is often done on the second echo of a double spin echo and is described as a *reduced bandwidth* acquisition. Note also that increasing the number of phase encoding steps with the

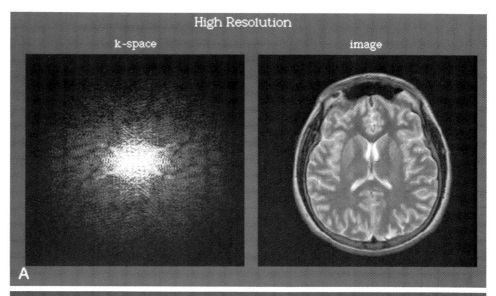

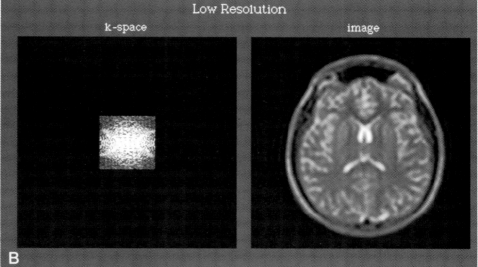

**FIGURE 9–15.** Resolution and field of view are determined by which points in *k*-space are measured (or sampled). **A,** A conventional high resolution image with normal *k*-space sampling. **B,** Only the central, low spatial frequencies are sampled, decreasing the resolution. **C,** Only every other point in *k*-space is sampled, decreasing the field of view and causing a wrap-around (or aliasing) artifact.

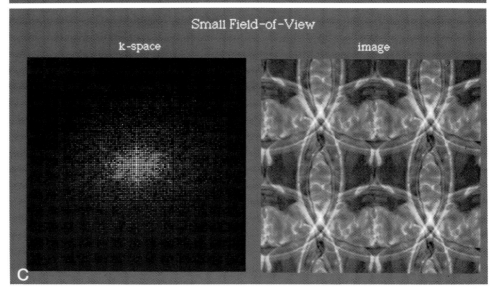

same $y$ resolution has the same effect as increasing the number of averages. That is, an image with 128 phase encoding steps and two averages and an image with twice the field of view (256 phase encoding steps) and one average have the same resolution, signal to noise ratio, and total imaging time, yet the second actually provides more information and will eliminate wrap-around problems by imaging a larger field of view. Often it is desirable to eliminate wrap-around problems along the frequency encoded axis by oversampling the data within the data collection window. For example, if $n_x$ is doubled and $\Delta t$ is halved, the field of view in $x$ is doubled without changing the total data collection time, the $x$ resolution, or the signal to noise ratio.

## Other Imaging Options

### Saturation Pulses

Presaturation is a useful way to suppress the signal of unwanted spins. Presaturation involves applying a selective 90 degree RF pulse followed by a strong gradient pulse before the imaging pulse sequence is started. In this way the chosen spins are tipped over and the signal is spoiled with the gradient pulse. If the imaging sequence is started (e.g., a standard spin echo) there will be very little recovery of magnetization of the presaturated spins so they will not contribute to the image. *Spatial presaturation* (e.g., above and below the desired image field of view) can be used to decrease wrap-around artifacts or prevent flow artifacts by suppressing the inflowing blood signal. *Frequency selective presaturation* can be used to suppress fat, exploiting the chemical shift difference of 3.5 ppm in resonant frequency between fat and water.

### Magnetization Transfer

A recent addition to MR is the use of magnetization transfer contrast, which makes use of the fact that in tissues the H being imaged consists of two exchanging pools: freely mobile water protons and restricted motion macromolecular protons. Although the center resonant frequencies of these two groups are the same, the restricted protons have a much shorter T2 and thus a much broader resonance. Consequently, the magnetization due to the restricted pool can be tipped by a much wider range of frequencies. An RF pulse applied slightly off-resonance thus will saturate the restricted protons but not affect the free protons. However, if the two pools exchange protons rapidly enough, the free protons also become saturated. As a result, there is additional tissue contrast when imaging the free pool that depends on the rate of exchange between the two pools in different tissues.[13]

## PRINCIPLES OF GRADIENT RECALLED ECHO IMAGING

Although SE imaging still is the standard for most clinical applications, a number of useful imaging techniques have been developed based on gradient recalled echoes.[14] In gradient recalled echo imaging there is only one RF pulse, and the flip angle may vary from 5 degrees to 90 degrees. The pulse sequence looks like the spin echo pulse sequence except that the 180 degree pulse and associated gradients are removed, and the sign of the $x$-compensation gradient is switched so that the gradient echo still will form. The term "gradient echo imaging" is somewhat unfortunate, because it suggests that this method uses gradient echoes instead of RF echoes. There is no RF echo in gradient recalled echo imaging, but as mentioned earlier, gradient echoes are an integral part of spin echo imaging as well. The difference would be better described in the following manner: spin echo imaging uses RF and gradient echoes, whereas gradient recalled echo imaging uses only gradient echoes. The primary advantage that comes from eliminating the 180 degree pulse is that TR can be made very short (even less than 10 msec) without causing significant RF heating in the patient.

With imaging times as short as a few seconds, motion artifacts due to respiration can be reduced significantly by collecting the entire image during one breath-hold. Alternatively, three-dimensional volume acquisitions can be collected in a few minutes. Rapid sequential images make it possible to follow the kinetics of administered contrast agents, opening an area of MR imaging studies analogous to nuclear medicine studies.

In addition to the advantages of short imaging times, gradient echo images show a unique sensitivity to the relaxation times T1 and T2, to magnetic field inhomogeneities (T2* effects) and chemical shift effects, and to motion (flow and diffusion). This sensitivity sometimes is merely a source of artifacts, but when exploited in a controlled way it can provide new sources of tissue contrast or methods for rapid quantitative measurements.

## Steady-State Free Precession

The bare bones of a gradient recalled echo imaging pulse sequence are simply a series of RF pulses, each with flip angle $\alpha$, separated by a repetition time TR. If TR>>T2, the physics of this situation is similar to that in the conventional spin echo pulse sequence (except the 180 degree refocusing pulse has been removed): the signal is composed only of transverse magnetization generated by the most recent RF pulse. However, for fast imaging, the TR usually is shorter than T2, which introduces a new feature. Each pulse still produces new transverse magnetization, but the transverse magnetization from previous RF pulses will not have decayed away completely. Different components of this previous transverse magnetization will have acquired different phases due to local field offsets (e.g., applied gradients, main field inhomogeneity) so that this old transverse magnetization may be incoherent. If these field offsets are the same during each TR period, however, the RF pulses will create echoes of the previous transverse magnetization at multiples of TR (Fig. 9–16). (Although 180 degree pulses produce the strongest echoes, smaller RF pulses also create echoes.) These echoes will add to the new transverse magnetization from the most recent RF pulse, creating a strong coherent signal immediately after each pulse. Also, the echoes combine to create a coherent signal just before each RF pulse.

After a number of pulses the magnetization will approach a steady state in which the signal pattern is repeated in the same way during each TR period. In this condition of *steady-state free precession* the coherent signals after the RF pulse ($M^+$) and before the RF pulse ($M^-$) both are

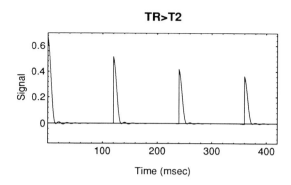

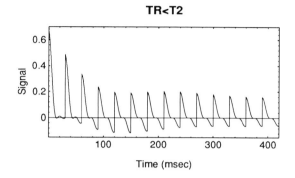

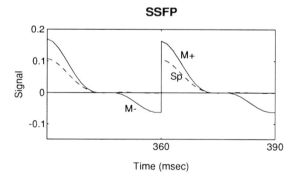

**FIGURE 9–16.** Steady-state free precession (SSFP). The development of the SSFP signal is illustrated for a series of 45 degree RF pulses applied to a sample with T2 = 60 msec for TR = 120 msec (top panel) and TR = 30 msec (middle panel). With TR > T2, each RF pulse generates a new signal, and after a number of pulses a steady-state is reached in which the signal produced after each pulse is the same. With TR < T2, each RF pulse still creates new transverse magnetization but also produces echoes of previously created transverse magnetization. The negative amplitude of the echoes means that the echo forms on the opposite axis from the initial free induction decay (e.g., if the free induction decay is on the $+y$ axis, the echo will be on the $-y$ axis). After a number of pulses the system approaches a steady state (bottom panel) in which a coherent signal forms both before ($M^-$) and after ($M^+$) each RF pulse. $M^-$ consists solely of echoes, whereas $M^+$ consists of echoes plus the most recent free induction decay. If the echoes are spoiled ($Sp$; dashed curve) the signal consists only of the most recent free induction decay. Fast gradient recalled echo imaging pulse sequences differ by whether the signal being imaged is the new transverse magnetization *(Sp)*, the echoes ($M^-$), or both ($M^+$).

constant. For long TR the echoes are severely attenuated by T2 decay and $M^-$ is not detectable, but as TR is shortened the $M^-$ signal becomes appreciable.

### Basic Types of Fast Imaging

Thus several sources of signal exist that can be imaged: the most recent transverse magnetization and echoes of previous transverse magnetization. The three basic types of fast imaging pulse sequence (spoiled, steady state $M^+$, steady state $M^-$) differ in how they use (or do not use) these potential signals (Fig. 9–17).

#### Spoiled (FLASH, Spoiled GRASS)

Random gradient pulses are added after data collection to spoil the echoes, so the signal is produced solely by the transverse magnetization created by the most recent RF pulse. In its current standard form, FLASH is a spoiled technique, because an additional variable gradient in $z$ (the slice selection axis) is added to the pulse sequence after data collection to act as a spoiler. The phase-encoding gra-

dient, which changes with each pulse, would serve to spoil the transverse magnetization over most of the image. However, because the phase-encoding gradient produces only slight phase changes near the center of the image, an additional variable gradient in $z$ must be added to the pulse sequence to provide spoiling over the entire image and avoid an artifactual brightening in the center where the echoes are not spoiled. To maintain uniform spoiling across the image, each phase encoding pulse is balanced by an equal but opposite pulse after data collection (a *rewinder* pulse). As an alternative to gradient spoiling, some systems use RF spoiling by varying the flip axis with each RF pulse. The magnetization then begins each TR period with a different phase angle and so ends each period with a different phase, preventing the formation of echoes. The spoiled pulse sequence will be referred to as FLASH in the following sections.

#### Steady-State $M^+$ (GRASS, FISP, FAST)

The phase encoding gradient is balanced to prevent partial spoiling, and the coherent signal after the RF pulse is used for imaging. This signal consists of the transverse

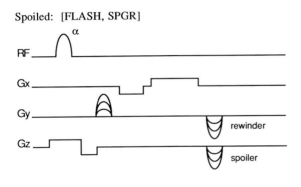

Spoiled: [FLASH, SPGR]

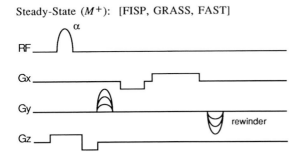

Steady-State ($M^+$): [FISP, GRASS, FAST]

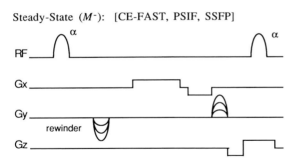

Steady-State ($M^-$): [CE-FAST, PSIF, SSFP]

**FIGURE 9–17.** Gradient recalled echo fast imaging pulse sequences. In a spoiled sequence the echoes are spoiled and only the free induction decay from the most recent RF pulse is imaged. In a steady-state sequence designed to image the magnetization after the RF pulse ($M^+$), the signal consists of both the most recent free induction decay and echoes of past free induction decays. In a steady-state sequence designed to image the magnetization before the RF pulse ($M^-$) the signal consists of only the echoes from previous free induction decays (the most recent free induction decay will not contribute to the signal until after the next RF pulse forms an echo).

magnetization from the most recent RF pulse plus echoes of the transverse magnetization from previous pulses. GRASS, FAST, and FISP are examples of steady-state techniques that image the $M^+$ signal, and in the following sections $M^+$ imaging is referred to as GRASS. When TR>>T2, the FLASH and GRASS methods produce similar images because the echoes are weak, but when TR<T2 the dependence of the signal on the tissue relaxation times is substantially different.

### Steady-State M⁻ (SSFP, CE-FAST, PSIF)

The coherent signal before the RF pulse is used for imaging. The pulse sequence is structured like the GRASS pulse sequence, except that it must run backward in time to image the signal before the RF pulse rather than the signal

after the RF pulse. The unbalanced portion of the slice selection gradient pulse immediately after the RF pulse dephases the most recently generated transverse magnetization, so that the coherent signal before the RF pulse consists solely of the echoes of transverse magnetization from previous RF pulses. SSFP, CE-FAST, and PSIF are examples of pulse sequences that image the $M^-$ signal, and in the following sections $M^-$ imaging is referred to as SSFP.

## Gradient Recalled Echo Imaging Signal and Contrast

### Dependence on Flip Angle

In conventional spin echo imaging, the pulse sequence parameters TR and TE are adjusted to control the signal intensity and, more importantly, the contrast in the image. In gradient recalled echo imaging, the TR is kept short (typically less than 30 msec) to minimize the imaging time and is not used for altering contrast. Fortunately, with gradient echo pulse sequences an additional parameter, the flip angle ($\alpha$),[14, 15] strongly affects the signal and contrast (Fig. 9–18).

Comparing first the two most commonly used methods, the FLASH and GRASS signals show some characteristic patterns. These two curves cross at the peak FLASH signal. This angle is called the *Ernst angle* ($\alpha_E$), and is given by

$$\cos \alpha_E = e^{-TR/T1}$$

For flip angles below the Ernst angle, the FLASH and GRASS signals are nearly identical and are primarily pro-

### Fast Imaging Signal Intensity

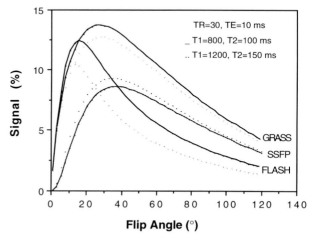

**FIGURE 9–18.** Fast gradient recalled echo imaging signal and contrast. The curves of signal versus flip angle were calculated for TR = 30 msec for the three types of gradient echo pulse sequence (FLASH, GRASS, SSFP). The signal is presented as a fraction of the fully relaxed magnetization. For each method, two curves are shown, one for a tissue with T1 = 800 msec and T2 = 100 msec, and one for T1 = 1200 msec and T2 = 150 msec, each with the same proton density. The GRASS and FLASH curves cross at the Ernst angle ($\alpha_E$). Below $\alpha_E$ there is little sensitivity to T1, and the images are proton density weighted. Above $\alpha_E$ the images are more T1 weighted. Although the signal is greater with GRASS than FLASH, contrast (the difference between the two curves) is better with FLASH. With SSFP contrast is reversed and thus is more T2 weighted.

ton density weighted. The reason the relaxation times do not affect the signal is that with small flip angles the longitudinal magnetization is disturbed only slightly, so recovery by T1 relaxation is relatively unimportant, and the echoes are weak. With larger flip angles, the GRASS signal can be substantially stronger, peaking at a larger flip angle than the FLASH signal. In this regime, the echoes of previous pulses make more of a contribution to the GRASS signal.

The contrast is qualitatively similar, but better (at least in the example in Fig. 9–18) with the FLASH signal. The reason for this is because for equal proton densities, contrast with FLASH is due entirely to T1 differences. T2 does not affect the steady state, because the echoes are spoiled, so the only T2 effect is in the decay between the RF pulse and the read-out period, and TE is assumed to be small. However, with the GRASS signal, echoes make an important contribution. A longer T2 leads to stronger echoes and a stronger signal, but a longer T1 leads to less recovery between RF pulses and a weaker signal. The normal positive correlation between these two relaxation times in vivo thus leads to conflicting contrast effects similar to those encountered in spin echo imaging. Therefore, although the signal with GRASS can be substantially larger than with the FLASH pulse sequence, the contrast is likely to be better with FLASH.

The SSFP signal is composed entirely of echoes from previous RF pulses (the new transverse magnetization produced by an RF pulse will not contribute to the signal until after the next RF pulse). This signal also suffers from the same conflict between T1 and T2 contrast, but the T2 weighting is much stronger than with the GRASS signal. As a result, the signal increases with increasing T1 and T2, so that the contrast pattern is more like traditional T2-weighted contrast than like T1-weighted contrast. However, the magnitude of the contrast still is much less than with the FLASH pulse sequence. Nevertheless, these curves were calculated for equal spin densities, and in practice, proton density often is correlated with T1 and T2 (higher proton density usually leads to longer relaxation times). This would tend to increase the contrast with SSFP, but decrease the contrast with GRASS and FLASH.

### T2* Effects

In addition to the relaxation time effects, gradient echo imaging is more sensitive to variation in the local magnetic field. Because there is no 180 degree refocusing pulse, as there is in SE imaging, any phase changes due to differences in the resonant frequency within a voxel will not be refocused during data collection. Such differences could be attributable to inhomogeneity of the main magnetic field, but even in a perfect magnet the inhomogeneity of the human body will produce field variations owing to *magnetic susceptibility* differences. Magnetic susceptibility is a measure of the degree to which a material becomes magnetized when placed in a magnetic field. The total field inside the material is due primarily to $B_0$, but a small contribution comes from the magnetized material itself. For this reason, field gradients can occur at the boundaries of dissimilar tissues (e.g., bone and soft tissue).

A spread of resonant frequencies within a voxel will lead to a spread of phase angles and a resulting loss in signal. This more rapid decay often is described by a transverse decay constant T2*, which is less than T2. This terminol-

ogy is convenient for characterizing these effects qualitatively, but caution should be used when interpreting T2* quantitatively. This form of the decay may not be a simple exponential, as T2 decay usually is. Also, the transverse decay rate that governs the steady-state signal discussed in the previous section is set by T2, not T2*, because the echoing processes discussed earlier refocus the effects of local field variations. T2* enters because the signal is measured not when the echoes occur (at the time of the RF pulses) but rather at a time (TE) from the echo. In a gradient recalled echo pulse sequence, TE is the time interval between the RF pulse and the gradient echo formed by the read-out gradient pulses. To minimize T2* signal loss, TE usually is kept short. With partial echo techniques the TE can be reduced to just a few milliseconds by shifting the gradient echo toward the beginning of the data collection window.

### Chemical Shift Effect

Gradient recalled echo imaging also exhibits a chemical shift effect because there is no 180 degree RF pulse to refocus phase differences due to the intrinsic difference in the resonant frequencies of water and fat. If a voxel contains both fat and water, the net signal will show oscillations in intensity as TE is changed and the fat and water come in and out of phase (Fig. 9–19). Each species will evolve at its natural resonant frequency for a time TE, so the phase difference between the two signals is $\Delta\phi = \Delta\omega TE$, with $\Delta\omega$ the angular frequency difference between fat and water. The chemical shift difference of fat and water is about 3.5 ppm, and the absolute frequency difference will be proportional to the field strength. For 0.5 T, the oscillation period in the signal versus TE curve is about 13.2 msec and at 1.5 T it is about 4.4 msec. In some situations, these effects will be the dominant source of image contrast, and the signal from a normal tissue with a mixture of fat and water (e.g., bone marrow) can be sup-

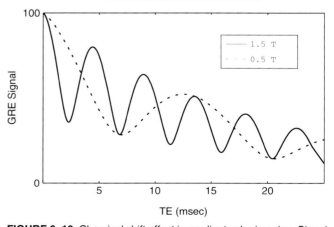

**GRE Chemical Shift Effect**

**FIGURE 9–19.** Chemical shift effect in gradient echo imaging. Signal decay curves for an imaging voxel that contains 30 per cent fat and 70 per cent water are shown for magnetic field strengths of 0.5 and 1.5 T. Because there is no 180 degree refocusing pulse, fat and water come in and out of phase as they precess at different frequencies for a time TE. Because the frequency difference is 3.5 ppm of the resonant frequency, the absolute difference is three times larger at the higher field.

pressed by choosing TE to be a time when fat and water are out of phase.

### Magnetization Preparation

In recent years a new feature has been added to the more conventional gradient recalled echo fast imaging pulse sequences. In the pulse sequences described earlier the magnetization is assumed to start at equilibrium and RF pulses were assumed to be applied for a sufficiently long time that a steady state is produced. (All of the earlier contrast calculations were based on the steady-state assumption.) However, another possibility is to quickly image magnetization that is not in a steady state and thereby produce different contrast in the image. This is done by applying a preparation pulse (e.g., a 180 degree pulse to produce contrast like an inversion recovery sequence) before beginning a series of low flip angle, very short TR (e.g., less than 10 msec) RF pulses for imaging. This process can be broken down further with a segmented $k$-space method by collecting only one half or one quarter of the data needed for an image and then giving another preparation pulse before continuing with the data collection.[16] With schemes like this the order in which the different phase encode steps are collected can affect the resulting image contrast.

### Three-Dimensional Volume Imaging

For clinical purposes it almost always is necessary to acquire images of an entire volume of tissue. Usually this is done by interleaving the pulse sequences, taking advantage of the fact that a substantial dead time exists after the pulse sequence has played out (which requires a little longer than TE) and when the pulse sequence is repeated on that slice (TR). In that dead time, the pulse sequence is started on another slice, and then another until the time TR has elapsed. Although a whole series of slices is acquired simultaneously, the pulse sequence still is essentially a single slice acquisition. An alternative method is true volume acquisition. With volume imaging no slice selection is done (or else a thick slab is excited) and the volume is divided into slices by phase-encoding along the $z$-axis as well as the $y$-axis (Fig. 9–20). The disadvantage of this approach is that many repetitions are required; for each $z$-phase encode step a full set of $y$-phase encode steps must be measured.

### Volume Imaging

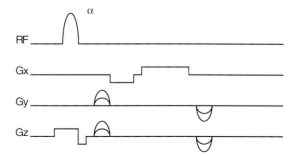

**FIGURE 9–20.** Volume imaging pulse sequence. The slice selective pulse excites a thick slab, and phase encoding is used on both the $y$ and $z$ axes. For each phase encode step in $y$ all of the $z$ phase encoding steps must be measured.

For 64 steps in $z$ and 128 steps in $y$, 8192 TR periods are required. For standard TRs used in spin echo imaging (200 to 4000 msec) the total imaging time is much too long. But with gradient recalled echo imaging, TR can be reduced to less than 10 msec, allowing volume acquisitions in just a few minutes.

Volume imaging has two important advantages over conventional two-dimensional imaging. First, the signal to noise ratio is improved substantially because signal is measured from each voxel on every pulse. With a conventional multislice interleaved acquisition, only a fraction of the total number of RF pulses hit a particular slice. Second, thinner sections can be achieved. With a multislice interleaved acquisition the slice thickness is determined by the slice selective RF pulse and is limited to 2 to 3 mm with conventional gradient strengths. With volume imaging, however, the sections in $z$ are determined by phase encoding, and the phase encoding pulse can be lengthened as needed to produce sections thinner than 1 mm. Signal to noise ratio is severely reduced because of the small voxel volumes, but the intrinsic high signal to noise ratio of the volume acquisition allows high resolution imaging with reasonable signal to noise ratio with an imaging time of 5 to 10 min.

### Flow Effects and MR Angiography

Gradient recalled echo imaging pulse sequences are the basis for most of the MR angiography techniques.[17–19] Two concepts are important for understanding flow effects in fast imaging: *signal saturation,* which produces bright vessels and dark tissue; and *flow compensation,* which corrects for artifacts and phase dispersion due to flow.

### Signal Saturation

With moderately large flip angles and short TR times, the steady-state signal generated is reduced substantially compared to the fully relaxed, long TR signal. To reach this saturated state, however, may require a series of RF pulses over a period longer than T1, and with short TR this could be many pulses. With slice selective imaging, any spins that enter the imaged plane by flow will be relatively unsaturated because they have not felt as many previous pulses as the surrounding stationary tissue. The blood signal, particularly in fast flowing vessels with rapid replacement, thus can be substantially stronger than the signal from the stationary tissue. Furthermore, no flow void artifact is present as in conventional spin echo imaging. In spin echo imaging, with a 90° and 180° pulse, any spins that move out of the selected slice during the interval between the two RF pulses will not contribute to the signal. With gradient echo imaging there is only one pulse, so even if spins subsequently move out of the selected slice they still will contribute to the signal. The large image contrast that can be produced between unsaturated blood and saturated stationary tissues is the basis of the time of flight MR angiography techniques.

### Phase Effects Due to Flow

To make use of the potential increased signal from flowing blood, the phase dispersion effects caused by flow through pulsed gradient fields must be corrected. Consider a pair of gradient pulses such as the compensation gradient

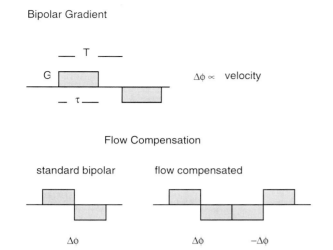

FIGURE 9–21. Phase changes due to flow. A bipolar pair of gradient pulses produces no net phase for stationary spins, but moving spins acquire a phase proportional to velocity. Flow-compensated gradient waveforms eliminate the phase change of spins moving with a constant velocity.

and the read-out gradient used in frequency encoding (Fig. 9–21). The initial compensating pulse is designed to balance exactly the first half of the read-out gradient, so that at the center of data collection all spins are back in phase. That is, the phase acquired by a spin during the first pulse will be exactly opposite to the phase acquired during the first half of the read-out gradient. However, if a spin moves a distance $\Delta x$ in the time between the two pulses, the phases will not balance, leaving a net phase offset at the center of data collection of $\Delta\phi = G\tau T\nu$, where $G$ is the gradient strength (Hz/cm), $\tau$ is the gradient duration, $T$ is the time between the start of the compensating gradient pulse and the start of the readout gradient, and $\nu$ is the velocity. This is just the phase difference resulting from the gradient pulse for two spins separated by a distance $\Delta x = \nu T$ (the distance moved in time $T$).

This effect is the basis for using a bipolar gradient pulse to encode velocity information in the phase of the signal and is used in the *phase contrast* MR angiography techniques. However, this same effect due to motion during application of the imaging gradients can lead to signal loss and artifacts. If a voxel in the blood vessel contains spins with a range of velocities, as it would in normal laminar or turbulent flow, the signals generated by these spins will have a range of phases, thus reducing the net signal. With pulsatile flow, these phase offsets will vary with each RF pulse, leading to motion artifacts along the phase encoding axis.

### Flow Compensation

Phase errors due to flow can be corrected in two ways. First, by minimizing the time $T$ between the compensation gradient and the readout gradient, these effects can be reduced. If the amplitude of the compensation gradient is then reduced, the gradient echo will occur nearer to the leading edge of the readout gradient, further reducing T and thus $\Delta\phi$. With such a *partial echo acquisition,* it often is possible to reduce the phase errors to an acceptable level, although reconstruction of images from these more limited data may require some additional processing.

The second solution to the problem is to add additional gradients to the pulse sequence that will compensate for constant velocity phase errors. With *flow compensated gradients* there effectively are two pairs of gradient pulses. A moving spin acquires a phase $+\Delta\phi$ from the first pair and a phase $-\Delta\phi$ from the second pair. As long as the velocity is constant there will be no net phase at the peak of the gradient echo. Further gradients can be added to compensate for acceleration (and higher derivatives), but in practice velocity compensation usually is sufficient.

By combining the effects of saturation of the signal from stationary tissue with flow compensation to preserve the large, unsaturated blood signal, fast imaging can produce angiograms of acceptable quality with high contrast.

## ARTIFACTS

Many image artifacts can arise when an MR imager is not working properly or is not shielded adequately from outside RF interference. A number of artifacts also can occur with a perfectly functioning MR system whenever one of the two basic implicit assumptions of MR imaging is violated. These assumptions are (1) when no field gradients are turned on, all spins have the same resonant frequency; and (2) each time the pulse sequence is repeated the same local signal is generated.

The first assumption is reflected in the way gradient fields are used for spatial localization, so that both the location of a selected slice and the position along the frequency encoded axis are determined by the precession frequency. Any intrinsic variation in the resonant frequency will lead to spatial distortions. A common example is the chemical shift artifact, in which the fat appears displaced from the water image along the frequency encoded axis because of the intrinsic 3.5 ppm difference in resonant frequency. This shift typically is one or two pixels in the image and can lead to characteristic artifacts at water-fat tissue boundaries: a dark edge where fat has been shifted out of the pixel or a bright edge where fat is shifted onto the adjacent water signal.

Intrinsic differences in precession frequency also arise when the magnetic field is not uniform. This could be due to intrinsic inhomogeneity of the magnet, but current systems usually are quite homogeneous. Instead, magnetic field variations usually are due to the nonuniformity of the human body and the resulting variation in magnetic susceptibility. Metallic implants, some cosmetics, and even tattoos can produce field variations and noticeable distortions of the image.[20] The basic susceptibility differences between air, water, and bone also can produce field nonuniformity at tissue interfaces, leading to subtle image distortions. In effect, the combination of the imaging gradients with intrinsic field variations alters the shape and location of the resolved voxels. For example, an intrinsic local field gradient that adds to the slice selection gradient will shift the position and decrease the thickness of the selected slice locally.

Spatial variations in the resonant frequency will lead to distortions along both the frequency encoded axis and the slice selection axis (e.g., the excited fat and the excited water actually lie in two planes, which are slightly displaced from one another in both $x$ and $z$). Phase encoding, however, is not affected by chemical shift or magnetic field variations. With phase encoding, the *y*-position of a local signal is encoded by the phase change from one repeat of the pulse sequence to the next, whereas with frequency encoding the *x*-position is determined by the phase change from one time sample to the next (i.e., by the frequency).

The second basic assumption of MR imaging is violated whenever the local MR signal changes during data acquisition. Patient motion (twisting, swallowing, and so forth), respiratory and cardiac motion, flowing blood, and cerebrospinal fluid pulsations all lead to a time-varying signal and artifacts in the image. Such motions have only a small effect on frequency encoding, because the data sampling occurs in a very short time (typically about 8 msec). However, the interval between phase encoding samples is much longer (TR), and there is time for substantial motion. Because one line in *k*-space is acquired with each phase encoding step, motion leads to an inconsistent set of data lines in *k*-space. Because each point in *k*-space corresponds to a simple wave pattern over the entire image plane, the image artifacts often are periodic and appear as ghosts shifted along the *y*-axis. It is important to remember that the spatial extent of the ghosts can be much larger than the spatial extent of the actual motion. For example, cardiac motion is limited to the vicinity of the heart, but the artifacts will propagate over the full width of the image.

## SUMMARY

In this chapter the physical principles of MR imaging are reviewed. Nuclei that possess an intrinsic magnetic moment (such as hydrogen) exhibit the phenomenon of nuclear magnetic resonance (NMR). When placed in a strong magnetic field, the nuclear magnetic moments tend to align with the field, creating a local equilibrium magnetization. A second, much weaker, magnetic field oscillating at the resonant frequency (the RF pulse) causes the magnetization to tip away from the main field direction and begin to precess. The precessing magnetization generates a signal in a nearby detector coil. Over time the magnetization relaxes back to equilibrium, and another RF pulse can be applied to generate another signal. The relaxation toward equilibrium is described by two time parameters: T1 is the time constant for relaxation of the longitudinal component of the magnetization, and T2 is the time constant for the transverse component.

MR imaging is based on the fact that the resonant frequency (or precession frequency) is directly proportional to the magnitude of the magnetic field. Gradient coils are used to alter the magnetic field in a controlled way so that the precession frequency varies in a linear fashion along a chosen spatial axis. The techniques of slice selection, frequency encoding, and phase encoding employ gradient pulses to encode the spatial location of the signal in the acquired NMR data. An image of the local magnetization is reconstructed from the data by a mathematical operation called the Fourier transform.

The image intensity is determined both by intrinsic properties of the tissue (e.g., proton density, relaxation times, and flow) and by the timing and amplitudes of the applied RF and gradient pulses (referred to as the pulse sequence). MR imaging is a highly flexible technique, and many pulse sequences are used to create images that differ substantially in signal to noise ratio, acquisition time, spatial resolution, and tissue contrast. Typical pulse sequences include spin echo, inversion recovery, and gradient recalled echo. In addition to providing high resolution anatomic images, MR imaging also is used for angiographic studies and quantitative flow measurements.

## References

1. Purcell EM, Torrey HC, Pound RV: Resonance absorption by nuclear magnetic moments in a solid. Phys Rev *69:*37, 1946.
2. Bloch F, Hansen WW, Packard M: Nuclear induction. Phys Rev *69:*127, 1946.
3. Abragam A: The Principles of Nuclear Magnetism. Oxford Clarendon Press, 1961.
4. Lauterbur PC: Image formation by induced local interaction: Examples employing nuclear magnetic resonance. Nature *242:*190, 1973.
5. Bottomley PA, Foster TH, Argersinger RE, et al: A review of normal tissue hydrogen NMR relaxation times and relaxation mechanisms from 1–100 MHz: Dependence on tissue type, NMR frequency, temperature, species, excision and age. Med Phys *11:*425, 1984.
6. Farrar TC, Becker ED: Pulse and Fourier Transform NMR, Introduction to Theory and Methods. New York, Academic Press, 1971.
7. Hahn EL: Spin echoes. Phys Rev *80:*580, 1950.
8. Wehrli FW, MacFall JR, Glover GH, et al: The dependence of nuclear magnetic resonance (NMR) image contrast on intrinsic and pulse sequence timing parameters. Magn Reson Imaging *2:*3, 1984.
9. Hendrick RE, Nelson TR, Hendee WR: Optimizing tissue contrast in magnetic resonance imaging. Magn Reson Imaging *2:*193, 1984.
10. Bracewell RN: The Fourier Transform and its Applications. New York, McGraw-Hill, 1986.
11. Listerud J, Einstein S, Outwater E, et al: First principles of fast spin echo. Magn Reson Q *8:*199, 1992.
12. Cohen MS, Weisskoff RM: Ultra-fast imaging. Magn Reson Imaging *9:*1, 1991.
13. Balaban RS, Ceckler TL: Magnetization transfer contrast in magnetic resonance imaging. Magn Reson Q *8:*116, 1992.
14. Wehrli FW: Fast scan magnetic resonance. Magn Reson Q *6:*165, 1990.
15. Buxton RB, Edelman RR, Rosen BR, et al: Contrast in rapid MR imaging: T1-weighted and T2-weighted imaging. J Comput Assist Tomogr *11:*7, 1987.
16. Chien D, Edelman RR: Ultrafast imaging using gradient echoes. Magn Reson Q *7:*31, 1991.
17. Finn JP, Goldmann A, Edelman RR: Magnetic resonance in the body. Magn Reson Q *8:*1, 1992.
18. Pelc NJ, Herfkens RJ, Shimakawa A, et al: Phase contrast cine magnetic resonance imaging. Magn Reson Q *7:*229, 1991.
19. Listerud J: First principles of magnetic resonance angiography. Magn Reson Q *7:*136, 1991.
20. Hendrick RE, Russ PD, Simon JH: MRI: Principles and Artifacts. New York, Raven Press, 1993.

# 10

# Magnetic Resonance Imaging: Practical Considerations

*Kevin W. McEnery, M.D., and*
*William A. Murphy, Jr., M.D.*

Since its introduction, magnetic resonance (MR) imaging has had an enormous impact on identification and understanding of the pathophysiology of musculoskeletal disease. As an imaging technology, it is ideally suited for the musculoskeletal system. The ability of MR imaging to demonstrate anatomic and physiologic details in multiple anatomic planes without the use of ionizing radiation continues to distinguish it from other imaging methods. It has enhanced the ability of the musculoskeletal radiologist to determine the exact extent of many soft tissue, bone, and joint conditions. MR imaging has assisted the clinician in the imaging of articulations including the knee, hip, shoulder, and wrist. It has replaced knee arthrography for the imaging of internal derangements and may do the same for wrist arthrography and tenography. In tumors, MR imaging continues to affect positively the routine management of bone and soft tissue tumors. In the determination and accurate identification of tumor margins, MR imaging enables limb salvage procedures to be effectively considered as permissible alternatives to amputation.

The general attributes that make MR imaging an important diagnostic method for the musculoskeletal system include (1) its great sensitivity to physical differences among tissue and fluids; (2) its ability to display these differences as tissue contrast; (3) its capacity to emphasize specific physical properties and manipulate them to accentuate tissue contrast; (4) the ability to select an imaging plane to complement the anatomic plane or pathologic features of interest; (5) its sensitivity to blood flow, which permits visualization of major blood vessels without the need for intravascular contrast agents; and (6) its apparent lack of biologic hazard.

Although MR imaging is particularly sensitive for detection of pathologic processes, it can be relatively nonspecific for determination of the cause of the abnormalities detected. MR images reflect the amount of water, fat, and mineral contained within the tissue of interest. As most pathologic processes manifest as altered morphology or edema (increased tissue free water), MR imaging allows detection of alterations. The cause of the detected abnormality, however, be it tumor, trauma, infection, or other insult, often cannot reliably be determined solely from the MR images. MR imaging has reinforced dependence upon the conventional radiograph, supplemented by clinical history, in the diagnosis and identification of musculoskeletal pathology. The conventional radiograph provides clues to the correct diag-

**TABLE 10–1. Relative MR Signal Intensity of Tissues**

| | T1-weighted | Proton Density–Weighted | T2-weighted |
|---|---|---|---|
| Cortical bone | Very low | Very low | Very low |
| Calcium | Very low | Very low | Very low |
| Yellow marrow | High | High | Intermediate |
| Red marrow | Low | Low | Intermediate |
| Tendon/ligament | Low | Low | Low |
| Fat | High | High | Intermediate |
| Muscle | Intermediate | Intermediate | Low |
| Most tumors | Intermediate | High | High |

noses, which are occult on MR images. Only a naive clinician interprets musculoskeletal MR studies without knowledge of conventional radiographic and clinical findings.

For musculoskeletal imaging, effective use of MR imaging is summarized in two words: signal intensity. Whether traditional spin echo, fast spin echo, or two-dimensional (2-D) or three-dimensional (3-D) gradient echo techniques are used, it is the signal intensity derived from the musculoskeletal tissue situated in a static magnetic field, reacting to external radiofrequency, that creates the images. Image quality and, therefore, diagnostic information are related to the magnitude of signal intensity detected after a given sequence of radiofrequency pulsations. In selection of MR imaging parameters, for every parameter change there are tradeoffs and compromises. Often the compromise is in the length of the examination. Effective musculoskeletal imaging involves maximizing image spatial resolution and signal intensity, and balancing this against the practical consideration of reasonable examination length.

MR images depend upon intrinsic tissue parameters that reflect tissue chemical characteristics (Table 10–1). Although phosphorus, nitrogen, and sodium nuclei may be imaged with MR, it is the distribution of hydrogen that is the basis of MR imaging. Even though practical MR imaging is limited to the hydrogen atom, the choice of imaging parameters is complex and crucial to the success of the MR imaging examination. For most purposes, pulse sequences for obtaining imaging data from the musculoskeletal system remain standard spin echo sequences. However, 2-D and 3-D gradient echo, inversion recovery, and fast spin echo techniques often are used. In addition, fat suppression sequences and enhancement of signal intensity provided by the supplementary use of intravascular administration of contrast agents further add to the ability to accentuate tissue contrast.

In image acquisition not only is the pulse sequence important, but other determinants of image quality such as slice thickness, slice spacing, pixel size (field of view), signal bandwidth, and imaging plane need to be considered. There are limitations to these parameters which are related to the specific imaging system employed. Factors inherent to the imaging system are magnetic field strength and gradient strength. In general, a higher field strength system has an advantage over a lower field strength system because of the greater tissue signal that can be obtained for a specific pulse sequence. The lesser tissue signal intensity delivered by a low-field system can be compensated by imaging repeated sequences. This strategy effectively increases the tissue signal, and therefore the image quality, but it also increases the examination length. The gradient strength of the imaging system is important, as it determines the minimum slice thickness that the system can practically distinguish. Steeper gradient strengths theoretically permit thinner slice selection.

The first crude MR images of the wrist were published by Hinshaw and colleagues in 1979.[1] Since then, the anatomy of the knee,[2] shoulder,[3] wrist,[4] elbow,[5] hip,[6] and ankle[7] has been redefined by their multiplanar cross-sectional appearance (Fig. 10–1). With the use of gradient echo techniques and specialized coils, improvement in resolution has been achieved. One study of finger interphalangeal joint anatomy reported a resolution of 200 × 100 microns.[8]

The goals of this chapter are to place MR imaging of the musculoskeletal system in perspective and to define the principles that make it uniquely suited for specific musculoskeletal imaging applications.

## GENERAL PRINCIPLES

In comparison with other methods, MR imaging remains an immature technology that almost certainly has yet to be exploited fully. However, there already are accepted imag-

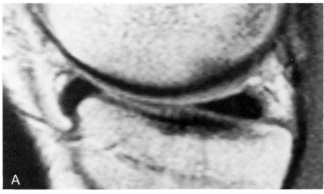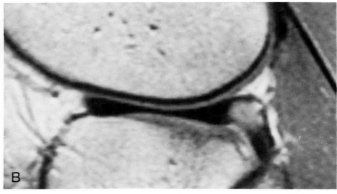

**FIGURE 10–1.** Normal menisci of the knee. Sagittal proton density–weighted (TR/TE, 2500/30) spin echo MR images.
**A** Medial meniscus.
**B** Lateral meniscus demonstrates posterior struts for passage of the popliteus tendon.

ing principles that allow radiologists to use this method effectively for musculoskeletal imaging. The primary aim of musculoskeletal MR imaging is to image the area of interest with the highest possible resolution and signal-to-noise ratio in the shortest examination time. A distinction should be made in determining if the examination is obtained for a ''routine'' indication, such as internal derangement of the knee, or is ordered for evaluation of a suspected bone or soft tissue mass. Examination time should not be an overriding issue in nonroutine applications of MR imaging. However, a routine examination of the knee generally can be completed effectively in 30 minutes or less and it is questionable whether additional pulse sequences are justified when a high sensitivity and specificity are possible with baseline sequences.

When performing MR imaging several choices and trade-offs must be considered. Prior to imaging, the decisions involve selection of the appropriate coil (e.g., body, knee, wrist), the correct anatomic plane (transaxial, coronal, sagittal, oblique), the appropriate slice thickness, the optimal slice spacing (contiguous or noncontiguous), the optimal pulse sequence, and the number of signal excitations to be averaged. In addition to standard spin echo sequences, pulse sequences that rely upon gradient echo techniques, including 2-D and 3-D (volume) acquisition, also are available. These can be supplemented by the use of fat saturation techniques, which are helpful in the evaluation of fat-containing tumors as well as joint derangements, especially those of the shoulder. The availability of gadolinium-enhanced examinations further increases the diagnostic power of MR imaging.

Given the infinite number of imaging parameters, protocols usually are chosen that maintain diagnostic imaging quality while balancing the demands of the patient throughput. These protocols depend on the type of magnet and the specific preferences of the individual radiologist. For most orthopedic examinations, standard imaging protocols usually are sufficient for an adequate examination. In the evaluation of bone and soft tissue tumors, protocols can serve as the initial guide, although the radiologist must tailor the examination based on analysis of the preliminary image data.

The general principles that have guided musculoskeletal MR imaging remain relatively unchanged from initial experience. First, the patient must be positioned in an optimal manner that places the area of interest in the center of the magnetic field. In this location, the magnetic field usually is the most homogeneous and affords the highest quality images. The major axis of the studied part should be parallel to one of the main orthogonal imaging planes, leading to images that can be oriented easily. Also, when images are required in an oblique plane (e.g., for assessment of the shoulder), it is easier technically to establish these nonorthogonal planes if the area of interest is maintained in an orthogonal orientation. The chosen position also must consider patient comfort. Precise patient position is meaningless if that position is uncomfortable and results in motion that decreases resolution and adversely affects the accuracy of the examination.

Second, it is important to select a surface coil that is optimized for the examination of the area of interest. Such coils are mandatory for high resolution musculoskeletal imaging and are available for the knee, shoulder, wrist, and temporomandibular joint. Imaging of the ankle usually is performed with the knee or head coil. For other areas, surface coils including those of the Helmholtz type provide a limited field of view but result in images of high anatomic detail. When imaging of an entire extremity is required, use of the body coil is necessary. With a surface coil, images 3 or 4 mm in thickness (or even less with gradient echo techniques) are possible. However, with the body coil thin section imaging is impractical, with images that are 5 to 8 mm in thickness being more typical.

Third, once a coil has been chosen, it is important to consider how slice thickness, acquisition magnification, and the number of signal acquisitions that are averaged influence signal intensity and resolution. Generally, a choice of thinner slices and greater magnification results in less signal but better in-plane resolution. The maximum resolution depends on several factors that are inherent to the imaging system. The higher the field strength, the greater the signal-to-noise ratio and therefore the smaller the field of view possible (Fig. 10–2). In addition, the gradient strength of the magnet provides potential limitations including the minimal field of view that can be maintained in order to allow an adequate signal-to-noise ratio. An additional factor to be considered is the bandwidth of signal sampling (Fig. 10–3). The lower the bandwidth, the higher the possible signal-to-noise ratio. The cost of a low signal bandwidth is a higher chemical shift artifact.[9]

Tissue contrast is determined by the pulse sequences employed. Spin echo sequences, whose contrast is dependent on both the T1 and the T2 effects of tissue, continue to be used most frequently and are the principal determinant of tissue contrast. While these sequences traditionally take a long time to acquire, they are the sequences to which other sequences are compared.

A final consideration is the use of contrast-enhancing chemical agents, specifically gadolinium compounds. These compounds can be delivered in an intravenous or intra-articular fashion. The purpose of intravenous administration of gadolinium is to enhance vascular tissues, much like the role of iodinated contrast agents used in CT scanning (Fig. 10–4). These agents shorten the T1 relaxation time, resulting in an increased signal intensity on T1-weighted images compared with that in nonenhanced images.

In routine orthopedic imaging there currently is no well-established role for routine use of such contrast agents. A potential role for intravenous administration of gadolinium compounds exists for tumor imaging. Also, there clearly is an important role for such contrast administration in the assessment of the postoperative back, in distinguishing scar tissue from recurrent disc herniation.[10] Reports of intra-articular injection of gadolinium compounds have appeared in the literature,[11–13] but this method currently is not yet officially approved by the Food and Drug Administration.

An often overlooked aspect of MR imaging is the manner in which the images are displayed. Unlike CT in which image window and level settings are constant, standard window and level settings for MR imaging do not exist, because the pixel values reflect the relative signal intensity within the series of images and therefore are not constant.

Safety considerations continue to be a constant concern with MR imaging. These relate to the presence of surgically implanted metallic objects such as aneurysm clips and pacemakers. As most MR imaging examinations are not emer-

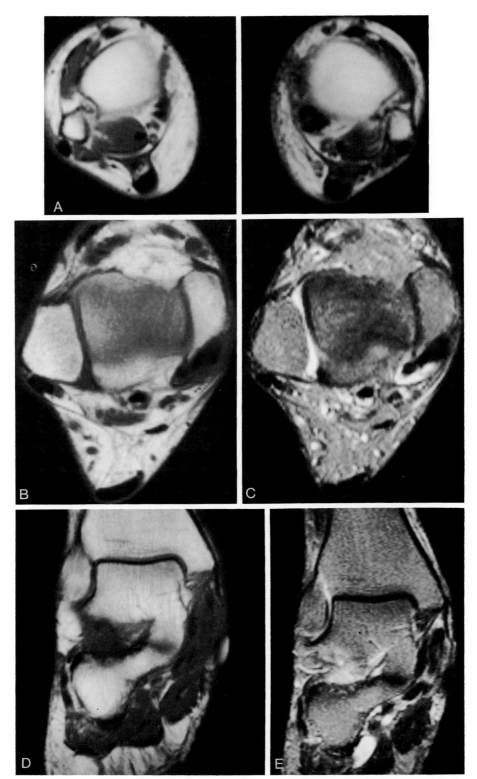

**FIGURE 10–2.** Effect of smaller field of view. Two different patients with abnormal tibialis posterior tendons. (Images photographed with the same relative magnification.) Effect of decreased field of view is to decrease pixel size and therefore increase anatomic resolution.

   **A** Patient with chronic left ankle pain. Transaxial T1-weighted (TR/TE, 600/20) spin echo MR image with both ankles included in imaging field of view. Note inhomogeneous signal and increased size of tibialis posterior tendon, on the left.

   **B–E** Second patient with persistent ankle pain after a fall.

   **B** Transaxial T1-weighted (TR/TE, 600/20) spin echo MR image demonstrates abnormal morphology of the tendon.

   **C** Transaxial T2-weighted (TR/TE, 2500/90) spin echo MR image shows altered tibialis posterior and flexor digitorum longus tendons, representing fluid within the tendon sheaths.

   **D,E** Coronal T1-weighted (TR/TE, 600/10) **(D)** and T2-weighted (TR/TE, 2500/90) **(E)** spin echo MR images reveal increased size and striations within the substance of the tibialis posterior tendon consistent with a type 1 tear. The appearance is difficult to distinguish from chronic tenosynovitis.

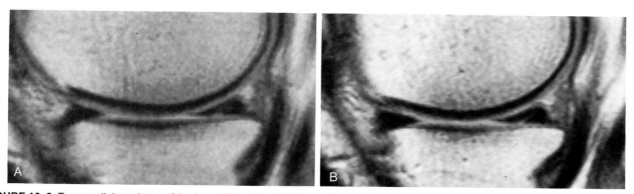

**FIGURE 10–3.** Torn medial meniscus of the knee: Effect of optimizing pulse sequence parameters.
  **A** Sagittal proton density–weighted (TR/TE, 2000/20) spin echo MR image.
  **B** Sagittal proton density–weighted (TR/TE, 2500/20) spin echo MR image with optimal bandwidth and improved presampling for tuning. These images were obtained during the same examination with the same T1 parameters and slice thickness. However, bandwidth was decreased and presampling was optimized to improve signal quality in **B.** The confidence in determining a meniscal tear is improved in **B.**

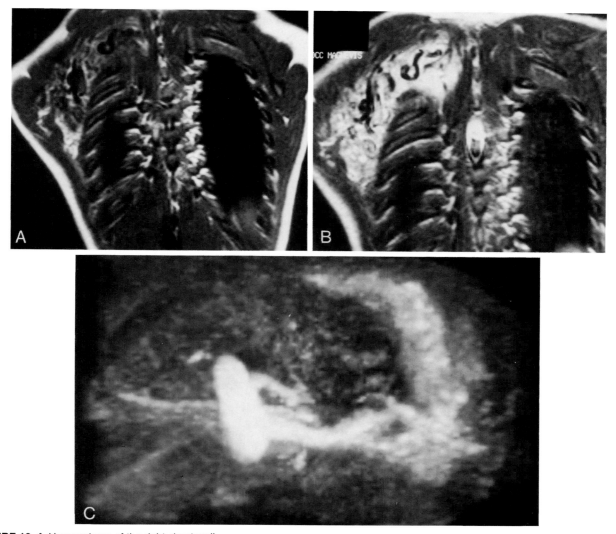

**FIGURE 10–4.** Hemangioma of the right chest wall.
  **A,B** Coronal T1-weighted (TR/TE, 500/15) spin echo MR image **(A)** and identical image after intravenous administration of a gadolinium compound **(B).** An inhomogeneous, low signal intensity soft tissue mass **(A)** shows intense gadolinium enhancement **(B)** consistent with a vascular tumor. Note serpentine-like structure, consistent with arterial vessels.
  **C** MR angiogram after gadolinium administration. In a view from the tip of the head looking downward, the aortic arch is seen, with vessels from the brachiocephalic artery supplying the intensely vascular mass.

gent, time can be taken to determine whether implanted surgical clips are contraindications to examination. MR imaging continues to have an unblemished record of safety for imaging patients with no prior surgical history. Some patients are claustrophobic when placed in the magnet. Relaxation devices such as music headphones can alleviate some concerns, and oral sedatives also are used. MR imaging has no known biologic long-term adverse effect.

## BONE MARROW IMAGING

MR imaging is exquisitely sensitive to changes in bone marrow composition. With few exceptions (aplastic anemia being the major one), all conditions that cause infiltration of marrow lengthen the T1 relaxation time locally and are detected by T1-weighted sequences. Pulse sequences such as short tau inversion recovery (STIR), gradient echo, and fat saturation and the intravenous administration of gadolinium compounds further supplement information derived from spin echo methods.

### Normal Marrow

In most appendicular skeletal sites and in adults, normal bone marrow has high signal intensity on all pulse sequences, related to the high proportion of fat. Marrow fat has the same signal intensity as subcutaneous fat. The signal intensity of the normal marrow appears uniform and homogeneous, except in specific anatomic locations where there is sufficient trabecular bone (load-bearing trabeculae in metaphyseal locations), cartilage (at the physeal plate), or fibrosis (the physeal scar following closure of the growth plate) to cause focally decreased signal intensity. The signal intensity of the marrow varies somewhat from patient to patient but usually is symmetric from one region to another in a given patient. In childhood, epiphyseal (or apophyseal) marrow has greater signal intensity than metaphyseal or diaphyseal marrow, a pattern that may persist in some adults.

It is important to recall that marrow comprises two major cell populations, fat cells and hematopoietic cells. The proportions of these cells vary according to age, anatomic location, and physiologic stimulation.[14–16] Marrow in infants is predominantly hematopoietic (red marrow). With skeletal growth and development, hematopoietic marrow is progressively replaced by fat (yellow marrow), with a proportionately smaller fraction of hematopoietic cells. The epiphyseal and apophyseal growth centers are composed predominantly of yellow marrow throughout life. Hematopoietic marrow tends to be most persistent at the proximal ends of the long tubular bones and in the osseous pelvis, vertebrae, and sternum. Physiologic stresses that require greater hematopoiesis will progressively recruit fatty marrow, reconverting it to red marrow. This can be documented in several hematologic diseases and in progressive skeletal metastases. Some types of anemias (sickle cell disease, thalassemia) may be associated with hyperplastic red marrow.

The patterns of signal intensity of marrow parallel these proportionate changes in yellow and red marrow fractionation and distribution. Fatty (or yellow) marrow has a high signal intensity on T1-weighted sequences, owing to the presence of fat protons. Hematopoietic (or red) marrow has a much lower signal intensity on T1-weighted sequences,

owing to the predominance of water protons. Thus, children tend to have high signal intensity in epiphyses and apophyses because of the large amount of fat and a somewhat lower signal intensity in the metadiaphyseal regions because of the greater amount of hematopoietic tissue. In the mature skeleton, the epiphysis, metaphysis, and diaphysis contain a more homogeneous distribution of cells and have more homogeneous signal intensity. The signal intensity at any time reflects the balance of yellow and red marrow. Overall, the trend is for the T1 relaxation times of marrow to become shorter with aging, as has been measured in the vertebral bodies of persons of various ages, indicating progressive fatty replacement.[17, 18]

With physiologic stresses that cause an increased fraction of hematopoietic (red) marrow, the signal intensity of such marrow on T1-weighted sequences diminishes[19] (Fig. 10–5). Likewise, in aplastic anemia, the observed signal intensity of the marrow is identical to that of otherwise normal yellow marrow so long as the fat fraction persists.[20]

Nearly all pathologic processes of the bone marrow cause lengthening of T1 times, thereby lowering the signal intensity of involved regions relative to surrounding fatty marrow. Thus, T1-weighted pulse sequences are recommended to detect bone marrow lesions and to characterize their extent, although these sequences do not provide diagnostic specificity (Fig. 10–6). T2-weighted images improve diagnostic specificity to a small extent. The appropriate diagnosis of a bone marrow disorder, however, is determined by analysis of the patient's history and the information obtained from the combination of diagnostic tests employed.

The availability of pulse sequences such as STIR and gradient echo has further increased the sensitivity of MR for marrow imaging. The STIR sequence is sensitive to bone marrow alterations because of its property to null the signal derived from fat and highlight any signal origination from other sources. In an individual with normal fat marrow, the STIR sequence causes the marrow to be absent of signal, becoming indistinguishable from cortical bone. Marrow edema is conspicuous with the STIR sequence. However, this sequence has limitations. It is very sensitive to magnetic field inhomogeneities as well as to patient movement, especially with high field strength systems.[21] The STIR sequence has been shown to be sensitive to the extent of tumor involvement in the marrow, but it may lead to an overestimation of this involvement.[21, 22]

Gradient echo images also have been employed to supplement spin echo images. Rather than depending upon the T1 or T2 properties of tissues, gradient echo images rely upon the T2* of imaged tissues.[23] These sequences are very sensitive to local field inhomogeneities, whether they relate to the magnet or arise within the patient. This sensitivity even applies to local field inhomogeneities caused by focal increases in trabecular bone density, as occur within the femoral neck.[23] Such inhomogeneity causes focal loss of signal intensity that may mimic a pathologic lesion or be misinterpreted as evidence of hematopoietic marrow.

### Pathologic Marrow

**Neoplasia.** Metastasis, plasma cell myeloma, leukemia, and lymphoma lead to the replacement of normal bone marrow, resulting in focally decreased signal intensity.[24–26]

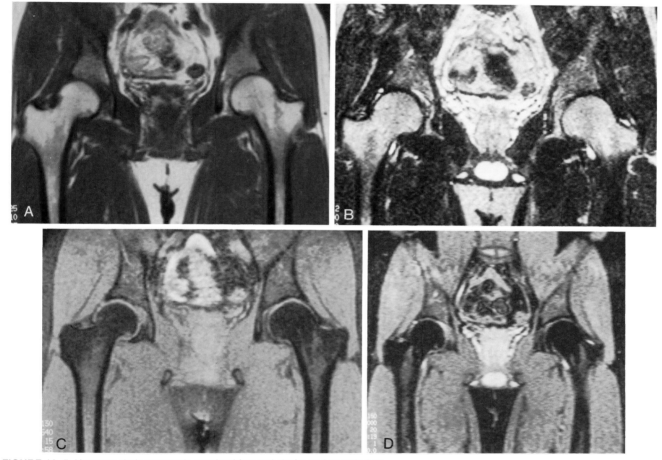

**FIGURE 10–5.** Hematopoietic marrow in proximal femoral shafts and acetabulum.

**A,B** Coronal T1-weighted (TR/TE, 525/10) **(A)** and T2-weighted (TR/TE, 2500/90) **(B)** spin echo MR images. Patchy low signal intensity in femoral shafts and homogeneous low signal intensity in acetabular roof are consistent with hematopoietic marrow hyperplasia. The femoral heads reveal predominantly fatty bone marrow.

**C,D** In a coronal T-weighted (TR/TE, 540/15) spin echo MR image with fat saturation **(C)** and a coronal inversion recovery image (TR/TE, 2000/20; inversion time, 50 msec) **(D)**, the contribution to signal intensity of the protons within fat is decreased. Areas of hematopoietic marrow demonstrate increased signal intensity in a distribution similar to that in **A** and **B.**

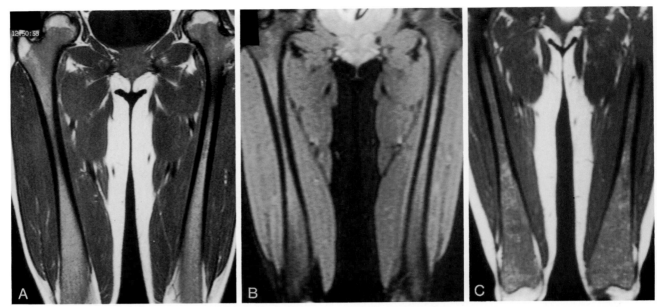

**FIGURE 10–6.** Bone marrow disorders: Gaucher's disease **(A,B)** and polycythemia vera **(C).**
 **A** Coronal T1-weighted (TR/TE, 600/20) spin echo MR image.
 **B** Coronal STIR (TR/TE, 2000/20; inversion time, 150 msec) image.
 **C** Coronal T1-weighted (TR/TE, 600/20) spin echo MR image.
 As the pathophysiology is similar in both these processes, the MR imaging appearances are the same. A relatively homogeneous low signal intensity is seen in the T1 images, reflecting replacement of normal marrow fat. In the STIR image, a homogeneous signal pattern of low signal intensity is seen. In all images, note the Erlenmeyer flask appearance of the distal portion of the femora.

These alterations are related primarily to replacement of the fat cells (with short T1 relaxation times) by tumor cells (with long T1 relaxation times), although other mechanisms including fat necrosis, new bone formation, and fibrosis, contribute to this decrease in signal intensity on T1-weighted pulse sequences.

T1-weighted pulse sequences are used appropriately for detection of tumor in marrow because the differences in contrast between normal marrow and areas of tumor infiltration are greatest with this imaging strategy. If tumor also involves the subcutaneous fat, T1-weighted sequences are optimal for similar reasons. As the repetition time (TR) or echo time (TE), or both, are prolonged, the signal intensities of marrow and tumor become more similar. Therefore, proton density– or T2-weighted sequences are not recommended for the detection of tumorous marrow. Conversely, tumor and muscle may have similar or identical signal intensity (and are difficult to differentiate) on T1-weighted sequences. With prolonged TR, TE, or both, the contrast differences between an extraosseous tumor mass and muscle are exaggerated because the T2 value of tumor is much longer than that of muscle. Thus, proton density– and T2-weighted sequences are useful to achieve this differentiation.

It is clear that MR imaging is a very sensitive method for the detection of malignant infiltration of bone marrow. In this regard, MR imaging is clearly more sensitive than conventional radiographs. It appears that MR imaging is superior to bone scintigraphy in the detection of local areas of marrow infiltration, particularly in patients with multiple myeloma. MR imaging is not well suited to the evaluation of the entire skeleton, however; when a rapid and effective method is required to survey all regions of the skeleton, scintigraphy using bone-seeking radiopharmaceutical agents is the technique of choice. In the assessment of focal areas of marrow infiltration, MR appears to be superior to CT for two major reasons: it provides better contrast resolution between normal bone marrow and tumor, and it allows direct imaging of the long axis of any bone.

Although MR imaging is highly sensitive to the detection of neoplastic involvement of the bone marrow, it must be considered a nonspecific technique. Various neoplastic and non-neoplastic processes characterized by marrow infiltration lead to similar alterations in T1 and T2 values. The differentiation of one type of tumor from another or of neoplasm from infection can be difficult.

**Osteomyelitis.** Owing to alterations in the signal intensity of the marrow cavity, MR imaging has been shown to be exquisitely sensitive to the detection of osteomyelitis.[27–30] As in the case of malignant infiltration, osteomyelitis results in the replacement of normal marrow by inflammatory cells and fluids that have longer T1 values than those of normal marrow and, hence, in decreased signal intensity on T1-weighted sequences and increased signal intensity on T2-weighted and STIR sequences. MR imaging also can assist in the assessment of patients with chronic infection, as focal areas of increased signal intensity are indicative of active infection.[31]

Unfortunately, MR imaging characteristics of osteomyelitis are not specific. In addition to infection, other processes that produce a decreased signal intensity in T1-weighted sequences include surgical alterations, malignant tumors, infarction, and fractures.[32, 33] Furthermore, it is not possible to differentiate a bone abscess from a sterile fluid collection (Fig. 10–7). The addition of T2-weighted sequences does not improve its specificity for the diagnosis of infection. Pyogenic and sterile abscesses, neoplasia, and fractures all result in prolonged T2 values and increased

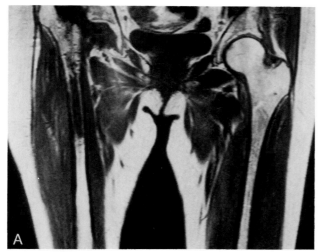

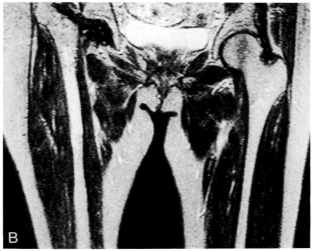

**FIGURE 10–7.** Sterile fluid collection in a patient following total hip replacement and antibiotic therapy. Coronal T1-weighted (TR/TE, 600/10) **(A)** and T2-weighted (TR/TE, 2500/90) **(B)** spin echo MR images. Note a linear band of dark signal intensity within the marrow cavity in **A** and high signal intensity in **B**. This confirms fluid within a cavity that remained following prosthesis removal. The presence of sterile fluid can be determined only by aspiration.

signal intensity of T2-weighted images. In the appropriate setting the typical appearance of fractures and infarction may help distinguish them from other entities.[33] The prolonged T2 values in osteomyelitis probably relate to increased fraction of water and blood in the infected area. The role of gadolinium enhancement in osteomyelitis is uncertain. One study of pediatric patients suggested that the presence of enhancement of signal intensity after the intravenous administration of gadolinium compounds can assist in the identification of areas of active infection, especially in the setting of chronic osteomyelitis.[34]

With regard to imaging strategy, T1-weighted sequences (that maximize contrast differences between normal and altered bone marrow) and images in the coronal and sagittal planes (that display the long axis of bone) are best able to delineate the intraosseous extent of the infection. These can then be supplemented by STIR sequences to accentuate focal marrow edema indicative of infection. In such instances, MR imaging accurately can confirm the presence

or absence of marrow abnormality and define the degree of medullary, cortical, and soft tissue involvement. An MR imaging examination showing only normal marrow is a good indication that osteomyelitis is absent.[27, 35]

A continuing controversy relates to techniques of assessment of the diabetic patient with symptoms of osteomyelitis involving the foot. MR imaging has proven sensitive for this diagnosis.[36] However, the specificity of this technique is diminished by the occurrence of neuropathic osteoarthropathy in patients with diabetes mellitus (Fig. 10–8). In this situation the neuropathic joint can lead to alterations in marrow signal intensity that simulate those of osteomyelitis, with decreased signal intensity on T1-weighted images and increased signal intensity on T2-weighted images.[37] It has been suggested that a pattern of decreased signal intensity on T1- and T2-weighted images adjacent to a joint space is indicative of a neuropathic joint.[38] In our experience, however, neuropathic joints can be associated with MR imaging findings that can clearly mimic those of osteomyelitis (Fig. 10–9). Radionuclide bone scanning suffers from the same lack of specificity, although supplemental agents such as gallium compounds and indium-labeled white blood cells may increase the diagnostic specificity and sensitivity. As such coordinated scintigraphic studies increase both the time and cost of scintigraphy, MR imaging may be more cost effective and time efficient. MR imaging also may allow detection of focal fluid collections (abscesses), which would not respond to conservative therapy and may warrant surgical intervention.

**Devascularization.** Devascularization of the bone marrow may result from a variety of insults, including fracture or dislocation, steroid therapy, sickle cell disease, hyperbaric pressure (caisson disease), and cellular infiltration (e.g., Gaucher's disease) (Fig. 10–10). Although the causative events may vary, the pathophysiologic processes are similar. Interruption of the blood supply leads to necrosis of trabeculae and marrow elements, and typically is followed by a reparative process in which injured tissue gradually is removed and replaced. The conversion of normal marrow rich in fat to necrotic marrow is characterized on MR imaging as a decrease in signal intensity on T1-weighted sequences.

The sensitivity of MR imaging in detecting devascularization of the bone marrow is best documented in processes that involve the femoral head, both in children (Legg-Calvé-Perthes disease) and in adults. In persons of all ages, the signal intensity derived from the normal bone marrow in the femoral head is high except in certain regions that normally possess lower signal intensity (physis, physeal scar, load-bearing trabeculae). In the femoral head (or other sites), devascularization leads to areas of low signal intensity surrounded by adjacent normal marrow of higher signal intensity. The diminution of signal intensity is independent of the selected pulse sequences, although intraosseous cysts or an adjacent joint effusion may lead to an increase in signal intensity as the TR and TE are prolonged. Therefore, the imaging protocol used for detection of ischemic marrow employs a T1-weighted pulse sequence that optimizes the contrast differences between the normal and the necrotic marrow fat. This sequence in children with Legg-Calvé-Perthes disease reveals focally decreased signal intensity in the epiphyseal ossification center. In adults, four basic patterns of femoral head devascularization (homogeneous, in-

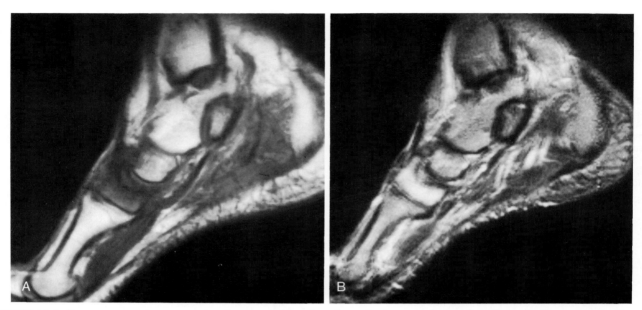

**FIGURE 10–8.** Bone marrow edema secondary to neuropathic osteoarthropathy in an adult diabetic patient with the onset of ankle pain without trauma. There was no detectable soft tissue swelling or ulceration. Plain film radiographs at time of the MR imaging examination were normal. The patient was treated with a protective cast, without antibiotics, with resolution of symptoms. Plain films six months later showed minimal neuropathic changes.

**A** Sagittal T1-weighted (TR/TE, 525/10) spin echo MR image. Decreased marrow signal is seen in the medial cuneiform bone and the ventral aspect of the navicular bone.

**B** Sagittal T2-weighted (TR/TE, 2500/90) spin echo MR image. Increased signal intensity is seen in areas corresponding to those in **A**, consistent with marrow edema.

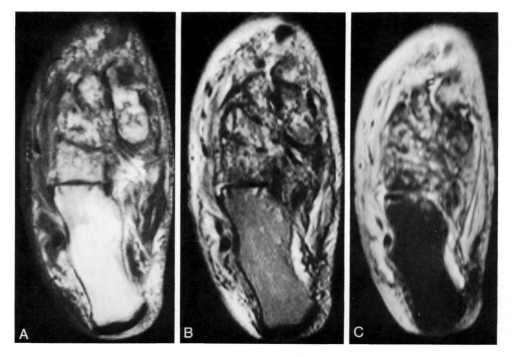

**FIGURE 10–9.** Osteomyelitis in the midfoot of a diabetic patient. A soft tissue ulceration (not shown) was present on the dorsum of the foot.

**A** Transaxial T1-weighted (TR/TE, 600/10) spin echo MR image. Note inhomogeneous, decreased signal intensity in the bones of the midfoot. Decreased signal intensity also is evident in the overlying soft tissues.

**B** Transaxial T2-weighted (TR/TE, 2000/90) spin echo MR image. Increased signal intensity is seen in the same distribution as in **A,** consistent with marrow edema. Overlying increased signal intensity is consistent with soft tissue edema. No drainable fluid collections are identified.

**C** Transaxial STIR (TR/TE, 2000/70; inversion time, 150 msec) MR image. Abnormal increased signal intensity within the bones of the midfoot and within the distal medial calcaneus also are consistent with marrow edema secondary to infection.

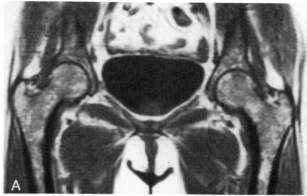

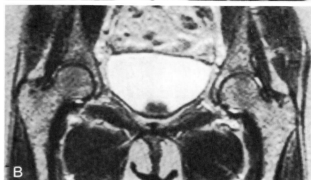

**FIGURE 10–10.** Diffuse marrow infarction in a patient with sickle cell disease.
  **A** Coronal T1-weighted (TR/TE, 600/20) spin echo MR image. Diffuse replacement of fat within the pelvis and femora has resulted in decreased signal intensity, reflecting diffuse marrow infarction. The femoral heads are normal.
  **B** Coronal T2-weighted (TR/TE, 2500/90) spin echo MR image. Patchy increased signal intensity in the marrow is evident.

homogeneous, band, and ring patterns) have been described. Individual patterns do not define the prognostic or therapeutic significance of the condition nor correlate with the clinical stages of the disease.

MR imaging clearly is more sensitive than conventional radiography in the detection of femoral head devascularization (Fig. 10–11). When radiographs are abnormal, MR imaging invariably is abnormal. More important, when radiographic findings appear normal or are equivocally abnormal, MR imaging commonly detects an abnormality. MR imaging is at least as sensitive as bone scintigraphy in the detection of femoral head devascularization. In instances in which the bone scan shows focally decreased or increased accumulation of the radionuclide, MR imaging invariably confirms the abnormality. Furthermore, when radionuclide studies appear normal or are indeterminate, MR may reveal an abnormality. Under these circumstances, a normal MR examination effectively excludes the presence of ischemic bone marrow.

Patients with a devascularized femoral head who undergo core decompression may return with persistent or new pain (Fig. 10–12). Accurate delineation of the cause of the pain is difficult, owing to the inability to distinguish between significant abnormalities in the bone marrow and postsurgical changes, even when both conventional radiographic and scintigraphic examinations are used. MR imaging seems effective in this determination. It shows the core decompression tracts as linear zones of low signal intensity surrounded by normal or abnormal marrow, and it demonstrates persistence, progression, regression, or resolution of devascularized marrow. The ability of MR imaging to allow differentiation among normal findings, postoperative abnormalities, and ischemic bone marrow is not shared by conventional radiography or radionuclide studies.[39] MR imag-

ing also may allow identification of those patients at risk for the development of collapse following core decompression by quantitating the amount of articular surface involved.[40] In one study, the most accurate prognostic sign of clinical outcome was the amount of the articular surface undermined by the zone of avascularity.[41]

MR imaging is sensitive to the detection of devascularization in many other sites of bone marrow, including the humeral head, the bones about the knee, and the carpal bones. In these sites, too, the MR imaging examination is superior to conventional radiography and radionuclide scanning for detection, characterization, and determination of the extent of the process. In most instances MR imaging does not allow identification of the specific cause of marrow devascularization; it reveals only an abnormal marrow (Fig. 10–13). Two factors improve its specificity, however. First, the clinical information and the results of other imaging studies usually limit the diagnostic possibilities. Second, additional pulse sequences may help to distinguish devascularized marrow from that involved in other marrow processes. On T2-weighted images, devascularized marrow remains of low signal intensity, whereas more hydrated tissue (as evident in neoplastic processes) is associated with increased signal intensity.

In practice, the sensitivity of MR imaging to the diagnosis of marrow devascularization exceeds that of conventional radiography and is at least equivalent to that of radionuclide methods. Asymptomatic or symptomatic bone marrow devascularization can be identified with MR imaging when results of other imaging methods appear normal or are equivocal. Furthermore, MR imaging may allow differentiation of devascularized regions from areas of reactive bone formation induced by surgical intervention.

The role of enhancement of signal intensity after the

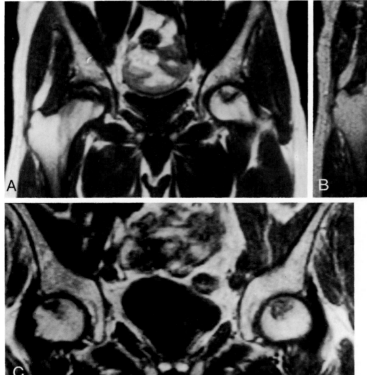

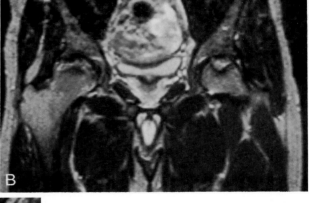

**FIGURE 10–11.** Osteonecrosis of the femoral heads in two patients.

**A,B** Coronal T1-weighted (TR/TE, 600/20) **(A)** and T2-weighted (TR/TE, 2500/90) **(B)** spin echo MR images. Bilateral osteonecrosis is manifested by marrow changes in the superior aspect of the femoral heads. These changes are more advanced in the right hip, with loss of the normal morphology of the femoral head. Radiographs demonstrated partial collapse of this femoral head. In the left hip, images demonstrate infarction that does not change the contour of the femoral head. The edema within the marrow, shown by increased signal intensity in **B**, suggests this is a relatively acute process.

**C** In a second patient, a coronal T1-weighted (TR/TE, 600/20) spin echo MR image demonstrates focal discrete marrow abnormality consistent with osteonecrosis of both femoral heads. There was no increased signal on T2-weighted images, suggesting a chronic process.

intravenous administration of gadolinium compounds in the assessment of suspected ischemic necrosis of bone has not been determined fully. In an animal study in which femoral heads were studied 3 hours after devascularization, the use of intravenous gadolinium administration and dynamic gradient echo imaging was more sensitive to the detection of the earliest perfusion alterations of necrosis, compared with T1-weighted or STIR images.[42] The clinical use of gadolinium in the early hours of avascularity remains questionable, however.

**Transient Osteopenia About the Hip.** This entity was initially described as a form of reflex sympathetic dystro-

phy. However, it subsequently has become known as transient osteoporosis of the hip.[43–45] The clinical presentation, seen more commonly in adults than in children,[46] is one of intense unilateral hip pain and limited range of motion.

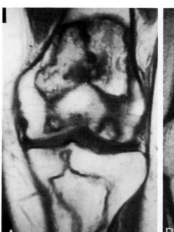

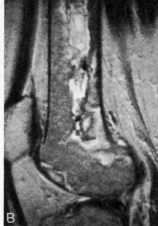

**FIGURE 10–13.** Bone marrow infarction in a patient seen following bone marrow transplant for leukemia, maintained on chronic immunosuppression therapy including steroid therapy.

**A** Coronal T1-weighted (TR/TE, 500/10) spin echo MR image.

**B** Sagittal T2-weighted (TR/TE, 2500/90) spin echo MR image.

MR imaging is sensitive to the changes in bone marrow associated with marrow infarction. This case demonstrates the typical appearance of bone marrow infarction with a linear pattern of dark signal intensity on the T1-weighted image that remains dark on the T2-weighted image but with an adjacent band of high signal intensity.

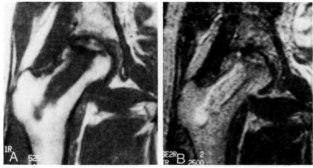

**FIGURE 10–12.** Marrow abnormality in the femoral neck following core decompression for osteonecrosis of the femoral head. Coronal T1-weighted (TR/TE, 525/10) **(A)** and T2-weighted (TR/TE, 2500/90) **(B)** spin echo MR images show wide areas of marrow abnormality in the femoral neck with decreased signal intensity in **A** and increased signal intensity in **B**. There is no evidence of marrow revascularization.

Plain film findings include minimal patchy osteopenia, but often such plain films are normal.[44] On MR images the symptomatic femoral head demonstrates diffuse decreased signal intensity on T1-weighted images consistent with marrow edema (Fig. 10–14). In some reported cases the symptoms spontaneously resolved with no residual effects noted six or more months after the original MR imaging examination. Several studies have indicated that in patients presenting with this diffuse type of marrow edema, conservative therapy results in spontaneous resolution. In patients undergoing biopsy, nonspecific changes are demonstrated—i.e., nonspecific inflammation consistent with marrow edema with no evidence of malignancy.[44, 47] One study of sequential MR imaging examinations noted a migratory pattern of marrow edema that differed from the process of progressive avascular necrosis.[48] However, there is a strong opinion that transient osteopenia is a precursor to avascular necrosis, and surgical intervention with core decompression is warranted.[49] This opinion is supported by results of animal studies.[50] Others have acknowledged that the process of transient osteoporosis cannot be distinguished from the initial presentation of avascular necrosis, and that core decompression limits the duration of symptoms in both disorders.[51]

## BONE TUMORS AND SOFT TISSUE MASSES

### General Considerations

Although much has been written regarding the ability of MR imaging to provide histologic diagnosis in cases of tumor, its prime role is the staging of musculoskeletal neoplasms.[52] Although certain musculoskeletal neoplasms have characteristic MR appearances, the imaging protocols must be designed, not to determine the histology, but rather to allow accurate staging of the tumor (Fig. 10–15). If local excision is considered, the exact margin of the tumor may be accurately assessed with MR imaging.

The most widely accepted system of staging for musculoskeletal tumors is that developed by Enneking and colleagues.[53] It is based upon a triad of tumor characteristics: the histologic grading (G), the site of tumor (T), and the presence or absence of distant metastasis (M) (Table 10–2). This staging system was developed prior to the widespread use of MR imaging and does not directly exploit its imaging capabilities. MR imaging contributes to the precise staging of lesions by allowing detection of extracompartmental involvement. In certain instances MR imaging is useful in showing extracompartmental extent that was not suspected based upon the plain film appearance. The staging of musculoskeletal neoplasms, especially sarcomas, also can be accomplished with the system advanced by the American Joint Committee for Cancer[54] (Table 10–3). This system stages musculoskeletal tumors based upon histologic grade, tumor size, regional lymph node involvement, and metastasis.[54] As applied to this staging system, MR imaging allows determination of the exact size of the lesion and the involvement of adjacent neurovascular structures in a manner that was not possible previously.

In these two staging systems, the dominant determinate of tumor stage is histology. Currently MR imaging contributes only to the substaging of the neoplasm based upon the determination of the size of the lesion. Other techniques such as nuclear medicine continue to serve as the primary screening methods for metastasis (see later discussion). In the future, these staging systems may evolve to incorporate the anatomic information derived from MR imaging. Ultimately, the true impact of MR imaging may relate to the successful use of limb salvaging surgery owing to the availability of anatomic information regarding exact tumor margins.

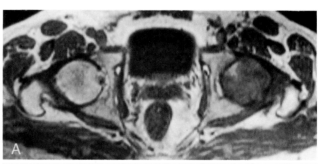
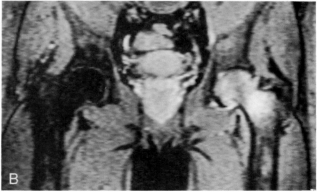

**FIGURE 10–14.** Transient osteopenia of the hip. This patient had a similar process in the right hip three years earlier. At the current time, he had left hip pain.

**A** A transaxial T1-weighted (TR/TE, 600/10) spin echo MR image shows low signal intensity in the left femoral head.

**B** A coronal STIR (TR/TE, 2000/20; inversion time, 150 msec) MR image reveals high signal intensity in the left femoral head and neck.

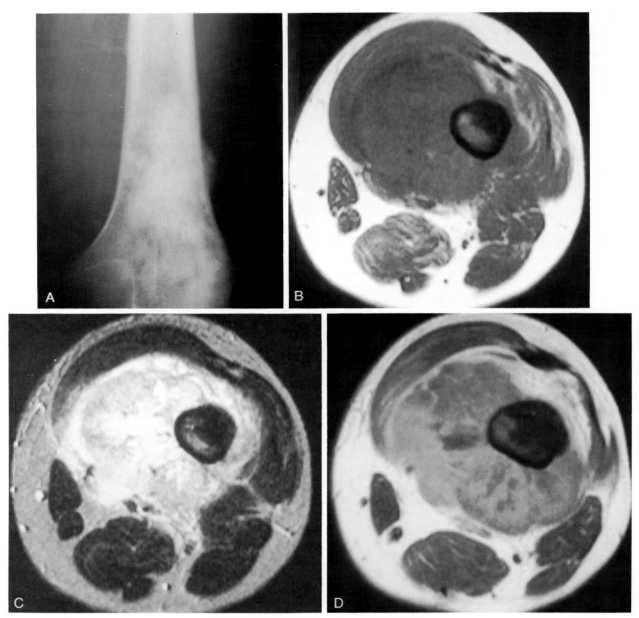

**FIGURE 10–15.** Osteosarcoma of the femur. A 19 year old man had an enlarging mass in the left distal thigh.

**A** On a plain radiograph, note a sclerotic lesion of the distal femur with soft tissue calcification. The diagnosis of osteosarcoma is suggested.

**B–D** Transaxial T1-weighted (TR/TE, 600/10) spin echo MR image **(B)**; transaxial T2-weighted (TR/TE, 2500/90) spin echo MR image **(C)**; transaxial T1-weighted (TR/TE, 600/10) spin echo MR image after the intravenous injection of a gadolinium compound **(D).** Note the soft tissue mass posterior and medial to the femur with low signal intensity in **B** and high signal intensity in **C.** The T2-weighted image demonstrates soft tissue edema (high signal) at the periphery of the mass and anteromedially. At this level the mass enhances with gadolinium **(D)**, with areas of diminished enhancement corresponding to ischemic or necrotic foci. Note the inability to determine the presence of calcification. The intraosseous portion of the tumor demonstrates low signal intensity on all images, corresponding to sclerosis demonstrated on the plain film.

## TABLE 10–2. Staging of Musculoskeletal Bone Neoplasms

| Stage | Grade | Site | Metastasis |
|-------|-------|------|------------|
| 1A | G1 | T1 | M0 |
| 1B | G1 | T2 | M0 |
| 2A | G2 | T1 | M0 |
| 2B | G2 | T2 | M0 |
| 3A | G1–2 | T1 | M1 |
| 3B | G1–2 | T2 | M1 |

G1 = low-grade histology; G2 = high-grade histology; T1 = intracompartmental lesion; G2 = extracompartmental lesion; M0 = no metastasis; M1 = metastasis.

As certain bone tumors have characteristic appearances on routine radiographs, such radiographs are fundamental to accurate diagnosis. Indeed, the presence of calcification is better determined with plain films than with MR imaging. In the context of staging, any bone lesion that has plain film evidence of periosteal involvement has extraosseous extension (Fig. 10–16). MR imaging, however, may demonstrate that a lesion believed to be confined to bone on the basis of routine radiography has local soft tissue extension, resulting in an increase in its tumor grade.

In the staging of musculoskeletal neoplasms, MR imaging is not the method of choice for the evaluation of metastasis. Radionuclide studies are sensitive to the detection of distant bone metastasis. MR imaging is best applied to the assessment of spinal metastasis. Furthermore, CT maintains a role in the assessment of both bone and soft tissue neoplasms. As MR imaging is insensitive to the presence of scattered calcification, CT remains the method of choice for detection of such calcifications. In addition, CT probably is more sensitive than MR imaging to the presence of cortical erosions by an extrinsic soft tissue mass (Fig. 10–17). As

some primary bone tumors, especially Ewing's sarcoma, have a known incidence of local spread within the affected bone, MR imaging protocols are useful in assessing an entire extremity to exclude skip metastasis proximal or distal to the site of the tumor.

In patients with musculoskeletal tumors, standard spin echo sequences with T1- and T2-weighting are the workhorse imaging sequences. Most lesions are of low signal intensity on T1-weighted images and of relatively high signal intensity on T2-weighted images. T1-weighted images provide high contrast at the lesion-marrow interface. T2-weighted sequences provide high contrast between the lesion and the surrounding muscle. Both T1- and T2-weighted images in two orthogonal planes are needed to assess tumor extent accurately. Gradient echo, STIR, and fat suppression MR images also can assist in discrimination of tumor and surrounding edema. In this regard, the most sensitive technique combines gadolinium enhancement with fat suppression (Fig. 10–18). This technique provides increased conspicuity of tumor spread and discrimination of tumor and edema. The value of gadolinium-enhanced techniques for the histologic characterization of tumors is not clear, however. Disagreement exists regarding whether tumors that enhance after contrast administration have a more aggressive histologic appearance. Gadolinium administration may be of aid during tissue sampling, allowing biopsy of portions of the tumor where there is increased vascularity, areas that may reflect more accurately the true histology of the lesion.[62]

## Benign and Malignant Bone Tumors

Preoperative characterization of bone tumors with MR imaging is a useful practice; however, patient age, radiographic appearance, and clinical history remain essential for accurate diagnosis. When radiographic characterization of

## TABLE 10–3. American Joint Committee for Cancer Staging System

| Stage | Grade | Size | Nodes | Metastasis |
|-------|-------|------|-------|------------|
| 1A | G1 | T1 | N0 | M0 |
| 1B | G1 | T2 | N0 | M0 |
| 2A | G2 | T1 | N0 | M0 |
| 2B | G2 | T2 | N0 | M0 |
| 3A | G3 | T1 | N0 | M0 |
| 3B | G3 | T2 | N0 | M0 |
| 3C | G1–3 | T1–2 | N1 | M0 |
| 4A | G1–3 | T3 | N0–1 | M0–1 |
| 4B | G1–3 | T1–3 | N0 | M1 |

Staging Determinates:

T = tumor size
- T1  <5 cm
- T2  >5 cm
- T3  involvement of adjacent bone or neurovascular bundle

N = lymph node
- N0  no lymph node involvement
- N1  lymph node involvement

M = metastatic disease
- M0  absent
- M1  present

G = histology grade
- G1  low grade
- G2  intermediate grade
- G3  high grade

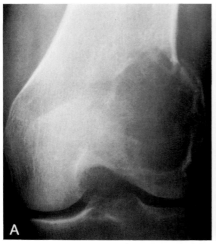 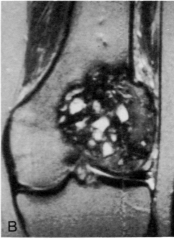

**FIGURE 10–16.** Giant cell tumor in a 45 year old woman with the acute onset of knee pain.

**A** On the routine radiograph an osteolytic lesion of the distal femur with a fracture is seen.

**B** A coronal T2-weighted (TR/TE, 2645/90) spin echo MR image demonstrates bowing of the lateral cortex, confirming extracortical extension. Medial extension of the tumor into the medial condyle also is evident. The tumor undermines the lateral articular cortex. A joint effusion is apparent.

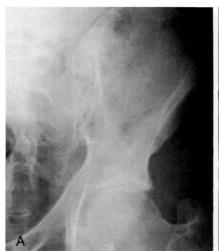 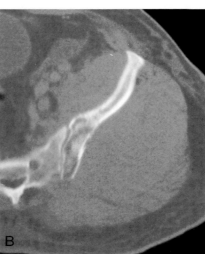 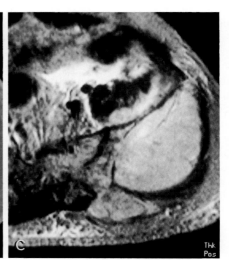

**FIGURE 10–17.** Lymphoma involving the left posterior iliac crest.

**A** On a plain radiograph subtle destruction of the left iliac crest is evident.

**B** On a transaxial CT scan a large soft tissue mass and permeative changes in the left ilium are consistent with a malignant tumor.

**C** Transaxial T2-weighted (TR/TE, 2500/90) spin echo MR image. The mass shows increased signal intensity, which is demarcated from muscle. Cortical discontinuity in the posterior aspect of the ilium is seen. Abnormal signal intensity in the left half of the sacrum confirms tumor extension.

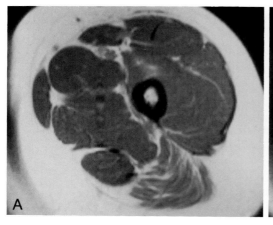 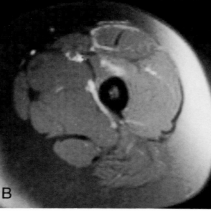

**FIGURE 10–18.** Osteosarcoma metastasis, gadolinium enhancement.

**A** Transaxial T1-weighted (TR/TE, 600/10) spin echo MR image after intravenous administration of gadolinium compound.

**B** Identical image with the addition of fat suppression. Both images demonstrate abnormal signal intensity in the vastus intermedius muscle. Note increased conspicuity of the enhancing area in the fat saturation image.

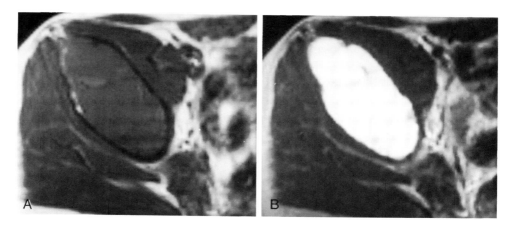

**FIGURE 10–19.** Aneurysmal bone cyst of the ilium. Transaxial T1-weighted (TR/TE, 600/15) **(A)** and T2-weighted (TR/TE, 2500/90) **(B)** spin echo MR images reveal an expansile lesion without extraosseous extension. The lesion is of low signal intensity in **A** and of high signal intensity in **B**. A fluid level also is evident in **A**.

the tumor is not clear, MR imaging can provide further information regarding tumor size. Characterization of the MR imaging findings as evidence of a benign or malignant bone tumor, however, leads to errors that adversely affect patient management.[55] Clearly, in most cases, data derived from MR imaging examinations in patients with bone tumors lack specificity.[56]

As an example, fluid levels, although commonly associated with aneurysmal bone cysts (Fig. 10–19), have been described in giant cell tumors, chondroblastomas, and telangiectatic osteosarcomas as well.[57] Peritumoral edema generally is associated with malignant tumors, including osteosarcoma and chondrosarcoma, or with giant cell tumors.[58] The presence of extensive soft tissue edema is a poor prognostic sign with a higher incidence of metastasis and poor response to chemotherapy.[61] Fibrous lesions tend to be of low signal intensity on all spin echo sequences, whereas cartilaginous lesions may demonstrate high signal intensity on T1-weighted images. Osteoid osteomas lead to MR imaging findings that resemble those of Ewing's tumor, osteonecrosis, stress fractures, and juvenile inflammatory arthritis.[59] Indeed, reactive soft tissue masses may surround an osteoid osteoma.[60]

Enhancement of signal intensity after gadolinium administration has been employed to assist in the tissue characterization. In one study, septal enhancement was identified in low-grade chondrosarcomas but not in osteochondromas.[63] In the management of osteosarcoma, gadolinium has been employed to predict[60] and to assess accurately the response to chemotherapy.[64, 65]

## Soft Tissue Masses

MR imaging has had a great effect on assessment and staging of soft tissue masses. Just as for bone tumors, however, in most instances MR imaging findings do not allow a specific histologic diagnosis. Most soft tissue lesions demonstrate low signal intensity on T1-weighted images and high signal intensity on T2-weighted images (Figs. 10–20 and 10–21). Lipomas are homogeneous in their signal intensity, which is identical to that of subcutaneous fat on all pulse sequences[66] (Fig. 10–22). A confident diagnosis of lipoma can be made when MR images demonstrate a homogeneous appearance and a well-circumscribed mass containing fat on all pulse sequences. When the fatty tumor is

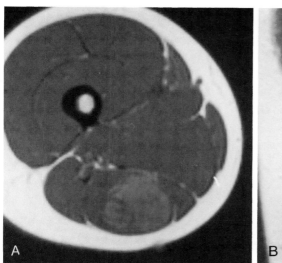
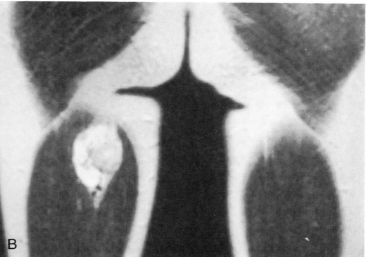

**FIGURE 10–20.** Alveolar soft part sarcoma. A 15 year old girl had a slowly growing mass in the thigh. A lobular mass in the gastrocnemius muscle is of low signal intensity in a transaxial T1-weighted (TR/TE, 500/10) spin echo MR image **(A)** and of high signal intensity in a coronal T2-weighted (TR/TE, 2500/90) spin echo MR image **(B).** The MR appearance lacks specificity.

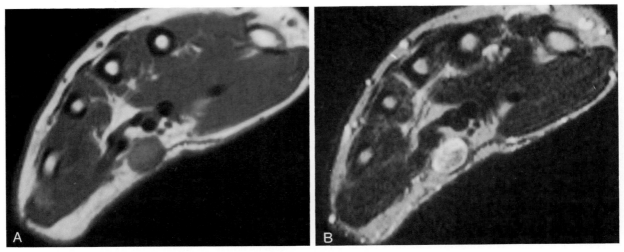

**FIGURE 10–21.** Hematoma anterior to the carpal tunnel simulating a tumor.
 **A** In a transaxial T1-weighted (TR/TE, 600/10) spin echo MR image, a well-circumscribed mass with slightly inhomogeneous low signal intensity is seen.
 **B** In a transaxial T2-weighted (TR/TR, 2500/90) spin echo MR image, the mass has increased signal intensity with a central area of low signal intensity. No surrounding soft tissue edema is evident.

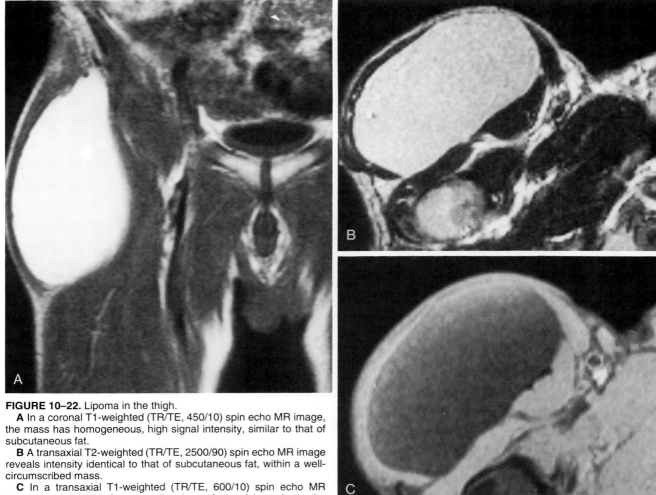

**FIGURE 10–22.** Lipoma in the thigh.
 **A** In a coronal T1-weighted (TR/TE, 450/10) spin echo MR image, the mass has homogeneous, high signal intensity, similar to that of subcutaneous fat.
 **B** A transaxial T2-weighted (TR/TE, 2500/90) spin echo MR image reveals intensity identical to that of subcutaneous fat, within a well-circumscribed mass.
 **C** In a transaxial T1-weighted (TR/TE, 600/10) spin echo MR image obtained with fat saturation, loss of signal intensity in the mass is seen.

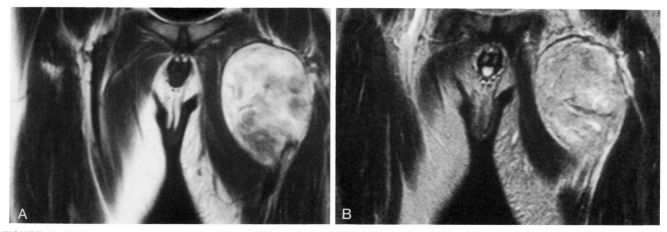

**FIGURE 10–23.** Liposarcoma in the left thigh. Coronal T1-weighted (TR/TE, 500/10) **(A)** and T2-weighted (TR/TE, 2800/90) **(B)** spin echo MR images show a well-circumscribed mass with inhomogeneous signal intensity.

heterogeneous in signal intensity, a liposarcoma should be considered (Fig. 10–23).

## TRAUMATIC ABNORMALITIES

### Soft Tissue Injury

Trauma to soft tissue results in a combination of hemorrhage and edema followed by healing and fibrosis. Generally, there is little need to image areas of soft tissue injury except when the injury causes a soft tissue mass, a tear of a ligament or tendon, or a cartilaginous lesion. MR imaging can be employed to locate and characterize hematomas and sites of soft tissue injury.[67] Clinical history is important, as early posttraumatic myositis ossificans can lead to MR imaging findings that simulate soft tissue sarcoma.[68, 69]

### Bone Injury

Most fractures are well evaluated with conventional radiography alone; those that occur in areas of complex anatomy, such as the spine or osseous pelvis, may be further delineated with CT.[70] MR imaging in trauma is useful in the identification of bone lesions that escape radiographic detection,[71–74] as it indicates those patients who may benefit from immobilization. The MR imaging appearance of a fracture may be nonspecific, of low signal intensity on T1-weighted images and high signal intensity on T2-weighted images (Fig. 10–24). STIR images, which demonstrate focal increased signal intensity in injured bone, probably offer the most sensitive evaluation of occult fracture.[75]

MR imaging is effective in the identification of fractures of the femoral neck when initial radiographs are normal.[76, 77] In the elderly patient with acute hip pain, MR imaging can

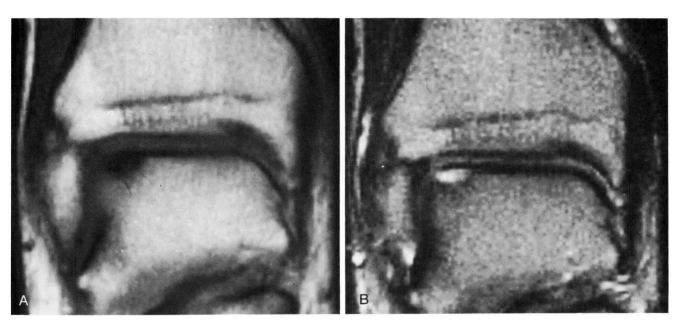

**FIGURE 10–24.** Osteochondral injury of the talar dome. Coronal T1-weighted (TR/TE, 600/10) **(A)** and coronal T2-weighted (TR/TE, 2500/90) spin echo MR images reveal a focal injury in the superolateral portion of the talar dome, with low signal intensity in **A** and high signal intensity in **B** consistent with marrow injury. The T2 image shows the overlying cartilage to be intact. Whether this injury will progress to osteochondritis dissecans cannot be determined.

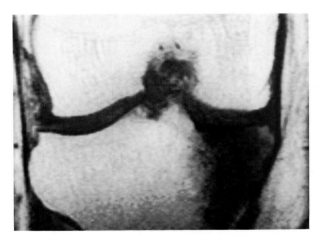

**FIGURE 10–25.** Marrow alterations in the medial tibial plateau in a patient with a tear of the anterior cruciate ligament. A coronal T1-weighted (TR/TE, 600/10) spin echo MR image demonstrates decreased signal intensity in the medial plateau consistent with marrow edema.

be a more cost-effective examination than scintigraphic methods in revealing such fractures. As marrow alterations appear almost immediately following fracture, when the MR examination is negative the cost of hospitalization is avoided.[78] In patients with fractures of the femoral neck, immediate surgical intervention reduces the length of hospitalization.

Posttraumatic marrow alterations detected with MR imaging may suggest associated ligamentous pathology (Fig. 10–25). For instance, an occult fracture in the lateral tibial plateau (Segond fracture) has a high association with tears of the anterior cruciate ligament.[79]

Stress fracture may be difficult to diagnose radiographically. Although scintigraphy is a valuable method for the identification of stress fractures, MR imaging also is useful, as it is a sensitive diagnostic test, allowing detection of reactive changes in marrow. A linear abnormality in an appropriate anatomic region on MR images is a relatively specific finding.[80] Care must be taken not to inappropriately

confuse the MR appearance of a stress fracture with that of a more aggressive lesion.[81]

## ABNORMALITIES OF SPECIFIC JOINTS

The impact of MR imaging upon the orthopedic management of traumatic abnormalities in various joints has been dramatic. In this regard, MR imaging has high sensitivity and specificity. Normal structures are delineated with great accuracy, and alterations of these structures are reflective of pathology. Some general comments regarding MR imaging of certain joints are included here, although the reader should refer to Chapter 70 for a more detailed analysis.

### Knee

MR imaging of the knee provides an accurate noninvasive view of meniscal and cruciate ligament pathology. The reported accuracy of MR imaging for the detection of cruciate ligament abnormalities is about 95 per cent. In evaluating the knee, structures of specific clinical significance include the medial and lateral menisci, anterior and posterior cruciate ligaments, and medial and lateral (fibular) collateral ligaments (Fig. 10–26).

MR imaging of the knee usually relies upon both sagittal and coronal images. Transaxial imaging alone is incapable of allowing full assessment of the menisci. Most centers rely upon a sagittal dual echo T2-weighted sequence supplemented with coronal T1- and T2-weighted sequences. The coronal T2-weighted sequence is particularly valuable in patients with recent knee injury. A 16 cm field of view with 4 mm slice thickness is employed, and a surface coil is mandatory. With these sequences, most standard knee examinations can be completed in 30 minutes or less.

Although spin echo sequences are the "gold standard" for MR imaging of the knee, other pulse sequences have been employed. These include gradient echo techniques (both 2-D and 3-D), inversion recovery sequences, and fat suppression techniques. Three-dimensional gradient echo

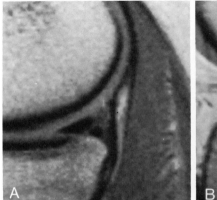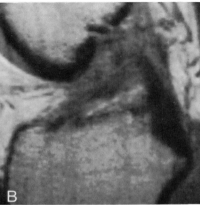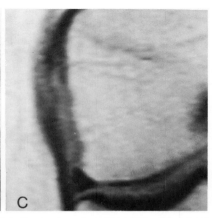

**FIGURE 10–26.** O'Donahue's unhappy triad—injuries to the medial meniscus, anterior cruciate ligament, and medial collateral ligament.

**A** A linear region of signal intensity in the posterior horn of the medial meniscus communicates with the inferior articular surface, confirming a tear, as seen in a sagittal proton density–weighted (TR/TE, 2500/20) spin echo MR image.

**B** A midline image from the same sagittal series shows abnormal architecture of the anterior cruciate ligament consistent with an acute tear.

**C** A coronal T1-weighted (TR/TE, 600/10) spin echo MR image demonstrates thinning of the medial collateral ligament with adjacent soft tissue edema.

techniques allow image reconstruction in almost an infinite number of planes.[82] These may be useful in evaluating the anterior cruciate ligament, as oblique sagittal images can be obtained parallel to the cruciate ligament, and the meniscus, as radial images of the meniscus can be acquired.[83]

MR imaging is accurate in the evaluation of meniscal injuries (Fig. 10–27). A meniscal grading system, using categories of grades I to III, is based on patterns of signal intensity.[84, 85] Grade I is characterized by a globular region of high signal intensity within the substance of the meniscus; grade II is characterized by a linear region of high signal intensity within the meniscus; and grade III is characterized by a region of high signal intensity that communicates with an articular surface. The initially proposed significance of grade II signal was to indicate a meniscus that had a potential to tear.[86–88] However, follow-up studies suggest that grade II patterns do not progress.[89] The practical question to be answered in all examinations is whether the identified intrameniscal signal communicates with an articular surface and therefore represents a tear.[90] Meniscal windowing has been suggested as a more accurate technique; however, some studies have questioned the value of this method.[91]

The normal anterior cruciate ligament is characterized by continuous fibers coursing in an oblique direction in the intercondylar notch. Discontinuity of these fibers signifies a tear. One secondary sign of a tear of the anterior cruciate ligament is anterior subluxation of the tibia.[92] The collateral ligaments are evaluated in a similar manner.

Patellar tracking examinations rely on gradient echo acquisition of images. As originally described, sequential images are obtained in the transaxial plane, with the knee imaged in varying degrees of passive flexion. The images are displayed in a cine loop.[93] With this technique, malalignment and abnormal tracking can be observed.[94, 95] Advancements in technique have focused upon studies of the dynamic range of motion with the knee working against a

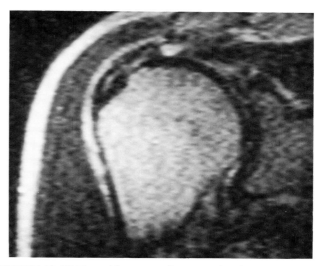

**FIGURE 10–28.** Tear of the supraspinatus tendon. A coronal oblique T2-weighted (TR/TE, 2500/90) spin echo MR image demonstrates a focal gap within the supraspinatus tendon, associated with increased signal intensity. Fluid also is present in the subdeltoid bursa.

force. Initial results with this technique suggest more accurate identification of patients with abnormal patellar motion, when compared with techniques performed without stress placed upon the knee.[96, 97]

### Shoulder

MR imaging of the shoulder is more challenging than that of the knee. This relates to the complexity of the joint and surrounding structures, especially the rotator cuff. Accurate interpretation of MR images requires an understanding of the normal appearance of the supraspinatus tendon and glenoid region.[98–100] Contributing to the difficulty of interpretation of MR images of the shoulder is the presence of ''magic angle'' effects. These effects occur in ligaments and tendons, in both the shoulder and ankle, when the fibers of the tendon are oriented approximately 55 degrees to the central plane of the magnet. This orientation leads to shortening of the apparent T1 time, resulting in an increase in signal intensity in the tendon, which simulates the appearance of a tear or tendinitis.[101–103]

MR imaging is accurate in the assessment of full-thickness tears of the supraspinatus tendon (Fig. 10–28), although difficulty is encountered in the accurate evaluation of partial-thickness tears of the rotator cuff. Specific signs of full-thickness tears include a gap in the tendon, associated retraction of the supraspinatus muscle, and fluid in the subdeltoid bursa. Like the knee, successful shoulder imaging requires a dedicated surface coil to increase diagnostic accuracy. Most protocols involve oblique coronal and oblique sagittal imaging planes, positioned parallel to and perpendicular to the supraspinatus tendon, respectively. These are supplemented by transaxial images. A small field of view with thin sections is essential. Spin echo sequences may be supplemented with fat saturation techniques to increase the sensitivity to diagnosis of partial tears of the rotator cuff. One report notes 100 per cent sensitivity and specificity for the diagnosis of partial tears when intra-articular gadolinium administration and fat saturation imaging were employed.[13]

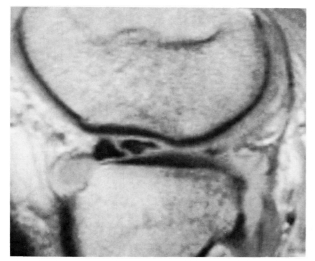

**FIGURE 10–27.** Bucket-handle tear of the lateral meniscus (flipped meniscus). A sagittal proton density–weighted (TR/TE, 2500/20) spin echo MR image demonstrates a "double anterior horn" of the lateral meniscus and an absent posterior horn of the lateral meniscus. The double anterior horn is caused by displacement of the posterior horn of the lateral meniscus, which now lies adjacent to the anterior horn.

The choice between MR imaging and CT arthrography of the shoulder is difficult to make. Both appear to have equal sensitivity for the diagnosis of full-thickness tears of the cuff. MR imaging may have more sensitivity in the evaluation of partial-thickness tears of the cuff whereas CT is better able to assess the appearance of labral cartilage. A recent review suggested that CT arthrography may become the examination of choice owing to its reduced cost when compared with MR imaging.[104]

## Ankle

MR imaging of the ankle has allowed more accurate assessment in patients with ankle pain. Studies have demonstrated the ability of MR imaging to demonstrate tendon abnormalities, including tears and tenosynovitis, with great accuracy. Specific structures that require assessment include the Achilles and tibialis posterior tendons.[105] The ankle ligaments are difficult to assess, given their oblique orientation. In one study, only anterior talofibular and calcaneofibular ligaments were identified reliably with MR imaging.[106] With the availability of high resolution 3-D gradient acquisition, it may be possible to improve visualization of ligamentous structures, especially the lateral and medial ligamentous complexes. It is likely that this information will be important in a select group of patients with ankle instability.

Anomalous muscles occur in the ankle, including accessory soleus, peroneus quartus, and flexor digitorum longus accessorius muscles[107–109] (Fig. 10–29). These can be imaged routinely with MR and must not be mistaken for soft tissue masses.

In contrast to knee imaging, the accepted universal MR protocol for ankle imaging has not been defined clearly. One reason is that the posterior ankle tendons have a curved

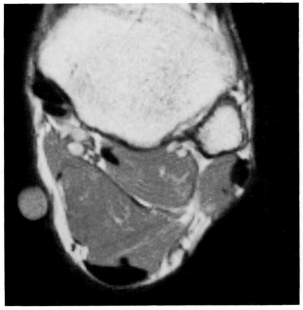

**FIGURE 10–29.** Accessory soleus muscle. A transaxial proton density–weighted (TR/TE, 2500/20) spin echo MR image demonstrates a soft tissue mass anterior to Achilles tendon corresponding to an accessory soleus muscle.

course around the medial and lateral malleoli and therefore are not parallel in their entirety to standard imaging planes. Disagreement exists as to whether the patient should be imaged in the prone or supine position. In our experience, prone positioning is not necessary, and the examination can effectively be performed in the supine position.

We have found that the most accurate diagnostic planes are the transaxial oblique and coronal planes. Some centers rely upon sagittal images. The slice thickness should be minimized, and T1- and T2-weighted images should be obtained in both planes. The field of view should be limited to one ankle. The tendons are relatively symmetric in a single patient and, with experience, a comparison study of the opposite ankle in a patient with unilateral symptoms is unwarranted.[110] With a small field of view, a more accurate assessment of tendon pathology usually is possible.

In assessing tendon integrity, one must be aware of the appearance of normal tendons. The tendons about the ankle should be of low signal intensity on all pulse sequences.[111] All tendons, with the exception of the Achilles tendon, are enclosed by a tendon sheath. The presence of fluid within the tendon sheath indicates inflammation or, more specifically, tenosynovitis. The MR imaging appearance of acute tenosynovitis is that of fluid within the tendon sheath with normal tendon morphology. In chronic tenosynovitis the tendon is increased in size and demonstrates an increase in signal intensity on both T1- and T2-weighted images. The use of gadolinium-enhanced tenography has been described.[12]

Abnormalities of the Achilles tendon on MR images have been well described.[112–114] The Achilles tendon is imaged optimally in the sagittal and transaxial planes. The specific clinical concern in assessment of the Achilles tendon is the degree of tendon injury, as extensive injuries are managed with surgery, and minimal injuries are treated conservatively with casting.

The tibialis posterior tendon is frequently injured, resulting in a progressive flat foot deformity. Injury to this tendon is graded on a three point scale.[115] In a grade I injury, the tendon is enlarged, owing to hemorrhage and edema. In a grade II injury the tendon is thinned, reflecting partially torn fibers. In grade III injuries, there is a gap between the torn ends of the tendon. In this classification system, an overlap exists in the MR appearance of a grade I injury and chronic tenosynovitis and often a reliable distinction between the two cannot be made.

## Elbow

MR imaging of the elbow has received limited attention in the literature.[5] Specific applications include evaluation of osteochondral injuries and abnormalities of the biceps tendon and ulnar collateral ligament.[116–118] With high resolution techniques, abnormalities of the ulnar and radial nerves are identifiable.[119] CT arthrography, however, may be superior to MR imaging in the evaluation of intra-articular bodies in the elbow joint. CT also is the diagnostic method of choice for evaluation of acute injuries.

Principles of MR imaging of the elbow are similar to those for other joints. A surface coil, a limited field of view, and thin sections in orthogonal planes are required. As specific elbow coils usually are not available, the shoulder or knee coil can be adapted for elbow imaging.

### Hip

The major indication for MR imaging of the hip is for detection of ischemic necrosis of the femoral head. Normal transaxial T1-weighted MR images effectively exclude the presence of ischemic necrosis. In most instances, the hip is imaged with the body coil, with a field of view that includes both hips. Some investigators prefer to image the hip with a surface coil, with the benefit of increased spatial resolution.

Additional indications for MR imaging of the hip include developmental dysplasia of the hip (particularly in infants in whom the femoral head is largely cartilaginous),[70] tumors, synovial processes, and infection.

### Wrist

The ability of MR imaging to assess wrist pathology continues to improve steadily. The resolution afforded by 3-D gradient echo techniques allows routine demonstration of intercarpal ligaments.[120, 121] MR imaging also allows assessment of the triangular fibrocartilage (TFC),[122–125] with reported accuracy of greater than 90 per cent in the detection of tears of the TFC.

### Temporomandibular Joint

MR imaging of the temporomandibular joint relies upon both static and cine studies. The use of dedicated surface coils allows imaging of both joints simultaneously.[126] Using thin sections, both acute and chronic alteration of the joint can be identified.[127, 128] MR imaging and arthrography, as well as arthroscopy, of the temporomandibular joint are addressed in Chapter 49.

### SPECIFIC ARTICULAR ABNORMALITIES

### Osteoarthritis

MR imaging has proven useful in assessment of osteoarthritis. This method is more sensitive to cartilage loss, the earliest sign of osteoarthritis, than are other techniques.[129, 130] However, the role of MR imaging in the management of osteoarthritis has yet to be determined.[131]

Analysis of patellofemoral cartilage with MR imaging has received the greatest attention. Although the transaxial plane appears most suited to this analysis, the optimal MR imaging sequence is not clear (see Chapter 70). Most sequences can detect advanced cartilage loss.[132, 133] However, the accuracy of these techniques has been questioned, and a clear consensus does not exist regarding the accuracy of MR imaging in the detection of subtle cartilage loss.[134–138]

### Synovial Inflammatory Disorders

In comparison with cartilage assessment, MR imaging has proven useful for the detection of synovial proliferation associated with inflammatory disorders such as rheumatoid arthritis[139–143] (Fig. 10–30). Typically, synovial inflammatory tissue is of low signal intensity on T1-weighted images and of intermediate to high signal intensity on T2-weighted images. It often is difficult to discriminate joint fluid from synovium. The use of intravenous gadolinium may help to clarify the problem, allowing evaluation of the extent of synovial proliferation and differentiation of it from normal tissue or joint fluid.[144, 145] Hypertrophied synovial tissue shows enhancement of signal intensity after intravenous administration of gadolinium, while joint fluid does not. The intensity of enhancement is thought to reflect the degree of inflammation.[146]

The exact role of MR imaging in management of rheumatoid arthritis has yet to be determined. Given its ability to detect abnormalities not apparent on radiographs, some authors have suggested that MR imaging may serve as a guide for therapeutic decisions, and that the technique may allow assessment of the response to disease-modifying agents.[147]

### MUSCLE ABNORMALITIES

### Normal Muscles

Although in most clinical practices assessment of muscle is not a common indication for MR imaging, abnormalities of muscle can be detected reliably. Both focal and diffuse abnormalities secondary to degeneration, inflammation, trauma, and neoplasm can be imaged.[61, 148–150] On all pulse sequences, normal muscle is of intermediate signal intensity. Therefore, normal muscle often can serve as a comparative standard or guide for determination of musculoskeletal pathology. As the signal intensity of muscle is distinctly

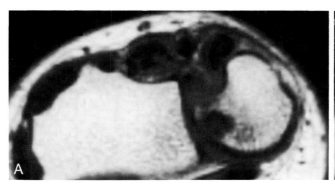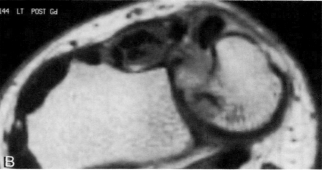

**FIGURE 10–30.** Rheumatoid arthritis of the wrist. Transaxial T1-weighted (TR/TE, 500/15) spin echo MR images obtained before **(A)** and immediately after **(B)** the intravenous administration of a gadolinium compound reveal abnormal tissue, particularly in the distal radioulnar joint, that is of low signal intensity in **A** and of higher signal intensity in **B**. The appearance is consistent with synovial hyperplasia. Erosion of the ulna also is demonstrated.

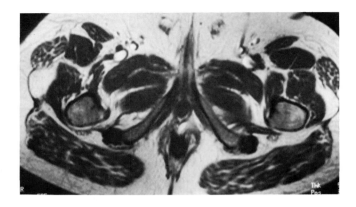

**FIGURE 10–31.** Muscle atrophy. A transaxial T1-weighted (TR/TE, 525/10) spin echo MR image shows inhomogeneous increased signal intensity consistent with fatty infiltration in the gluteal, iliacus, and psoas muscles.

different from that of fat, intermuscular fat planes usually are readily defined, and specific muscle groups are identified easily. As muscle is a dynamic organ, physiologic changes can be detected with MR imaging. In exercised muscle, there is an increase in the T2 relaxation time.[151–154]

### Pathologic Muscles

Because many muscle disorders are characterized by fatty infiltration, diseased muscles can be detected with MR imaging[155, 156] (Fig. 10–31). Chronic myopathies, including muscular dystrophy, can reveal patterns of diffuse atrophy.[155] Similar atrophy may be indicative of chronically denervated muscle. Acute inflammation, such as occurs in dermatomyositis, is demonstrated as muscle edema.[157] The distribution of myopathy is well delineated with MR imaging; more severe involvement occurs in patients with congenital myopathy, compared with those with muscular dystrophy or polymyositis.[158] MR imaging also can be employed to determine the response of muscle to therapeutic intervention, with a return of normal signal intensity correlating to therapeutic success.[159]

In the imaging of acute traumatic muscle pathology, athletic injuries are manifested as hemorrhage and edema within the affected muscle.[160] MR imaging also can be employed to assess the resolution of the injury, including the development of fibrosis or fatty infiltration.[161, 162] MR imaging of these abnormalities requires images of high resolution and sequences such as STIR imaging optimized for the detection of edema.[163, 164] The ability of MR imaging to allow identification of acute muscle alterations in an otherwise undamaged muscle may be inadequate with current techniques.[165]

### CHEMICAL SHIFT IMAGING AND SPECTROSCOPY

As noted earlier, MR imaging is sensitive but not specific in determining the tissue composition of detected neoplasms. T1- and T2-weighted images allow localization of the tumor mass, and the T2-weighted images provide visualization of the body's response to that tumor, usually manifested as soft tissue edema. Whereas MR imaging reflects the density of water protons within the imaged tissue, MR spectroscopy gauges the chemical composition of the tissue. This biochemical composition provides functional information to potentially complement the anatomic information provided by standard MR imaging.

With MR spectroscopy, the two chemical spectra that appear to have the greater clinical potential are $^1$H and $^{31}$P. In spite of the abundance of $^1$H (water) in tissues, most efforts have focused on $^{31}$P. The phosphorus spectrum can be created from chemical shift frequencies of the major phosphate metabolites. This requires a high field strength and can be accomplished at 1.5 T, although experimental 4 T magnets designed specifically for spectroscopy also have been utilized.[166] Peaks for $^{31}$P adenosine triphosphate (ATP), phosphocreatine (PCr), and inorganic phosphate (Pi) are resolved. Phosphodiester (PDE) and phosphomonoester (PME) peaks also have been identified, and tracking the changes in these metabolites may have a role in the assessment of musculoskeletal tumors. A characteristic spectral peak for adenosine diphosphate (ADP) is not resolved, owing to its low concentration and overlap with ATP. The relative concentration of these metabolites can be measured and pH values determined from the location of the Pi and PCr peaks.[167, 168]

A strategy that shows promise is the direct coupling of MR imaging and MR spectroscopy. This involves acquiring the MR imaging examination and then employing the same localization information to determine the magnetic spectra of specific locations within the tissue.[169, 170] This technique may prove useful for assessment of tumor response to chemotherapy.[171] The combined procedure also has been employed to localize individual muscle groups and their response to exercise and injury.[172, 173]

Phosphorus spectroscopy is performed on skeletal muscle or other musculoskeletal tissues to study normal energy metabolism, to characterize energy metabolism in disease, and to monitor the success or failure of various therapeutic regimens.[174–180]

The spectra for resting, exercising, and recovering muscle have been well described and are similar among persons of all ages. During exercise, PCr decreases as it provides the source to maintain ATP levels, resulting in an elevation of Pi. This is associated with acidification (decreased pH) owing to lactate production from glycolysis. During recovery following exercise, PCr rises rapidly and pH returns to normal.[181] Spectra from a variety of muscular disorders have been generated, and some have been recognized as specific for certain diseases.[175, 182]

In tumor imaging, two main applications of spectroscopy have evolved. The first involves prospectively evaluating the metabolism of tumors to predict their potential response to chemotherapy. The second is a direct evaluation of the response of tumors to chemotherapy.[168, 183] Bone tumors have altered metabolism, which manifests as changes in the spectral peaks, as compared with non-neoplastic processes or normal tissues. Relative elevation of PME and Pi peaks appears to be a marker of tumor activity. Several investigations have shown promising results in using phosphorus spectra to distinguish normal from neoplastic musculoskeletal tissue.[170, 176, 184–188]

Although the pace of developments in MR spectroscopy has not matched the rapid advances made in anatomic MR imaging, progress nonetheless is being made. Further studies and investigation are needed to determine the role of this technology in clinical imaging and patient management.

## SUMMARY

As MR imaging continues to mature, it is reasonable to postulate that applications of MR imaging also will evolve. Radiologists involved in musculoskeletal MR imaging must be aware of the optimal sequences available. In an era of cost containment, however, every imaging technique will be judged by its clinical as well as its cost effectiveness.

### References

1. Hinshaw WS, Andrew ER, Bottomley PA, et al: An in vivo study of the forearm and hand by thin section NMR imaging. Br J Radiol 52:36, 1979.
2. Reicher MA, Rauschning W, Gold RH, et al: High resolution magnetic resolution imaging of the knee joint: normal anatomy. AJR 145:895, 1985.
3. Middleton WD, Kneeland JB, Carrera GF, et al: High-resolution imaging of the normal rotator cuff. AJR 148:559, 1987.
4. Mesgarzadeh M, Schneck CD, Bonakdarpour A: Carpal tunnel: MR imaging. Part I. Normal anatomy. Radiology 171:743, 1989.
5. Bunnell DH, Fisher DA, Bassett LW, et al: Elbow joint: normal anatomy on MR images. Radiology 165:527, 1987.
6. Bassett LW, Ullis K, Seeger LL, et al: Anatomy of the hip: correlation of coronal and sagittal cadaver cryomicrosections with magnetic resonance images. Surg Radiol Anat 13:301, 1991.
7. Schneck CD, Mesgarzadeh M, Bonakdarpour A, et al: MR imaging of the most commonly injured ankle ligaments. Part I. Normal anatomy. Radiology 184:499, 1992.
8. Fry ME, Jacoby RK, Hutton CW, et al: High-resolution magnetic resonance imaging of the interphalangeal joints of the hand. Skel Radiol 20:273, 1991.
9. Wong EC, Jesmanowicz A, Hyde JS: High-resolution, short echo time MR imaging of the fingers and wrist with a local gradient coil. Radiology 181:393, 1991.
10. Ross JS, Delamarter R, Hueftle MG, et al: Gadolinium-DTPA-enhanced MR imaging of the postoperative lumbar spine: time course and mechanism of enhancement. AJR 152:825, 1989.
11. Engel A: Magnetic resonance knee arthrography. Enhanced contrast by gadolinium complex in the rabbit and in humans. Acta Orthop Scand (Suppl) 240:1, 1990.
12. Mayer DP, Jay RM, Schoenhaus H, et al: Magnetic resonance arthrography of the ankle. J Foot Surg 31:584, 1992.
13. Palmer WE, Brown JH, Rosenthal DI: Rotator cuff: evaluation with fat-suppressed MR arthrography. Radiology 188:683, 1993.
14. Vogler JB, Murphy WA: Bone marrow imaging. Radiology 168:679, 1988.
15. Ricci C, Cova M, Kang YS, et al: Normal age-related patterns of cellular and fatty bone marrow distribution in the axial skeleton: MR imaging study. Radiology 177:83, 1990.
16. Zawin JK, Jaramillo D: Conversion of bone marrow in the humerus, sternum, and clavicle: changes with age on MR images. Radiology 188:159, 1993.
17. Dooms GC, Fisher MR, Hricak H, et al: Bone marrow imaging: Magnetic resonance studies related to age and sex. Radiology 155:429, 1985.
18. Richards MA, Webb JA, Jewell SE, et al: In-vivo measurement of spin lattice relaxation time (T1) of bone marrow in healthy volunteers: the effects of age and sex. Br J Radiol 61:30, 1988.
19. Kangarloo H, Dietrich RB, Taira RT, et al: MR imaging of bone marrow in children. J Comput Assist Tomogr 10:205, 1986.
20. Kaplan PA, Asleson RJ, Klassen LW, et al: Bone marrow patterns in aplastic anemia: Observations with 1.5-T MR imaging. Radiology 164:441, 1987.
21. Jones KM, Unger EC, Granstrom P, et al: Bone marrow imaging using STIR at 0.5 and 1.5 T. Magn Res Imag 10:169, 1992.
22. Golfieri R, Baddeley H, Pringle JS, et al: The role of the STIR sequence in magnetic resonance imaging examination of bone tumours. Br J Radiol 63:251, 1990.
23. Sebag GH, Moore SG: Effect of trabecular bone on the appearance of marrow in gradient-echo imaging of the appendicular skeleton. Radiology 174:855, 1990.
24. Daffner RH, Lupetin AR, Dash N, et al: MRI in the detection of malignant infiltration of the bone marrow. AJR 146:353, 1986.
25. Libshitz HI, Malthouse SR, Cunningham D, et al: Multiple myeloma: appearance at MR imaging. Radiology 182:833, 1992.
26. Thomsen C, Sorensen PG, Karle H, et al: Prolonged bone marrow T1-relaxation in acute leukaemia. In vivo tissue characterization by magnetic resonance imaging. Magn Res Imag 5:251, 1987.
27. Berquist TH, Brown ML, Fitzgerald RH, et al: Magnetic resonance imaging: Application in musculoskeletal infection. Magn Res Imag 3:219, 1985.
28. Beltran J, Noto AM, McGhee RB, et al: Infections of the musculoskeletal system: High-field strength MR imaging. Radiology 164:449, 1987.
29. Tang JS, Gold RH, Bassett LW, et al: Musculoskeletal infection of the extremities: evaluation with MR imaging. Radiology 166:205, 1988.
30. Unger E, Moldofsky P, Gatenby R, et al: Diagnosis of osteomyelitis by MR imaging. AJR 150:605, 1988.
31. Mason MD, Zlatkin MB, Esterhai JL, et al: Chronic complicated osteomyelitis of the lower extremity: evaluation with MR imaging. Radiology 173:355, 1989.
32. Murphy WA, Totty WG: Musculoskeletal magnetic resonance imaging. Magn Reson Ann 2:1, 1986.
33. Erdman WA, Tamburro F, Jayson HT, et al: Osteomyelitis: characteristics and pitfalls of diagnosis with MR imaging. Radiology 180:533, 1991.
34. Dangman BC, Hoffer FA, Rand FF, et al: Osteomyelitis in children: gadolinium-enhanced MR imaging. Radiology 182:743, 1992.
35. Yuh WT, Corson JD, Baraniewski HM, et al: Osteomyelitis of the foot in diabetic patients: evaluation with plain film. 99mTc-MDP bone scintigraphy and MR imaging. AJR 152:795, 1989.
36. Wang A, Weinstein D, Greenfield L, et al: MRI and diabetic foot infections. Magn Res Imag 8:805, 1990.
37. Seabold JE, Flickinger FW, Kao SC, et al: Indium-111-leukocyte/technetium-99m-MDP bone and magnetic resonance imaging: difficulty of diagnosing osteomyelitis in patients with neuropathic osteoarthropathy. J Nucl Med 31:549, 1990.
38. Beltran J, Campanini DS, Knight C, et al: The diabetic foot: magnetic resonance imaging evaluation. Skel Radiol 19:37, 1990.
39. Chan TW, Dalinka MK, Steinberg ME, et al: MRI appearance of femoral head osteonecrosis following core decompression and bone grafting. Skel Radiol 20:103, 1991.
40. Beltran J, Knight CT, Zuelzer WA, et al: Core decompression for avascular necrosis of the femoral head: correlation between long-term results and preoperative MR staging. Radiology 175:533, 1990.
41. Lafforgue P, Dahan E, Chagnaud C, et al: Early-stage avascular necrosis of the femoral head: MR imaging for prognosis in 31 cases with at least 2 years of follow-up. Radiology 187:199, 1993.
42. Nadel SN, Debatin JF, Richardson WJ, et al: Detection of acute avascular necrosis of the femoral head in dogs: dynamic contrast-enhanced MR imaging vs. spin-echo and STIR sequences. AJR 159:1255, 1992.
43. Alarcon GS, Sanders C, Daniel WW: Transient osteoporosis of the hip: magnetic resonance imaging. J Rheumatol 14:1184, 1987.
44. Wilson AJ, Murphy WA, Hardy DC, et al: Transient osteoporosis: transient bone marrow edema? Radiology 167:757, 1988.
45. Bloem JL: Transient osteoporosis of the hip: MR imaging. Radiology 167:753, 1988.
46. Pay NT, Singer WS, Bartal E: Hip pain in three children accompanied by transient abnormal findings on MR images. Radiology 171:147, 1989.
47. Potter H, Moran M, Schneider R, et al: Magnetic resonance imaging in diagnosis of transient osteoporosis of the hip. Clin Orthop 280:223, 1992.
48. Hauzeur JP, Hanquinet S, Gevenois PA, et al: Study of magnetic resonance imaging in transient osteoporosis of the hip. J Rheumatol 18:1211, 1991.
49. Neuhold A, Hofmann S, Engel A, et al: Bone marrow edema of the hip: MR findings after core decompression. J Comput Assist Tomogr 16:951, 1992.
50. LiK C, Hiette P: Contrast-enhanced fat saturation magnetic resonance imaging for studying the pathophysiology of osteonecrosis of the hips. Skel Radiol 21:375, 1992.
51. Hofmann S, Engel A, Neuhold A, et al: Bone-marrow oedema syndrome and

transient osteoporosis of the hip. An MRI-controlled study of treatment by core decompression. J Bone Joint Surg [Br] 75:210, 1993.

52. Berquist TH: Magnetic resonance imaging of primary skeletal neoplasms. Radiol Clin North Am 31:411, 1993.

53. Enneking W: Staging of musculoskeletal neoplasms. Skel Radiol 13:183, 1985.

54. Russell WO, Cohel J, Enzinger FM: Clinical and pathological staging system for soft tissue sarcomas. Cancer 40:1562, 1977.

55. Kransdorf MJ, Jelinek JS, Moser RP Jr: Imaging of soft tissue tumors. Radiol Clin North Am 31:359, 1993.

56. Varma DG, Ayala AG, Carrasco CH, et al: Chondrosarcoma: MR imaging with pathologic correlation. Radiographics 12:687, 1992.

57. Burr BA, Resnick D, Syklawer R, et al: Fluid-fluid levels in a unicameral bone cyst: CT and MR findings. J Comput Assist Tomogr 17:134, 1993.

58. Golfieri R, Baddeley H, Pringle JS, et al: Primary bone tumors. MR morphologic appearance correlated with pathologic examinations. Acta Radiol 32:290, 1991.

59. Goldman AB, Schneider R, Pavlov H: Osteoid osteomas of the femoral neck: report of four cases evaluated with isotopic bone scanning. CT and MR imaging. Radiology 186:227, 1993.

60. Woods ER, Martel W, Mandell SH, et al: Reactive soft-tissue mass associated with osteoid osteoma: correlation of MR imaging features with pathologic findings. Radiology 186:221, 1993.

61. Hanna SL, Fletcher BD, Parham DM, et al: Muscle edema in musculoskeletal tumors: MR imaging characteristics and clinical significance. J Magn Res Imag 1:441, 1991.

62. Rubin SJ, Feldman F, Dick HM, et al: Heterogeneous in vivo MR images of soft tissue tumors: guide to gross specimen sampling. Magn Res Imag 10:351, 1992.

63. Geirnaerdt MJ, Bloem JL, Eulderink F, et al: Cartilaginous tumors: correlation of gadolinium-enhanced MR imaging and histopathologic findings. Radiology 186:813, 1993.

64. deBaere T, Vanel D, Shapeero LG, et al. Osteosarcoma after chemotherapy: evaluation with contrast material-enhanced subtraction MR imaging. Radiology 185:587, 1992.

65. Fletcher BD: Response of osteosarcoma and Ewing sarcoma to chemotherapy: imaging evaluation. AJR 157:825, 1991.

66. Roth D, Widelec J, Ramon F, et al: Adipose tumors of soft tissues. J Belge Radiol 75:321, 1992.

67. Deutsch AL, Mink JH: Magnetic resonance imaging of musculoskeletal injuries. Radiol Clin North Am 27:983, 1989.

68. Ehara S, Nakasato T, Tamakawa Y, et al: MRI of myositis ossificans circumscripta. Clin Imaging 15:130, 1991.

69. Kransdorf MJ, Meis JM, Jelinek JS: Myositis ossificans: MR appearance with radiologic-pathologic correlation. AJR 157:1243, 1991.

70. Lang P, Genant HK, Jergesen HE, et al: Imaging of the hip joint. Computed tomography versus magnetic resonance imaging. Clin Orthop 274:135, 1992.

71. Yao L, Lee JK: Occult intraosseous fracture: detection with MR imaging. Radiology 167:749, 1988.

72. Mink JH, Deutsch AL: Occult cartilage and bone injuries of the knee: detection, classification, and assessment with MR imaging. Radiology 170:823, 1989.

73. Berger PE, Ofstein RA, Jackson DW, et al: MRI demonstration of radiographically occult fractures: what have we been missing? RadioGraphics 9:407, 1989.

74. Deutsch AL, Mink JH, Shellock FG: Magnetic resonance imaging of injuries to bone and articular cartilage. Emphasis on radiographically occult abnormalities. Orthop Rev 19:66, 1990.

75. Meyers SP, Wiener SN: Magnetic resonance imaging features of fractures using the short tau inversion recovery (STIR) sequence: correlation with radiographic findings. Skel Radiol 20:499, 1991.

76. Deutsch AL, Mink JH, Waxman AD: Occult fractures of the proximal femur: MR imaging. Radiology 170:113, 1989.

77. Quinn SF, McCarthy JL: Prospective evaluation of patients with suspected hip fracture and indeterminate radiographs: use of T1-weighted MR images. Radiology 187:469, 1993.

78. Rizzo PF, Gould ES, Lyden JP, et al: Diagnosis of occult fractures about the hip. Magnetic resonance imaging compared with bone-scanning. J Bone Joint Surg [Am] 75:395, 1993.

79. Weber WN, Neumann CH, Barakos JA, et al: Lateral tibial rim (Segond) fractures: MR imaging characteristics. Radiology 180:731, 1991.

80. Lee JK, Yao L: Stress fractures: MR imaging. Radiology 169:217, 1988.

81. Hayes CW, Conway WF, Sundaram M: Misleading aggressive MR imaging appearance of some benign musculoskeletal lesions. RadioGraphics 12:1119, 1993.

82. Gay SB, Chen NC, Burch JJ, et al: Multiplanar reconstruction in magnetic resonance evaluation of the knee. Comparison with film magnetic resonance interpretation. Invest Radiol 28:142, 1993.

83. Buckwalter KA, Pennes DR: Anterior cruciate ligament: oblique sagittal MR imaging. Radiology 175:276, 1990.

84. Lotysch M, Mink J, Crues JV, et al: Magnetic resonance imaging in the detection of meniscal injuries. Magn Res Imag 4:94, 1986.

85. Crues JV, Mink J, Levy TL, et al: Meniscal tears of the knee: accuracy of magnetic resonance imaging. Radiology 164:445, 1987.

86. Dillon EH, Pope CF, Jokl P, et al: The clinical significance of stage 2 meniscal abnormalities on magnetic resonance knee images. Magn Res Imag 8:411, 1990.

87. Negendank WG, Fernandez-Madrid FR, Heilbrun LK, et al: Magnetic resonance imaging of meniscal degeneration in asymptomatic knees. J Orthop Res 8:311, 1990.

88. Kaplan PA, Nelson NL, Garvin KL, et al: MR of the knee: the significance of high signal in the meniscus that does not clearly extend to the surface. AJR 156:333, 1991.

89. Dillon EH, Pope CF, Jokl P, et al: Follow-up of grade 2 meniscal abnormalities in the stable knee. Radiology 181:849, 1991.

90. DeSmet AA, Norris MA, Yandow DR, et al: MR diagnosis of meniscal tears of the knee: importance of high signal in the meniscus that extends to the surface. AJR 161:101, 1993.

91. Buckwalter KA, Braunstein EM, Janizek DB, et al: MR imaging of meniscal tears: narrow versus conventional window width photography. Radiology 187:827, 1993.

92. Vahey TN, Hunt JE, Shelbourne KD: Anterior translocation of the tibia at MR imaging: a secondary sign of anterior cruciate ligament tear. Radiology 187:817, 1993.

93. Shellock FG, Mink JH, Fox JM: Patellofemoral joint: kinematic MR imaging to assess tracking abnormalities. Radiology 168:551, 1988.

94. Shellock FG, Mink JH, Deutsch AL, et al: Patellar tracking abnormalities: clinical experience with kinematic MR imaging in 130 patients. Radiology 172:799, 1989.

95. Kujala UM, Osterman K, Kormano M, et al: Patellofemoral relationships in recurrent patellar dislocation. J Bone Joint Surg [Br] 71:788, 1989.

96. Shellock FG, Mink JH, Deutsch AL, et al: Patellofemoral joint: identification of abnormalities with active-movement, "unloaded" versus "loaded" kinematic MR imaging techniques. Radiology 188:575, 1993.

97. Brossmann J, Muhle C, Schroder C, et al: Patellar tracking patterns during active and passive knee extension: evaluation with motion-triggered cine MR imaging. Radiology 187:205, 1993.

98. Mirowitz SA: Normal rotator cuff: MR imaging with conventional and fat-suppression techniques. Radiology 180:735, 1991.

99. Coumas JM, Waite RJ, Goss TP, et al: CT and MR evaluation of the labral capsular ligamentous complex of the shoulder. AJR 158:591, 1992.

100. Liou JT, Wilson AJ, Totty WG, et al: The normal shoulder: common variations that simulate pathologic conditions at MR imaging. Radiology 186:435, 1993.

101. Fullerton GD, Cameron IL, Ord VA: Orientation of tendons in the magnetic field and its effect on T2 relaxation times. Radiology 155:433, 1985.

102. Erickson SJ, Cox IH, Hyde JS, et al: Effect of tendon orientation on MR imaging signal intensity: a manifestation of the "magic angle" phenomenon. Radiology 181:389, 1991.

103. Erickson SJ, Prost RW, Timins ME: The "magic angle" effect: background physics and clinical relevance [editorial]. Radiology 188:23, 1993.

104. Stiles RG, Otte MT: Imaging of the shoulder. Radiology 188:603, 1993.

105. Cheung Y, Rosenberg ZS, Magee T, et al: Normal anatomy and pathologic conditions of ankle tendons: current imaging techniques. RadioGraphics 12:429, 1992.

106. Beltran J, Munchow AM, Khabiri H, et al: Ligaments of the lateral aspect of the ankle and sinus tarsi: an MR imaging study. Radiology 177:455, 1990.

107. Ekstrom JE, Shuman WP, Mack LA: MR imaging of accessory soleus muscle. J Comput Assist Tomogr 14:239, 1990.

108. Buschmann WR, Cheung Y, Jahss MH: Magnetic resonance imaging of anomalous leg muscles: accessory soleus, peroneus quartus and the flexor digitorum longus accessorius. Foot Ankle 12:109, 1991.

109. Paul MA, Imanse J, Golding RP, et al: Accessory soleus muscle mimicking a soft tissue tumor. A report of 2 patients. Acta Orthop Scand 62:609, 1991.

110. Erickson SJ, Rosengarten JL: MR imaging of the forefoot: normal anatomic findings. AJR 160:565, 1993.

111. Cardone BW, Erickson SJ, Hartog BD, et al: MRI of injury to the lateral collateral ligamentous complex of the ankle. J Comput Assist Tomogr 17:102, 1993.

112. Daffner RH, Reimer BL, Lupetin ARE, et al: Magnetic resonance imaging in acute tendon ruptures. Skel Radiol 15:619, 1986.

113. Beltran J, Noto AM, Mosure JC, et al: Ankle: Surface coil imaging at 1.5 T. Radiology 161:203, 1986.

114. Quinn SF, Murray WT, Clark RA, et al: Achilles tendon: MR imaging at 1.5 T. Radiology 164:767, 1987.

115. Rosenberg ZS, Cheung Y, Jahss MH, et al: Rupture of posterior tibial tendon: CT and MR imaging with surgical correlation. Radiology 169:229, 1988.

116. Murphy BJ: MR imaging of the elbow. Radiology 184:525, 1992.

117. Mirowitz SA, London SL: Ulnar collateral ligament injury in baseball pitchers: MR imaging evaluation. Radiology 185:573, 1992.

118. Ho CP, Sartoris DJ: Magnetic resonance imaging of the elbow. Rheum Dis Clin North Am 17:705, 1991.

119. Rosenberg ZS, Beltran J, Cheung YY, et al: The elbow: MR features of nerve disorders. Radiology 188:235, 1993.

120. Smith DK: Volar carpal ligaments of the wrist: normal appearance on multiplanar reconstructions of three-dimensional Fourier transform MR imaging. AJR 161:353, 1993.

121. Smith DK: Dorsal carpal ligaments of the wrist: normal appearance on multi-planar reconstructions of three-dimensional Fourier transform MR imaging. AJR 161:119, 1993.

122. Golimbu CN, Firooznia H, Melone CP Jr, et al: Tears of the triangular fibrocartilage of the wrist: MR imaging. Radiology 173:731, 1989.

123. Schweitzer ME, Brahme SK, Hodler J, et al: Chronic wrist pain: spin-echo and short tau inversion recovery MR imaging and conventional and MR arthrography. Radiology 182:205, 1992.

124. Cerofolini E, Luchetti R, Pederzini L, et al.: MR evaluation of triangular fibrocartilage complex tears in the wrist: comparison with arthrography and arthroscopy. J Comput Assist Tomogr 14:963, 1990.

125. Zlatkin MB, Chao PC, Osterman AL, et al: Chronic wrist pain: evaluation with high-resolution MR imaging. Radiology 173:723, 1989.

126. Wright SM, Wright RM: Bilateral MR imaging with switched mutually coupled receiver coils. Radiology 170:249, 1989.

127. Schellhas KP: Internal derangement of the temporomandibular joint: radiologic staging with clinical, surgical, and pathologic correlation. Magn Res Imag 7:495, 1989.

128. Schellhas KP, Wilkes CH, Fritts HM, et al: Temporomandibular joint: MR imaging of internal derangements and postoperative changes. AJR 150:381, 1988.

129. Chan WP, Lang P, Stevens MP, et al: Osteoarthritis of the knee: comparison of radiography, CT, and MR imaging to assess extent and severity. AJR 157:799, 1991.

130. McAlindon TE, Watt I, McCrae F, et al: Magnetic resonance imaging in osteoarthritis of the knee: correlation with radiographic and scintigraphic findings. Ann Rheum Dis 50:14, 1991.

131. Martel W, Adler RS, Chan K, et al: Overview: new methods in imaging osteoarthritis. J Rheumatol (Suppl) 27:32, 1991.

132. Conway WF, Hayes CW, Loughran T, et al: Cross-sectional imaging of the patellofemoral joint and surrounding structures. RadioGraphics 11:195, 1991.

133. DeSmet AA, Monu JU, Fisher DR, et al: Signs of patellar chondromalacia on sagittal T2-weighted magnetic resonance imaging. Skel Radiol 21:103, 1992.

134. Adam G, Nolte-Ernsting C, Prescher A, et al: Experimental hyaline cartilage lesions: two-dimensional spin-echo versus three-dimensional gradient-echo MR imaging. J Magn Res Imag 1:665, 1991.

135. Hodler J, Trudell D, Pathria MN, et al: Width of the articular cartilage of the hip: quantification by using fat suppression spin-echo MR imaging in cadavers. AJR 159:351, 1992.

136. Hodler J, Berthiaume MJ, Schweitzer ME, et al: Knee joint hyaline cartilage defects: a comparative study of MR and anatomic sections. J Comput Assist Tomogr 16:597, 1992.

137. Heron CW, Calvert PT: Three-dimensional gradient-echo MR imaging of the knee: comparison with arthroscopy in 100 patients. Radiology 183:839, 1992.

138. Recht MP, Kramer J, Marcelis S, et al: Abnormalities of articular cartilage in the knee: analysis of available MR techniques. Radiology 187:473, 1993.

139. Brown DG, Edwards NL, Greer JM, et al: Magnetic resonance imaging in patients with inflammatory arthritis of the knee. Clin Rheumatol 9:73, 1990.

140. Corvetta A, Giovagnoni A, Baldelli S, et al: MR imaging of rheumatoid hand lesions: comparison with conventional radiology in 31 patients. Clin Exp Rheumatol 10:217, 1992.

141. Rubens DJ, Blebea JS, Totterman SM, et al: Rheumatoid arthritis: evaluation of wrist extensor tendons with clinical examination versus MR imaging—a preliminary report. Radiology 187:831, 1993.

142. Jorgensen C, Cyteval C, Anaya JM, et al: Sensitivity of magnetic resonance imaging of the wrist in very early rheumatoid arthritis. Clin Exp Rheumatol 11:163, 1993.

143. Schweitzer ME, Falk A, Pathria M, et al: MR imaging of the knee: can changes in the intracapsular fat pads be used as a sign of synovial proliferation in the presence of an effusion? AJR 160:823, 1993.

144. Kursunoglu-Brahme S, Riccio T, Weisman MH, et al: Rheumatoid knee: role of gadopentetate-enhanced MR imaging. Radiology 176:831, 1990.

145. Bjorkengren AG, Geborek P, Rydholm U, et al: MR imaging of the knee in acute rheumatoid arthritis: synovial uptake of gadolinium-DTPA. AJR 155:329, 1990.

146. Konig H, Sieper J, Wolf KJ: Rheumatoid arthritis: evaluation of hypervascular and fibrous pannus with dynamic MR imaging enhanced with Gd-DTPA. Radiology 176:473, 1990.

147. Jaffe IA: New approaches to the management of rheumatoid arthritis. J Rheumatol 19:2, 1992.

148. Fisher MR, Dooms GC, Hricak H, et al: Magnetic resonance imaging of the normal and pathologic muscular system. Magn Res Imag 4:491, 1986.

149. Schedel H, Reimers CD, Nagele M, et al: Imaging techniques in myotonic dystrophy. A comparative study of ultrasound, computed tomography and magnetic resonance imaging of skeletal muscles. Europ J Radiol 15:230, 1992.

150. Metzler JP, Fleckenstein JL, Vuitch F, et al: Skeletal muscle lymphoma: MRI evaluation. Magn Res Imag 10:491, 1992.

151. Fleckenstein JL, Canby RC, Parkey RW, et al: Acute effects of exercise on MR imaging of skeletal muscle in normal volunteers. AJR 151:231, 1988.

152. Fisher MJ, Meyer RA, Adams GR, et al: Direct relationship between proton T2 and exercise intensity in skeletal muscle MR images. Invest Radiol 25:480, 1990.

153. deKerviler E, Leroy-Willig A, Jehenson P, et al: Exercise-induced muscle modifications: study of healthy subjects and patients with metabolic myopathies with MR imaging and P-31 spectroscopy. Radiology 181:259, 1991.

154. Shellock FG, Fukunaga T, Mink JH, et al: Exertional muscle injury: evaluation of concentric versus eccentric actions with serial MR imaging. Radiology 179:659, 1991.

155. Kuriyama M, Hayakawa K, Konishi Y, et al: MR imaging of myopathy. Comput Med Imaging Graph 13:329, 1989.

156. Lamminen AE, Tanttu JI, Sepponen RE, et al: Magnetic resonance of diseased skeletal muscle: combined T1 measurement and chemical shift imaging. Br J Radiol 63:591, 1990.

157. Hernandez RJ, Keim DR, Sullivan DB, et al: Magnetic resonance imaging appearance of the muscles in childhood dermatomyositis. J Pediatr 117:546, 1990.

158. Lamminen AE: Magnetic resonance imaging of primary skeletal muscle diseases: patterns of distribution and severity of involvement. Br J Radiol 63:946, 1990.

159. Hernandez RJ, Sullivan DB, Chenevert TL, et al: MR imaging in children with dermatomyositis: musculoskeletal findings and correlation with clinical and laboratory findings. AJR 161:359, 1993.

160. Fleckenstein JL, Weatherall PT, Parkey RW, et al: Sports-related muscle injuries: evaluation with MR imaging. Radiology 172:793, 1989.

161. DeSmet AA, Fisher DR, Heiner JP, et al: Magnetic resonance imaging of muscle tears. Skel Radiol 19:283, 1990.

162. Fleckenstein JL, Shellock FG: Exertional muscle injuries: magnetic resonance imaging evaluation. Top Magn Res Imag 3:50, 1991.

163. Greco A, McNamara MT, Escher RM, et al: Spin-echo and STIR MR imaging of sports-related muscle injuries at 1.5 T. J Comput Assist Tomogr 15:994, 1991.

164. Hernandez RJ, Keim DR, Chenevert TL, et al: Fat-suppressed MR imaging of myositis. Radiology 182:217, 1992.

165. Fleckenstein JL, Watumull D, Conner KE, et al: Denervated human skeletal muscle: MR imaging evaluation. Radiology 187:213, 1993.

166. Barfuss H, Fischer H, Hentschel D, et al: In vivo magnetic resonance imaging and spectroscopy of humans with a 4 T whole-body magnet. NMR Biomed 3:31, 1990.

167. Cohen JS: Phospholipid and energy metabolism of cancer cells monitored by 31-P magnetic resonance sspectroscopy: possible clinical significance. Mayo Clin Proc 63:1199, 1988.

168. Lenkinski RE, Schnall MD: Magnetic resonance spectroscopy. In ME Kricun (Ed): Imaging of Bone Tumors. Philadelphia, W.B. Saunders Co, 1993.

169. Lenkinski RE, Holland GA, Allman T, et al: Integrated MR imaging and spectroscopy with chemical shift imaging of P-31 at 1.5 T: initial clinical experience. Radiology 169:201, 1988.

170. Shinkwin MA, Lenkinski RE, Daly JM, et al: Integrated magnetic resonance imaging and phosphorus spectroscopy of soft tissue tumors. Cancer 67:1849, 1991.

171. Dewhirst MW, Sostman HD, Leopold KA, et al: Soft-tissue sarcomas: MR imaging and MR spectroscopy for prognosis and therapy monitoring. Work in progress. Radiology 174:847, 1990.

172. Fleckenstein JL, Bertocci LA, Nunnally RL, et al: Exercise-enhanced MR imaging of variations in forearm muscle anatomy and use: importance in MR spectroscopy. AJR 153:693, 1989.

173. Kariya Y, Itoh M, Nakamura T, et al: Magnetic resonance imaging and spectroscopy of thigh muscles in cruciate ligament insufficiency. Acta Orthop Scand 60:322, 1989.

174. Vock P, Hoppeler H, Hartl W, et al: Combined use of magnetic resonance imaging (MRI) and spectroscopy (MRS) by whole body magnets in studying skeletal muscle morphology and metabolism. Invest Radiol 20:486, 1985.

175. Newman RJ: Clinical applications of nuclear magnetic resonance spectroscopy: A review. J Roy Soc Med 77:774, 1984.

176. Nidecker AC, Muller S, Aue WP, et al: Extremity bone tumors: Evaluation by P-31 MR spectroscopy. Radiology 157:167, 1985.

177. Burt CT, Koutcher J, Roberts JT, et al: Magnetic resonance spectroscopy of the musculoskeletal system. Radiol Clin North Am 24:321, 1986.

178. Redmond OM, Stack JP, Dervan PA, et al: Osteosarcoma: use of MR imaging and MR spectroscopy in clinical decision making. Radiology 172:811, 1989.

179. Lenkinski RE, Listerud J, Shinkwin MA, et al. Magnetic resonance imaging and magnetic resonance spectroscopy of bone tumors and bone marrow disease. Invest Radiol 24:1006, 1989.

180. Norris SL, Gober JR, Haywood LJ, et al: Altered muscle metabolism shown by magnetic resonance spectroscopy in sickle cell disease with leg ulcers. Magn Res Imag 11:119, 1993.

181. Cresshull I, Dawson MJ, Edwards RHT, et al: Human muscle analyzed by $^{31}$P nuclear magnetic resonance in intact subjects. J Physiol 317:18, 1981.

182. Park JH, Vansant JP, Kumar NG, et al: Dermatomyositis: correlative MR imaging and P-31 MR spectroscopy for quantitative characterization of inflammatory disease. Radiology 177:473, 1990.

183. Daly PF, Cohan JS: Magnetic resonance spectroscopy of tumors and potential in vivo clinical applications: a review. Cancer Res 49:770, 1989.

184. Ross B, Helsper JT, Cox J, et al: Osteosarcoma and other neoplasms of bone.

Magnetic resonance spectroscopy to monitor therapy. Arch Surg *122:*1464, 1987.

185. Bryant DJ, Bydder GM, Case HA, et al: Use of phosphorus-31 MR spectroscopy to monitor response to chemotherapy in non-Hodgkin lymphoma. J Comput Assist Tomogr *12:*770, 1988.

186. Redmond OM, Stack JP, Dervan PA, et al: Osteosarcoma: Use of MR imaging and MR spectroscopy in clinical decision making. Radiology *172:*811, 1989.

187. Negendank WG, Crowley MG, Ryan JR, et al: Bone and soft-tissue lesions: diagnosis with combined H-1 MR imaging and P-31 MR spectroscopy. Radiology *173:*181, 1989.

188. Zlatkin MB, Lenkinski RE, Shinkwin M, et al: Combined MR imaging and spectroscopy of bone and soft tissue tumors. J Comput Assist Tomogr *14:*1, 1990.

# 11

# Diagnostic Ultrasonography

*Laurence A. Mack, M.D., and*
*William Scheible, M.D.*

The development of high frequency linear array real-time transducers has dramatically increased the capabilities of ultrasonography in the evaluation of the musculoskeletal system. This group of devices shares common characteristics of excellent near-field resolution, electronic focusing, and very high transducer frequency (7 to 10 megahertz [MHz]). These qualities are especially important in imaging tendons and muscles, which often are superficial and whose internal architecture commonly is parallel to the transducer surface. Real-time transducers allow vastly increased flexibility in varying the plane of section in comparison to older sonographic techniques. Although the role of diagnostic ultrasonography in problems related to bone, joint, and soft tissue is somewhat limited compared with CT and MR imaging, the situations are increasing in which the technique offers significant information, usually with less discomfort, risk, cost, and time expenditure than alternative radiographic or isotopic procedures.

## FUNDAMENTAL PHYSICS

The heart of ultrasonographic imaging technology is the transducer. A transducer converts electrical energy to sound energy and back again. Crystalline materials can be physically deformed by an electrical current, resulting in the production of sound waves. Sound waves returning from the body then deform the transducer crystal similarly to produce an electrical current. The property of crystals that exhibit this behavior is called the piezoelectric effect, and it forms the cornerstone for the clinical applications of ultrasonography. The transducer acts as a receiver for approximately 999/1000 of any time period, having been operative only instantaneously as a sender of sound waves.

In clinical use, the emitted sound waves have a frequency of 2.25 to 10 MHz; 1 MHz equals one million cycles per second (cps). These frequencies are far above the range of human hearing, which has an upper limit of approximately 20,000 cps. Frequency is inversely related to wavelength and to the depth of penetration into a given material. A higher frequency transducer (10 MHz, for example) is capable of penetrating into soft tissue only a few centimeters. Conversely, the higher the frequency, the better the resolution capability. Because of their superficial location, most musculoskeletal problems are better imaged with higher frequency instruments.

The transducer usually is placed directly on the skin of the patient. A suitable acoustic coupling agent, most often an aqueous gel, is applied to the skin surface to create a gas-free pathway for sound waves. Scanning planes are variable. In most applications, the structure under evaluation should be imaged parallel and transverse to the axis of its fibers.

The interaction of propagated sound waves with tissue interfaces in the body is a second key consideration in sonographic imaging. Whenever the sound beam encounters an interface between tissues of different acoustic impedance, reflection or refraction occurs. It is the waves reflected back to the transducer crystal and converted into electrical input that are recorded and displayed as ultrasonographic images. Early imaging with ultrasound technology was termed "bistable" because display essentially was an all-or-none phenomenon. Diagnostic information provided by this technique was limited to definition of boundaries of organs or lesions and to characterization of fluid and solid structures. Bistable display has been replaced by gray-scale technology, which allows returning echoes of different intensities to be displayed with varying shades of gray that provide information about organ parenchyma.

Initial reports in musculoskeletal ultrasonography used static scanners. Such devices are cumbersome and difficult to use. The complex, mechanical nature of the scanning gantries limited available planes of section and precluded dynamic assessment of structures. Such instruments have been replaced by real-time scanners. Real-time can be considered the sonographic equivalent of radiographic fluoroscopy because it allows the creation of multiple images per second and thus allows the observation and recording of dynamic events.

Commercially available units use a variety of techniques to acquire their information. Mechanical sector scanners produce high quality images but are limited by suboptimal superficial resolution as a result of near-field artifact and a narrow superficial image field. They are, in addition, prone to producing artifact. Because only small portions of parallel tendon fibers in the center of the image have the specular reflection geometry, an artifactual heterogeneity of the tendons may be observed.

High resolution linear array transducers are best applied to musculoskeletal examination. Transducers of 7 to 10 MHz are preferable to those of lower frequency. Lower frequency (3.5 to 5 MHz) transducers may be required for adequate tissue penetration in the examination of deeper structures. Compared with mechanical transducers, linear array transducers demonstrate superior near resolution. In addition, their broad superficial field of view is helpful in evaluating superficial abnormalities, and a greater portion of the parallel tendon and muscle fibers will fulfill the specular reflection condition that best delineates pathologic structure and avoids artifact.

Techniques to evaluate and display blood flow also have been developed. Pulsed Doppler sonography permits the interrogation of blood vessels to determine the direction and character of flow. Newer computer techniques now permit display of Doppler information simultaneously with gray-scale data by use of color. Different colors are used to indicate direction and mean velocity of movement. Such color Doppler images allow rapid and precise localization of vessels for pulsed Doppler evaluation, characterization of vascular distribution, and semiquantitative assessment of flow volume.

## PRINCIPLES OF CLINICAL ULTRASONOGRAPHY

Descriptive terminology in diagnostic ultrasonography is relatively straightforward. Lesions are characterized as being either cystic or solid. Cystic structures are typified by any fluid-filled mass such as a renal cyst, a pancreatic pseudocyst, or a normal organ such as the distended urinary bladder. Cystic organs or masses are echo-free. Because their fluid nature does not impede the transmission of sound, a strong buildup of echoes, often called posterior acoustic enhancement, is seen deep to the area. Solid masses and the parenchyma of most organs exhibit a variable pattern of middle amplitude gray tones. The liver parenchyma, the nongravid uterus, and the thyroid gland are examples. Many neoplasms and inflammatory masses show a complex echographic appearance, containing both solid and fluid elements. This usually is a manifestation of tissue necrosis, hemorrhage, or inflammatory debris, but the inherent cystic or solid character of the lesion can be ascertained by knowledge of these physical principles.

Deterrents to successful ultrasonography are air and bone because the vast majority of acoustic energy is reflected by these media. For this reason, much of the thorax is blind to ultrasonography. Likewise, intestinal gas sometimes hinders examinations of the abdomen and retroperitoneum. This feature can be used to advantage in the assessment of bone architecture for the detection of subtle contour abnormalities caused by fracture.[1]

The earliest use of diagnostic ultrasonography was in the differentiation of cystic from solid mass lesions that had been detected by clinical or radiographic examinations. Although this still is an important task for sonography, distinction between cystic and solid is only one feature of tissue characterization. Analysis of gray-scale patterns sometimes allows anticipation of the histologic makeup of a given lesion. Fat, for example, tends to be highly echogenic. On the other hand, lymphoma and some neurogenic tumors, although solid on pathologic examination, may be hypoechoic, mimicking the findings in cysts. Unfortunately, although experimental work with tissue characterization has been extant for years, no truly reliable or practical measurements exist to grant ultrasonography meaningful tissue specificity.

Several unique properties of ultrasonography make the technique particularly useful. It is noninvasive and painless to the patient. It generally is less expensive and performed more rapidly than alternative studies. The risks associated with iodinated contrast material are eliminated. So far as is known, pulsed ultrasound beams in clinically useful power settings and frequencies have no deleterious effect on somatic or genetic cells.[2, 3] Sonography is well suited to sequential follow-up studies to determine response to a particular therapeutic regimen. Because it allows localization of lesions in three dimensions, sonography is a useful technique for guiding percutaneous aspiration or biopsy and for mapping radiation portals.

## CLINICAL USE IN BONE, JOINT, AND SOFT TISSUE DISEASES

### Popliteal Space

The use of ultrasonography for evaluating various swellings in the popliteal space gained acceptance early. Because the fluid-solid distinction was accomplished easily even by early instruments and because popliteal cysts and popliteal artery aneurysms constitute the majority of masses in this area, sonography frequently has been used in diagnosing these lesions.

Popliteal cysts (Baker's cysts) arise in knee joints that have a communication between the knee joint and the gastrocnemiosemimembranosus bursa as well as an intra-articular abnormality to produce an effusion capable of distending the joint.[4-7] The gastrocnemiosemimembranosus bursa is situated between the medial head of the gastrocnemius muscle and the semimembranosus muscle more laterally.[8, 9] Anatomic connection between the bursa and the knee joint is present in about 50 per cent of normal persons. The bursa is lined with synovium continuous with that in the joint space.

A joint effusion is a response to a number of abnormalities of the knee. As a component in the genesis of popliteal cysts, effusions most often are related to the synovial proliferation of rheumatoid arthritis or to traumatic internal derangements of the knee joint. Popliteal cysts also have been described in patients with osteoarthritis, gout, Reiter's syndrome, pigmented villonodular synovitis, and osteochondritis dissecans.[5]

In the past, arthrography was the most important tool in the diagnosis of popliteal cyst. Arthrographic success rates for detecting popliteal cysts are variable, with cited figures ranging from 7 to 42 per cent.[4] However, several problems were associated with this technique. It is thought that, in many instances, a check valve mechanism limits flow of synovial fluid to one direction.[6] As a result, contrast arthrography might fail to detect some popliteal cysts.[4] It also has been noted that flexion of the knee can collapse the suprapatellar bursa, forcing fluid into the gastrocnemiosemimembranosus bursa.[8] In this circumstance, arthrographic filling of the distended bursa can lead to a false diagnosis of popliteal cyst. Because many of these patients are likely to be asymptomatic,[10] any arthrographic diagnosis of popliteal cyst should be substantiated by sonography. Conversely, any sonographically diagnosed popliteal cyst probably is clinically significant.[10] Lack of anatomic continuity between the knee joint and the gastrocnemiosemimembranosus bursa prevents arthrographic demonstration of a significant number of cysts. Also, the contrast agent may not fill the entire cyst because of fibrin clots, adhesions, and loculations.

The sonographic appearance of popliteal cysts consists of a smooth-walled cystic mass visualized medially in the popliteal fossa (Fig. 11–1). Variable amounts of septation, debris, or pannus may be seen within the cyst. Color Doppler sonography may be helpful in differentiating cysts from the popliteal artery, which lies more centrally within the popliteal fossa. The size threshold for sonographic identification of popliteal cysts should be less than 1 cm, partic-

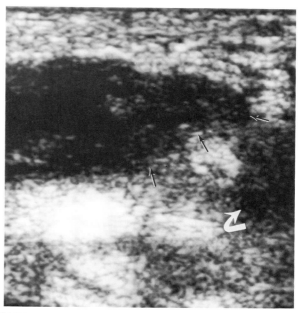

**FIGURE 11–2.** Ruptured Baker's cyst. A longitudinal prone scan in a patient with ruptured Baker's cyst demonstrates loss of sharp margination at the inferior aspect of the popliteal cyst (arrows) and adjacent soft tissue edema (curved arrow). Note debris within the popliteal cyst.

ularly with the use of higher frequency transducers. The size of the cyst on sonography may differ from that visualized on arthrography. Incomplete opacification, filling defects from clot or debris, and distention from gas and contrast agent may account for these differences.

Rupture of a popliteal cyst or hemorrhage into the cyst can lead to a clinical picture that closely mimics deep venous thrombophlebitis.[9, 11, 12] Compression of the popliteal vein by the cyst also can produce physical signs resembling thrombophlebitis.[13] The distinction between a popliteal cyst and thrombophlebitis is an important one to make, as anticoagulant therapy is required in the latter instance and is not without hazard. Ultrasonography has been a valuable aid in this clinical setting.[5, 7, 14-16] Loss of normal sharp margins along the inferior aspect of the cyst and superficial fluid spaces with surrounding edema are the most common findings associated with rupture (Fig. 11–2).[17] Sonography may fail to detect some ruptured cysts that have decompressed.

Ultrasonography also may be helpful in patients in whom the synovial membrane herniates through a weakened posterior capsule of the knee joint. This probably occurs in those persons who lack anatomic communication between the joint space and the gastrocnemiosemimembranosus bursa; therefore, when rupture occurs, a pseudocapsule forms to contain fluid.[9] These collections most often are located between the gastrocnemius and the soleus muscles.

It is important to remember that not every swelling in this area is secondary to a popliteal cyst, and sonography conveniently can exclude other causes, such as a popliteal artery aneurysm, soft tissue tumor, or abscess.[6, 7, 14] Aneurysms of the popliteal artery are the most frequent of the peripheral arterial aneurysms.[18] Atheromatous disease is causative in the vast majority of cases, and a significant number of patients have coexisting cardiovascular disease,

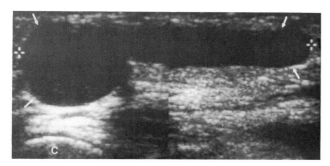

**FIGURE 11–1.** Popliteal cyst. Longitudinal scan of the popliteal fossa shows a cystic fluid-filled mass in the proximal part of the calf (arrows). The patient is prone with head to viewer's left. *C,* Femoral condyle.

including abdominal aortic aneurysm.[18–20] The lesions are bilateral in up to 59 per cent of cases, although involvement of only one side may be evident clinically.[18, 20, 21] Popliteal artery aneurysms commonly are associated with thromboembolic complications, including thrombosis, venous occlusion, ulceration and gangrene, and peripheral embolization.[18, 21–24] A 3 per cent prevalence of limb loss has been cited for untreated popliteal artery aneurysms.[18] Up to 15 per cent of patients may have associated popliteal vein thrombosis, thus being at risk for pulmonary embolism.[25]

The ultrasonographic diagnosis of popliteal artery aneurysm is relatively straightforward as long as continuity of the mass with a proximal and distal vessel can be ascertained.[22] This occasionally may be difficult when the popliteal artery is exceedingly tortuous.[19] Use of color and pulsed Doppler techniques has greatly enhanced diagnostic capabilities in this application by facilitating vascular identification. Thus, angiography, the traditional method for diagnosing and evaluating popliteal artery aneurysms, is not necessary to establish the diagnosis.[18, 20] In addition, arteriography suffers from several limitations that are overcome by ultrasonography.[21, 22, 26, 27] Many patients with popliteal artery aneurysms have diffuse vascular disease, and compromised proximal inflow may preclude visualization of the popliteal artery. Thrombus within an aneurysm, easily documented by sonography, is not well seen with arteriography, which opacifies only the patent lumen carrying flowing blood. Thrombus is considered by some clinicians to be an indication for surgery.[26, 27] Clinical diagnosis is not always straightforward, as in cases in which pulsation is absent because of a thrombosed aneurysm.[14]

Because of the high rate of complications in untreated popliteal artery aneurysms, elective surgical correction is recommended for most patients.[18, 22, 23] A sensitive, noninvasive screening procedure is necessary, and ultrasonography is thought by some investigators to be more accurate than either clinical or arteriographic evaluation.[22, 23, 26, 27] The size of the normal popliteal artery has been determined in control groups, and ultrasonography yields accurate measurements because there is no magnification distortion.[26, 27] In addition to the ability of sonography to detect aneurysms and thrombus within them, the technique easily accomplishes a survey of the other leg for clinically silent aneurysms.

Ultrasonography has been recommended as a screening procedure for patients with rheumatoid arthritis who have painful or asymptomatic swelling of the popliteal space.[6, 28] Because structural integrity of the knee joint is not an issue in these patients, the risks, discomfort, and costs of arthrography can be avoided. Moreover, ultrasonography is a particularly attractive means of performing serial noninvasive studies to monitor response to various therapeutic endeavors.[6, 29] Popliteal cysts probably are best treated by anterior synovectomy, as recurrences and sinus tracts are not rare after attempts at cyst removal only.[6, 30] Synovial ablation with radioisotopes also has been advocated, with ultrasonography used in an effort to diagnose synovial thickening prior to the onset of radiographic bony changes.[29]

## Knee

The role of ultrasonography in the evaluation of the knee has been diminished by MR imaging. However, sonography may be helpful in evaluating specific problems when results of other examinations are not definitive. Investigations have centered on the sonographic evaluation of cartilage. In a series of patients with osteoarthritis, ultrasonography was shown to be capable of measuring the thickness of articular cartilage and of assessing its surface characteristics.[31] However, with increasing severity of disease, the sharp interface between cartilage and soft tissue is blurred, making measurement of cartilage thickness more difficult. In one report, the sonographic features that were best at distinguishing normal from abnormal cartilage were loss of cartilage hypoechogenicity and decrease in the sharpness of the anterior cartilage margin.[32] Similar findings were reported by Brussaard and associates.[33] Small areas of osteochondritis dissecans also can be visualized as contour changes in the bony margin of the femoral condyle.[34] Internal echogenicity of such defects may vary, depending on the degree of calcification of the fragment. In one of 25 reported cases, a loose osteochondral fragment was visualized, suggesting a future application of the technique.[34]

Real-time ultrasonography is capable of showing the posterior horns of the medial and lateral menisci, which are injured most frequently yet are the most difficult to see at arthroscopy.[35] The normal meniscus appears as a triangular hyperechoic structure. Tears are visualized as hypoechoic linear defects within this structure. Vertical concentric tears as small as 2 mm and horizontal tears as small as 4 mm have been seen consistently in vitro.[36] The clinical utility of this technique has not been evaluated systematically, however.

Meniscal cysts are a common cause of masses in locations that are atypical for simple popliteal cysts.[37] Such cysts are most common in the third decade of life, in men, on the right side, and in the lateral meniscus.[38] The vast majority of meniscal cysts are associated with tears of the menisci.[39, 40] Because of tightly adherent medial collateral ligaments, medial cysts may lie at some distance from the meniscus.[41] Lateral cysts usually are found adjacent to the underlying meniscal lesion.

Several reports have described the sonographic appearance of meniscal cysts.[38, 41, 42] Meniscal cysts are easily identified sonographically as fluid-containing spaces superficial to the menisci and collateral ligaments (Fig. 11–3). By acting as an acoustic standoff, the cyst also may enhance the ability to visualize the underlying meniscal tear. Meniscal cysts must be differentiated from ganglion cysts and hypoechoic neural tumors, which may occur in similar locations.

## Patellar Tendon

Jumper's knee, a term describing a group of conditions that constitute the most common cause of extra-articular knee pain,[43] is seen in persons whose activities involve frequent, vigorous use of the extensor mechanism of the knee. Athletic activities that include repetitive jumping, running, or kicking are involved most often.[44] Jumper's knee is thought to be caused by multiple partial fiber tears of the patellar tendon that lead to degeneration, necrosis, or fibrosis rather than to be the result of a primary inflammatory lesion.[45]

When scanned longitudinally, the normal patellar tendon is visualized as a linear structure of medium echogenicity

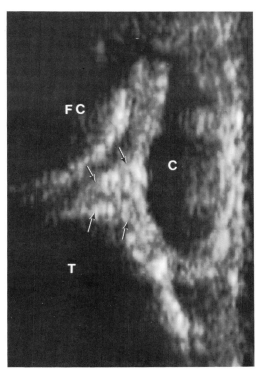

**FIGURE 11–3.** Meniscal cyst. Coronal scan of the lateral aspect of the knee demonstrates a meniscal cyst *(C)* just superficial to the posterior horn of the lateral meniscus (arrows). *FC,* Femoral condyle; *T,* tibia.

deep to more echogenic subcutaneous fat and the hypoechoic serous pretibial bursa.[46] Deep to the tendon, a second anechoic bursa may be seen. The internal architecture is similar to that of other tendons, with parallel echogenic fibers and homogeneous density. Some reports describe a slight decrease in echogenicity in normal sedentary persons at the superior attachment, where the tendon is very slightly larger in diameter.[46] Other investigators have failed to observe this finding.[47] In athletic persons, the patellar tendon may assume a more conical configuration with broadening of this superior attachment.[46]

Seventy-seven to 90 per cent of abnormalities in patellar tendinitis are visualized at the proximal attachment of the tendon (Fig. 11–4).[45, 47] In early stages of disease, the tendon appears enlarged secondary to edema.[43] Such enlargement most often is diffuse. If the inflammatory process continues, the tendon becomes heterogeneous in its internal architecture with areas of central hypoechogenicity being the most common sonographic finding. However, hyperechoic foci occasionally may be seen. Such focal areas correlate closely with areas of abnormal tendon observed at surgery and correlate well with abnormalities visualized on CT scans and MR images.[45] Pathologic findings in these areas of focal abnormality include mucoid degeneration, granulation tissue, and intratendinous hematomas.[46] In the final stages of long-standing disease, the tendinous margins become irregular and the normal tendon architecture is disrupted by fibrosis and scarring.[43] Postoperatively, findings similar to those in long-standing tendinitis may be noted with the margin of the tendon being less well defined than in the preoperative patient. Excellent correlation of sonographic features and pathologic findings at surgery has been

reported with very few false-positive and false-negative examinations.[45–48] Sonography also has been reported to be helpful in the preoperative localization of lesions.

In pediatric patients with extra-articular knee pain, characteristic sonographic findings in Osgood-Schlatter's disease have been reported. Although this condition usually is diagnosed clinically or by soft tissue radiography, sonography may play a role in less characteristic clinical presentations. De Flaviis and coworkers divided sonographic findings into four groups.[42] The most common presentation was fragmentation of the ossification center of the tibial tuberosity with a decrease in echogenicity. Swelling of the cartilage and subcutaneous tissue also was noted in 20 per cent of cases. Patellar tendon swelling and fluid in the infrapatellar bursa are less common findings. Similar findings were reported by Lanning and Heikkinen and Laine and coworkers, who also noted characteristic elevation of a thin fragment of the tibial tuberosity in 25 per cent of cases.[49, 50]

## Hip

The painful hip frequently is a diagnostic challenge because of the protean causes of such pain, both intrinsic and referred from other sites. Ultrasonography can be used as a screening procedure to document the presence of intra-articular fluid.[51, 52] Percutaneous needle aspiration of the effusion, with or without concurrent arthrography, can guide further therapy effectively.

Disease processes in the femoral triangle must be distinguished from pathologic bone or joint lesions in the adjacent hip. Abscess, hematoma, cellulitis, thrombophlebitis, aneurysm, and lymphadenopathy can be manifested in nonspecific and overlapping ways. Sonography often can differentiate among these conditions and, if necessary, affords a convenient method to guide percutaneous aspiration or biopsy of possibly abnormal areas.[53] Processes of vascular origin must be separated from those of other causes with important implications for contemplated surgery.[54] Direct visualization of venous thrombosis is possible with diagnostic sonography.[55, 56] Prompt institution of anticoagulant or antibiotic therapy, or both, often is effective and can obviate surgery.

Fluid collections within the iliopsoas bursa often are associated with the synovitis that accompanies many arthritides. Distention of this space causes pain that is easily confused with other conditions and can produce a mass effect in the pelvis. Sonography aids in establishing this diagnosis, which can be confirmed by subsequent hip arthrography.[57]

Developmental dysplasia of the hip is present in approximately 1 per cent of newborns, and roughly 0.1 per cent of neonates have frank dislocation.[58] Developmental dysplasia of the hip is more frequent in girls than in boys, in infants born with breech presentation, in firstborn infants, and in pregnancies complicated by oligohydramnios. Timely treatment generally has excellent results, underscoring the need for prompt and accurate diagnosis. Although clinical evaluation by an experienced pediatrician is reliable, many cases are not straightforward. In the past, plain film radiography frequently has been used to evaluate infants suspected of having developmental dysplasia of the hip, but this method is beset with numerous potential pitfalls.[59] Sequential radiographic examinations often are necessary dur-

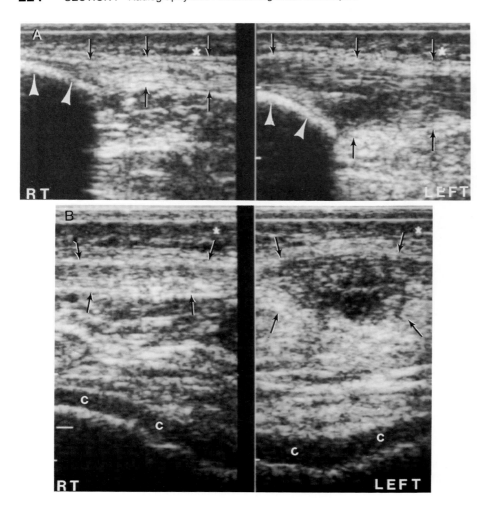

**FIGURE 11–4.** Patellar tendinitis.

**A** Longitudinal scans of the patellar tendon in the right and left knees demonstrate normal appearance on the right side (arrows). On the left, the tendon is thickened and of decreased echogenicity. Arrowheads indicate patellar surface.

**B** Transverse images of the right and left knees in the same patient demonstrate heterogeneity of internal architecture of the affected patellar tendon (arrows) in the left knee. Note the hypoechoic cartilage on the femoral condyle (C). At surgery the hypoechoic region proved to be an area of mucoid degeneration. The patellar tendon in the right knee (arrows) is normal.

ing the course of treatment, with the obviously undesirable effect of exposure to additional radiation.

Ultrasonography has an important role in the diagnosis of developmental dysplasia of the hip.[60, 61] Early reports used articulated-arm B-scanners, and although the results were encouraging, the technical hurdles encountered in obtaining reproducible images were thought by most radiologists to be considerable. Real-time evaluation with high-resolution mechanical sector and linear array transducers has proved to be a simpler and more easily learned technique.[58, 62–65] Graf proposed a complex static, nonstress technique.[66] Using coronal images, the shape of the acetabulum and the position of the femoral head are assessed. Harcke and Grissom, Novick, and others have proposed a dynamic stress technique.[67, 68] Using this technique, the hip is visualized in coronal and transverse images (Fig. 11–5). Movement of the femoral head with various stress maneuvers is evaluated. The thickness of the acetabular cartilage can be determined. Increased thickness of the cartilage has been suggested as an early sign of dysplasia.[69] Using either method, excellent results have been reported with low rates of false-negative and false-positive examinations.

The femoral head is cartilaginous and does not ossify until about 3 to 6 months after birth. This is at once a limitation for radiography and a boon for ultrasonography. The anatomic relationship of the capital femoral epiphysis to the acetabulum can be ascertained easily and precisely

with sonography. The cartilaginous acetabular labrum is a crucial determinant of these relationships, and only sonography can visualize this structure directly.[65] In two clinical reports, sonography proved to be reliable in diagnosing abnormally positioned hips in infants.[58, 63] Importantly, ultrasonic examinations can be carried out during the course of treatment while the child is immobilized in a splint or cast. In fact, sonography yielded information to alter the treatment plan in nearly one fourth of the cases in one series.[63]

Sonographic evaluation of children with Legg-Calvé-Perthes disease has been reported.[70, 71] Close correlation between the sonographic appearance of the femoral head and the radiographic appearance was noted. Of interest is the observation that new bone formation during the healing phase may be documented earlier by ultrasonography than by conventional techniques.

## Shoulder

Shoulder pain and weakness on elevation of the arm are common clinical problems. In patients over 40 years of age, rotator cuff disease is a frequent cause. Rotator cuff fibers may fail a few at a time, giving rise to a clinical presentation that often is misinterpreted as bursitis or tendinitis. Failure of large groups of cuff fibers leads to sudden weakness of elevation and external rotation of the arm. In addi-

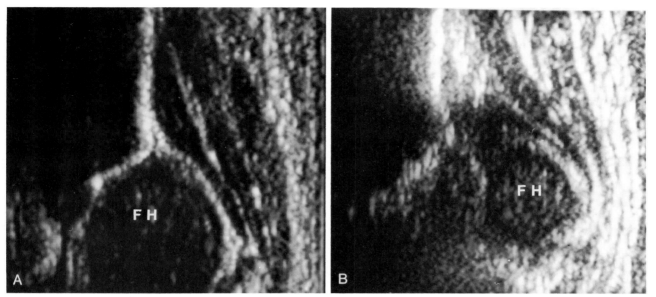

**FIGURE 11–5.** Developmental dysplasia of the hip. Coronal scans in a normal infant **(A)** and in an infant with hip dysplasia **(B)** demonstrate lateral dislocation of the femoral head (FH) in **B**. (Courtesy of W. Winters, M.D., Seattle, Washington.)

tion to pain and weakness, rotator cuff disease may lead to symptomatic abrasion against the undersurface of the coracoacromial arch with painful crepitance.

An initial report by Seltzer and coworkers demonstrated that articulated-arm scanners could visualize the rotator cuff.[51] Farrar and associates, in 1983, described the use of real-time mechanical sector scanners for examination of the cuff tendons.[72] Numerous more recent reports using high-resolution linear array real-time ultrasonography have demonstrated that sonography may serve as an alternative means of examining the rotator cuff.[73–76] Several different techniques for examination of the rotator cuff have been described.[76, 77] All share the underlying principle of attempting to examine the tendons in two orthogonal planes whenever possible.

After the suggestion of Middleton, previously published criteria for diagnosis of rotator cuff tears can be categorized into four groups: (1) nonvisualization of the cuff, (2) localized absence or focal nonvisualization, (3) discontinuity, and (4) focal abnormal echogenicity.[78] The efficacy of these criteria are supported in a report by Weiner and Seitz.[79]

No cuff tendon will be visualized in patients with large or massive rotator cuff tears (Figs. 11–6 and 11–7). The absence of cuff tendon allows the subdeltoid bursa, which may be quite thickened in this context, to directly approximate the surface of the humeral head or humeral articular cartilage. Joint and bursal effusions commonly accompany

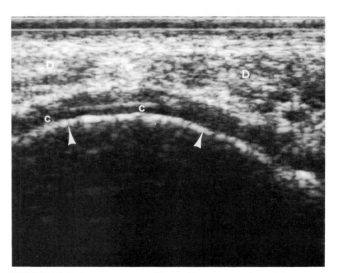

**FIGURE 11–6.** Normal shoulder. Sonogram perpendicular to the long axis of the supraspinatus tendon *(SS)*. The tendon is of measurable thickness as it courses over the humeral head (arrowheads). Note the deltoid muscle *(D)* and biceps tendon (arrow).

**FIGURE 11–7.** Large rotator cuff tear. Transverse view of the supraspinatus tendon similar to that in Figure 11–6 demonstrates absence of the supraspinatus tendon. Arrowheads indicate humeral head; *C,* humeral cartilage; *D,* deltoid muscle.

large tears and are seen along the biceps tendon and lateral to the greater tuberosity, respectively. Large tears of the supraspinatus tendon may extend posteriorly to involve the infraspinatus tendon or anteriorly to involve the biceps tendon and the subscapularis tendon.

Smaller full-thickness tears will appear as localized absence of the cuff with the subdeltoid bursa touching the humeral surface. This results in loss of the normal anterior arc of the subdeltoid bursa and the development of focal concavity. The most common location of such smaller tears is the anterolateral portion of the supraspinatus tendon in the "critical zone." Even smaller tears will appear as a discontinuity of the cuff filled with hypoechoic joint fluid or hyperechoic reactive tissue highlighting the defect (Fig. 11–8). Small cuff lesions often are best visualized during extension and internal rotation of the arm. A small amount of bursal fluid commonly is present in these smaller tears and may be the only sonographic finding with the arm in neutral position.

Abnormalities of cuff echogenicity may be diffuse or focal. Diffuse abnormality of cuff echogenicity is an unreliable sonographic sign for cuff tear but may indicate diffuse cuff inflammation or fibrosis. Although diffuse abnormality of cuff echogenicity is unreliable in detection of full-thickness tears, significant disparity of cuff thickness suggests cuff attrition. Significant degrees of cuff attrition are associated with partial-thickness tears and also suggest that progressive cuff changes are present. Focal abnormal echogenicity from granulation tissue, hypertrophied synovium, and hemorrhage has been associated with small full- and partial-thickness tears.[76] More recently, the visualization of either a focal intratendinous hypoechoic or dominant echogenic focus has been suggested as an additional criterion for diagnosis of partial-thickness tears.[79]

In addition to the major criteria that were just described, several minor sonographic findings have proved helpful in the authors' experience. Subdeltoid bursal effusion, concavity of the subdeltoid bursal contour, elevation of the humeral head relative to the acromion, and obliteration of the space normally occupied by the supraspinatus tendon all are associated with defects in the cuff.[80]

Sonography also plays an important role in the evaluation of patients who have had an acromioplasty and especially in those who have had a surgical repair of a full-thickness tear.[81, 82] Postoperatively the tendons of the cuff, especially the supraspinatus, often are echogenic and thinned when compared with those in the contralateral normal shoulder.[81, 82] Harryman and associates demonstrated a high rate of recurrent rotator cuff tear, noting recurrences in 20 per cent of patients in whom a defect limited to the supraspinatus tendon was repaired and in more than 50 per cent of those patients who preoperatively had had large tears involving more than the supraspinatus tendon.[83] Because such tears often are large and multiple tendons frequently are involved, they most often appear sonographically as total absence of the cuff (Fig. 11–9). It may be difficult to differentiate small recurrent tears from the appearances created when only a small amount of cuff tendon

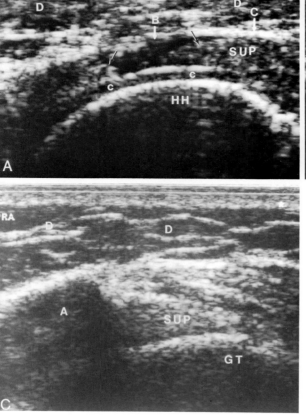

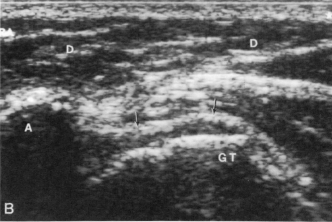

**FIGURE 11–8.** Small rotator cuff tear.

**A** Transverse view of the supraspinatus muscle demonstrates a small tear (arrows) filled with joint fluid. HH, Humeral head; *C*, humeral cartilage; *D*, deltoid muscle; *SUP*, residual supraspinatus tendon.

**B** A view perpendicular to **A** (longitudinal to the supraspinatus tendon) demonstrates absence of the normal tendon (arrows). *GT*, Greater tuberosity; *A*, acromion.

**C** A scan posterior to **B** through the normal portion of the supraspinatus tendon demonstrates its characteristic beak-shape.

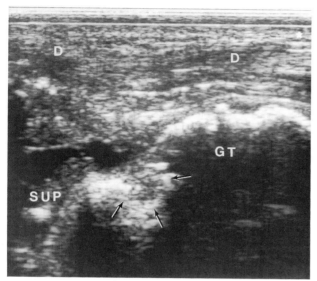

**FIGURE 11–9.** Recurrent rotator cuff tear. A scan longitudinal to the supraspinatus tendon in a patient in whom a rotator cuff repair had been performed demonstrates recurrent tear with retraction of the cuff *(SUP)*. Note the bony defect created by the reimplantation trough (arrows) and the absence of the normal echoes of the subdeltoid bursa. *GT*, Greater tuberosity; *D*, deltoid muscle.

remains to be reattached, unless baseline scans are available in the immediate postoperative period. Mack and associates reported that sonography allowed confirmation of all instances of recurrent cuff tear diagnosed at surgery and also allowed confirmation of 10 of 11 intact tendons.[84] Crass and associates reported similar results when sonography was compared with surgical findings.[82]

Diagnosis of fracture in the adult humerus is a new application for ultrasonography. In this role, the bony contour is evaluated for abnormal shape or discontinuity (Fig. 11–10). The overlying supraspinatus tendon may be thickened as a result of edema or hemorrhage. Fat may be seen within the joint as a highly echogenic joint effusion that

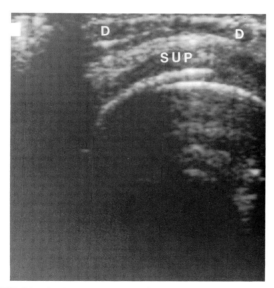

**FIGURE 11–10.** Humeral fracture. Scan transverse to the plane of the supraspinatus tendon *(SUP)* demonstrates discontinuity of the humeral head in a patient with a subtle greater tuberosity fracture. *D*, deltoid muscle.

exhibits a characteristic swirling appearance on joint motion. Such findings correspond to a fat-fluid level that may be seen with other imaging techniques. Patten and coworkers demonstrated that such fractures could be readily seen by ultrasound.[1] In 42 per cent of patients the fractures were not visible on initial plain films. In a limited number of cases, degenerative changes and calcific tendinitis mimicked characteristic findings of fracture. Therefore, these authors recommended that all positive sonograms be followed by further radiologic evaluation.

Common diagnostic pitfalls include inadequate transducer positioning and failure to maintain proper transducer orientation with respect to tendon fibers, causing tendons to appear artifactually heterogeneous. The use of multiple focal zones may hide characteristic acoustic shadows created by areas of calcific tendinitis. Patient-related factors, including truncal obesity and large subdeltoid bursal effusions, may limit diagnostic information available from scans.

A number of authors have reported greater than 90 per cent sensitivity and specificity in the evaluation of the rotator cuff prior to surgical intervention. However, other groups have had less success with this technique. The sonographic criteria used, the patient population studied, the diagnostic information desired, and operator experience and interest are crucial factors in explaining the wide variation in published results.[73–78, 84–88]

### Ankle and Foot

Injuries to the Achilles tendon are common in both athletes and in undertrained, middle-aged patients who exert themselves acutely. Because of its superficial location, clinical examination often is sufficient to allow diagnosis of acute disruption of the tendon. However, in 20 to 30 per cent of cases, the clinical diagnosis may be incorrect. Ultrasonography also has been found to be useful in patients with tendinitis and those in whom xanthomas secondary to familial hypercholesterolemia are suspected.

The Achilles tendon is best examined with the patient prone and with the feet extending beyond the table. Use of an acoustic standoff helps compensate for the geometry of the region. The normal tendon appears in longitudinal section as a superficial, hyperechoic structure surrounded by the echogenic peritenon.[89] In transverse section, the tendon is elliptical in shape, with broadening in its more caudal aspects. Deep to the tendon, the preachilles fat pat is visualized as an area of low heterogeneous echogenicity. Superficial to the tendon at its insertion to the calcaneus, the superficial bursa may be observed when distended by fluid but not when normal.[90] A second bursa can be visualized deep to the calcaneal attachment.

Complete rupture of the Achilles tendon appears as discontinuity with retraction of the upper fragment, small amounts of adjacent fluid, and an echogenic clot in the tear (Fig. 11–11). Use of the Thompson maneuver may be helpful in demonstrating disruption of the tendon. Partial tears have been described as hypoechoic areas within the tendon or as heterogeneity of tendon echogenicity.[91] The sonographic appearance of tendinitis is more controversial. Neuhold and coworkers described increased diameter with preservation of normal architecture.[91] Fornage found similar thickening with a decrease in echogenicity over the asymptomatic, contralateral side in 86 per cent of cases.[89] Mathie-

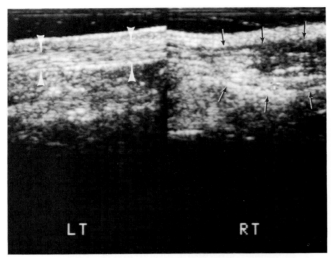

**FIGURE 11–11.** Achilles tendon rupture. Paired longitudinal images demonstrate disruption of the right Achilles tendon (arrows) with edema and clot. The patient is prone and the head is to the viewer's left. Arrowheads indicate the normal left Achilles tendon.

son and coworkers were not able to confirm these findings.[90] In patients who had had tendon repair, scans initially demonstrated tendon enlargement, with areas of increased echogenicity within the tendon from suture material and adjacent to the tendon from presumed inflammation. These findings resolve in the majority of patients.[92]

In patients with heterozygous familial hypercholesterolemia, the Achilles tendon is the most common location for xanthomas. These lesions appear as thickening of the tendon, with a decrease in overall echogenicity in 89 per cent of cases.[93] Focal areas of heterogeneous echogenicity also may be seen. In 86% of cases in one series, the sonogram was positive when clinical examination had failed to detect abnormality.[93]

### Hand, Wrist, and Elbow

Fornage and associates demonstrated that the normal tendons of the hand could be visualized by ultrasonography.[94] The echogenicity of these structures was somewhat variable depending on the frequency of transducers used and the geometry of imaging.[95] The sonographic features of masses of the hand and fingers, including synovial cysts, angiomas, and glomus tumors, have been described. Synovial cysts are hypoechoic, angiomas are minimally hyperechoic, and the remainder of focal masses are very hyperechoic in echogenicity. Inflammatory abnormalities, including foreign bodies and tenosynovitis, also can be visualized with ultrasonography. Jeffrey and associates reported eight patients with acute suppurative tenosynovitis.[96] The affected tendons were 25 per cent larger than contralateral structures. In five of six cases, hypoechoic areas adjacent to symptomatic tendons contained purulent material.

Although MR imaging has become the primary imaging method in the evaluation of the wrist for carpal tunnel syndrome, some features of the disease can be visualized using ultrasonography. Buchberger and associates reported visualizing the normal superficial and deep flexor tendons of the wrist.[97] The median nerve also could be seen as an oval echogenic structure. In symptomatic patients, the nerve

was increased in area on transverse sections at the level of the pisiform, and palmar bowing of the flexor retinaculum also was noted. Sonographic findings in tenosynovitis of the wrist have been described by Gooding, who noted fluid surrounding the tendons with mild increased echogenicity of tendons.[98] Other authors have suggested that inflammation leads to a decrease in tendon echogenicity.[97] Differences in technical factors may explain this disparity. Ganglion cysts of the wrist may be seen as well-marginated hypoechoic structures that can be differentiated from other abnormalities such as lipomas or aneurysms (Fig. 11–12).[99]

Normal anatomy of the elbow as visualized by sonography has been described by Barr and Babcock.[100] In seven views, they were able to image the structures of the elbow in patients over a wide range of ages, from several months to 45 years. Because sonography allows visualization of cartilage that may not be visible with radiography, ultrasonography has been found to be particularly helpful in infants and children. The sonographic findings in transphyseal fractures, joint effusions, and cellulitis have been described.[101] Characteristic findings in tennis elbow have been reported, consisting of hypoechoic extratendinous collections in muscle tears, fluid collections adjacent to the carpi radialis brevis in bursitis, and alterations of tendon echogenicity and size in enthesopathy and tendinitis.[102]

### Tumors of Bone and Soft Tissue

Modern gray-scale methodology has contributed greatly to the depiction of normal soft tissue anatomy of the trunk and extremities.[103, 104] Intramuscular fascial planes are defined clearly, and the muscles themselves are composed of uniform, low amplitude echoes. Using this anatomic information, sonography allows differentiation between true mass and muscular hernias, muscular asymmetry, hematoma, or other causes of palpable abnormalities.[105]

Ultrasonography may serve as a correlative imaging method in the evaluation of tumors of musculoskeletal origin.[106–110] Sonographic assessment of lesions arising in the extremities as well as the axial skeleton, pelvis, retroperi-

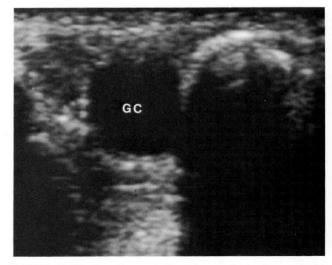

**FIGURE 11–12.** Ganglion cyst. Scan in a patient with a palpable dorsal mass demonstrates a well-marginated hypoechoic structure (GC) adjacent to bone.

toneum, trunk, and abdominal wall has been described (Fig. 11–13).[94, 111–117] Although sonography easily catalogues mass lesions into cystic or solid groupings, little histologic specificity is obtained from the sonographic appearances alone.[118, 119] In fact, strict adherence to usually reliable sonographic criteria can result in interpretive errors. Soft tissue tumors of neural or nerve sheath origin can mimic the findings classically associated with cystic lesions, even though these are solid neoplasms.[120, 121] Fatty tissue often is extremely echogenic, and lipomatous tumors can appear quite dense on gray-scale sonograms.[122] Neoplasms of lymphatic origin typically contain extensive cystic areas (Fig. 11–14).[111, 113] Highly vascular tumors, such as hemangiomas, also can have numerous fluid regions. Color Doppler imaging may be helpful in defining vascular anatomy associated with such lesions.

Because many of these lesions either arise from bone or involve bone secondarily, and because ultrasonography has negligible success in visualizing intraosseous structures, the role of sonography in this setting is limited. However, this technique may be helpful in the evaluation of cartilage-bone relationships in cases of osteochondroma. As in other applications, cartilage appears as a hypoechoic layer superficial to the high-level echoes generated by bone, and the cartilage cap may be measured accurately.[123] Malghem and coworkers have described the use of ultrasonography in differentiating benign from malignant osteochondromas by measuring the thickness of the cartilage cap in patients with symptomatic osteochondromas.[124] They recommend using a thickness of the cartilage cap of less than 1 cm as an indicator of a benign lesion, greater than 2 cm as indicative of malignant transformation, and 1 to 2 cm as indefinite in the differentiation of benign and malignant tumors. In addition, bursal formation overlying the osteochondroma may be detected.

Once the presence of a lesion is identified, sonography can be employed as a means of monitoring the response of any extraosseous tumor bulk to therapeutic regimens.[106, 107, 125] Enlargement of a tumor mass can be the result of

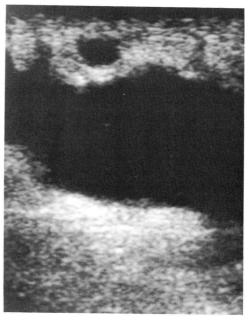

**FIGURE 11–14.** Lymphangioma. Scan of the forearm demonstrates complex fluid spaces in this patient with invasive lymphangioma.

hemorrhage or necrosis rather than tumor growth, a distinction sonography can make.[119] After resection, ultrasonography can be used to monitor recurrence of lesions. Recurrent tumors can be detected with a sensitivity of 87 per cent, and lesions as small as 5 mm can be visualized.[126] The technique is well suited to sequential examinations and generally is reproducible if care is taken to establish reference landmarks. Pretreatment tumor mapping with ultrasonography has been used to guide radiotherapy portals.[107] Finally, sonography offers a rapid and accurate method of localizing a soft tissue mass for percutaneous biopsy.[108, 127] Areas of hemorrhage or necrosis have poor cytologic yield, and the needle can be directed to more appropriate regions for sampling.

### Infections of Bone and Soft Tissue

Detection of abscesses remains a challenging task for diagnostic imaging. Ultrasonography frequently is called upon in this situation, and when the suggestive area is located superficially, as in the extremity or abdominal wall, the technique is quite successful. Demonstration of intraabdominal and retroperitoneal abscesses also is feasible, although correlative radiographic or isotopic studies often are necessary for diagnosis.[128]

Sonographic features of soft tissue abscesses vary considerably.[119, 129–131] A typical abscess contains predominantly fluid but often has debris as well that is manifested as fine, low-level echoes within the cystic mass. This material sometimes accumulates in the dependent portion of the abscess, a phenomenon that can be documented by changing the patient's position. The margins of an abscess usually are indistinct in contrast to simple cysts. The anechoic or hypoechoic regions often are surrounded by regions of increased echogenicity representing an adjacent inflammatory reaction (Fig. 11–15).[132] Many abscesses, notably chronic or partially treated lesions, are complex in

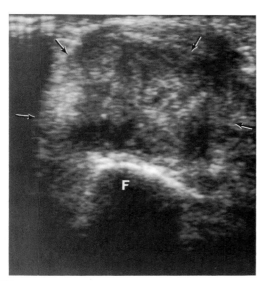

**FIGURE 11–13.** Malignant fibrous histiocytoma. Transverse scan of the thigh demonstrates a well-marginated mass (arrows) of heterogeneous echogenicity. *F*, Femoral shaft.

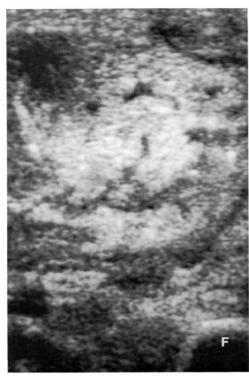

**FIGURE 11–15.** Cellulitis. Transverse scan of the thigh demonstrates an area of increased echogenicity with disruption of normal muscle architecture. The soft tissue process is separated from bone. *F,* femoral shaft.

appearance and can even be difficult to distinguish from surrounding soft tissue. Gas-containing abscesses can be quite echogenic on sonograms, an appearance thought to be a result of the numerous highly reflective interfaces engendered by ''microbubbles.''[131]

Despite the variable sonographic appearance of abscesses and the considerable overlap with other lesions, including hematomas and tumors, sonography is of significant diagnostic aid in this clinical problem.[133] Cellulitis can be treated effectively with antibiotics, but abscesses frequently require percutaneous or open surgical drainage. Segregation of abscess from simple cellulitis of the extremity can be accomplished with sonography.[14] This capability can be extended to encompass the abdominal wall, trunk, and neck. Paravertebral abscesses are present in a significant percentage of patients with infections of the spine.[134] The presence of a paraspinous abscess often is difficult to establish with conventional radiography, and as a rule ultrasonography, CT scanning, and MR imaging are more successful.

Sonographic guidance for percutaneous needle aspiration of various lesions has proved to be quite satisfactory for aspiration or continuous drainage of abscesses.[127, 132, 135–137] This approach can spare a number of patients the risk and expense of surgical intervention.[138] Importantly, sonography is an objective means of monitoring the response of a given inflammatory lesion to appropriate therapy.

Characteristic sonographic findings have been described in osteomyelitis. Although such infections characteristically begin in the medullary region of bone, they rapidly progress to involve adjacent soft tissues.[139] Visualization of anechoic fluid collections adjacent to bone has been described by

several investigators as highly suggestive of osteomyelitis.[139–141] Elevation of the periosteum also may be visualized. In pediatric patients, periosteal elevation of greater than 2 mm was associated with subperiosteal pus in 16 of 18 patients.[141] When present, disruption of the bony cortex can be demonstrated and sequestra may be seen.[142] Clinically, it may be difficult to distinguish between cellulitis and osteomyelitis. Demonstration of soft tissue between bone and a fluid collection is helpful in this clinical circumstance in suggesting cellulitis as a cause.[139]

## Foreign Bodies

Foreign bodies in the soft tissues, especially in the hands and feet, pose a challenging diagnostic problem. Even if they are radiopaque, conventional radiographs do not provide three-dimensional localization. Sonographic detection depends on differences in acoustic impedance between adjacent tissues and the foreign body (Fig. 11–16). Because all reported foreign bodies are hyperechoic, they are best visualized in slightly hypoechoic tissues such as subcutaneous fat, muscle, or inflammatory tissue.[143] While in older reports, acoustic standoffs such as Kitecko were used to improve near-field resolution, newer devices with improved electronic focusing make the use of standoffs unnecessary. In vitro experiments have demonstrated the utility of sonography in detecting a variety of foreign bodies of 5 mm or less in size, including those of wood, glass, steel and plastic.[144, 145] When foreign bodies are imaged end-on with large angles of incidence with respect to the acoustic beam, their size may be underestimated.[146] Whenever possible, the foreign body should be imaged perpendicular to its suspected position on the basis of mechanism of injury.

High levels of accuracy have been reported in several clinical series.[143, 147, 148] Rare false-negative examinations have been encountered in cases with recent surgery in which residual soft tissue air makes detection of small foreign bodies difficult. Once the foreign body has been localized, removal may be accomplished under direct sonographic visualization.[148]

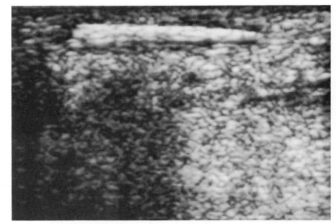

**FIGURE 11–16.** Foreign body. Scan of the foot demonstrates a foreign body as hyperechoic compared with adjacent soft tissue. The plain films were negative. A splinter later was removed with sonographic localization.

## Miscellaneous Soft Tissue Conditions

Skin thickening is a feature of many dermatologic and nondermatologic conditions. Close correlation was found between early A-mode sonography and radiography in the measurement of skin thickness.[149] Scleredema is an unusual hypertrophy of the dermis peculiar to diabetic patients. High-frequency (10 MHz) real-time instruments are capable of distinguishing among epidermis, dermis, subcutaneous fat, and muscle.[150] Thus, sonography might be useful for the quantitative assessment of the natural history or response to treatment of diseases that affect dermal thickness. Similarly, the thickness of the heel pad is known to be increased in conditions such as acromegaly and long-term phenytoin (Dilantin) therapy. Sonography can be used as a quick and accurate mode to measure the heel pad.[151] Sonographic quantification of loss of soft tissue mass in the foot might be able to predict those diabetic patients at risk of developing ulcerations.[152]

Children with various forms of muscular dystrophy showed changes in the echo texture of the quadriceps muscle when surveyed with sonograms of the leg.[153] It might be feasible on the basis of sonograms to differentiate children with true neuromuscular disease from those with non-neuromuscular hypertonia.

## Spine

Early attempts to measure the dimensions of the lumbar spinal canal with ultrasonography met with somewhat conflicting results and claims.[154–157] With the advent of high-resolution CT scanners and MR imaging, these cumbersome sonographic methods have become of only historical interest. Some success has been achieved in the diagnosis of disc herniation by ultrasonic scanning via an anterior approach through the disc space.[158] Problems with identifying the precise level being surveyed would seem to limit this technique.

Occult spinal dysraphism in infants can result in the insidious development of lower extremity sensorimotor changes, gait disturbances, foot deformities, and bowel and bladder dysfunction. Early diagnosis allows corrective surgery for the tethered cord syndrome to halt or prevent these complications altogether. In about one half of the children so affected, the spinal defect is signaled by a cutaneous marker, such as hairy nevi, hemangiomas, or sinus tracts. Children at risk can be screened with sonography for cord tethering because in the first year of life, ossification of the posterior elements of the spine is incomplete. This provides a window for scanning from a posterior approach.[159–161] The spinal cord and abnormalities affecting it can be imaged with striking clarity. A positive sonogram sometimes can obviate invasive preoperative examinations, such as myelography, a difficult and potentially hazardous procedure in this age group. Infants with obvious defects of the caudal spine also can be evaluated by sonography to further clarify the nature of their lesions. For example, the presence of neural tissue within a myelomeningocele sac can be documented (Fig. 11–17).[162, 163]

## Intraoperative Spine Sonography

Considerable advances have been made in neurosurgery of the spinal cord, in part related to the development of intraoperative sonographic techniques.[164–167] With appropriate care to maintain sterile conditions, many real-time sonographic systems can be adapted for use in the operating room, and instruments now exist that are designed specifically for this purpose.

One of the major advantages of sonography is delineation of the extent of a particular problem prior to opening the dura, thus reducing the time and risk of a surgical procedure. Also, processes anterior to the spinal cord, an area normally not seen without manipulation of the cord, can be identified easily.[165, 168, 169] On-line monitoring of the

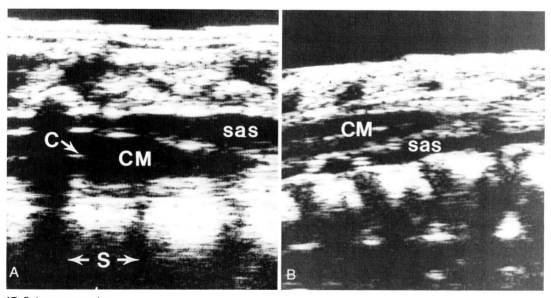

**FIGURE 11–17.** Spine sonography.
**A** Normal infant spine. The conus medullaris *(CM)* lies dependent within the subarachnoid space *(sas)* and tapers normally in the midlumbar canal. Observe the central canal of the cord *(C)* and shadowing from the posterior elements *(S)*.
**B** Tethered cord. The conus medullaris *(CM)* is fixed in a dorsal position within the subarachnoid space *(sas)*. On real-time examination, a lack of motion can be documented as well.

surgical procedure provides valuable information in tumor surgery.[165, 167, 168, 170] Localization and drainage of intramedullary cysts and syrinxes, whether idiopathic or related to trauma or adjacent neoplasms, are relatively straightforward with ultrasonic guidance.[164, 171–174] Effectiveness of decompression can be assessed prior to terminating the operation.

Additional applications of intraoperative spine sonography include evaluation of patients with trauma. Identification of bone fragments, foreign bodies, and cord compression and determination of spinal alignment can be accomplished with sonography.[169, 175–177] The ultimate goals of operative intervention in these patients are relief of neural compression and stabilization of the vertebral column. The adequacy of cord decompression and Harrington rod placement can be monitored, and any necessary adjustments can be made instantaneously.[175, 176] Operation time and manipulation of the cord thus are minimized. It is quite likely that intraoperative sonography will become an integral component of spinal surgery.

### Metabolic Disease

The parathyroid glands are intimately involved in calcium homeostasis and thereby exert considerable influence on bone metabolism. It is the parathyroid glands themselves, however, rather than the osseous changes, that are of interest to sonographers. True primary hyperparathyroidism almost always is the result of a single hyperfunctioning benign adenoma of the parathyroid gland. Rarely is multiglandular hyperplasia or parathyroid carcinoma involved. Hyperplasia typically is seen in patients with long-standing renal insufficiency, and the differentiation of primary from secondary hyperparathyroidism usually can be made on clinical grounds.

Normal parathyroid glands measure approximately 3 × 4 × 5 mm and, until the advent of high-resolution real-time sonography, had by and large evaded all attempts to image them. Early work by Sample and coworkers, using antiquated articulated arm B-scanners, demonstrated the feasibility of using ultrasonography to detect parathyroid gland enlargement in the neck.[178] A positive sonogram was a reliable test; this has been substantiated by other investigators using state-of-the-art high-resolution real-time systems.[179–181] If documentation of parathyroid gland enlargement is important for diagnosis and management, ultrasonography now is accepted as the procedure of choice. Accuracy rates of approximately 90 per cent have been reported from several centers.[179–181]

On sonograms, parathyroid adenomas and hyperplastic glands appear identical, which is not surprising because they have the same appearance histologically as well. The lesions are well circumscribed, often ovoid, and hypoechoic relative to adjacent thyroid glandular tissue (Fig. 11–18).

Preoperative localization of the adenoma has the potential to shorten the time required for a neck exploration by allowing a unilateral neck dissection for solitary adenoma in patients with primary hyperparathyroidism. Ultrasonographic localization can be equally helpful in patients with recurrent or persistent hyperparathyroidism after initial surgery.[182] These patients present many difficulties to the surgeon because of the anatomic disruption that occurs during initial exploration of the neck.

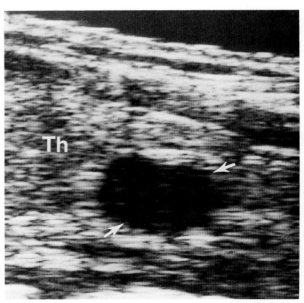

**FIGURE 11–18.** Parathyroid adenoma. This longitudinal sonogram through the lower pole of the thyroid gland *(Th)* confirms the presence of a 1 cm hypoechoic mass (arrows) deep to the thyroid. Either adenoma or hyperplasia could produce this appearance.

Should sonography fail to confirm parathyroid gland enlargement in the neck, CT scanning, MR imaging, and thallium-technetium scans may be useful.[183–185] Approximately 5 per cent of the population harbors ectopic parathyroid tissue, which usually is situated in the superior mediastinum along the embryologic pathway of thymic descent.

In most instances, sonographic confirmation of an enlarged parathyroid gland is sufficient grounds to proceed with surgery. Occasionally, tissue confirmation is desired and percutaneous needle aspiration biopsy can be accomplished with sonographic guidance.[186, 187] Gland ablation by injection of absolute ethanol has been proposed as a means of enhancing the results of pharmacologic treatment in patients with secondary hyperparathyroidism.[188]

### Hemophilia and Altered Coagulability States

A significant population is at risk for hemorrhage, either from primary blood dyscrasias or from secondary alterations in clotting mechanisms. The latter circumstance frequently is iatrogenic, as many patients are placed on anticoagulant medication. The relative ease with which ultrasonography detects fluid collections such as hematomas makes this an attractive method for evaluating these patients. Sonography has proved efficacious in this clinical problem, both in diagnosing areas of hemorrhage and in following the natural history of the bleeding (Fig. 11–19).[189–192]

Rectus sheath hematoma is a specific clinical entity that is misdiagnosed in as many as 60 per cent of cases.[193, 194] Signs and symptoms often mimic acute abdominal or pelvic conditions, such as intestinal obstruction or hernia, twisted ovarian cyst, or perivesicular inflammatory disease. Factors predisposing to rectus sheath hematoma include violent muscular contraction (cough, sneeze, exercise), pregnancy and labor, tension on the abdominal wall (ascites, obesity), blood dyscrasias, and anticoagulant therapy.[193] Conserva-

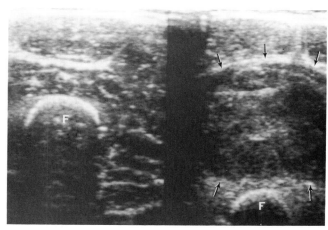

**FIGURE 11–19.** Thigh hematoma. Paired transverse images of the thigh demonstrate a hematoma (arrows) of the left vastus intermedius muscle. *F,* Femoral shaft.

tive treatment is recommended and entails analgesia, compresses, and rest. Surgery is to be avoided.[194] The sonographic appearance of rectus sheath hematoma is characteristic and consists of an ellipsoid or spindle-shaped fluid collection in the superficial anterior abdominal wall.[195–197] The tight boundaries of the rectus sheath confine the bleeding, and the process does not cross the midline unless it occurs low, where the posterior portion of the sheath is deficient.

Iliopsoas hematoma is a common complication of hemophilia.[198, 199] A somewhat typical syndrome of pain and nerve deficit occurs with bleeding isolated to the closed iliacus compartment that contains the femoral nerve. The psoas fascia is looser and allows more extensive hemorrhage to take place. When this occurs on the right side, differentiation from acute appendicitis may be difficult clinically. Sonography is capable of detecting hemorrhage in both of these muscle compartments.[190, 199, 200]

Hemorrhage into the wall of the intestine or into the root of the mesentery also is a complication of altered coagulability. Intramural intestinal hematoma exhibits somewhat characteristic, albeit nonspecific, sonographic features.[201] The diagnosis of occult mesenteric hematoma often is very difficult. Sonography allows identification of this lesion and may establish its origin as separate from neighboring parenchymal organs.[202]

Depending on the age and chronicity of the hemorrhage, hematomas display a spectrum of appearances on grayscale sonograms.[189, 191, 203] When fresh and composed of liquid blood, a hematoma is homogeneous and appears virtually echo-free.[189] Internal echoes appear when a clot begins to organize and then fragment, resulting in a more complex sonographic appearance. Liquefaction of a clot then may lead once again to a variable fluid pattern on sonography. This inconstant pattern causes difficulty in attempting to predict the age of a given collection of blood.[203] Considerable overlap exists, with similar features demonstrated by abscesses or tumors, for example. Nonetheless, the appropriate clinical setting generally allows an accurate diagnosis, and the real task of diagnostic ultrasonography is to allow detection of an abnormality in the circumstance that often escapes conventional radiographic approaches. By enabling an accurate diagnosis to be made, sonography

can eliminate the need for a more elaborate and perhaps invasive workup.

## Pleural and Pericardial Disease

Systemic rheumatologic diseases such as rheumatoid arthritis and lupus erythematosus affect the pleural and pericardial surfaces. Detection of fluid in either location is accomplished readily with ultrasonography.

Air and bone, the major constituents of the thorax, both interfere with transmission of sound waves and thereby limit the usefulness of ultrasonography in the chest. Pleural fluid usually accumulates adjacent to the chest wall, however, and displaces the lung away from the transducer. Consequently, sonography can be used to confirm the presence of pleural fluid and assist thoracentesis.[204–211] This is especially true for loculated or small collections and in cases in which the position of the hemidiaphragm is crucial information. As little as 5 ml of pleural fluid can be detected.[206, 210] Because the visceral pleural surface can be identified, pneumothorax has been an infrequent complication when sonography is used to guide thoracentesis.[208, 211, 212]

Although in theory a distinction of fluid collections from solid lesions should be made easily by sonography and in fact usually is, sonographic features alone have poor predictive value regarding the success of fluid retrieval.[205, 208, 210] Organizing effusions may appear echo-free yet defy aspiration. Conversely, many complex-appearing pleural collections yield fluid. One finding that indicates free-flowing fluid is the demonstration of a change in position or configuration of the collection when the patient's position is changed. Other observations unique to real-time imaging further increase the predictive value of sonography. Any pleural collection that changes shape with patient respiration or that exhibits septations that move is likely to contain retrievable fluid.[213] Because of the greater flexibility, shorter scan times, and portability of real-time systems compared with their static B-scan counterparts, they can contribute clinically relevant information in a large percentage of patients.[214]

Any radiographic opaque area that abuts on the chest wall can be investigated by ultrasonography.[210, 215] Some solid lesions, such as pulmonary Hodgkin's disease, are difficult to distinguish from fluid collections.[216]

Clinically overt rheumatoid heart disease is rare.[217] The echographically determined frequency of pericardial effusion is approximately 15 to 30 per cent.[218, 219] Seldom is the effusion hemodynamically significant. Likewise, indices of left ventricular function may show mild abnormalities but rarely is there clinical manifestation of left ventricular depression. Echocardiographic abnormalities have been identified in scleroderma and related diseases as well.[220]

## SUMMARY

In this chapter, a review is provided of the musculoskeletal applications of diagnostic ultrasonography. Although alternative techniques such as CT scanning and MR imaging have influenced dramatically the manner in which ultrasonography is employed, the benefits of diagnostic ultrasonography, which include less cost and time expenditure and less patient discomfort, ensure that its place in clinical imaging is secure. Advances in transducer technology have expanded its applicability to the assessment of many structures, particularly those that are situated superficially. The orthopedic and rheumatologic disorders that can be assessed with ultrasonographic imaging include traumatic, metabolic, degenerative, infectious, and neoplastic processes.

## References

1. Patten RM, Mack LA, Wang KY, et al: Nondisplaced fractures of the greater tuberosity of the humerus: Sonographic detection. Radiology 182:201, 1992.
2. Baker ML, Dalrymple GV: Biological effects of diagnostic ultrasound: A review. Radiology 126:479, 1978.
3. Ziskin MC: Ultrasonic bioeffects and their clinical relevance: An overview. Clin Diagn Ultrasound 16:1, 1985.
4. Wolfe RD, Colloff B: Popliteal cysts: An arthrographic study and review of the literature. J Bone Joint Surg [Am] 54:1057, 1972.
5. McDonald DG, Leopold GR: Ultrasound B-scanning in the differentiation of Baker's cyst and thrombophlebitis. Br J Radiol 45:729, 1972.
6. Moore CP, Sarti DA, Louie JS: Ultrasonographic demonstration of popliteal cysts in rheumatoid arthritis: A non-invasive technique. Arthritis Rheum 18:577, 1975.
7. Carpenter JR, Hattery RR, Hunder GG, et al: Ultrasound evaluation of the popliteal space: Comparison with arthrography and physical examination. Mayo Clin Proc 51:498, 1976.
8. Doppman JL: Baker's cyst and the normal gastrocnemio-semi-membranosus bursa. AJR 94:646, 1965.
9. Pastershank SP, Mitchell DM: Knee joint bursal abnormalities in rheumatoid arthritis. J Can Assoc Radiol 28:199, 1977.
10. Hermann G, Yeh H-C, Lehr-Janus C, et al: Diagnosis of popliteal cyst: Double-contrast arthrography and sonography. AJR 137:369, 1981.
11. Good AE: Rheumatoid arthritis, Baker's cyst, and thrombophlebitis. Arthritis Rheum 7:56, 1964.
12. Schmidt MC, Workman JB, Barth WF: Dissection or rupture of a popliteal cyst: A syndrome mimicking thrombophlebitis in rheumatic diseases. Arch Intern Med 134:694, 1974.
13. Swett HA, Jaffe RB, McIff EB: Popliteal cysts: Presentation as thrombophlebitis. Radiology 115:613, 1975.
14. Lawson TL, Mittler S: Ultrasonic evaluation of extremity soft-tissue lesions with arthrographic correlation. J Can Assoc Radiol 29:58, 1978.
15. Rudikoff JC, Lynch JJ, Phillips E, et al: Ultrasound diagnosis of Baker cyst. JAMA 235:1054, 1976.
16. Ambanelli U, Manganelli P, Nervetti A, et al: Demonstration of articular effusions and popliteal cysts with ultrasound. J Rheumatol 3:134, 1976.
17. Gompels BM, Darlington LG: Evaluation of popliteal cysts and painful calves with ultrasonography: Comparison with arthrography. Ann Rheum Dis 41:355, 1982.
18. Wychulis AR, Spittell JA, Wallace RB: Popliteal aneurysms. Surgery 68:942, 1970.
19. Sarti DA, Louie JS, Lindstrom RR, et al: Ultrasonic diagnosis of a popliteal artery aneurysm. Radiology 121:707, 1976.
20. Chitwood WR, Stocks LH, Wolfe WG: Popliteal artery aneurysms: Past and present. Arch Surg 113:1078, 1978.
21. Silver TM, Washburn RL, Stanley JC, et al: Gray scale ultrasound evaluation of popliteal artery aneurysms. AJR 129:1003, 1977.
22. Scott WW, Scott PP, Sanders RC: B-scan ultrasound in the diagnosis of popliteal aneurysms. Surgery 81:436, 1977.
23. Collins GJ, Rich NM, Phillips J, et al: Ultrasound diagnosis of popliteal arterial aneurysms. Am Surg 42:853, 1976.
24. Sprayregen S: Popliteal vein displacement by popliteal artery aneurysms: Report of two cases. AJR 132:838, 1979.
25. Giustra PE, Root JA, Mason SE, et al: Popliteal vein thrombosis secondary to popliteal artery aneurysm. AJR 130:25, 1978.
26. Davis RP, Neiman HL, Yao JST, et al: Ultrasound scan in diagnosis of peripheral aneurysms. Arch Surg 112:55, 1977.
27. Neiman HL, Yao JST, Silver TM: Gray-scale ultrasound diagnosis of peripheral arterial aneurysms. Radiology 130:413, 1979.
28. Baumann D, Kremer H: Arthrography and sonography in the diagnosis of Baker's cysts. ROFO 127:463, 1977.
29. Cooperberg PL, Tsang I, Truelove L, et al: Gray scale ultrasound in the evaluation of rheumatoid arthritis of the knee. Radiology 126:759, 1978.
30. Meire HB, Lindsay DJ, Swinson DR, et al: Comparison of ultrasound and positive contrast arthrography in the diagnosis of popliteal and calf swellings. Ann Rheum Dis 33:221, 1974.
31. Aisen AM, McCune WJ, MacGuire A, et al: Sonographic evaluation of the cartilage of the knee. Radiology 153:781, 1984.
32. McCune WJ, Dedrick DK, Aisen AM, et al: Sonographic evaluation of osteoarthritic femoral condylar cartilage. Correlation with operative findings. Clin Orthop 254:230, 1990.
33. Brussaard C, Naudts P, De Schepper A: Ultrasonographic diagnosis of chondromalacia of the femoropatellar joint. J Belge Radiol 74:303, 1991.
34. Gregersen HE, Rasmussen OS: Ultrasonography of osteochondritis dissecans of the knee. Acta Radiol 30:552, 1989.
35. Selby B, Richardson ML, Montana MA, et al: High resolution sonography of the menisci of the knee. Invest Radiol 21:332, 1986.
36. Selby B, Richardson ML, Nelson BD, et al: Sonography in the detection of meniscal injuries of the knee: Evaluation in cadavers. AJR 149:549, 1987.
37. Burk DL Jr, Dalinka MK, Kanal E, et al: Meniscal and ganglion cysts of the knee: MR evaluation. AJR 150:331, 1988.
38. Peetrons P, Allaer D, Jeanmart L: Cysts of semilunar cartilages of the knee: A new approach by ultrasound imaging. J Ultrasound Med 9:333, 1990.
39. Barrie HJ: The pathogenesis and significance of meniscal cysts. J Bone Joint Surg [Br] 61:184, 1979.
40. Ferrer-Roca O, Vilalta C: Lesions of the meniscus. Part II. Horizontal cleavages and lateral cysts. Clin Orthop 146:301, 1980.
41. Coral A, van Holsbeeck M, Adler RS: Imaging of meniscal cyst of the knee in three cases. Skel Radiol 18:451, 1989.
42. De Flaviis L, Nessi R, Scaglione P, et al: Ultrasonic diagnosis of Osgood-Schlatter and Sinding-Johansson diseases of the knee. Skel Radiol 18:193, 1989.
43. Fritchy D, de Gautard R: Jumper's knee and ultrasonography. Am J Sports Med 16:637, 1988.
44. Davies SG, Baudouin CJ, King JB, et al: Ultrasound, computed tomography and magnetic resonance imaging in patellar tendinitis. Clin Radiol 43:52, 1991.
45. Kälebo P, Swärd L, Karlsson J, et al: Ultrasonography in the detection of partial patellar ligament ruptures (jumper's knee). Skel Radiol 20:285, 1991.
46. Fornage BD, Rifkin MD, Touche DH, et al: Sonography of the patellar tendon: Preliminary observations. AJR 143:179, 1984.
47. Myllymäki T, Bondestam S, Suramo I, et al: Ultrasonography of jumper's knee. Acta Radiol 31:147, 1990.
48. King JB, Perry DJ, Mourad K, et al: Lesions of the patellar ligament. J Bone Joint Surg [Br] 72:46, 1990.
49. Lanning P, Heikkinen E: Ultrasonic features of the Osgood-Schlatter lesion. J Pediatr Orthop 11:538, 1991.
50. Laine KR, Harjula A, Peltokallio P: Ultrasound in the evaluation of the knee and patellar regions. J Ultrasound Med 6:33, 1987.
51. Seltzer SE, Finberg HJ, Weissman BN: Arthrosonography: Technique, sonographic anatomy, and pathology. Invest Radiol 15:19, 1980.
52. Wilson DJ, Green DJ, MacLarnon JC: Arthrosonography of the painful hip. Clin Radiol 35:17, 1984.
53. Gitschlag KF, Sandler MA, Madrazo BL, et al: Disease in the femoral triangle: Sonographic appearance. AJR 139:515, 1982.
54. Wales LR, Azose AA: Saphenous varix: Ultrasonic diagnosis. J Ultrasound Med 4:143, 1985.
55. Wing V, Scheible W: Sonography of jugular vein thrombosis. AJR 140:333, 1983.
56. Raghavendra BN, Rosen RJ, Lam S, et al: Deep venous thrombosis: Detection by high-resolution real-time ultrasonography. Radiology 152:789, 1984.
57. Janus C, Hermann G: Enlargement of the iliopsoas bursa: Unusual cause of cystic mass on pelvic sonogram. J Clin Ultrasound 10:133, 1982.
58. Harcke HT, Clarke NMP, Lee MS, et al: Examination of the infant hip with real-time ultrasonography. J Ultrasound Med 3:131, 1984.
59. Blank E: Some effects of position on the roentgenographic diagnosis of dislocation of the infant hip. Skel Radiol 7:59, 1981.
60. Graf R: The ultrasonic image of the acetabular rim in infants: An experimental and clinical investigation. Arch Orthop Trauma Surg 99:35, 1981.
61. Graf R: New possibilities for the diagnosis of congenital hip joint dislocation by ultrasonography. J Pediatr Orthop 3:354, 1983.
62. Novick G, Ghelman B, Schneider M: Sonography of the neonatal and infant hip. AJR 141:639, 1983.
63. Boal DKB, Schwenkter EP: The infant hip: Assessment with real-time US. Radiology 157:667, 1985.
64. Morin C, Harcke HT, MacEwen GD: The infant hip: Real-time US assessment of acetabular development. Radiology 157:673, 1985.
65. Keller MS, Chawla HS: Sonographic delineation of the neonatal acetabular labrum. J Ultrasound Med 4:501, 1985.
66. Graf R: Fundamentals of sonographic diagnosis of infant hip dysplasia. J Pediatr Orthop 4:735, 1984.
67. Harcke HT, Grissom LE: Performing dynamic sonography of the infant hip. AJR 155:837, 1990.
68. Novick GS: Sonography in pediatric hip disorders. Radiol Clin North Am 26:29, 1988.
69. Soboleski DA, Babyn P: Sonographic diagnosis of developmental dysplasia of the hip: Importance of increased thickness of acetabular cartilage. AJR 161:839, 1993.
70. Naumann T, Kollmannsberger A, Fischer M, et al: Ultrasonographic evaluation of Legg-Calvé-Perthes disease based on sonoanatomic criteria and the application of new measuring techniques. Eur J Radiol 15:101, 1992.
71. Wirth T, LaQuesne GW, Paterson DC: Ultrasonography in Legg-Calvé-Perthes disease. Pediatr Radiol 22:498, 1992.
72. Farrar IL, Matsen FA 3rd, Rogers JV, et al: Dynamic sonographic study of lesion of the rotator cuff. American Academy of Orthopedic Surgeons 50th Annual Meeting, Anaheim, CA, March 1983.
73. Mack LA, Matsen FA, Kilcoyne RF, et al: Ultrasound evaluation of the rotator cuff. Radiology 157:205, 1985.
74. Middleton WD, Reenus WR, Totty WF, et al: Ultrasonographic evaluation of the rotator cuff and biceps tendon. J Bone Joint Surg [Am] 68:440, 1986.

75. Mack LA, Gannon MK, Kilcoyne JF, et al: Sonographic evaluation of the rotator cuff. Accuracy in patients without prior surgery. Clin Orthop 234:21, 1988.
76. Crass JR, Craig EV, Feinberg SB: Ultrasonography of rotator cuff tears: A review of 500 diagnostic studies. J Clin Ultrasound 16:313, 1988.
77. Miller CL, Karasick D, Kurtz AB, et al: Limited sensitivity of ultrasound for the detection of rotator cuff tear. Skel Radiol 18:179, 1989.
78. Middleton WD: Status of rotator cuff sonography. Radiology 173:307, 1989.
79. Weiner SN, Seitz WH: Sonography of the shoulder in patients with tears of the rotator cuff: Accuracy and value for selecting surgical options. AJR 160:103, 1993.
80. Middleton WD: Ultrasonography of the shoulder. Radiol Clin North Am 30:927, 1992.
81. Mack LA, Nyberg DA, Matsen FR, et al: Sonography of the postoperative shoulder. AJR 150:1089, 1988.
82. Crass JR, Craig EV, Feinberg SB: Sonography of the postoperative rotator cuff. AJR 146:561, 1986.
83. Harryman DDT 2d, Mack LA, Wang KY, et al: Rotator cuff repair: Correlation of functional results with cuff integrity. J Bone Joint Surg [Am] 73:982, 1991.
84. Mack LA, Nyberg DA, Matsen FA 3d: Sonographic evaluation of the rotator cuff. Radiol Clin North Am 26:161, 1988.
85. Hodler J, Fretz CJ, Terrier F, et al: Rotator cuff tears: Correlation of sonographic and surgical findings. Radiology 169:791, 1988.
86. Brandt TD, Cardone BW, Grant TH, et al: Rotator cuff sonography: A reassessment. Radiology 169:791, 1989.
87. Furtschegge A, Resch H: Value of ultrasonography in preoperative diagnosis of rotator cuff tears and postoperative follow-up. Eur J Radiol 8:69, 1988.
88. Soble MG, Kaye AD, Guay RC: Rotator cuff tear: Clinical experience with sonographic detection. Radiology 173:319, 1989.
89. Fornage BD: Achilles tendon: US examination. Radiology 159:759, 1986.
90. Mathieson JR, Connell DG, Cooperberg PL, et al: Sonography of the Achilles tendon and adjacent bursae. AJR 151:127, 1984.
91. Neuhold A, Stiskal M, Kainberger F, et al: Degenerative Achilles tendon disease: Assessment by magnetic resonance and ultrasonography. Eur J Radiol 14:213, 1992.
92. Maffulli N, Dymond NP, Regine R: Surgical repair of ruptured Achilles tendon in sportsmen and sedentary patients: A longitudinal ultrasound assessment. Int J Sports Med 11:78, 1990.
93. Ebeling T, Farin P, Pyörälä K: Ultrasonography in the detection of Achilles tendon xanthomata in heterozygous familial hypercholesterolemia. Atherosclerosis 97:217, 1992.
94. Fornage BD, Schernberg FL, Rifkin MD: Ultrasound examination of the hand. Radiology 155:785, 1985.
95. Fornage BD, Rifkin MD: Ultrasound examination of the hand (letter to the editor). Radiology 160:853, 1986.
96. Jeffrey RB Jr, Laing FC, Schechter WP, et al: Acute suppurative tenosynovitis of the hand: Diagnosis with US. Radiology 162:741, 1987.
97. Buchberger W, Schon G, Strasser K, et al: High-resolution ultrasonography of the carpal tunnel. J Ultrasound Med 10:531, 1991.
98. Gooding GAW: Tenosynovitis of the wrist. J Ultrasound Med 7:225, 1988.
99. Paivansalo M, Jalovaara P: Ultrasound findings of ganglions of the wrist. Eur J Radiol 13:178, 1991.
100. Barr LL, Babcock DS: Sonography of the normal elbow. AJR 157:793, 1991.
101. Markowitz RL, Davidson RS, Harty MP, et al: Sonography of the elbow in infants and children. AJR 159:829, 1992.
102. Maffulli N, Regine R, Carrillo F, et al: Tennis elbow: An ultrasonographic study in tennis players. Br J Sports Med 24:151, 1990.
103. Lenkey JL, Skolnick ML, Slasky BS, et al: Evaluation of the lower extremities. J Clin Ultrasound 9:413, 1981.
104. Slasky BS, Lenkey JL, Skolnick ML, et al: Sonography of soft tissues of extremities and trunk. Semin Ultrasound 4:288, 1982.
105. Sintzoff SA Jr, Gillard I, Van Gansbeke D, et al: Ultrasound evaluation of soft tissue tumors. J Belge Radiol 75:276, 1992.
106. Bernardino ME, Jing BS, Thomas JL, et al: The extremity soft-tissue lesion: A comparative study of ultrasound, computed tomography, and xeroradiography. Radiology 139:53, 1981.
107. deSantos LA, Goldstein HM: Ultrasonography in tumors arising from the spine and bony pelvis. AJR 129:1061, 1977.
108. Zornoza J, Bernardino ME, Ordonez NG: Percutaneous needle biopsy of soft tissue tumors guided by ultrasound and computed tomography. Skel Radiol 9:33, 1982.
109. Yiu-Chiu VS, Chiu LC: Complementary value of ultrasound and computed tomography in the evaluation of musculoskeletal masses. RadioGraphics 3:46, 1983.
110. Totty WG: Radiographic evaluation of soft tissue sarcomas. Orthop Rev 14:257, 1985.
111. Gilsanz V, Yeh HC, Baron MG: Multiple lymphangiomas of the neck, axilla, mediastinum, and bones in an adult. Radiology 120:161, 1976.
112. Miller WB, Melson GL: Abdominal wall endometrioma. AJR 132:467, 1979.
113. Leonidas JC, Brill PW, Bhan I, et al: Cystic retroperitoneal lymphangioma in infants and children. Radiology 127:203, 1978.
114. El-Khoury GY, Bassett GS: Symptomatic bursa formation with osteochondromas. AJR 133:895, 1979.
115. Reuter KL, Raptopoulos V, DeGirolami U, et al: Ultrasonography of a plexiform neurofibroma of the popliteal fossa. J Ultrasound Med 1:209, 1982.
116. Hanson RD, Hunter TB, Haber K: Ultrasonographic appearance of anterior abdominal wall desmoid tumors. J Ultrasound Med 2:141, 1983.
117. Fornage BD, Schernberg FL, Rifkin MD, et al: Sonographic diagnosis of glomus tumor of the finger. J Ultrasound Med 3:523, 1984.
118. Goldberg BB: Ultrasonic evaluation of superficial masses. J Clin Ultrasound 3:91, 1975.
119. Gooding GAW, Herzog KA, Laing FC, et al: Ultrasonographic assessment of neck masses. J Clin Ultrasound 5:248, 1977.
120. Chinn DH, Filly RA, Callen PW: Unusual ultrasonographic appearance of a solid schwannoma. J Clin Ultrasound 10:243, 1982.
121. Hoddick WK, Callen PW, Filly RA, et al: Ultrasound evaluation of benign sciatic nerve sheath tumors. J Ultrasound Med 3:505, 1984.
122. Behan M, Kazam E: The echographic characteristics of fatty tissues and tumors. Radiology 129:143, 1978.
123. Prayer LM, Kropej DH, Wimberger DM, et al: High-resolution real-time sonography and MR imaging in assessment of osteocartilaginous exostoses. Acta Radiol 32:393, 1991.
124. Malghem J, Vande Berg B, Noël H, et al: Benign osteochondromas and exostotic chondrosarcomas: Evaluation of cartilage cap thickness by ultrasound. Skel Radiol 21:33, 1992.
125. Levine E, Lee KR, Neff JR, et al: Comparison of computed tomography and other imaging modalities in the evaluation of musculoskeletal tumors. Radiology 131:431, 1979.
126. Pino G, Conzi GF, Murolo C, et al: Sonographic evaluation of local recurrences of soft tissue sarcomas. J Ultrasound Med 12:23, 1993.
127. Holm HH, Pedersen JF, Kristensen JK, et al: Ultrasonically guided percutaneous puncture. Radiol Clin North Am 13:493, 1975.
128. Korobkin M, Callen PW, Filly RA, et al: Comparison of computed tomography, ultrasonography, and gallium-67 scanning in the evaluation of suspected abdominal abscess. Radiology 129:89, 1978.
129. Weiner CI, Diaconis JN: Primary abdominal wall abscess diagnosed by ultrasound. Arch Surg 110:341, 1975.
130. Doust BD, Quiroz F, Stewart JM: Ultrasonic distinction of abscesses from other intra-abdominal fluid collections. Radiology 125:213, 1977.
131. Kressel HY, Filly RA: Ultrasonographic appearance of gas-containing abscesses in the abdomen. AJR 130:71, 1978.
132. vanSonnenberg E, Wittich GR, Casola G, et al: Sonography of thigh abscess: Detection, diagnosis, and drainage. AJR 149:769, 1987.
133. Yeh H-C, Rabinowitz JG: Ultrasonography of the extremities and pelvic girdle and correlation with computed tomography. Radiology 143:519, 1982.
134. Allen EH, Cosgrove D, Millard FJC: The radiological changes in infections of the spine and their diagnostic value. Clin Radiol 29:31, 1978.
135. Smith EH, Bartrum RJ: Ultrasonically guided percutaneous aspiration of abscesses. AJR 122:308, 1974.
136. vanSonnenberg E, Ferrucci JT Jr, Mueller PR, et al: Percutaneous drainage of abscesses and fluid collections: Technique, results, and applications. Radiology 142:1, 1982.
137. Clark RA, Towbin R: Abscess drainage with CT and ultrasound guidance. Radiol Clin North Am 21:445, 1983.
138. Yousefzadeh DK, Schumann EM, Mulligan GM, et al: The role of imaging modalities in diagnosis and management of pyomyositis. Skel Radiol 8:285, 1982.
139. Abiri MM, Kirpekar M, Ablow RC: Osteomyelitis: Detection with US. Radiology 172:509, 1989.
140. Bar-Ziv J, Barki Y, Maroko A, et al: Rib osteomyelitis in children. Early radiologic and ultrasonic findings. Pediatr Radiol 15:315, 1985.
141. Howard CB, Einhorn M, Dagan R, et al: Ultrasound in diagnosis and management of acute haematogenous osteomyelitis in children. J Bone Joint Surg [Br] 75:79, 1993.
142. Williamson SL, Seibert JJ, Glasier CM, et al: Ultrasound in advanced pediatric osteomyelitis. Pediatr Radiol 21:288, 1991.
143. Fornage BD, Schernberg FL: Sonographic diagnosis of foreign bodies of the distal extremities. AJR 147:567, 1986.
144. Little CM, Parker MG, Callowich MC, et al: The ultrasonic detection of soft tissue foreign bodies. Invest Radiol 21:275, 1986.
145. Gooding GAW, Hardiman T, Sumers M, et al: Sonography of the hand and foot in foreign body detection. J Ultrasound Med 6:441, 1987.
146. Coombs CJ, Mutimer KL, Slattery PG, et al: Hide and seek: Pre-operative ultrasonic localization of non radio-opaque foreign bodies. Aust NZ J Surg 60:989, 1990.
147. Banerjee B, Das RK: Sonographic detection of foreign bodies of the extremities. Br J Radiol 64:107, 1991.
148. Shiels WE II, Babcock DS, Wilson JL, et al: Localization and guided removal of soft-tissue foreign bodies with sonography. AJR 155:1277, 1990.
149. Alexander H, Miller DL: Determining skin thickness with pulsed ultrasound. J Invest Dermatol 72:17, 1979.
150. Cole GW, Handler SJ, Burnett K: The ultrasonic evaluation of skin thickness in scleredema. J Clin Ultrasound 9:501, 1981.
151. Gooding GAW, Stress RM, Graf PM, et al: Heel pad thickness: Determination by high-resolution ultrasonography. J Ultrasound Med 4:173, 1985.
152. Gooding GAW, Stress RM, Graf PM, et al: Sonography of the sole of the foot. Invest Radiol 21:45, 1986.
153. Heckmatt JZ, Leeman S, Dubowitz V: Ultrasound imaging in the diagnosis of muscle disease. J Pediatr 101:656, 1982.
154. Porter RW, Wicks M, Ottewell D: Measurement of the spinal canal by diagnostic ultrasound. J Bone Joint Surg [Br] 60:481, 1978.

155. Finlay D, Stockdale HR, Lewin E: An appraisal of the use of diagnostic ultrasound to quantify the lumbar spinal canal. Br J Radiol 54:870, 1981.

156. Hibbert CS, Delaygue C, McGlen B, et al: Measurement of the lumbar spinal canal by diagnostic ultrasound. Br J Radiol 54:905, 1981.

157. Kadziolka R, Asztely M, Hansson T, et al: Ultrasonic measurement of the lumbar spinal canal. J Bone Joint Surg [Br] 63:504, 1981.

158. Portela LA: Sonography of the normal and abnormal intact lumbar spinal canal. AJR 144:386, 1985.

159. Scheible W, James HE, Leopold GR, et al: Occult spinal dysraphism in infants: Screening with high-resolution real-time ultrasound. Radiology 146:743, 1983.

160. James HE, Scheible W, Kerber C, et al: Comparison of high-resolution real-time ultrasonography and high-resolution computed tomography in an infant with spinal dysraphism. Neurosurgery 13:301, 1983.

161. Raghavendra BN, Epstein FJ, Pinto RS, et al: The tethered spinal cord: Diagnosis by high-resolution real-time ultrasound. Radiology 149:123, 1983.

162. Naidich TP, McLone DG, Shkolnik A, et al: Sonographic evaluation of caudal spine anomalies in children. AJNR 4:661, 1983.

163. Naidich TP, Fernbach SK, McLone DG, et al: Sonography of the caudal spine and back: Congenital anomalies in children. AJNR 5:221, 1984.

164. Dohrmann GJ, Rubin JM: Intraoperative ultrasound imaging of the spinal cord: Syringomyelia, cysts, and tumors—a preliminary report. Surg Neurol 18:395, 1982.

165. Rubin JM, Dohrmann GJ: Work in progress. Intraoperative ultrasonography of the spine. Radiology 146:173, 1983.

166. Quencer RM, Montalvo BM: Normal intraoperative spinal sonography. AJR 143:1301, 1984.

167. Quencer RM, Montalvo BM, Green BA, et al: Intraoperative spinal sonography of soft-tissue masses of the spinal cord and spinal canal. AJR 143:1307, 1984.

168. Knake JE, Chandler WF, McGillicuddy JE, et al: Intraoperative sonography of intraspinal tumors: Initial experience. AJNR 4:1199, 1983.

169. Montalvo BM, Quencer RM, Green BA, et al: Intraoperative sonography in spinal trauma. Radiology 153:125, 1984.

170. Avila NA, Shawker TH, Choyke PL, et al: Cerebellar and spinal hemangioblastomas: Evaluation with intraoperative gray-scale and color Doppler flow US. Radiology 188:143, 1993.

171. Rubin JM, Dohrmann GJ: The spine and spinal cord during neurosurgical operations: Real-time ultrasonography. Radiology 155:197, 1985.

172. Quencer RM, Morse BMM, Green BA, et al: Intraoperative spinal sonography: Adjunct to metrizamide CT in the assessment and surgical decompression of post-traumatic spinal cord cysts. AJR 142:593, 1984.

173. Hutchins WW, Vogelzang RL, Neiman HL, et al: Differentiation of tumor from syringohydromyelia: Intraoperative neurosonography of the spinal cord. Radiology 151:171, 1984.

174. Kochan JP, Quencer RM: Imaging of cystic and cavitary lesions of the spinal cord and canal. The value of MR and intraoperative sonography. Radiol Clin North Am 29:867, 1991.

175. Quencer RM, Montalvo BM, Eismont FJ, et al: Intraoperative spinal sonography in thoracic and lumbar fractures: Evaluation of Harrington rod instrumentation. AJR 145:343, 1985.

176. McGahan JP, Benson D, Chehrazi B, et al: Intraoperative sonographic monitoring of reduction of thoracolumbar burst fractures. AJR 145:1229, 1985.

177. Mirvis SE, Geisler FH: Intraoperative sonography of cervical spinal cord injury: Results in 30 patients. AJR 155:603, 1990.

178. Sample WF, Mitchell SP, Bledsoe RC: Parathyroid ultrasonography. Radiology 127:485, 1978.

179. Scheible W, Deutsch AL, Leopold GR: Parathyroid adenoma: Accuracy of preoperative localization by high-resolution real-time sonography. J Clin Ultrasound 9:325, 1981.

180. Simeone JF, Mueller PR, Ferrucci JT Jr, et al: High-resolution real-time sonography of the parathyroid. Radiology 141:745, 1981.

181. Reading CC, Charboneau JW, James EM, et al: High-resolution parathyroid sonography. AJR 139:539, 1982.

182. Reading CC, Charboneau JW, James EM, et al: Postoperative parathyroid high-frequency sonography: Evaluation of persistent or recurrent hyperparathyroidism. AJR 144:399, 1985.

183. Doppman JL, Krudy AG, Brennan MF, et al: CT appearance of enlarged parathyroid glands in the posterior superior mediastinum. J Comput Assist Tomogr 6:1099, 1982.

184. Park CH, Intenzo C, Cohn HE: Dual-tracer imaging for localization of parathyroid lesions. Clin Nucl Med 11:237, 1986.

185. Kang YS, Rosen K, Clark OH, et al: Localization of abnormal parathyroid glands of the mediastinum with MR imaging. Radiology 189:137, 1993.

186. Solbiati L, Montali G, Croce F, et al: Parathyroid tumors detected by fine-needle aspiration biopsy under ultrasonic guidance. Radiology 148:793, 1983.

187. Gooding GAW, Clark OH, Stark DD, et al: Parathyroid aspiration biopsy under

188. Solbiati L, Giangrande A, DePra L, et al: Percutaneous ethanol injection of parathyroid tumors under US guidance: Treatment for secondary hyperparathyroidism. Radiology 155:607, 1985.

189. Kaplan GN, Sanders RC: B-scan ultrasound in the management of patients with occult abdominal hematomas. J Clin Ultrasound 1:5, 1973.

190. Nowotny C, Niessner H, Thaler E, et al: Sonography: A method for localization of hematomas in hemophiliacs. Haemostatis 5:129, 1976.

191. Thomas JL, Cunningham JJ: Echographic detection and characterization of abdominal hemorrhages in patients with altered coagulation states. Arch Intern Med 138:1392, 1978.

192. Shirkhoda A, Mauro MA, Staab EV, et al: Soft tissue hemorrhage in hemophiliac patients: Computed tomography and ultrasound study. Radiology 147:811, 1983.

193. Spitz HB, Wyatt GM: Rectus sheath hematoma. J Clin Ultrasound 5:413, 1977.

194. Titone C, Lipsius M, Krakauer JS: ''Spontaneous'' hematoma of the rectus abdominis muscle: Critical review of 50 cases with emphasis on early diagnosis and treatment. Surgery 72:568, 1972.

195. Hamilton JV, Flinn G, Haynie CC, et al: Diagnosis of rectus sheath hematoma by B-mode ultrasound: A case report. Am J Obstet Gynecol 125:562, 1976.

196. Kaftori JK, Rosenberger A, Pollack S, et al: Rectus sheath hematoma: Ultrasonographic diagnosis. AJR 128:283, 1977.

197. Wyatt GM, Spitz HB: Ultrasound in the diagnosis of rectus sheath hematoma. JAMA 241:1499, 1979.

198. Goodfellow J, Fearn CBD, Matthews JM: Iliacus haematoma: A common complication of haemophilia. J Bone Joint Surg [Br] 49:748, 1967.

199. Forbes CD, Moule B, Grant M, et al: Bilateral pseudotumors of the pelvis in a patient with Christmas disease. AJR 121:173, 1974.

200. Kumari S, Fulco JD, Karayalcin G, et al: Gray scale ultrasound: Evaluation of iliopsoas hematomas in hemophiliacs. AJR 133:103, 1979.

201. Lee TG, Brickman FE, Avecilla LS: Ultrasound diagnosis of intramural intestinal hematoma. J Clin Ultrasound 5:423, 1977.

202. Fon GT, Hunter TB, Haber K: Utility of ultrasound for diagnosis of mesenteric hematoma. AJR 134:381, 1980.

203. Wicks JD, Silver TM, Bree RL: Gray scale features of hematomas: An ultrasonic spectrum. AJR 131:977, 1978.

204. Sandweiss DA, Hanson JC, Gosink BB, et al: Ultrasound in diagnosis, localization, and treatment of loculated pleural empyema. Ann Intern Med 82:50, 1975.

205. Doust BD, Baum JK, Maklad NF, et al: Ultrasonic evaluation of pleural opacities. Radiology 114:135, 1975.

206. Gryminski J, Krakowka P, Lypacewicz G: The diagnosis of pleural effusion by ultrasonic and radiologic techniques. Chest 70:33, 1976.

207. Ravin CE: Thoracocentesis of loculated pleural effusions using grey scale ultrasonic guidance. Chest 71:666, 1977.

208. Laing FC, Filly RA: Problems in the application of ultrasonography for the evaluation of pleural opacities. Radiology 126:211, 1978.

209. Adams FV, Galati V: M-mode ultrasonic localization of pleural effusion. JAMA 239:1761, 1978.

210. Hirsch JH, Carter SJ, Chikos PM, et al: Ultrasonic evaluation of radiographic opacities of the chest. AJR 130:1153, 1978.

211. Edell SL: Pleural effusion aspiration with ultrasound. Clin Radiol 29:377, 1978.

212. Harnsberger HR, Lee TG, Mukuno DH: Rapid, inexpensive real-time directed thoracentesis. Radiology 146:545, 1983.

213. Marks WM, Filly RA, Callen PW: Real-time evaluation of pleural lesions: New observations regarding the probability of obtaining free fluid. Radiology 142:163, 1982.

214. Hirsch JH, Rogers JV, Mack LA: Real-time sonography of pleural opacities. AJR 136:297, 1981.

215. Wolson AH: Ultrasonic evaluation of intrathoracic masses. J Clin Ultrasound 4:269, 1976.

216. Shin MS, Gray PW: Pitfalls in ultrasonic detection of pleural fluid. J Clin Ultrasound 6:421, 1978.

217. Burney DP, Martin CE, Thomas CS, et al: Rheumatoid pericarditis: Clinical significance and operative management. J Thorac Cardiovasc Surg 77:511, 1979.

218. Hernandez-Lopez E, Chahine RA, Anastassiades P, et al: Echocardiographic study of the cardiac involvement in rheumatoid arthritis. Chest 72:52, 1977.

219. MacDonald WJ, Crawford MH, Klippel JH, et al: Echocardiographic assessment of cardiac structure and function in patients with rheumatoid arthritis. Am J Med 63:890, 1977.

220. Gottdiener JS, Moutsopoulos HM, Decker JL: Echocardiographic identification of cardiac abnormality in scleroderma and related disorders. Am J Med 66:391, 1979.

# 12

# Imaging Techniques in Intraspinal Diseases

*Victor Haughton, M.D.*

This chapter describes the more important imaging techniques that can be used to evaluate the spine or spinal cord, or both. As the subject is extensive and complex, only an overview of such techniques is provided, and the reader is encouraged to consult other available textbooks[1-11] for a complete discussion of neuroradiologic imaging.

The most common disorders of spinal joints that are referred to radiologists by neurologists or neurosurgeons are osteoarthritis of the facet joints and intervertebral disc degeneration causing myelopathy, radiculopathy, low back pain, or sciatica. The differential diagnosis of such clinical manifestations often includes many other spinal conditions, such as neoplasms, cysts, and infections. The techniques of and indications for the commonly used imaging procedures are described briefly, after which the characteristic imaging abnormalities of the common osseous and articular disorders of the spine are illustrated.

## IMAGING TECHNIQUES

The primary diagnostic methods used to evaluate the spine are routine radiography, CT, MR imaging, conventional tomography, nuclear isotope imaging, ultrasonography, myelography, and angiography. Each of these methods is considered in the following discussion, with the exception of ultrasonography, which is described in Chapter 11, and routine radiography, discussed in Chapters 1 and 40.

## Computed Tomography

CT is a versatile imaging technique that has been used to demonstrate almost every type of pathologic condition of the spine. Because the transaxial tomographic sections that typically are employed are thin (1 or several millimeters thick), CT is suited to examining only short segments of the spine. Long spinal segments are examined more effectively with conventional radiography or tomography, MR imaging, or myelography.

**Indications.** CT is effective for evaluating any pathologic process that has been localized to a short segment of the spine by clinical or routine radiographic abnormalities. In the investigation of low back pain, CT is an effective imaging method, and it is performed simply and safely as an outpatient procedure. It has greater sensitivity in the diagnosis of discal herniation or facet joint disease and less radiation exposure than myelography or conventional radiography. For cervical radiculopathy, CT is an efficient and effective study. CT serves as a complementary study to routine radiography or myelography in the delineation of fractures in patients who have had spinal trauma. CT may be used as a primary or supplementary technique in the assessment of congenital, neoplastic, or infectious diseases.

**Techniques.** State-of-the-art CT scanning for the spine includes spiral and conventional slice selection, a slice thickness that varies from 1 to 5 mm, reconstruction algorithms optimized for bone and soft tissue depiction, and three-dimensional reformatting. The technical factors that are optimal for a CT examination depend on the precise clinical situation. When maximal soft tissue contrast is needed, high mA, a long scan time, a relatively larger pixel size, and thicker slice collimation are selected, whereas for maximal spatial resolution in high contrast tissue, thinner slices, smaller pixels, and high detail reconstruction algorithms are used (Fig. 12–1). In almost all instances, an accurate, detailed localizer image is required to select the plane and the location of the transaxial sections of the spine. Many display modes are available for CT data, including magnification techniques, image reformation in a secondary plane, and pseudo–three-dimensional image display (Fig. 12–2). A more detailed discussion of CT techniques is given in Chapter 8.

In the examination of the lumbar spine, sufficient contrast resolution must be available to detect discal fragments (which are slightly more dense than the dural sac), and sufficient spatial resolution is required to demonstrate osseous detail about the facet joints. A localizer image in the lateral projection, and sometimes in the frontal projection, is obtained to facilitate selection of appropriate CT levels and gantry angles for examining the region of interest. The anatomic configuration of the neural foramina, intervertebral discs, and facet joints is displayed optimally when the plane of the CT section parallels that of the closest vertebral endplates. The orthodox CT techniques for the lumbar spine rely on a sequence of images for each intervertebral disc level that is to be imaged. On a lateral localizer image, a cursor is aligned with the axis of the midportion of the intervertebral disc (Fig. 12–3A). A series of contiguous 5 mm thick images with this same axis is programmed beginning 15 mm above the cursor location and ending 15 mm below it (Fig. 12–3B). With this technique, it is evident that some overlap of the CT slices is present posteriorly, whereas anteriorly there may be small gaps in the continuity of the CT slices (Fig. 12–3B).

In the examination of the cervical (or thoracic) intervertebral discs, different CT parameters must be chosen, as, in this region, the intervertebral discs are thinner and the epidural fat is sparser, increasing the need for high contrast resolution. The localizer image is used to identify the intervertebral disc space (Fig. 12–4). A cursor line is constructed along the axis of the midportion of the disc, and a series of 1.0 or 1.5 mm thick images is obtained at, above, and below this level (Fig. 12–4). Most frequently, the C5-C6 and C6-C7 spinal levels are studied. In some instances, it may be necessary to place material of water density around the patient's neck to improve the image quality.[12] The shoulder should be withdrawn from the scanning area

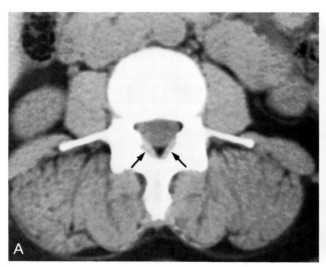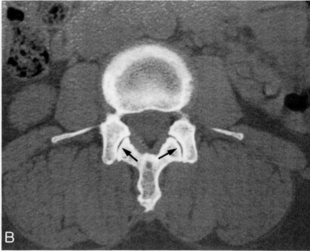

**FIGURE 12–1.** Comparison of techniques optimized to show soft tissue **(A)** and bone **(B)** in the lower lumbar spine.
 **A** In a 5 mm thick slice with high mAs and narrow window, soft tissues such as the ligamentum flavum (arrows) and dural sac are demonstrated.
 **B** With a 1.5 mm thick slice, a high detail reconstruction algorithm, and a wide window, the osseous anatomy, including the facet joints (arrows), is demonstrated optimally.

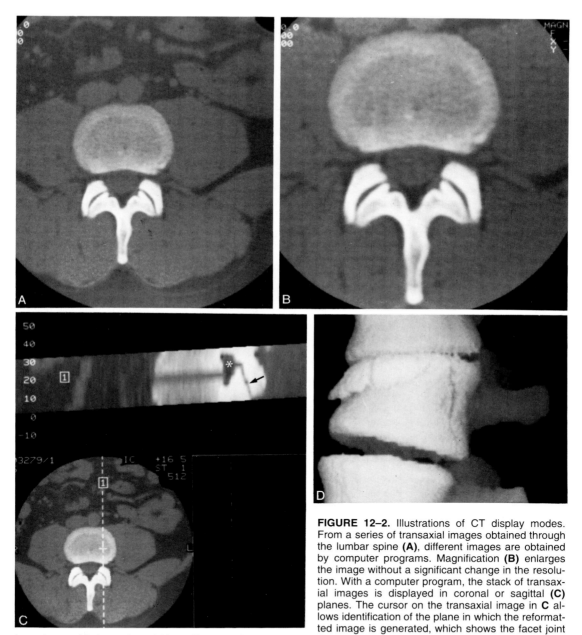

**FIGURE 12–2.** Illustrations of CT display modes. From a series of transaxial images obtained through the lumbar spine **(A)**, different images are obtained by computer programs. Magnification **(B)** enlarges the image without a significant change in the resolution. With a computer program, the stack of transaxial images is displayed in coronal or sagittal **(C)** planes. The cursor on the transaxial image in **C** allows identification of the plane in which the reformatted image is generated, which shows the facet joint (arrow), neural foramen (asterisk), and intervertebral disc space. The stack of transaxial images also may be displayed in a simulated three-dimensional format **(D)**. In **D**, a comminuted compression fracture of a lumbar vertebra is illustrated.

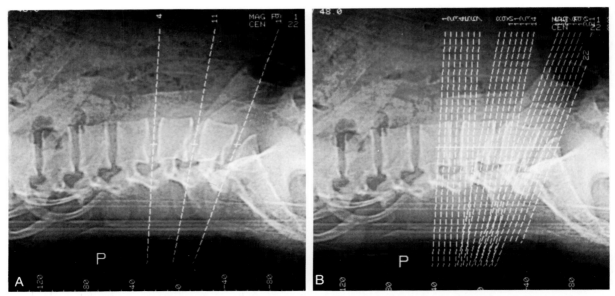

**FIGURE 12–3.** The localizer view of the lumbar spine used to select the levels of the transaxial slices to be obtained. In **A**, the planes of the lower three lumbar intervertebral discs have been identified. In **B**, a series of slices has been selected, which includes one slice through each of the selected intervertebral discs and slices 5, 10, and 15 mm above and below the center of the disc space. Note that the images completely encompass the neural foramina and spine except for small wedges.

as much as possible to reduce imaging artifacts. The patient should be instructed to hold the breath and not to swallow or move during collection of the CT image data.

When the intervertebral discs or facet joints are not the primary area of interest, different imaging parameters may be more effective. For example, in studying a suspected vertebral fracture, thin contiguous CT scans without a change in gantry angle are obtained so that image reformation in a sagittal, coronal, or oblique plane is facilitated. Data acquisition using low mAs, which shortens the examination time, suffices when spatial resolution is more important than contrast resolution. When the soft tissues are to be studied, a high mAs technique and relatively thicker CT slices are used.

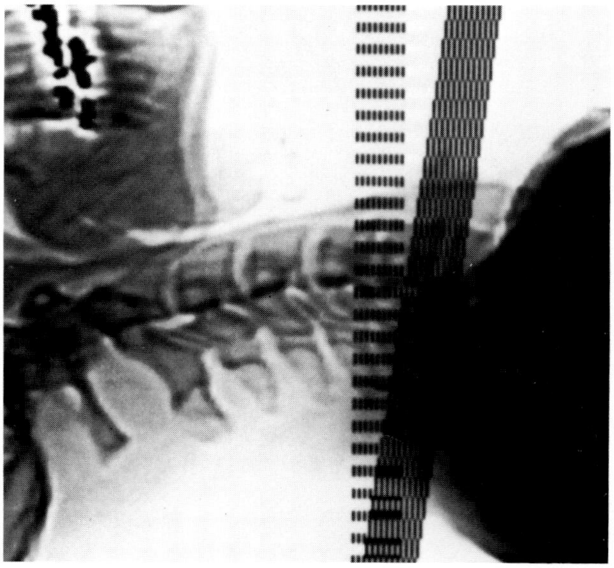

The injection of an aqueous contrast medium into the subarachnoid space can be used to improve the visualization of intrathecal structures (Fig. 12–5). This can be achieved in several ways. One technique, which is referred to as the low dose myelogram, consists of 5 ml of the contrast agent (in a concentration of about 170 mg of iodine per milliliter) that is injected either by a C1-C2 puncture or by a lumbar puncture, depending on which spinal level is closer to the region of interest. The contrast medium then is dispersed by tilting the patient appropriately so that gravity causes the medium to move in the less viscous cerebrospinal fluid. The patient then is placed immediately in the CT scanner. Alternatively, CT is performed after myelography. The precise interval of time between the two examinations that ensures optimal evaluation depends on which portion of the spine is being studied. CT scanning usually is delayed 4 to 6 hours after a lumbar myelogram, and it is accomplished immediately after a cervical myelogram.

**FIGURE 12–4.** A localizer view of the cervical spine used to select levels for studying the C5-C6 and C6-C7 intervertebral discs. A series of slices was selected, which includes the intervertebral disc and neural foramina.

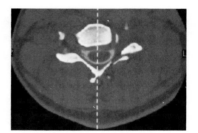

**FIGURE 12–5.** Intrathecal contrast enhancement to facilitate visualization of the subarachnoid space and the spinal cord. The relationship of the spinal cord to the fractured cervical spine is demonstrated effectively in the transaxial image because intrathecal contrast medium was added to the subarachnoid space. The technique also is called low dose myelography.

The intravenous injection of contrast material is a rarely required but potentially effective supplement to the CT examination of the spine. The meninges, the nerve root sleeves, the epidural venous plexuses, and regions with epidural scar tissue increase substantially in radiodensity after such intravenous injection (Fig. 12–6). Usually a series of images is obtained before and after the administration of the contrast medium, which is infused as rapidly as possible (5 to 10 min generally is required for the infusion process). As the patient is likely to move between the two series of images, a second localizer scan is acquired prior to the second series to ensure that an identical sequence of images is obtained. This facilitates comparison of the two sets of images.

## Magnetic Resonance Imaging

The major advantages of MR imaging relate to its non-invasiveness, versatility, and sensitivity. Its major disadvantage is a relatively high cost. During the MR imaging examination of patients with metallic implants or prostheses, imaging artifacts or local tissue damage (due to heating of the metal) may be encountered. Cardiac pacemakers may malfunction in the magnetic field. Patients on life support

and monitoring systems likewise should not be subjected to MR imaging.

**Indications.** MR imaging has replaced many CT and myelographic studies and has become the primary imaging method for most spinal lesions. Providing sagittal images noninvasively of the entire spinal column in one acquisition, it serves as an excellent screening study. With detailed, multiplanar slices, and multiple means of adjusting contrast, it has excellent sensitivity and specificity. Specialized hardware and acquisitions are used for spinal imaging, including surface coils for each region of the spine, fast acquisition times (which minimize motion and artifact), and fat suppression.

**Techniques.** As with CT, specific technical parameters, including location and thickness of the individual scans, must be selected for MR imaging on the basis of the precise clinical questions that require answers. The choice of an imaging plane is more complex with MR imaging than with CT, as direct sagittal or coronal image acquisition is possible with MR imaging but not with CT. In most instances, sagittal MR images of the spine are used, supplemented with transaxial scans at specified levels. The choice of a field of view and a matrix size as well as other parameters is guided by the desire to provide anatomic detail in the

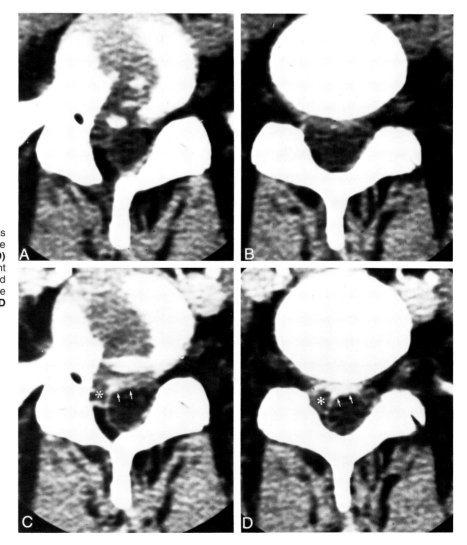

**FIGURE 12–6.** CT analysis using intravenous administration of contrast material. CT of the lumbar spine without **(A, B)** and with **(C, D)** intravenous contrast enhancement in a patient with previous laminectomy. Scar (arrows) and a herniated disc fragment (asterisks) are shown. **A** and **C** are at same level; **B** and **D** are at same level.

shortest possible image acquisition time. The diagnostic information provided by MR imaging is influenced considerably by the size or strength of the magnet, specific technical factors, including the magnetic pulse sequence used, and the availability of various types of receiver coils. For spinal imaging, specially designed small surface receiver coils provide more detailed images by suppressing the signal noise originating from areas outside the region of interest and by matching the region of interest to the viewing matrix.

In MR imaging, pulses of radiofrequency energy are used to measure the density of hydrogen nuclei (proton density) in a tissue. The process of restoring the magnetic vector along the static magnetic field after the pulses have ceased is termed relaxation. Relaxation times of tissue components are of great importance in MR imaging. Two relaxation times can be distinguished: T1 or longitudinal, and T2 or transverse. Pulse sequences can be chosen in such a way that the image is dominated either by the proton density or by one or both of the relaxation times.[10] Whereas in CT only a single image is obtained, in MR imaging the operator adjusts the imaging parameters systematically to obtain a series of images containing different information. A single image rarely provides sufficient information for diagnostic purposes.

A long interval between the excitation pulses (TR) combined with a short interval of the refocusing pulses (TE) produces an image in which contrast depends mainly on proton density; a long TR and a long TE produce a T2-weighted image; and a short TR and a short TE produce a relatively T1-weighted image. In T1-weighted images the signal from fat is intense (white), that from spinal cord is intermediate, and that from cerebrospinal fluid (CSF) is

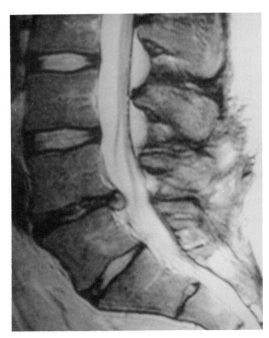

**FIGURE 12–8.** MR imaging. A sagittal T2-weighted (TR/TE, 3214/102) (fast) spin echo image shows disc degeneration (manifested as decreased signal intensity) and a disc herniation at the L4-L5 spinal level. The spinal cord and nerve roots are well shown.

weak (black). Figures 12–7 and 12–8 provide examples of T1-weighted and T2-weighted MR images. In T2-weighted images CSF has a more intense signal than the spinal cord or fat (Fig. 12–9).

Both T1- and T2-weighted images are of value in investigations of spinal disorders. With T1 weighting, the contours of the spinal cord can be distinguished easily from the surrounding CSF. Because bone and CSF are not well distinguished in T1-weighted images, however, osteophytes compressing the subarachnoid space are not identified easily. In T2-weighted images, the high intensity signal of the subarachnoid space contrasts with the lower intensity signal of osseous structures. The spinal cord is demonstrated less effectively in T2-weighted images because of the inferior signal-to-noise ratio and the intense signal from the CSF. For diastematomyelia, syringomyelia, or intramedullary neoplasms, the T1-weighted images usually are definitive. For multiple sclerosis involving the spinal cord or for characterization of some neoplasms, the T2-weighted sequence is useful. In general, however, a combination of T1- and T2-weighted images is used.

Contrast enhancement is used in many spinal MR imaging studies. With intravenous contrast medium, tumors and non-neoplastic processes are demonstrated. Contrast medium may help demonstrate the extent of tumor. In discitis, contrast medium provides confirmatory evidence of the inflammation in the disc and the paraspinal abscess or inflammation. In postoperative differentiation of scar from recurrent herniated disc, contrast enhancement in spinal nerves has been detected, suggesting wallerian degeneration and abnormal capillary permeability. Enhancement is seen normally in spinal nerve ganglia. Contrast medium has been used to demonstrate diffusion of solutes into the intervertebral disc. In the spinal cord, enhancement may be seen

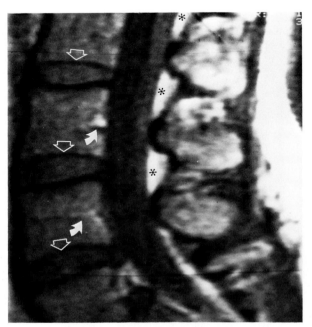

**FIGURE 12–7.** MR imaging. A T1-weighted spin echo MR image of the lumbar spine (TR/TE, 500/20). Note the basivertebral vein (curved arrows), epidural fat (asterisks) posterior to the subarachnoid space, and intervertebral discs (open arrows). Behind the epidural fat, the low signal intensity ligamentum flavum and interspinous ligaments are seen.

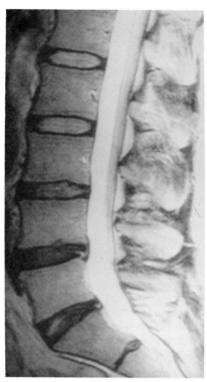

**FIGURE 12–9.** MR imaging. A sagittal T2-weighted (TR/TE, 3287/102) spin echo image shows disc, spinal canal, and vertebral morphology. Note the decreased signal intensity in the degenerating lower three lumbar intervertebral discs. In two of the discs, small tears are visible in the posterior anulus fibrosus.

secondary to demyelination, infarction, or vascular engorgement as well as neoplasm. Fat suppression technique often is used with contrast medium in spinal imaging to eliminate the high signal intensity of the spinal epidural fat.

Gradient echo and fast spin echo MR imaging has been used effectively in the spine. With gradient echo images, because of the speed of acquisition and capability of imaging moving tissues accurately, artifacts from CSF motion are minimized. Other artifacts are produced. Fast spin echo images have been used effectively in spine imaging because of their short acquisition time. Signal intensity from the intervertebral discs is less with fast spin echo technique than conventional spin echo or gradient echo technique (Fig. 12–9).

For a more detailed description of MR imaging techniques, see Chapters 9 and 10.

**Contrast Media.** Contrast agents used in MR imaging differ somewhat in purpose from those used in diagnostic radiology. MR imaging contrast agents are used both to distinguish tissue components with identical signal characteristics and to shorten the relaxation times. In addition, radiographic contrast agents are involved directly in the imaging process, whereas in MR imaging the enhancement is indirect.[10] Shortened relaxation times lead to a stronger signal in T1-weighted images and a signal of lower intensity in T2-weighted images.

Paramagnetic contrast media have had excellent safety profiles with very rare serious reactions. An ionic and two nonionic chelates of gadolinium have been marketed for use with MR imaging.

## Myelography

Prior to the development of CT and MR imaging, myelography was the most important neuroradiologic technique for examination of the spine. This technique involves the opacification of the subarachnoid space with contrast material.

**Indications.** Although it is a safe and effective method for demonstrating the subarachnoid space, spinal cord, and nerve root sheaths, myelography is more costly and more invasive than CT or MR imaging, which may be performed on an outpatient basis. Myelography is indicated in patients with cervical radiculopathy, especially if the results of a cervical CT or MR scan are ambiguous. For evaluation of spinal cord disorders, however, MR imaging is preferred. Myelography may be used for confirming a complete block of the subarachnoid space. The technique is useful in detecting cysts within the spinal cord or subarachnoid space, as contrast material will demonstrate the cystic nature of the process and its communication with the subarachnoid space. Currently myelography also is used in investigating persistent low back pain after laminectomy, a symptom that is not evaluated effectively by any single technique.

**Contrast Media.** The contrast media for myelography include gas (room air, carbon dioxide, oxygen), water-soluble (aqueous) iodinated media (metrizamide, iopamidol, iohexol, iotrol), and oily contrast media (iophendylate). The water-soluble media, at present the standard choice for most myelographic studies, have major advantages in that they produce ideal opacification and faithfully demonstrate the subarachnoid space and intrathecal structures (Fig. 12–10). The only contraindication to their use is the rare allergy to the aqueous contrast media. The side effects of aqueous media include nausea, vomiting, headache, changes in affect and cognition, and hallucinations. Side effects usually appear between 6 and 12 hours after myelography when the concentration of dye in the cerebral cisterns approaches a maximum. By the time the contrast medium has been completely excreted in the urine—that is, at 24 hours—side effects have resolved. The only serious complication reported is seizures, the frequency of which is approximately 0.1 per cent for metrizamide and lower for the other aqueous myelographic media recently introduced: iopamidol, iohexol, and iotrol. In patients with a known low seizure threshold (epilepsy or alcoholism), aqueous myelographic contrast media should be used cautiously. The package insert for metrizamide cautions against myelography in patients with multiple sclerosis, whose conditions have been observed to deteriorate either spontaneously or after myelography.

Although iophendylate (Pantopaque) does not often produce acute side effects, it does cause arachnoiditis when it remains in the subarachnoid space. Therefore, Pantopaque has essentially been replaced by water-soluble contrast media for myelography. Pantopaque also demonstrates the subarachnoid space less effectively because it is immiscible with CSF. It is unsuitably radiodense for myelography or for CT. Although the aqueous media are removed physiologically from the subarachnoid space, Pantopaque must be aspirated through an 18 gauge needle.

Gas is an effective and safe contrast material for studying the spinal cord but requires pluridirectional tomography and special expertise on the part of the examiner. Except for the

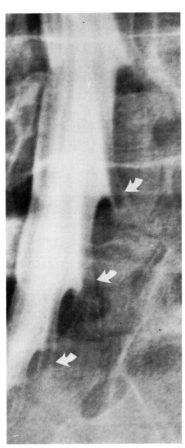

**FIGURE 12–10.** Myelography. Oblique radiograph during a lumbar myelogram with an aqueous contrast medium, demonstrating normal opacification of root sheaths (arrows).

risks associated with cannulating the subarachnoid space, there are no contraindications to the use of intrathecal gas. The side effects of gas myelography include disagreeable paresthesias and often severe headache. Except when MR imaging is not available or is contraindicated, gas myelography at present has no important indications.

**Techniques.** The basic technique for myelography with water-soluble, gaseous, or oily contrast media includes cannulation of the subarachnoid space with either a C1-C2 or a lumbar puncture. For the cervical route a 20, 22, or 25 gauge needle is placed with fluoroscopic or radiographic monitoring between the C1 and C2 vertebrae approximately two thirds the distance from the anterior to the posterior margins of the spinal cord. Use of careful technique by experienced personnel will minimize the risk of damaging the vertebral artery or spinal cord with the needle tip. When the contrast medium is injected through the needle, the patient should be prone, with the neck mildly extended and the fluoroscopic table nearly flat to create a trap into which the contrast medium will pool. Radiographs in posteroanterior, oblique, and lateral projections are obtained without moving the patient to minimize the mixing and diffusion of the contrast medium.

If the contrast medium is to be moved with the aid of gravity from one region in the spinal canal to another, turbulent flow, mixing, and diffusion must be avoided to maintain adequate concentration of the contrast medium

and to minimize side effects. For example, to study the thoracic region after a cervical myelogram, the patient is rolled into a lateral decubitus position with the head elevated slightly, after which the head of the table is elevated 10 to 15 degrees for 1 min. If the patient then is rolled supine and the table is returned to a horizontal position, the contrast medium is trapped in the thoracic subarachnoid space. Excellent anteroposterior and lateral radiographs of the spinal cord can then be obtained. If a lumbar examination is needed, the patient again is rolled into the decubitus position, the head of the table is elevated 10 to 15 degrees above horizontal for another minute, and the patient then is turned to the prone position. Radiographs of the lumbar region in posteroanterior, lateral, and oblique projections are obtained (Fig. 12–10). For the oblique lumbar myelographic films, the patient may be rolled because mixing does not usually occur once the contrast medium is in the lumbar subarachnoid space. Low voltage (60 to 70 kV) and precise collimation are important for optimal results.

The contrast agent also may be administered by lumbar puncture, especially when the primary objective is a lumbar myelographic study. The most effective technique, which has negligible risk, is to pass a 20, 22, or 25 gauge needle in the midline between the L3 and L4 spinous processes into the thecal sac.

When Pantopaque myelography is undertaken, a sufficiently large needle (18 gauge) is required to permit injection and removal of the very viscous, oily contrast medium. Sufficient Pantopaque (6 to 12 ml) must be injected to opacify the caudal end of the lumbar sac as high as the L3-L4 interspace. When the thoracic or cervical region (Fig. 12–11) is to be evaluated, either large volumes of contrast medium are injected or the patient is tilted, with fluoroscopic monitoring, to permit the contrast material to flow by gravity into the other regions. Pantopaque usually is not administered by a C1-C2 puncture because its removal by this route is difficult. Pantopaque is contraindicated if the subarachnoid space contains bloody CSF.

Myelographic techniques must be modified if gas is to be used as the contrast material. The first step is to place the patient in a lateral decubitus position with pillows and sponges placed so that the spine is as parallel to the table top as possible. The patient must be comfortable to minimize voluntary movements. The subarachnoid space may be cannulated by a lumbar puncture, in which case 30 to 50 ml of CSF is removed prior to injecting the gas, or by a C1-C2 puncture. The head of the table then is tilted 20 degrees downward and oxygen, filtered room air, or carbon dioxide is injected until the desired region of the spinal canal is filled with gas. Successive filling of the lumbar, thoracic, and cervical spine can be monitored by asking the patient to report the sensations he or she feels or by obtaining a conventional tomographic section. Usually 40 ml is required to fill the lumbar subarachnoid space, 60 ml to fill the thoracic region, and about 80 ml to completely fill the spinal subarachnoid space to the cervicomedullary junction. Thin pluridirectional tomographic images (see discussion later in this chapter) with tight collimation are obtained of the area of interest (Fig. 12–12). If lumbar puncture was performed, gas is allowed to escape through the needle, and after filming is complete, the needle is removed. The patient is returned to the hospital ward with instructions not to elevate his or her head above the torso for 16 hours.

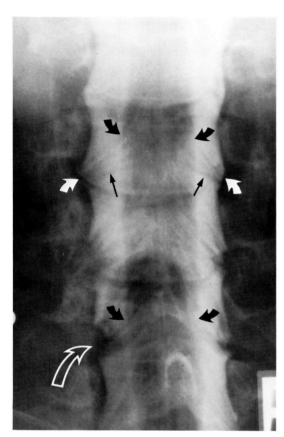

**FIGURE 12–11.** Cervical myelogram. The spinal cord (curved black arrows) and nerve roots (straight black arrows and curved white arrows) are normal. The root sheaths fill normally except on the right at C6-C7, where a disc herniation deforms the root sheath (open arrow).

## Single Photon Emission Computed Tomography

There are several skeletal applications for single photon emission CT (SPECT), and it may be used as an adjunct to conventional bone scanning. In comparison with planar images, SPECT provides increased contrast resolution (because the tomographic technique excludes the noise from tissues outside the plane of imaging) but inferior spatial resolution. Therefore, SPECT is a supplement to rather than a replacement of conventional bone scanning.

**Indications.** Although it rarely allows differentiation among the abnormalities produced by trauma, infection, osteoarthritis, and spondylolysis, SPECT has been used to distinguish effectively between active and inactive processes in the spine and may allow differentiation of a symptomatic and an asymptomatic spondylolysis. Increased activity in a pars interarticularis detected on SPECT correlated well with the presence of pain in one series of patients with spondylolysis.[13] A negative SPECT study suggested that a pars interarticularis defect was asymptomatic. Conventional planar bone scanning is less effective in localizing activity to the pars interarticularis because the lumbar vertebral body and posterior neural arch are not distinguished easily.

**Techniques.** For adults, 25 mCi of $^{99m}$Tc-medronate is injected intravenously. Two to 3 hours later the patient is placed supine in a straight and symmetric position on the imaging table with the arms folded and out of the area to be imaged. The use of pillows under the knees and other means to ensure the patient's comfort helps obtain an optimal study. A gamma camera with a circular 400 mm field of view rotates 360 degrees, acquiring 64 projections in 21 min, during which time the patient must be completely immobile to eliminate motion artifact. A $64 \times 64$ matrix is used and acquisition time is 20 sec per projection. Artifacts due to incomplete angular sampling, nonuniformity of the gamma camera, variations in the center of rotation, or gantry instability are minimal. After 9 point spatial smoothing of each of the 64 projections, tomographic images approximately 6 mm thick are obtained by back projection.[13] Three or four sets of SPECT images are obtained prior to the acquisition of conventional planar images (500,000 counts).

## Spinal Angiography

As a result of the development of selective catheterization of the intercostal and lumbar arteries, the anterior

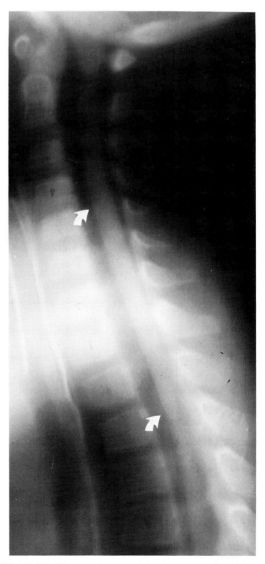

**FIGURE 12–12.** Gas myelogram. On the conventional tomogram, the cervical and upper thoracic spinal cord (arrows) is demonstrated.

spinal artery can be visualized safely and effectively. The major indications for spinal arteriography are vascular malformations or tumors involving the spinal cord, dura, spine, or subarachnoid space (Fig. 12–13).[14–16] Spinal angiography may be performed to evaluate the feasibility of embolizing a vascular malformation or a tumor prior to surgery. Some surgeons request spinal arteriography prior to spinal surgery to locate the artery of Adamkiewicz and thereby prevent its injury during the surgical procedure. In addition to the general contraindications of angiography, compression of the anterior spinal artery, which may lead to an ascending paralysis if the artery were to be opacified, represents a specific contraindication to spinal arteriography. Complications of the procedure are rare.

Spinal angiography usually is performed with a small (No. 5 French) catheter via the transfemoral route. The tip is tapered and the catheter is shaped so that the intercostal and lumbar arteries can be entered selectively and then injected with contrast medium. Only the narrow tip of the catheter enters the origin of the intercostal or lumbar vessel. One to 2 ml of contrast medium is injected while high resolution magnification radiographs are obtained during a 10 sec period using a conventional film changer or digital subtraction technique.

### Miscellaneous Techniques

**Discography.** Discography is not purely an imaging technique because symptoms produced during the test are

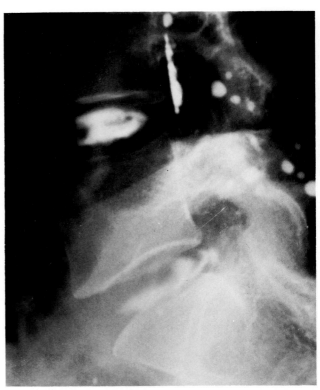

**FIGURE 12–14.** Normal findings on a discogram are evident with contrast medium seen in the L4-L5 disc interspace, centrally and without extravasation. The L5-S1 interspace shows abnormal findings, with extravasation of the contrast medium posteriorly. (Courtesy of B. Ghelman, M.D., New York, New York.)

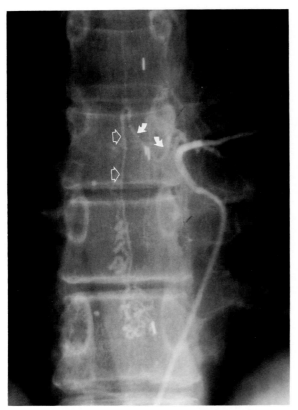

**FIGURE 12–13.** Spinal arteriogram demonstrating an arteriovenous malformation. By means of a catheter in an intercostal artery, a radiculomedullary artery (solid arrows) is opacified, which causes filling of the anterior spinal artery (open arrows). The distal tangle of vessels represents the malformation.

considered to have as much diagnostic value as the radiographs obtained.[17–19] Despite some enthusiastic advocates, this technique never gained wide acceptance by radiologists. The major indication of discography is the further evaluation of neck or low back pain after more routine tests have been nondiagnostic. It also has been used to document the accurate placement of a needle in the nucleus pulposus prior to the injection of chymopapain.

Numerous modifications of the basic discography technique have been described. By one of several routes, small gauge needles are placed with fluoroscopic monitoring into the nucleus pulposus of the selected disc or discs, most commonly in the lower lumbar or lower cervical spine. In some protocols, a local anesthetic agent or saline solution is injected with firm manual pressure into the nucleus pulposus while the patient's symptoms and the amount of fluid injected are monitored. More than 1 ml of fluid entering the disc or pain that duplicates the patient's presenting complaint is considered a positive sign of a herniation of the intervertebral disc or other pathologic condition of the disc. Radiographs are obtained to demonstrate the location of the injected contrast medium and the pattern of opacification, findings that are considered by some authorities to be diagnostic for various types of discal lesions. A small amount of contrast medium contained entirely within the nucleus pulposus suggests an intact anulus fibrosus (Fig. 12–14). Radiographic demonstration of contrast medium leaking outside the anulus fibrosus indicates a tear of the anulus, which may be present with or without a nuclear herniation.

**Epidural Venography.** The cervical or lumbar epidural venous plexus can be opacified by an injection of contrast medium into the ascending lumbar vein or directly into the medullary cavity of a vertebral body (epidural venography) (Fig. 12–15).[20–24] The primary indication for epidural venography has been suspected herniated disc or spinal stenosis that was not detected by myelography. The diagnostic accuracy of the test has varied from poor (because of technical difficulties in achieved venous filling) to good (when patients were selected carefully and excellent opacification was obtained). The risks of epidural venography are approximately the same as those for angiography. CT scanning and MR imaging, which provide the means of detecting myelographically silent lateral disc herniations without contrast medium or cannulation, have made epidural venography obsolete.

**Epidurography.** CT and MR imaging which provide direct visualization of the epidural space, have essentially replaced epidurography, in which opacification of the epidural space with an aqueous contrast medium is accomplished.[25] In the past, the primary indication for the procedure was detection of herniated lumbar intervertebral discs that were not demonstrated by myelography. The procedure involved the placement of a needle or catheter in the epidural space, the injection of a few milliliters of aqueous contrast medium, and the obtaining of radiographs to visualize the contrast medium as it diffused into the epidural space (Fig. 12–16). Disc fragments that obstructed the flow of contrast medium in the spinal canal or within the neural foramen were demonstrated as filling defects. Few compli-

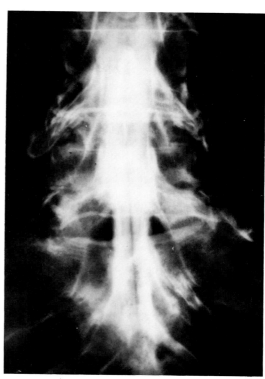

**FIGURE 12–16.** Epidurogram. Contrast medium injected into the epidural space surrounds the root sheaths in each neural foramen.

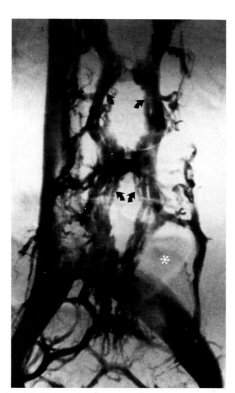

**FIGURE 12–15.** Epidural venogram. The lumbar vertebral plexus and vena cava are opacified via the ascending lumbar veins. The anterior internal vertebral veins (arrows) fill normally. Failure to fill the radicular veins at the left L5-S1 level (asterisk) is related to a herniated disc.

cations were reported. In selected cases, when technically adequate examinations were obtained, herniated discs were demonstrated effectively.

**Pluridirectional Tomography.** MR imaging and CT have caused a decline in the use of pluridirectional spinal tomography. The radiation dose from pluridirectional tomography is 10 to 30 centigrays (cGy) (rad), compared with about 4 cGy for CT. With pluridirectional tomography (Fig. 12–12), images that demonstrate bone detail in 1.0 mm thick sagittal or coronal sections with a resolution of 0.1 mm are possible.

Pluridirectional tomography is indicated when direct sagittal or coronal images of the spinal osseous structures are needed. Trauma is one such indication because vertebral alignment, transverse fractures, and anatomic relationships of the facet joints can be shown effectively. Conventional tomography may be useful when combined with myelography, especially if gas is used as the contrast material.

With regard to technique, the patient is placed on the examining table so that the desired plane of section is nearly horizontal (supine position for coronal sections, decubitus position for sagittal sections). Bolsters, tape, and pillows are used to make the patient comfortable and immobile. The motion is selected (hypocycloidal or spiral) for 1 mm thick tomographic images. Levels also are selected using scout projections, after which images are obtained at 3 mm intervals for most spinal examinations.

## FACET JOINT DISEASES

Because routine radiographs and myelography have only a minor role in diagnosing facet joint disease, the use of

CT and MR imaging in the diagnosis of facet joint degeneration is emphasized in this section. Articular cartilage destruction, subarticular bone erosion, and even hyperostosis are identified most effectively by CT. MR imaging allows visualization of the articular cartilage (Fig. 12–17) and demonstrates encroachment of the superior articular process on the neural foramen (the superior articular facet syndrome) (Fig. 12–18). Hydrarthrosis, which produces a characteristic high intensity signal on the long TR, long TE images, and compression of the dural sac and neural foramina by hypertrophic changes are among other degenerative changes that can be demonstrated by MR imaging.

## Degeneration

Lumbar facet joint degeneration, especially in the later stages, is a significant cause of local or radiating pain.[26–32] Five stages of degeneration of facet joints have been described on the basis of pathologic examinations of the spine: synovitis, joint capsule laxity, articular cartilage destruction, subarticular erosions, and hyperostosis. This pathologic classification is useful radiologically, although not every stage can be detected or categorized conveniently by means of CT or MR imaging.

**Synovitis and Capsular Laxity.** No imaging criteria have been described for detecting the first and second stages of degeneration. The first stage, synovitis, is characterized by hyperemia and inflammatory cell infiltration within the synovium and the capsule of the facet joint. Neither CT nor MR imaging has sufficient resolution to detect inflammation confined to the narrow capsule. MR imaging may be used to detect a hydrarthrosis, however, which in T2-weighted images appears as a high intensity signal within this joint space. The clinical significance of the hydrarthrosis or its relationship to synovitis is uncertain.

The second stage of degeneration is characterized by

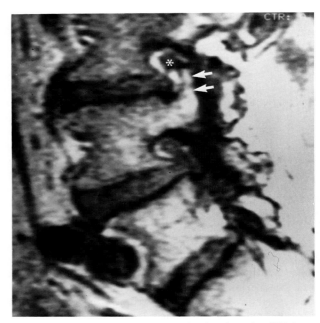

**FIGURE 12–18.** Parasagittal T1-weighted spin echo MR image through the lumbar neural foramina demonstrating the superior articular facet syndrome. The L4 superior process (arrows) encroaches on the neural foramen, with obliteration of most of the fat and compression of the spinal nerve (asterisk). At the L4-L5 level, the neural foramen is narrowed owing to disc degeneration.

laxity of the capsule. The vacuum phenomenon (Fig. 12–19), which is a frequent CT finding in patients with sciatica, may be the result of this abnormal laxity[32] and is presumed to be related to accumulation of dissolved nitrogen derived from the blood stream. In most cases, other evidence of degeneration is found in association with nitrogen within the facet joint.

**Articular Cartilage Destruction.** The third stage of degeneration is characterized by thinning of the articular cartilage that lines the superior and inferior articular processes.[32] In normal lumbar facet joints, the superior and inferior articular cortical surfaces are separated by a distance of 2 to 4 mm, which represents the thickness of the two cartilaginous layers. A narrowed distance between the superior and inferior articular processes in a CT scan signifies erosion of the cartilage (Fig. 12–20). Because the lumbar facet joints normally are oriented in a nearly vertical plane, partial volume averaging is a minimal factor, especially when thin slices are used.

Facet joints with articular cartilage thinning (or subarticular bone erosions) frequently are associated with sciatic or low back pain.[32] The stimulation of naked nerve endings within the facet joints may be experienced by the patient as pain in the distribution of the sciatic nerve, simulating sciatica or a herniated intervertebral disc clinically. Injection of facet joints with an anesthetic agent and steroid preparation is a way of evaluating the association of the facet joints and pain,[27, 28] as the relief of the patient's pain by such an injection suggests that the joint is indeed the source of pain. Routine radiographic or MR images are poor alternatives to CT scans for demonstrating facet joint degeneration. If they are obtained with fluoroscopic monitoring to ensure that the central beam is aligned with the plane of the joint, radiographs may demonstrate articular cartilage destruction, but

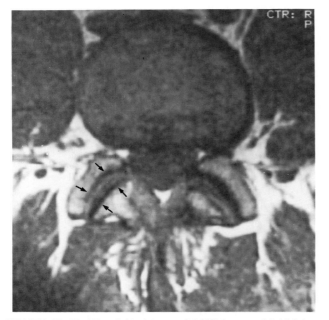

**FIGURE 12–17.** T1-weighted transaxial MR image of L4-L5 facet joints. Cartilage is visualized between the articular cortices of the superior and inferior articular processes (arrows).

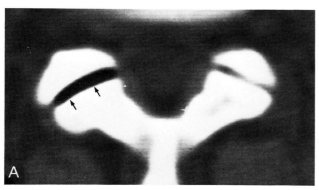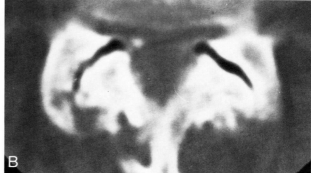

**FIGURE 12–19.** Two examples of gas accumulation (vacuum phenomenon) in the lumbar facet joints. In **A**, the facet joints appear relatively normal except for the gas (arrows) present in the right facet joint. In **B**, severely degenerated facet joints are accompanied by vacuum phenomena.

without the accuracy or simplicity of CT. MR imaging may show the articular cartilage but, as yet, not with sufficient detail to document early facet arthropathy. SPECT imaging often is capable of diagnosing facet arthropathy, but it usually is not included in the diagnostic evaluation.

**Subarticular Bone Erosion.** The fourth stage of degeneration, subarticular bone erosion, is characterized by changes in the cortical bone adjacent to the facet joint. As the articular cartilage is eroded, the cortical bone is exposed to the synovial fluid, which may cause osseous resorption, either in the articular processes or in the adjacent laminae. The CT manifestations of these erosions are irregularities of the articular cortical surfaces or cysts within the adjacent bone (Fig. 12–21). In some cases gas within the joint space fills these erosions, suggesting that there is free communication between them and the articular cavity. The CT demonstration of a gas collection between the ligamentum flavum and the lamina suggests the presence of a synovial cyst that has dissected behind the ligamentum flavum. Bone sclerosis frequently accompanies subarticular erosions and, in some cases, obliterates the medullary cavity of the articular processes and even the laminae.

**Hyperostosis.** The final stage of degeneration is hyperostosis, which refers both to the transformation of spongy medullary bone into dense bone and to the formation of osteophytes, findings that are well demonstrated with CT (Fig. 12–22). Osteophytes that develop from the medial surface of the articular processes may narrow the spinal canal or the neural foramina and produce sciatic pain by compressing a spinal nerve. Facet joint injections are nei-

ther highly effective nor easily achieved in this stage of articular degeneration.

Hyperostosis may be detected on routine anteroposterior, oblique, or lateral radiographs, although the relationship of the osteophytes to the spinal nerves and dural sac is better delineated with CT and parasagittal MR images (see Fig. 12–18).

Degenerative calcifications in the capsule of the facet joints and the adjacent ligamentum flavum (Fig. 12–23) are findings that resemble hyperostosis; their pathogenesis and clinical significance are uncertain.[32]

Facet joint disease can be detected myelographically. When the facet joints are sufficiently hypertrophic, the myelogram reveals that the dural sac is deformed, espe-

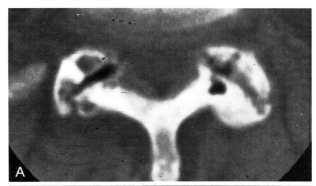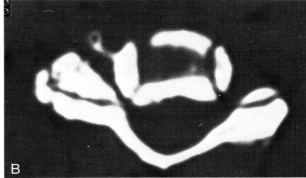

**FIGURE 12–21.** Examples of subarticular bone erosions demonstrated by CT in the lumbar facet joints **(A)** and cervical facet joints **(B)**. In **A**, severe subarticular bone erosions are present, some of which have filled with gas that developed as a result of the vacuum phenomenon in the adjacent joints.

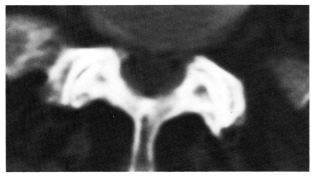

**FIGURE 12–20.** An example of articular cartilage destruction in both apophyseal joints related to osteoarthritis.

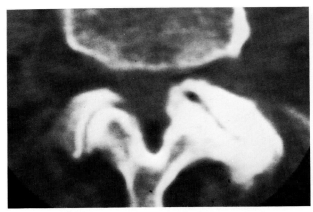

**FIGURE 12–22.** An example of a hyperostotic lumbar facet joint. The superior and inferior articular facets on the left side have hypertrophied and caused narrowing of the neural foramen.

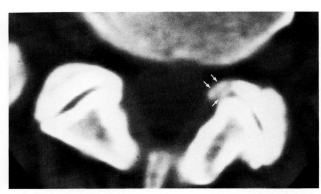

**FIGURE 12–23.** Calcifications (arrows) in the capsule and synovium of the facet joint and contiguous ligamentum flavum are observed. (From Carrera GF, et al: Radiology *134*:145, 1981.)

cially along its posterolateral aspect, a finding that is best visualized in the oblique films. This type of deformity usually can be distinguished accurately from that of disc degeneration by its location. A large impression on the posterolateral border of the dural sac at L4-L5 suggests a synovial cyst (Fig. 12–24).

MR imaging may reveal degenerative changes in the facet joints, with destruction of cartilage and sclerosis in the adjacent subcortical bone. The higher signal intensity associated with cartilage in the facet joint is replaced by low signal intensity. In cases of hydrarthrosis of the facet joints, a region with the signal intensity of fluid is present in the joint.

**Synovial Cysts.** Synovial cysts are uncommon lesions that develop in degenerated facet joints, most frequently at the L4-L5 spinal level, by herniation of synovium and synovial fluid through the joint capsule or by differentiation of synovial cells derived from the degenerating cartilage or the joint capsule, or both.[33] Pathologically, these cysts consist of fibrous tissue with synovium-lined spaces. Their clinical manifestations usually are related to the associated facet joint degeneration: low back or sciatic pain, usually

without positive mechanical signs or electromyographic evidence of root compression.

The CT findings of a synovial cyst usually are sufficiently characteristic that a precise diagnosis can be made (Fig. 12–25). Those synovial cysts that are medial to the ligamentum flavum at the L4-L5 spinal level appear as nearly round structures that displace epidural fat and may indent the dural sac. The capsule of the cyst usually is noticeably denser than the fluid contents (Fig. 12–25). In 75 per cent of synovial cysts, capsular calcification is present. In some cases the fluid in the cyst is replaced with gas, which probably enters the cyst after collecting in the degenerated joint (Fig. 12–26). In serial CT studies the cyst may appear to be filled alternately with gas and with fluid, and it may enlarge or collapse spontaneously. Those synovial cysts that lie between the ligamentum flavum and the lamina or lateral to the facet joint may be more difficult to recognize except when they are filled with gas. In any of these locations, synovial cysts almost invariably are associated with articular cartilage destruction and subarticular bone erosion in the adjacent apophyseal joint.

Synovial cysts may be difficult to demonstrate with MR

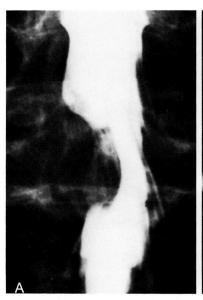
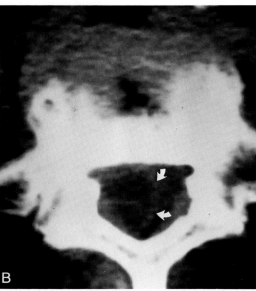

**FIGURE 12–24.** Synovial cyst. The myelogram **(A)** demonstrates a synovial cyst of the right L5-S1 facet joint producing an extradural defect. CT **(B)** shows that the capsule of the cyst (arrows) is denser than epidural fat or CSF.

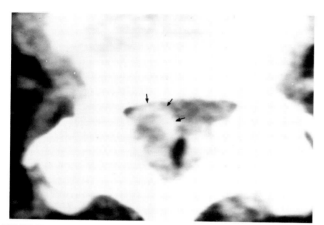

**FIGURE 12–25.** An example of a synovial cyst (arrows) of the right L4-L5 facet joint demonstrated by CT. Note that the capsule of the cyst is calcified.

imaging as the cyst fluid has a signal intensity similar to that of CSF and the thin capsule may be inconspicuous. A rounded capsule of low signal intensity adjacent to a degenerated facet joint indicates the presence of a synovial cyst. Contrast enhanced T1-weighted spin echo MR images are effective for demonstrating the capsule of a synovial cyst, which usually enhances markedly.

### Ankylosing Spondylitis

Although rheumatoid diseases causing facet joint changes are described in detail elsewhere in this book, it is appropriate to discuss ankylosing spondylitis briefly, which characteristically affects the facet joints of the spine earlier and more severely than other synovial joints, and which not uncommonly has neurologic complications.[34, 35] In addition to destruction of the facet joints, ankylosing spondylitis may produce a conus medullaris syndrome, related to a meningeal inflammatory process causing dense adhesive arachnoiditis. As a result, the nerve roots become embedded in the thickened arachnoid, and diverticula developing from the dural sac erode the neural arch and vertebral bodies.

The CT findings in the conus medullaris syndrome of ankylosing spondylitis usually are diagnostic (Fig. 12–27). Transaxial sections in the plane of the intervertebral disc show the absence of cartilage and the disorganized cortical articular surface in the region of the facet joint. Ossification of the anulus fibrosus and osteopenia of the vertebral bodies also are typical. Bone erosions in the laminae, articular processes, or vertebral body in the lumbar spine are seen (Fig. 12–28). With an intrathecal contrast medium, the nature of the osseous erosions is clarified, owing to opacification of the diverticula. On contrast enhanced CT as well as on myelography, the nerve roots are conspicuously absent from within the dural sac because of the adhesive arachnoiditis.

MR effectively shows the diverticula and erosions of the laminae and vertebrae, the squaring of the vertebral bodies, and clumping or adherence of nerve roots to the dural sac.

Another complication of ankylosing spondylitis that warrants CT imaging is fracture.[36] In the bamboo spine of ankylosing spondylitis, fractures often extend through the intervertebral disc space and neural arch, involving the pars interarticularis near the facet joints (Fig. 12–29). In a patient with advanced ankylosing spondylitis, a cleft in the neural arch more likely represents a fracture than a facet joint.

### Trauma

Unstable fractures involving the facet joints or adjacent pars interarticularis, especially in the cervical spine, may be difficult to demonstrate by routine radiographs.[37–44] These unstable injuries include "perched," locked, and distracted facet joints and pars interarticularis fractures.[42, 43] When the cervical facet joints are perched, CT shows the superior and inferior articular processes in different transaxial cuts so that an abnormally slender lateral mass without a joint space is demonstrated (Fig. 12–30). When the cervical facet joints are locked, the superior articular process can be identified posterior to the inferior articular process. The convex surfaces of the semilunar articular processes appose each other in locked facet joints (Fig. 12–31), whereas the flat articular surfaces face in opposite directions. In the presence of distracted facet joints, CT shows an abnormally wide joint space, which usually contains blood (Fig. 12–

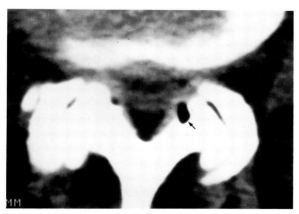

**FIGURE 12–26.** Synovial cyst. A gas-filled synovial cyst (arrow) of the left L4-L5 facet joint. Such cysts may extend between the ligamentum flavum and lamina, frequently producing erosions of the lamina and sometimes filling with gas.

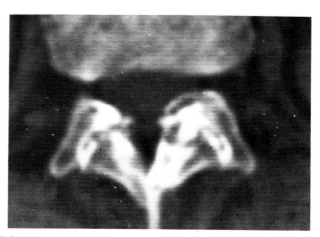

**FIGURE 12–27.** CT appearance of the facet joints in ankylosing spondylitis. The articular cartilage is destroyed.

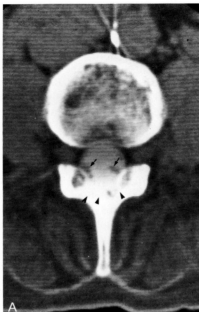

**FIGURE 12–28.** Ankylosing spondylitis. The CT examination **(A)**, which was enhanced with an intrathecal aqueous contrast medium, demonstrates only a few nerve roots (arrows) because the remainder adhere to the dural sac. The lamina is eroded by diverticula of the dural sac (arrowheads). Myelography **(B)** in the same patient shows the diverticula (arrows) arising from the dural sac.

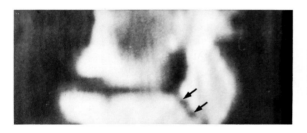

**FIGURE 12–29.** Ankylosing spondylitis with spinal fracture. Reformatted parasagittal CT image through the pars interarticularis shows a fracture associated with ankylosing spondylitis. The fracture line (arrows) has a superficial resemblance to a facet joint.

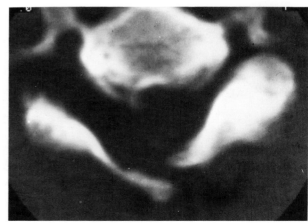

**FIGURE 12–30.** CT in a perched right facet joint. The right lateral mass appears more slender than the left lateral mass because the left inferior articular process sits atop the superior articular process.

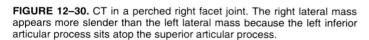

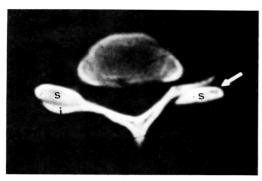

**FIGURE 12–31.** Locked cervical facet joints shown by CT. The superior articular process (s) on the left (arrow) lies behind the inferior articular process (i). (From Yetkin Z, et al: AJNR *6*:633, 1985.)

32). Sagittal MR images effectively show dislocations but not all fractures, and they demonstrate the effect of the dislocation on the spinal cord or subarachnoid space (see Chapter 69).

## INTERVERTEBRAL DISC DISEASES

### Degenerative Disease

The degenerative processes that affect the intervertebral disc include lengthening and weakening of the fibers in the anulus fibrosus and loss of water and protein from the nucleus pulposus. If the anular fibers are sufficiently weakened, they rupture, allowing the nucleus pulposus to herniate. Retention of a herniated nucleus pulposus fragment behind the posterior longitudinal ligament is called a subligamentous herniation. A herniated fragment that has penetrated the posterior longitudinal ligament as well is called a sequestered or free fragment. Partial rupture of the anulus fibrosus with escape of nuclear material into the medial rings of the anulus is called a protruded disc. Ninety per cent of herniated intervertebral discs occur at the L4-L5 or L5-S1 disc level and the majority of the remainder at the L3-L4 spinal level. If the anulus fibrosus ruptures without herniation of the nucleus pulposus, a bulging anulus fibrosus develops. The slack inner layers bulge centripetally, and the outer layers bulge centrifugally, with the result that the intervertebral disc has a larger cross section, the nucleus pulposus has a smaller cross section, and the interspace is diminished in height. A radial tear of the anulus without herniation, also called simple disc rupture, is more common in older persons than a radial tear with herniation of the nucleus pulposus.

**Herniated Disc.** The CT and MR imaging characteristics of a herniated nucleus pulposus in the lumbar spine have been described and verified in numerous studies.[45–57] A subligamentous herniation produces focal, curvilinear extension of the disc margin beyond that of the adjacent vertebral body, with displacement of fat in the epidural space. The restraining effect of the posterior longitudinal ligament causes the borders of the herniated disc to appear smooth (Fig. 12–33). The fragment may appear to displace, compress, or obscure a spinal nerve. The nuclear fragment usually has a density on CT scans similar to that of the intervertebral disc (70 to 110 Hounsfield units [HU]) or a signal intensity in MR images similar to that of cartilage in the intervertebral disc (Fig. 12–34). CT frequently demonstrates calcification or ossification (Figs. 12–35 and 12–36), especially in the margin of the fragment; less commonly, gas is seen within the nuclear fragment (Figs. 12–36 and 12–37).

Disc herniations that are larger than 1 cm in diameter

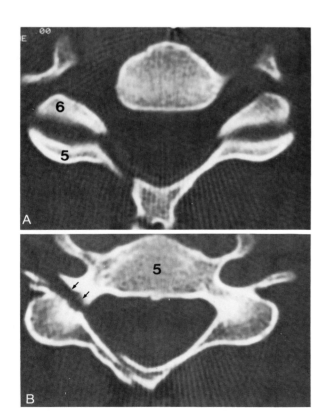

**FIGURE 12–32.** Distracted C5-C6 right facet joint **(A)** associated with a fracture (arrows in **B**) of the pars interarticularis of C5.

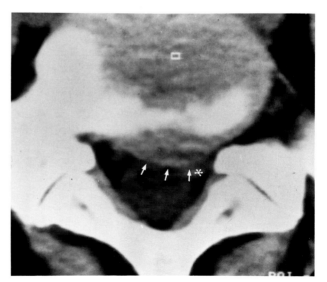

**FIGURE 12–33.** Subligamentous herniated nucleus pulposus. Transaxial CT scan shows a smooth, focal, curvilinear displacement (arrows) of the disc margin at L5-S1. The dural sac and left S1 root sheath (asterisk) are displaced. (From Haughton VM, et al: Radiology *142*:103, 1982.)

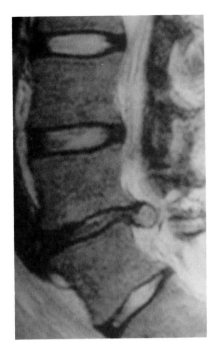

**FIGURE 12–34.** Sagittal T2-weighted (TR/TE, 3214/102) fast spin echo MR image showing a herniated L4-L5 intervertebral disc.

**FIGURE 12–35.** Herniated nuclear fragment (asterisk) with a dense rim of calcification. The S1 root sheath (arrows) and dural sac are displaced.

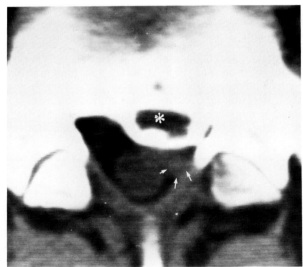

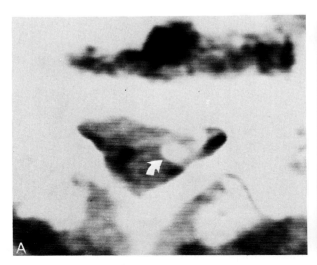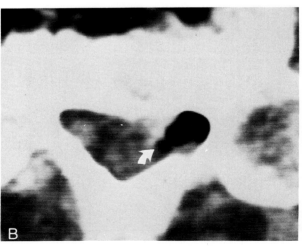

**FIGURE 12–36.** Herniated L5-S1 disc (arrows) containing both calcification **(A)** and gas **(B)**.

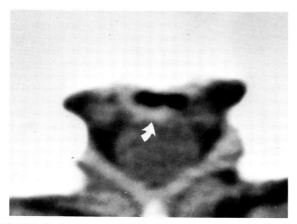

**FIGURE 12–37.** Central L5-S1 herniation (arrow) containing gas.

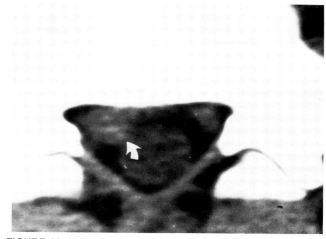

**FIGURE 12–39.** Free fragment of disc (arrow), 10 mm below the L5-S1 intervertebral disc, obscuring the right S1 root sheath. The density of the fragment is greater than that of the dural sac or contralateral root sheath.

usually signify rupture through the posterior longitudinal ligament, producing a free or sequestered fragment that has a different CT or MR imaging appearance than that associated with subligamentous herniations.[46, 49, 51, 58, 59] Fragments that are free but still adjacent to the intervertebral disc have an irregular contour (Fig. 12–38), with a density or signal intensity comparable to that of the intervertebral disc; gas or calcium is unusual in a free fragment. Of diagnostic importance, when the free fragment has migrated away from the intervertebral disc, the disc margin itself may appear entirely normal. The migrated free fragment may appear as a rounded, oblong, or irregular mass (Figs. 12–39 to 12–42). If it is in contact with the dural sac, the fragment may resemble on CT scans an anomalous or cystic root sheath except for its greater density. On MR images, root sheaths and disc fragments do not resemble each other. With CT, a free disc fragment also may resemble an epidural neoplasm except that the disc fragment usually has a higher density (70 to 110 HU) than a neoplasm (20 to 60 HU), and the latter more typically is accompanied by bone erosion. It has been emphasized repeatedly that free fragments are a contraindication to chymopapain treatment as

the enzyme injected into the nucleus pulposus will not reach the fragment that is outside the posterior longitudinal ligament but will leak into the epidural space.

CT and MR imaging have had a great impact in the detection of extreme lateral disc herniations, which occupy a position lateral to the neural foramen[45, 47] and are difficult to delineate with myelography. These nuclear fragments displace fat in and adjacent to the neural foramen and obscure the exiting spinal nerve (Fig. 12–43). Representing up to 16 per cent of all herniated discs, the far lateral herniations distort the spinal nerve lateral to the root sheath. Differentiation of an extreme lateral herniation from the less common neurofibroma may be difficult, although bone erosion associated with a foraminal mass is more suggestive of a neoplasm.

The detection of cervical[60–62] and thoracic[63] disc herniations requires careful CT or MR imaging analysis. In the cervical spine, those levels at which disc degeneration is

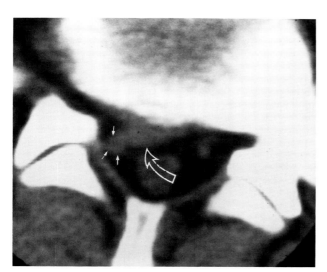

**FIGURE 12–38.** Sequestered disc fragment. A portion of the herniated nucleus pulposus (curved arrow) lies outside the anulus fibrosus, where it compresses the right S1 nerve root (small arrows).

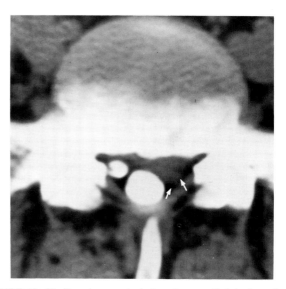

**FIGURE 12–40.** Free fragment of disc shown with intrathecally enhanced CT. The left root sheath of S1 fails to opacify because a disc fragment (arrows) compresses it.

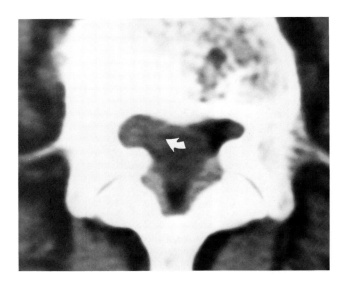

**FIGURE 12–41.** Free disc fragment in the right L5 lateral recess. The fragment (arrow) is denser than the dural sac, and it displaces the fat from the lateral recess.

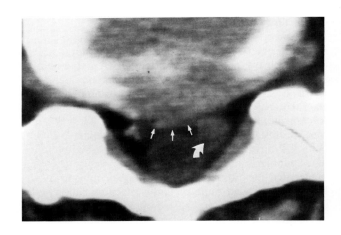

**FIGURE 12–42.** A combination of subligamentous (small arrows) and free (large arrow) disc fragments. The free fragment, compressing the left S1 root sheath, was the cause of the patient's symptoms.

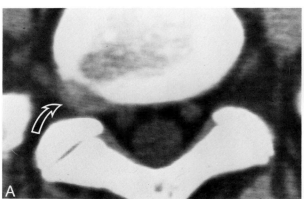

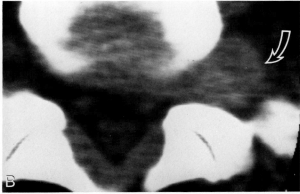

**FIGURE 12–43.** Extreme lateral disc herniations. In **A**, a herniation (arrow) displaces the fat and right fifth nerve root sheath in the right L5-S1 neural foramen. In **B**, a large far lateral fragment (arrow) resembles a benign tumor. (From Williams AL, et al: AJR *39*:345, 1982. Copyright 1982, American Roentgen Ray Society.)

most frequent, C5-C6 and C6-C7, frequently are obscured by artifacts created by the shoulders in the field of view. The narrow dimension of the cervical intervertebral discs and the paucity of adjacent epidural fat increase the need for thinner slices and high contrast resolution. Furthermore, in contrast to lumbar nerve roots, cervical roots occupy the inferior (caudal) portion of the neural foramen; therefore, cervical disc herniations producing radicular symptoms occupy the foramen at or below the level of the uncovertebral joint. Lateral disc herniations are not common in the cervical region because of the presence of the uncinate processes. Calcification in herniated cervical discs is common, but gas is not.

The CT or MR imaging criteria allowing diagnosis of a cervical disc herniation are similar to those used in the detection of a herniation in the lumbar spine.[64] A focal abnormality of the disc margin encroaching on the neural foramen or spinal canal (Fig. 12–44) is seen. In symptomatic cases, either the cervical nerve root sheath is compressed or the spinal cord is deformed, and detection of the latter abnormality with CT can be aided by the use of intrathecal contrast material (Fig. 12–45).

Myelography demonstrates intervertebral disc disease by means of indirect signs, particularly a characteristic change in the contour of the opacified dural sac or root sheath. Those disc herniations that fail to alter the adjacent dural sac or the nerve root sheath will escape myelographic detection; extreme lateral discal herniations and some at the L5-S1 spinal level are representative of this group. The identification of a disc herniation with myelography requires a careful examination using multiple projections. In the lateral myelographic projection, an angular indentation of the dural sac or a "double density" is a sign of a herniated disc (Fig. 12–46). In an anteroposterior projection, the dural sac may be asymmetric. Oblique views usually show the herniated disc deforming the anterolateral surface of the dural sac (Fig. 12–46), in contrast to the impression caused by an abnormal facet joint, which affects the posterolateral margin of the dural sac. The most reliable myelographic indication of a herniated disc is shortening and "trumpeting" of a nerve root sheath, in which the

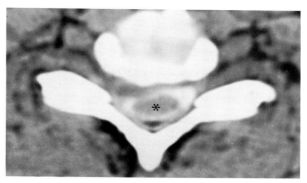

**FIGURE 12–45.** Herniated C6-C7 disc using CT with intrathecal enhancement. The spinal cord (asterisk) and subarachnoid space are deformed by the herniation.

nerve root itself appears widened because it is either edematous or compressed and elevated (Fig. 12–46). This relatively specific sign of disc herniation should be distinguished from root sheath amputation without widening of the nerve, a combination of findings that may reflect arachnoid fibrosis.

Disc herniations can be detected effectively by MR imaging[65–69] using criteria that are similar to those employed for CT. A focally abnormal disc margin that displaces a spinal nerve and fat in the spinal canal or neural foramen is typical (Figs. 12–47 and 12–48). T1-weighted spin echo MR images may be used in the transaxial or sagittal plane to identify this abnormal disc margin. T2-weighted spin echo images also are useful, despite a poorer signal-to-noise ratio, because compression of the dural sac is demonstrated easily in this sequence, in which CSF has a substantially higher signal intensity than bone. MR imaging also may show changes within the herniated intervertebral disc. In many cases of herniated disc, MR imaging reveals a radial tear of the anulus as a thin tongue of higher signal intensity in this region of the disc that normally is of low signal intensity. It may show diminished signal intensity in the degenerating disc from which the herniated fragment originated. Furthermore, MR imaging may show enhancement of the margin of the herniated disc when paramagnetic contrast medium is given intravenously, either because granulation tissue is located adjacent to the fragment or because contrast medium has diffused from the epidural plexus into the disc.

Thoracic disc herniations manifested by myelopathy are studied more effectively by MR or myelography, both of which provide a faster way of screening the entire thoracic subarachnoid space, than by CT. Myelography, which has been supplanted by MR imaging because of its noninvasiveness, is very sensitive in detecting herniated thoracic discs that indent the anterior subarachnoid space. Usually the thoracic disc herniations that are symptomatic can be shown myelographically to displace the spinal cord posteriorly and sometimes even indent it (Fig. 12–49). Gas and water-soluble contrast media are well suited to thoracic myelography. The MR imaging characteristics of thoracic disc herniations include an abnormal signal intensity from the discs, most evident on the T2-weighted images, and a disc margin that protrudes into the spinal canal and displaces or at least touches the spinal cord (Fig. 12–50). Both

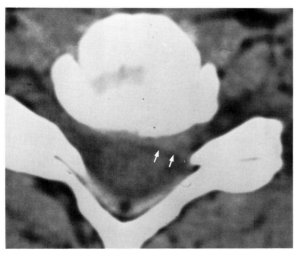

**FIGURE 12–44.** Herniated left C5-C6 cervical disc (arrows) demonstrated by CT without contrast medium.

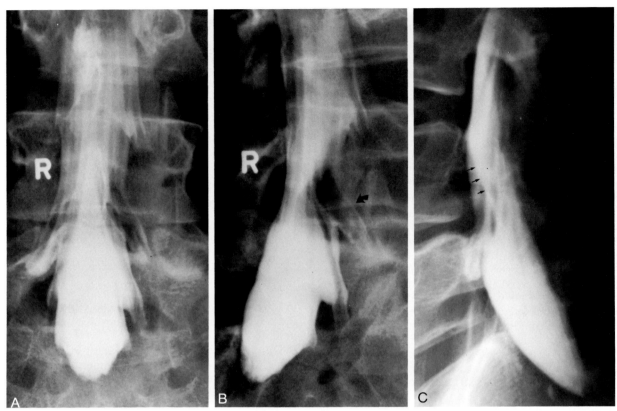

**FIGURE 12–46.** Lumbar myelogram with aqueous contrast medium demonstrating an L4-L5 herniated disc. The anteroposterior radiograph **(A)** shows slight asymmetry of the dural sac. The dural sac deformity is more pronounced in the oblique film **(B)**, which also shows the widening or "trumpeting" of the left L5 nerve root sheath (arrow). The lateral film **(C)** shows the double density (arrows) caused by the herniated disc fragment displacing the dural sac asymmetrically.

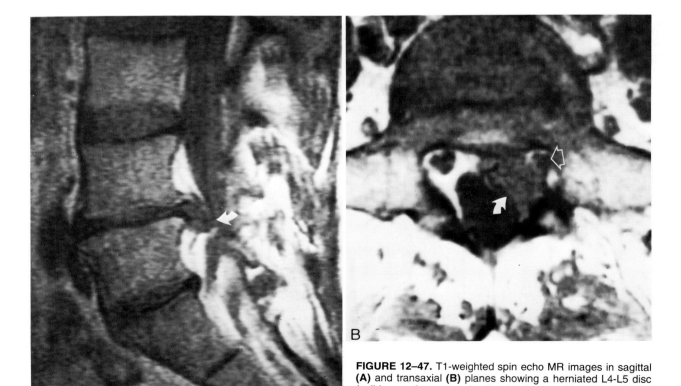

**FIGURE 12–47.** T1-weighted spin echo MR images in sagittal **(A)** and transaxial **(B)** planes showing a herniated L4-L5 disc (solid arrows) compressing the dural sac and left L5 root (open arrow).

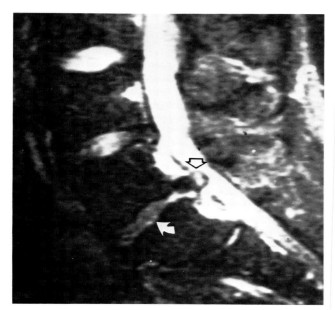

**FIGURE 12–48.** Herniated L5-S1 disc (open arrow), demonstrated by a T2-weighted spin echo MR image. The diminished signal intensity from the L5-S1 disc (solid arrow) is a nonspecific finding.

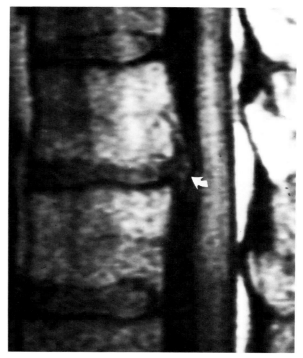

**FIGURE 12–50.** T1-weighted spin echo MR image demonstrating a herniated thoracic disc (arrow).

signs are detected easily in long TR, long TE image sequences, in which CSF has an intense signal.

**Bulging Anulus Fibrosus.** With CT, the hallmark of the bulging anulus fibrosus is a disc margin that extends in all directions beyond the adjacent vertebral endplates (Fig. 12–51).[44] The disc extension generally is symmetric, except when scoliosis is present, in which case the disc prominence usually is greater on the concave side of the spinal curvature. The normally straight or concave posterior border of the intervertebral disc either is maintained or becomes convex. Calcification in the periphery of the disc due

to degenerative changes in Sharpey's fibers and a vacuum phenomenon in the nucleus pulposus (and, rarely, in the anulus fibrosus) are additional CT characteristics. The displaced posterior margin of the intervertebral disc leads to narrowing of the spinal canal and the neural foramina; the epidural fat may be diminished and the dural sac displaced posteriorly by the bulging disc.

The myelographic appearance of the dural sac in the presence of a bulging anulus fibrosus also is characteristic.[70] In the lateral projection, a curvilinear, thumbprint-like impression on the opacified ventral dural sac, often at multiple levels, is evident (Fig. 12–52). This deformity lacks

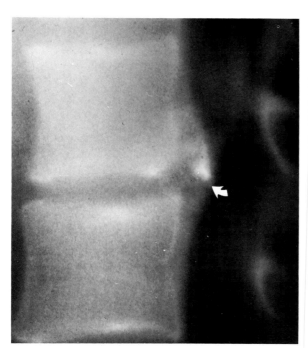

**FIGURE 12–49.** Gas myelogram with tomography demonstrating a herniated thoracic disc (arrow).

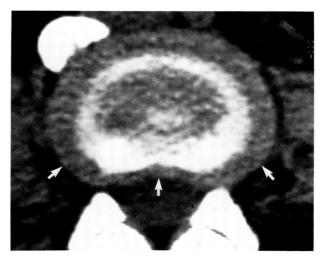

**FIGURE 12–51.** Bulging intervertebral disc. The anulus fibrosus (arrows) extends beyond the adjacent vertebral endplate in all directions, although the normal concavity of the posterior disc margin is preserved.

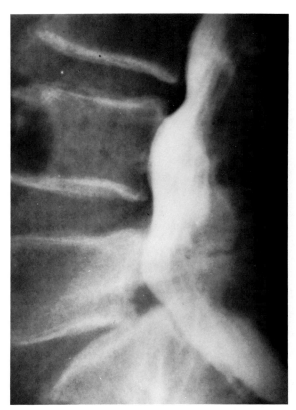

**FIGURE 12–52.** Characteristic myelographic findings in bulging intervertebral discs. The dural sac is indented on its anterior surface by the anulus fibrosus at multiple levels. In addition, the sac is indented posteriorly at L3-L4 and L5-S1 by degenerated facet joints.

the angularity and tenting or the double density appearance that accompanies a herniated disc. Anteroposterior projections reveal symmetric deformity of the lateral margin of the dural sac secondary to the elevation produced by the disc margin. Only rarely do bulging discs displace, compress, or amputate the root sheaths.

Diminished signal intensity on T2-weighted spin echo MR images has been reported as a nonspecific sign of disc degeneration that may accompany a bulging (or herniated) intervertebral disc.[66] In some cases, MR imaging also shows a radial tear of the anulus fibrosus in cases of a bulging anulus (Fig. 12–53), although discography shows these tears more effectively. When paramagnetic contrast medium is given intravenously, enhancement of signal intensity may be noted in the radial tear, presumably related to the ingrowth of granulation tissue.

**Spinal Stenosis.** Narrowing of the spinal canal may be a complication of a variety of degenerative processes of the spine (see Chapter 40). Osteophytes about the apophyseal joints and thickening or hypertrophy of the ligamenta flava are examples of degenerative changes that lead to spinal stenosis.[71, 72] Normally 2 to 3 mm thick, the ligamentum flavum exceeds 5 mm in thickness in pathologic cases, leading to displacement of epidural fat in the spinal canal and compression of the dural sac. CT and MR imaging effectively demonstrate such ligamentous hypertrophy, and in some cases calcification also may be detected in the ligamentum flavum or in the posterior longitudinal ligament.[73–76]

CT, MR imaging, or myelography may be used alone or in combination to evaluate patients with suspected spinal stenosis,[77] allowing assessment of the site and extent of stenosis and identification of any degenerative changes in the facet joints, discs, and ligamentum flavum, as well as developmental abnormalities, such as short pedicles or thick laminae.[78, 79] In symptomatic spinal stenosis, the spinal canal (central stenosis) or foramen (lateral stenosis) is narrowed to such a degree that the spinal cord, root sheath, or dural sac is compressed (Fig. 12–54). A canal less than 1.5 sq cm in area or a lateral recess less than 3 mm deep has been considered a sign of stenosis.[80, 81] Obliteration of the epidural fat usually is a reliable sign of spinal stenosis on CT scans or MR images, except in those rare cases (for example, Cushing's disease) in which the fat itself acts as a mass that compresses the dural sac. The myelographic diagnosis of spinal stenosis is based on compression of the dural sac or a root sheath.

### Inflammatory Disease

The term discitis is used to describe inflammation of the intervertebral disc.[80–86] An infectious cause is suggested but proved in only a fraction of cases. With CT, the characteristic finding of discitis is multiple erosions of similar size, occurring in the osseous endplates on either side of the affected intervertebral disc space at an early stage of the disease (Fig. 12–55). Almost invariably, a soft tissue mass also is seen, extending from the disc into the spinal canal and centrifugally into the perispinal tissues. Fragments of disc material may be demonstrated in the spinal canal and neural foramina. In later stages, collapse of the disc space and bone sclerosis are evident.

MR imaging is a sensitive and specific technique in the diagnosis of discitis.[66, 87] Abnormalities are detected on MR

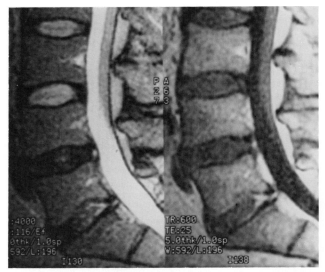

**FIGURE 12–53.** MR images (sagittal plane) demonstrating bulging of the L5-S1 and L4-L5 discs. The T2-weighted (TR/TE, 4000/116) spin echo image (left) shows diminished signal intensity in the lower lumbar discs. In the posterior anulus of L5-S1, the tongue of higher signal intensity tissue represents the radial tear. On the contrast enhanced T1-weighted (TR/TE, 600/25) spin echo image (right), the tear in the anulus enhances because of the granulation tissue present in it.

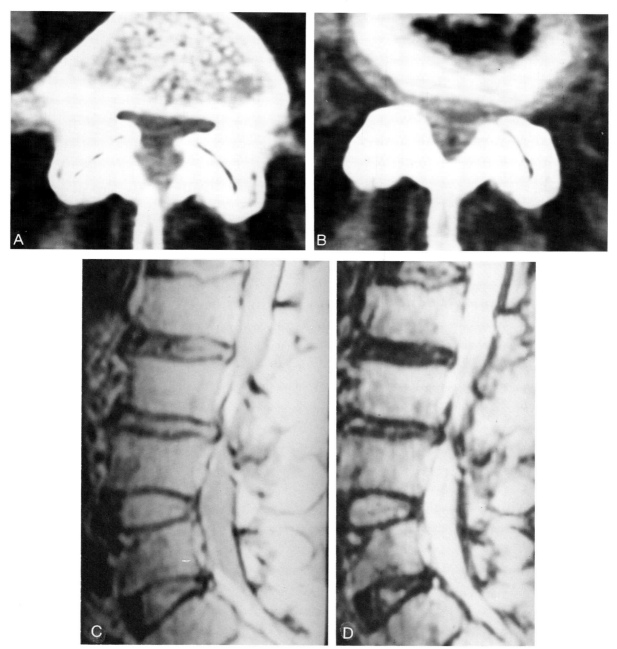

**FIGURE 12–54.** Examples of spinal stenosis.
   **A, B** CT scanning. In **A**, the central canal and lateral recesses are narrowed by facet joint degeneration. In **B**, a thick ligamentum flavum and bulging anulus fibrosus compress the dural sac.
   **C, D** In MR images with proton density-weighting **(C)** and T2-weighting **(D)**, the severely stenotic spinal canal at L3-L4 is shown. A mildly bulging disc together with the thickened ligamentum flavum nearly obliterates the spinal canal.

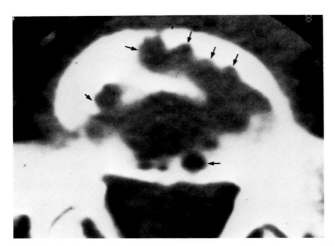

**FIGURE 12–55.** Multiple focal erosions (arrows) of the L5 vertebral endplate are characteristic of discitis. Some of the erosions are confluent.

images (Fig. 12–56) earlier than on plain radiographs or scintigraphs. MR imaging demonstrates the compression of the dural sac and the epidural inflammatory mass or abscess that occur.[88] Tuberculous infections may destroy the intervertebral disc less rapidly than purulent infections while affecting multiple adjacent vertebrae. A paravertebral abscess cavity characteristically occurs.[89]

A second condition, which may be inflammatory, relates to calcification of the intervertebral disc, particularly in the cervical spine of children.[83, 84] Although not uniformly symptomatic, this self-limited disorder has been associated with pain, fever, and decreased motion of the neck. Herniation of the calcified fragment leading to a myelopathy has been documented in some patients.

## Miscellaneous Disc Abnormalities

**Cartilaginous (Schmorl's) Node.** Displacement of a portion of the nucleus pulposus through the cartilaginous and osseous vertebral endplates into the vertebral spongiosa is a common finding of questionable clinical significance in older patients. The CT appearance, which usually is diagnostic, includes a defect in the spongy bone, often surrounded by a sclerotic rim of variable thickness (Fig. 12–57). The appearance of a cartilaginous node on MR images also is diagnostic. When gadolinium compounds are injected intravenously, enhancement of signal intensity about Schmorl's node may be seen.

**Limbus Vertebra.** A characteristic defect in the vertebral body is produced by herniation of a portion of the nucleus pulposus beneath the ring apophysis before its fusion with the vertebral body. The limbus vertebra is thought to result from trauma occurring at a time when the junction of the ring apophysis and vertebral body is weaker than the anulus fibrosus. CT scans and MR images show the distorted interface between the intervertebral disc and the adjacent vertebral body (Fig. 12–58).

**Ruptured Ring Apophysis.** Trauma with axial compressive loading of the spine, especially in young male patients, produces a characteristic type of fracture, in which a wedge-shaped fragment of the endplate is dislodged and displaced posteriorly (see Chapter 69). In routine radiographs, the thin linear silhouette of the displaced ring apophysis may be detected within the spinal canal. With CT the fracture line in the osseous endplate is displayed more effectively, and the ring apophysis within the spinal canal also is shown (Fig. 12–59). MR also shows the distorted intervertebral disc in these cases. The displaced fragment of the ring apophysis usually appears as a region of low signal intensity in the spinal canal.

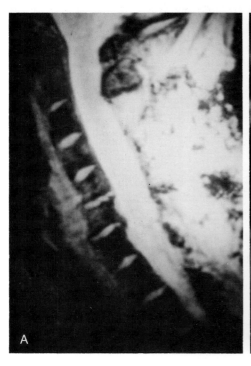
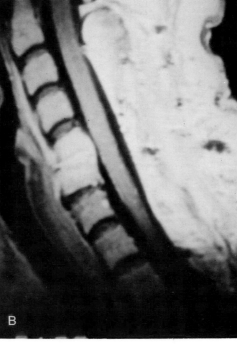

**FIGURE 12–56.** Discitis. MR images demonstrating typical findings in discitis. The T2-weighted image **(A)** demonstrates increased signal intensity in the C5 and C6 vertebral bodies and intervening disc space. The T1-weighted image obtained after the intravenous administration of contrast medium **(B)** demonstrates marked enhancement in the C5 and C6 vertebrae, intervening disc, and soft tissues ventral to the infected disc.

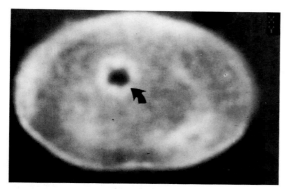

**FIGURE 12–57.** Cartilaginous (Schmorl's) node (arrow) producing a lucent defect in the vertebral endplate surrounded by sclerosis. (Reproduced by permission from Haughton VM, Williams AL: Computed Tomography of the Spine. St. Louis, 1982, The CV Mosby Co.)

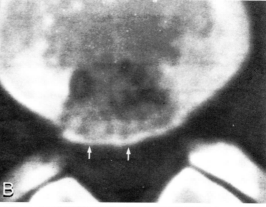

**FIGURE 12–58.** Limbus vertebra demonstrated by CT as a defect in the vertebral endplate (arrow) and ring apophysis.

## UNCOVERTEBRAL JOINT DISEASES

A unique anatomic feature of the cervical spine is the uncovertebral joint, the space between one cervical vertebral body and the uncinate processes that project superiorly from the next lower cervical vertebral body. These processes lie lateral to the intervertebral disc in the upper cervical spine and posterolateral to the discs in the lower cervical spine. A small cleft may appear in the disc material in the uncovertebral joint. Degeneration of the uncovertebral joint, producing radiculopathy, is common in patients with cervical spondylosis; subluxation of the joint is a common finding in unstable cervical spine fractures.

### Degeneration

With degeneration of the intervertebral disc and loss of disc space height, the uncinate process assumes an abnormal relationship with the adjacent vertebral body. The clefts that develop in the nucleus pulposus as a result of disc degeneration extend into the uncovertebral portion of the disc. The remodeling that results from the abnormal anatomic relationship leads to hyperostosis of the uncinate process and adjacent vertebral body. These changes can be detected radiographically (see Chapter 40) or with more

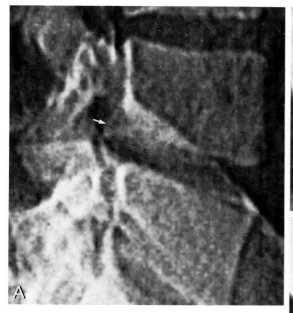

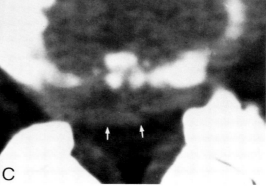

**FIGURE 12–59.** Traumatic avulsion of the L4-L5 ring apophysis and rupture of the intervertebral disc. The localizer view **(A)** shows the ring apophysis (arrow) displaced into the spinal canal. Transaxial CT scans show the fragment of vertebral endplate and ring apophysis (arrows in **B**) and the disc margin (arrows in **C**) displaced posteriorly.

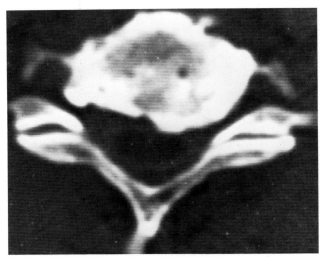

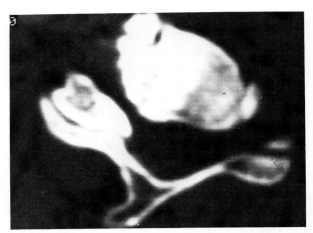

**FIGURE 12–61.** Hyperostosis about the right uncovertebral joint of C5-C6.

**FIGURE 12–60.** Hypertrophic changes in the left uncinate process of C6 due to uncovertebral joint degeneration. The left neural foramen is narrowed.

accuracy by CT. The latter method reveals both the hypertrophic and the destructive changes that accompany degeneration in the uncovertebral joints (Figs. 12–60 and 12–61). Erosions may be demonstrated in the cortical bone of the uncinate process or adjacent vertebral body, and sclerosis may be seen in the adjacent spongy bone. As the uncinate process hypertrophies, the neural foramen (especially the caudal portion, which the spinal nerve roots occupy) is narrowed, and compression of the spinal nerves may occur.

Transaxial MR images may show uncovertebral joint changes that encroach on the neural foramen. Myelography is not as sensitive or specific for demonstrating uncovertebral joint changes.

### Trauma

Although isolated fractures of the uncovertebral joints are rare, the rotation or slippage of one vertebral body on another that may accompany unstable fractures commonly causes a diastasis of the uncovertebral joints.[42, 43] In fact, after trauma, asymmetry of the normally symmetric uncovertebral joints should prompt a thorough inspection of the spine to exclude a subtle, unstable fracture (Fig. 12–62).

## OSSEOUS ABNORMALITIES

### Neoplasms

CT, angiography, pluridirectional tomography, and MR imaging may be used to visualize the primary bone tumors that involve the spine. In most cases these tumors are detected efficiently by routine radiographic screening, although additional imaging methods may be useful in characterizing some of these tumors.[90–94] For example, CT effectively demonstrates the radiolucent nidus within a sclerotic lesion resulting from an osteoid osteoma, the mixed osteolytic and osteosclerotic pattern of an osteoblastoma, expansion of bone in an aneurysmal bone cyst or giant cell tumor, the permeative pattern of bone destruction of an osteosarcoma, or the osteolysis of plasma cell myeloma (Fig. 12–63). Angiography in aneurysmal bone cysts may be useful in demonstrating the typical exuberant neovascularity and in selecting patients for embolization.

Most primary bone tumors in the spine appear as regions of low signal intensity on T1-weighted spin echo MR images and of high signal intensity on T2-weighted spin echo MR images. Hemorrhagic tumors, however, will have a different and often diagnostic appearance, and vertebral hemangiomos usually are associated with high signal intensity on T1-weighted spin echo MR images. The intravenous

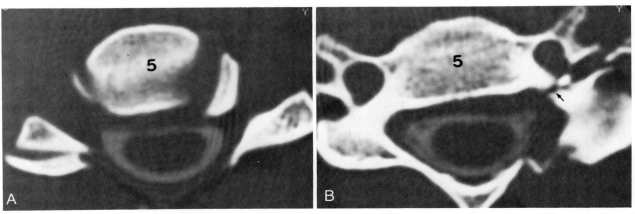

**FIGURE 12–62.** Distraction of the left C5-C6 uncovertebral joint due to a C5 pars interarticularis fracture. In **A**, note the asymmetry of the uncovertebral joints. The fracture (arrow in **B**) is demonstrated in an adjacent transaxial scan.

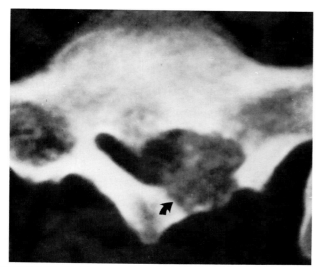

**FIGURE 12–63.** Plasma cell myeloma (arrow) destroying the neural arch of S1.

administration of a gadolinium contrast agent, when combined with fat suppression techniques, is effective in demonstrating intraosseous tumors of the spine. When fat suppression techniques are not employed, however, the enhancement of signal intensity within the tumor resulting from the administration of a gadolinium chelate may lead to diagnostic difficulty as the tumor becomes isointense with the adjacent marrow.

MR imaging is sensitive for detecting metastatic involvement of the vertebral column, in which the characteristic signal intensity from the bone marrow is replaced by the usually lower intensity signal of the tumor. Because of the weak MR signal arising from cortical bone, osteoclastic or osteoblastic changes are not demonstrated effectively by MR imaging. Invasion of the epidural space, however, can be delineated by displacement of epidural fat.

### Trauma

Routine radiographs, which are available readily, inexpensive, and efficient for screening large segments of the spinal column, are the primary diagnostic studies in most cases of spinal trauma.[44] They are insensitive, however, for detecting certain types of fracture. Because of overlying bony silhouettes, undisplaced neural arch fractures are difficult to detect with conventional radiographs. Vertically oriented fractures that are nearly perpendicular to the central ray and rotatory subluxations—for example, C1 on C2—also are demonstrated ineffectively by routine radiographs. Therefore, conventional tomographic images or CT scans often are used to supplement routine radiographs in patients with spinal trauma. CT is effective in demonstrating vertically oriented fractures. Therefore, it is sensitive for most fractures through the neural arch and articular pillars and for many vertebral body fractures as well. Furthermore, it confirms narrowing of the central spinal canal due to displacement of fracture fragments resulting from, for example, a comminuted ''burst'' fracture of a vertebral body (Fig. 12–64). CT also is capable of demonstrating soft tissue injuries, such as a traumatically herniated interverte-

bral disc, epidural hematoma compressing the spinal cord,[87, 95] or avulsion of cervical nerve roots (Fig. 12–65).

Pluridirectional tomography is useful for demonstrating transversely oriented fractures, especially those not detected by routine radiographs because of overlying structures. For example, an undisplaced fracture of the base of the odontoid process, which may be overlooked on routine radiographs, can be shown definitively with pluridirectional tomography. Conventional tomography also may be useful for demonstrating the alignment of the facet joints or the vertebral bodies when plain radiographs have been inconclusive, as is common at the C7-T1 spinal level. MR imaging, which does not show bone detail and cannot be used with many life support systems, is not an important ancillary diagnostic technique for spinal fractures.

Myelography has few applications in cases of spinal trauma, especially in the acute stage. One conventional indication for myelography is in evaluating the degree of spinal cord or nerve root compression produced by a fracture or dislocation. Another indication is the detection of a syringomyelia resulting from a spinal cord injury.

Provided that the patients do not have implanted ferrous metal devices, MR imaging provides an efficient and more effective alternative to myelography in patients with trauma to the spinal cord (Fig. 12–66). MR imaging is useful for evaluating patients with suspected spinal cord disruption, edema secondary to trauma (central cord syndrome), hydromyelia, epidural hematoma, disruption of the interspinous ligaments, or traumatic herniated disc[96, 97] (Fig. 12–66).

### Neural Arch Defects

It is important to differentiate the several types of neural arch defects from facet joints or acute fractures. Such defects include retrosomatic clefts, pars interarticularis defects (spondylolysis), retroisthmic defects, synchondroses, and spina bifida occulta.[98–104] These defects usually are shown by CT or plain radiographs; some pars interarticularis defects also are demonstrated by MR imaging.

The retrosomatic cleft is a rare defect in the pedicles near their junction with the vertebral body.[98] It is found primarily in women, who often have low grade back pain. The adjacent intervertebral disc space may be narrowed. In CT images the cleft usually has irregular, sclerotic margins (Fig. 12–67). Retrosomatic clefts often are associated with other types of defects, such as a contralateral spondylolysis.

Spondylolytic defects in the pars interarticularis have an uncertain pathogenesis (see Chapter 67). The rarity of the defects in young children suggests they are acquired rather

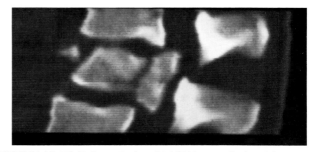

**FIGURE 12–64.** Reformatted sagittal CT image of a burst fracture of the L2 vertebral body.

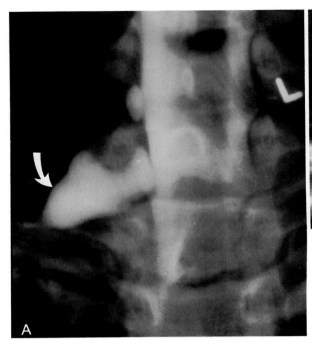
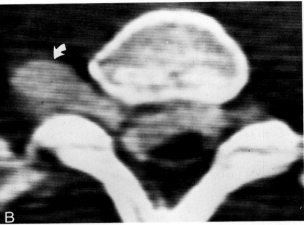

**FIGURE 12–65.** Avulsed cervical nerve root and traumatic meningocele (arrows) demonstrated by myelography (A) and subsequent CT (B).

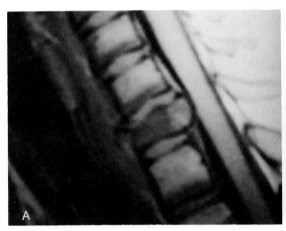
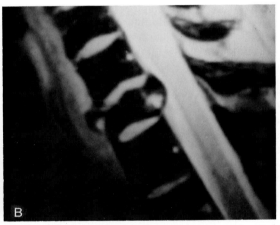

**FIGURE 12–66.** Sagittal T1-weighted (A) and T2-weighted (B) spin echo MR images in a patient with a burst fracture of C7. The relationship of the fragments to the spinal cord can be evaluated. No spinal cord edema is evident in this case.

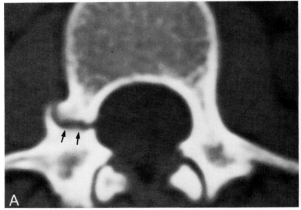
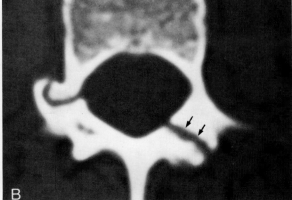

**FIGURE 12–67.** Transaxial CT scans show a retrosomatic cleft (arrows in A) in the pedicle of L2. A slightly lower section from the same patient shows a pars interarticularis defect in the contralateral neural arch (arrows in B). (From Johansen JG, et al: Radiology *148*:447, 1983.)

than congenital and presumably related to acute trauma or, more commonly, chronic stress. Although detection of pars interarticularis defects by plain radiographs is efficient, some cases are not seen because of overlying shadows or an unfavorable angle of the central x-ray beam with respect to the plane of the defect. Therefore, defects are detected in some patients by CT after a negative routine radiographic or myelographic examination.

The CT appearances of spondylolysis are characteristic (Fig. 12–68). The pars interarticularis defects may be so smooth, uniform, and linear that they give the appearance of normal facet joints.[100] An analysis of the contiguous slices will reveal that the facet joints separate neural arches of adjacent vertebrae, whereas the cleft divides one neural arch, usually that of L5. In some cases the defect may be irregular and sclerotic, simulating degenerated facet joints.[100] In other cases the defect may be unilateral, with a sclerotic pars interarticularis on the opposite side. The most common appearance of spondylolysis, however, is an elongated, thin isthmus of the neural arch containing irregular defects, especially in L5 (Fig. 12–68). Spondylolisthesis and elongation of the anteroposterior diameter of the spinal canal are characteristic.

The retroisthmic defect is rare.[99] It has been reported as an incidental finding, usually in women, and often associated with other defects of the neural arch. Unlike the pars defect or retrosomatic cleft, the retroisthmic defect is located posterior to the pars interarticularis. It is thought to be a congenital abnormality containing fibrous tissue that does not ossify. In CT scans it appears as a thin cleft without sclerotic margins posterior to the neural arch (Fig. 12–69).

A synchondrosis may be confused with a neural arch cleft. As the vertebra ossifies from three centers (two in the neural arch and one in the vertebral body), osseous defects (synchondroses) become evident between the centers. Synchondroses are seen in the first decade of life and are located anterior to the sites of retrosomatic clefts. Their borders are sharp, straight, and uniform, with no evidence of bone sclerosis (Fig. 12–70).

The most common and least significant type of neural arch cleft is spina bifida occulta. It is composed of nonossifying fibrous tissue in the midline between the two halves

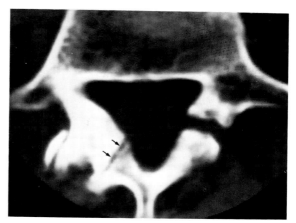

**FIGURE 12–69.** Retroisthmic defect (arrows) in the right L5 neural arch. A pars interarticularis defect is present in the left neural arch. (From Johansen JG, et al: AJNR *5*:835, 1984.)

of the neural arch. Differentiation from fracture usually is easy because of the midline location and corticated margins of spina bifida occulta.

Congenital absence of a pedicle produces a large defect in a neural arch. These defects have been detected in the cervical, thoracic or lumbar region.[101–103]

## SPINAL CORD AND MENINGEAL DISEASES

### Mass Lesions

To evaluate processes affecting the spinal cord and meninges, MR imaging has become the primary tool. In MR images, processes intrinsic and extrinsic to the cord that produce spinal cord signs are shown effectively noninvasively. Myelography has the disadvantage that it may cause progression of neurologic findings in some patients with spinal cord compression. CT has the disadvantage that affected spinal levels first must be identified by clinical examination or MR imaging.

Mass lesions involving the spine usually are classified as extradural, extramedullary-intradural, or intramedullary. Most extradural tumors are malignant and the majority involve the osseous spinal column. The extramedullary-intra-

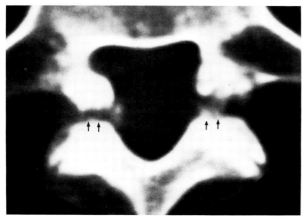

**FIGURE 12–68.** An example of bilateral spondylolytic (pars interarticularis) defects (arrows). (From Grogan JP, et al: Spondylolysis studied with computed tomography. Radiology *145*:737, 1982.)

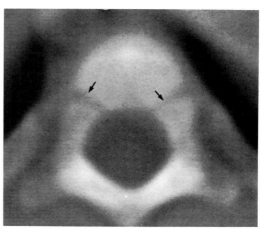

**FIGURE 12–70.** Synchondroses (arrows) in a thoracic vertebra of a 6 year old child.

dural lesions typically are benign schwannomas and meningiomas. Intramedullary processes include benign cysts, degenerative processes, and malignant tumors. In this section, imaging of processes in each region is discussed. Other texts can be consulted for more detailed discussions.[11]

**Extradural Lesions.** MR imaging is the primary imaging method for evaluation of suspected extradural lesions affecting the spinal cord. MR images show the spinal cord effectively. With specially designed coils, such as phased-array, a sagittal image of the entire spinal cord can be obtained in a few minutes.

The majority of extradural masses that affect the spinal cord are metastases to the vertebral column. Characteristically, osseous metastases that replace the fatty marrow normally present in the vertebra produce an area of abnormally low signal intensity in T1-weighted spin echo MR images and of abnormally high signal intensity in T2-weighted spin echo images. MR imaging is reported to be effective in distinguishing pathologic fractures from benign compression fractures[105] but it is not definitive in all cases. A useful adjunct to the T1- and T2-weighted images in uncertain cases is contrast enhanced T1-weighted fat suppressed images, which show metastatic foci as regions of high signal intensity or enhancement.

Epidural masses that affect the spinal cord but not the spinal column also are effectively shown by MR imaging. T1- or T2-weighted sagittal or transaxial images may reveal narrowing of the subarachnoid space. The contrast enhanced, fat suppressed image also may demonstrate the epidural lesions (which enhance). Lymphoma, usually characterized by spread over several spinal segments, is a common tumor that enters into the differential diagnosis of epidural masses. Differentiation between the numerous neoplasms that affect the epidural space or vertebral column by MR imaging is inexact. MR imaging, however, allows differentiation of neoplasm from degenerative processes affecting the spinal cord.

With the advent of fast imaging and specially designed spine coils MR imaging has become the primary imaging method for examining patients with suspected spinal cord compression.

The myelographic signs of epidural or vertebral metastases (or other malignant neoplasms) are narrowing or complete obliteration of the subarachnoid space and blocking of the flow of the contrast medium. The ventral, lateral, or dorsal surface of the dura may be affected.

**Extramedullary-Intradural Lesions.** Although meningiomas and schwannomas (Fig. 12–71) constitute the great majority of tumors that occur in this location, epidural and spinal cord tumors that grow exophytically into the subarachnoid space also are included in the differential diagnosis of extramedullary-intradural processes.

MR imaging essentially has replaced CT scanning and myelography in the evaluation of extramedullary-intradural tumors. Tumors in this space, which displace CSF, are detected readily on sagittal, coronal, or transaxial images. On T1-weighted images, meningiomas and schwannomas are of higher signal intensity than CSF. On T2-weighted images, they are of lower signal intensity than CSF.[106, 107] After intravenous administration of a paramagnetic contrast medium, meningiomas and schwannomas show marked, usually uniform, enhancement. Differentiation of schwan-

noma and meningioma by MR imaging usually is accurate. Schwannomas have a relationship to the spinal nerves in the cervical, thoracic or lumbar spine, often enlarging neural foramina. Meningiomas may calcify (with foci of persistently low signal intensity), may develop in the cervical or thoracic spine, and usually have a slightly lower signal intensity than schwannomas on T2-weighted images. Less common extramedullary-intradural lesions may not be distinguished easily from meningiomas and schwannomas. Suspected spread of tumor along the pia, meningeal carcinomatosis, has a characteristic appearance with MR imaging. Contrast enhancement is considered essential for detection of tumor along the pia, leading to a ''sugar-coated'' appearance (Fig. 12–72).[108, 109]

Extramedullary-intradural tumors, which enlarge the subarachnoid space by displacing the spinal cord and replacing CSF with solid tissue, have a characteristic myelographic appearance; a cap or meniscus with sharp, smooth, curvilinear borders and displacement of the spinal cord usually are evident provided that several projections are obtained during the myelogram. Meningiomas usually occur posterior to the thoracic cord, especially in women; schwannomas frequently are found in the neural foramen at any level, often in patients with von Recklinghausen's disease. The myelographic distinction between meningiomas and neurofibromas generally is not reliable.

CT is effective for detecting extramedullary-intradural lesions only if the lesions have first been localized by either radiographic, myelographic, or clinical examination. In the demonstration of the mass and the displaced spinal cord, CT performed after the introduction of intrathecal contrast medium is preferred. Intravenous administration of a contrast agent during the CT examination also is useful, leading to enhancement of either a schwannoma or a meningioma. Calcification sufficient to be detected by CT is uncommon in meningioma and rare in schwannoma. Hyperostosis has been delineated by CT or routine radiography in a few cases of meningioma of the spine; pressure erosion involving the pedicles, adjacent vertebral bodies, or neural arches is detected in schwannomas involving the neural foramen (Fig. 12–71).

**Intramedullary Lesions.** The processes that commonly affect the spinal cord include neoplasms, such as an astrocytoma, ependymoma, and, rarely, hemangioblastoma or lipoma; cysts, such as syringomyelia or hydromyelia; and non-neoplastic conditions, such as myelomalacia, demyelination, arteriovenous malformation, and atrophy. Although these conditions may involve the long spinal tracts in similar ways, the clinical history and physical examination often provide some specific clues as to the cause; however, imaging studies usually are required to establish a definitive diagnosis.[104, 110–113]

MR imaging is the technique of choice for evaluating intramedullary processes, and it detects both changes in cord caliber and changes in signal intensity from within the cord. Neoplasms characteristically enlarge the cord. Astrocytomas, ependymomas, and hemangioblastomas produce a region of prolonged T1 (lower signal intensity on T1-weighted images) and prolonged T2 (higher intensity on T2-weighted images) within the cord. The borders between the normal cord and the neoplasm usually are indistinct and irregular (Figs. 12–73 and 12–74). The majority of spinal cord tumors are of nearly homogeneous signal intensity,

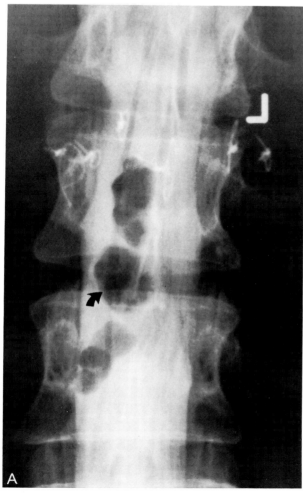

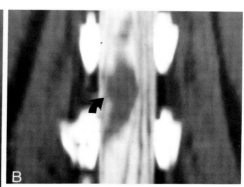

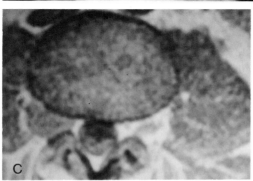

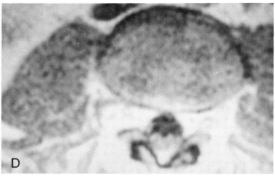

**FIGURE 12–71.** Imaging in spinal schwanno-mas.

**A, B** A large mass (arrows) is identified in a myelogram **(A)** and a coronal reformatted CT image **(B)**.

**C, D** In another patient, transaxial MR images obtained before **(C)** and after **(D)** gadopentetate dimeglumine administration reveal a mass in the right neural foramen, which enhances mark-edly.

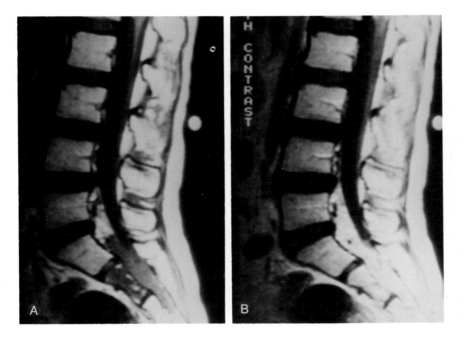

**FIGURE 12–72.** Parasagittal T1-weighted spin echo MR images obtained prior to **(A)** and after **(B)** intravenous contrast medium administration in a patient with pial and osseous metastases. Note that in the unenhanced T1-weighted image **(A)**, the S1 metastasis is evident. After contrast medium administration **(B)**, the small tumor nodules along the conus are conspicuous. In this image, the S1 metastasis is obscured owing to its enhancement. With fat suppression, metastases to the vertebrae are not obscured when intravenous contrast medium is administered.

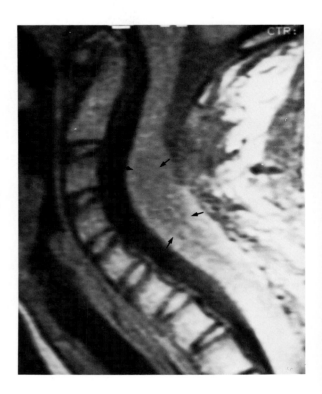

**FIGURE 12–73.** Sagittal T1-weighted spin echo MR image illustrating a cervical cord astrocytoma. The spinal canal and cord are enlarged. Within the widened spinal cord, an indistinct region of diminished signal intensity corresponding to the tumor is identified (arrows).

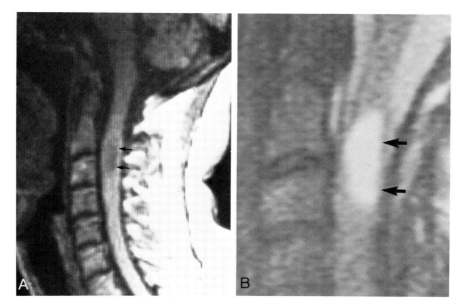

**FIGURE 12–74.** Sagittal T1-weighted **(A)** and T2-weighted **(B)** spin echo MR images of a cervical ependymoma (arrows). The signal intensity of the tumor differs from that of the cerebrospinal fluid.

which is intermediate between those of CSF and spinal cord. In the highly vascular tumors, such as hemangioblastoma, abnormal blood vessels may be demonstrated as regions of low signal intensity. Calcification, which occurs rarely in intramedullary neoplasms, is difficult to distinguish by MR imaging. Cystic areas in some tumors appear as regions of more prolonged T1 and T2 values. Hemorrhage has a characteristic high intensity signal on T1- and T2-weighted images. Fat in a lipoma has a characteristic high intensity signal on T1-weighted images and a low intensity signal on T2-weighted images and, often, a narrow chemical shift artifact of low signal intensity at its interface with the spinal cord or CSF.

MR imaging detects and characterizes syringomyelia or hydromyelia effectively.[114] In the ependymal cell–lined hydromyelia or the glial cell–lined syringomyelia, MR images characteristically show a homogeneous intramedullary process that is sharply demarcated from the spinal cord, with a prolonged T1 and T2 similar to that of CSF (Fig. 12–75). In various pulse sequences, therefore, the cyst cavities are isointense with CSF. Even small posttraumatic cysts that are difficult to detect with myelography or CT are readily identified in MR images (Fig. 12–76). The rare cysts that contain proteinaceous fluid having T1 and T2 relaxations similar to those of the spinal cord are difficult to distinguish with MR imaging. The majority of intramedullary cysts expand the spinal cord.

The differential diagnosis of a syrinx includes both neoplasms and myelomalacia. In contrast to spinal cord cysts, neoplasms have poorly defined boundaries with regard to the adjacent spinal cord and usually a signal intensity intermediate between those of CSF and spinal cord. An intramedullary process that is not isointense with CSF is either a neoplasm or a cyst with proteinaceous fluid.

Myelomalacia, demyelination, viral myelitis, and multiple sclerosis may produce a region of prolonged T1 and T2 within the spinal cord. In these conditions, the signal intensity rarely is the same as that of CSF, and the spinal cord is not expanded. In most instances, myelomalacia may be differentiated from a cyst because its borders are indistinct

and its signal intensity differs from that of CSF. Flaccid cysts that do not enlarge the silhouette of the spinal cord may be difficult to distinguish from myelomalacia, however, and conventional CT or myelography may be indicated after the MR imaging examination. Myelomalacia is more easily differentiated from a neoplasm, which usually expands the spinal cord.

Spinal cord atrophy has numerous causes, including

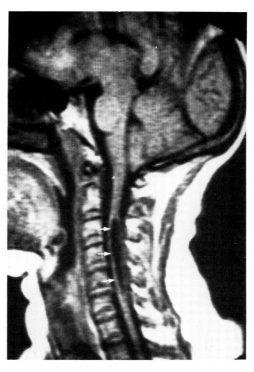

**FIGURE 12–75.** MR imaging in hydromyelia. A sagittal T1-weighted spin echo image shows a well-defined process (arrows) in the cervical cord at the C3-C5 spinal levels, which is isointense with CSF. The downward displacement of the cerebellar tonsils and inferior cerebellar vermis indicates an associated Chiari malformation.

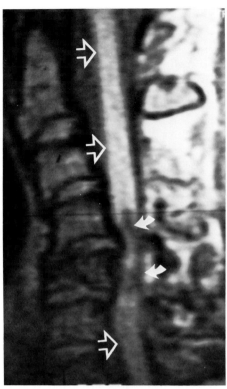

**FIGURE 12–76.** Traumatic syringomyelia shown by T1-weighted spin echo MR imaging. The fracture-dislocation of the cervical vertebrae and a low intensity process (solid arrows) in the spinal cord (open arrows) are shown.

trauma, degeneration, ischemia, infarction, and irradiation. Atrophy can be detected by myelography or contrast-enhanced CT, but because MR imaging demonstrates the contours of the spinal cord effectively and noninvasively it has replaced the other techniques. Various patterns of atrophy have been recognized.[104]

Myelography is slightly less sensitive than MR imaging for demonstrating intramedullary lesions. Because most spinal tumors and some cysts expand the spinal cord, their presence is detected easily in the opacified subarachnoid space. Cysts that communicate freely with the subarachnoid space have a characteristic myelographic appearance because of their opacification, although other cysts that do not become opacified, either immediately or by the time of delayed radiographic imaging, have a nonspecific appearance that may suggest neoplasm. When a tumor produces a complete block of the subarachnoid space, myelographic evaluation is incomplete unless an injection of contrast medium is made both above and below the lesion.

CT usually is not used as a primary diagnostic tool if a spinal cord tumor or cyst is suspected because myelography and MR imaging are more efficient in detecting and analyzing expansion of the spinal cord. If CT is used in the evaluation of spinal cord tumors, it is employed in combination with or as an adjunct to myelography (Figs. 12–77 and 12–78). CT may confirm myelographic findings in these cases and demonstrate penetration of contrast medium into an abnormal cord.

## Congenital Malformations

Congenital malformations of the spinal cord commonly are associated with additional osseous and articular abnormalities in spinal and extraspinal sites.[114–117] Two important types of malformations are described in the following discussion.

**Chiari Malformation.** The Chiari II or Arnold-Chiari malformation is characterized by a myelomeningocele and caudal displacement of the cerebellar tonsils and hindbrain. It has many other associated abnormalities, such as a large massa intermedia, a deformed anterior commissure, a beaked quadrigeminal plate, and absence of the falx cerebelli.[118] The spinal malformation also may cause abnormalities in growth or development of the lower extremities.

MR imaging is the procedure of choice for evaluating patients with a suspected Chiari malformation. The sagittal images demonstrate the developmental abnormalities in the posterior fossa (Fig. 12–75) and cerebrum and the anatomic relationships of the meningocele, spinal cord, filum terminale, and nerve roots. Lipomas or lipomeningoceles, which commonly accompany the malformation, are well shown by sagittal MR images with short TR and short TE, in

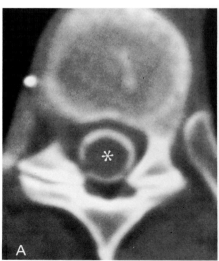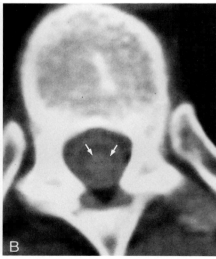

**FIGURE 12–77.** CT in syringomyelia. An image obtained immediately after opacification of the subarachnoid space **(A)** shows an enlarged spinal cord (asterisk). A delayed image **(B)** demonstrates the contrast medium (arrows) in the spinal cord.

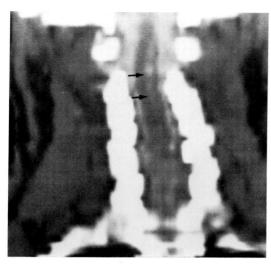

**FIGURE 12–78.** Intrathecally enhanced CT in syringomyelia. The reformatted coronal image shows contrast medium within the spinal cord (arrows).

which fat yields a high intensity signal. The contents of the dural sac are effectively demonstrated, especially in long TR, long TE images, in which CSF yields a high intensity signal.

CT also may be used to evaluate Chiari malformations. The unenhanced CT images show obliteration of the cisterna magna by the ectopic cerebellar tonsils, medulla, or cerebellar vermis.[118] In the lumbar region, the low density tissue associated with a lipoma, the dural sac protruding through the posterior elements of the spinal canal, and the low termination of the spinal cord are detected with high resolution CT technique, often aided by sagittal reformatted images. After the administration of intrathecal contrast material, CT may demonstrate the filling defect created by the cerebellar tonsils in the subarachnoid space at the cranial

end of the spinal canal and the relationship of the spinal cord, nerve roots, and meningocele in the lumbar spine.

Myelography represents an alternative method of diagnosing Chiari malformations. A C1-C2 puncture carries a higher risk in patients with Chiari malformations because the tonsils may fill the subarachnoid space at the craniospinal junction and make atraumatic cannulation of the subarachnoid space difficult. Puncture of the subarachnoid space in the lumbar region also carries a higher risk of trauma because of the anomalously low and dorsal position of the spinal cord that commonly accompanies a meningocele. Nonetheless, myelography generally can be performed without complications in patients with the Chiari malformation. Myelography is sensitive in demonstrating the caudal displacement of the cerebellar tonsils, the meningocele, and the precise position of the spinal cord, but it is less effective in defining the abnormal nerve roots and the frequently associated lipoma involving the filum terminale.

**Dysraphism.** Dysraphism includes all the congenital malformations of the spine that are thought to result from defective closure of the neural tube. One type of dysraphism that commonly has associated deformities in the lower extremities is diastematomyelia. Indirect signs of diastematomyelia that may be detected with conventional radiography include scoliosis, narrowing of intervertebral disc spaces, widening of the interpediculate distances, and, in some cases, a spicule of bone dividing the spinal canal (Fig. 12–79). These signs are not sensitive, as many cases of diastematomyelia involve only the spinal cord or meninges.

CT and MR imaging, which show the malformed spinal cord and meninges directly, demonstrate the hemicords of diastematomyelia effectively (Fig. 12–80), even in the large fraction of cases without osseous abnormalities. The nerve roots, which originate only from one lateral margin of the hemicords, are better demonstrated if intrathecal contrast medium is used with CT. MR imaging is particularly useful in demonstrating syrinxes, which commonly complicate di-

**FIGURE 12–79.** Diastematomyelia.

**A** A conventional anteroposterior radiograph of the lumbar spine demonstrates widening of the interpediculate distance, a decreased intervertebral disc space between L1 and L2, and a bony spicule overlying the center of the spinal canal (arrow).

**B** A lateral conventional tomogram obtained during gas myelography confirms the narrowing of the intervertebral disc space (solid arrow) and allows identification of the spicule (open arrow) that bisected the spinal cord.

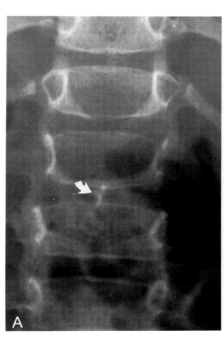
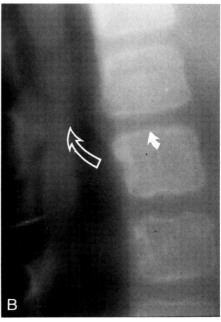

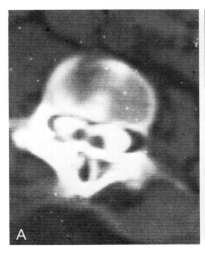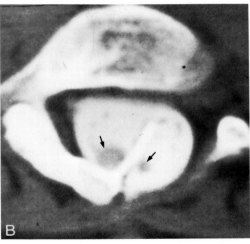

**FIGURE 12–80.** CT with intrathecal enhancement in diastematomyelia. The transaxial image in **A** shows division of the spinal cord into two unequal halves. At a lower level **(B)**, the osseous spicule is demonstrated between the two hemicords (arrows). (From Arredondo F, et al: Radiology *136*:685, 1980.)

astematomyelia. Thickening or lipomatous infiltration of the filum terminale, meningocele, and lipomeningocele, each of which are common in diastematomyelia, are shown well by MR imaging and CT.

### Arachnoiditis and Postlaminectomy Scars

Although the name suggests inflammation of the arachnoid membrane, arachnoiditis encountered in clinical practice is characterized more by a fibrotic reaction in the meninges than by inflammatory cell infiltration. Clinically arachnoiditis may produce pain and weakness in the distribution of the affected nerves. As arachnoiditis progresses, the nerves of the cauda equina first become adherent to the dural sac and then are incorporated into and compressed by dense fibrous tissue. Arachnoiditis may be precipitated by intrathecal contrast media, especially Pantopaque or iocarmate, intrathecal anesthetics, blood, infections such as tuberculosis or syphilis, or spinal surgery. An idiopathic arachnoiditis ossificans also is recognized.[120]

Contrast enhanced CT is an effective way of demonstrating the changes of arachnoiditis. The subarachnoid space in the intrathecally enhanced images appears devoid of nerve roots because they have been incorporated into the dural sac (Fig. 12–81). It may accompany laminectomy and epidural scarring, in which case the epidural fat is replaced with a more or less amorphous homogeneous tissue, usually with a density of about 40 HU. With intravenous contrast medium, the thickened dura and epidural fibrosis are enhanced, resulting in increased density.

Arachnoiditis has characteristic myelographic features. The deficiency of nerve roots within the opacified subarachnoid space may be evident. More obvious are the irregular, asymmetric distortions of the dural margin, which lacks an anatomic relationship to the disc space. Often the residual Pantopaque that caused the arachnoiditis may be evident. In postsurgical cases, the proximity of the dural irregularity to the laminectomy defect is evident.

MR imaging of the spine may demonstrate changes of arachnoiditis, but with less sensitivity than CT.[121] T1-weighted transaxial or sagittal MR images may show clumping or an irregular course of nerve roots in the thecal sac. On T2-weighted images, the nerve roots may be less apparent because of the high signal intensity of CSF. After

intravenous administration of contrast medium, slight enhancement of the dural sac may be observed or, less regularly, marked enhancement of a nerve root. In cases of arachnoiditis secondary to Pantopaque myelography, Pantopaque may be evident as a region of high signal intensity on T1-weighted MR images. In postlaminectomy patients, MR imaging is the technique of choice for distinguishing epidural scar and recurrent herniated disc.[122–124] MR images after the intravenous administration of contrast medium show more enhancement in the epidural scar than in the recurrent disc fragment.[125–127] Scar tissue enhancement is a function of the age of the scar, the dose and type of contrast medium that is used, and the duration of elapsed time between the injection of contrast material and the imaging examination.[55, 127]

### SUMMARY

This chapter has provided an overview of the more important imaging techniques that are employed in the evaluation of intraspinal diseases. Routine radiography, CT scanning, MR imaging, myelography, and SPECT are used in the analysis of disorders of the facet joints, intervertebral discs, uncovertebral articulations, vertebrae, spinal cord,

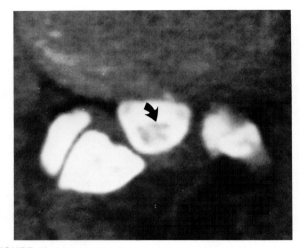

**FIGURE 12–81.** Intrathecally enhanced CT demonstrating clumping of the nerve roots (arrow) in arachnoiditis.

and meninges. The interested reader should refer to additional chapters of this book dealing with degenerative diseases of the spine (Chapter 40), spinal trauma (Chapter 69), and tumors (Chapters 83 and 85), and infections (Chapter 65) of the spine.

## References

1. Post MJD: Computed Tomography of the Spine. Baltimore, Williams & Wilkins, 1984.
2. Latchaw RE: Computed Tomography of the Head, Neck and Spine. Chicago, Year Book Medical Publishers, 1985.
3. Shapiro RE: Myelography. 4th Ed. Chicago, Year Book Medical Publishers, 1984.
4. Gonzales CF, Grossman CB, Masdev JC: Head and Spine Imaging. New York, Wiley, 1985.
5. Haughton VM, Williams AL: Computed Tomography of the Spine. St Louis, CV Mosby, 1982.
6. Newton TH, Potts DG (Eds): Computed Tomography of the Spine and Spinal Cord. San Anselmo, CA, Clavadel Press, 1983.
7. Partain CL, James AE Jr, Rollo FD, et al: Nuclear Magnetic Resonance Imaging. Philadelphia, WB Saunders Co, 1985.
8. Haughton VM, Williams AL: Computed Tomography of the Spine. St Louis, CV Mosby, 1982.
9. Haughton VM: Computed Tomography of the Spine. In VM Haughton (Ed): Contemporary Issues in Computed Tomography, Vol. 2. New York, Churchill Livingstone, 1983.
10. Valk J, MacLean C, Algra PR: Basic Principles of Nuclear Magnetic Resonance Imaging. Amsterdam, Elsevier, 1985.
11. Atlas SW: Magnetic Resonance Imaging of the Brain and Spine. New York, Raven Press, 1991.
12. Orrison WW, Johansen JG, Eldevik OP, et al: Optimal computed-tomographic techniques for cervical spine imaging. AJR 144:180, 1982.
13. Collier B, Johnson RP, Carrera GF, et al: Painful spondylolysis or spondylolisthesis studied by single photon emission computed tomography. Radiology 154:207, 1985.
14. DiChiro G, Doppman J, Ommaya AK: Selective arteriography of arteriovenous aneurysms of spinal cord. Radiology 88:1065, 1967.
15. DiChiro G, Doppman JL, Ommaya AK: Radiology of spinal cord arteriovenous malformations. Prog Neurol Surg 4:329, 1971.
16. Djindjian R, Hurth M, Howdart R: Angiography of the Spinal Cord. Paris, Masson, 1970.
17. Collis JS Jr, Gardner WS: Lumbar discography, an analysis of 1,000 cases. J Neurosurg 19:452, 1962.
18. Kieffer SA, Stadlan EM, Mohandas A, et al: Discographic anatomic correlation of developmental changes with age in the intervertebral disc. Acta Radiol [Diagn] (Stockh) 9:733, 1979.
19. Fernstrom V: A discographic study of ruptured lumbar intervertebral discs. Acta Chir Scand Suppl 258:11, 1960.
20. Dell CW Jr, Coel MN, Igrelgi RJ: Ascending lumbar venography in lumbar disc disease. J Bone Joint Surg [Am] 59:159, 1977.
21. Drasin GF, Daffner RH, Sexton RF, et al: Epidural venography: Diagnosis of herniated lumbar intervertebral disc and other disease of the epidural space. AJR 126:1010, 1976.
22. Gashaler R, Holgate RC: Lumbar epidural venography in diagnosis of disc herniations. AJR 112:992, 1976.
23. Hatten HP Jr: Lumbar epidurography with metrizamide: Review of 65 cases employing a pure Seldinger technique with caudal approach through the sacral notch and selective nerve root sheath injection. Radiology 137:129, 1980.
24. Kirkaldy-Willis MW, Prebraum HW: Epidural venography in the diagnosis of lumbar disc disease. Surg Neurol 5:287, 1976.
25. Luyondijhs W, Van Voorthosen AE: Contrast examination of the spinal epidural space. Acta Radiol [Diagn] (Stockh) 5:1051, 1966.
26. Carrera GF, Williams AL, Haughton VM: Computed tomography in sciatica. Radiology 137:433, 1980.
27. Carrera GF: Lumbar facet joint injection in low back pain and sciatica: Description of technique. Radiology 137:661, 1980.
28. Carrera GF: Lumbar facet joint infection in low back pain and sciatica: Preliminary results. Radiology 137:665, 1980.
29. Lefkowitz DM, Quencer RM: Vacuum facet phenomenon: A computed tomographic sign of degenerative spondylolisthesis. Radiology 144:562, 1982.
30. Badgely C: The articular facets in relation to low back and sciatic radiation. J Bone Joint Surg 23:481, 1941.
31. Ghormley RL: Low back pain with special reference to the articular facets with presentation of an operative procedure. JAMA 101:1773, 1933.
32. Carrera GF, Haughton VM, Syvertsen A, et al: Computed tomography of lumbar facet joints. Radiology 134:145, 1981.
33. Hemminghytt S, Daniels DL, Williams AL, et al: Intraspinal synovial cysts: Natural history and diagnosis by CT. Radiology 145:375, 1982.
34. Grossman H, Gray R, St Louis EL: CT of long standing ankylosing spondylitis with cauda equina syndrome. AJNR 4:1077, 1983.
35. Russell ML, Gordan DA, Ogryzlo MA, et al: The cauda equina syndrome of ankylosing spondylitis. Ann Intern Med 78:551, 1979.
36. Weinstein PR, Karpman RR, Gall EP, et al: Spinal cord injury, spinal fracture, and spinal stenosis in ankylosing spondylitis (Abstr). Radiology 148:597, 1983.
37. Brant-Zawadzki M, Miller EM, Federle MP: CT in the evaluation of spine trauma. AJR 136:369, 1981.
38. O'Callaghan JP, Ullrich CG, Yuan HA, et al: CT of facet distraction in flexion injuries of the thoracolumbar spine: The "naked" facet. AJR 134:563, 1980.
39. Swartz JD, Puleo S: Fractures of the C-1 vertebra: Report of two cases documented with computed tomography (Abstr). Radiology 151:830, 1984.
40. Brant-Zawadzki M, Jeffrey RB Jr, Minagi H, et al: High resolution CT of thoracolumbar fractures. AJR 138:699, 1982.
41. Lee C, Kim KS, Rogers LF: Sagittal fracture of the cervical vertebral body. AJR 139:55, 1982.
42. Yetkin Z, Osborn AG, Giles DS, et al: Uncovertebral and facet joint dislocations in cervical articular pillar fractures: CT evaluation. AJNR 6:633, 1985.
43. Pech P, Kilgore DP, Pojunas KW, et al: Cervical spinal fractures: CT detection. Radiology 157:117, 1985.
44. Williams AL, Haughton VM, Meyer GA, et al: Computed tomographic appearance of the bulging annulus. Radiology 142:403, 1982.
45. Williams AL, Haughton VM, Daniels DL, et al: CT recognition of lateral lumbar disk herniation. AJR 139:345, 1982.
46. Williams AL, Haughton VM, Daniels DL, et al: Differential CT diagnosis of extruded nuclear pulposus. Radiology 148:141, 1983.
47. Novetsky GJ, Berlin L, Epstein AJ, et al: Extraforaminal herniated disk: Detection by computed tomography. AJNR 3:653, 1982.
48. Eldevik OP, Dugstad G, Orrison WW, et al: Effect of clinical bias on the interpretation of myelography and spinal computed tomography. Radiology 145:85, 1982.
49. Dillon WP, Kaseff LG, Knackstedt VE, et al: Computed tomography and differential diagnosis of the extruded lumbar disc. J Comput Assist Tomogr 7:969, 1983.
50. Firooznia H, Benjamin V, Kricheff II, et al: CT of lumbar spine disk herniation: Correlation with surgical findings. AJNR 5:91, 1984.
51. Fries JW, Abodeely DAA, Vijungco J, et al: Computed tomography of herniated and extruded nucleus pulposus. J Comput Assist Tomogr 6:874, 1982.
52. Risius B, Modic MT, Hardy RJ Jr, et al: Sector computed tomographic spine scanning in the diagnosis of lumbar nerve root entrapment. Radiology 143:109, 1982.
53. Haughton VM, Eldevik OP, Magnaes B, et al: Prospective comparison of computed tomography and myelography in the diagnosis of herniated lumbar disks. Radiology 142:103, 1982.
54. Anand AK, Lee BCP: Plain and metrizamide CT of lumbar disk disease: Comparison with myelography. AJNR 3:567, 1982.
55. Ross JS, Modic MT, Masaryk TJ, et al: Assessment of extradural degenerative disease with Gd-DTPA enhanced MR imaging. AJR 154:151, 1990.
56. Ross JS, Tkach JA, Van Dyhe C, et al: Clinical MR imaging of degenerative spinal disease: pulse sequences, gradient echo techniques and contrast agents. J Magn Reson Imaging 1:29, 1991.
57. Grenier N, Greselle JF, Downs C, et al: MR imaging of foramina and extraforaminal lumbar disc herniations. J Comput Assist Tomogr 14:243, 1990.
58. Yousem DM, Atlas SW, Goldberg HI, et al: Degenerative narrowing of the cervical spine neural foramina: Evaluation with high resolution 3DFT gradient-echo MR imaging. AJR 156:1229, 1991.
59. Ross JS, Ruggieri PM, Tkach JA, et al: Gd-DTPA enhanced 3D MR imaging of cervical degenerative disc disease: Initial experience. AJNR 13:127, 1992.
60. Daniels DL, Grogan JP, Johansen JG, et al: Cervical radiculopathy: Computed tomography and myelography compared. Radiology 151:109, 1984.
61. Russell EJ, D'Angelo CM, Zimmerman RD, et al: Cervical disc herniation: CT demonstration after contrast enhancement. Radiology 152:703, 1984.
62. Miyasaka K, Isu T, Iwasaki Y, et al: High resolution computed tomography in the diagnosis of cervical disc disease (Abstr). Radiology 150:862, 1984.
63. Hochman MS, Pena C, Remmez R: Calcified herniated thoracic disc diagnosed by CT: A case report. J Neurosurg 52:722, 1980.
64. Landman JA, Hoffman JC Jr, Braun IF, et al: Value of computed tomographic myelography in the recognition of cervical herniated disk. AJNR 5:391, 1984.
65. Modic MT, Pavlicek W, Weinstein MA, et al: Magnetic resonance imaging of intervertebral disc disease. Radiology 152:103, 1984.
66. Modic MT, Pavilcek W, Weinstein MA, et al: Magnetic resonance imaging of intervertebral disk disease: Clinical and pulse sequence considerations. Radiology 152:103, 1984.
67. Moon KL Jr, Genant HK, Helms CA, et al: Musculoskeletal applications of nuclear magnetic resonance. Radiology 147:161, 1983.
68. Chafetz NI, Genant HK, Moon KL, et al: Recognition of lumbar disk herniation with NMR. AJR 141:1153, 1983.
69. Modic MT, Weinstein MA, Pavlicek W, et al: Nuclear magnetic resonance imaging of the spine. Radiology 148:757, 1983.
70. Kieffer SA, Sherry RG, Wellenstein DE, et al: Bulging lumbar intervertebral disc: Myelographic differentiation from herniated disc with nerve root compression. AJNR 3:51, 1982.
71. Brown HA: Enlargement of the ligamentum flavum: A cause of low back pain with sciatic radiation. J Bone Joint Surg 20:325, 1938.
72. Yong-Hing K, Reilly J, Kirkaldy-Willis WH: The ligamentum flavum. Spine 1:226, 1976.
73. Ono K, Ota H, Tada K, et al: Ossified posterior longitudinal ligament. Spine 2:126, 1977.
74. Williams DM, Gabrielsen TO, Latack JT: Ossification in the caudal attachments of the ligamentum flavum: An anatomic and computed tomographic study. Radiology 145:693, 1982.

75. Williams DM, Gabrielsen TO, Latack JT, et al: Ossification in the cephalic attachment of the ligamentum flavum: An anatomical and CT study. Radiology *150*:423, 1984.

76. Malghem JJ, Nagent de Deuxchaisnes C, Rombouts-Lindemans C, et al: Ossification of posterior longitudinal ligament of the cervical spine: Report of a case with computed tomographic study and associated with Forestier's disease (Abstr). Radiology *135*:814, 1980.

77. McAfee PC, Ullrich CG, Levinsohn EM, et al: Computed tomography in degenerative lumbar spinal stenosis: The value of multiplanar reconstruction. RadioGraphics *2*:529, 1982.

78. Edwards MK, Harwood-Nash DC, Fitz CR, et al: CT metrizamide myelography of the cervical spine in Morquio syndrome. AJNR *3*:666, 1982.

79. Morgan DF, Young RF: Spinal neurological complications of achondroplasia (Abstr). Radiology *137*:889, 1980.

80. Price AC, Allen JH, Eggers FM, et al: Intervertebral disc space infection: CT changes. Radiology *149*:725, 1983.

81. Mikhael MA, Ciric IS, Tarkington JA, et al: Neuroradiologic evaluation of lateral recess syndrome. Radiology *140*:97, 1981.

82. Agula LA, Piraino DW, Modic MT, et al: The intranuclear cleft of the intervertebral disc: Magnetic resonance imaging. Radiology *155*:155, 1985.

83. Sartoris DJ, Moskowitz PS, Kaufman RA, et al: Childhood diskitis: Computed tomographic findings. Radiology *149*:701, 1983.

84. Blomquist HK, Lindquist M, Mattsson S: Calcification of intervertebral discs in childhood. Pediatr Radiol *8*:23, 1979.

85. Price AC, Allen JH, Eggers FM, et al: Intervertebral disk-space infection: CT changes. Radiology *149*:725, 1983.

86. Hermann G, Mendelson DS, Cohen BA, et al: Role of computed tomography in the diagnosis of infectious spondylitis (Abstr). Radiology *152*:860, 1984.

87. Post MJD, Seminer DS, Quencer RM: CT diagnosis of spinal epidural hematoma. AJNR *3*:190, 1982.

88. Post MJD, Sze G, Quencer RM: Gadolinium enhanced MR in spinal infection. J Comput Assist Tomogr *14*:721, 1990.

89. Sharif HJ, Clark DC, Aabed MY, et al: Granulomatous spinal infections. Radiology *177*:101, 1990.

90. Haney P, Gellad F, Swartz J: Aneurysmal bone cyst of the spine: Computed tomographic appearance. J Comput Tomogr *7*:322, 1983.

91. Haney P, Gellad F, Swartz J: Aneurysmal bone cyst of the spine: Computed tomographic appearance (Abstr). Radiology *151*:830, 1984.

92. Omojola MF, Fox AJ, Vinuela FV: Computed tomographic metrizamide myelography in the evaluation of thoracic spinal osteoblastoma. AJNR *3*:670, 1982.

93. Meyer JE, Lepke RA, Lindfors KK, et al: Chordomas: Their CT appearance in the cervical, thoracic and lumbar spine. Radiology *153*:693, 1984.

94. Helms A, Genant HK: Computed tomography in the early detection of skeletal involvement with multiple myeloma (Abstr). Radiology *148*:888, 1983.

95. Levitan LH, Wiens CW: Chronic lumbar extradural hematoma: CT findings. Radiology *148*:707, 1983.

96. Kerslaki RW, Jaspan T, Worthington BS: Magnetic resonance imaging of spinal trauma. Br J Radiol *64*:386, 1991.

97. Schweitzer ME, Cervilla V, Resnick D: Acute cervical trauma: Correlation of MR imaging findings with neurologic deficit. Radiology *179*:287, 1991.

98. Johansen JG, McCarty DJ, Haughton VM: Retrosomatic clefts: Computed tomographic appearance. Radiology *148*:447, 1983.

99. Johansen JG, Haughton VM, Hemminghytt S: The CT appearance of retroisthmic clefts. AJNR *5*:835, 1984.

100. Grogan JP, Hemminghytt S, Williams AL, et al: Spondylolysis studied with computed tomography. Radiology *145*:737, 1982.

101. Manaster BJ, Normal A: CT diagnosis of thoracic pedicle aplasia. J Comput Assist Tomogr *7*:1090, 1983.

102. Kish KK, Wilner HI: Spondylolysis of C2: CT and plain film findings. J Comput Assist Tomogr *70*:517, 1983.

103. Brugman E, Palmers Y, Staelens B: Congenital absence of a pedicle in the cervical spine: A new approach with CT scan. Neuroradiology *17*:121, 1979.

104. Mawad ME, Hilal SK, Fetell MR, et al: Patterns of spinal cord atrophy by metrizamide CT. AJNR *4*:611, 1983.

105. Yuh WTC, Fisher DJ, Mayer-Yuh NA, et al: Review of the use of high-dose gadoteridol in the magnetic resonance evaluation of central nervous system tumors. Invest Radiol *27*:539, 1992.

106. Demachis H, Takashima T, Kadoya M, et al: MR imaging of spinal neurinomas in the pathological correlation. J Comput Assist Tomogr *14*:250, 1990.

107. Holtas S: MR imaging of spinal neurofibromatosis. Acta Radiol *32*:279, 1991.

108. Sze G: MR imaging of the spinal cord: Current status and future advances. AJR *159*:149, 1992.

109. Blews DE, Wang H, Kumar AJ, et al: Intradural spinal metastases in pediatric patients with primary intracranial neoplasms: Gd-DTPA enhanced MR versus CT myelography. J Comput Assist Tomogr *14*:730, 1990.

110. DiChiro G, Doppman JL, Dwyer AJ, et al: Tumors and arteriovenous malformations of the cord using MR. Radiology *165*:689, 1985.

111. Modic MT, Weinstein MA, Pavlicek W, et al: Magnetic resonance imaging of the cervical spine: Technical and clinical observations. AJR *141*:1129, 1983.

112. Kan S, Fox AJ, Vinuela F, et al: Delayed CT metrizamide enhancement of syringomyelia secondary to tumor. AJNR *4*:73, 1983.

113. Quencer RM: Needle aspiration of intramedullary and intradural extramedullary masses of the spinal canal. Radiology *134*:115, 1980.

114. Pojunas KW, Williams AL, Daniels DL, et al: Syringomyelia and hydromyelia: Magnetic resonance evaluation. Radiology *153*:679, 1984.

115. Arredondo F, Haughton VM, Hemmy DC, et al: The computed tomographic appearance of the spinal cord in diastematomyelia. Radiology *136*:685, 1980.

116. Naidich TP, McLone DG, Mutluer S: New understanding of dorsal dysraphism with lipoma (lipomyeloschisis): Radiologic evaluation and surgical correction. AJR *140*:1065, 1983.

117. Naidich TP, Harwood-Nash DC, McLone DG: Radiology of spinal dysraphism. Clin Neurosurg *30*:341, 1983.

118. Naidich TP, McLone DG, Fulling KH: Chiari malformations. Part IV. The hindbrain. Neuroradiology *25*:179, 1983.

119. Barthelemy CR: Arachnoiditis ossificans. J Comput Assist Tomogr *6*:809, 1982.

120. Johnson CE, Sze G: Benign lumbar arachnoiditis: MR imaging with gadopentetate dimeglumine. AJNR *11*:763, 1990.

121. Ross JS, Modic MT, Masaryk TJ, et al: Assessment of extradural degenerative disease with Gd-DTPA enhanced MR imaging: Correlation with surgical and pathologic findings. AJR *154*:151, 1990.

122. Bundschuh CV, Stein L, Slusser JH, et al: Distinguishing between scar and recurrent herniated disc in postoperative patients: Value of contrast enhanced CT and MR imaging. AJNR *11*:949, 1990.

123. Ross JS: Magnetic resonance assessment of the postoperative spine: Degenerative disc disease. Radiol Clin North Am *29*:793, 1991.

124. Haughton VM, Nguyen C, Ho KC, et al: An experimental study of contrast enhancement in post-laminectomy epidural fibrosis. AJNR (in press).

125. Glichstein MF, Sussman SK: Time-dependent scar enhancement in magnetic resonance imaging of the postoperative lumbar spine. Radiology *20*:333, 1991.

126. Ibrahim MA, Jesmanowicz A, Hyde JS, et al: Contrast enhancement in normal intervertebral discs: time and dose dependence. AJNR (in press).

127. Ross JS, Masaryk TJ, Schroeder M, et al: MR imaging of the post-operative lumbar spine. AJNR *11*:771, 1990.

# 13

# Arthrography, Tenography, and Bursography

*Donald Resnick, M.D.*

In the past, contrast opacification of joint cavities (arthrography), tendon sheaths (tenography), and bursae (bursography) has been a frequently employed and often useful procedure for evaluation of joints and surrounding tissues. The indications for such contrast opacification have diminished significantly in recent years owing to refinements in other diagnostic methods, particularly MR imaging. This chapter summarizes the indications, techniques, and normal and abnormal findings of this examination at specific locations in the body, although arthrographic abnormalities in patients with joint prostheses are described in Chapter 19.

Owing to the increasing importance of diagnostic assessment of internal derangements of joints and to the ever increasing application of MR imaging to this assessment, Chapter 70 of this textbook is devoted to a complete discussion of this topic. Some anatomic and arthrographic features related to internal articular derangements, therefore, are repeated in Chapter 70. It is the author's opinion, however, that a chapter devoted to arthrography, tenography, and bursography, despite the decreasing importance of these procedures, remains appropriate for a textbook devoted to diagnostic imaging.

## OVERVIEW

Arthrography is an established diagnostic technique that has undergone remarkable changes during the last 30 years. Although original descriptions virtually were confined to the examination of the knee and the supplementary use of plain film radiography, arthrography subsequently was applied to the evaluation of many different joints and was coupled with each succeeding technologic advancement, including fluoroscopy, conventional and computed tomography, digital radiography, and MR imaging. An increasing number of scientific papers appeared that described refinements in arthrographic technique and newer applications of the examination, and entire books dealing with arthrography in general and arthrography of individual joints became available.[371–375] The introduction of MR imaging and of arthroscopy and arthroscopic surgery[698] in recent years has led to significant modifications in arthrography, particularly with regard to the type of examinations being performed; the technique remains popular in many areas of the United States and throughout the world.[699]

The types of arthrographic examinations performed as well as their indications vary from one institution to another and have undergone considerable change in the last 15 years. Up to that time, evaluation of meniscal lesions represented the single most frequent reason for performing arthrography. Although knee arthrograms still are commonly obtained, their number has decreased dramatically in many hospitals owing to the increasing popularity of MR imaging and arthroscopy. Knee arthrography currently is employed in institutions in which MR imaging is not available, in the examination of obese patients or of those in whom MR imaging is contraindicated, and, in some instances, as a primary diagnostic technique (e.g., the assessment of meniscal abnormalities in patients who have had previous meniscal surgery). Glenohumeral joint arthrography and, more recently, subacromial bursography have become more popular, related to mounting interest in the alterations of the glenoid labrum that accompany shoulder instability and in the shoulder impingement syndrome.

Such alterations, however, also can be studied with MR imaging. Initially designed to evaluate the changes of rheumatoid arthritis, wrist arthrography currently is employed most typically to delineate injuries of the intercarpal ligaments and triangular fibrocartilage.

In the past 25 years, orthopedic surgery also has undergone dramatic modifications, with a new emphasis placed on arthroplasties of the hip and knee as well as other sites. Arthrographic evaluation of joint prostheses has been a natural consequence of this changing emphasis in articular surgery, and aspiration with subsequent contrast opacification of articulations containing prosthetic replacements represents an important component of the workload in many radiology departments (see Chapter 19).

Although arthrography of the ankle and elbow has undergone less change, arthrography of the temporomandibular joint and tenography in the hand and foot have become more commonplace.[700] The ability of the arthrogram to provide direct evidence regarding the integrity of the meniscus in the temporomandibular joint as well as the realization that alterations in this integrity and aberrations of meniscal position produce significant clinical manifestations explains the popularity of this procedure, although this examination too has been influenced by the newer technologies, such as multiplanar and three-dimensional CT and MR imaging (see Chapters 8, 9, 10, and 49).

## CONTRAST AGENTS AND TECHNIQUES

The choice of a specific contrast material is influenced directly by the type of and indications for arthrography. Various radiopaque and radiolucent (air or carbon dioxide) contrast media exist that can be used separately as a single contrast technique (radiopaque contrast material or air alone) or combined as a double contrast technique (radiopaque material and air together), depending on the clinical situation. Single contrast examination with positive contrast material is suitable for the investigation of synovial inflammation or proliferation, synovial cyst formation, ligamentous and capsular injury, adhesive capsulitis, and painful joint prostheses, especially in the hip and knee.[376] Single contrast examination (sometimes combined with conventional tomography or CT) with positive contrast material or air is the technique of choice for the identification of intraarticular osteocartilaginous bodies, although double contrast examination using small amounts of radiopaque contrast material occasionally is used, particularly in a small or tight articulation, such as the elbow or ankle. With regard to the menisci of the knee, the benefits of single versus double contrast technique are debated in the literature, although most experienced arthrographers prefer the latter. Double contrast arthrography also is superior to the single contrast study for the analysis of the rotator cuff and glenoid surface in the shoulder.

The usual radiopaque material that is used for arthrography is a water-soluble contrast agent such as meglumine diatrizoate (Renografin-M 60) or diatrizoate sodium (Hypaque Sodium 50%), although investigators have indicated that other water-soluble contrast agents,[377] nonionic dimers,[378, 662, 701, 702] and perfluorocarbon compounds[379] may be superior with regard to better image quality or fewer adverse effects, or both. Histologic abnormalities in the synovial membrane are encountered after the injection of most of these agents and, in experimental situations, consist of mild focal proliferation of surface synovial cells, stromal mononuclear cells, and eosinophils, and dilation and congestion of vascular channels[380] (Fig. 13–1). In humans, histologic abnormalities also are consistent with a low grade synovial inflammatory process and may be accompanied by eosinophilia in the synovial fluid.[381, 382] Although such abnormalities may explain postprocedural pain, discomfort, and swelling, other factors also may be important, including the additional influx of fluid into an already distended joint in response to hyperosmolar positive contrast material[383, 384, 645] and synovial inflammation, as in rheumatoid arthritis, that may have preceded the arthrographic examination.

Although early examiners used carbon dioxide as the negative contrast material, room air is used by most arthrographers today and, in fact, may be preferable,[385, 386] causing less patient discomfort, perhaps related to a less dramatic decrease in the pH of the joint fluid.[369]

## JOINT PUNCTURE, ASPIRATION, AND REASPIRATION

The technique for joint puncture varies according to the specific articulation being examined and is summarized in appropriate sections of this chapter. Fluoroscopic monitoring of the procedure ensures successful introduction of the needle and provides additional insight into joint mechanics and associated osseous or soft tissue abnormalities.

Aspiration of joint contents prior to arthrography is a recommended practice for most examinations, especially those of the knee, in which sizeable effusions lead to deterioration in the image detail provided by the contrast medium; it also provides fluid samples that can be inspected immediately for "wear" particles[370] and can be transported to the laboratory, when necessary, for more detailed analysis. Such aspiration becomes mandatory when the possibility of infection is being considered, as in patients with painful joint prostheses. Although the bactericidal or bacteriostatic effect of the iodinated contrast medium is influenced by a number of factors, including the chemical composition of the contrast agent, the type of bacteria, and the pH of the fluid,[387–389] it generally is recommended that joint fluid be collected prior to the instillation of the contrast material. When fluid cannot be recovered easily, nonbacteriostatic sterile saline solution can be introduced into the joint and reaspirated. As it also has been determined that lidocaine has a significant antibacterial effect,[389] this agent should be used very prudently during diagnostic puncture of a possibly septic joint and should not enter into contact with the bacteriologic specimen.

Removal of the positive contrast material or air, or both, from the joint at the termination of the examination is attempted by a minority of arthrographers but generally is not necessary. Reaspiration increases the length of the procedure, involves added patient discomfort, and has a theoretical risk of introducing infection.[385] It is not recommended by this author.

## ADMINISTRATION OF EPINEPHRINE

The administration of epinephrine has been shown to be effective in increasing the quality of the arthrograms, par-

ticularly those of the knee. Epinephrine reduces simultaneously the egress of contrast material from the joint and the influx of body fluid through the synovial membrane into the joint so that its addition to the injection solution enhances and prolongs the sharpness of the image provided by the contrast material.[376] This provides important additional time during which supplementary radiography, fluoroscopy, conventional tomography, or CT scanning may be performed. Although it is possible that intra-articular epinephrine has a direct irritant effect on the synovium or that it enhances indirectly any irritant effect of the positive contrast medium by prolonging the latter's contact time with the synovium,[383, 682] this is not documented and, if true, might be offset by a decrease or delay in joint distention caused by the epinephrine. In general, 0.2 to 0.3 ml of 1:1000 epinephrine is used in the evaluation of large articulations, such as the knee and glenohumeral joint, and 0.15 ml is used in smaller articulations, such as the elbow and ankle.

## FILM SUBTRACTION TECHNIQUES

Film subtraction techniques are useful in the evaluation of painful joint prostheses, especially in the hip and knee (see Chapter 19). Methylmethacrylate cement impregnated with barium has been used in the fixation of the acetabular and femoral components during total hip arthroplasty and of the femoral, tibial, and, possibly, patellar components during total knee arthroplasty. The barium impregnated cement appears on conventional radiographs as a radiodense region that facilitates the delineation of abnormal radiolucent gaps at the interface of cement and bone, metal, or polyethylene. Arthrography with radiopaque contrast material further documents the presence of these gaps, which, when extensive, indicate prosthetic loosening with or without infection. Unfortunately, during arthrography, the contrast material, which extends between cement and bone or metal, is obscured by the radiopacity of the cement itself. Because of this, subtraction technique may be necessary.

Although the standard method of film subtraction (Fig. 13–2) involves the preparation of a subtraction mask from the initial scout radiograph and the superimposition of this mask on each of the succeeding films obtained during the administration of the contrast material, digital radiographic equipment represents a newer method that may be employed to perform subtraction arthrography.[390, 683] This technique, which is described more completely elsewhere in this chapter, can correct for patient movement, allows rapid sequential images to be obtained, and can be processed in a positive or negative mode (Fig. 13–3). Digital subtraction arthrography is most useful when applied to the evaluation of the wrist, allowing the examiner to monitor the sites of abnormal communication of one compartment with another.[391, 684]

## POSTEXERCISE AND STRESS VIEWS

Application of stress is fundamental to the success of certain arthrographic examinations, such as those of the knee (see later discussion). It also is a useful technique in the arthrographic evaluation of ligamentous injuries of the ankle, wrist, and first metacarpophalangeal joint.

In some situations, properly performed arthrography in-

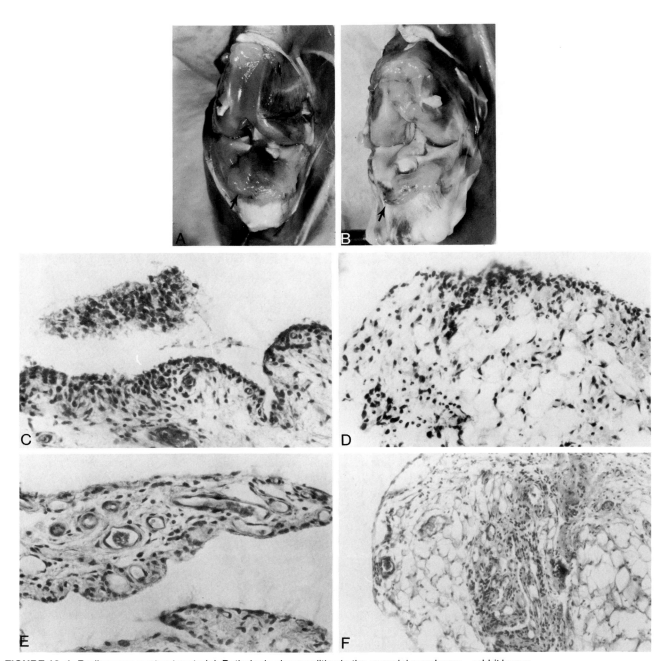

**FIGURE 13–1.** Radiopaque contrast material: Pathologic abnormalities in the synovial membrane—rabbit knees.

**A** Meglumine diatrizoate (Renografin-M 60, Squibb). Two hours after 1.5 ml of Renografin was injected, observe edematous and hemorrhagic synovial tissue (arrow).

**B** Diatrizoate sodium (Hypaque Sodium 50%, Winthrop). Twenty-four hours after the intra-articular injection of 1.5 ml of Hypaque, the synovium is contracted and adherent (arrow).

**C, D** Meglumine diatrizoate. Two hours **(C)** and 24 hours **(D)** after Renografin injection, histologic abnormalities are apparent in the knee. In **C,** observe proliferation and hypertrophy of synovial cells and dilated, congested vessels. In **D,** focal proliferation of surface synovial cells and stromal infiltration by mononuclear cells, eosinophils, and a few mast cells are seen.

**E, F** Diatrizoate sodium. Two hours **(E)** after injection of Hypaque, marked dilation and congestion of the vessels are evident. Eosinophils are visible beneath the synovial surface and in the stroma. Twenty-four hours **(F)** after the injection, findings include dilation and congestion of vessels with marked mononuclear cell and eosinophil infiltration.

(From Pastershank SP, et al: Radiology *143*:331, 1982.)

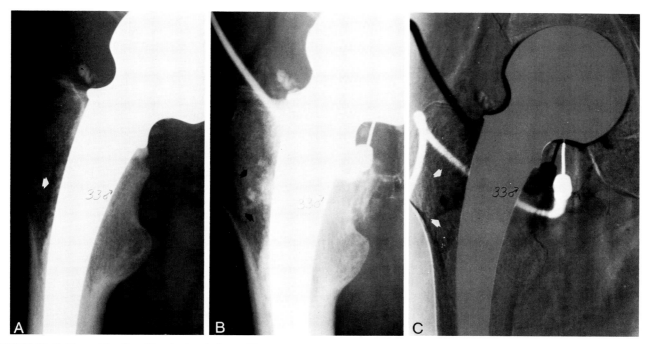

**FIGURE 13–2.** Film subtraction: Standard technique—Thompson prosthesis.

**A** The conventional film shows poor definition of the bone-cement interface (arrow).

**B** A radiograph obtained after the injection of 5 ml of radiopaque contrast material reveals a collection of the material at the bone-cement interface (arrows) and lymphatic filling.

**C** A subtraction film confirms the presence of contrast medium at the bone-cement interface (arrows) in this patient with an infected prosthesis.

(From Guerra J Jr, Resnick D: Appl Radiol, Mar–April 1984, p 83.)

cludes filming before and after passive or active movement of the joint. As an example, the arthrographic diagnosis of disruption of the rotator cuff of the shoulder may be possible only on those views obtained after movement or exercise of the glenohumeral joint. It still is advisable as a routine to obtain preexercise radiographs or fluoroscopic spot films owing to the deterioration of the sharpness of the contrast material and its soft tissue extravasation on those films obtained after articular movement.

## CONVENTIONAL AND COMPUTED TOMOGRAPHY

Conventional tomography is being employed increasingly in the arthrographic evaluation of certain joints, such as the elbow and ankle, in which overlapping and confusing lines exist and in which osteochondral fractures and intra-articular bodies may be hidden. Furthermore, many osteochondral fracture sites may not be tangential to the radiographic beam in the usual projections. In some instances, conventional arthrotomography may be the only means of demonstrating contrast medium tracking between an incompletely healed osteochondral fracture and the parent bone.

CT combined with arthrography has been used to assess chondral defects in some joints. It is useful for finding cartilaginous abnormalities in the anteroinferior glenoid rim (Bankart deformity) of the shoulder that have occurred subsequent to anterior dislocation or for finding a chondral fracture in the hip, particularly in association with pelvic disruption. The technique also is valuable in the detection of osteochondral bodies in any joint.

## INTRA-ARTICULAR PRESSURE RECORDING

The continual monitoring of changes in intra-articular pressure during the injection of increasing volumes of contrast fluid provides information regarding total articular capacity and compliance of the joint capsule. It may be accomplished by connecting the injection needle to a Hewlett-Packard pressure transducer and Hewlett-Packard strip-chart recorder using an air-free manometer tubing system. When this equipment is combined with a pump that infuses fluid at a fixed rate, accurate measurements of intra-articular pressure can be expected.

Although such measurements from the joint cavity have been used mainly in experimental situations, certain clinical applications of the technique are apparent. The determination of intra-articular pressure during arthrography of the glenohumeral joint can provide pressure versus volume curves that deviate from the biphasic shape of the normal curve in patients with complete disruption of the rotator cuff (in which pressure readings remain depressed owing to free passage of fluid from the articular cavity to the subacromial bursa) and in those with adhesive capsulitis (in which there appears an abnormal increase in intra-articular pressure at all injection volumes).[392, 726] As the arthrographic diagnosis of adhesive capsulitis in this location as well as elsewhere, such as the hip, wrist, and ankle, is based primarily on a "tight" feel due to increased resistance during the injection process, analysis of pressure-volume relationships provides a more precise means of establishing the presence and severity of the condition.

Intracapsular pressure monitoring during arthrographic evaluation of painful joint prostheses also may have clinical

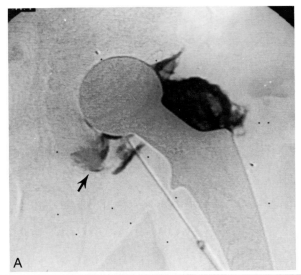

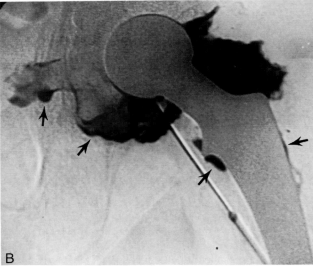

**FIGURE 13–3.** Film subtraction: Digital technique—total hip arthroplasty. Subtraction images obtained after the injection of 5 ml **(A)** and 15 ml **(B)** of contrast agent readily allow identification of abnormal collections of the contrast material (arrows). (From Resnick D, et al: Invest Radiol *19*:434, 1984.)

importance[393] (Fig. 13–4). It allows the identification of the specific pressure within the joint at which contrast material insinuates itself into the bone-cement or the prosthesis-cement interface, or both. It is reasonable to assume that abnormal leakage of contrast material that becomes evident at lower intra-articular pressure is more significant than that at higher pressure, and that such extravasation appearing almost immediately at extremely low intra-articular pressure indicates grossly loose prostheses. This technique also allows identification of postoperative adhesive capsulitis, characterized by small intra-articular capacity and rapid elevation of joint pressure during the infusion of fluid.

## COMPLICATIONS

Arthrography is considered a safe procedure. Initial reports describing pneumoarthrography included occasional examples of complications, such as pain, swelling, and sub-

cutaneous emphysema.[307, 308] The most serious complication was reported by Kleinberg in 1927.[309] In this report, a 19 year old youth was subjected to pneumoarthrography of the knee because of a possible intra-articular fragment. The needle had been inserted in a less than careful fashion, after which it was connected to an oxygen tank and oxygen was administered. The patient immediately complained of chest pain and a feeling of "dying." He subsequently became pulseless with widely dilated pupils, absent respirations, and an inaudible heart beat. At this point, the patient was "apparently dead." Resuscitation and intracardiac injection of epinephrine revived the patient and he was discharged from the hospital 10 days after the procedure. Because a knee radiograph obtained shortly after the procedure failed to reveal intra-articular or periarticular gas, it was suggested that a stream of oxygen was forced directly into the bloodstream, occluding vessels in the lungs and producing cardiac failure.

As currently performed, arthrography rarely is associated with significant complications. Newberg and associates[394] conducted a survey of 57 radiologists experienced in arthrography who had performed more than 126,000 arthrographic procedures. There were no deaths, three cases of infection, and 61 cases of hives. Other acute reactions, all of which were extremely rare, included hypotension, seizures, air embolism, and laryngeal edema. More frequently, mild pain and discomfort are encountered during the procedure. Subsequent to it, synovitis with pain and swelling occasionally is apparent, particularly in patients with preexisting synovial inflammation. This complication generally is transient, disappearing within a day or two. Joint sepsis rarely is observed if proper sterile technique is employed. A vasovagal response may result in temporary lightheadedness and hypotension, but these symptoms quickly disappear.

Hypersensitivity reaction to iodinated contrast agent rarely is observed. Although the potential problem exists of performing arthrography in a patient who has had a previously documented reaction to contrast material, the examination generally is accomplished in such persons without precipitating recurrent reactions.[394] Although pretreatment commonly is recommended in this situation,[395] it does not definitively prevent a reaction. An alternative approach is to perform arthrography using air alone,[396] particularly in patients with a history of previous reaction to contrast material who exhibit great apprehension or reluctance regarding the examination.

## WRIST AND HAND

### Arthrography of the Wrist

Arthrography of the wrist (Tables 13–1 and 13–2) is a safe procedure, which sometimes is useful in the diagnosis of traumatic and other articular disorders.[1–5, 397, 398, 703]

### Technique (Fig. 13–5)

The standard arthrographic technique is well described. Under fluoroscopic control, a 22 gauge, 1.5 inch long needle is introduced into the wrist from a dorsal approach. Most often, the radiocarpal compartment is the site of injection, although other compartments of the wrist may be studied (see later discussion). For a radiocarpal joint arthro-

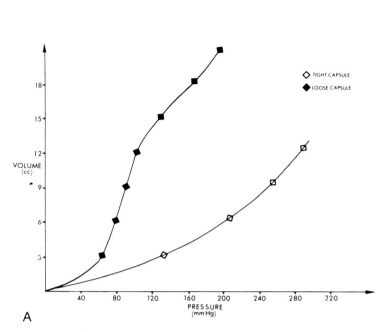

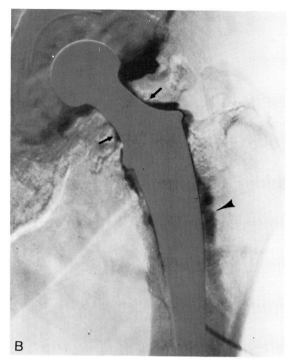

**FIGURE 13–4.** Intra-articular pressure recording: Postoperative hip joint.

**A** Pressure recording in patients with normal capsular compliance and with adhesive capsulitis. In two different patients with painful hips after total joint replacement, the pressure versus volume curves indicate a more rapid rise in intra-articular pressure associated with adhesive capsulitis (tight capsule).

**B** Adhesive capsulitis. This subtraction radiograph obtained after the injection of 12 ml of the contrast agent (intra-articular pressure greater than 360 mm Hg) shows a constricted capsule (arrows) and the abnormal accumulation of the contrast material at the bone-cement and metal-cement interfaces on the femoral side of the joint. Permeation of a segment of the lateral femoral cement mantle by the contrast agent (arrowhead) is seen.

gram, the needle is guided under the radial lip, entering the radiocarpal compartment between the scaphoid and the radius. Occasionally, this compartment must be entered at the junction of scaphoid, lunate, and radius, but at this site, care must be taken not to place the needle too far distally, such that the scapholunate interosseous ligament is violated. A total of 1.5 to 2.5 ml of 60 per cent meglumine diatrizoate (Renografin) is administered. Posteroanterior, lateral, and oblique radiographs are obtained before and after mild exercise.

In recent years, several modifications in this technique have been emphasized. Fluoroscopic monitoring combined with sequential spot filming or videotaping during the injection of contrast material allows more precise delineation of sites of abnormal compartmental communication.[399, 400, 705] Magnification radiography, analysis of joint motion, and application of stress are additional techniques that have

been advocated for more definitive diagnosis.[400, 401] Conventional tomography or CT scanning after the introduction of the contrast agent has allowed the identification of exact sites of perforation of the triangular fibrocartilage[402, 704] as well as ligamentous disruption and cartilage loss,[403] although the procedure significantly prolongs the time of the examination. Selective injection of the midcarpal compartment, rather than the radiocarpal compartment, has been introduced as a superior method for analysis of the scapholunate and lunotriquetral ligaments,[404] owing to less obscuration by the contrast material although, alone, it will not allow identification of a tear of the triangular fibrocartilage in the presence of intact intercarpal ligaments (see later discussion).[663]

Digital arthrography can be used successfully in the examination of the wrist. The technique combines the advantages of fluoroscopic monitoring and videotaping and provides the examiner with the opportunity to view the dynamics of the injection process in both the positive and the negative mode.[391, 684, 706–708] The technique used involves an initial test exposure and subsequent multiple exposures

**TABLE 13–1. Wrist Arthrography: Key to Numbers Used to Identify Structures**

1. Radiocarpal compartment
2. Inferior radioulnar compartment
3. Prestyloid recess
4. Extensor tendons and sheaths
5. Lymphatics
6. Midcarpal compartment
7. Common carpometacarpal compartment
8. Volar radial recesses
9. Pisiform-triquetral compartment

**TABLE 13–2. Indications for Wrist Arthrography**

Evaluation of:
Presence and extent of synovial inflammation
Injuries to the triangular fibrocartilage, interosseous ligaments, and joint capsule
Soft tissue masses

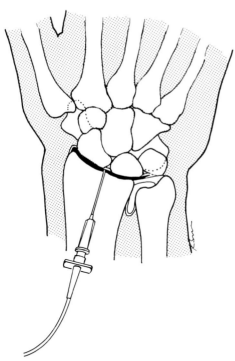

**FIGURE 13–5.** Wrist arthrography: Technique. Radiocarpal joint injection. A needle is introduced into the radiocarpal compartment from a dorsal approach and 1.5 to 2.5 ml of contrast material is injected.

obtained at the rate of approximately one exposure each second for 20 to 30 sec during the administration of the contrast agent (Fig. 13–6). An image acquired before the appearance of the contrast medium is used as a mask that is subtracted from the remaining frames in the run. Subtraction images are displayed in real time during the procedure and are reviewed in a closed-loop movie format at the conclusion of the study. Sandbags placed on the patient's forearm prevent significant movement; slight degrees of wrist motion produce artifacts that generally can be eliminated altogether by reregistration of the digitized image. The digital technique has many other advantages, including the ability to subtract the carpal bones from the sequential images, providing a clear view of the distribution of the contrast material during the injection process. Furthermore, if more than one wrist compartment is injected (see following discussion), digital technique with subtracted images can eliminate any contrast material that had resulted from previous opacification of other compartments.[707, 708]

In recent years, great interest has developed regarding the technique of three-compartment wrist arthrography, in which separate injections into the radiocarpal, midcarpal, and inferior radioulnar compartments are employed. This method was popularized by Levinsohn and colleagues.[709–711] The rationale for this technique was based on the existence of abnormalities involving only the proximal surface of the triangular fibrocartilage or of disruptions of this fibrocartilage or the interosseous ligaments of the wrist that allowed passage of contrast material in only one direction and not the other; such abnormalities might not be detected with radiocarpal arthrography alone. Other investigators have

questioned the need for multicompartmental arthrography of the wrist and have emphasized the importance of full distention of the radiocarpal compartment (or other compartments) to ensure visualization of all sites of compartmental communication.[712, 713]

Based on an analysis of reported data, three-compartment wrist arthrography represents the most reliable arthrographic method in the detection of communications among the various compartments of the wrist. The procedure, however, is more time consuming than single compartment arthrography. Furthermore, it is not clear if those tears of the triangular fibrocartilage or interosseous ligaments in the proximal carpal row that allow contrast material to pass in only one direction are clinically significant. Indeed, communications among the compartments of the wrist have been documented in asymptomatic persons, and identical arthrographic abnormalities may be encountered when bilateral wrist examinations are performed and comparison is made between the symptomatic and asymptomatic sides.[714] Some reports have indicated that arthrographic results correlate better with ulnar-sided rather than radial-sided pain.[715]

### Normal Wrist Arthrogram (Figs. 13–7 and 13–8)

Contrast opacification of the radiocarpal compartment reveals a concave sac with smooth synovial surfaces extending between the distal end of the radius and proximal carpal row. The prestyloid recess appears as a finger-like projection that approaches the ulnar styloid process from the ulnar limit of the radiocarpal joint. One or more volar radial recesses are located beneath the distal end of the radius.

If the midcarpal joint is injected, contrast material normally will extend proximally between the scaphoid and lunate and between the lunate and triquetrum to the level of the scapholunate and lunotriquetral interosseous ligaments. It will extend distally into the common carpometacarpal and intermetacarpal compartments. If the distal radioulnar joint is injected, contrast material sits like a cap on the articular surface of the ulna.[716] A small diverticulum extending into the proximal surface of the triangular fibrocartilage has been reported as a normal variation.[717]

As indicated in Chapter 22, communication between the radiocarpal compartment and other compartments in the wrist during arthrography may be observed in "normal" persons or cadavers. The radiocarpal compartment may communicate with the midcarpal compartment in 13 to 47 per cent of the population and with the inferior radioulnar compartment in 7 to 35 per cent.[2, 3, 6] The prevalence of these findings increases in older persons.[405] Arthrographic communication between the radiocarpal and pisiform-triquetral compartments is frequent, particularly with forceful injection of contrast material into either compartment.[5, 7] It is observed in more than 50 per cent of cases.[405] Arthrographic communication between the pisiform-triquetral and midcarpal compartments, however, is considered abnormal.[684]

Opacification of tendon sheaths and lymphatics generally is not observed in "normal" wrist arthrograms,[2] although Trentham and associates[6] indicated that tendon sheath visualization may be apparent in 6 per cent of such normal examinations.

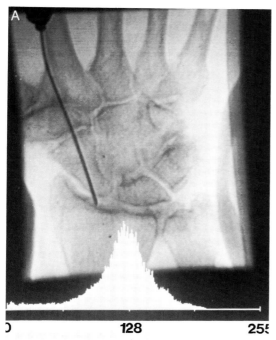

**FIGURE 13–6.** Wrist arthrography: Digital technique—cadaver. Radiocarpal joint injection.

**A** A test exposure is obtained prior to the introduction of the contrast material and is evaluated by computer algorithm to ensure adequate radiographic technique.

**B, C** Subtraction images are shown after the injection of 0.5 ml **(B)** and 1.0 ml **(C)** of the contrast agent into the radiocarpal joint. In **B,** there is slight irregularity of the contrast agent in the radial aspect of the radiocarpal joint (1). In **C,** most of the radiocarpal compartment (1) has been opacified and filling of the inferior radioulnar joint (2) is occurring through a small defect in the triangular fibrocartilage (arrowhead).

**D, E** Coronal sections of the wrist confirm minimal irregularity of the articular cartilage of the radius and scaphoid (arrow) and a perforation in the triangular fibrocartilage (arrowhead).

**(B, E** From Resnick D, et al: AJR *142*:1187, 1984. Copyright 1984, American Roentgen Ray Society.)

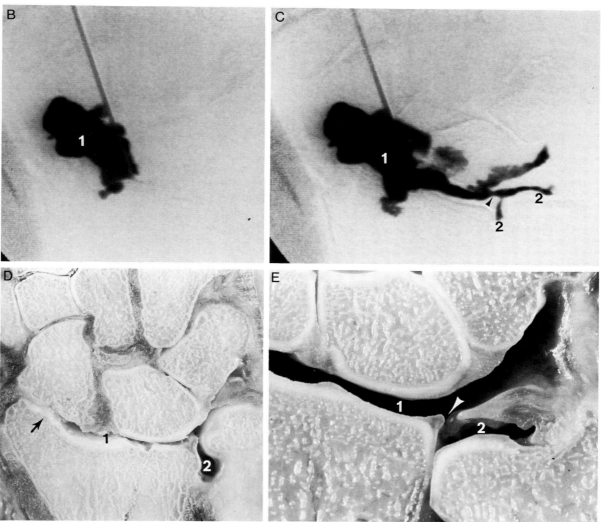

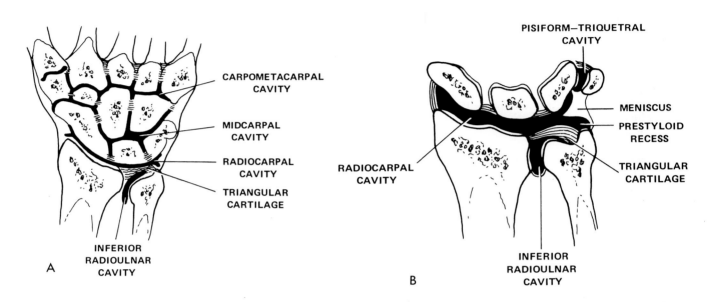

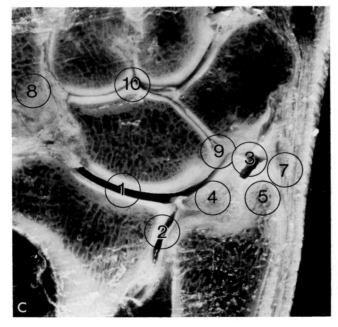

**FIGURE 13–7.** Wrist arthrography: Normal anatomy.

**A** Drawing of a coronal section of the wrist. Observe the radiocarpal cavity, which is separated from the inferior radioulnar cavity by the triangular fibrocartilage, and from the midcarpal cavity by interosseous ligaments extending between bones of the proximal carpal row. A (common) carpometacarpal cavity is indicated between the bones of the distal carpal row and bases of the four ulnar metacarpals. This compartment extends distally between the metacarpal bases as intermetacarpal compartments. The first carpometacarpal compartment also is indicated between the trapezium and base of the first metacarpal.

**B** Detailed drawing of the radiocarpal compartment. Note its C shape, with a Y-shaped ulnar limit produced by the meniscus. The proximal limb or diverticulum at the ulnar limit of the radiocarpal compartment is the prestyloid recess, which is intimate with the ulnar styloid. The distal limb extends along the triquetrum and may, in some instances, communicate with the pisiform-triquetral compartment.

**C** Coronal section of cadaveric wrist. Identified structures are the radiocarpal compartment (1), inferior radioulnar compartment (2), prestyloid recess (3), triangular fibrocartilage (4), ulnar styloid (5), ulnar collateral ligament (7), scaphoid (8), interosseous ligament between lunate and triquetrum (9), and midcarpal compartment (10).

**(B, C** From Resnick D: Radiology *113*:331, 1974.)

## Rheumatoid Arthritis (Figs. 13–9 and 13–10)

Injection of contrast material into the radiocarpal compartment in patients with rheumatoid arthritis reveals certain abnormalities.[2, 5, 6, 8] The most characteristic changes are corrugated irregularity of the contrast material (25 to 90 per cent) and opacification of lymphatic vessels (30 to 38 per cent). These two findings are not specific for rheumatoid arthritis but are reliable indicators of synovial inflammation. The corrugated pattern suggests villous hypertrophy of the synovial membrane and may be evident initially at specific sites in the radiocarpal compartment, such as the prestyloid or volar radial recesses.[8, 9] The basis of the lymphatic filling is not entirely known. The synovial membrane contains lymphatics, particularly along the volar aspect of the wrist. Synovial inflammation and hypertrophy in rheumatoid arthritis and related disorders may increase the permeability of the synovial membrane, allowing greater and more rapid absorption of contrast material by both vascular and lymphatic channels. This has been substantiated by radioisotopic studies revealing more rapid clearance of contrast material from rheumatoid joints than from traumatic articulations.[10] Lymphatic hyperplasia is well recognized in rheumatoid arthritis,[11] and lymphatic filling has been observed in other rheumatoid joints during arthrography.[12, 13] Lymphatic filling occasionally may be seen in normal persons with overdistention of the articular cavity during arthrography of the wrist or other joints.

Communication between the radiocarpal compartment and other compartments in the rheumatoid wrist is frequent. This communication, which may occur between radiocarpal and midcarpal compartments (35 to 70 per cent), radiocarpal and inferior radioulnar compartments (55 to 70 per cent), radiocarpal and common carpometacarpal compartments (53 per cent), and radiocarpal and pisiform-triquetral compartments (50 per cent), lacks specificity as a finding of rheumatoid arthritis because of its common occurrence in normal persons[2, 3, 6] and in patients with other types of articular disease.[5]

Tendon sheath visualization after radiocarpal compartment arthrography is observed in 20 to 28 per cent of rheumatoid wrists, presumably related to inflammatory synovial tissue or pannus within the articular cavity and tendon sheaths. This visualization is observed more frequently on the dorsum of the wrist related to filling of the sheaths about the extensor tendons. Tendon sheath visualization is not a reliable indicator of rheumatoid arthritis because of its occasional occurrence in other articular diseases[5] and normal persons.[6]

In summary, wrist arthrography in patients with rheumatoid arthritis reveals certain abnormalities that suggest the presence of synovial inflammation. These abnormalities, particularly a corrugated synovial pattern and lymphatic filling, are not specific for rheumatoid arthritis, as they occur in other disorders with predominant synovial hypertrophy. Wrist arthrography may be helpful in indicating the presence and extent of synovial inflammation and its response to treatment (Table 13–3), although MR imaging is a superior technique in this regard (see Chapters 25 and 70).

### Trauma

The assessment of injury to the triangular fibrocartilage complex and interosseous carpal ligaments represents the major indication for wrist arthrography today, although MR imaging also is useful in this assessment (see Chapter 70).

Arthrographic abnormalities occurring after wrist trauma include compartmental communications, tendon sheath visualization, and mild synovial irregularity.[4, 5, 14, 335, 407, 408] These abnormalities may follow a single traumatic episode or relate to repetitive trauma. In this latter situation, occupational trauma, such as occurs in pneumatic drillers or boxers, may produce similar arthrographic alterations[5] (Fig. 13–11).

The pattern of compartmental communication depends on the site of trauma. With injuries to the triangular fibrocartilage or ulnar styloid, communication between the radiocarpal and inferior radioulnar compartments is observed (Fig. 13–12). In these instances, the capsule about the inferior radioulnar joint also may be disrupted, with soft tissue extravasation of contrast material. With scaphoid fractures or injuries to the interosseous ligaments between the bones of the proximal carpal row, communication between the radiocarpal and midcarpal compartments is seen (Figs. 13–13 to 13–15). Direct arthrographic opacification of other compartments of the wrist or tissue extravasation[408] may delineate capsular injuries (Fig. 13–16).

Synovial irregularity is absent or localized on wrist arthrograms after trauma.[5] Tendon sheath communication may be observed but lymphatic filling generally is absent. Contrast material that enters the substance of a ligament is consistent with rupture.[409] Osteocartilaginous fragments produce intra-articular filling defects.[410, 411]

Wrist arthrography has a definite role in allowing identification of the cause of the patient's symptoms and signs after trauma. This role is better established in instances of ulnar-sided pain and in young persons, in whom compart-

*Text continued on page 297*

**TABLE 13–3. Frequency of Arthrographic Abnormalities in Arthritic Disorders of the Wrist**

| Disorder | Abnormality | | | | |
| | Synovial Irregularity | | Lymphatic Filling | Compartment Communication | Tendon Communication |
| | *Corrugated* | *Noncorrugated* | | | |
| --- | --- | --- | --- | --- | --- |
| Rheumatoid arthritis | + + + | | + + | + + + | + |
| Posttraumatic arthritis | | + | − | + + | + |
| Rheumatoid variant disorders | + + + | | + + | + + + | − |
| Neuropathic disease | | + + | − | + + | + |
| Occupation-induced arthritis | + + | | + | + + | − |
| Gout | + + | | + | + + | + |
| Septic arthritis | + + | | + + | + + | + |

+ = Mild abnormalities; + + = moderate abnormalities; + + + = severe abnormalities; − = no abnormality.

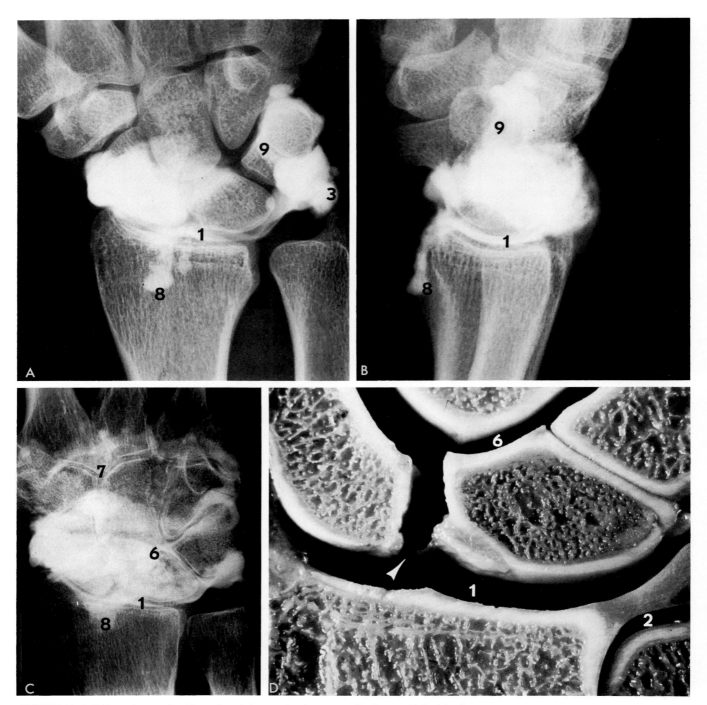

**FIGURE 13–8.** Wrist arthrography: Normal and abnormal arthrograms. Radiocarpal joint injection.

**A, B** Frontal and lateral views. Observe the contrast-filled radiocarpal compartment (1), which is communicating with the pisiform-triquetral compartment (9). Also note the prestyloid recess (3) and volar radial recesses (8).

**C, D** Radiocarpal–midcarpal compartment communication. A frontal radiograph after opacification of the radiocarpal compartment (1) reveals its communication with the midcarpal (6) and common carpometacarpal (7) compartments. This communication is possible when a defect exists in the interosseous ligaments extending between bones of the proximal carpal row. On a photograph of a coronal section of the cadaveric wrist, observe disruption of the scapholunate ligament (arrowhead). The inferior radioulnar compartment (2) and volar radial recesses (8) also are indicated.

*Illustration continued on opposite page*

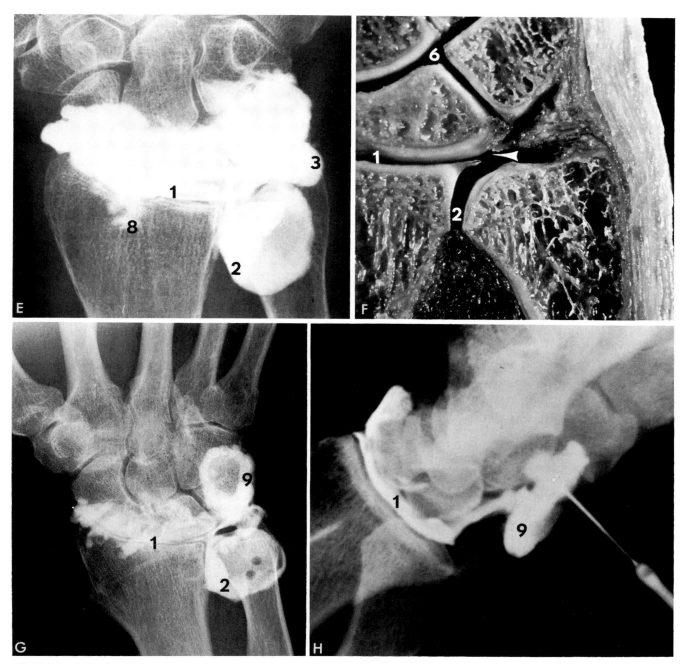

**FIGURE 13–8** Continued

**E, F** Radiocarpal–inferior radioulnar compartment communication. A frontal radiograph after opacification of the radiocarpal compartment (1) reveals its communication with the inferior radioulnar compartment (2). This communication is possible when a defect exists in the triangular fibrocartilage. Such a defect (arrowhead) is illustrated on a photograph of a coronal section of the wrist. Other indicated structures are the midcarpal compartment (6), volar radial recesses (8), and prestyloid recess (3).

**G, H** Radiocarpal compartment–pisiform-triquetral compartment communication. A frontal radiograph after introduction of contrast material into the radiocarpal compartment (1) demonstrates its communication with the pisiform-triquetral compartment (9) and inferior radioulnar compartment (2). On an oblique radiograph in another patient, a needle has been inserted into the pisiform-triquetral compartment (9). Overdistention of this cavity allows contrast material to flow into the radiocarpal compartment (1).

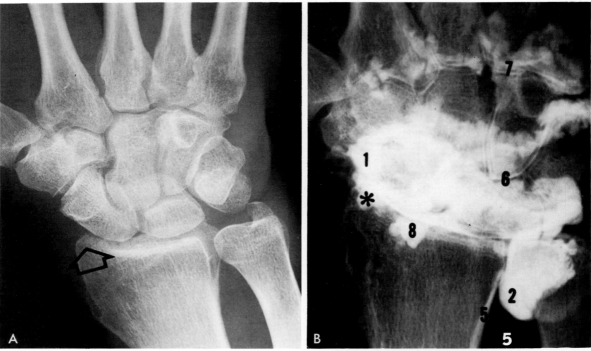

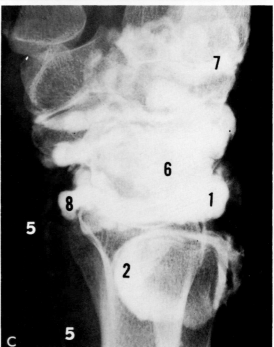

**FIGURE 13–9.** Wrist arthrography: Rheumatoid arthritis.

**A** On the initial film, a small erosion of the radial styloid is evident (arrow).

**B, C** Posteroanterior **(B)** and oblique **(C)** views after radiocarpal joint arthrography demonstrate severe synovial irregularity or corrugation (asterisk), radiocarpal compartment (1) communication with the inferior radioulnar (2), midcarpal (6), and common carpometacarpal (7) compartments, lymphatic filling (5), and prominent volar radial recesses (8).

(From Resnick D: Radiology *113*:331, 1974.)

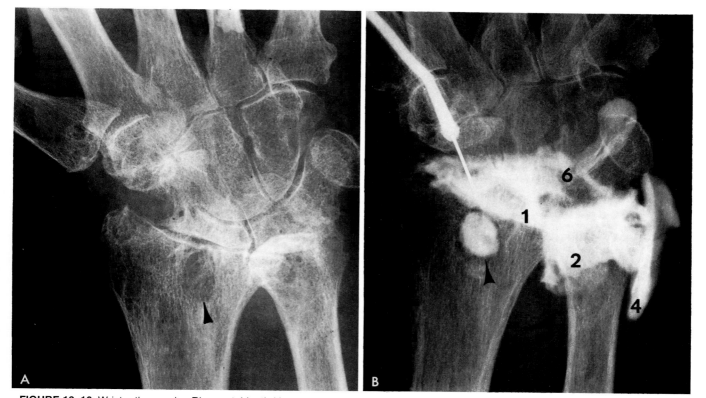

**FIGURE 13–10.** Wrist arthrography: Rheumatoid arthritis.

  **A** The initial film demonstrates severe rheumatoid involvement of the wrist with erosions, subchondral cysts (arrowhead), and subluxation.

  **B** After radiocarpal compartment (1) arthrography, observe filling of the inferior radioulnar (2) and midcarpal (6) compartments and opacification of the extensor carpi ulnaris tendon sheath (4) and radial cyst (arrowhead). The synovium is slightly irregular.

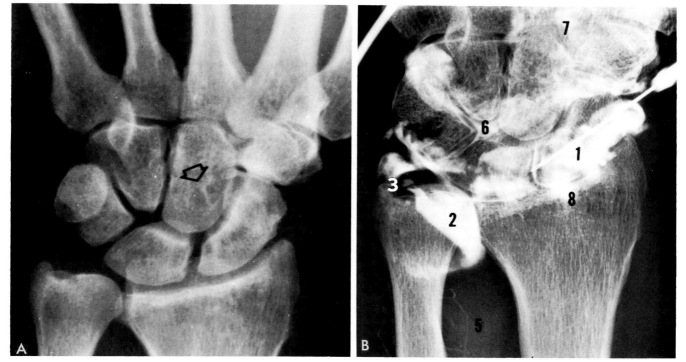

**FIGURE 13–11.** Wrist arthrography: Occupational trauma—driller's disease. This 61 year old man had worked as a pneumatic driller for 35 years and had intermittent wrist pain and swelling.

  **A** The initial film reveals extensive cystic abnormality throughout the carpal bones (arrow).

  **B** After opacification of the radiocarpal compartment (1), contrast material outlines the inferior radioulnar (2), midcarpal (6), and common carpometacarpal (7) compartments, volar radial recesses (8), prestyloid recess (3), and lymphatics (5).

  (From Resnick D: Radiology *113*:331, 1974.)

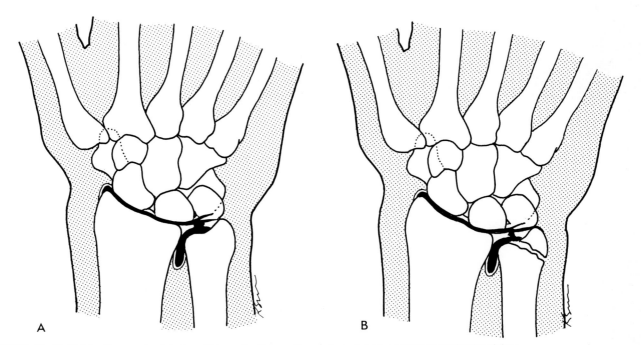

**FIGURE 13–12.** Wrist arthrography: Injuries of triangular fibrocartilage, ulnar styloid, and inferior radioulnar joints.

    **A, B** Diagrams indicate the pattern of compartmental communication that may be seen after isolated injury to the triangular fibrocartilage **(A)** or ulnar styloid **(B).** In both instances, contrast material introduced into the radiocarpal compartment will opacify the inferior radioulnar compartment through defects in the triangular fibrocartilage.

*Illustration continued on opposite page*

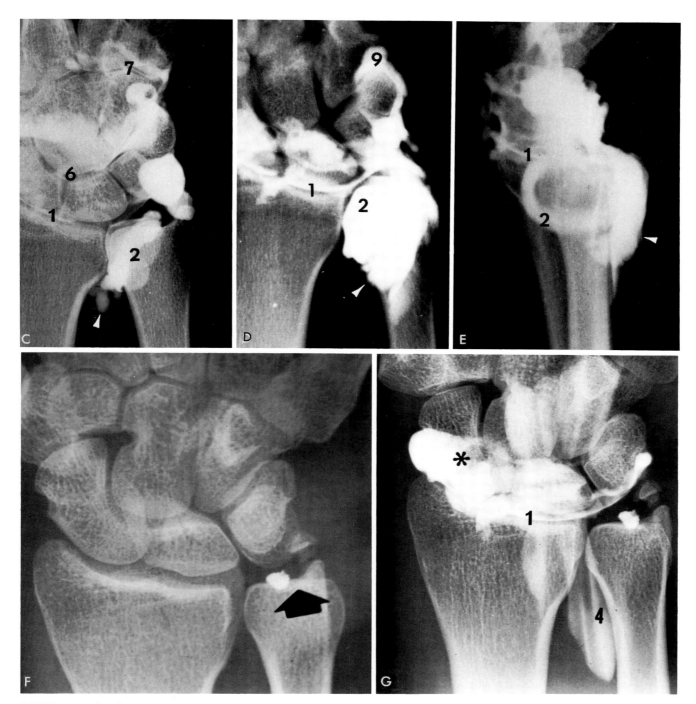

**FIGURE 13–12** *Continued*

**C** Triangular fibrocartilage injury. This young man developed pain over the distal end of the ulna after an injury. A radiocarpal joint arthrogram reveals communication between the radiocarpal compartment (1) and inferior radioulnar compartment (2). The midcarpal (6) and common carpometacarpal (7) compartments also are opacified. Small contrast-filled diverticula near the proximal aspect of the inferior radioulnar joint (arrowhead) may indicate a capsular tear.

**D, E** Triangular fibrocartilage and inferior radioulnar capsular injury. Another young patient with significant disability after an accident. Frontal **(D)** and lateral **(E)** radiographs after radiocarpal joint arthrography reveal communication of the radiocarpal compartment (1) with the inferior radioulnar (2) as well as the pisiform-triquetral compartment (9). Note soft tissue extravasation of contrast material from the inferior radioulnar compartment (arrowheads), indicating a capsular tear.

**F, G** Ulnar styloid injury. The initial film indicates a previous fracture of the ulnar styloid and a metallic fragment (arrow). The radiocarpal joint arthrogram outlines contrast material within the radiocarpal compartment (1), which is smooth in outline, opacification of extensor tendon sheaths (4), and a cartilaginous loose body (asterisk) producing a persistent filling defect.

**(F, G,** From Resnick D: Radiology *13*:331, 1974.)

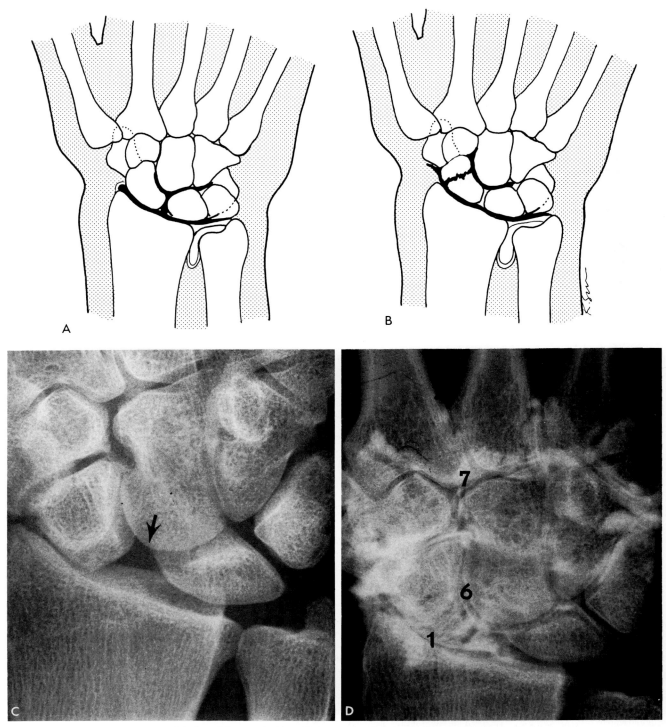

**FIGURE 13–13.** Wrist arthrography: Injuries of the scaphoid and interosseous ligaments of the proximal carpal row.

**A, B** Injury to the interosseous ligament between scaphoid and lunate **(A)** allows communication between the radiocarpal and midcarpal compartments. Similar communication may occur through a fracture of the scaphoid **(B).**

**C, D** Scapholunate dissociation with disruption of the scapholunate ligament. The initial film **(C)** reveals widening of the scapholunate space (arrow) and foreshortening of the scaphoid. Secondary degenerative joint disease of the radiocarpal compartment is seen. After radiocarpal joint arthrography **(D)** contrast material has flowed from the radiocarpal compartment (1) into the midcarpal (6) and common carpometacarpal (7) compartments. Contrast material overlies the scapholunate space.

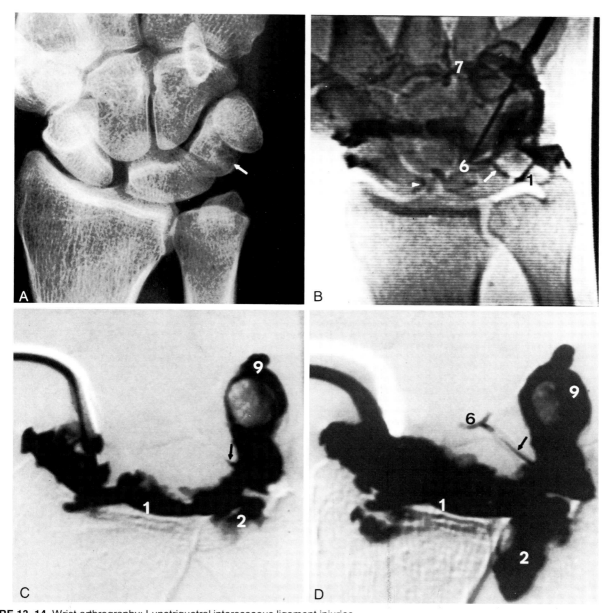

**FIGURE 13–14.** Wrist arthrography: Lunotriquetral interosseous ligament injuries.

**A, B** In this patient, the initial radiograph **(A)** reveals subtle loss of parallelism between the apposing surfaces of the lunate and the triquetrum and cystic changes in the triquetrum (arrow). The scapholunate space is abnormally wide. In **B,** a midcarpal compartment (6) injection of contrast material shows communication with the radiocarpal compartment (1) via the space between the lunate and the triquetrum (arrow). Although the contrast agent flows normally between the distal portions of the scaphoid and the lunate (arrowhead), it did not reach the radiocarpal compartment in this area. The common carpometacarpal (7) compartment also is opacified.

**C, D** In a cadaver, subtraction images are provided after the injection of 1.0 ml **(C)** and 2.0 ml **(D)** of contrast material into the radiocarpal compartment (1). In **C,** opacification of this compartment, the inferior radioulnar compartment (2) (indicating a tear of the triangular fibrocartilage), and the pisiform-triquetral compartment (9) is seen. A small amount of contrast agent is present in the space between the lunate and triquetrum (arrow). In **D,** opacification of the midcarpal compartment (6) has begun through a tear in the lunotriquetral interosseous ligament (arrow).

**(C, D,** From Resnick D, et al: AJR *142*:1187, 1984. Copyright 1984, American Roentgen Ray Society.)

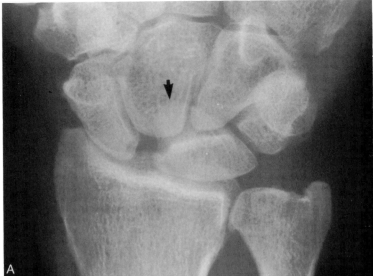

**FIGURE 13–15.** Wrist arthrography: Scapholunate and lunotriquetral ligament injuries.

**A** The initial radiograph shows widening between the scaphoid and lunate bones and dorsal tilting of the lunate with its volar border (arrow) located too far distally.

**B** An initial subtraction image after injection of the midcarpal joint (6) shows abnormal communication of this compartment with the radiocarpal compartment (1) through the lunotriquetral space (arrowhead), indicative of a tear of the lunotriquetral interosseous ligament. At this stage, the flow of contrast material between the scaphoid and lunate bones (arrow) is a normal finding.

**C** A subsequent subtraction image confirms also the presence of a scapholunate interosseous ligament tear as contrast material now has reached the radiocarpal joint (1) through the space between the scaphoid and lunate (arrow).

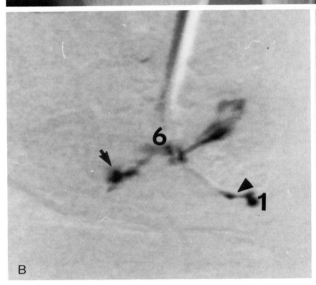

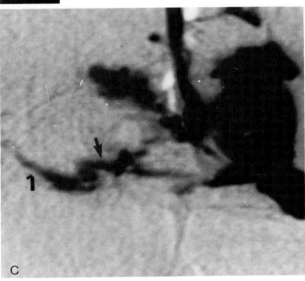

**FIGURE 13–16.** Wrist arthrography: Injury of the capsule about the first carpometacarpal joint. After direct opacification of this compartment, extravasation of contrast material on the radial aspect of the wrist (arrow) indicated a capsular injury.

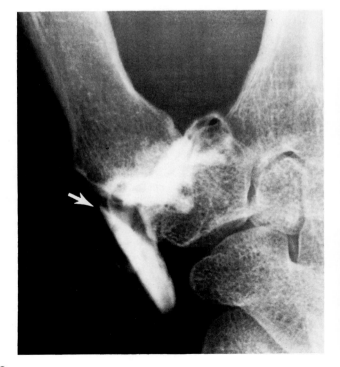

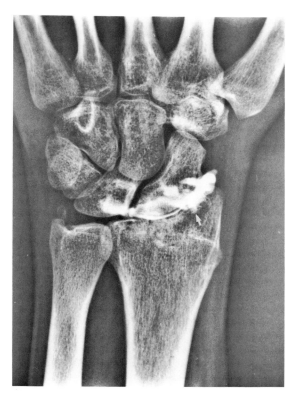

**FIGURE 13–17.** Wrist arthrography: Adhesive capsulitis. In this 20 year old man, only 0.5 ml of contrast material could be introduced into the radiocarpal joint. Observe incomplete filling of this compartment and small volar recesses (arrow). Note evidence of remote fractures of the radius and ulnar styloid.
(From Maloney MD, et al: Radiology *167*:187, 1988.)

mental communication may provide presumptive evidence of the site of soft tissue injury when initial radiographs are normal. In older patients, the frequency of such communication in asymptomatic persons limits the value of wrist arthrography. In the elderly, degeneration of the scapholunate or lunotriquetral interosseous ligament or triangular fibrocartilage allows communication among various compartments of the wrist.[718] In this regard, the association of degenerative perforations of both the lunotriquetral interosseous ligament and the triangular fibrocartilage, especially in persons with a long ulna, or ulnar plus variance, is well known.

The technique of wrist arthrography also is applicable to the acutely injured patient with a fracture of the distal portion of the radius, in whom the integrity of the triangular fibrocartilage is unknown,[412] or with a complex carpal dislocation when information is required regarding the specific sites of ligamentous disruption.[413] Furthermore, in instances of remote injury, the technique may be useful; the identification of contrast material within the fracture line of a previously disrupted scaphoid bone indicates the absence of osseous union.[646]

## Adhesive Capsulitis

Although the occurrence of adhesive capsulitis in the shoulder, hip, and ankle is relatively well known, that involving the wrist has received very little attention. In two articles, Maloney, Hanson, and their coworkers[719, 720] described 10 patients in whom persistent pain and limited range of motion in the wrist developed after trauma. Radio-

carpal joint arthrography showed decreased capacity, small volar and prestyloid recesses, and adhesions preventing complete opacification of the joint (Fig. 13–17). Extravasation of contrast material along the needle track also was evident. Closed manipulation of the wrist under general anesthesia may lead to clinical improvement.

### Other Articular Disorders

Arthrographic alterations in patients with other articular disorders are consistent with the pathogenesis of these disease processes. Reported findings in gout are compartmental and tendon sheath communications, lymphatic visualization, and synovial irregularity.[6] In this disease, communication between the radiocarpal and inferior radioulnar compartments is unusual, whereas communication between the radiocarpal and midcarpal compartments is more common (Fig. 13–18). Lymphatic visualization and corrugated synovial irregularity simulate the findings of rheumatoid arthritis.

It is expected that wrist arthrography in patients with rheumatoid variant disorders, such as psoriasis, Reiter's syndrome, and ankylosing spondylitis, would reveal abnormalities similar to those of rheumatoid arthritis. This has been documented in patients with ankylosing spondylitis, in whom wrist arthrograms demonstrate corrugated synovial irregularity, lymphatic filling, and compartmental and tendon sheath communication[5] (Fig. 13–19). In neuropathic osteoarthropathy, reported findings are noncorrugated synovial irregularity and compartmental and tendon sheath communication[5] (Fig. 13–20). In this disorder, localized

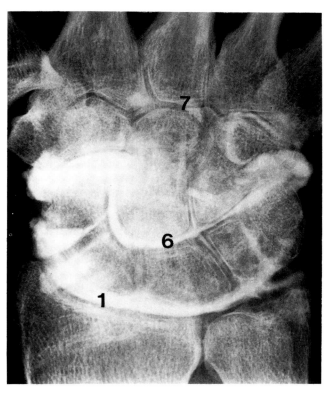

**FIGURE 13–18.** Wrist arthrography: Gouty arthritis. A radiocarpal joint arthrogram in a patient with gout demonstrates communication between the radiocarpal (1), midcarpal (6), and common carpometacarpal (7) compartments. The inferior radioulnar compartment does not opacify. The degree of synovial irregularity is mild.

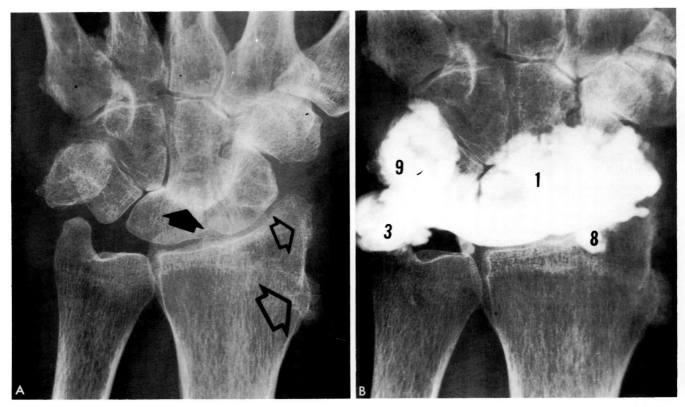

**FIGURE 13–19.** Wrist arthrography: Ankylosing spondylitis. A middle-aged man with ankylosing spondylitis and peripheral joint disease. On clinical examination, marked synovitis of the wrist was evident.

**A** The initial film demonstrates mild osteoporosis, irregular new bone formation in the distal portion of the radius (open arrows), and midcarpal joint space narrowing (solid arrow).

**B** A frontal view after radiocarpal joint arthrography indicates mild to severe corrugated synovial irregularity within the radiocarpal compartment (1), pisiform-triquetral compartment (9), prestyloid recess (3), and volar radial recesses (8).

(From Resnick D: Radiology *113*:331, 1974.)

synovial inflammation related to areas at which the synovial membrane is reflected over abnormal bone or intra-articular pieces of cartilage and bone, some embedded in the membrane itself, produces contrast irregularity. Compartmental and tendon sheath visualization is expected in neuropathic osteoarthropathy as a consequence of capsular and soft tissue disruption.

Wrist arthrography in patients with septic arthritis allows documentation of intra-articular needle placement for aspiration of joint contents. Subsequent contrast opacification will reveal findings similar to those of rheumatoid arthritis.[5]

### Evaluation of Soft Tissue Masses

Although wrist arthrography can provide useful information for the surgeon who is evaluating a patient with an adjacent soft tissue mass,[5, 15, 16, 414] such evaluation is accomplished far better by MR imaging (see Chapters 70 and 95). These masses may represent synovial cysts, ganglion cysts, or enlarged tendon sheaths.

In the evaluation of wrist ganglia, contrast material injected directly into the swelling may fail to opacify the wrist, whereas contrast material injected into the wrist may reveal its communication with the soft tissue mass[15, 703] (Fig. 13–21). This phenomenon of a "one-way valve" between the ganglion and articular cavity is similar to that noted

with synovial cysts about any articulation. It therefore is logical to first inject the joint itself. This usually will demonstrate the site of communication with filling of the soft tissue mass, although, in some cases, it is necessary to decompress the cyst initially. If, in fact, an arthrogram does not opacify the cystic mass, a second injection directly into the mass can be attempted.

Synovial cysts or herniations about the wrist are particularly frequent in rheumatoid arthritis, although they may accompany other articular disorders[16] (Fig. 13–22). As elsewhere, these cysts contain synovial fluid and may result from elevation of intra-articular pressure.

Cystic swelling about the wrist can indicate an enlarged tendon sheath (Fig. 13–23). In this situation, contrast opacification of the wrist may reveal communication with the sheath, allowing accurate diagnosis.[5]

### Arthrography of the Metacarpophalangeal and Interphalangeal Joints of the Hand

Arthrography of the metacarpophalangeal and interphalangeal joints is not performed commonly. Occasionally it may be useful in defining the extent of articular involvement in joint diseases, such as rheumatoid arthritis, or in delineating the presence and type of articular injury.

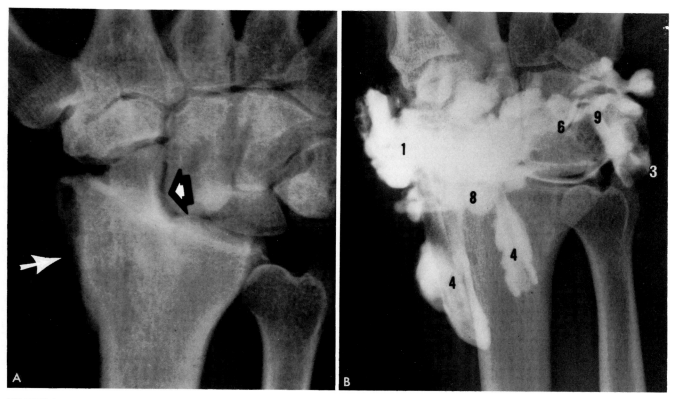

**FIGURE 13–20.** Wrist arthrography: Neuropathic osteoarthropathy. This 49 year old man had severe diabetes, peripheral neuropathy, and probable neuropathic disease of the wrist as well as the ipsilateral elbow and shoulder.

**A** The plain film indicates extensive sclerosis of the distal portion of the radius and scaphoid (arrows) and extreme joint space narrowing. Although the deformity of the distal end of the radius suggested a previous fracture, the patient denied a history of trauma.

**B** The radiocarpal joint arthrogram reveals localized synovial irregularity and capsular disruption of the radiocarpal compartment (1), communication with the midcarpal (6) and pisiform-triquetral (9) compartments, prominent volar radial recesses (8), opacification of the extensor tendon sheaths (4), and a persistent filling defect in the prestyloid recess (3).

(From Resnick D: Radiology *113*:331, 1974.)

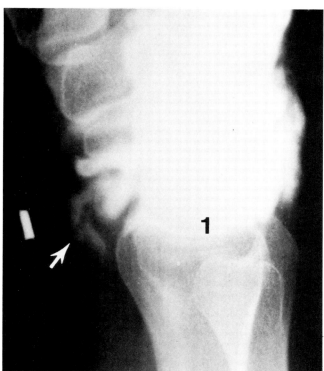

**FIGURE 13–21.** Wrist arthrography: Ganglion. After injection of contrast material into the radiocarpal compartment (1), a volar ganglion has opacified (arrow beneath metal marker), whose origin could be traced to the scapholunate space at surgery. Other wrist compartments also have filled with contrast material.

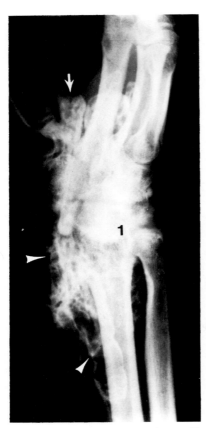

**FIGURE 13–22.** Wrist arthrography: Synovial cyst. After injection of the radiocarpal compartment (1) in this patient with rheumatoid arthritis, a large contrast-filled volar synovial cyst can be seen (arrowheads), which communicates with tendon sheaths (arrow).
(Courtesy of the late J. Bowerman, M.D., Baltimore, Maryland.)

### Technique (Fig. 13–24)

Injection of the metacarpophalangeal joint of the second, third, fourth, or fifth digit is best attempted under fluoroscopy with the digit flexed as much as 90 degrees.[17] The space between the metacarpal head and proximal phalanx then can be palpated and entered with a 22 or 26 gauge needle from a dorsolateral approach, adjacent to the extensor tendon. One to 1.5 ml of contrast material (Renografin) is injected. An alternative method consists of injecting the metacarpophalangeal joint with the finger in extension by inserting the needle from a radial (lateral) approach between the extensor apparatus and the articular surface. Injection of the first metacarpophalangeal joint is performed under fluoroscopic control from a dorsoradial approach with a 22 or 26 gauge needle, utilizing 1 to 1.5 ml of contrast material.[18-20]

Injection of the proximal interphalangeal or distal interphalangeal joints of the four medial digits and the interphalangeal joint of the thumb is accomplished under fluoroscopy from a dorsolateral approach adjacent to the extensor tendon using a 26 gauge needle and 0.5 to 1 ml of contrast material.

Modifications of metacarpophalangeal and interphalangeal joint arthrography include the use of double-contrast technique (radiopaque contrast media and air) and magnification.[415]

### Normal Arthrogram (Fig. 13–25)

Contrast opacification of the metacarpophalangeal joint reveals a linear collection between the metacarpal head and proximal phalanx with proximal recesses or extensions at the radial, ulnar, dorsal, and volar aspects of the joint. The volar part of the joint capsule has a triangular structure, like

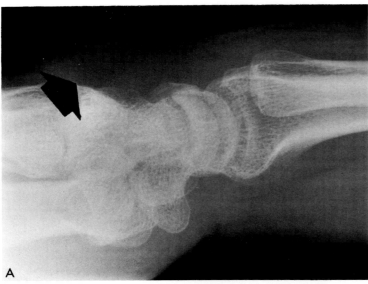
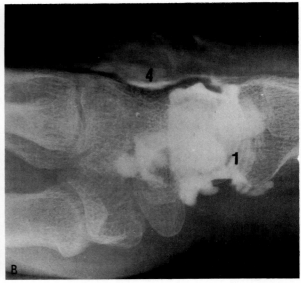

**FIGURE 13–23.** Wrist arthrography: Enlarged tendon sheath. A 28 year old man had a painful mass on the dorsum of the wrist. After radiography and arthrography, surgery was performed. At operation, 3 to 5 cm of hypertrophied gray synovium was noted in the extensor tendon sheaths. Microscopic evaluation demonstrated chronic synovial inflammation with cellular infiltration by lymphocytes and plasma cells as well as noncaseating granulomas.
  **A** The initial film reveals considerable soft tissue swelling on the dorsum of the wrist (arrow).
  **B** The radiocarpal joint arthrogram demonstrates communication of the radiocarpal compartment (1) with an irregular extensor tendon sheath (4).

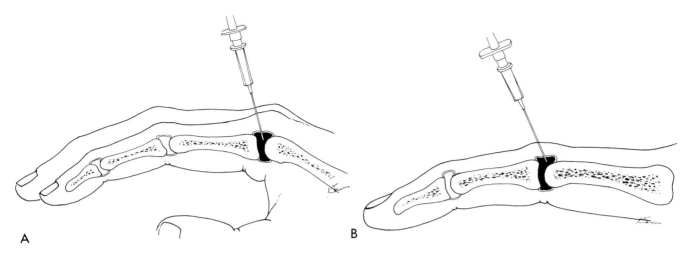

**FIGURE 13–24.** Metacarpophalangeal and interphalangeal joint arthrography: Technique. Injection into either the metacarpophalangeal **(A)** or interphalangeal **(B)** joints of the hand is best accomplished from a dorsal approach under fluoroscopic control.

a meniscus, which occupies the space between the articular surfaces.[415] At the first metacarpophalangeal joint, large proximal dorsal and volar recesses again are evident (10 to 20 mm in length), whereas the distal recesses are smaller (1 to 5 mm in length). The collateral ligaments produce small indentations at the joint line. Arthrography of the interphalangeal joints produces a similar pattern, with contrast material between the phalanges, larger proximal and smaller distal recesses, and waistlike defects at the sides related to the collateral ligaments.

### Abnormal Arthrogram

In rheumatoid arthritis and other synovial disorders, arthrographic findings include an irregular corrugated pattern of contrast material, enlarged articular cavities, perforations or retractions of the joint capsule, cartilage lesions, and lymphatic filling[21, 22] (Fig. 13–26).

After injury, opacification of the articular cavity may reveal disruption of the capsule and adjacent ligaments with soft tissue extravasation of contrast material. Opacification is particularly helpful at the first metacarpophalangeal joint in the evaluation of injuries on the ulnar aspect of the articulation, the gamekeeper's thumb[18–20, 23–26] (Fig. 13–27). In this clinical situation, damage to the ulnar collateral and accessory collateral ligaments, volar plate, and capsule may be observed. Arthrographic findings include extravasation of variable size along the ulnar aspect of the joint[18–20] and a filling defect produced by interposition of the dorsal aponeurosis between the torn ligament and its phalangeal attachment.[19, 20, 25] These findings may be associated with plain film abnormalities, such as fractures of the proximal phalanx and stress film changes of increased joint laxity, although arthrographic alterations may be the only radiographic abnormalities.

## Tenography and Bursography of the Hand and Wrist

Contrast opacification of tendon sheaths (tenography) and bursae (bursography) is a relatively simple radiographic procedure with limited clinical application. Tenography in rheumatoid arthritis allows accurate appraisal of the distribution and extent of synovial involvement of the tendon sheaths on the volar or dorsal aspect of the hand and wrist.[27–29] Outlining the synovial sheaths within the carpal tunnel may demonstrate local mechanical factors producing the carpal tunnel syndrome,[30] whereas visualization of sheaths or bursae on the volar aspect of the hand and wrist may provide insight into the pathogenesis and appearance of infections.[31] Most of these potential applications of tenography and bursography are better accomplished with MR imaging, however.

### Technique (Fig. 13–28)

Evaluation of flexor tendon sheaths of the fingers is accomplished by injecting 0.5 to 3 ml of Renografin.[30] A 22 gauge, 1.5 inch needle is introduced under fluoroscopy through the palmar skin overlying the distal one third of the proximal phalanx of the second through fifth digits. The needle is advanced in a proximal direction until increased resistance is encountered when the tip enters the tendon. The needle is withdrawn slightly, creating a sudden drop in resistance, and is advanced at a more shallow angle within the sheath. The injection of the sheath of the flexor pollicis longus is accomplished by flexing the terminal phalanx of the thumb, palpating the tendon, and inserting the needle directly into the sheath.

Contrast opacification of the extensor tendon sheaths on the dorsum of the wrist can be accomplished by palpating the tendons and advancing the needle into the sheath through the dorsal carpal ligament.[30]

Direct puncture of the bursae on the volar aspect of the wrist has been described. Five milliliters of contrast material can be injected into the ulnar bursa, outlining its normal communication with the digital flexor tendon sheaths.[32, 33]

### Normal Tenogram

**Digital Flexor Tendon Sheaths** (Fig. 13–29). The flexor tendons of the fingers, the sublimis digitorum and profundus digitorum, are enveloped by digital sheaths from a line of insertion of the flexor profundus to a line 1 cm proximal to the proximal border of the deep transverse ligament.[34] This arrangement, which is not constant, is most frequent in the index, middle, and ring fingers.[35] Any of these three

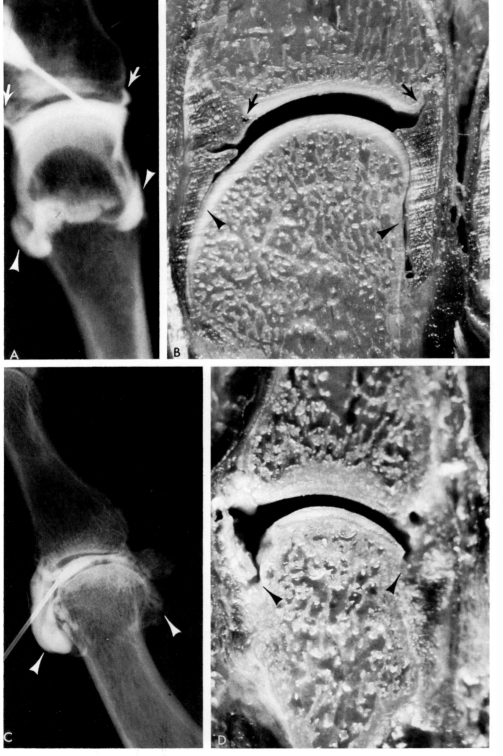

**FIGURE 13–25.** Metacarpophalangeal and interphalangeal joint arthrography: Normal arthrogram.

**A, B** Second metacarpophalangeal joint. Contrast opacification of this articulation reveals a smooth layer of radiopaque material between the metacarpal head and proximal phalanx and prominent proximal recesses (arrowheads) compared to distal recesses (arrows). A coronal section through the joint demonstrates the large proximal extent of the articular cavity (arrowheads) compared to the distal extent (arrows).

**C, D** First metacarpophalangeal joint. Contrast opacification of this articulation outlines a smooth synovial cavity with large proximal volar and dorsal recesses (arrowheads). On a coronal section, the extent of the proximal recesses can be seen (arrowheads).

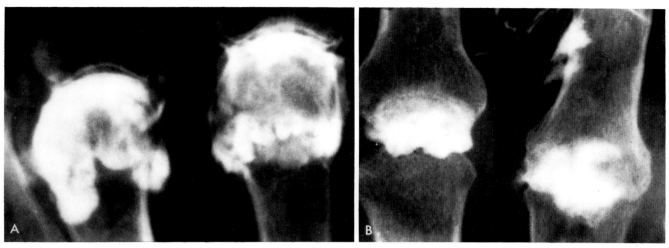

**FIGURE 13–26.** Metacarpophalangeal joint arthrography: Rheumatoid arthritis. In two patients with rheumatoid arthritis, opacification of the metacarpophalangeal joints demonstrates irregularity and filling defects consistent with synovial inflammation **(A)** and decreased joint capacity consistent with synovial fibrosis **(B)**. (Courtesy of M. Laval-Jeantet, M.D., Paris, France.)

sheaths may extend to the wrist.[36] The flexor sheath of the thumb extends from the terminal phalanx to a point 2 to 3 cm proximal to the proximal volar crease of the wrist, although on occasion a septum separates proximal and distal halves of the sheath.[35] The synovial sheath of the little finger also commences at its terminal phalanx. It may end near the deep transverse ligament or continue into the palm, expanding to envelop the adjacent tendons of the second, third, and fourth fingers.[34, 35, 37, 38]

**Synovial Sacs of the Palm** (Fig. 13–30). Communication between the individual digital tendon sheaths and synovial sacs or bursae in the palm is not constant[36]; most frequently, such continuation is noted involving the first digit. Not uncommonly the digital sheath of the fifth finger also continues into the palm.[35] Such communication is uncommon in the second, third, and fourth fingers.

The ulnar bursa on the medial aspect of the palm comprises three communicating invaginations[34, 35]; a superficial extension lies in front of the flexor sublimis, a middle one lies between the tendons of the sublimis and the profundus, and a deep extension is found behind the flexor profundus. The bursa, beginning at the proximal end of the digital sheaths, spreads out proximally, overlying the third, fourth, and fifth metacarpals. A statistical analysis of the tendon sheath patterns in the hand using air insufflation techniques in 367 cases demonstrated that the ulnar bursa communicated with the sheaths of the little finger in 81 per cent, of the index finger in 5.1 per cent, of the middle finger in 4.0 per cent, and of the ring finger in 3.5 per cent of cases.[36]

The radial bursa is the expanded proximal continuation of the digital sheath of the flexor pollicis longus muscle. It is found on the radial aspect of the palm overlying the second metacarpal. It continues proximally along the volar radial aspect of the wrist, terminating about 2 cm above the transverse carpal ligament.[34]

Intercommunications between the ulnar and radial bursae may be noted in 50 per cent of cases. Such connection is made via intermediate bursae. These accessory synovial sacs may be posterior in location, between the carpal canal and flexor profundus digitorum of the index finger, or, less commonly, anterior in location, between the superficial and

deep tendons of the index finger. A separate carpal sheath that does not communicate with either radial or ulnar bursa may be found enveloping the index flexor tendons.[34] Additionally, a small synovial sac may enclose the tendon of the flexor carpi radialis as it passes under the crest of the trapezium.[34]

**Carpal Tunnel** (Fig. 13–31). Tendons, vessels, and nerves passing from the forearm to the hand must traverse a canal on the volar surface of the wrist formed between a deep excavation on the undersurface of the carpal bones and the transverse volar carpal ligament. The latter extends in the wrist from the radial side (inserting on the trapezium, scaphoid, and occasionally the radial styloid) to the ulnar side (inserting into the pisiform and hook of the hamate). On its radial aspect, a small opening in the volar carpal ligament as it bridges the trapezium produces a tunnel for the flexor carpi radialis tendon. Through the canal proper, which is triangular in transverse section, pass the digital flexor tendons and sheaths and the median nerve. Compression of the latter may result in the carpal tunnel syndrome; this may be associated with local or systemic diseases[39, 40] (see Chapter 77).

**Extensor Tendon Sheaths** (Fig. 13–32). Several synovial sheaths are located in the dorsum of the wrist beneath the dorsal carpal ligament; they extend for a short distance proximal and distal to that ligament. By insular attachments of the dorsal carpal ligament on the posterior and lateral surfaces of the radius and ulna, six distinct avenues are created for transport of ligamentous structures. The most medial compartment (sixth compartment) contains the extensor carpi ulnaris tendon and sheath (4 to 5 cm long), lying at the dorsomedial aspect of the distal ulna. In the fifth compartment, a long sheath (6 to 7 cm long) covers the extensor digiti quinti proprius, which lies in close proximity to and may communicate with the inferior radioulnar joint. The fourth compartment on the posteromedial aspect of the radius contains a large sheath (5 to 6 cm long) enclosing the tendons of the extensor digitorum communis and the extensor indicis proprius. In the third compartment are the sheath (6 to 7 cm long) and tendon of the extensor pollicis longus. The sheath may extend as far distally as the

*Text continued on page 309*

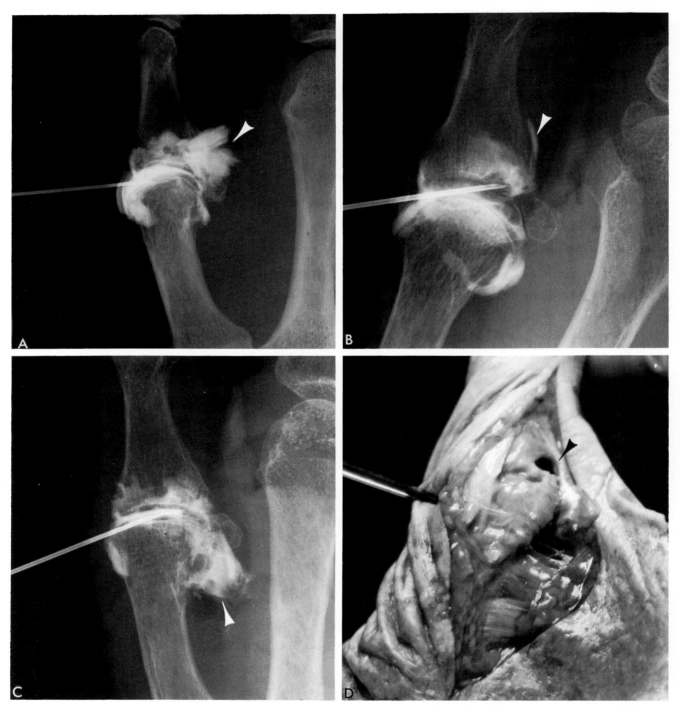

**FIGURE 13–27.** Metacarpophalangeal joint arthrography: Gamekeeper's thumb. After injury to the ulnar aspect of the first metacarpophalangeal joint, arthrography may reveal extravasation of contrast material.

**A–C** In these three cadavers, note the various patterns of contrast extravasation (arrowheads) along the ulnar side of the metacarpal head and proximal phalanx.

**D** A photograph of a dissection of cadaver in **C** outlines the space between the avulsed ligament and its origin on the proximal phalanx (arrowhead).

(From Resnick D, Danzig L: AJR *126*:1046, 1976. Copyright 1976. American Roentgen Ray Society.)

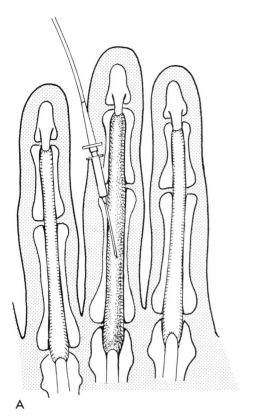

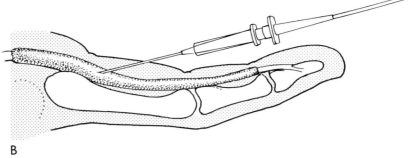

**FIGURE 13–28.** Tenography of the hand and wrist: Technique of injecting the distal flexor tendon sheaths. A palmar approach is used and a 22 gauge needle is placed within the sheath at the approximate level of the midportion of the proximal phalanx.

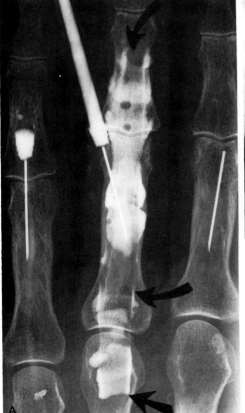

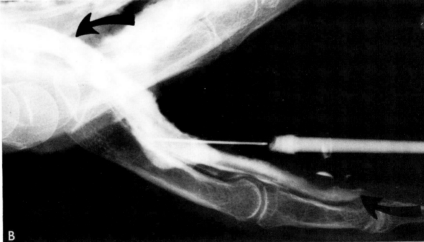

**FIGURE 13–29.** Tenography of the hand and wrist: Normal tenogram of the digital flexor tendon sheaths. Contrast medium within the synovial sheath (arrows) extends from a site close to the distal interphalangeal joint to another site proximal to the metacarpophalangeal joint. No communication with the palmar synovial sacs is seen. (From Resnick D: AJR *124*:44, 1975. Copyright 1975. American Roentgen Ray Society.)

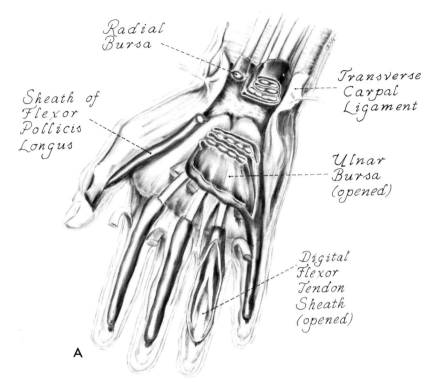

*Radial Bursa*

*Sheath of Flexor Pollicis Longus*

*Transverse Carpal Ligament*

*Ulnar Bursa (opened)*

*Digital Flexor Tendon Sheath (opened)*

A

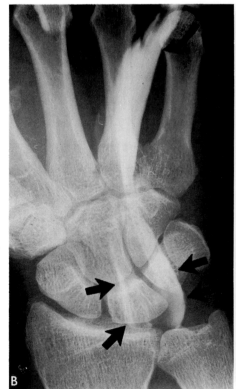

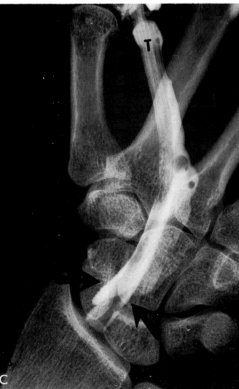

**FIGURE 13–30.** Tenography of the hand and wrist: Normal appearance of synovial sacs of the palm.

**A** The digital flexor tendon sheaths of the second through fourth fingers terminate proximal to the metacarpophalangeal joint. That of the fifth finger communicates with the ulnar bursa. The sheath of the flexor pollicis longus is continuous with the radial bursa. Note the three invaginations of the ulnar bursa and, in this drawing, absence of communication between radial and ulnar bursae.

**B** Injection of the digital sheath of the fifth finger (curved arrow) reveals communication with the ulnar bursa (straight arrows).

**C** The synovial sheath of the flexor pollicis longus (T) is continuous with the radial bursa (arrows).

*Illustration continued on opposite page*

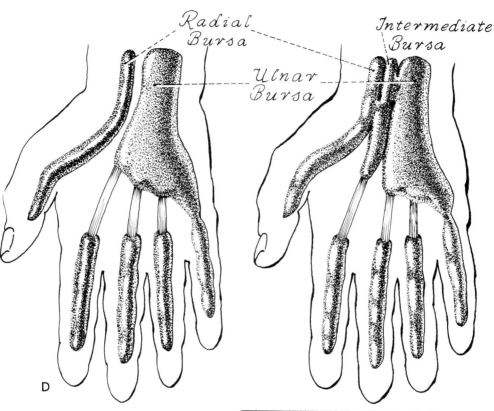

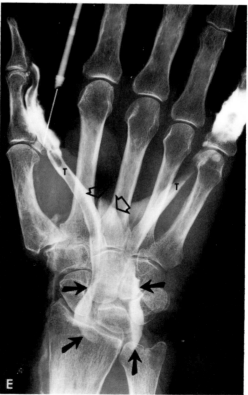

**FIGURE 13–30** *Continued*

**D** The radial and ulnar bursae may be separate, distinct cavities or may communicate via intermediate bursae.

**E** The digital flexor sheaths of the first and fifth fingers (T) extend into the wrist. A large palmar sac (solid arrows) consists of communicating radial and ulnar bursae. An intermediate bursa (open arrows) is recognizable.

(From Resnick D: AJR *124*:44, 1975. Copyright 1975, American Roentgen Ray Society.)

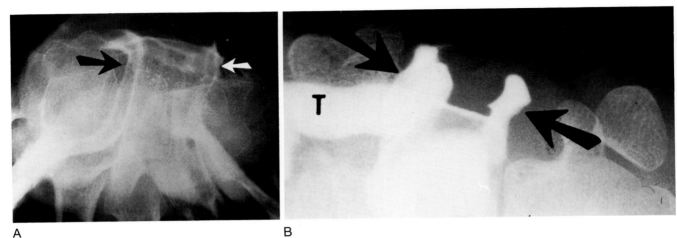

A                                          B

**FIGURE 13–31.** Tenography of the hand and wrist: Normal appearance of the carpal tunnel.
  **A** Contrast medium within the communicating radial and ulnar bursae delineates many flexor tendons within the carpal tunnel (arrows).
  **B** An injection of the sheath of the flexor pollicis longus (T) outlines a noncommunicating radial bursa (arrows) within the carpal tunnel.
(From Resnick D: AJR *124*:44, 1975. Copyright 1975. American Roentgen Ray Society.)

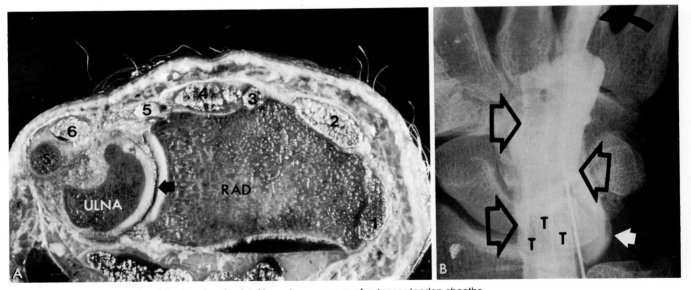

**FIGURE 13–32.** Tenography of the hand and wrist: Normal appearance of extensor tendon sheaths.
  **A** A transverse cross section through the distal portion of the radius (RAD), ulna, ulnar styloid (S), and inferior radioulnar joint (arrow) reveals the six compartments of the extensor tendons and sheaths.
  **B** An injection has been made into the sheath (open arrows) enclosing the tendons (T) of the extensor digitorum communis and extensor indicis proprius. Previous injection of the flexor digiti minimi brevis sheath of the fifth finger (curved arrow) introduced contrast material, which continued into the ulnar bursa (straight arrow).
  (From Resnick D: AJR *124*:44, 1975. Copyright 1975, American Roentgen Ray Society.)

trapezium or first metacarpal bone. Lateral to this in the second compartment are sheaths (5 to 6 cm long) covering the extensor carpi radialis longus and extensor carpi radialis brevis, which may communicate with the sheath of the extensor pollicis longus. Finally, a compartment along the lateral aspect of the radius (first compartment) contains a common synovial sheath (5 to 6 cm long) enclosing the abductor pollicis longus and extensor pollicis brevis.

### Abnormal Tenogram

Rheumatoid arthritis and related disorders are associated with inflammation of the synovium-lined tendon sheaths and tendons. Effusions related to fluid production within the sheaths may produce distention, and villous hypertrophy of the synovial lining can lead to thickening and irregularity of the tendon sheath wall, a nodular corrugated pattern of the contrast material and, on some occasions, interference with normal communicating pathways.[27-29] Displacement of the sheaths and lymphatic filling may occur.[22, 28] Sacculations and pseudodiverticula of the sheath may be outlined.[22, 29] Although tenography is not particularly beneficial in establishing a diagnosis of rheumatoid arthritis, as the presence of this disease generally is apparent on clinical examination, this procedure, by outlining the extent of synovial disease, may aid the surgeon who is contemplating operative intervention and the internist who is evaluating a therapeutic regimen. MR imaging provides similar information.

The tendon sheaths and bursae represent an important pathway for dissemination of infections in the hand.[31, 37] Their selective catheterization and visualization may be useful in detecting the extent of tissue contamination and in providing an understanding of the infectious process. Furthermore, in selected cases of carpal tunnel syndrome, tenography may reveal displacement of synovial sheaths by neighboring masses or edema. Finally, the injection of contrast material containing a small amount of lidocaine into an abnormal tendon sheath may lead to relief of clinical manifestations, confirming the origin of specific clinical findings (Fig. 13–33).[416]

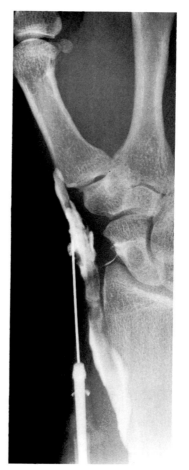

**FIGURE 13–33.** Tenography of the hand and wrist: Tenosynovitis. Contrast material mixed with lidocaine has been injected into the most lateral extensor compartment in a patient with de Quervain's syndrome. Prompt relief of pain ensued.

## ELBOW

### Elbow Arthrography

Arthrography of the elbow (Table 13–4) is not a commonly performed procedure.[336] Although it is a safe, relatively easy examination that may be used to outline the nature and extent of intra-articular disorders and the cause of adjacent soft tissue masses,[41-46] such disorders and masses are better evaluated with MR imaging.

### Technique (Fig. 13–34)

The patient is seated adjacent to the radiographic table and the elbow is flexed to approximately 90 degrees, semi-pronated, and positioned beneath the fluoroscope. With an

#### TABLE 13–4. Indications for Elbow Arthrography

Evaluation of:
    Presence and extent of synovial inflammation
    Intra-articular cartilaginous and osseous bodies
    Soft tissue masses
    Trauma in children

opaque metal marker, a mark is placed over the articular cavity between the radial head and capitulum of the humerus for appropriate localization. Six to 10 ml of contrast material alone (60 per cent Renografin), 0.5 to 1 ml of contrast material plus 6 to 10 ml of air, or 8 to 12 ml of air alone is used for injection, depending on the indication for the study. The injection of contrast material alone is particularly useful for outlining the presence and extent of synovial disorders, capsular integrity, and synovial cysts, whereas the double contrast study with contrast material and air or the single contrast study with air alone may be superior in demonstrating cartilaginous and osseous defects and free intra-articular bodies.[41, 310] After injection, fluoroscopic spot films and anteroposterior, oblique, and lateral radiographs are obtained, supplemented with conventional tomography or CT scanning when necessary.[311, 417, 685]

### Normal Elbow Arthrogram (Fig. 13–35)

On frontal radiographs, a thin layer of contrast material or air is observed between the humerus, radius, and ulna. A periradial prolongation or recess is apparent about the proximal portion of the radius, which is indented where the annular ligament surrounds the bone. Proximal extension of contrast material along the anterior surface of the humerus may resemble the ears of a rabbit, the ''Bugs Bunny''

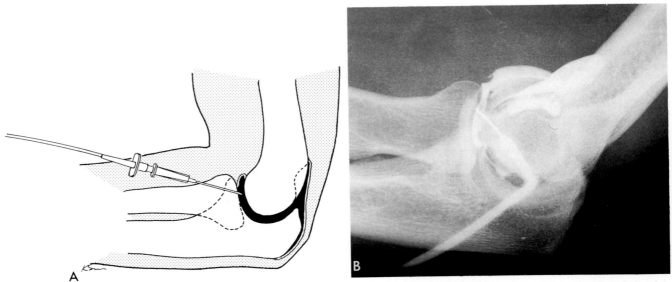

**FIGURE 13–34.** Elbow arthrography: Technique. Under fluoroscopic control, a needle is directed between the radial head and capitulum into the elbow joint from a lateral (radial) approach.

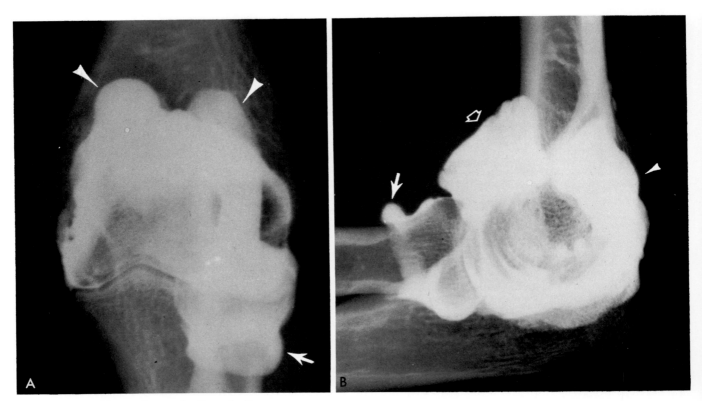

**FIGURE 13–35.** Elbow arthrography: Normal arthrogram.

**A** Anteroposterior radiograph. Observe the thin layer of contrast material between humerus and ulna, the proximal extension of material in front of the humerus resembling the ears of a rabbit (arrowheads), and the periradial or annular recess (arrow).

**B** Lateral radiograph. Note the periradial or annular recess (arrow), the coronoid or anterior recess (open arrow), and the olecranon or posterior recess (arrowhead).

sign.[22] On a lateral radiograph, the periradial or annular recess again is apparent. In addition, coronoid (anterior) and olecranon (posterior) recesses are seen. The borders of all recesses and the remainder of the articular cavity appear smooth in configuration, with two exceptions: The anterior border of the coronoid recess may be slightly wrinkled in flexion, and the medial border adjacent to the collateral ligament is irregular.[41] Smooth articular cartilage is observed on the humerus, radial head, and ulna; it is of uniform thickness except for a portion of the trochlear notch of the ulna, which lacks cartilage.

### Abnormal Elbow Arthrogram

**Rheumatoid Arthritis and Other Synovial Disorders.** Synovial inflammation with hypertrophy and villous transformation accounts for an irregular outline of contrast material, which may be apparent in rheumatoid arthritis[47] (Fig. 13–36) and disorders such as juvenile chronic polyarthritis,[22] ankylosing spondylitis, neuropathic osteoarthropathy (Fig. 13–37), and septic arthritis. Lymphatic visualization is common and capsular distention, sacculation, and cystic swelling may be observed.[22, 30] Capsular rupture and synovial cyst formation also are seen.[48–50, 421, 422] Cysts, which may become large, occur anteriorly, medially, laterally, or even posteriorly over the olecranon and are more frequent in patients with elbow flexion contractures. These cysts most frequently occur when the articulation itself is involved extensively in the rheumatoid process, but on occasion they may represent a relatively early sign of the disease. Altered dynamics at the proximal radioulnar joint and elbow may be contributing factors in the production of these cysts, and the caput ulnae syndrome frequently is apparent in the ipsilateral wrist.[48, 51] Cysts in the antecubital fossa may produce swelling of the forearm and compress the interosseous nerve.[16]

Nodular filling defects within the contrast-filled elbow joint may represent hypertrophied synovium, as in rheumatoid arthritis, or synovial masses associated with pigmented villonodular synovitis and idiopathic synovial (osteo)chondromatosis (Fig. 13–38).

**Trauma.** Opacification of the traumatized elbow joint, particularly after the introduction of air or air and contrast material, may reveal cartilaginous and osseous defects associated with osteochondritis dissecans (transchondral fractures). In these instances, contrast medium may dissect beneath the adjacent osseous fragment or reveal loose or embedded bodies elsewhere in the joint cavity,[41] although it is suggested that conventional tomography alone is as useful as arthrography or arthrotomography in the diagnosis of most intra-articular bodies.[417] Computed arthrotomography also may be used (Fig. 13–39). Localized areas of synovial irregularity, capsular rupture, and soft tissue dissection of contrast material are additional arthrographic findings following elbow trauma.[45, 418, 419] Intra-articular hematomas may be evident.[46] Following gunshot injury of the elbow, metallic fragments may produce a lead arthrogram.[52]

It appears that elbow arthrography is more useful in the evaluation of trauma in children than in adults.[420, 721] The developing anatomy of the immature elbow is complex, and injuries to its unossified cartilaginous areas may escape detection on routine radiographs. Opacification of the joint with contrast material may allow detection of infractions in the cartilage, due to leakage of the contrast agent along the

fracture line, and thereby provide a more accurate classification of the growth plate injury. The technique also may delineate any rotation of the fracture components, cartilaginous spurs, and intra-articular chondral bodies.[420, 686] The advantages of elbow arthrography, in comparison to MR imaging, in this clinical setting have not been established.

### Olecranon Bursography

Injection of the olecranon bursa is accomplished readily and may delineate the nature of soft tissue masses in this area.[53]

### Technique (Fig. 13–40)

The olecranon bursa lies superficially like a cap about the olecranon process. Under fluoroscopy with the elbow flexed, a needle is placed into the bursa approximately 2 cm distal to the tip of the olecranon. Several milliliters of contrast material may be injected.

### Normal and Abnormal Olecranon Bursogram (Fig. 13–41)

A half-moon–shaped collection of contrast material is identified on the normal olecranon bursogram.[22, 53] In rheumatoid arthritis and related disorders, sacculation, distention, or protrusion along the dorsal aspect of the forearm can be identified and intrabursal nodules are seen. The olecranon bursa may communicate with the elbow joint under these abnormal conditions.

## SHOULDER

### Arthrography of the Glenohumeral Joint

Contrast opacification of the glenohumeral joint (Table 13–5) as an aid to the diagnosis of rotator cuff tear, adhesive capsulitis, previous dislocation, articular disease, and bicipital tendon abnormalities has been a subject of a great number of articles.[54–64, 722] The examination is performed readily and the arthrographic findings are reliable.[358, 423] The major question that arises, however, relates to the relative benefit of arthrography of the glenohumeral joint compared with MR imaging (see Chapter 70),[728, 731] as well as with ultrasonography (see Chapter 11)[729] and arthroscopy.[730]

### Technique (Fig. 13–42)

Two basic techniques have been advocated for glenohumeral joint arthrography: single contrast examination and double contrast examination. Modifications of these techniques, including digital arthrography[727] and conventional and computed arthrotomography, are necessary in certain situations (see later discussion).

**Single Contrast Examination.** After preliminary radiographs of the shoulder are obtained, the patient is positioned

**TABLE 13–5. Indications for Glenohumeral Joint Arthrography**

| Evaluation of: |
| --- |
| Rotator cuff tears |
| Adhesive capsulitis |
| Bicipital tendon abnormalities |
| Previous dislocations |
| Presence and extent of synovial inflammation |

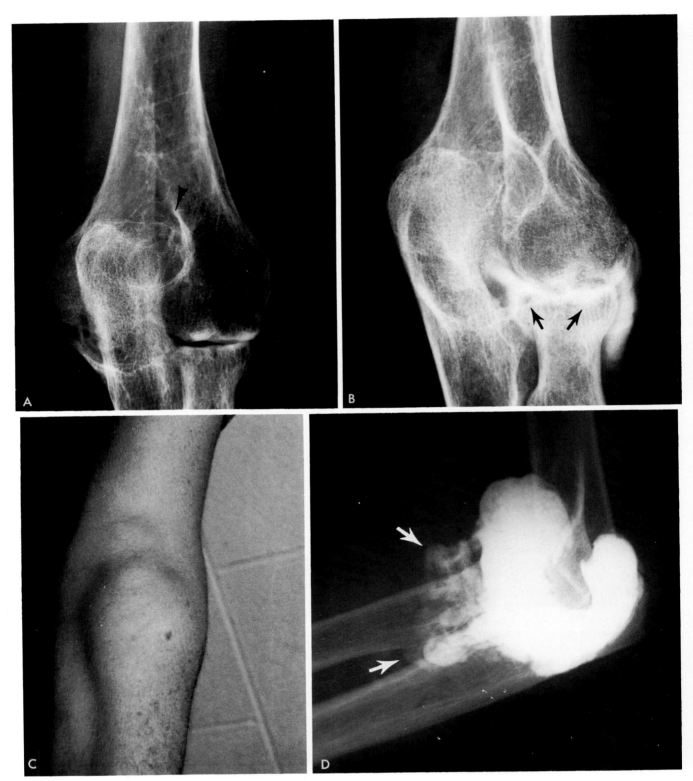

**FIGURE 13–36.** Elbow arthrography: Rheumatoid arthritis.

   **A, B** Plain film **(A)** and arthrogram **(B)** in a patient with long-standing rheumatoid arthritis. The initial radiograph reveals joint space narrowing, erosion, sclerosis, and a large cystic lesion of the distal portion of the humerus (arrowhead). The arthrogram indicates a reduced articular volume due to synovial fibrosis. Only a small amount of contrast material could be introduced, which flows between the distal end of the humerus and radial head (arrows).

   **C, D** Clinical photograph **(C)** and arthrogram **(D)** from a 50 year old man with rheumatoid arthritis and a periarticular mass due to a synovial cyst. The photograph reveals the mass on the anterior surface of the elbow. The arthrogram outlines the distal cystic dilation of the articular cavity with irregular synovium (arrows).

   **(C, D,** From Ehrlich GE: J Bone Joint Surg [Am] *54*:165, 1972.)

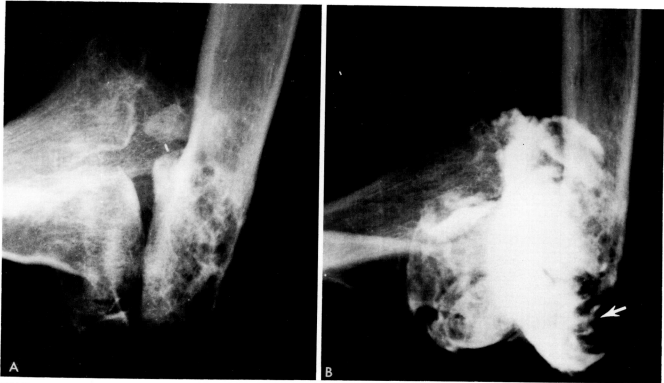

**FIGURE 13–37.** Elbow arthrography: Neuropathic osteoarthropathy.
   **A** The plain film outlines severe flattening of the distal portion of the humerus, deformity of the ulna and radial head, sclerosis, fragmentation, and subluxation.
   **B** Arthrography confirms the presence of articular deformity. The synovium is moderately corrugated or irregular in outline, particularly proximally (arrow). Some filling defects relate to intra-articular osseous bodies.

**FIGURE 13–38.** Elbow arthrography: Idiopathic synovial (osteo)chondromatosis. A lateral view after arthrography delineates irregular nodular filling defects (arrowheads), which represent cartilaginous foci resulting from synovial metaplasia.

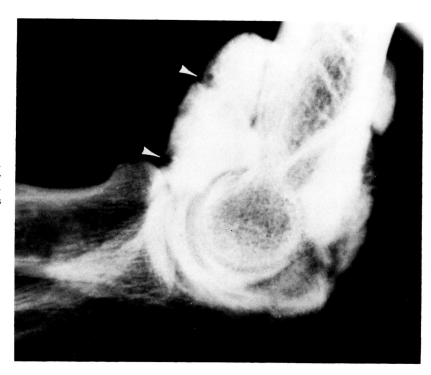

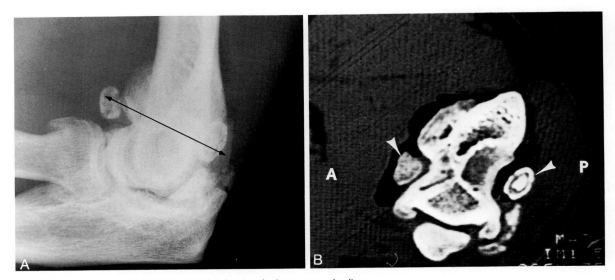

**FIGURE 13–39.** Elbow computed arthrotomography: Intra-articular osseous bodies.
   **A** The initial radiograph reveals multiple osseous bodies both in front of and behind the distal portion of the humerus.
   **B** After the introduction of 10 ml of air, a transaxial CT scan at the approximate level indicated in **A** confirms the intra-articular location of several of the bodies (arrowheads). A, Anterior; P, posterior.

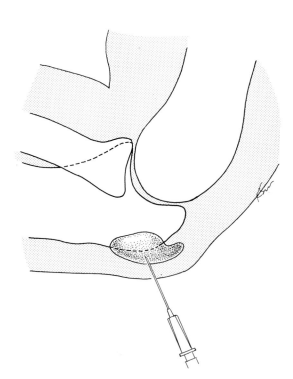

**FIGURE 13–40.** Olecranon bursography: Technique. A needle is inserted into the bursa approximately 2 cm distal to the olecranon tip.

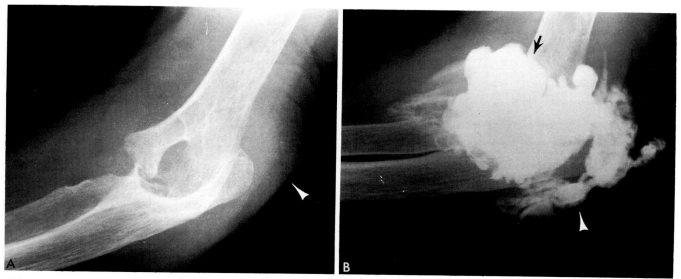

**FIGURE 13–41.** Olecranon bursography: Rheumatoid arthritis. This patient had a swollen olecranon bursa.
  **A** An initial radiograph outlines the soft tissue swelling over the ulnar olecranon (arrowhead) and severe destruction of the elbow joint.
  **B** After injection of the bursa (arrowhead), contrast material flowed into the elbow joint (arrow). Observe the enlarged articular and bursal cavities and the nodular, corrugated synovium.

supine under the fluoroscope with the hand in external rotation, anchored with a sandbag. Some radiographers advocate an oblique position, but the anteroposterior position generally is preferred.[65] A lead marker is placed over the subchondral border of the humerus (medial margin) at the junction of the middle and distal thirds of the glenoid cavity, although a grid may be used rather than a lead marker.[66] A 3 inch, 18 or 20 gauge spinal needle is inserted in a vertical direction toward the glenohumeral joint under fluoroscopic guidance. The needle may contact the extreme medial margin of the humeral head, at which point it is elevated slightly and directed more medially, or it may pass directly into the articular cavity. Ten to 15 ml of 60 per cent Renografin is injected, which, with accurate needle placement, should flow away from the needle tip. The needle is withdrawn and, after mild exercise of the shoulder, anteroposterior radiographs are obtained in internal and external rotation, and axillary and tangential bicipital groove radiographs also are obtained. This series of radiographs is repeated after moderate exercise of the shoulder.

**Double Contrast Examination.** More recently, double contrast shoulder arthrography has been advocated using approximately 1 to 4 ml of Renografin and 10 to 15 ml of air.[67, 68, 374] The needle placement is performed in a manner identical to that outlined previously. After injection and withdrawal of the needle, the patient is placed upright with a 2.3 kg (5 lb) sandbag in his or her hand. Radiographs in internal and external rotation are obtained with or without a spot film device. The patient then is returned to the supine position and internal rotation, external rotation, axillary, and bicipital groove films are made. These radiographs can be repeated after mild exercise of the shoulder. The proponents of the double contrast technique observe that, with this technique, the width of the rotator cuff tear and the integrity of cuff tendons can be assessed, allowing the surgeon to plan the operative technique more accurately. Furthermore, the internal structures of the joint, including the glenoid labrum, are better identified.[337]

The author has used both single and double contrast arthrography and agrees that the double contrast study is superior, although it is more difficult to interpret, requiring a good deal of experience. In addition, the author believes that approximately 2 ml of lidocaine should be injected with the contrast material during shoulder arthrography, as

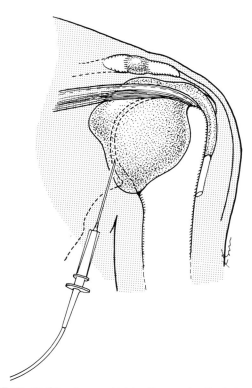

**FIGURE 13–42.** Glenohumeral joint arthrography: Technique (schematic drawing). An anterior approach is used. A needle is inserted into the joint at the level of the junction of the middle and lower thirds of the glenoid cavity.

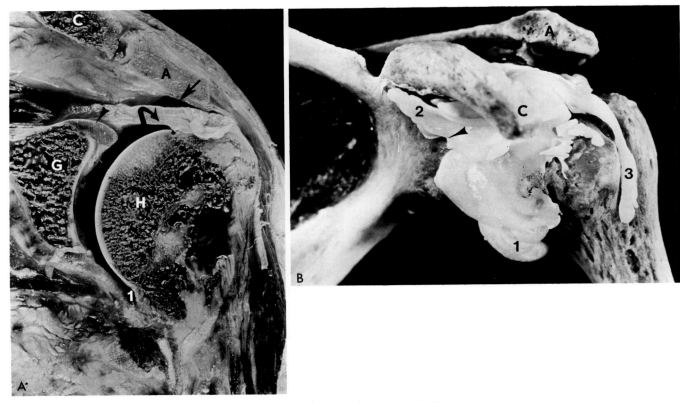

**FIGURE 13–43.** Glenohumeral joint arthrography: Anatomy and normal single contrast arthrogram.

**A** Coronal section of the glenohumeral joint. Observe the glenoid (G), humeral head (H), distal end of the clavicle (C), acromion (A), subacromial (subdeltoid) bursa (straight arrow), rotator cuff (curved arrow), and glenoid labrum (arrowhead). The joint cavity is seen extending inferiorly as the axillary pouch (1). (From Armbuster T et al: AJR *129*:667, 1977. Copyright 1977, American Roentgen Ray Society.)

**B** Anterior view of macerated specimen after glenohumeral joint arthrography using methylmethacrylate. A model of the distended joint has been created. Note the axillary pouch (1), subscapular recess (2), indentation between these latter two structures (arrowhead), bicipital tendon sheath (long head of the biceps) (3), acromion (A), and coracoid process (C).

*Illustration continued on opposite page*

this procedure may be associated with mild immediate or delayed discomfort.[383, 384]

### Normal Glenohumeral Joint Arthrogram
(Figs. 13–43 and 13–44)

Contrast material is identified between the humeral head and the glenoid. In external rotation, the contrast substance ends abruptly laterally at the anatomic neck of the humerus. In this view, an axillary pouch may be opacified on the undersurface of the humeral head. In internal rotation, a prominent subscapular recess is observed overlying the glenoid and lateral scapular region. The axillary and subscapular recesses are not a continuous sac, as a definite indentation is observed between them. The tendon of the long head of the biceps is visible as a radiolucent filling defect within the articular cavity and can be traced for a variable distance within the contrast-filled tendon sheath into the bicipital groove and along the metaphysis of the humerus.

In the axillary view, contrast material is identified between the glenoid cavity and humeral head, anterior to the scapula (subscapular recess), and within the bicipital tendon sheath. The cartilaginous surfaces of glenoid and humerus, as well as the glenoid labrum, are seen. In this projection, contrast material should not overlie the surgical neck of the humerus. The tangential view of the bicipital groove demonstrates an oval filling defect within the contrast-filled sheath, representing the biceps tendon.

### Complete and Incomplete Tears of the Rotator Cuff

Tears in the rotator cuff musculature may involve the entire thickness of the cuff (complete tear) or a portion of the cuff (incomplete or partial tear). Their causes and pathogenesis are discussed in Chapter 70. Although the diagnosis of a chronic, complete tear of the rotator cuff musculature may be made on the basis of plain radiographic alterations, acute disruptions commonly are undetectable by conventional radiography, requiring additional techniques for diagnosis.[428] Arthrography remains one of the most popular accessory techniques in this regard despite recent interest in the application of MR imaging and ultrasonography to the diagnosis of rotator cuff abnormalities[425, 426, 647, 664–666] (see Chapters 11 and 70). Double contrast glenohumeral joint arthrography is the preferred arthrographic technique in this clinical situation with suggested modifications, including the application of stress,[429] the supplementary use of conventional tomography or CT scanning,[430, 687] and the monitoring of intra-articular pressure.[392]

**Complete Tear** (Fig. 13–45). In this situation, abnormal communication exists between the glenohumeral joint cavity and the subacromial (subdeltoid) bursa. Contrast material can be identified within the bursa as a large collection superior and lateral to the greater tuberosity and adjacent to the undersurface of the acromion. The contrast material in

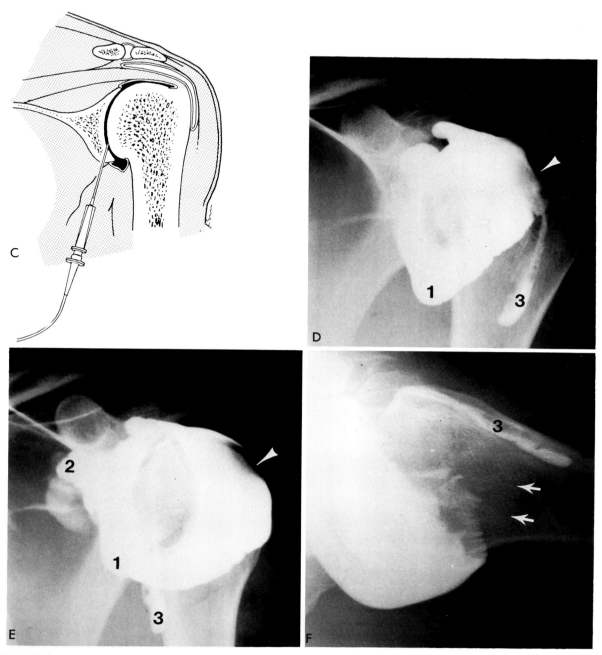

**FIGURE 13–43** *Continued*

**C** Diagram of normal arthrogram. Observe that the contrast material flows up to the greater tuberosity, below the rotator cuff.

**D** Normal arthrogram: External rotation. Visualized structures include the axillary pouch (1) and bicipital tendon sheath (3). Note that the subscapular recess is not well seen and the contrast material ends abruptly laterally at the anatomic neck of the humerus (arrowhead).

**E** Normal arthrogram: Internal rotation. Observe the prominent subscapular recess (2), axillary pouch (1), and bicipital tendon sheath (3). The articular cartilage of the humeral head is well seen (arrowhead). Minimal extravasation of contrast material has occurred in the axilla near the injection site.

**F** Normal arthrogram: Axillary view. Observe the bicipital tendon (3) and the absence of contrast material over the surgical neck of the humerus (arrows).

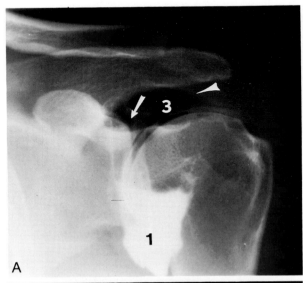

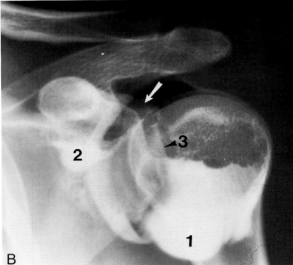

**FIGURE 13–44.** Glenohumeral joint arthrography: Normal double contrast arthrogram (upright projections).

**A** Normal arthrogram: External rotation. Visualized structures include the axillary pouch (1), bicipital tendon (3), glenoid fibrocartilage (arrow), and articular cartilage of the humeral head. The distended articular cavity (arrowhead) above the bicipital tendon should not be misinterpreted as filling of the subacromial (subdeltoid) bursa.

**B** Normal arthrogram: Internal rotation. Visualized structures include the subscapular recess (2), axillary pouch (1), bicipital tendon (3), glenoid fibrocartilage (arrow), and articular cartilage of the humeral head.

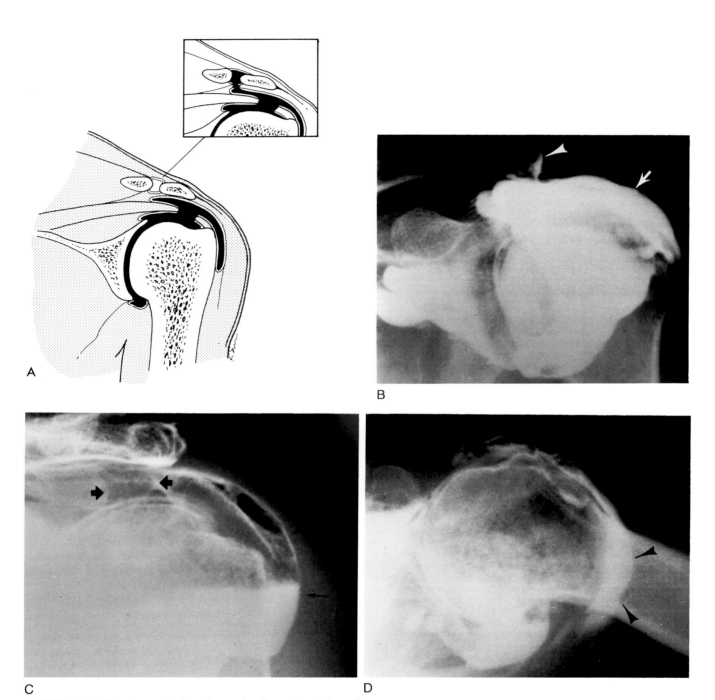

C                                              D

**FIGURE 13–45.** Glenohumeral joint arthrography: Complete rotator cuff tear.

  **A** The arthrographic findings of a complete tear of the rotator cuff. Contrast material extends from the glenohumeral joint through the rotator cuff into the subacromial (subdeltoid) bursa. The inset reveals contrast material extending from the glenohumeral joint through the rotator cuff into the subacromial bursa, and from there into the acromioclavicular joint.

  **B** Single contrast arthrography. In this patient with a rotator cuff tear, contrast material in the subdeltoid bursa (arrow) has led to opacification of the acromioclavicular joint (arrowhead).

  **C, D** Double contrast arthrography. The external rotation view **(C)** demonstrates that contrast material has extended from the glenohumeral joint into the subacromial (subdeltoid) bursa (thin arrows). The width of the tear of the rotator cuff can be seen (between heavy arrows). In another patient with a rotator cuff tear, an axillary view **(D)** reveals a "saddle-bag" configuration, with contrast material overlying the surgical neck of the humerus (arrowheads). **(C,** Courtesy of J. Mink, M.D., Los Angeles, California.)

the bursa is separated from the articular cavity by a lucent area of varying size, representing the rotator cuff itself. If the musculature is thick, this lucent region is quite large, whereas if the musculature is atrophic, it is small or even absent. In the presence of a complete rotator cuff tear, contrast material is identified as a "saddle-bag" radiodense area across the surgical neck of the humerus on the axillary view. In some patients with complete tears, the contrast material will pass from the subacromial bursa into the acromioclavicular joint.[427, 667, 724]

Using double contrast shoulder arthrography, the degree of degeneration of the torn rotator cuff can be recognized.[68, 648, 725] Furthermore, the width of the tear itself is identified. The location of the disrupted tendons is apparent as the tendinous ends are coated by positive contrast material. In some patients, the torn rotator cuff tendons are either absent or consist of only a few small pieces, prohibiting adequate surgical repair or, at the very least, requiring an alternative method of surgery.[69–71]

Killoran and associates[54] have emphasized three potential sources of error in the diagnosis of a complete rotator cuff tear: Inadequate distribution of opaque material within the joint may prevent adequate visualization of the subacromial bursa; the contrast-filled sheath of the biceps tendon may project slightly lateral to the greater tuberosity on external rotation, simulating filling of the subacromial bursa; and inadvertent bursal injection may simulate a complete tear unless it is recognized that the articular cavity is not opacified. Although it is the subacromial bursa that usually is entered, direct injection of the subcoracoid bursa also is possible[424, 723] (Fig. 13–46).

Arthrography also has been used after operative repair of a torn rotator cuff. Results indicate that a watertight closure

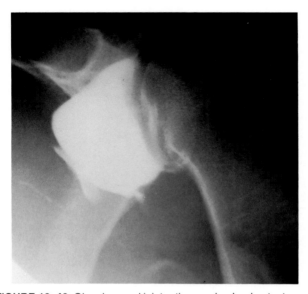

**FIGURE 13–46.** Glenohumeral joint arthrography: Inadvertent opacification of the subcoracoid bursa. The well-circumscribed collection of contrast material beneath the coracoid process conforms in size and configuration to the subcoracoid bursa, generally located between the subscapularis tendon below and the coracoid process and combined tendon of the short head of the biceps and coracobrachialis above. This bursa usually is separate from the subacromial bursa, communicating with it in approximately 10 per cent of people. (Courtesy of G. Greenway, M.D., Dallas, Texas.)

of the glenohumeral joint is accomplished infrequently and is not necessary for a good functional result.[668]

**Incomplete Tear** (Figs. 13–47 and 13–48). A partial tear may involve the deep surface of the rotator cuff, the superficial surface, or the interior substance of the tendon. Tears within the substance of the cuff generally will escape arthrographic detection but may not require operative repair.[72] Tears involving the superior surface of the cuff also will not be demonstrated on glenohumeral joint arthrography, although they rarely may be seen with direct subacromial bursography.[64, 732] Tears on the inferior surface of the rotator cuff can be diagnosed on arthrography. In these cases, an irregular circular or linear collection of contrast material may be identified above the opacified joint cavity, near the anatomic neck of the humerus.[54, 68] The intact superficial fibers of the rotator cuff prevent opacification of the subacromial bursa.[64] A false negative arthrogram in the presence of a partial tear of the rotator cuff can indicate that the tear is too small for recognition or that a fibrous nodule has occluded the defect.

### Adhesive Capsulitis

Glenohumeral joint arthrography has been used in the diagnosis and treatment of adhesive capsulitis.[73, 74, 431, 733–738]

**Diagnosis** (Fig. 13–49). Adhesive capsulitis prevents normal distention of the glenohumeral joint. Its pathologic basis is unknown; the condition may relate to capsular thickening,[75] contracture of the coracohumeral ligament and rotator interval,[739] adhesions between the capsule and bicipital tendon,[76] and adhesions in the subacromial bursa and beneath the coracoid process.[77] Adhesive capsulitis generally follows shoulder trauma, either to the soft tissues or to the osseous structures.[78] Usually, the entire joint capsule is involved, abnormalities being detected initially in the fibrous layer of the capsule, with obliteration of dependent recesses. Adhesive capsulitis has been described in other joints as well,[79] including the ankle, hip, and wrist.

Arthrography is considered by most investigators, although not all,[432] as a reliable means of detecting adhesive capsulitis. Single contrast (radiopaque contrast agent) technique is preferable,[649] and simultaneous determination of the intra-articular pressure has been described.[392] The main arthrographic abnormality in adhesive capsulitis of the glenohumeral joint is a joint of low capacity evidenced by increased resistance to injection and a "tight" feel. Only a small amount of fluid (5 to 8 ml) may be injected successfully, and when the hand is released from the plunger, the fluid may quickly return to the syringe. The subscapular and axillary recesses are small or absent. Filling of the bicipital tendon sheath is variable; in some cases it appears normal, whereas in others it fills poorly or not at all, or contrast material may leak from the sheath. Contrast agent also commonly leaks elsewhere in the joint, particularly from the subscapular recess. An additional finding is irregularity of the capsular insertion.

**Treatment** (Fig. 13–50). Joint distention during arthrography, the "brisement" procedure,[74] may aid in treatment of this condition,[312] although its benefits are controversial.[737, 738] This technique requires slow, intermittent injection of larger and larger volumes of contrast material (mixed with saline solution, corticosteroids, and lidocaine), allowing some of the fluid to return into the syringe after each injection. The patient is instructed to move the arm

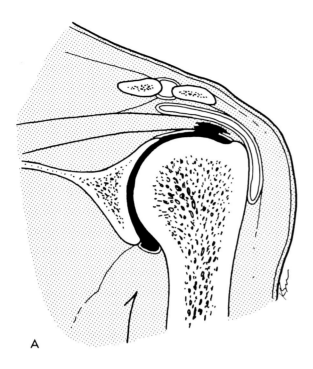

A

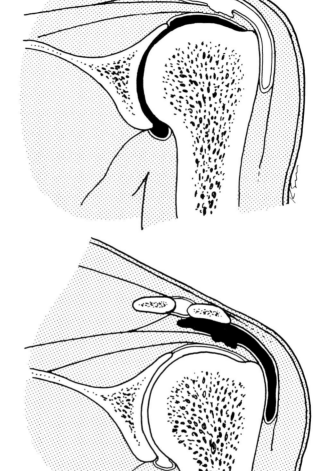

B

**FIGURE 13–47.** Glenohumeral joint arthrography: Incomplete rotator cuff tear.

**A** Diagram illustrating that a tear on the undersurface of the rotator cuff can produce an irregular collection of contrast material after opacification of the glenohumeral joint.

**B** In the presence of a partial tear on the superior surface of the rotator cuff, glenohumeral joint arthrography (top drawing) is unrewarding. Subacromial bursography (lower drawing) may demonstrate an irregular collection of contrast material.

**C** A double contrast arthrogram reveals a partial tear (arrowhead) on the undersurface of the rotator cuff. (Courtesy of J. Mink, M.D., Los Angeles, California.)

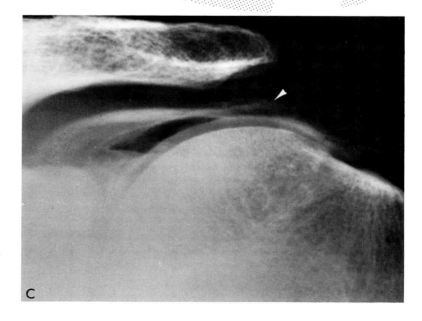

C

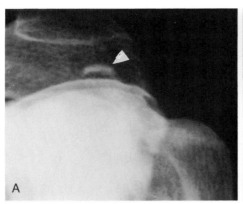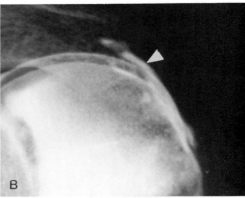

**FIGURE 13–48.** Glenohumeral joint arthrography: Incomplete rotator cuff tear. External **(A)** and internal **(B)** rotation views show contrast material (arrowheads) extending into the undersurface of the rotator cuff in this single contrast arthrogram.

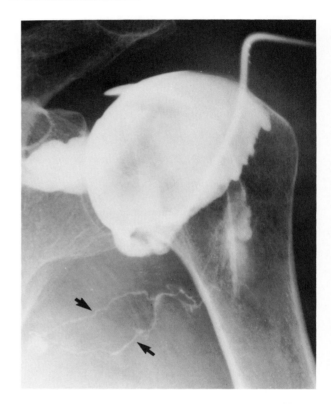

**FIGURE 13–49.** Glenohumeral joint arthrography: Diagnosis of adhesive capsulitis. After the introduction of 10 ml of contrast material, the patient complained of pain and it was difficult to inject any additional amount of the solution. Note the "tight-looking" articulation with a small axillary recess and opacification of lymphatic channels (arrows).

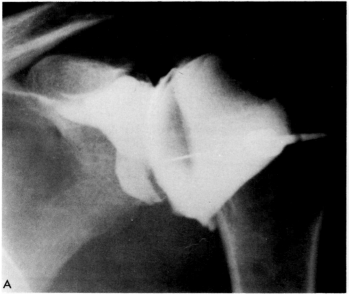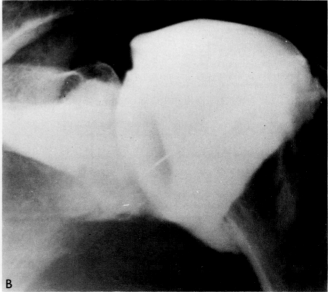

**FIGURE 13–50.** Glenohumeral joint arthrography: Treatment of adhesive capsulitis. Radiographs exposed during the brisement procedure indicate joint distention in a patient with adhesive capsulitis after injection of 15 ml **(A)** and 50 ml **(B)** of contrast material.

carefully during the procedure. In some patients, 100 ml of fluid eventually may be injected, although free extravasation, particularly at the subscapular recess or the bicipital tendon sheath, frequently occurs with extensive distention, and the procedure is halted. Postprocedural physical therapy is mandatory. The author's investigation with this technique in approximately 50 patients has revealed favorable results. With severe capsular restriction, the brisement procedure is less beneficial, and in all patients, symptoms may return, requiring repeated examinations. The technique also has been applied to the treatment of adhesive capsulitis in other locations, such as the wrist[719] and hip,[650] with inconstant therapeutic results.

### Abnormalities of the Bicipital Tendon
#### (Figs. 13–51 to 13–53)

Certain abnormalities of the bicipital tendon, such as complete rupture, are easy to recognize clinically and do not require arthrography for documentation, whereas others may produce nonspecific shoulder symptoms and signs, in which case arthrography indeed can be helpful.[313] These latter abnormalities include partial tears, dislocation, and tenosynovitis. In such cases, however, MR imaging appears to be a superior technique (see Chapter 70).

In the normal glenohumeral joint arthrogram, visualization of the tendon sheath and tendon of the long head of the biceps is not constant. Therefore, although the absence of visualization indeed may represent a tear of the biceps, it is not a reliable sign. Occasionally, after exercise, the tendon sheath will be seen when it was not apparent on preexercise films. Furthermore, leakage of contrast material from the biceps sleeve can be seen in normal persons,[54] although some investigators regard it as a sign of disruption of the transverse bicipital ligament,[55, 59] rupture of the bicipital tendon itself,[56] or overdistention of the articular cavity.[80]

Considering the wide variation in the arthrographic appearance of the bicipital tendon and sheath in normal persons, the radiologist must not rely too heavily on the arthrogram in establishing the existence of a significant abnormality, and, in fact, the precise role of this method in comparison to others, such as MR imaging and ultrasonography,[651, 664, 669] in the diagnosis of alterations of the biceps tendon apparatus has been questioned. Still, when a complete bicipital tendon rupture is apparent clinically, arthrography may confirm the diagnosis, demonstrating distortion of the synovial sheath and failing to identify the tendon within the opacified sheath. The arthrographic diagnosis of complete rupture is more accurate in cases of acute tears; with less acute ruptures, shrinkage of adjacent tissues may obscure the abnormal findings.[61] Incomplete tears of the bicipital tendon produce increased width of the tendon and distortion of the synovial sheath.[68] Medial (or, more rarely, posterior[740]) dislocation of the tendon and sheath from their normal positions in the intertubercular groove can be suggested when the positions of these structures do not change on the internal and external rotation radiographs.[68] This finding can be verified on the bicipital groove radiograph.[433] It also can be detected with computed arthrotomography.

### Abnormalities Occurring After Previous Dislocations (Fig. 13–54)

Anterior dislocations of the glenohumeral joint are associated with soft tissue damage. As the dislocating humeral head moves anteriorly, it detaches or lifts the articular capsule from the glenoid and neck of the scapula, producing an abnormal recess of variable size between the subscapular and axillary recesses. On arthrography, the abnormal recess fills with contrast material, obscuring the indentation that normally is present between the subscapular and axillary recesses. This finding is more evident on radiographs taken in internal rotation.

Additional findings related to anterior dislocation are injuries of cartilage and bone. The Bankart deformity involves an avulsion or compression defect of the anteroinferior rim of the glenoid and may be purely cartilaginous in nature.[81] The arthrogram, particularly when obtained with double contrast technique, may outline the cartilaginous abnormalities about the glenoid labrum[314] (see subsequent discussion). The second defect associated with previous anterior dislocation is a Hill-Sachs compression deformity on the posterolateral aspect of the humeral head. This finding generally is evident on plain films but may require arthrography for demonstration if the defect is small or involves only cartilage.

In recent years, the application of conventional[314, 434–437, 688] and computed[438–441, 670, 741–746] arthrotomography to the diagnosis of abnormalities in the unstable shoulder has been emphasized (see also Chapter 70). In many patients with recurrent dislocations, the history alone allows accurate diagnosis; in others, however, particularly those with the more common problem of recurrent subluxations, nonspecific shoulder pain and disability are encountered. Routine radiography and conventional arthrography are helpful in some cases, but the delineation of internal joint structures requires that conventional tomography or CT scanning be performed after the introduction of air or of contrast material and air into the joint.

The assessment of the integrity of the fibrocartilaginous labrum has been emphasized in patients with shoulder instability. Although the use of arthroscopy in this assessment has become increasingly popular, and, in the hands of some examiners, the technique is highly accurate,[442–444] it is an invasive and expensive procedure that requires general anesthesia. Conventional or computed arthrotomography represents a more ideal screening technique.

Thin-section conventional arthrotomography can be accomplished in two ways (prone oblique or supine oblique patient position), each giving a different perspective of the labrum and both requiring considerable experience and expertise on the part of the examiner and meticulous positioning of the patient. Such patients may be positioned in a prone oblique manner, with the affected shoulder facing downward and the neck flexed, with the opposite shoulder moved slightly forward to avoid overlap with the side of interest and the scapula on the involved side directed perpendicular to the table top.[314] Alternatively, a supine oblique position can be used, with the injured shoulder closest to the table.[434] The described techniques of conventional arthrotomography also differ somewhat with regard to the amount of contrast agent that is advocated. In general, 1 or 2 ml of radiopaque contrast material and 10 to 15 ml of air are instilled into the joint.

Computed arthrotomography is accomplished after the injection of 10 to 15 ml of air with or without 1 ml of radiopaque contrast material. The patients are examined in the supine position with their arms positioned by their sides

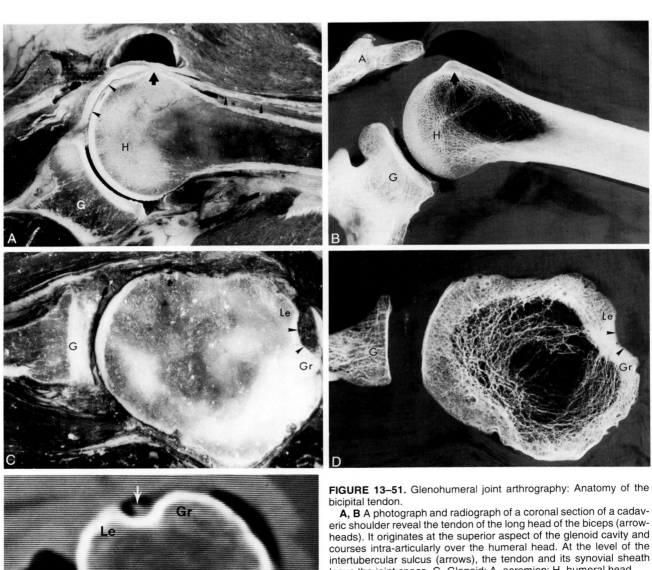

**FIGURE 13–51.** Glenohumeral joint arthrography: Anatomy of the bicipital tendon.

**A, B** A photograph and radiograph of a coronal section of a cadaveric shoulder reveal the tendon of the long head of the biceps (arrowheads). It originates at the superior aspect of the glenoid cavity and courses intra-articularly over the humeral head. At the level of the intertubercular sulcus (arrows), the tendon and its synovial sheath leave the joint space. G, Glenoid; A, acromion; H, humeral head.

**C, D** A photograph and radiograph of a transverse section of a cadaveric shoulder at the level of the intertubercular sulcus (arrowheads) reveal that the latter is bordered by the greater tuberosity (Gr) posteriorly, the lesser tuberosity (Le) anteriorly, and the transverse humeral ligament laterally. G, Glenoid.

**E** A transaxial CT scan at the level of the intertubercular sulcus after the administration of intra-articular air shows the bicipital tendon (arrow) in its normal position within the sulcus. Gr, Greater tuberosity; Le, lesser tuberosity.

(**A–D,** From Cone RO, et al: AJR *141*:781, 1983. Copyright 1983, American Roentgen Ray Society.)

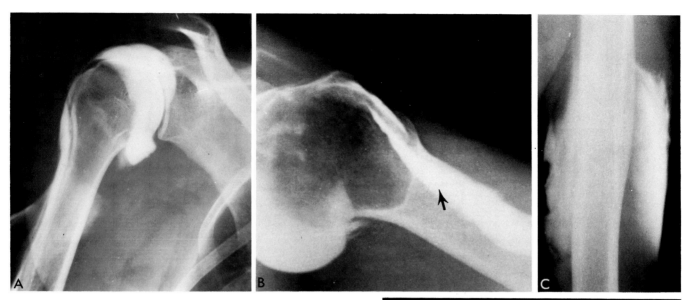

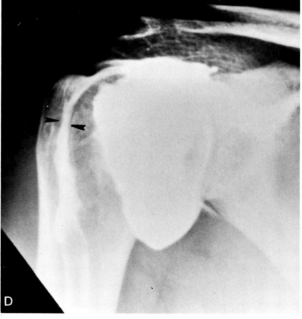

**FIGURE 13–52.** Glenohumeral joint arthrography: Abnormalities of the bicipital tendon.

**A** Tear of the transverse bicipital ligament. Note contrast extension for a considerable distance along the course of the bicipital tendon with soft tissue extravasation. (Courtesy of J. Mink, M.D., Los Angeles, California.)

**B, C** Bicipital tendon rupture. Axillary **(B)** and frontal **(C)** views in a patient with known rupture of the bicipital tendon reveal contrast material extension along the course of the bicipital tendon and extravasation into the soft tissues of the arm. The normal lucency of the bicipital tendon itself is not seen within the contrast-filled sheath (arrow).

**D** Bicipital tendon rupture. This view with the humerus in external rotation shows collapse of the bicipital tendon sheath (arrowheads) with absence of the normal radiolucent shadow of the tendon in this region. (Courtesy of A. B. Goldman, M.D., New York, New York.)

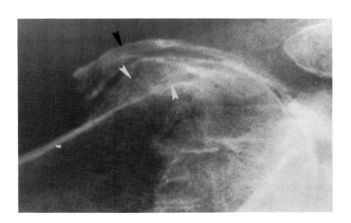

**FIGURE 13–53.** Glenohumeral joint arthrography: Abnormalities of the bicipital tendon—dislocation of the tendon. On a modified axillary view of the shoulder, the contrast-filled tendon sheath and tendon (black arrowhead) are displaced from the intertubercular sulcus (white arrowheads). (Courtesy of A. B. Goldman, M.D., New York, New York.)

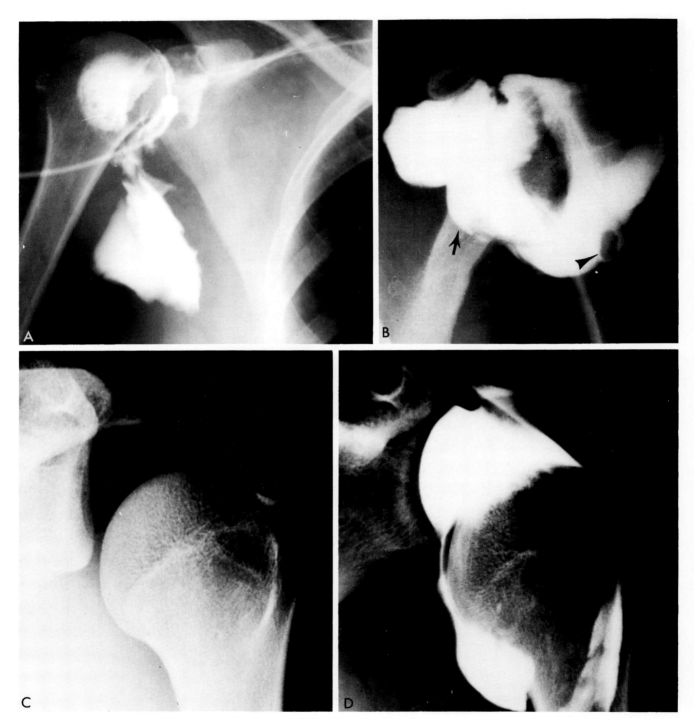

**FIGURE 13–54.** Glenohumeral joint arthrography: Previous dislocation and subluxation.

   **A** After an acute anterior dislocation of the glenohumeral joint with an associated fracture of the greater tuberosity, arthrography outlines an anterior capsular tear with soft tissue extension of contrast material. (Courtesy of J. Mink, M.D., Los Angeles, California.)

   **B** In a patient with previous anterior dislocations of the glenohumeral joint, arthrography demonstrates an abnormal recess (arrow) between the axillary pouch and subscapular recess and an intra-articular body (arrowhead).

   **C, D** In a patient with voluntary inferior subluxation of the glenohumeral joint, the initial film **(C)** reveals the depressed position of the humeral head with respect to the glenoid. Arthrography **(D)** outlines the distorted joint cavity and stretched bicipital tendon.

and their shoulders in a neutral attitude or in slight internal rotation; to distend the posterior capsule optimally with air, external rotation of the shoulder can be used.[440, 742] Either 5 ml collimation and 3 mm table incrementation or continuous 3 mm sections are used, and an average of 15 scans is sufficient. Reformatted coronal or sagittal images rarely are required.

The interpretation of the images obtained with either conventional or computed arthrotomography requires knowledge of the cross-sectional appearance of the normal humeral head and glenoid region of the scapula (Fig. 13–55). The head of the humerus essentially is round and smooth on superior sections taken at the level of the coracoid process, which is the appropriate level for evaluation of a Hill-Sachs lesion; the smooth appearance changes to an irregular one at the level of the cartilage-bone junction in the neck of the humerus, where a constant constriction or concavity is evident between the greater tuberosity and the humeral head itself. Owing to the presence of this normal constriction, a Hill-Sachs lesion is diagnosed most reliably when a contour abnormality is seen on the uppermost transverse sections of the humeral head.[787] The bicipital groove, located between the greater and lesser tuberosities of the humerus, varies considerably in both depth and configuration.[445]

The articular surface of the glenoid fossa is gently concave and covered by hyaline cartilage, which normally is thinner at the center than at the periphery. On cross section, the posterior margin of the fossa appears larger and more rounded than the more pointed anterior margin. The inclination of the fossa is characterized by mild retroversion superiorly, changing to slight anteversion on progressively caudal sections. The glenoid labrum is a fibrous structure that is firmly attached to the edge of the fossa, thereby adding depth and contributing to the stability of the joint. Disruption of the integrity of the labrum, most commonly involving the anterior and inferior portions, is the most frequent form of derangement in recurrent shoulder dislocations, and it is not uncommon for the superior portion to become partially detached from the underlying glenoid with increasing age in normal persons.[446] In cross section, the labrum usually appears essentially triangular. Variations in the shape of the anterior and posterior portions of the labrum are frequent, however, in asymptomatic persons and create considerable diagnostic difficulty in the interpretation of computed arthrotomograms or, for that matter, MR images (see Chapter 70). On conventional arthrotomography, the anterior portion often is longer and more pointed than the posterior portion, which frequently appears slightly larger, more rounded, and smoother. On computed arthrotomograms, the anterior portion most commonly has a smoothly rounded apex, although on occasion the apex is pointed and closely resembles the appearance on conventional arthrotomograms. The base of the labrum abuts on the articular cartilage of the glenoid, somewhat analogous to the meniscus in the knee. Air or contrast material normally may track between the base of the labrum and the cartilage and should not be mistaken for evidence of partial detachment.[440]

The fibrous capsule of the glenohumeral joint is loose and redundant. Posteriorly and inferiorly, it is continuous with the capsular border of the labrum and adjacent bones; anteriorly and superiorly, its relationship to the labrum is affected by the subscapularis recess or bursa, which lies between the subscapularis muscle and the scapula, with the precise anterior insertion of the capsule in relation to the labrum being described differently by different investigators.[347, 446, 447] Uhthoff and Piscopo,[448] in a study of 52 fetal and embryonic shoulders, found that the anterior capsule attached to the labrum or close to it in 77 per cent of cases and, in the remaining 23 per cent, it inserted into the neck of the scapula, thus creating a pouch (see Chapter 70).

The subscapularis bursa is one of two constant recesses in the fibrous capsule; the other is the axillary recess, which projects between the scapula and the neck of the humerus. Anteriorly, the capsule becomes thickened, forming the superior, middle, and inferior glenohumeral ligaments, which vary in both configuration and degree of development.[446, 447] Of these structures, which course from the humeral head to converge on the anterior margin of the glenoid fossa, the superior ligament is identified most commonly. It may be seen in an intracapsular position along the superior portion of the joint where it inserts into the labrum, near the attachment of the bicipital tendon.[446] The subscapularis bursa communicates with the joint through an opening between the superior and middle glenohumeral ligaments,[447] or between the middle and inferior glenohumeral ligaments, or at both sites, and its size varies according to the degree of development of the middle glenohumeral ligament. When the ligament is well developed, the bursa is small and the muscle is closely applied to the surface of the scapula; conversely, when the ligament is poorly developed, the bursa is capacious and the muscle is displaced anteriorly,[446] described by several authors as representing a less stable anterior capsular mechanism.[446, 449–451] Turkel and collaborators[452] have demonstrated that the inferior glenohumeral ligament is the strongest of the three and plays a primary role in anteroinferior stability. The tendon of the long head of the bicipital muscle arises from the superior and posterior portions of the labrum, traverses the glenohumeral joint superiorly, and then extends inferiorly within the bicipital groove to leave the joint in front of the humeral neck.

Abnormalities of the glenoid labrum depicted on conventional or computed arthrotomography include foreshortening or thinning or contrast imbibition along its free margin (Figs. 13–56 and 13–57). The labrum also may be completely detached, along with one or more of the glenohumeral ligaments. Such detachment of the superior limit of the glenoid labrum is a distinctive lesion that has been designated superior labral anterior to posterior tear, or the SLAP lesion (see Chapter 70). An osseous Bankart lesion typically is visualized as an elevation of a small sliver of bone and irregularity of the adjacent glenoid rim. A depression along the posterolateral aspect of the humeral head is indicative of a Hill-Sachs lesion. Additional abnormalities that can be detected include intra-articular osteocartilaginous bodies and subluxation or dislocation of the bicipital tendon, which, in rare instances when displaced in a posterior direction,[740] may block concentric reduction of the humeral head after an anterior glenohumeral joint dislocation[453] (Fig. 13–58). Differentiation of an abnormally enlarged anterior capsular contour from a normal variant is difficult on the basis of the cross-sectional display.[440] Some investigators, however, report success in differentiating normal and abnormal anterior capsular configurations.[670]

Both conventional and computed arthrotomographic

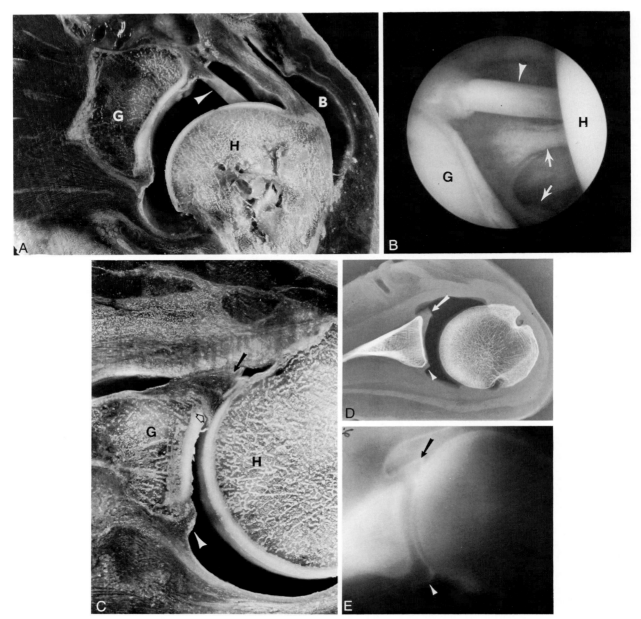

**FIGURE 13–55.** Glenohumeral joint arthrography: Normal joint anatomy.

   **A** A coronal section of a cadaveric shoulder after the introduction of air into the glenohumeral joint shows the articular cartilage of the glenoid cavity (G) and humeral head (H). Note the long head of the bicipital tendon (arrowhead) arising from the supraglenoid tubercle. The subacromial (subdeltoid) bursa is identified (B).

   **B** Arthroscopy reveals the long head of the bicipital tendon (arrowhead) attaching to the supraglenoid tubercle. The superior and middle glenohumeral ligaments are indicated (arrows). G, Glenoid cavity; H, humeral head.

   **C** A transverse section through a distended glenohumeral joint in a cadaver shows the articular cartilage of the glenoid cavity (G) and the humeral head (H). The anterior (solid arrow) and posterior (arrowhead) portions of the glenoid labrum are indicated. Note that the anterior portion of the glenoid labrum is triangular and more pointed than the posterior portion, which is more rounded and smoother. Observe also that there exists a potential space (open arrow) where the base of the labrum abuts on the articular cartilage of the glenoid cavity.

   **D** A radiograph of a similar section to that shown in **C** delineates the normal anterior (arrow) and posterior (arrowhead) portions of the glenoid labrum. This is similar to the appearance observed with computed arthrotomography.

   **E** Conventional arthrotomography shows similar characteristics of the anterior (arrow) and posterior (arrowhead) portions of the glenoid labrum.

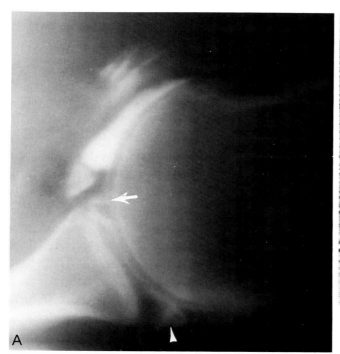

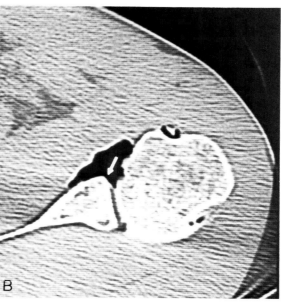

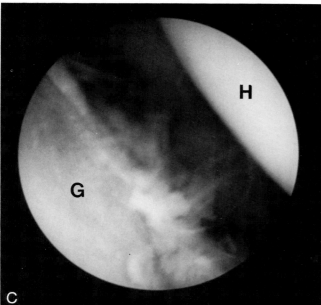

**FIGURE 13–56.** Glenohumeral joint arthrography: Glenoid labrum abnormalities.

**A** Conventional arthrotomography delineates a tear of the anterior portion of the glenoid labrum (arrow) and imbibition of contrast material in the posterior portion of the labrum (arrowhead).

**B** Computed arthrotomography shows complete detachment of the anterior portion of the glenoid labrum (arrow). The anterior portion of the capsule is redundant.

**C** Arthroscopy demonstrates a frayed and irregular appearance of the anterior portion of the labrum. G, Glenoid cavity; H, humeral head.

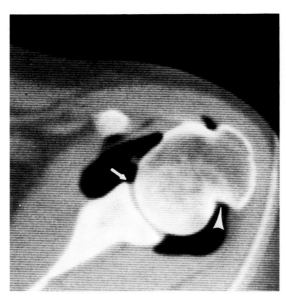

**FIGURE 13–57.** Glenohumeral joint arthrography: Glenoid labrum and humeral head abnormalities. Computed arthrotomography of the glenohumeral joint reveals a Hill-Sachs lesion (arrowhead) as well as absence of the anterior portion of the glenoid labrum (arrow).

studies are reported to be highly accurate. With regard to their series using conventional arthrotomography, Braunstein and O'Connor[434] accurately characterized the anterior labral abnormality seen in all nine of their patients; however, no patients with normal arthrograms were explored, and thus no data on false negatives are available. Of the 21 patients with surgical confirmation reported by McGlynn and coworkers,[437] the labrum was accurately characterized as normal or abnormal in all cases, and there were no false positives or false negatives. Pappas and collaborators[436] ex-

amined 46 patients with prone oblique conventional arthrotomography; 18 patients with positive findings and three normal subjects had operative intervention in which the accuracy of the interpretations was confirmed. In an analysis of 55 patients undergoing conventional arthrotomography, Deutsch and coworkers[440] found that the technique classified the status of the labrum in 13 of the 16 patients who had surgery or arthroscopy (sensitivity, 86 per cent; accuracy, 81 per cent).

Reported studies also have underscored the accuracy of computed arthrotomography. In an investigation of 10 patients, Shuman and others[439] observed that, on the basis of surgical confirmation of the findings, computed arthrotomography correctly characterized the labrum as abnormal in five persons and normal in one. Kinnard and collaborators[438] reported that of 10 patients undergoing computed arthrotomography for evaluation of shoulder instability, three had labral abnormalities that were confirmed at surgery. Deutsch and colleagues,[440] in an investigation of 81 patients with computed arthrotomography, found that the examination accurately characterized the glenoid labrum as normal, abnormal, or detached in 38 of the 44 patients who had surgery or arthroscopy (sensitivity, 96 per cent; accuracy, 86 per cent). Hill-Sachs defects were seen in 20 of 29 patients with anterior labral abnormalities, and bicipital tendon abnormalities were evident in six patients. Excellent results with computed arthrotomography also were reported by Pennes and colleagues[742] and Wilson and coworkers,[743] and the technique has been employed successfully in the analysis of patients with recurrent shoulder dislocation after surgical repair.[745]

Although both computed and conventional arthrotomography are well applied to the evaluation of patients with shoulder instability, the former appears superior at this time because it is more comprehensive, requires less technical

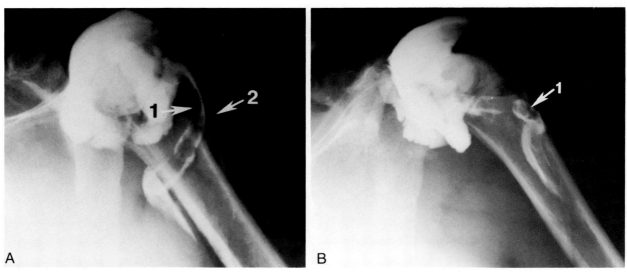

**FIGURE 13–58.** Glenohumeral joint arthrography: Posterior displacement of the long head of the bicipital tendon. This 41 year old man sustained an anterior dislocation of the glenohumeral joint that was manipulated and "reduced." Three months later, he had marked restriction of both active and passive motion of the shoulder. An arthrogram of the glenohumeral joint was performed.

**A** In internal rotation of the humerus, the dislocated long head of the bicipital tendon is seen in an unusual position (1). A bone fragment also is evident (2).

**B** In external rotation of the humerus, motion is restricted by the posteriorly displaced long head of the bicipital tendon (1). At surgery, the latter was released from its origin and tenodesis in the bicipital groove was performed, reestablishing full shoulder motion.

(From Freeland AE, Higgins RW: Orthopedics 8:468, 1985.)

expertise and radiation exposure, and is tolerated better by patients in pain.[440] It also has the capability of allowing examination of both shoulders at once. Its advantages, however, in comparison with those of standard MR imaging or MR arthrography are not so clear, and all such techniques have definite limitations owing to the variability in the size and shape of the normal glenoid labrum (see Chapter 70).

### Rheumatoid Arthritis and Other Synovial Disorders (Figs. 13–59 and 13–60)

Synovial, cartilaginous, osseous, and soft tissue changes of rheumatoid involvement of the glenohumeral joint can be identified on arthrography.[82–85] These findings include a corrugated, enlarged synovial cavity, nodular filling defects, cartilage loss, contrast filling of osseous erosions, lymphatic filling, enlarging axillary lymph nodes, capsulitis with a restricted joint cavity, and rotator cuff tear. The last-mentioned abnormality, reported by DeSmet and coworkers[82] in 5 of 13 patients with rheumatoid arthritis (38 per cent), probably is related to erosion of the inner aspect of the tendon by the inflamed synovium.[83] It should be expected that other disorders characterized by synovial inflammation also could lead to rupture of the rotator cuff, a speculation that is substantiated by observation of this complication in septic arthritis of the glenohumeral joint.[86] In the presence of a rotator cuff tear in patients with rheumatoid arthritis,

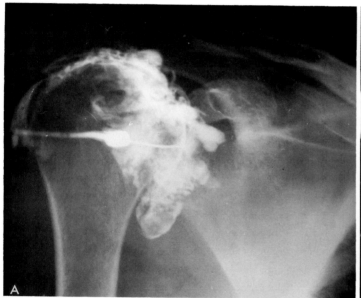
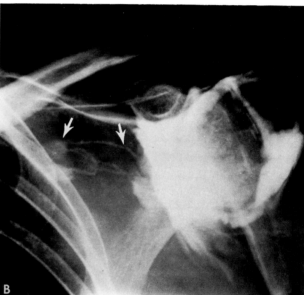
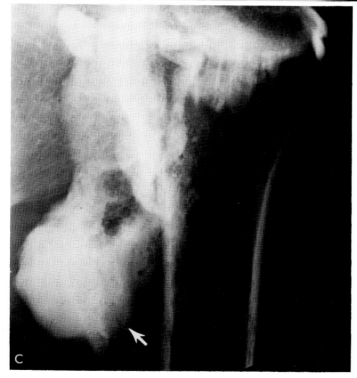

**FIGURE 13–59.** Glenohumeral joint arthrography: Rheumatoid arthritis.

**A** Contrast opacification of the articular cavity reveals a corrugated synovial pattern with nodular filling defects. The rotator cuff also was abnormal. (Courtesy of J. Mink, M.D., Los Angeles, California.)

**B** In another patient, adhesive capsulitis is present with nonvisualization of the normal axillary pouch and subscapular recess. Observe filling of the lymphatic vessels (arrows).

**C** A large axillary synovial cyst (arrow) can be seen in a third patient with rheumatoid arthritis.

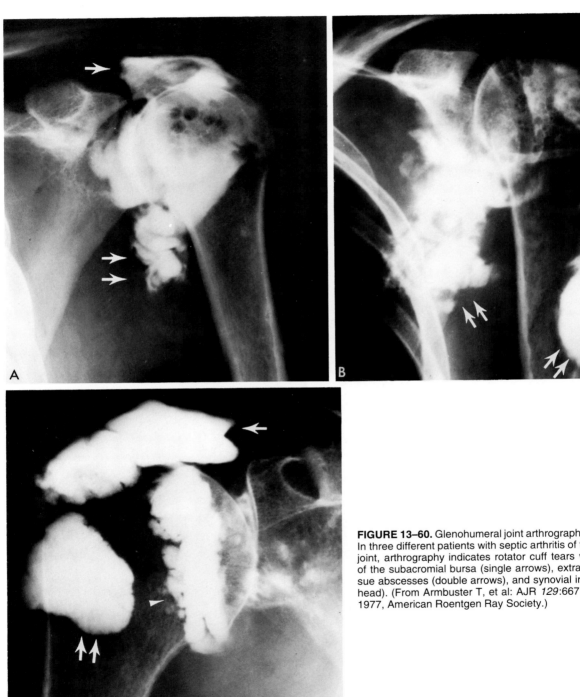

**FIGURE 13–60.** Glenohumeral joint arthrography: Septic arthritis. In three different patients with septic arthritis of the glenohumeral joint, arthrography indicates rotator cuff tears with opacification of the subacromial bursa (single arrows), extra-articular soft tissue abscesses (double arrows), and synovial irregularity (arrowhead). (From Armbuster T, et al: AJR *129*:667, 1977. Copyright 1977, American Roentgen Ray Society.)

arthrography of the glenohumeral joint may lead to opacification of an enlarged subacromial bursa containing radiolucent masses.[87] These masses represent lobulated fatty tissue, which may be attached to the synovial lining.

In rheumatoid arthritis and other synovial disorders, synovial cysts about the glenohumeral joint may be documented by arthrography, as these cysts frequently communicate with the joint cavity.[454] They may be filled with blood.[88]

Septic arthritis of the glenohumeral joint may lead to synovial irregularity and capsular and rotator cuff rupture, with the formation of soft tissue abscesses.[86] These abscesses appear as irregular contrast-filled cavities on glenohumeral joint arthrography.

Percutaneous catheter drainage has been suggested as a technique that can be applied to the treatment of septic arthritis of the glenohumeral joint,[455, 747] as well as other articulations such as the hip.[747] Fluoroscopy is used to monitor the placement of one or more catheters in the articulation, and their tips should be positioned in the most dependent portions of the joint (posterior with the patient in the supine position) to facilitate adequate drainage.

## Subacromial (Subdeltoid) Bursography

Although the subacromial bursa occasionally is injected inadvertently during attempted glenohumeral joint arthrography, it is only a potential space in normal persons so that direct, purposeful opacification of this structure in the absence of subacromial bursal changes is difficult (Fig. 13–61). This is unfortunate, as there are practical reasons for performing subacromial bursography. First, contrast filling of this bursa will delineate the superior surface of the rotator cuff musculature and, when coupled with subsequent conventional tomography, can delineate partial-thickness tears of the cuff that begin on its external or superior surface.[732] Second, subacromial bursography may identify a small bursa in association with adhesive capsulitis,[338] and the inclusion of lidocaine and corticosteroid preparation in the injection solution may provide diagnostic and therapeutic benefit in patients with adhesive bursitis. Third, the soft tissues in the superior aspect of the joint are affected in the shoulder impingement syndrome[456–459]; although the diagnosis of this condition generally is provided by the clinical examination, which reveals a painful and restricted arc of

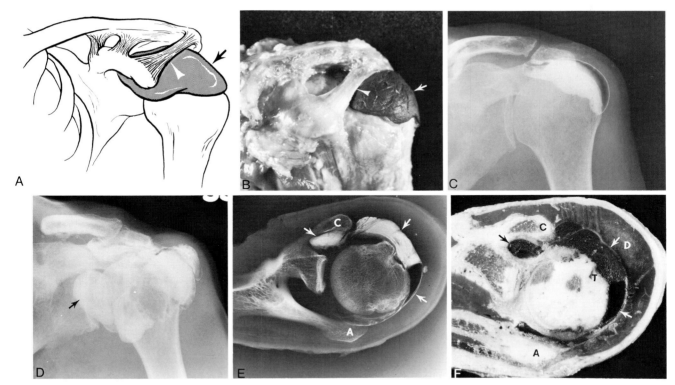

**FIGURE 13–61.** Subacromial bursography: Anatomy and normal bursogram.
   **A** A drawing reveals the subacromial bursa (arrow) sitting like a cap above the humeral head. Observe its relationship to the coracoacromial ligament (arrowhead) extending from the coracoid process anteriorly to the acromion posteriorly.
   **B** An anterior view of a dissected shoulder reveals the subacromial bursa (arrow) filled with latex and the coracoacromial ligament (arrowhead).
   **C** The normal subacromial bursa has been opacified with air and radiopaque contrast material. It is smooth and extends beneath the acromion process.
   **D** In another cadaver, a large subacromial (subdeltoid) bursa contains air and radiopaque contrast material. A subcoracoid extension (arrow) overlies the joint space, but there is no contrast material within the articular cavity.
   **E, F** A radiograph and photograph of a transverse section of the shoulder illustrated in **D** show the coracoid process (C), the acromion (A), the subacromial bursa (arrows) with medial extension behind the coracoid process, the bicipital tendon (T) in the bicipital groove, and the deltoid muscle (D).
   (**C, E, F,** From Strizak AM, et al: J Bone Joint Surg [Am] *64*:196, 1982.)

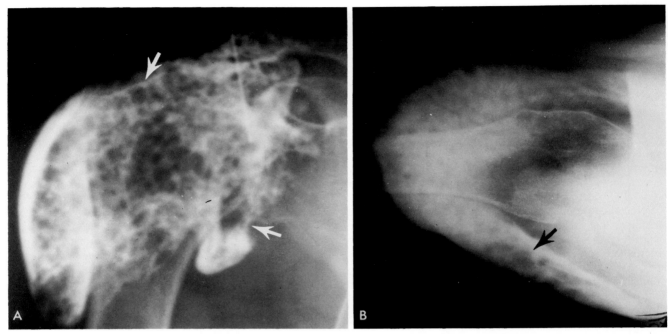

**FIGURE 13–62.** Subacromial bursography: Rheumatoid arthritis. Frontal **(A)** and axillary **(B)** views reveal an enlarged subacromial bursa with innumerable nodular filling defects (arrows). (Courtesy of W. J. Weston, M.D., Lower Hutt, New Zealand.)

shoulder motion, supplemented with conventional radiography and fluoroscopy (see Chapter 3), opacification of the subacromial bursa can provide additional documentation of the syndrome's presence.[457] Finally, the degree of primary bursal abnormality accompanying rheumatoid arthritis or other synovial disorders is defined by this procedure (Fig. 13–62).

Although a superolateral approach can be used to insert a needle directly into the subacromial bursa, the author prefers an anterior technique.[460] The patient is placed supine on the fluoroscopy table, and a point approximately in the middle of the anterior margin of the acromion is identified. A 22 gauge spinal needle is advanced vertically until its tip contacts the edge of the acromion; the needle then is displaced slightly caudally (immediately below the inferior surface of the bone), still maintaining its vertical orientation while advancing it more deeply, parallel to the undersurface of the acromion, in an anteroposterior direction (Fig. 13–63). As the tip of the needle passes the margin of the acromion, a gentle popping sound indicates that it has extended through the coracoacromial ligament into the subacromial bursa. Alternatively, the needle can be advanced until it contacts the posterior, descending portion of the bone.[457] At that time, a syringe filled with air is connected with a tube to the needle and the latter gradually is removed while the examiner maintains firm pressure on the plunger of the syringe. At the point at which the needle tip is free in the bursa, resistance to injection decreases sharply, and a small amount of air can be introduced. Visualization of the air as a curvilinear radiolucent collection lateral to the greater tuberosity of the humerus confirms the intrabursal location of the needle tip. Single contrast (2 to 4 ml of radiopaque contrast material) or double contrast (1 ml of radiopaque contrast material and 5 to 10 ml of air) technique can be used, and 1 or 2 ml of lidocaine (Xylocaine)

or bupivacaine (Marcaine) or a steroid preparation (methylprednisolone sodium succinate [Solu-Medrol], 65 mg), or both, can be added to the injection solution.

Positive bursographic findings include a thin vertical collection of contrast material within the outer portion of the rotator cuff in instances of partial tear of the cuff; a small, contracted irregular bursal sac in cases of adhesive bursitis (Fig. 13–64A); and pooling of the contrast material in the lateral (subdeltoid) portion of the subacromial bursa during abduction of the externally rotated arm in instances of the shoulder impingement syndrome (Fig. 13–64B). Bursotomography occasionally is required in the diagnosis of some of these conditions, particularly a partial-thickness tear of the rotator cuff musculature.

## Arthrography of the Acromioclavicular Joint

A previous report has outlined normal arthrographic findings of the acromioclavicular joint.[89] The technique involves puncturing the joint from the superior aspect under fluoroscopy, using a 21 gauge needle (Fig. 13–65). One milliliter of contrast material will reveal an L-shaped articular cavity with a horizontal limb extending beneath the distal end of the clavicle. Although acromioclavicular joint arthrography in rheumatoid arthritis conceivably could outline the degree of synovial irregularity, cartilaginous, discal, and osseous destruction, and the presence of a synovial cyst, there appears to be little clinical application for this procedure in rheumatoid arthritis. A report has indicated that arthrography may provide useful information in dislocation of the acromioclavicular joint, however.[315] Leakage of contrast medium around the articulation and in the direction of the coracoid process may provide information regarding the severity of the injury to the ligaments.

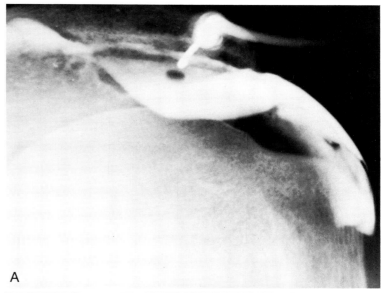

**FIGURE 13–63.** Subacromial bursography: Technique of examination.

**A** Note the position of the needle. It is advanced in a posterior direction immediately beneath the acromion process. Contrast medium outlines the smooth confines of the bursa.

**B** Conventional tomography can be used in conjunction with the bursogram to define the characteristics of the superior surface of the rotator cuff. In this case, the study was accomplished after a normal arthrogram of the glenohumeral joint.

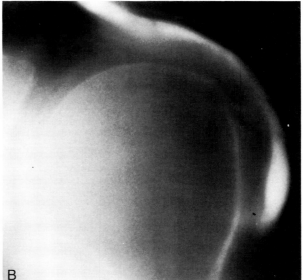

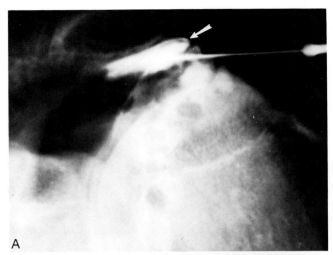

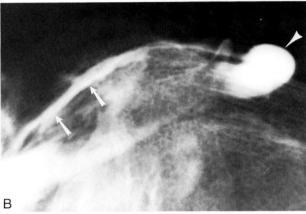

**FIGURE 13–64.** Subacromial bursography: Abnormal findings.

**A** Adhesive bursitis. After glenohumeral joint arthrography, direct opacification of a contracted subacromial bursa (arrow) is accomplished. The instillation of a corticosteroid preparation into the bursa in such cases can produce beneficial clinical results.

**B** Shoulder impingement syndrome. Direct opacification of the subacromial bursa reveals that, as the patient elevates his arm, the contrast agent pools in the lateral portion of the bursa (arrowhead), with only a small amount of contrast material present in the medial portion (arrows). (From Cone RO III, et al: Radiology *150*:29, 1984.)

## HIP

### Arthrography of the Hip

Although most descriptions of hip arthrography record its application in the investigation of patients with painful prostheses (which is discussed elsewhere in this book), this procedure also may be utilized in patients with congenital, traumatic, and articular disorders (Table 13–6).

#### TABLE 13–6. Indications for Hip Arthrography

Evaluation of:
Developmental dysplasia of the hip
Septic arthritis and osteomyelitis with epiphyseal separation
Epiphyseal dysplasia and osteonecrosis
Certain synovial disorders
Soft tissue masses
Trauma

### Technique (Fig. 13–66)

Many techniques exist for puncturing the hip joint. Some use a direct or angulated anterior approach,[90–93] whereas others describe lateral,[748] superior,[94] or inferior[95, 316] approaches. The technique will vary somewhat in adults and in children. Fluoroscopy is mandatory.[96]

The author uses an anterior approach in performing hip arthrography. The patient is placed supine on the table with the legs stabilized in internal rotation by sandbags or a traction device. After preliminary films are obtained, the femoral artery is palpated in the groin and a metal marker is placed 2 cm lateral and 2 cm distal to this point. The position of the marker is checked under the fluoroscope; it should lie near the medial margin of the femoral neck. After skin preparation and adequate local anesthesia, an 18 gauge, 3 inch spinal needle is inserted in a superior direction with fluoroscopic guidance to contact the bone at the junction of the medial aspect of the femoral head and neck. This position is checked by turning the patient into a steep oblique projection. A joint aspirate may be sent to the laboratory; if no fluid is obtained, nonbacteriostatic saline solution is injected and then recovered, to be sent for analysis. Ten to 15 ml of contrast medium (60 per cent Renografin) then is injected, and the needle is withdrawn. Anteroposterior radiographs in internal and external rotation, a frog-leg view, and true lateral radiographs are obtained before and after mild exercise.

In infants and children, an anterolateral subphyseal plate site is ideal for contacting the bone.[96] This metaphyseal location is within the joint capsule yet distant from the femoral vessels, cartilaginous femoral head, and growth plate. Some arthrographers prefer an anteromedial or inferomedial approach.[461] Approximately 1.5 to 2 ml is injected in infants and 5 to 8 ml in adolescents.[462] Some investigators prefer to document the intra-articular location of the needle tip by injecting a small amount of air; air emboli may complicate this testing strategy.[463]

In performing hip arthrography in patients with joint prostheses, subtraction arthrography frequently is necessary so that contrast material can be differentiated from the radiopaque acrylic cement that is used to fix the prosthesis in place.[97] As indicated previously, conventional or digital techniques can be used to create the subtracted images.[390, 463, 749, 750] In patients who have been treated with Girdlestone arthroplasty, intracapsular placement of the needle is best accomplished from an anterior approach with needle advancement to the midpoint of the intertrochanteric line.[751]

Additional modifications with regard to hip arthrography include its supplementation with conventional tomography or CT scanning and the incorporation of pressure monitoring within the joint during or after the injection of the contrast material.[393, 464]

### Normal Hip Arthrogram (Fig. 13–67)

The normal hip arthrogram in adults consists of the following structures. The recess capitus is a thin, smooth collection of contrast material between the articular surfaces of acetabulum and femoral head.[98, 99] This recess is interrupted only at the site where the ligamentum teres enters the fovea centralis of the femoral head. The ligamentum transversum produces a radiolucent defect adjacent to the inferior rim of the acetabulum. An inferior articular recess

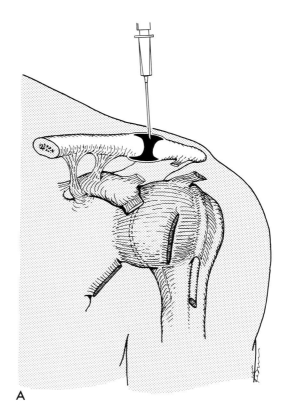

**FIGURE 13–65.** Arthrography of the acromioclavicular joint: Technique and normal arthrogram.

   **A** The joint is punctured from the superior aspect.

   **B** In a cadaver, the normal contrast-filled articular cavity (arrow) is viewed in an inferosuperior radiographic projection. (Courtesy of W. J. Weston, M.D., Lower Hutt, New Zealand.)

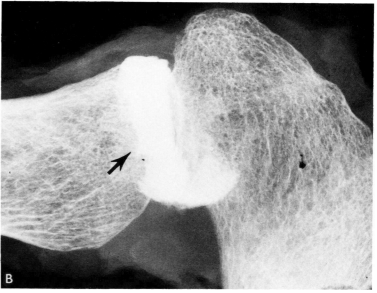

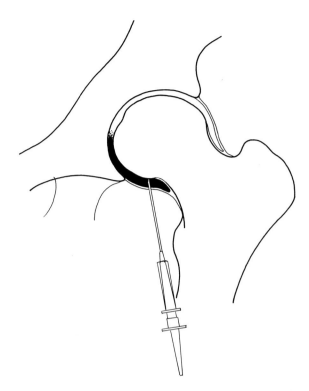

**FIGURE 13–66.** Hip arthrography: Technique. The needle is inserted from an anterior approach and directed superiorly so as to contact the osseous surface at the junction of the femoral head and femoral neck.

**FIGURE 13–67.** Hip arthrography: Normal arthrogram. The recess capitus (rc) is a thin, smooth collection of contrast medium between opposing articular surfaces and is interrupted only where the ligamentum teres (double arrows) enters the fovea centralis of the femoral head. The ligamentum transversum (lt) is seen as a radiolucent defect adjacent to the inferior rim of the acetabulum. The ligamentum teres bridges the acetabular notch and effectively deepens the acetabulum. The inferior articular recess (iar) forms a pouch at the inferior base of the femoral head below the acetabular notch and ligamentum transversum. The superior articular recess (sar) extends cephalad around the acetabular labrum (lab). The acetabular labrum is seen as a triangular radiolucent area adjacent to the superolateral lip of the acetabulum. The zona orbicularis (zo) is a circumferential lucent band around the femoral neck, which changes configuration with rotation of the femur. The recess colli superior (rcs) and recess colli inferior (rci) are poolings of contrast material at the apex and base of the intertrochanteric line and are the most caudal extensions of the synovial membrane. (From Guerra J Jr, et al: Radiology *128*:11, 1978.)

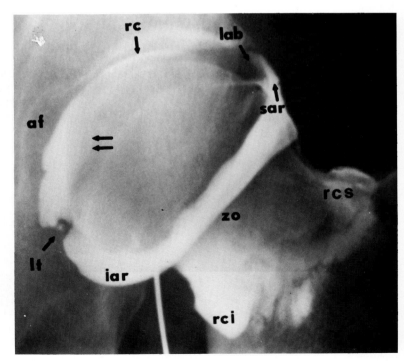

exists as a pouch at the inferior base of the femoral head below the acetabular notch and ligamentum transversum. The superior articular recess extends cephalad around the acetabular labrum. The latter appears as a triangular radiolucent area adjacent to the superolateral lip of the acetabulum. The zona orbicularis is a circumferential lucent band around the femoral neck, which changes configuration during femoral rotation. The recess colli superior and recess colli inferior are poolings of contrast material beneath the zona orbicularis and the apex and base of the intertrochanteric line.

In children, similar arthrographic features are apparent.[96] The cartilaginous tissue around the femoral head is abundant in amount, reflecting both articular cartilage and that portion of the femoral head that is not yet ossified.

### Developmental Dysplasia of the Hip (Fig. 13–68)

In infants, hip arthrography may be useful in the evaluation of developmental dysplasia of the hip (see Chapter 86), although generally it is not essential for diagnosing the condition.[92, 94, 95, 100, 101] Conventional arthrography is considered adequate by most investigators, although some advocate video-arthrography.[101] Ultrasonography and MR imaging are competitive diagnostic techniques.

In infants with developmental dysplasia of the hip, the cartilaginous limbus will be apparent as a filling defect beneath the displaced head of the femur. In this situation, the head will deform or compress the limbus and the ligamentum teres is stretched, leading from the inferior margin of the acetabulum to the fovea of the dislocated femoral head. The capsule also is stretched around the head, and the opacified hip joint will have an hourglass configuration.[100]

The hip arthrogram may be used to evaluate the adequacy of reduction of a dislocated femoral head, particularly in the older infant or child.[95] In this situation, an inverted limbus may be interposed between the acetabulum and head, preventing complete reduction. Arthrography will outline the inverted limbus, and pooling of contrast material may be identified between the femoral head and medial acetabular wall. This information may aid the orthopedic surgeon in determining the need for surgery and in planning the operative procedure.

It should be emphasized that, owing to the unossified nature of the cartilaginous femoral head in the newborn, the differentiation of developmental dysplasia of the hip from infectious (see subsequent discussion) and traumatic epiphyseal separation is extremely difficult or impossible on the basis of routine radiography. Arthrography will document that the femoral head is situated in the acetabulum in cases of epiphysiolysis and, therefore, it is essential in this differential diagnosis.[465, 466]

### Septic Arthritis in Infants (Figs. 13–69 to 13–71)

Hip arthrography is useful in the clinical setting of neonatal sepsis and an apparent dislocation of the femoral head.[105] In this situation, it is impossible to determine the exact position of the unossified femoral head on initial radiographs. Two possibilities exist: The hip indeed is dislocated, or there is a pathologic epiphyseal separation related to osteomyelitis with a normal relationship between cartilaginous head and acetabulum. A hip arthrogram will allow aspiration of joint contents and documentation of the position of the femoral head. The diagnosis of true dislo-

cation or epiphyseal separation then can be made accurately.

Glassberg and Ozonoff[106] also have emphasized the use of arthrography in septic arthritis of the hip. This technique allows accurate placement of the needle for aspiration and assessment of the degree of cartilaginous destruction.

### Epiphyseal Dysplasia, Legg-Calvé-Perthes Disease, and Related Conditions (Fig. 13–72)

Hip arthrography has been employed to investigate the pathogenesis of multiple epiphyseal dysplasia and spondyloepiphyseal dysplasia.[107] Although the study does not allow differentiation among the various dysplasias, it does reveal that the cartilaginous head generally is smooth despite the presence of irregular fragmented ossific densities within the femoral head, suggesting that these disorders relate to faulty, incomplete, or delayed epiphyseal ossification. The integrity of the articular cartilage also can be evaluated by using hip arthrography.

Hip arthrography may have more immediate clinical benefit in evaluating patients with Legg-Calvé-Perthes disease.[91, 109–111] In this condition, one arthrographic finding is an absolute enlargement of the femoral head related to hyperplasia of the epiphyseal cartilage. This finding suggests that the apparent noncontact of femoral head and medial acetabulum noted on initial plain film radiography in this condition is, in reality, related to cartilaginous hyperplasia,[110] so that subluxation is not present. This method of identifying the true position of the cartilaginous head may allow the surgeon to determine which position of the hip will be best during treatment of the condition. Bilateral hip arthrograms may be necessary in these persons, enabling normal and abnormal sides to be compared.[359] MR imaging also can be used in the assessment of hip involvement in Legg-Calvé-Perthes disease (see Chapter 81).

Arthrography in patients with transient synovitis of the hip has outlined similar thickening of articular cartilage.[110] Because many investigators suggest that synovitis may be etiologically related to Legg-Calvé-Perthes disease, the observation that synovitis can lead to cartilaginous hyperplasia is significant.

Arthrography of the hip in Legg-Calvé-Perthes disease also has been used to demonstrate the existence of an osteochondral fragment.[330] This uncommon complication relates to the presence of an unhealed necrotic fragment, which appears separate from the remainder of the femoral head. The arthrogram will delineate whether the necrotic fragment is loose; in this case, contrast material introduced into the hip will dissect under the osteochondral fragment.

### Trauma

In addition to traumatic epiphysiolysis, arthrography has been employed to investigate other posttraumatic abnormalities of the hip. In patients with single or recurrent anterior[467] or posterior[468] dislocations of the femoral head, hip arthrography alone or in combination with CT[752] may outline distortion of or defects in the joint capsule, tears of the ligamentum teres, and intra-articular osteocartilaginous bodies.

After injury[469] or surgery,[393] or on an idiopathic basis,[470] capsular constriction (adhesive capsulitis) may appear in the hip, although it is more widely recognized in the shoulder and ankle. In such cases, plain films generally are un-

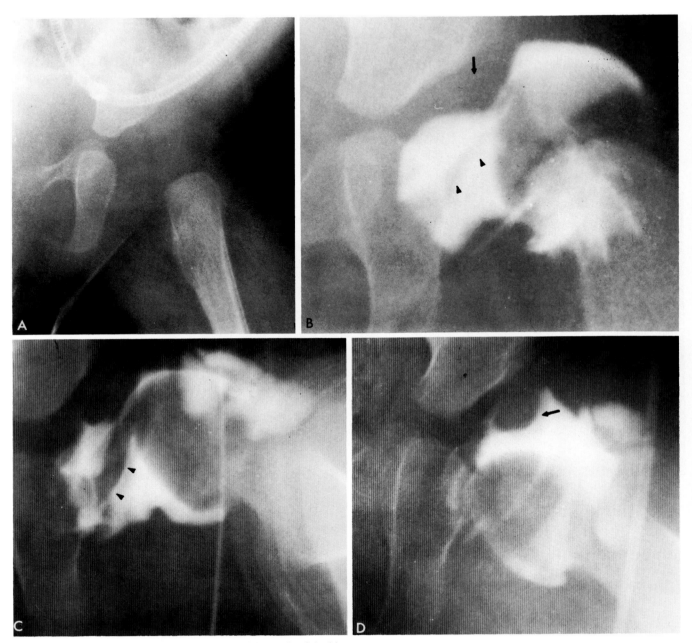

**FIGURE 13–68.** Hip arthrography: Developmental dysplasia of the hip.

**A, B** A 2 month old infant with hip dislocation. The initial film **(A)** reveals the lateral position of the femur with respect to the acetabulum. The arthrogram **(B)** obtained in neutral position outlines the radiolucent cartilaginous femoral head, a deformed limbus (arrow) between the displaced femoral head and acetabulum, and a stretched ligamentum teres (arrowheads). Because of the stretched capsule, the opacified hip joint has an hourglass configuration.

**C, D** A 1 year old infant with hip dislocation. On an initial arthrographic view **(C)**, observe the dislocated femoral head and stretched ligamentum teres (arrowheads). In another view obtained with 45 degrees of abduction, flexion, and traction **(D)**, the limbus appears inverted (arrow).

(From Kaye JJ, et al: Radiology *114*:671, 1975.)

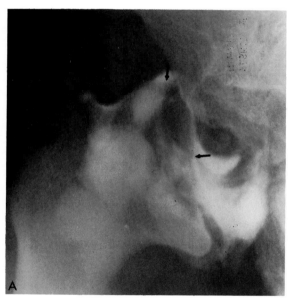 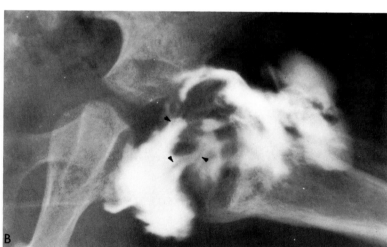

**FIGURE 13–69.** Hip arthrography: Septic arthritis.

**A** In a male infant with septic dislocation of the femoral head, an arthrogram reveals severe cartilaginous deformity with a triangular cartilaginous head (arrows). Normal recesses are absent.

**B** In another male infant with septic dislocation of the femoral head, lateral subluxation and synovial adhesions with a swirled appearance of contrast material (arrowheads) are evident.

(**A, B,** From Glassberg GB, Ozonoff MB: Radiology *128*:151, 1978.)

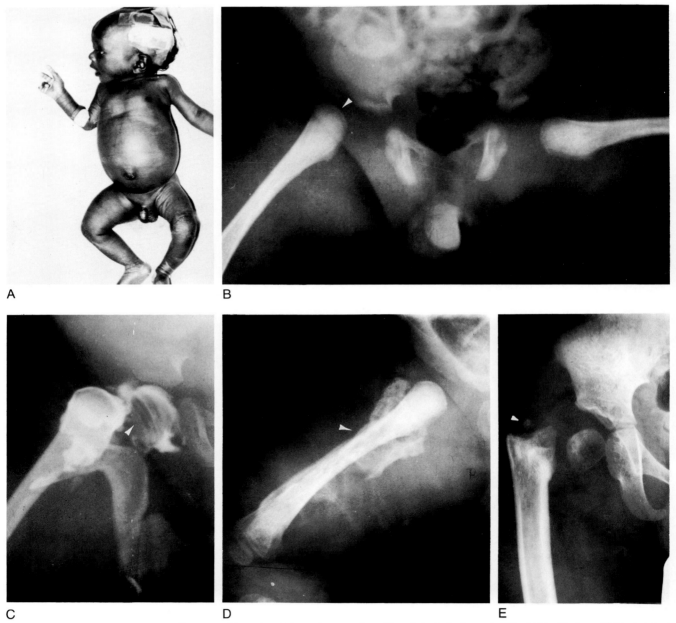

**FIGURE 13–70.** Hip arthrography: Osteomyelitis with epiphyseal separation. The clinical photograph **(A)** of this 10 day old black infant demonstrates a swollen right leg, held in abduction and flexion. An initial radiograph **(B)** reveals an apparent "dislocation" of the right hip because of the laterally displaced femoral metaphysis (arrowhead). An arthrogram **(C)** obtained 4 days later outlines a radiolucent femoral head (arrowhead), which is in normal position with respect to the acetabulum, and a displaced femoral metaphysis indicating an epiphyseal separation. Several weeks later **(D)** after treatment with a hip spica, metaphyseal bone destruction (arrowhead) indicates the presence of osteomyelitis. **E,** Radiograph made at 37 months of age delineates residual changes of the femoral metaphysis, varus deformity, a deformed and partially ossified femoral head within the acetabulum, acetabular flattening, and a small ossification center of the greater trochanter (arrowhead). **(A–D,** From Kaye JJ, et al: Radiology *114*:674, 1975.)

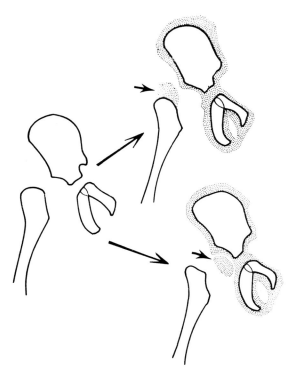

**FIGURE 13–71.** Hip arthrography: Septic arthritis versus osteomyelitis with epiphyseal separation. In either case, an initial radiograph (on left) will indicate a displaced metaphysis with respect to the acetabulum. With a true dislocation (top right) the cartilaginous epiphysis is displaced laterally (arrow). With an epiphyseal separation (bottom right) the femoral head is placed normally in the acetabulum (arrow) (cartilaginous areas are stippled).

(From Kaye JJ, et al: Radiology *114*:674, 1975.)

remarkable or show nonspecific findings, including osteopenia or intra-articular osseous bodies. Accurate diagnosis is accomplished with arthrography, during which a low capacity of the joint cavity is demonstrated. Difficulty injecting as little as 8 ml of contrast material into the hip is encountered, owing to a rapid rise in intra-articular pressure. The normal articular recesses are obliterated. On histologic inspection of the joint capsule, a chronic inflammatory reaction with fibrosis is seen, which has caused it to adhere to the femoral neck.[469]

In a review of 13 patients with adhesive capsulitis of the hip, Lequesne and collaborators[470] defined two categories of the disease: secondary capsular constriction accompanying synovial (osteo)chondromatosis or an osteoid osteoma; and primary or idiopathic capsular constriction occurring in the absence of additional articular abnormalities, which was self-limiting, resolving in periods varying from 3 to 18 months. In all cases, arthrography documented the low intra-articular capacity (no more than 10 ml of contrast material could be injected) and the absence of opacification of normal joint recesses.

Tears and deformities of the acetabular labrum have been recorded following trauma,[471] and cyst formation (ganglia) in the labrum has been identified.[472, 689, 753] Routine radiography may reveal gas-containing soft tissue masses, and during arthrography, contrast material may extend from the joint into the labral tear and ganglion. This condition is recognized as a complication of chronic acetabular dysplasia.

### Articular Disorders (Figs. 13–73 to 13–75)

Contrast opacification of the hip may allow more accurate diagnosis of a variety of articular disorders. In idio-

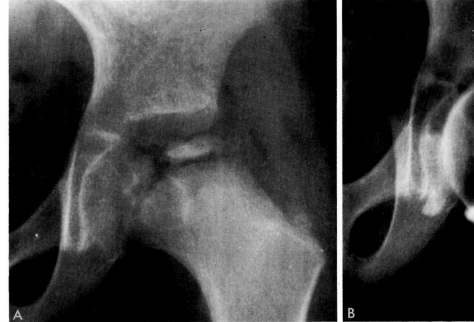
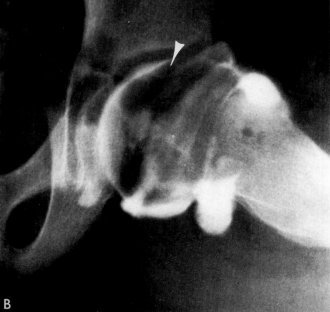

**FIGURE 13–72.** Hip arthrography: Legg-Calvé-Perthes disease.
 **A** On the initial film, epiphyseal fragmentation and metaphyseal irregularity are apparent.
 **B** Arthrographic image in hip abduction indicates a relatively smooth radiolucent cartilaginous head (arrowhead), which is well covered by the acetabulum.

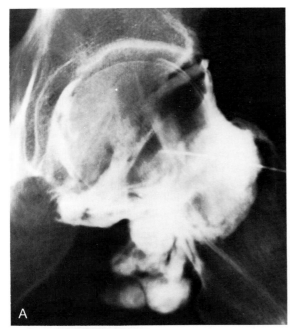

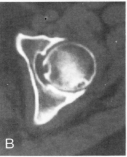

**FIGURE 13–73.** Hip arthrography: Pigmented villonodular synovitis. The initial radiograph of the hip (not shown) in this 57 year old woman revealed a normal joint space and cystic areas in the femoral head and neck.

**A** Aspiration of the joint revealed brown discoloration of the synovial fluid, and arthrography documents an enlarged and irregular joint cavity with small, medial collections or pools of contrast material.

**B** A transaxial CT scan shows the well-defined cysts in the femoral head, each possessing a slightly sclerotic margin, and minimal narrowing of the posterior portion of the joint. Surgery confirmed the diagnosis of pigmented villonodular synovitis.

(Courtesy of V. Vint, M.D., San Diego, California.)

pathic synovial (osteo)chondromatosis or pigmented villonodular synovitis, the extent of synovial and capsular abnormality can be determined in this fashion.[112] This is important not only in outlining the severity of the disorder but also in establishing the correct diagnosis when plain films are not conclusive. In patients with septic arthritis, hip arthrography provides a technique for aspiration and culture and also a means of evaluating cartilaginous, osseous, and synovial abnormalities.

### Synovial Cysts

Hip arthrography in rheumatoid arthritis and other synovial disorders will reveal the degree of intra-articular alterations and the presence or absence of communicating synovial cysts (Fig. 13–76). Opacification of the iliopsoas bursa may be identified and, although this is apparent in 15

per cent of normal hips,[113] communication of the hip and iliopsoas bursa in the presence of intra-articular diseases such as osteoarthritis, rheumatoid arthritis, pigmented villonodular synovitis, infection, calcium pyrophosphate dihydrate crystal deposition disease, and idiopathic synovial (osteo)chondromatosis may lead to bursal enlargement, producing a mass in the ilioinguinal region that may simulate a hernia and cause obstruction of the femoral vein.[114, 115] A second potential communication that may allow decompression of a hip joint with elevated intra-articular pressure exists at the crossing of the iliofemoral and iliopubic ligaments, at which point fluid may dissect into the fat plane of the obturator externus muscle.[98]

Of the 15 or more synovium-lined bursae that have been described about the hip, it is the iliopsoas bursa (also termed the iliopectineal, iliofemoral, iliac, or subpsoas bursa) that deserves emphasis in any discussion of synovial cysts in this region. Measuring approximately 3 to 7 cm long and 2 to 4 cm wide and extending from the inguinal ligament to the lesser trochanter of the femur, the iliopsoas bursa is present in about 98 per cent of adults. It communicates with the hip joint via an aperture ranging in diameter from 1 mm to 3 cm, and enlargement of this channel in the 15 per cent of normal adults who possess this aperture or creation of a communicating pathway in those adults who do not is an expected consequence of virtually any disease process of the hip that leads to an elevation of intra-articular pressure (Fig. 13–77). This phenomenon is somewhat less frequent in children, owing to a decreased prevalence of normal communication between the iliopsoas bursa and the hip.

The iliopsoas bursa is bounded anteriorly by the iliopsoas muscle and posteriorly by the pectineal eminence and the thin portion of the capsule of the hip joint.[473] Its lateral border is the iliofemoral ligament and its medial border is the cotyloid ligament; its superior border is the inguinal ligament and its inferior border is the pubofemoral ligament.[473] When distended, a painless or painful soft tissue mass is created, possibly accompanied by shortening of the stride related to avoidance of hyperextension, flexion of the hip and knee with external rotation of the thigh, weakness of the extremity, and point tenderness inferior to the inguinal ligament and 2 cm lateral to the femoral artery. The mass itself may compress the adjacent neurovascular structures, rarely causing secondary venous obstruction with distal edema, displace pelvic organs, become secondarily infected or traumatized, or induce an abducted gait. In the absence of a clear-cut history of arthritis, the patient with an enlarged iliopsoas bursa initially may be evaluated by a general surgeon, who easily may misinterpret the mass and its associated symptoms and signs as evidence of an inguinal hernia, aneurysm of the femoral artery, undescended testicle, varices, adenopathy, or solid neoplasm. Arteriographic evaluation may lead to inadvertent puncture of the bursa or, at the time of operation, the enlarged synovium-lined structure may present a puzzle to the surgeon, who was anticipating some other disease process.[474] Accurate preoperative diagnosis is provided by arthrography of the hip (which may be combined with CT), direct opacification of the bursa, ultrasonography, MR imaging, or CT alone.[473, 475–477, 479]

Although other bursae about the hip represent potential sites for inflammation and mass formation with or without associated changes in the joint, the frequency of involve-

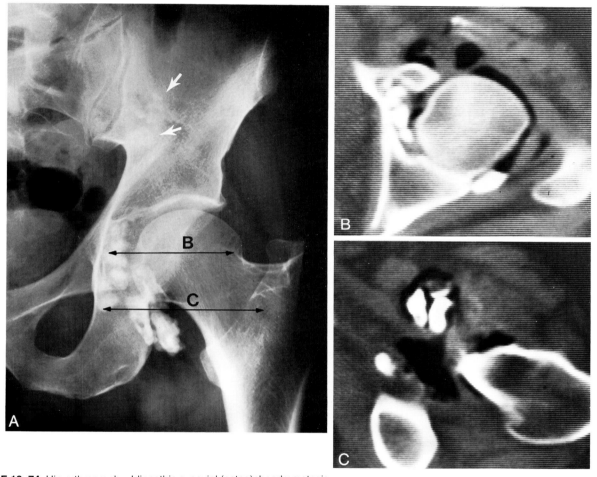

**FIGURE 13–74.** Hip arthrography: Idiopathic synovial (osteo)chondromatosis.

 **A** An initial radiograph reveals multiple calcified or ossified collections in the acetabular fossa that are extending medially and inferiorly, in the distribution of the iliopsoas bursa. Note the additional subtle calcified collections near the sacroiliac joint (arrows).

 **B, C** After the introduction of air into the hip, two transaxial CT scans at the levels indicated in **A** document the intra-articular location **(B)** and intrabursal location **(C)** of the bodies. Histologic confirmation of idiopathic synovial (osteo)chondromatosis was obtained.

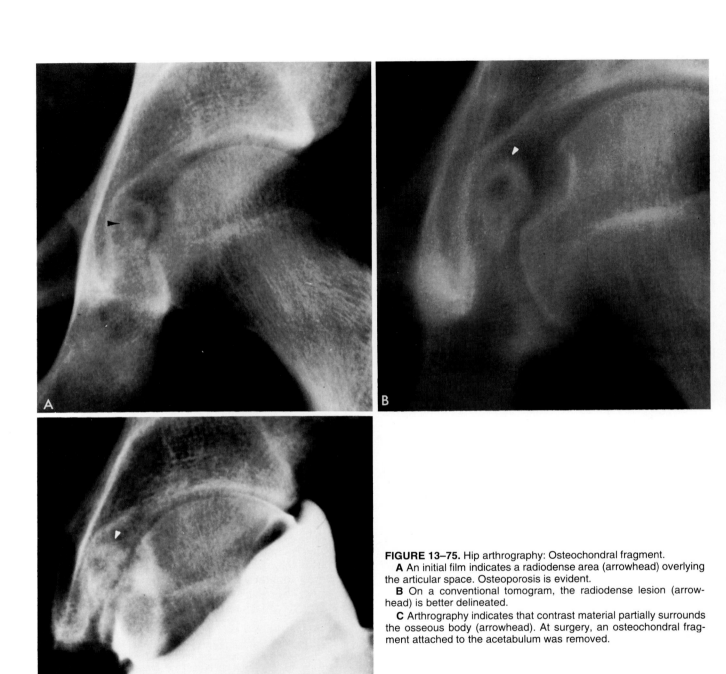

**FIGURE 13–75.** Hip arthrography: Osteochondral fragment.

**A** An initial film indicates a radiodense area (arrowhead) overlying the articular space. Osteoporosis is evident.

**B** On a conventional tomogram, the radiodense lesion (arrowhead) is better delineated.

**C** Arthrography indicates that contrast material partially surrounds the osseous body (arrowhead). At surgery, an osteochondral fragment attached to the acetabulum was removed.

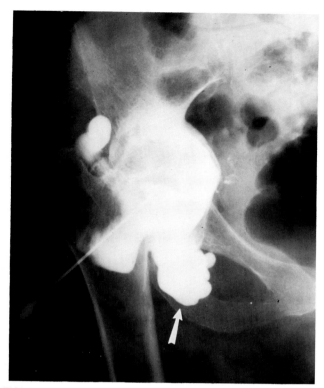

**FIGURE 13–76.** Hip arthrography: Rheumatoid arthritis and synovial cyst formation. In this 65 year old woman with rheumatoid arthritis and an apparent "femoral hernia," arthrography indicates that the clinically evident soft tissue mass is related to a synovial cyst (arrow). Observe the sacculation of the articular cavity and a protrusio acetabuli defect.

ment and the severity of the accompanying clinical manifestations are less.[754, 755] Arthrography of the native hip or, more commonly, one containing prostheses may demonstrate opacification of bursae about the greater trochanter, ischiotrochanteric bursae, or cystlike collections or abscesses not corresponding to any anatomic structure (see Chapter 19);[756] and overdistention of the articular cavity during this procedure can lead to iatrogenic rupture of the capsule, with a feathery pattern of extravastion of the contrast material.[473] The direction of such extravasation is variable, including into the retropsoas region,[478] and the contrast agent may extend for a considerable distance.

With regard to the imaging strategy that is used to evaluate suspected synovial cysts about the hip, ultrasonography should be performed after conventional radiography in the setting of a probable groin mass or other suggestive clinical manifestations. If a nonpulsatile fluid collection without Doppler evidence of flow is demonstrated, this technique then can be used for diagnostic aspiration of its contents. Fluid analysis should distinguish a synovial cyst or iliopsoas bursitis from a lymphocele, abscess, or hematoma. Subsequent injection of contrast material may opacify the hip joint, confirming the diagnosis; if not, hip arthrography, CT scanning, or MR imaging may be desirable for delineation of potential articular communication if surgery is being contemplated. The results of conservative management can be followed noninvasively with either ultrasonography or CT. In general, arteriography and lymphangiography have no place in the present-day diagnosis of suspected disease of synovial origin about the hip joint.

## Snapping Hip Syndrome

A variety of causes have been implicated in the hip pain associated with an audible snapping. Intra-articular abnormalities, including single or multiple osteocartilaginous bodies, typically result in a faint sound associated with true femoral-acetabular motion; extra-articular causes often are characterized by a loud snap and, in some cases, a sudden jump of the fascia lata or gluteus maximus over the greater trochanter as the hip moves in a well-delineated fashion.[480] Other proposed causes have included slipping of the iliopsoas tendon over the iliopectineal eminence[481] and of the iliofemoral ligaments over the anterior portion of the hip capsule.[482]

Several studies[480, 483, 757–759] have confirmed that subluxation of the iliopsoas tendon is one cause of a snapping hip. Iliopsoas bursography[483, 758, 759] or hip arthrography in which the iliopsoas bursa also is opacified[480] confirms the changing position of the iliopsoas tendon and its displacement over the iliopectineal line during flexion and extension of the hip. An abrupt change in the position of the tendon coincident with the audible sound and palpable snap is observed.

## KNEE

### Arthrography of the Knee

Despite the recent challenge presented by arthroscopy and newer imaging techniques such as CT and MR imaging, the role of arthrography is most established for abnormalities of the knee, as it is useful in evaluating this joint in a variety of clinical situations[116, 652, 760, 761] (Table 13–7). The technique of examination has evolved through the years; single contrast examination using air and oxygen[117] or radiopaque substances[118, 119] has been replaced, in large part, by double contrast examination using air and radiopaque contrast material,[120] which is preferable for evaluation of subtle meniscal and articular cartilage abnormalities. Some studies, however, indicate that comparable results can be obtained with either technique.[317] In recent years computed arthrotomography (or CT alone) has been introduced in the evaluation of a number of knee problems, including chondromalacia of the patella, cruciate ligament injuries, and even meniscal abnormalities. Today, however, the gold standard for the noninvasive assessment of internal derangements of the knee is MR imaging (see Chapter 70), which largely has replaced knee arthrography in many institutions.

**TABLE 13–7. Indications for Knee Arthrography**

| |
|---|
| Evaluation of: |
| Meniscal tears, cysts, and ossicles |
| Discoid menisci |
| Postmeniscectomy syndromes |
| Ligamentous injuries |
| Transchondral fractures |
| Chondromalacia patellae |
| Degenerative joint disease |
| Intra-articular osseous and cartilaginous bodies |
| Synovial disorders |
| Blount's disease |
| Soft tissue masses |

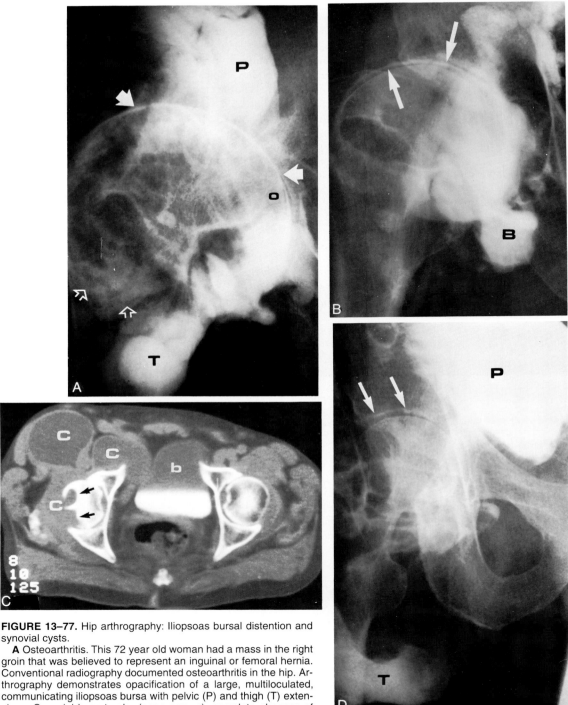

**FIGURE 13–77.** Hip arthrography: Iliopsoas bursal distention and synovial cysts.

**A** Osteoarthritis. This 72 year old woman had a mass in the right groin that was believed to represent an inguinal or femoral hernia. Conventional radiography documented osteoarthritis in the hip. Arthrography demonstrates opacification of a large, multiloculated, communicating iliopsoas bursa with pelvic (P) and thigh (T) extensions. Synovial hypertrophy (open arrows), complete absence of articular cartilage (solid arrows), osteophytosis (O), and flattening of the femoral head indicate advanced degenerative joint disease.

**B** Legg-Calvé-Perthes disease. In a 71 year old woman with a history of Legg-Calvé-Perthes disease resulting in coxa magna and secondary osteoarthritis, a right inguinal mass suggested a neoplasm. The arthrogram of the hip reveals simultaneous filling of the iliopsoas bursa (B), which lies inferomedial to the articulation. Additional findings are thinning of the femoral and acetabular cartilage (arrows), enlargement and flattening of the femoral head, and nodal opacification from a prior lymphangiogram.

**C, D** Rheumatoid arthritis. A CT scan **(C)** was obtained in the evaluation of swelling in the right groin of a middle-aged man with rheumatoid arthritis. The transaxial scan reveals several collections of fluid density (C) around and anterior to the right hip joint, one of which extends into the pelvis with leftward displacement of the urinary bladder (b). Bone erosions also are apparent (arrows). At surgery, an intraoperative contrast study **(D)** demonstrates opacification of both intrapelvic (P) and thigh (T) portions of the extensive multiloculated cysts. There is no contrast material within the hip joint itself (arrows).

(**A–C,** From Sartoris DJ, et al: Skel Radiol *14*:85, 1985.)

## Technique (Fig. 13–78)

Two double contrast examination techniques (horizontal beam and fluoroscopic) have been advocated,[120, 121] although at present the fluoroscopic technique virtually has replaced horizontal beam radiography. The knee is punctured from a medial or lateral approach with a 20 gauge needle and all intra-articular fluid is aspirated. If a previous patellectomy has been performed, an anterior approach is used with the patient sitting on the edge of the table.[484]

The fluoroscopic technique relies on vertical imaging with fluoroscopy.[122, 123] Its main advantage is direct monitoring of the menisci during the examination, allowing ideal tangential positioning. After puncture of the joint and aspiration of joint contents, 2 to 5 ml of contrast material (60 per cent Renografin) and 30 ml of air are injected. Some investigators have used carbon dioxide in place of air,[122] although recent evidence suggests that this causes more postprocedural pain, owing to a decrease in joint pH.[369] The patient then exercises moderately and is placed beneath the fluoroscopic unit. Nine to 18 exposures are made of each meniscus, using slight changes in position and appropriate leg traction. A variety of traction devices have been described to provide appropriate varus and valgus stress during the examination.[124–129, 339, 340, 485] After fluoroscopy, overhead films or spot films are taken to evaluate articular cartilage and cruciate ligaments and to determine whether a popliteal cyst is present.

The foremost key to the success of the fluoroscopic technique of knee arthrography is the examination of all parts of both menisci. To accomplish this, fluoroscopic spot filming should be begun with the patient in one lateral position and continued through the oblique and frontal positions until the patient is in the opposite lateral attitude. This procedure then is repeated for the opposite meniscus. Although the patient generally is examined in the prone position, obtaining additional spot films with the patient supine sometimes is helpful.[486, 487] Stereoscopic spot filming has been described,[488] but generally it is not required. The success of knee arthrography also depends on spot filming being accomplished with the meniscus projected clear of the femoral and tibial articular surfaces. This is facilitated by raising and lowering the leg until the cartilage in the tibia is seen in a tangential fashion. Adequate stress placed on the knee is fundamental to arthrographic success and should be accomplished without excessive twisting of the leg, a procedure that may produce buckling of the meniscus. Finally, palpation and massaging of the knee with a gloved hand during fluoroscopic monitoring allow analysis of joint recesses and the suprapatellar pouch and aid in the diagnosis of abnormal synovial folds, masses, and intra-articular osteocartilaginous bodies.

Radiographic tubes with small focal spots are essential for quality films. A 0.6 mm focal spot is satisfactory, although a 0.3 mm focal spot tube will produce superior images. Proper coning of the x-ray beam is mandatory, and the resulting images can be displayed on the film with a 4 on 1, 6 on 1, or 9 on 1 format. These should be numbered consecutively, usually proceeding from the posterior aspect of the meniscus to the anterior aspect.

It is imperative that most of the intra-articular fluid be aspirated.[671] This may require a joint puncture with an 18 gauge needle when the aspirate is thick. When considerable intra-articular fluid is present, contrast coating of the menisci is less than ideal, and subtle tears will be missed. Removed fluid also can be studied.[370] The presence of wear particles in the synovial fluid, consisting of cartilaginous fragments, is strongly indicative of significant intra-articular pathology.[370, 489, 490] Although characterization of the specific nature of these particles requires cytologic analysis of the filtered synovial fluid[489] or even ferrography,[490] gross inspection of the synovial fluid removed at the time of arthrography provides data that can support a positive arthrographic diagnosis.[370]

The examination must be performed in a rapid (albeit not rushed) manner, as the contrast coating will deteriorate as time elapses. The meniscus that is suspected to be injured should be examined first.

The addition of intra-articular epinephrine (0.2 ml of 1:1000 solution) may enhance meniscal visualization by causing vasoconstriction of synovial vessels, decreasing both the amount of contrast material absorbed from the joint cavity and the amount of intra-articular fluid formed.

Certain overhead films have been recommended after the procedure. These are obtained to evaluate the cruciate ligaments, articular cartilage, and synovial cavity. Lateral radiographs obtained in a cross-table supine projection and sitting position with one leg over the side of the table are useful. Anteroposterior views also are helpful, and delayed films have been recommended.[130, 341] Special projections to evaluate the cruciate ligaments (which also may require conventional tomography or CT scanning) may be used. These are discussed later in this chapter.

### Normal Knee Arthrogram (Fig. 13–79)

**Medial Meniscus** (Fig. 13–80). The medial meniscus is identified as a sharply defined, soft tissue triangular shadow. Its posterior horn usually is large, averaging 14 mm wide.[119] Its midportion is somewhat smaller, whereas the anterior horn usually is the smallest portion of the medial meniscus, averaging 6 mm wide.[119] Occasionally the anterior horn may be larger than the midportion of the medial meniscus.[131] The peripheral surface of the medial meniscus is firmly attached to the medial collateral ligament. Certain normal recesses about the medial meniscus produce focal pouchlike collections of air and contrast material.[132, 133] A superior recess frequently is present above the posterior horn of the medial meniscus. A posterior inferior recess is less common, although the presence of such a recess beneath the anterior horn of the medial meniscus is more frequent. These inferior recesses beneath the medial meniscus generally are small, and some regard recesses that are greater than 2 mm in size as abnormal.[134] The anterior part of the medial meniscus is covered with the base of the infrapatellar fat pad, making evaluation of this region more difficult.

**Lateral Meniscus** (Fig. 13–81). The lateral meniscus is more circular in configuration than the medial meniscus. It too is projected as a sharply defined triangular radiodense area surrounded by air and contrast material. It changes little in size from its anterior to its posterior horn, averaging 10 mm wide.[135] Inferior recesses are frequent beneath both the anterior and the posterior horns of the lateral meniscus. The anterior horn is attached to the lateral portion of the capsule, but the posterior horn of the lateral meniscus is

*Text continued on page 354*

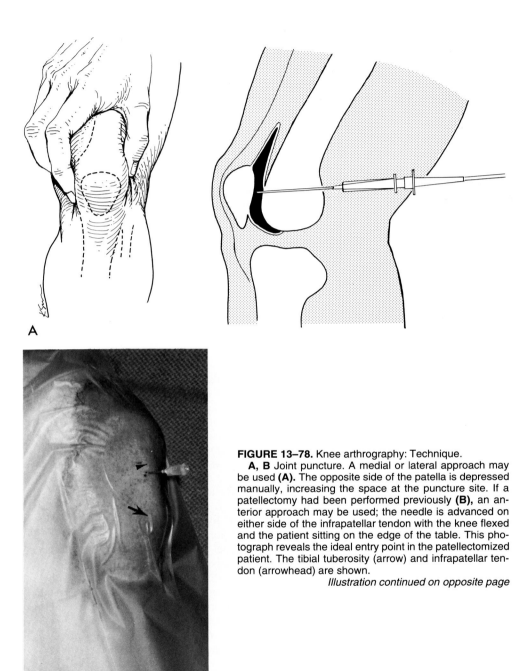

**FIGURE 13–78.** Knee arthrography: Technique.

**A, B** Joint puncture. A medial or lateral approach may be used **(A).** The opposite side of the patella is depressed manually, increasing the space at the puncture site. If a patellectomy had been performed previously **(B),** an anterior approach may be used; the needle is advanced on either side of the infrapatellar tendon with the knee flexed and the patient sitting on the edge of the table. This photograph reveals the ideal entry point in the patellectomized patient. The tibial tuberosity (arrow) and infrapatellar tendon (arrowhead) are shown.

*Illustration continued on opposite page*

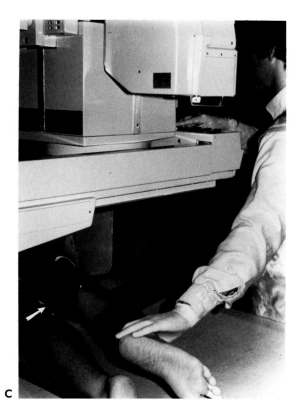

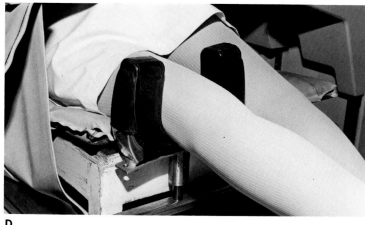

**FIGURE 13–78** *Continued*

C Fluoroscopic technique. In this photograph, the patient is positioned for evaluation of the anterior portion of the lateral meniscus. The metal brace (arrow) is used for appropriate stress. Other stress devices also are available.

D Fluoroscopic technique. Application of stress can be provided by various methods. In this illustration, the knee is held between padded supports that are connected to a crosspiece on the table. The patient is lying on a board. (Courtesy of I. Martin, M.D., and P. Stoner, M.D., London, England.)

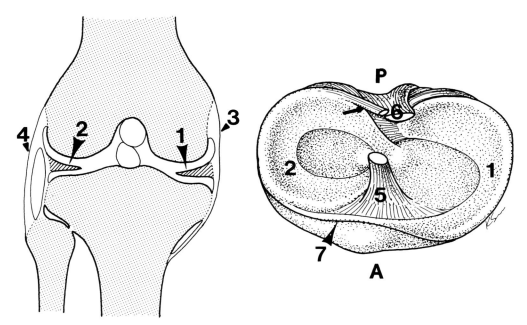

**FIGURE 13–79.** Knee arthrography: Pertinent anatomy. Coronal section (on left) and view of the upper portion of the tibia (on right). A, Anterior; P, posterior. Visualized structures are the medial meniscus (1), lateral meniscus (2), medial collateral ligament (3), fibular collateral ligament (4), anterior cruciate ligament (5), posterior cruciate ligament (6), transverse ligament of the knee (7), and slip, or meniscofemoral ligament, extending from the lateral meniscus close to the posterior cruciate ligament (arrow). Observe the relatively large posterior horn of the medial meniscus and its firm attachment to the medial collateral ligament and the more circular configuration of the lateral meniscus, with its relatively uniform size.

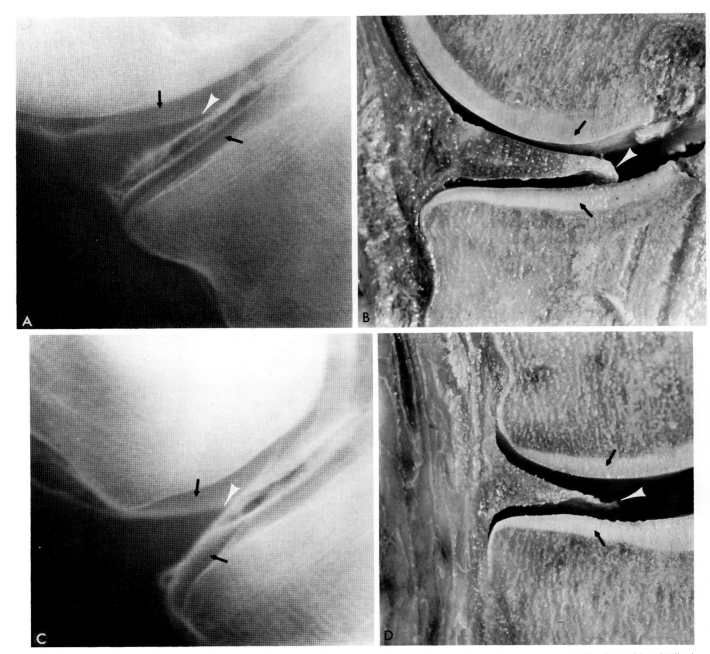

**FIGURE 13–80.** Knee arthrography: Anatomy and normal arthrography of the medial meniscus (arthrograms and pie-shaped longitudinal sections).

**A, B** Posterior horn of the medial meniscus. This segment is relatively large, extending for a considerable distance into the articular cavity (arrowheads). The adjacent articular recesses are small. The articular cartilage (arrows) is smooth.

**C, D** Midportion of the medial meniscus. This segment does not extend as far into the joint (arrowheads). The articular cartilage again appears normal (arrows).

*Illustration continued on opposite page*

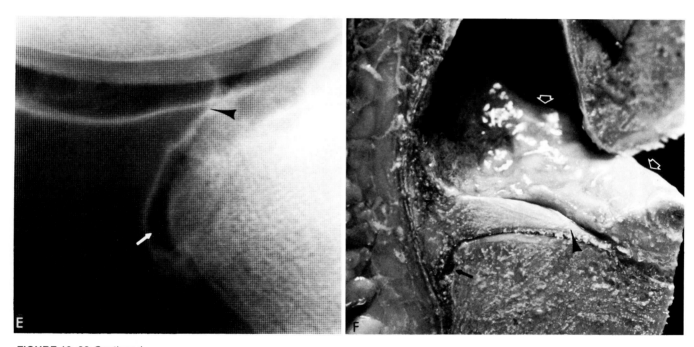

**FIGURE 13–80** *Continued*
**E, F** Anterior horn of the medial meniscus. The size of this segment is variable (arrowheads). Note the fat pad that overlies the meniscus (open arrows). An inferior recess is visualized (solid arrows).

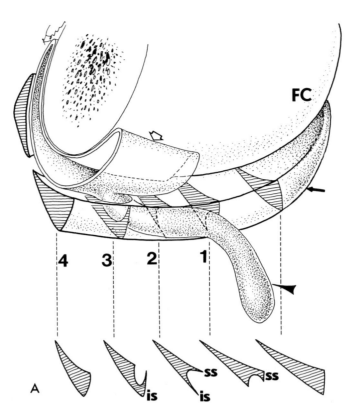

**FIGURE 13–81.** Knee arthrography: Anatomy and normal arthrography of the lateral meniscus—arthrograms and pie-shaped longitudinal sections.

**A** Diagrammatic representation of the posterolateral aspect of the knee joint demonstrates relationships of the lateral meniscus (solid arrow) and popliteus tendon sheath (arrowhead). The most posterior aspect of the femoral condyle (FC) and synovial reflection (open arrow) are indicated. The popliteus muscle originates posteriorly and inferiorly on the tibia and extends obliquely, anteriorly, and superiorly to insert on the lateral aspect of the femur. The popliteus tendon enters the joint close to the posterior and lateral aspects of the meniscus and passes through an oblique tunnel. Anteroinferior and posterosuperior to the intra-articular portion of the popliteus tendon are recesses, which fill with contrast medium during arthrography. Two bands of connective tissue, termed struts or fascicles, connect the posterior horn of the lateral meniscus to the joint capsule around the popliteal tendon sheath. Classically, (1) the more posterior aspect of the lateral meniscus will reveal an intact superior strut (ss); (2) a slightly more anterior section will reveal both superior strut (ss) and inferior strut (is); (3) a more anterior section will reveal only an inferior strut (is); and (4) a still further anterior section (midportion of the lateral meniscus) will depict an intact meniscus with no visible popliteal tendon sheath.

**B, C** Posterior aspect of the lateral meniscus (section 2). In this arthrogram and longitudinal section, observe the popliteus tendon sheath (arrowheads), lateral meniscus (arrows), superior strut (ss), and inferior strut (is). The latter strut has been disrupted in the preparation of this section.

**D, E** Slightly more anterior aspect of the lateral meniscus (section 3). In this arthrogram and longitudinal section, note the popliteus tendon sheath (arrowheads), lateral meniscus (arrows), and inferior strut (is). A thin superior strut is visible on the arthrogram but is absent on the section.

**F, G** Anterior horn of the lateral meniscus. In this arthrogram and longitudinal section, the meniscus (solid arrows) is well shown. Observe the articular cartilage (arrowheads) and prominent recesses (open arrows).

*Illustration continued on opposite page*

separated from the capsule by the synovial sheath of the popliteus tendon. This sheath fills with air and contrast material and overlies the peripheral portion of the posterior horn of the lateral meniscus, producing variable arthrographic findings, which have received great attention.[133, 136–139, 331, 332, 342] Two delicate bands of connective tissue, termed struts or fascicles, connect the posterior horn of the lateral meniscus to the joint capsule around the popliteal tendon sheath. In any one view of this portion of the lateral meniscus, two struts may be observed with the intervening sheath, one strut may be apparent in conjunction with the sheath, or the sheath may be observed without visualization of either strut. Classically, however, arthrography of the most posterior aspect of the lateral meniscus will reveal an intact superior strut; a slightly more anterior view will re-

veal both struts, and a more anterior projection will reveal an inferior strut. The variability in appearance of the fascicles or struts of the lateral meniscus combined with the presence of an overlying air-filled tendon sheath makes difficult the evaluation of the posterior horn of the lateral meniscus. Narrowing, compression, or absence of the popliteus tendon sheath, however, may indicate tears of the lateral meniscus, discoid menisci, adhesive capsulitis, prior surgery, or a rare congenital abnormality.[342]

### Meniscal Abnormalities

**Meniscal Tear.** Arthrography remains a highly accurate technique for the evaluation of a number of meniscal abnormalities, including tears, and is the preferred method of some radiologists despite the application of CT,[653, 654, 672]

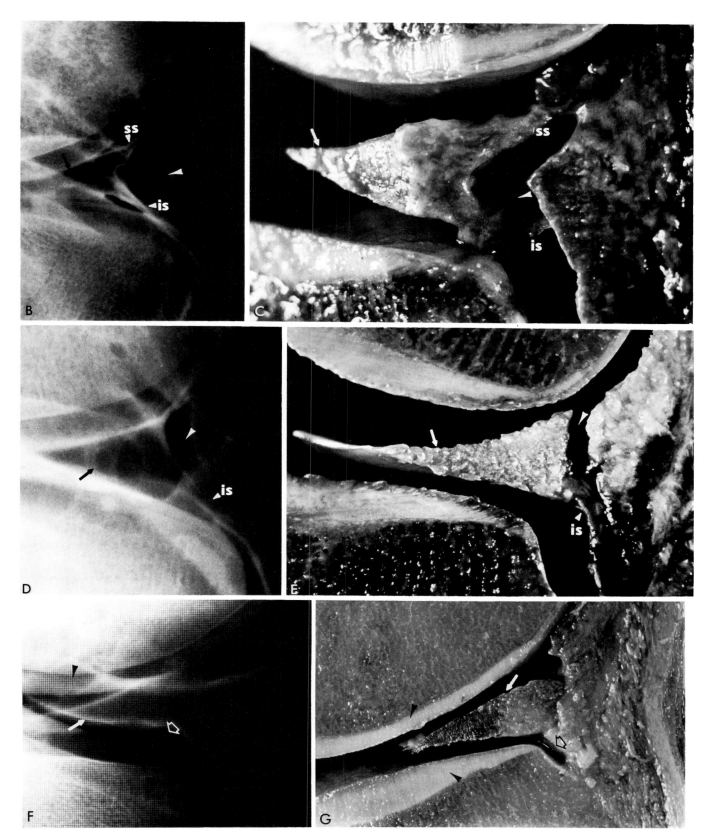

**FIGURE 13–81** *Continued*

MR imaging,[655, 656, 673, 674, 690–692, 762] and ultrasonography[675] to the assessment of lesions of the menisci. The arthrographic appearance of meniscal tears in both adults[116, 121, 122, 134, 140–142, 318, 694, 762] and children[143–145] has been well described. A classification of types of meniscal tears has been used,[121, 369] although specification of a particular type of tear during arthrography often is impossible and, even when possible, may have little clinical significance. The location of the tear in one aspect of the meniscus is of greater significance. A meniscal tear is more frequent on the medial side, involving particularly the posterior horn of the medial meniscus. The lateral meniscal tear most commonly involves the anterior horn.

*Vertical Concentric Tear* (Fig. 13–82). A vertical radiodense line extending through the meniscus will be observed. The inner fragment may be displaced, producing a bucket-handle tear, and may lodge in the central portion of the joint, where it may or may not be identified during arthrography.[491, 676]

*Vertical Radial Tear* (Fig. 13–83). A vertical tear along the inner contour of the meniscus will produce a contrast-coated inner meniscal margin and a blunted meniscal shadow.

*Horizontal Tear* (Fig. 13–84). Horizontal tears, which are observed more frequently in older persons,[146] also may be present in younger patients without producing symptoms.[147] A radiopaque line of contrast material is apparent overlying the meniscal shadow, extending to the superior or inferior surface. The meniscus may lose its wedge-shaped configuration.

*Combined Tears.* Combinations of any of the meniscal alterations can be observed.

**Meniscal Cyst** (Fig. 13–85). Meniscal cysts are multiloculated collections of mucinous material of unknown cause that have predilection for the lateral aspect of the knee.[148–151, 693] They usually occur in young men, with an average age of 30 years, but they have been reported in children as well as in elderly patients.[763] Meniscal cysts tend to be larger on the medial side of the knee and, in any location, may produce pain and swelling.[763] Most observers believe that these cysts develop after trauma, although others consider that degenerative or congenital factors may be important. The cysts generally are located at the peripheral meniscal margin and do not communicate with the joint cavity. In this location, they may produce few or no arthrographic changes. Cysts that are located more centrally may distort the menisci[492] or may be opacified because of articular communication. In fact, delayed radiographs obtained after arthrography may reveal such communication.[320] Meniscal cysts frequently occur after meniscectomy. Rarely, they may erode bone[321] or contain gas.[657]

Gross and microscopic studies of excised menisci may reveal a surprisingly high (7 per cent) percentage of associated cysts.[319, 361] These menisci commonly reveal horizontal tears, and tracks may be identified leading from the tear to the cysts.[343, 493] These facts, coupled with the observation that fluid within the cyst histochemically resembles synovial fluid, suggest that a pumping mechanism may exist that propels synovial fluid through the tears into the surrounding soft tissue, creating meniscal cysts. Thus, the cysts may not arise from primary myxoid degeneration.

**Discoid Meniscus** (Fig. 13–86). A discoid meniscus has an altered shape. It is broad and disc-like rather than semilunar in appearance although intermediate varieties of discoid menisci have been described.[152] These include the slab type (flat, circular meniscus), biconcave type (biconcave disc, thinner in its central portion), wedge type (large but normally tapered meniscus), anterior type (enlarged anterior horn), forme fruste (slightly enlarged meniscus), and grossly torn type (too deformed for accurate classification). A discoid lateral meniscus[153–158, 494] is much more common than a discoid medial meniscus.[157–164, 495–497, 658]

The reported frequency of discoid lateral menisci varies from 0 to 16 per cent,[152, 165, 764] although occasionally a higher frequency, determined by arthrography in children[143, 166] or by direct inspection during meniscectomy,[154, 157, 167] is cited. The usual age of patients at the time of clinical presentation is between 15 and 35 years, and men are affected more frequently. These patients commonly have symptoms of a torn cartilage. Bilateral discoid menisci and a familial occurrence of an abnormal meniscal shape[168] also have been noted.

An embryologic explanation for discoid menisci has not yet been determined. During development, undifferentiated mesenchymal tissue exists between the cartilaginous precursors of bone. This tissue subsequently cavitates, producing an articular cavity. In some joints, a portion of the mesenchyme exists as fibrocartilaginous discs or menisci. In knee development, under normal circumstances, undifferentiated mesenchyme evolves into fetal cartilage, which by the tenth week is semilunar in shape, closely resembling the adult meniscus.[155, 162] This normal sequence of embryologic development, therefore, does not contain a stage in which either the medial or the lateral meniscus is discoid[498]; the appearance of such a meniscus in a child or adult cannot occur through persistence of a fetal stage. Of interest, however, is the demonstration of discoid menisci as normal findings in various vertebrates.[677]

Kaplan[155] has postulated that the discoid lateral meniscus is acquired after birth as a result of an abnormal attachment of its posterior horn to the tibial plateau. He suggested that a primary abnormality of the inferior strut or fascicle will

*Text continued on page 362*

---

**FIGURE 13–82.** Knee arthrography: Vertical concentric meniscal tear.

**A** Vertical concentric (bucket-handle) tears. The medial meniscus is viewed from above with the posterior horn located superiorly. The vertical tear can be seen and the inner fragment is displaced centrally (arrow). The arthrographic appearance will depend on the specific site of the tear. A view of the posterior aspect of the meniscus (1) will be normal. Slightly more anteriorly (2) a vertical tear will be apparent with minimal displacement of the fragment. At positions 3 and 4, an amputated meniscal shadow will be apparent. At position 5, significant displacement of the inner fragment is observed. The anterior horn of the meniscus (6) will appear normal.

**B, C** Vertical concentric tears—two examples of medial meniscal abnormalities. Observe the contrast- or air-filled linear shadows (arrowheads) in the meniscus. A popliteal cyst is evident (arrows).

**D, E** Vertical concentric tears—bucket-handle type. An arthrogram and photograph of a gross specimen from two different patients. The arthrogram outlines amputation of the medial meniscus (arrow) with a displaced inner fragment (arrowhead) located in the central portion of the joint. The gross photograph of a torn medial meniscus (posterior horn on top; anterior horn on bottom) demonstrates the amputated meniscus (arrow) and a displaced inner fragment (arrowhead).

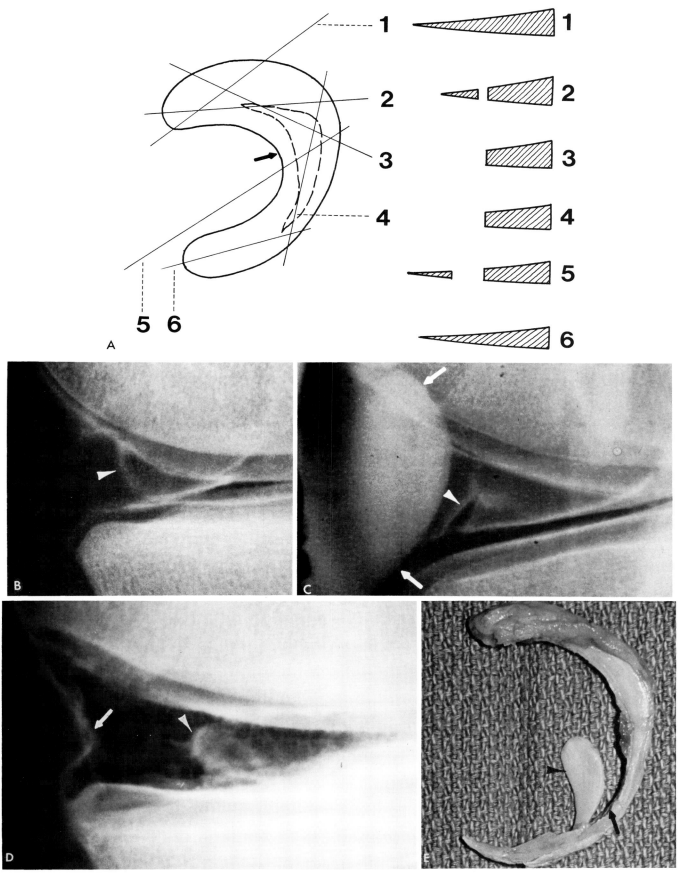

**FIGURE 13–82** *See legend on opposite page*

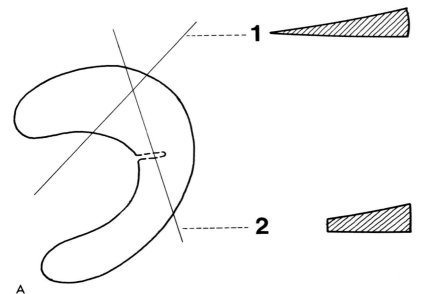

**FIGURE 13–83.** Knee arthrography: Vertical radial meniscal tear.

**A** The medial meniscus is viewed from above. Its posterior horn is located superiorly. A vertical radial tear is evident on the inner contour of the meniscus. Some arthrographic views (1) will appear normal, whereas others passing through the tear (2) will reveal a blunted, contrast-coated meniscal shadow.

**B** An arthrogram demonstrates such a radial tear (arrowhead) of the medial meniscus.

**C** In a different patient, the radial component (arrowhead) of the tear in the medial meniscus is evident. Elsewhere, the tear is more complex.

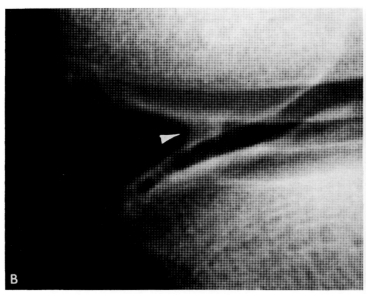

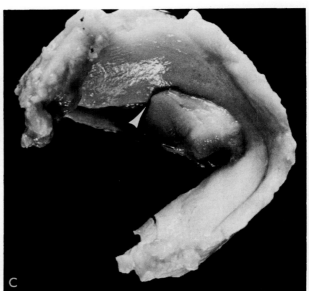

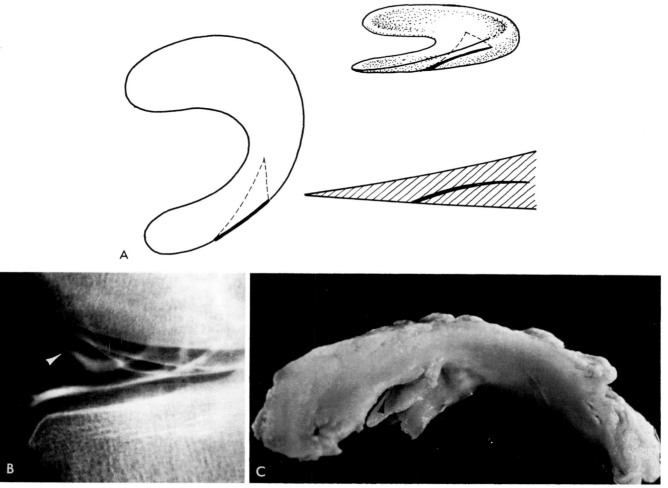

**FIGURE 13–84.** Knee arthrography: Horizontal meniscal tear.

**A** The medial meniscus is viewed from above (drawing on left), in front (drawing on top right), and in longitudinal section (drawing on bottom right). The extent and appearance of the tear can be appreciated.

**B, C** An arthrogram and photograph of a gross specimen in a patient with a horizontal tear of the medial meniscus. Note the tear (arrowheads), which is filled with contrast material on the arthrogram.

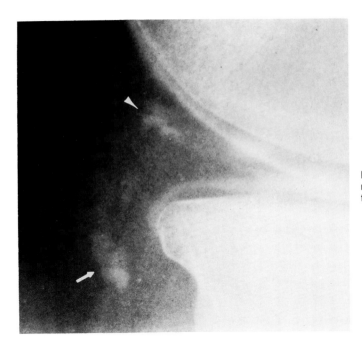

**FIGURE 13–85.** Knee arthrography: Meniscal cyst. A cyst of the medial meniscus is opacified (arrow) and associated with a horizontal tear of the meniscus (arrowhead).

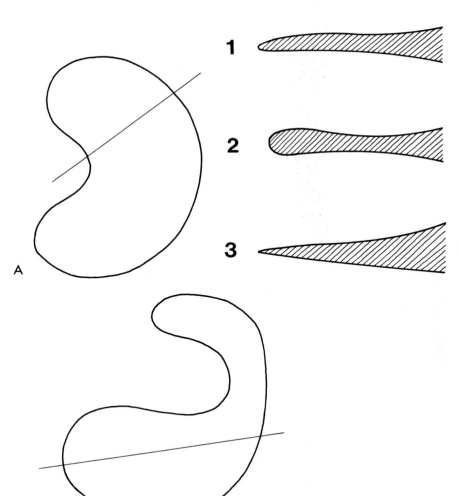

**FIGURE 13–86.** Knee arthrography: Discoid meniscus.

**A, B** Types of discoid menisci include the slab type (1), biconcave type (2), wedge type (3), and anterior type (4).

*Illustration continued on opposite page*

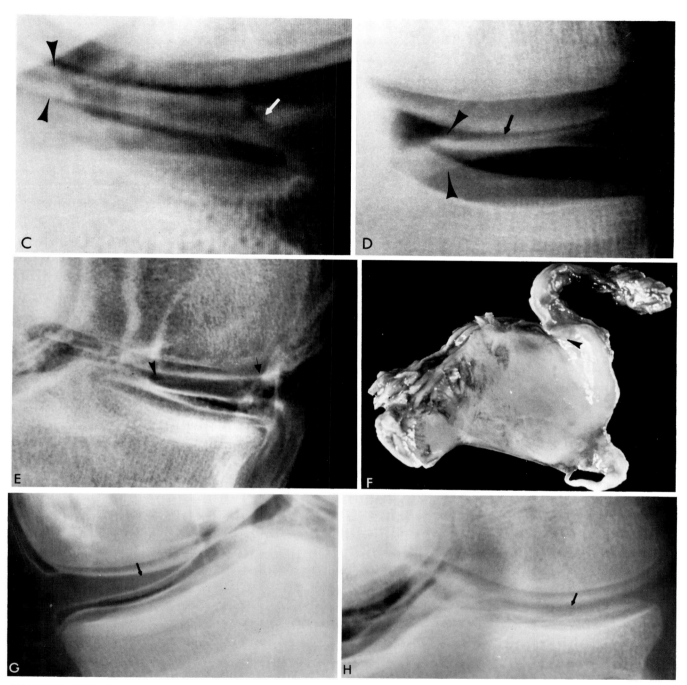

**FIGURE 13–86** *Continued*

  **C** Discoid lateral meniscus (slab type) with tear. Observe that the meniscus extends far into the joint cavity (arrowheads). A vertical tear is evident (arrow).

  **D** Discoid lateral meniscus (biconcave type). The central extension (arrowheads) and the thinner central portion (arrow) of the meniscus are observed.

  **E, F** Discoid medial meniscus (slab type). The preoperative arthrogram demonstrates the discoid meniscus extending far into the central portion of the joint (arrowhead), with a peripheral tear (arrow). The specimen photograph confirms the discoid medial meniscus with a peripheral tear (arrowhead).

  **G** Discoid medial meniscus (wedge type). An apparently intact discoid meniscus (arrow) is noted.

  **H** Discoid medial meniscus (slab type). During compression of the medial compartment of the knee, a discoid medial meniscus (arrow) is interposed between the tibia and the femur, preventing contact between the articular cartilages.

  (**E–H,** From Resnick D, et al: Radiology *121*:575, 1976.)

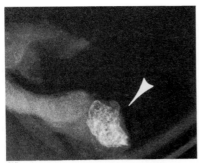

**FIGURE 13–87.** Knee arthrography: Meniscal ossicle. A radiograph of a removed medial meniscus reveals a meniscal ossicle (arrowhead), which simulated an intra-articular osseous body on the initial plain films of the knee.

leave a lateral meniscus attached posteriorly only by the meniscofemoral ligament (ligament of Wrisberg) and eventually will produce a discoid meniscus because of repetitive abnormal mediolateral and anteroposterior movement of the meniscus, with subsequent enlargement and thickening of meniscal tissue. Other investigators have noted that this strut frequently is poorly visualized or definitely abnormal in many patients with discoid lateral menisci, observations that lend support to Kaplan's theory.[152] Investigations have documented that a complete type of discoid lateral meniscus with intact ligamentous attachments, which generally is asymptomatic,[494] also exists.

Initial plain films in patients with discoid menisci generally are unrewarding, although widening of the articular space in the ipsilateral compartment of the knee documented by weight-bearing radiography, a high fibular head, a "cupped" tibial plateau,[499] and an abnormally shaped lateral malleolus have been observed in patients with discoid lateral menisci. A discoid medial meniscus may be associated with irregularity of the medial margin of the proximal tibial epiphysis.[333] Arthrography reveals the abnormally large and elongated meniscus, frequently extending to the intercondylar notch. The margins of the body of the meniscus are relatively parallel rather than converging in configuration. An associated meniscal tear frequently is observed.[322]

**Meniscal Ossicle** (Figs. 13–87 to 13–89). Meniscal ossicles represent foci of ossification within the menisci. They rarely are observed in the human knee,[169–173, 500] although they are a normal finding in the knees of certain rodents.[174] Ossicles represent hyaline cartilage enclosing lamellar and cancellous bone and marrow. Their origin in humans is controversial; some investigators believe they are vestigial structures,[171, 174] whereas others suggest they are acquired after trauma.[169, 500] Patients with knee ossicles may be asymptomatic or have local pain and swelling.[788]

Initial films reveal ossification of variable shape in the anterior or posterior portion of either the medial or the lateral meniscus.[344] The most common site is the posterior horn of the medial meniscus. Thus, the radiodense region generally is located centrally within the articular space. Arthrography confirms the location of the ossification within the meniscus.[173] The meniscus itself may be normal, contain associated tears,[169–171, 323] or be discoid in type.[175]

Meniscal ossicles must be differentiated from other causes of articular radiodensities, particularly intra-articular

osteochondral fragments. These latter fragments are not located centrally, may move in location from one examination to another, or may appear in the joint recesses. If a meniscal ossicle produces considerable symptoms, requiring meniscectomy, radiography of the removed meniscus will document the intrameniscal location of the ossification.

**Meniscectomy.** Significant changes in the surgical management of meniscal abnormalities in the knee are the consequence of two major factors: the increasing awareness that the menisci have weight-bearing capacity and transmit an important component of the load during daily physical activities[501, 502]; and the current popularity of arthroscopic surgery (see Chapter 70). Meniscectomy is no longer considered a harmless operation, because of the documentation of progressive damage of the articular cartilage after removal of the meniscus,[183–185, 346, 503] although similar degenerative changes are encountered when a severely torn meniscus is left in place.[504] The advocacy of partial rather than total meniscectomy appears to represent a philosophy midway between one that recommends complete removal of all damaged menisci and one that suggests a conservative approach to all meniscal injuries. Results after partial meniscectomy accomplished by open or arthroscopic surgery have been promising[505–507] and depend on the type and location of the meniscal tear and the integrity of the remaining portions of the joint. Retention of the peripheral one third of the meniscus provides stress protection to the outer and middle regions of the ipsilateral compartment of the knee, and its salvage then appears to be physiologically sensible.[501] Spontaneous healing of a tear in the peripheral (or central) portion of the meniscus[508, 509] occurs from an ingrowth of connective tissue and is consistent with anatomic studies indicating a relatively abundant vascular supply to the outer meniscal substance[510, 511] (Fig. 13–90). A peripheral vascular synovial fringe extends a short distance over both the femoral and the tibial surfaces of the menisci, except in the posterolateral region of the lateral meniscus, but it does not contribute any vessels to the meniscal stroma[510]; a vascular response originating from the perimeniscal vessels and peripheral synovial fringe is fundamental to the production of a fibrovascular scar at the site of a torn meniscus, emphasizing that the outer blood supply to the meniscus is sufficient to effect a reparative process in those meniscal lesions with which it communicates.[512]

A total meniscectomy involves the removal of the entire

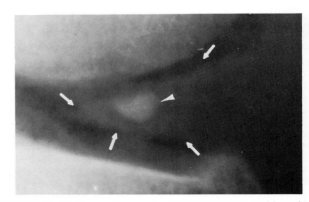

**FIGURE 13–88.** Knee arthrography: Meniscal ossicle. In this patient, an arthrogram using air alone confirms that an ossicle (arrowhead) is located in the anterior horn of the lateral meniscus (arrows).

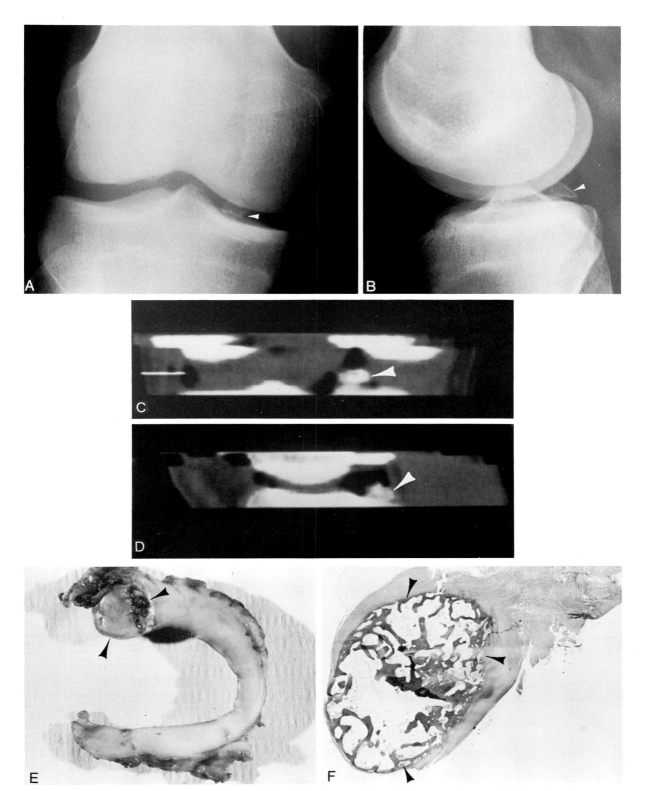

**FIGURE 13–89.** Knee arthrography: Meniscal ossicle. This 20 year old man injured his knee playing basketball and, during the next year, noted pain, clicking, and popping.

**A, B** The frontal and lateral radiographs reveal a bone fragment (arrowheads) in the distribution of the posterior horn of the medial meniscus.

**C, D** Computed arthrotomography with coronal **(C)** and sagittal **(D)** image reformation demonstrates the ossicle (arrowheads) in the medial meniscus. At surgery, a small tear of the medial meniscus and an ossicle in the posterior horn of this meniscus were observed. There was slight erosion of bone adjacent to the ossicle.

**E, F** In a different patient, an ossicle (arrowheads) in the posterior horn of the medial meniscus is evident.

(Courtesy of G. Greenway, M.D., Dallas, Texas.)

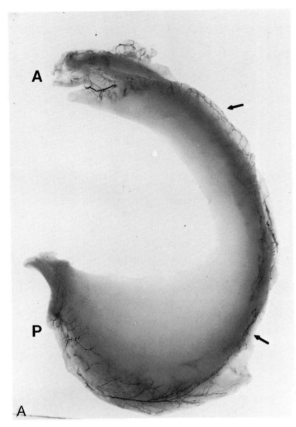

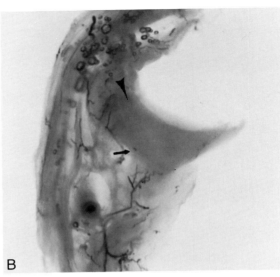

**FIGURE 13–90.** Knee arthrography: Meniscal blood supply.

**A** Medial meniscus. Note the peripheral arterial blood supply (arrows) and the avascular inner zone. A, Anterior; P, posterior.

**B** Medial meniscus. A cross section shows a blood vessel in the central zone of the meniscus (arrow) and absence of blood supply in the superior (arrowhead) and inferior surfaces of the meniscus.

(From Danzig L, et al: Clin Orthop *172*:271, 1983.)

meniscus from its capsular attachment. A partial meniscectomy may involve the removal of the anterior two thirds of the abnormal meniscus, deliberately leaving the posterior horn in place (Fig. 13–91); or, alternatively, the torn portion of the meniscus may be removed, leaving the remainder of the meniscus intact. After complete meniscectomy, fibrous regeneration of the meniscus occurs within 6 weeks to 3

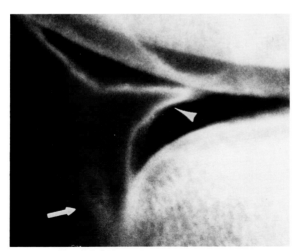

**FIGURE 13–91.** Knee arthrography: Retained fragment after meniscectomy. This patient described recurrent symptoms after a partial medial meniscectomy. A retained posterior horn is apparent (arrowhead). A small collection of contrast material (arrow) may represent a partial separation of the meniscus from the medial collateral ligament.

months.[176] The regenerated meniscus is thinner and narrower than a normal meniscus, with a decreased surface area and diminished mobility. Tears through regenerated menisci, although reported,[177, 178] are rare.

Plain film radiographic findings after meniscectomy may include flattening of the ipsilateral femoral condyle, a spur projecting inferiorly from the margin of the femoral condyle at the meniscectomy site, and joint space narrowing.[344, 345] Arthrographic evaluation after complete or partial meniscectomy may reveal a retained fragment, a regenerated meniscus, a tear of the opposite meniscus, or additional abnormalities.[179–182]

***Retained Fragment.*** The retained posterior horn after incomplete meniscectomy will resemble a normal posterior horn, although it may be irregular or contain an obvious tear (Fig. 13–91). After the removal of the inner fragment of a bucket-handle tear, the retained peripheral fragment will appear as a truncated shadow with rough, irregular surfaces.[180]

***Regenerated Meniscus.*** With regeneration of the meniscus, a small triangular shadow resembling an equilateral or isosceles triangle is observed, varying from 2 to 7 mm wide.[180] It possesses smooth, well-defined margins but is not associated with adjacent normal recesses at the meniscocapsular junction.

***Tear of Opposite Meniscus.*** Arthrographic findings in this situation are no different from those associated with meniscal tears in patients who have not undergone meniscectomy. The torn meniscus may have been overlooked on preoperative arthrography or may have occurred after surgery.

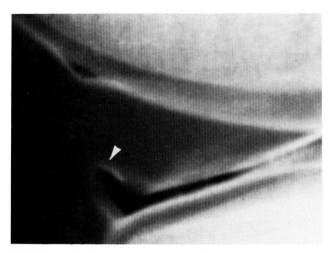

**FIGURE 13–92.** Knee arthrography: Mobile meniscus. A prominent inferior recess (arrowhead) beneath the posterior horn of the medial meniscus may lead to hypermobility, with clinical symptoms and signs.

*Additional Abnormalities.* A variety of additional causes exist for postmeniscectomy pain, including ligament injury, loose bodies, and cartilage ulceration. Some of these causes are unrelated to the previous meniscal surgery, whereas others, such as degenerative joint disease, may occur with increased frequency after meniscectomy.[183, 184, 346] Radiographic evidence of degenerative joint disease has been noted in 85 per cent of knees within 10 years after meniscectomy.[185] Other investigators reported such changes in 23 to 62 per cent of knees,[183, 186, 187] but the frequency will depend on the length of postoperative clinical follow-up and the type of surgery,[188] as well as other factors.

**Miscellaneous Meniscal Abnormalities.** The diagnosis of a hypermobile meniscus is open to question.[116] An abnormally mobile meniscus could conceivably occur when adjacent recesses are greater than 2 mm in size (Fig. 13–92), with the exception of the inferior recess about the anterior horn of the lateral meniscus, which frequently is prominent in normal persons.[134] Hypermobility also may be associated with previous peripheral meniscal tears or detachment.

One type of peripheral meniscal tear that has been emphasized is disruption of the meniscotibial (coronary) ligament.[513] This ligament is a band of fibrous tissue connecting the menisci peripherally to the tibia and appears to be important in maintaining an intimate relationship between the menisci and the tibial plateaus. A tear of the meniscotibial ligament, which is much more frequent on the medial side of the joint, leads to abnormal elevation of the meniscus from the tibial surface without its separating completely from the joint capsule (Fig. 13–93).

**Meniscal Abnormalities in Children.** Compared with their frequency in adolescents and adults, meniscal tears are uncommon in children.[514, 515, 786] Lateral meniscal lesions are more frequent in this age group than in adults, and a tendency for peripheral detachment of the meniscus in children has been noted.[515] Also, owing to their vascularity, histologic characteristics, biochemical composition, and physical properties, the developing menisci may have greater reparative ability than the menisci of either adolescents or adults,

underscoring the importance of preservation of some or all of a traumatized meniscus in a child.[498]

### Ligamentous Injury

**Collateral Ligament Tears** (Fig. 13–94). Injuries of the collateral ligaments may produce plain film radiographic findings, including widening of the joint space during varus or valgus stress and calcification, particularly near the femoral site of attachment of the medial collateral ligament (Pellegrini-Stieda syndrome). Recent tears of the collateral ligaments may be documented by arthrography, although MR imaging is a far more effective diagnostic method (see Chapter 70). Contrast material introduced into the joint space will extravasate into the adjacent soft tissues. This finding is more readily apparent on the medial aspect of the knee, where a linear radiodense region may indicate a contrast-coated outer margin of the medial collateral ligament. Lateral (fibular) collateral ligament injuries are more difficult to diagnose on arthrography because of the normal distance between the joint capsule and lateral collateral ligament.[134] As noted previously, an elevated meniscus and an enlarged synovial fold between the tibial margin and meniscus may indicate a tear of the coronary ligament.[116, 513]

**Cruciate Ligament Injuries** (Fig. 13–95). Several arthrographic techniques have been employed for the evaluation of cruciate ligament injuries, with varying degrees of success. Initial techniques using double contrast arthrography were accurate in less than 50 per cent of cases,[121, 122] stimulating investigation with modified methods of examination. Some investigations report success using a lateral view of the knee, flexed to 90 degrees over the edge of the table[189] or elevated above the table,[516] or employing single positive contrast examinations.[517] Others indicate approximately 75 to 90 per cent accuracy in diagnosing anterior cruciate ligament tears using conventional tomography.[190] This technique is improved if tomographic exposures are obtained immediately after injection, although this is time consuming, delaying the meniscal examination.

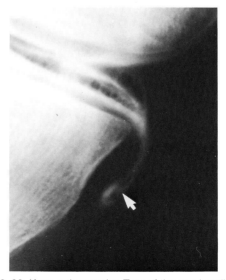

**FIGURE 13–93.** Knee arthrography: Tear of the meniscotibial (coronary) ligament. Observe elevation of the medial meniscus with an abnormal collection of contrast material extending inferiorly (arrow). (Courtesy of C. Chen, M.D., Taipei, Taiwan.)

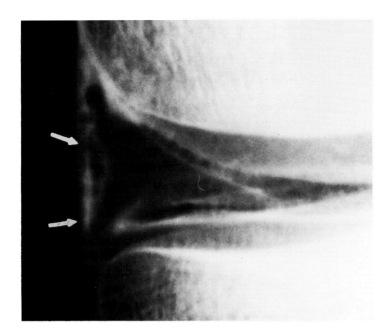

**FIGURE 13–94.** Knee arthrography: Collateral ligament injuries. A tear of the medial collateral ligament allows contrast material to pass from the articular cavity into the soft tissues, outlining the lateral aspect of the ligament (arrows).

In a series of articles, Pavlov and collaborators[191, 192, 518–520] have emphasized the role of double contrast arthrography in the evaluation of the cruciate ligaments. Although the study of the cruciate ligaments can be accomplished after the investigation of the menisci, it is better employed before the menisci are studied, immediately after the introduction of radiopaque contrast material, air, and epinephrine. The knee is passively flexed and extended several times with the patient in the supine, sitting, and prone positions, and attention then is directed to the anterior cruciate ligament. Two types of images are obtained: a horizontal cross-table lateral radiograph and fluoroscopic spot films. In both instances, the anterior cruciate ligament is examined while being tensed with a simulated ''anterior drawer'' maneuver. For the horizontal cross-table lateral radiograph, the patient sits with the legs flexed between 45 and 75 degrees over the side of the table, and the proximal end of the tibia is pushed anteriorly with respect to the femoral condyles by a firm pillow located behind the calf. An overpenetrated cross-table lateral radiograph is exposed while the patient holds a grid cassette adjacent to the medial aspect of the knee. After this, the patient lies on his or her side with the affected knee dependent and flexed 45 to 75 degrees. A stress band extends around the calf from the side of the table that is in front of the knee, and the examiner pulls the distal part of the leg posteriorly against the stress band. Although a properly performed cruciate ligament examination takes only 1 or 2 min and is not incompatible with subsequent and adequate investigation of the menisci, it must be done carefully and meticulously. When accomplished by an experienced arthrographer, the accuracy of the technique surpasses 90 per cent,[518] although similar accuracy has been reported from the clinical examination alone.[521] Of course, arthrography also allows the identification of meniscal lesions that commonly accompany injuries of the anterior cruciate ligament.[522]

The fundamental arthrographic criterion of a normal anterior cruciate ligament is an anterior synovial surface that is ''ruler-straight'' on one or both of these radiographs.[518]

The ligament is considered to be lax but intact if the anterior synovial surface is bowed and concave anteriorly. The arthrographic abnormalities associated with disruption of the anterior cruciate ligament are more definite when simultaneous visualization of the posterior cruciate ligament is accomplished (decreasing the likelihood of technical inadequacies) and include nonvisualization, a wavy, lumpy, or acutely angulated anterior surface, irregularity of the inferior attachment of the ligament, pooling of the contrast medium in the usual location of the ligament, and visualization of the plica synovialis infrapatellaris (the infrapatellar synovial fold, which otherwise is easily misinterpreted as evidence of a normal anterior cruciate ligament).[190–193, 518–520] It should be emphasized that the abnormal findings frequently are subtle, requiring of the examiner a good deal of experience and knowledge.[659]

An alternative approach to the diagnosis of tears of cruciate ligaments is provided by CT alone or in combination with arthrography of the knee[324, 523–527] (Fig. 13–96). Although CT also has been used to evaluate the menisci,[528, 529] this clinical application is less defined, and both applications will require reevaluation in the years ahead owing to the capability of MR imaging to demonstrate soft tissue structures.[690–692]

Prior descriptions of the CT technique that is required to evaluate the cruciate ligaments have been conflicting not only with respect to the need for intra-articular contrast material but also with respect to whether the contrast material should be radiopaque material, air, or both. There is no uniform agreement regarding the position of the knee in the CT gantry, the necessity for angulation of the gantry, or the benefit of reformatted or even three-dimensional images. The author prefers to examine the patient in the supine position with his or her knee flexed 20 to 30 degrees and believes that two-dimensional sagittal and coronal reconstruction of the image data is essential for correct diagnosis.

MR imaging has influenced dramatically the diagnostic strategy employed to evaluate the ligaments of the knee and

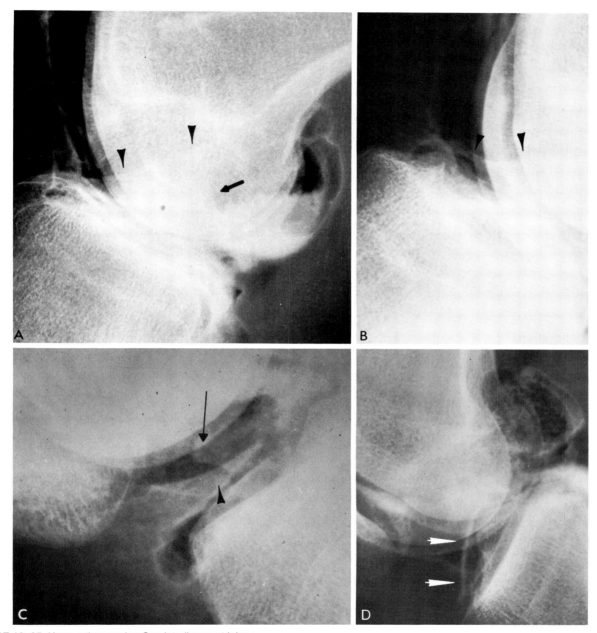

**FIGURE 13–95.** Knee arthrography: Cruciate ligament injury.

**A** On this lateral view, the anterior cruciate (arrowheads) and posterior cruciate (arrow) ligaments are seen. Note their normal appearance and smooth contour.

**B** A torn anterior cruciate ligament is evident (arrowheads). Note the irregular coating and bowed appearance of the torn ligament.

**C** In another patient, an intra-articular body (arrow) represents a contracted anterior portion of the detached anterior cruciate ligament. The meniscal shadow (arrowhead) also can be seen.

**(B, C,** From Dalinka MK, et al: CRC Crit Rev Radiol Sci *5*:1, 1973.)

**D** Infrapatellar synovial fold. On the lateral view **(D),** coating of the infrapatellar synovial fold (arrows) simulates an intact anterior cruciate ligament.

**(D,** From Dalinka MK, Garofola J: AJR *127*:589, 1976. Copyright 1976, American Roentgen Ray Society.)

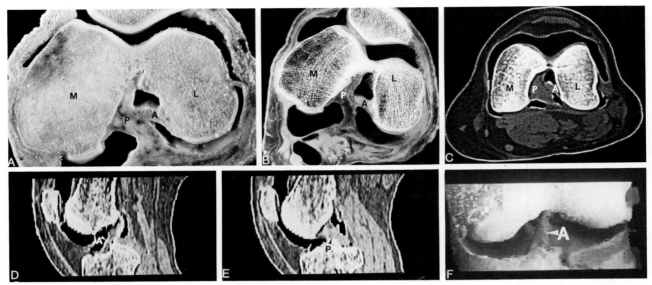

**FIGURE 13–96.** Knee arthrography: Normal cruciate ligaments using computed arthrotomography.

**A–C** A photograph **(A)** and radiograph **(B)** of a transverse section of a cadaveric knee following the instillation of intra-articular air and a transaxial CT scan **(C)** of the intact specimen show the normal anterior (A) and posterior (P) cruciate ligaments. M, medial femoral condyle; L, lateral femoral condyle.

**D, E** Reconstructed sagittal CT images of the normal anterior cruciate ligament (A) and normal posterior cruciate ligament (P) are shown.

**F** A three-dimensional CT image displays the normal anterior cruciate ligament (A).

other joints (see Chapter 70).[530, 531] Early studies indicated that tears of the anterior and posterior cruciate ligaments and the collateral ligaments could be identified accurately by this technique, owing to an altered signal and an abnormal position or configuration of the affected ligament.[531] Such studies also confirmed that meniscal abnormalities could be detected with MR imaging.[692] These diagnostic considerations are discussed in detail in Chapter 70.

### Lesions of Articular Cartilage

Contrast material within the joint cavity allows visualization of portions of articular cartilage. Because of the differences in shape of the articular surfaces of the femur and tibia, the tibial cartilage is evaluated more completely than the femoral cartilage. Knee arthrography with conventional tomography may improve visualization of cartilaginous surfaces.[194] Abnormalities such as osteochondral fracture (osteochondritis dissecans) and chondromalacia may be identified, although the latter is better studied with computed arthrotomography and MR imaging. Cartilage thinning associated with degenerative joint disease is discussed later in this chapter.

**Osteochondral Fracture (Osteochondritis Dissecans)** (Fig. 13–97). Transchondral fractures exist where tangential shearing forces are applied to the articular surface. In the knee, such fractures are most frequent on the lateral surface of the medial femoral condyle, although they may be noted elsewhere as well. The fracture fragment may consist of cartilage, cartilage and bone, or bone alone. It may remain in situ with relatively normal overlying cartilage, become depressed with an indentation of the articular surface, or become detached, existing as a loose body in the articular cavity or as an attached body at a distant synovial site (Fig. 13–98)

Arthrography will allow evaluation of the cartilaginous or osseous surface, or both, at the fracture site.[195, 196] Contrast medium may outline a normal, swollen, or depressed cartilaginous surface, or it may dissect beneath the osteochondral fragment. The relative integrity of the cartilaginous surface can influence the need for and choice of surgical procedure.

The detection of intra-articular osteochondral bodies accompanying osteochondritis dissecans or other disorders may require the combination of arthrography and conventional tomography or CT scanning[532] (Fig. 13–99). The author prefers computed arthrotomography, employing large amounts of intra-articular air, with or without a small amount of radiopaque contrast material, and closely spaced transaxial CT scans with the patient supine or prone, depending on the location of the fragments. Care must be exercised so that the tibial spines are not misinterpreted as evidence of abnormal intra-articular osseous bodies.[532]

**Chondromalacia.** The role of arthrography in the diagnosis of chondromalacia of the patella has been the subject of debate. Most observers regard its role as minor or nonexistent,[134, 197, 533] although others are more optimistic.[198, 199] The posterior surface of the patella is V-shaped, with medial and lateral facets separated by an osseous ridge. Routine lateral projections during arthrography demonstrate only a small amount of the patellar cartilaginous surface, that near the apex of the ridge. Axial projections increase the cartilaginous area that can be visualized, and oblique projections that are tangential to the medial and lateral facets may further improve this visualization.[325] If overhead and fluoroscopic filming is accomplished using lateral, oblique, and axial positions supplemented with conventional tomography or CT scanning, the diagnosis of chondromalacia indeed may be substantiated by arthrography in

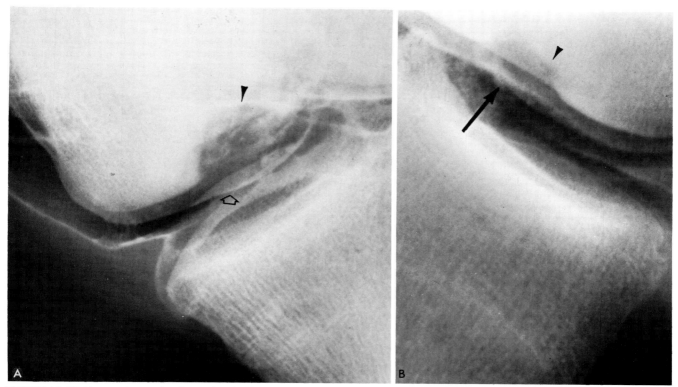

**FIGURE 13–97.** Knee arthrography: Osteochondral fractures. Two examples of osteochondral fractures (arrowheads) evaluated with arthrography. One **(A)** demonstrates swollen articular cartilage over the lesion (open arrow), and the other **(B)** reveals irregular cartilaginous thinning (solid arrow). (**A,** From Wershba M, et al: Clin Orthop *107*:81, 1975; **B,** courtesy of M. K. Dalinka, M.D., Philadelphia, Pennsylvania).

some patients.[362, 534–536] (Fig. 13–100). Whether arthrographic diagnosis will ever be more accurate than clinical diagnosis of the disorder remains to be seen. Furthermore, MR imaging has proved to be far more effective in this regard than arthrography.

On arthrography, chondromalacia produces absorption or imbibition of contrast material by the patellar cartilage. Nodular elevation, fissuring, or diminution of the cartilaginous surface may be apparent.

## Evaluation of Additional Bone or Soft Tissue Injuries

**Quadriceps Tendon Rupture** (Fig. 13–101). The plain film radiographic findings associated with quadriceps tendon rupture have been summarized.[200] These include a suprapatellar soft tissue mass representing the retracted proximal portion of the disrupted tendon, absence of the normal quadriceps soft tissue shadow, effusion, and calcification or

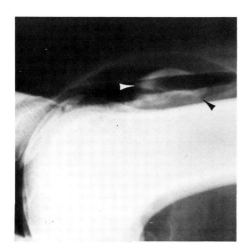

**FIGURE 13–98.** Knee arthrography: Chondral fragment. After an injury, this patient continued to have pain and swelling of the knee. Plain films were unremarkable except for the presence of an effusion. After arthrography, a lateral film reveals a large contrast-coated cartilaginous fragment in the suprapatellar pouch (arrowheads).

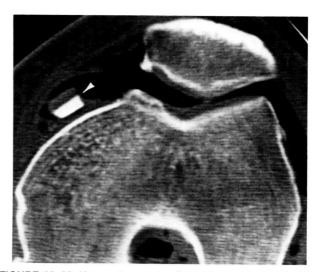

**FIGURE 13–99.** Knee arthrography: Osteochondral fragment. After the introduction of air into the knee joint, a transaxial CT scan reveals the fragment (arrowhead), consisting of cartilage and bone, in the medial aspect of the joint.

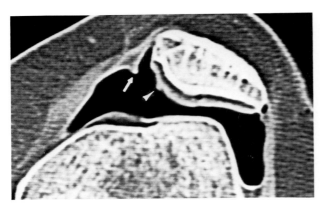

**FIGURE 13–100.** Knee arthrography: Chondromalacia patellae. A transaxial image during computed arthrotomography using air and a small amount of radiopaque contrast material shows cartilage fibrillation (arrowhead) and imbibition of contrast material, especially at the junction of the medial and most medial (odd) facets of the patella, consistent with chondromalacia patellae. A small medial plica (arrow) also is evident. As it is difficult to judge patellar position when large amounts of air or contrast material are placed in the joint, the diagnosis of patellar subluxation is better accomplished with CT alone or with MR imaging.

ossification within portions of an avulsed patellar fragment. Arthrography in partial[201] or complete[202] quadriceps tendon rupture will substantiate the clinical and radiographic diagnosis. Contrast material introduced into the knee joint will extend outside the quadriceps tendon[537] and may reveal communication with the prepatellar or infrapatellar bursa.

**Suprapatellar Bursa Rupture.** Rupture of the suprapatellar bursa has been described.[203, 765] Arthrographic findings include collection of contrast material near the apex of the bursa, with dissection into the thigh.

**Tibial Plateau Fracture.** Arthrography in patients with previous tibial plateau fractures has been employed to delineate the integrity of the cartilaginous surface.[204]

**Miscellaneous Injury** (Fig. 13–102). After injury, adhesions may occasionally divide the articulation into two separate cavities. An inflammatory synovitis occurring after trauma or other conditions can result in thickening of normal synovial folds or plicae, producing divisions of the articular space and clinical manifestations[102–104, 108] (see following discussion).

### Synovial Plicae

The term "synovial plicae" refers to remnants of synovial tissue that in early development originally divided the joint into three separate compartments, and which may be found normally in the adult knee.[102–104, 108, 538–544] Usually of no consequence, these structures may become pathologically thickened and lead to symptoms mimicking arthritis, injuries involving the meniscus, and other common internal derangements of the knee. In addition, persistence of these structures in their embryonic form, as complete septa, may cause a variety of intra-articular compartmental syndromes.

The synovial cavity of the adult knee is the most extensive and complex in the body, and it represents in its final form the end result of a sequence of developmental steps that have been studied extensively. In the embryo of 7 weeks' gestation, the tibial and femoral cartilages are separated by unchondrified blastema, which becomes thinned to form a discrete disc or intermediate zone.[545] As the joint

continues to grow, and prior to the development of the fibrous joint capsule, adjacent mesenchyme becomes incorporated into an intra-articular position. This embryonic mesenchyme gives rise to the menisci and cruciate ligaments at approximately 8 weeks of development.[545] It generally is agreed that cavities are not seen in the previously solid embryonic synovial mesenchyme until approximately 9 weeks of embryogenesis. Originally, three compartments are partitioned by septa of embryonic synovium: a superior femoropatellar compartment and two inferior femorotibial compartments.[546] These primitive cavities enlarge by proliferation of the lining tissue and extend into the middle portion of the blastemal intermediate zone. At this time, the cavities are irregular in outline and frequently contain strands of tissue, and their lining bears little resemblance to the typical synovial tissue of the adult.[545] Progressive involution of these mesenchymal septa leads to the formation of a single joint space by approximately 12 weeks.[545] Persistence of any portion of these embryonic partitions constitutes a synovial plica. These synovial remnants can be encountered in 18 to 60 per cent of adult knees, a frequency that largely may reflect the diligence and persistence of the examiner.[540, 541]

The three most commonly encountered plicae are classified according to the partitions from which they took origin, as suprapatellar, medial patellar, and infrapatellar (Fig. 13–103). Of these, the infrapatellar plica is most frequent, followed by the suprapatellar plica, and, after that, the medial plica.[541] Each of these septa varies widely in size and shape,

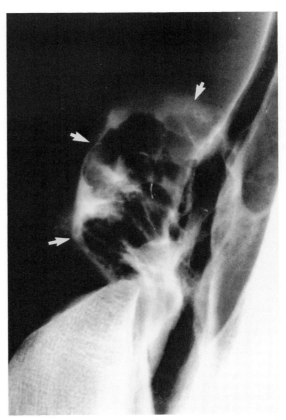

**FIGURE 13–101.** Knee arthrography: Rupture of the quadriceps tendon. Arthrography in this 58 year old man with recent trauma shows anterior extravasation of contrast material (arrows) consistent with a partial disruption of the quadriceps tendon.

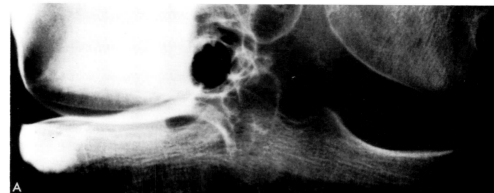

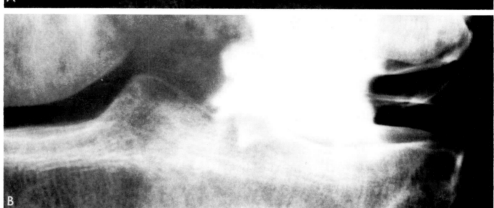

**FIGURE 13–102.** Knee arthrography: Articular adhesions. This man had sustained a gunshot wound to the knee, producing a femoral fracture and articular adhesions. Separate injections into the medial **(A)** and lateral **(B)** compartments were necessary to opacify the entire articular cavity. These arthrographic findings may indicate the presence of a hypertrophied synovial plica.

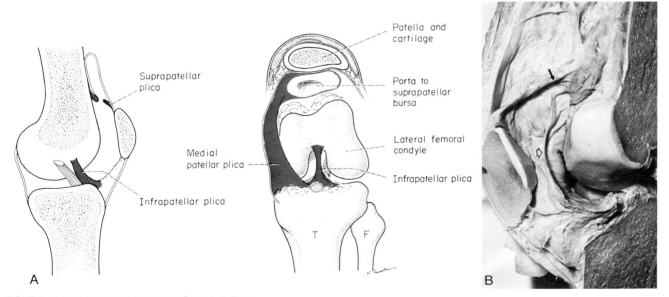

**FIGURE 13–103.** Knee arthrography: Synovial plicae.
 **A** A schematic drawing depicts the three most commonly encountered synovial plicae.
 **B** A sagittal section through the knee demonstrates the suprapatellar plica (solid arrow) and the medial patellar plica (open arrow). (From Deutsch AL, et al: Radiology *141*:627, 1981.)

and various combinations may exist simultaneously. Their identification can be accomplished by arthrography,[538, 547, 548, 766] computed arthrotomography,[549, 767] MR imaging (see Chapter 70), or arthroscopy,[543, 544, 554–557] depending on their location and size.

The suprapatellar plica, or plica synovialis suprapatellaris, represents a remnant of the embryonic septum that divides the suprapatellar cavity from the medial and lateral joint compartments. This synovial fold may vary widely in the adult and most commonly takes one of the following three forms: (1) an intact septum completely dividing the suprapatellar pouch from the remainder of the knee; (2) an intact septum except for a variably sized, centrally placed diaphragm known as the porta; and (3) a variably sized, crescent-shaped fold arising medially from the undersurface of the quadriceps tendon above the level of the patella and extending inferiorly to insert along the medial edge of the knee joint[103, 546] (Fig. 13–104).

On double contrast arthrograms, the suprapatellar plica is best visualized on the lateral view with the knee in full extension. This position allows for complete distention of the suprapatellar pouch. The plica is seen as a thin, delicate fold obliquely crossing the suprapatellar pouch to insert near the patella. On fluoroscopy, it is readily pliable, moving easily with flexion and extension of the knee. With computed arthrotomography, this plica most commonly appears as a fine line parallel to the medial wall of the joint.[549]

The medial patellar plica has been referred to variously as a wedge, a band, or a shelf.[102, 766] This synovial remnant has its origin on the medial wall of the knee joint, near the suprapatellar plica, and courses obliquely downward relative to the patella, to insert into the synovium, which covers

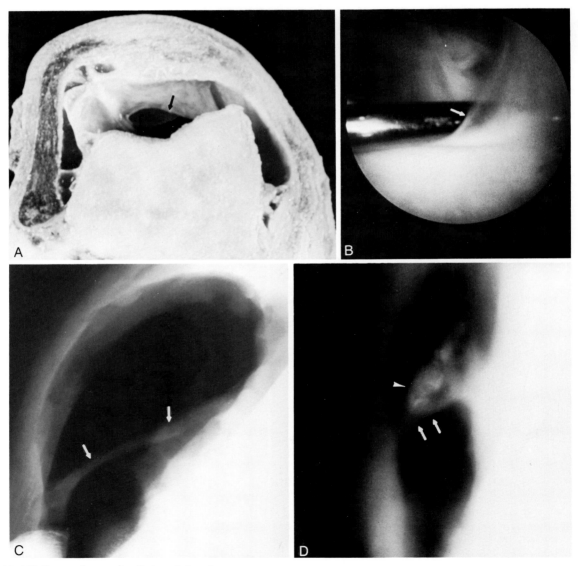

**FIGURE 13–104.** Knee arthrography: Suprapatellar plica.

   **A** A transverse section through the suprapatellar pouch in a cadaver demonstrates the plica and prominent porta (arrow).

   **B** An arthroscopic view of a suprapatellar plica (arrow) in a patient.

   **C, D** Two examples of the appearance of suprapatellar plicae (arrows) during arthrography. In **D**, an arthrotomogram, observe that intra-articular osteocartilaginous bodies (arrowhead) are trapped above the plica.

   (**A, B,** From Deutsch AL, et al: Radiology *141*:627, 1981.)

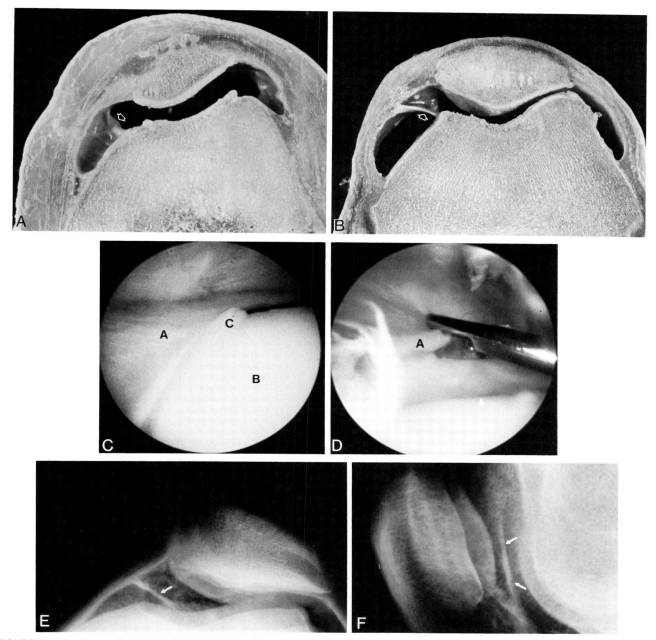

**FIGURE 13–105.** Knee arthrography: Medial patellar plica.

**A, B** Transverse sections through cadaveric knee joints at the level of the patella demonstrate medial patellar plicae (arrows). (From Deutsch AL, et al: Radiology *141*:630, 1981.)

**C, D** Arthroscopy reveals the characteristics of a symptomatic medial patellar plica. In **C,** the plica (A) is "bowstrung" over the femoral condyle (B) in flexion, with localized chondromalacia (C) of the articular surface of the femur. In **D,** the medial patellar plica (A) is resected using basket forceps. (From Richmond JC, McGinty JB: Clin Orthop *178*:185, 1983.)

**E, F** Arthrographic demonstration of a medial patellar plica (arrows) is provided on axial and near-lateral projections.

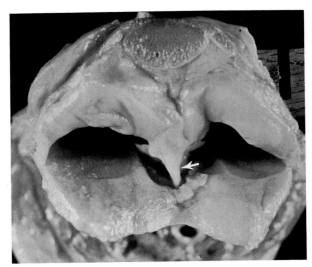

**FIGURE 13–106.** Knee arthrography: Infrapatellar plica. A transverse section of a cadaveric knee through the level of the intercondylar notch allows optimal visualization of the course of the infrapatellar plica (arrow) with the patella retracted anteriorly and superiorly. (From Deutsch AL, et al: Radiology *141*:631, 1981.)

the infrapatellar fat pad (Fig. 13–105). Its inner edge may be rounded, sharp, or smooth, or it may contain small fenestrations.[102] Its configuration varies with knee position, lying transverse to the femur with the knee extended and parallel to the axis of the femur with the joint flexed.

Arthrographic demonstration of the medial patellar plica depends on careful technique and the inclusion of axial views of the patellofemoral compartment.[548, 550, 551] On the axial projections, this plica is seen as a flat, lucent region lying just anterior to the medial femoral condyle in the medial aspect of the patellofemoral joint. In an almost lateral projection, with the knee in slight internal rotation, the medial patellar plica appears as a stringlike radiolucent line superimposed on the superior part of the medial femoral condyle, extending from the suprapatellar bursa to the infrapatellar fat pad.[550] Computed arthrotomography delineates the location and the thickness of this plica.[549, 767]

The infrapatellar plica, or ligamentum mucosum, represents a vestige of the membranous partition that once separated the medial and lateral embryonic compartments of the knee.[538] It often is fan-shaped, with a narrow femoral margin in the intercondylar notch, widening as it descends through the inferior joint space to attach distally to the inferior and medial aspects of the patellar articular cartilage (Fig. 13–106). From there the plica continues as two fringelike alar folds to cover the infrapatellar fat and separate the synovium from the ligamentum patellae.[108] Its course parallels that of the anterior cruciate ligament, which is located just posterior to it. The course and position of the plica change with increasing flexion of the knee because the site of insertion into the intercondylar fossa is displaced. On rare occasions, the infrapatellar plica may be double, or it may persist into adult life as an intact septum, although it is encountered more commonly as a fenestrated septum or series of fibrous bands in the adult knee.[102, 108]

The infrapatellar plica can be identified on double contrast arthrography on both the lateral and the intercondylar views. Because of their anatomic relationship, the infrapatellar plica easily may be confused with the anterior cruciate

ligament, resulting in an incorrect diagnosis in patients with complete disruption of the anterior cruciate ligament.[193]

Symptomatic plicae are encountered most commonly in what has been referred to as the "plica syndrome."[102, 103, 108, 540, 542] In this syndrome, the medial patellar plica, which normally exists as a fine, thin, flexible fold of synovium of little clinical significance, becomes pathologically thickened and symptomatic.[552-558, 660] Among the postulated factors in the initiation of a traumatic synovitis leading to secondary abnormalities within the plicae are trauma, strenuous exercise, osteochondritis dissecans, injuries to the meniscus, and intra-articular osteocartilaginous bodies. Regardless of the inciting event, when inflammation exists with edema and thickening, fibrous repair may result in increasing collagenization and progressive loss of elasticity.[540] With continued thickening, the plica becomes relatively unpliable and no longer glides normally but snaps against the underlying femoral condyle. Repeated irritation and abrasion result in erosive changes of the articular cartilage of the condyle or even the patella.[552, 553]

The diagnosis may be suspected from the history and physical examination. Classically, the patient relates an episode of blunt or twisting trauma followed by the development of a joint effusion. Excessive stress precipitates a dull, aching pain medial to the patella, which is aggravated by flexion. A clicking sensation without locking or giving way is another common clinical complaint. A palpable or audible snap may occur on knee movement, and a symptomatic plica may be palpated as a tender, bandlike structure parallel to the medial border of the patella. In some cases, a pathologic plica may simulate primary monoarticular arthritis.[559] Alternatively, in rheumatoid arthritis and in other conditions in which a chronic synovial inflammatory process is present, the plicae may become irregularly thickened.

Although much attention has focused on the plica syndrome, these embryonic remnants may manifest themselves in another clinically significant manner. Both the suprapatellar and infrapatellar plicae may persist in their entirety and lead to complete compartmentalization of the knee joint. Failure of the suprapatellar partition to involute may produce an entirely separate suprapatellar bursa.[103, 538, 560, 561] Clinically, the bursa may be manifested as a mass in the suprapatellar area, which is cystic or rubbery and firm on palpation.[103, 546] This may be recognized on double contrast arthrography by the appearance of either a small suprapatellar space or an extrinsic compression on the suprapatellar pouch[538, 561] (Fig. 13–107). CT or MR imaging may be of value in further characterizing the nature of the mass and its relation to the knee joint. Documentation of a separate bursa is of considerable importance in planning an optimal surgical approach; in this regard, a case has been described in which osteocartilaginous bodies in a separate suprapatellar bursa could not be located by using an infrapatellar surgical incision.[546] Documentation of a separate bursa also is important in the management of penetrating wounds with acute suppurative bursitis, in which rupture of the partitioning membrane may unnecessarily contaminate the joint.[546]

Persistence of the infrapatellar plica in its entirety will divide the knee joint into separate medial and lateral compartments.[563] The author has encountered this finding in several patients who have had a history of previous trauma with healed supracondylar fractures.[538] This fact suggests that trauma may initiate either fibrous thickening and hy-

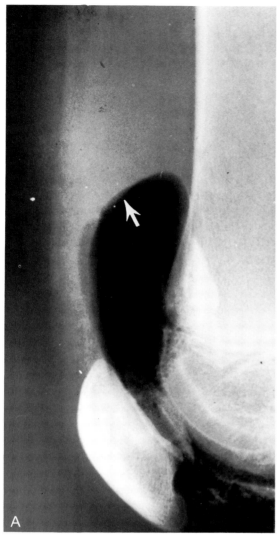

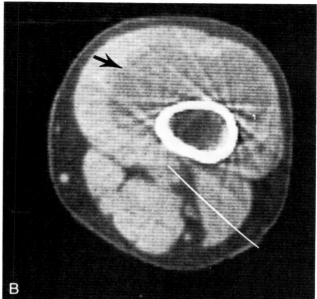

**FIGURE 13–107.** Knee arthrography: Noncommunicating suprapatellar pouch cyst.

**A** A lateral view from a double contrast knee arthrogram demonstrates minimal extrinsic impression on the suprapatellar pouch (arrow).

**B** A transaxial CT scan through the femoral diaphysis at a level cephalad to the suprapatellar pouch reveals a large cystic structure (arrow) not visualized during arthrography.

(From Deutsch AL, et al: Radiology *141*:632, 1981.)

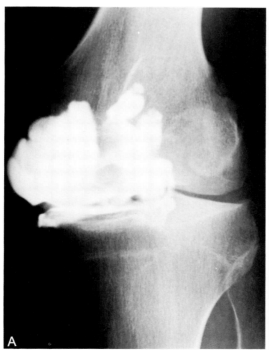

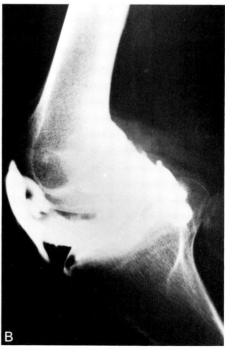

**FIGURE 13–108.** Knee arthrography: Compartmentalization of the knee in the nail-patella syndrome. Frontal **(A)** and lateral **(B)** views after the initial injection of contrast material into the medial aspect of the joint demonstrate a well-demarcated and independent medial compartment. (From Deutsch AL, et al: Radiology *141*:633, 1981.)

pertrophy of the infrapatellar plica or intra-articular fibrosis, leading to abnormal compartmentalization of the joint. Of interest, similar compartmentalization has been identified in hereditary onycho-osteoarthrodysplasia (the nail-patella syndrome)[538] (Fig. 13–108). The probable relation, however, between anomalies of the patella and aberrations in joint development remains incompletely understood.[562]

### Articular Disorders (Table 13–8)

**Degenerative Joint Disease** (Fig. 13–109). Contrast examination of the knee in patients with degenerative joint disease delineates abnormalities of the articular cartilage and menisci and the presence of intra-articular osseous bodies and popliteal cysts.[197] Arthrography in these persons, however, does have certain limitations: Proper positioning during arthrography in the elderly patient with degenerative disease can be extremely difficult and time consuming; tangential portions of the cartilaginous surface are the only areas that are visualized adequately; and evaluation of femoropatellar disease is difficult, as the patellar cartilage is

**TABLE 13–8. Causes of Multiple Filling Defects on Knee Arthrograms**

| |
|---|
| Rheumatoid arthritis |
| Pigmented villonodular synovitis |
| Idiopathic synovial (osteo)chondromatosis |
| Hemangioma, angioma |
| Lipoma arborescens |

not well shown. Despite these shortcomings, arthrography may delineate generalized cartilaginous thinning or localized cartilaginous defects. A rough, irregular surface with imbibition of contrast material may be apparent.

Compared with routine and weight-bearing radiographic films, arthrography adds little additional information regarding alterations in the more involved femorotibial compartment.[197] In the less involved (contralateral) compartment, arthrography may reveal information regarding cartilaginous integrity not obtainable by these other examinations. In both femorotibial compartments as well as in

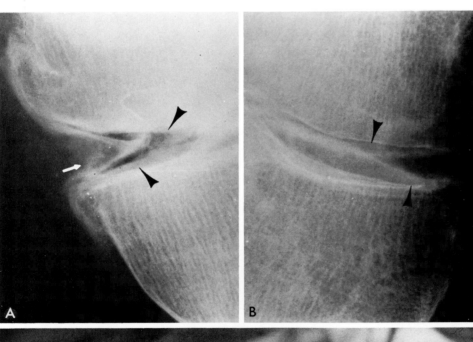

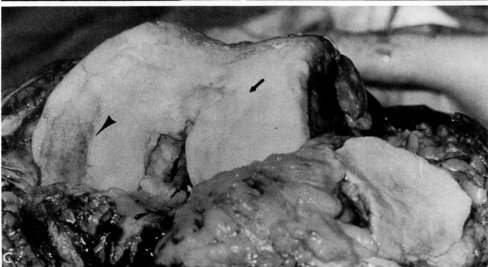

**FIGURE 13–109.** Knee arthrography: Degenerative joint disease. A 56 year old man had left knee pain for 15 years. Initial films revealed more significant changes in the medial femorotibial compartment than in the lateral femorotibial compartment. Arthrography was performed.

**A** In the medial compartment, findings included severe denudation of articular cartilage on both femur and tibia (arrowheads). The medial meniscus is swollen, with an incomplete vertical tear (arrow) and an irregular inner contour.

**B** In the lateral compartment, moderate thinning of articular cartilage can be seen (arrowheads), although the meniscus appears normal. Radionuclide examination confirmed the presence of both medial and lateral compartment abnormalities.

**C** During a total knee replacement, severe abnormalities of the medial compartment (arrowhead) and moderate abnormalities of the lateral compartment (arrow) were detected on the anterior surface of the femur.

the patellofemoral compartment, cartilaginous alterations are better defined with MR imaging (see Chapters 39 and 70).

Meniscal alterations in patients with degenerative joint disease can include acute tears, similar in appearance to those occurring in patients without degenerative joint disease, or degenerative tears. These latter tears appear as swollen, irregular meniscal surfaces with fragmented inner contours and imbibition of contrast material. Horizontal collections of contrast material within the involved meniscus represent degenerative crevices.

Loose or attached bodies in degenerative joint disease may be detected on arthrography. They result from surface disintegration or osteophyte fragmentation. These intra-articular osseous bodies may remain free in the joint cavity or attach at a distant synovial site.

Synovial cyst formation may complicate degenerative joint disease as well as other disorders. This complication is discussed later in this chapter.

**Rheumatoid Arthritis** (Fig. 13–110). Arthrographic findings have been documented in the knee in rheumatoid arthritis.[205–208, 564, 565] These include enlargement of the joint cavity or suprapatellar pouch, nodular irregularity or corrugation of the synovial membrane, filling defects within the joint cavity, lymphatic filling,[10, 12, 13, 207, 326] destruction of hyaline cartilage and fibrocartilage,[565] and synovial cyst formation. After synovectomy, these findings may be less marked, although they frequently recur, often as early as 3 months after surgery.

**Pigmented Villonodular Synovitis** (Figs. 13–111 and 13–112). The knee arthrogram in diffuse pigmented villonodular synovitis reveals an enlarged synovial cavity, irregular synovial outline with ''laking'' or pooling of contrast material, and nodular filling defects.[209–211]

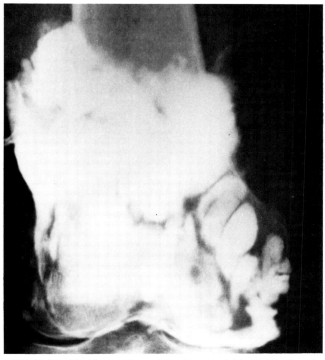

**FIGURE 13–110.** Knee arthrography: Rheumatoid arthritis. Nodular and linear irregularity and pooling of contrast material reflect synovial hypertrophy.

Arthrographic alterations associated with localized nodular synovitis of the knee may include a masslike lesion coated with contrast material.[212] Identification of such a mass is important, as patients with this lesion may have symptoms and signs that suggest a mechanical problem.[213] Differential diagnosis of such a mass includes an enlarged infrapatellar fat pad, sometimes termed Hoffa's disease,[214] an intra-articular ganglion arising from the alar fold of synovium,[215] an uncalcified intra-articular body, and other rare synovial tumors, such as fibromas, hemangiomas, and giant cell tumors.[363]

**Idiopathic Synovial (Osteo)Chondromatosis** (Fig. 13–113). Knee arthrography in idiopathic synovial (osteo)chondromatosis reveals an enlarged synovial cavity and multiple small, sharply defined filling defects.[216, 217] Occasionally larger defects are apparent. The nodular lesions of idiopathic synovial (osteo)chondromatosis are better defined than those of pigmented villonodular synovitis.

**Lipoma Arborescens.** Lipoma arborescens is a rare intra-articular lesion of unknown cause, most commonly located in the knee, consisting of focal deposits of fat beneath the swollen synovial lining.[218] Arthrography reveals numerous moderately well defined defects of variable size.[219, 365, 768, 769] Rarely, true lipomas may produce filling defects in the opacified knee.[327] With both conditions, however, computed arthrotomography and MR imaging allow a more precise diagnosis, owing to the distinctive x-ray attenuation value (with computed arthrotomography) and signal intensity characteristics (with MR imaging) of adipose tissue (see Chapter 70).

**Synovial Hemangioma.** Hemangiomas of the synovial membrane occur most frequently in the knee, although they also are apparent in other joints, as well as in synovial tendon sheaths.[220–222] Initial radiographs may reveal soft tissue masses, calcified phleboliths, and a hemophilia-like arthropathy with osteoporosis and epiphyseal enlargement (see Chapter 63).[223] Arthrography may reveal single or multiple radiolucent defects, and arteriography will outline hypervascular tumors.[224] A synovial angioma may have a similar arthrographic appearance.[225]

**Hemophilia.** Reported arthrographic findings of the knee in hemophilia are synovial irregularity, focal areas of cartilage thinning, and osseous irregularities covered by relatively normal cartilage (see Chapter 63).[116, 226]

## Blount's Disease (Fig. 13–114)

Dalinka and coworkers[227] suggested that arthrography in patients with Blount's disease (tibia vara) reveals information that is necessary to evaluate and manage these patients. The plain film findings in this condition are well known and include varus deformity of the proximal portion of the tibia, cortical thickening of the medial tibial shaft, and the presence of a bony excrescence on the posteromedial aspect of the proximal tibial metaphysis (see Chapter 81). The medial aspect of the proximal tibia appears depressed. Arthrography allows analysis of the integrity of the unossified cartilage above the medial tibial plateau, information that can assist the surgeon.[228] If this cartilage is normal, a valgus osteotomy correcting the angular deformity is sufficient treatment; if significant cartilaginous depression is evident, additional surgery may be required to control ligament laxity, including elevation of the tibial plateau.

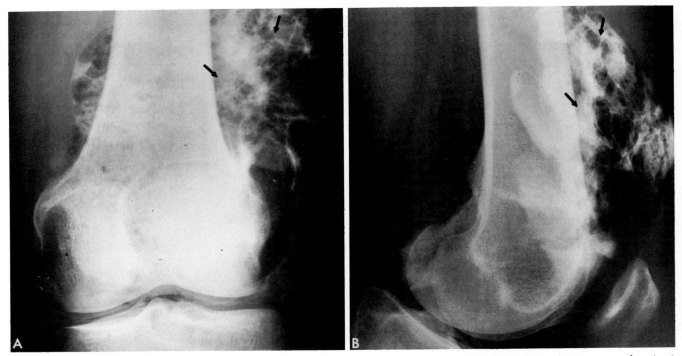

**FIGURE 13–111.** Knee arthrography: Diffuse pigmented villonodular synovitis. Observe the irregular distribution and appearance of contrast material (arrows) in the suprapatellar pouch. (From Dalinka MK, et al: CRC Crit Rev Radiol Sci 5:1, 1973.)

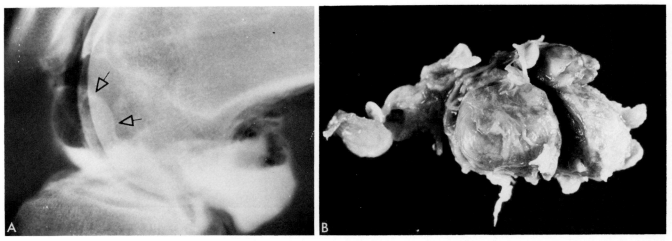

**FIGURE 13–112.** Knee arthrography: Localized nodular synovitis. This 25 year old man complained of a popping sensation in his knee with intermittent locking. Arthrography **(A)** reveals a prominence in the region of the infrapatellar fat pad (arrows). A photograph **(B)** of the removed and sectioned specimen reveals a fibrous, well-circumscribed mass.

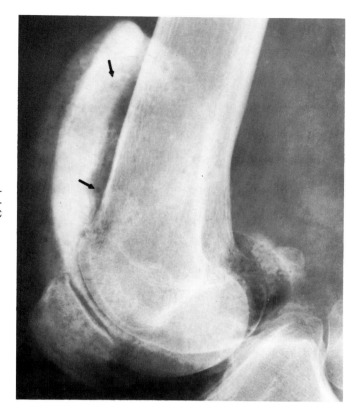

**FIGURE 13–113.** Knee arthrography: Idiopathic synovial (osteo)-chondromatosis. Observe multiple sharply defined filling defects (arrows) throughout the articular cavity. (From Dalinka MK, et al: CRC Crit Rev Radiol Sci *5*:1, 1973.)

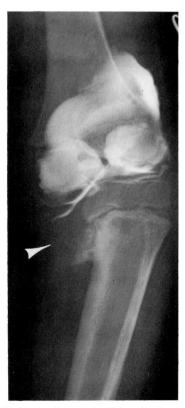

**FIGURE 13–114.** Knee arthrography: Blount's disease. In this 5 year old child, knee arthrography reveals depression of epiphyseal cartilage and metaphyseal bone (arrowhead), with stress fractures of the metaphysis. A tibial osteotomy was performed, which was unsuccessful. (From Dalinka MK, et al: Radiology *113*:161, 1974.)

## Synovial Cysts

Synovial cysts about the knee are most frequent in the popliteal region, where communication between the joint and normal posterior bursae can be identified.[229–232] The most commonly involved bursa is the gastrocnemiosemi-membranosus bursa,[566–568] located posterior to the medial femoral condyle between the tendons of the gastrocnemius and semimembranosus muscles, with an additional portion anterior to the medial head of the gastrocnemius. The anterior limit of this bursa abuts on the posterior surface of the joint capsule and is relatively thin.[229] Communication between the bursa and the knee joint occurs in 35 to 55 per cent of cadavers[229, 231] and increases in frequency with advancing age. This communication occurs via a transverse slit, usually between 15 to 20 mm long.[229] The opening may be covered with a fibrous membrane in approximately 70 per cent of cases.[229]

Swelling of this posterior bursa is termed a Baker's cyst.[233, 569] The cause of such cysts is not entirely clear, and various theories have been proposed: (1) Herniation of the synovial membrane of the knee through a weak area in the posterior joint capsule; (2) rupture of the posterior joint capsule with extravasation of fluid into the soft tissues and secondary encapsulation; and (3) rupture of the posterior joint capsule producing communication with a normally occurring posterior bursa. Of these theories, the third theory seems most probable,[220–231, 234, 235] as direct observation rarely has documented a synovial herniation from the knee into a normal bursa or a popliteal cyst completely separated from the articular cavity.

The presence of a slit between articular cavity and posterior bursa may be responsible for a ball-valve mechanism

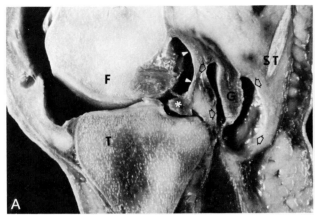
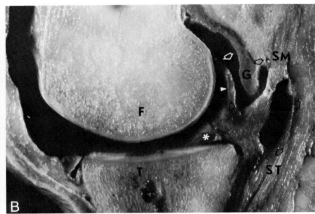
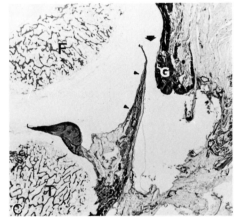

**FIGURE 13–115.** Knee arthrography: Anatomy of the posterior bursae—photographs and a photomicrograph of sagittal sections through the knee of a cadaveric specimen.

**A** Sagittal section through the knee at the level of the medial femoral condyle near the intercondylar notch. F, Femur; T, tibia; asterisk, posterior horn of medial meniscus. The anterior margin of the band of tissue directly posterior to the medial femoral condyle is the knee joint capsule (arrowheads). The posterior margin of this same band of tissue is the anterior margin of the gastrocnemiosemimembranosus bursa (arrows), which lies anterior to the medial head of the gastrocnemius muscle (G). The semimembranosus muscle is not seen in this section. The semitendinosus muscle (ST) is seen more posteriorly, with the posterior margin of the bursa (arrows) opposed to it.

**B** A sagittal section through the medial femoral condyle 1 cm medial to **A**. A transverse slit (white arrowhead) represents communication between the knee joint and the gastrocnemiosemimembranosus bursa (open arrows). The opening is oriented cranially and arises about 2 cm inferiorly to the most superior aspect of the posterior joint capsule. The semimembranosus muscle (SM) courses obliquely posterior to the medial head of the gastrocnemius muscle (G). The semitendinosus muscle (ST) forms the posterior margin of the gastrocnemiosemimembranosus bursa. Arrowhead, Knee joint capsule; asterisk, posterior horn of medial meniscus.

**C** Photomicrograph (×1) of a sagittal section at the level of the medial femoral condyle. The transverse slit (solid arrow) is readily apparent. The membranous septum could not be seen. G, Medial head of the gastrocnemius muscle; open arrows, gastrocnemiosemimembranosus bursa; arrowheads, posterior joint capsule.

(From Guerra J Jr, et al: AJR *136*:593, 1981. Copyright 1981, American Roentgen Ray Society.)

that has been noted in conjunction with synovial cysts[236, 237, 350]; fluid introduced into a cyst may not enter the joint cavity (Fig. 13–115). Because of this one-way directional flow, arthrography rather than bursography is more accurate in defining the extent of a cyst and its connection with a neighboring joint. This ball-valve mechanism, however, is not present invariably. Rauschning and collaborators[568] have divided popliteal cysts into those with a true one-way valve (approximately 50 per cent of cases) and those in which unimpeded flow of fluid occurs in both directions; a strong positive correlation was found between the presence of a valve mechanism and the absence of articular disorders, and between the absence of a valve mechanism and the presence of joint effusions and disease.

In addition to the gastrocnemiosemimembranosus bursa, a second posterior bursa is located beneath the popliteal tendon,[232, 770] which communicates less frequently with the joint. A third posterior bursa exists between the medial head of the gastrocnemius and the distal end of the biceps. A weak point occurs laterally beneath the popliteal tendon, which may represent an extended popliteal tendon sheath.[16, 232] Furthermore, communication may exist between the knee and proximal tibiofibular joint cavity in 10 per cent of adults. Occasionally, anterior, medial, and lateral synovial cysts also may be observed.[238, 347, 570–573] In

fact, synovial cysts may extend simultaneously in more than one direction.[678]

Any of these synovial cysts may enlarge, producing a mass with or without pain. Rupture of a cyst is associated with soft tissue extravasation of fluid contents. Ruptures occurring posteriorly can simulate a compartment syndrome or thrombophlebitis,[348] and, in fact, two or more of these conditions can coexist.[239–241, 328, 594, 771] Giant synovial cysts can extend into the calf, ankle, heel, and thigh.[242–245, 572, 574]

Conventional radiography usually provides nonspecific evidence of a synovial cyst. A joint effusion and a soft tissue mass are evident in some cases, although the latter abnormality may be difficult to distinguish from normal soft tissue structures. Occasionally, intrabursal osteocartilaginous bodies or radiolucent collections, calcification in the bursal wall, or bone erosions are seen.[575–578]

Arthrography of the knee is an accurate method of diagnosing synovial cysts,[246–251] although some investigators also recommend ultrasonic[252–257, 579–583] or isotopic[258, 584–586] examination in this clinical situation. CT appears of little value in diagnosing these cysts in most cases, although this examination is useful in the evaluation of a suspected synovial cyst when its position is atypical or when it is not opacified on arthrography.[259, 587–589] MR imaging of such cysts may provide the most detailed information regarding the distribution and extent of the process and the degree of synovial inflammation (see Chapter 70).[590]

Routine overhead films after injection of contrast material usually will reveal the synovial cyst, although specialized techniques may be helpful, including radiography after bandage wrapping of the suprapatellar pouch, exercise, and standing. Knee flexion will accentuate filling of the posterior bursae,[251] probably related to widening of the communicating slit between bursa and joint cavity and compression of the suprapatellar pouch between the quadriceps tendon and anterior surface of the femur. Cineradiography will document the to-and-fro movement of fluid between these two structures, although demonstration of a small posterior synovial cyst, particularly during knee flexion, may not indicate a pathologic situation and must be differentiated from the normal bulging of the posterior capsule of the knee joint that occurs in this position.[230]

The arthrographic appearance of an abnormal synovial cyst will vary.[593] In most instances, a well-defined, lobulated structure filled with air and radiopaque contrast material will be revealed. It may have an irregular surface related to hypertrophy of its synovial lining and be associated with adjacent lymphatic filling. Alternatively, the entire cyst or a portion of it may rupture,[260, 261] with extravasation of contrast material into soft tissues posteriorly, or, less commonly, superiorly or anteriorly.[238, 247, 250, 571, 572, 591] Sinus tracts leading from the cyst to the skin surface may be encountered.[592]

Any inflammatory, degenerative, traumatic, or neoplastic condition that produces a knee effusion can lead to synovial cyst formation[569] (Fig. 13–116). These conditions include rheumatoid arthritis, degenerative joint disease, gout, pigmented villonodular synovitis, and idiopathic synovial (osteo)chondromatosis, as well as other localized or systemic articular conditions. In the absence of any obvious cause,

the radiologist must search diligently for meniscal abnormality. Synovial cysts may be noted in children with juvenile chronic polyarthritis[262] (Fig. 13–117) or on a familial basis.[263] In children, popliteal cysts appear to have a much better prognosis than in adults, and the frequency of noncommunicating cysts is higher.[569] Surgical removal of synovial cysts without treatment of the underlying articular disease process rarely is successful, as the cyst will recur.[349, 364]

The differential diagnosis of synovial cysts about the knee includes a variety of neoplasms of soft tissue or bone origin,[595–597] thrombophlebitis and hematomas,[598, 599] varicose veins, aneurysms, and other conditions. The simultaneous occurrence of synovial cysts and some of these disorders is well known, especially with regard to venous thrombosis, thrombophlebitis, and cystic degeneration of the popliteal artery.[600–602]

### Accuracy of Knee Arthrography

The accuracy of this examination in detecting abnormalities of the knee, particularly meniscal alterations, depends primarily on the quality of the study and the expertise of the observer.[603–606] In the hands of a skilled radiologist, the accuracy rate of diagnosing medial meniscal tears in patients who have these tears documented at surgery may reach 99 per cent; similarly, the accuracy in diagnosing lateral meniscal tears can approximate 93 per cent.[134] False-negative arthrograms in patients with meniscal tears or false-positive arthrograms in patients without tears are rare if the examination is performed carefully by experienced radiologists.[329] Because arthrography can be a safe and reliable procedure in diagnosing meniscal abnormalities, it should be preferred over arthroscopy in this clinical situation, or, at the very least, should be combined with arthroscopy.[351–353, 694] Arthroscopy appears to be more accurate for

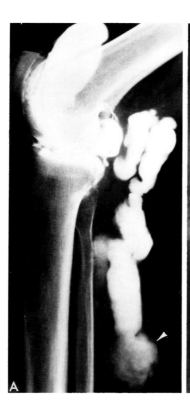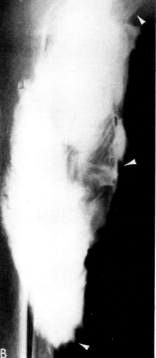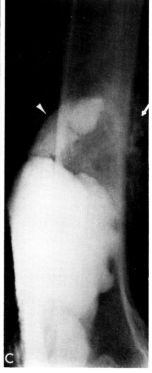

**FIGURE 13–116.** Knee arthrography: Synovial cyst formation.

**A** Rheumatoid arthritis. A typical large popliteal cyst extending into the calf is filled with contrast material. It is slightly irregular in contour, particularly inferiorly (arrowhead), which may reflect synovial inflammation. No free extravasation into the soft tissues is seen.

**B** Rheumatoid arthritis. Another popliteal cyst extends behind the tibia. It has an irregular, feathery appearance (arrowheads) consistent with tissue extravasation.

**C** Rheumatoid arthritis. Extension of suprapatellar pouch. On this lateral view of the pouch following arthrography, note the cystic extension superiorly (arrowhead) with adjacent lymphatic filling (arrow).

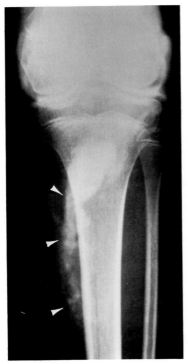

**FIGURE 13–117.** Knee arthrography: Synovial cyst formation. Juvenile chronic arthritis. A large synovial cyst (arrowheads) extends inferiorly from the knee in this child. (Courtesy of N. Ghaed, M.D., Denver, Colorado.)

meniscal lesions involving the central edge and anterior horn; arthrography is more sensitive to midbody and peripheral meniscal tears. The arthrographic diagnosis of other conditions, such as cruciate lesions and chondromalacia, is less accurate. At the present time, CT,[528, 529] and scintigraphy[607] have little or no role in the evaluation of meniscal lesions. MR imaging, however, currently is the

**TABLE 13–9. Indications for Ankle Arthrography**

Evaluation of:
    Ligamentous injuries
    Transchondral fractures
    Intra-articular osseous and cartilaginous bodies
    Adhesive capsulitis

most effective, noninvasive technique for the analysis of meniscal as well as ligamentous abnormalities of the knee (see Chapter 70).

## ANKLE AND FOOT

### Ankle Arthrography (Table 13–9)

Injuries of the ankle are a common problem and may lead to considerable disability. Orthopedic surgeons do not agree on the proper mode of therapy for treatment of ankle ligament "sprains"; some recommend surgical intervention, whereas others advocate conservative treatment. It is because of this disagreement that the number of requests for ankle arthrography varies from one institution to another, the procedure being used particularly by physicians who believe in operative treatment of ankle sprains. Contrast opacification of the ankle allows identification and delineation of ligamentous injuries and can be combined effectively with routine and stress radiography of the ankle.

#### Technique (Fig. 13–118)

Arthrographic technique[264–266, 772–774] has been well described. Ideally, the examination should be performed within a few days of the acute injury as blood and tissue adhesions about the ligamentous tear may result in false-negative examinations or subtle abnormalities if the procedure is delayed.[264, 265, 695]

The procedure is accomplished under fluoroscopic control with the patient in the recumbent position. Both supine

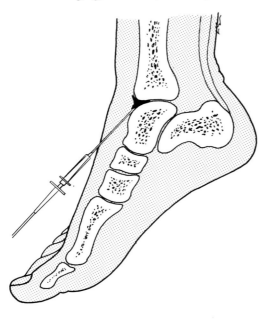
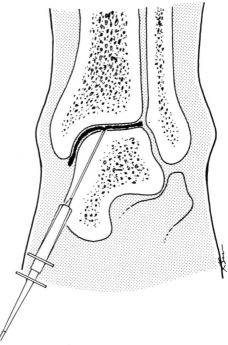

**FIGURE 13–118.** Ankle arthrography: Technique. A needle is inserted from an anterior approach into the tibiotalar joint.

and lateral fluoroscopy may be necessary. A metal marker is placed over the anteromedial portion of the ankle, approximately 1 cm below the joint line. A 20 gauge, 1.5 inch needle is introduced into the ankle under fluoroscopic guidance after cleaning the skin and applying a local anesthetic. Six to 10 ml of 60 per cent Renografin is injected, which may be mixed with approximately 1 ml of lidocaine. The needle is withdrawn and radiographs are exposed in anteroposterior, oblique, and lateral projections after mild exercise of the ankle. Stress radiographs also may be obtained.

## Normal Ankle Arthrogram (Fig. 13–119)

Under normal circumstances, ankle arthrography results in opacification of the articular cavity without evidence of extra-articular leak except for filling of the tendon sheath of the flexor hallucis longus or the flexor digitorum longus, or both, in approximately 20 per cent of patients.[264–268] The posterior subtalar joint will be opacified in approximately 10 per cent of patients. All other patterns of contrast extravasation are regarded as abnormal.

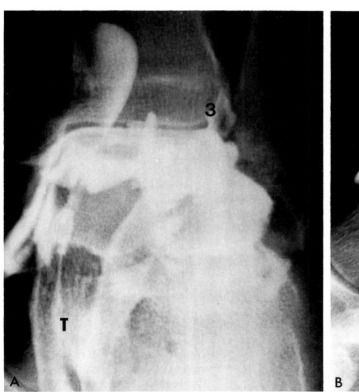

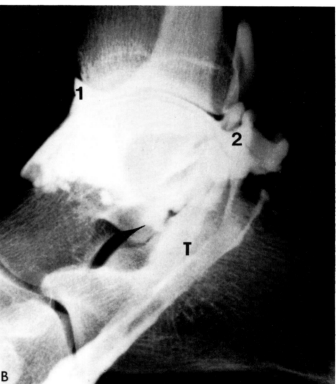

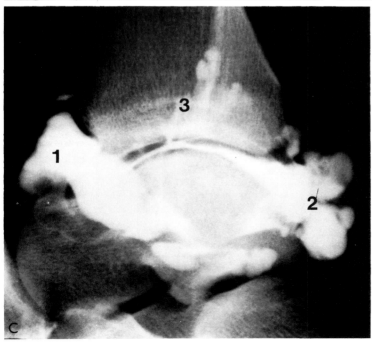

**FIGURE 13–119.** Ankle arthrography. Normal arthrogram.

**A, B** Anteroposterior **(A)** and lateral **(B)** views. The tibiotalar joint has been opacified. Note the normal recesses: anterior recess (1), posterior recess (2), and syndesmotic recess (3). Filling of the medial tendon sheaths (T) and posterior subtalar joint (arrowhead) is a normal finding.

**C** Lateral view from another patient showing prominent (but normal) anterior (1), posterior (2), and syndesmotic (3) recesses.

The normal ankle arthrogram reveals three recesses. In the region of the syndesmosis between distal portions of the tibia and fibula, a small vertical recess, best delineated on oblique radiographs, 1 to 2.5 cm high and approximately 4 mm wide can be observed.[267] Additional anterior and posterior recesses are best observed on lateral radiographs. All three recesses should be smooth and well delineated.

### Ligamentous Injuries (Figs. 13–120 and 13–121)

Arthrographic abnormalities associated with ligamentous injuries have been well described[264–274, 608, 773] and require an understanding of pertinent anatomy of the ankle.[275]

**Anterior Talofibular Ligament Injury.** The anterior talofibular ligament extends from the anterior surface of the distal portion of the fibula to the talar neck. It is most susceptible to injury. With tears, contrast material will be seen both inferior and lateral to the distal end of the fibula on frontal radiographs and anterior to the distal part of the fibula on lateral radiographs. Occasionally, on anteroposterior views, the contrast material will overlie the syndesmosis.

**Calcaneofibular Ligament Injury.** The calcaneofibular ligament, a strong ligament, originates from the posterior aspect of the distal portion of the fibula and inserts on the superior aspect of the calcaneus. When this ligament is torn, contrast material fills the peroneal tendon sheaths as the inner aspect of the sheaths also is torn.[609–613] Tears of the calcaneofibular ligament are associated with tears of the anterior talofibular ligament,[354] so that the arthrographic findings of both ligament injuries are apparent. A third ligament, the posterior talofibular ligament, also may be injured in these instances.

Contrast opacification of the peroneal tendon sheaths, although always an abnormal finding on ankle arthrograms,[610] is not specific for calcaneofibular ligament disruption.[609] Isolated filling of these sheaths is most compatible with a new or old injury to this ligament, whereas such filling combined with leakage of contrast material distal and lateral to the lateral malleolus suggests combined ruptures of the anterior talofibular and calcaneofibular ligaments or an anterior talofibular ligament rupture associated with disruption of the peroneal tendon sheaths. Opacification of the sheaths may be prevented by blood or fibrin clot so that false-negative arthrograms are encountered.[609, 613]

**Distal Anterior Tibiofibular Ligament Injury.** This structure extends from the anterior and lateral aspects of the distal portion of the tibia to the adjacent anterior portion of the distal fibular end. After injury to this ligament, extravasation of contrast material occurs between distal tibia and fibula, beyond the syndesmotic recess. Its arthrographic appearance may simulate that of capsular rupture.[614]

**Deltoid Ligament Injury.** The deltoid ligament originates from the medial malleolus and extends to the talus and calcaneus. With tears of the deltoid ligament, contrast material extravasates beyond the medial confines of the joint.

The amount of extravasation of contrast material occurring after tears of any of these ligaments depends on many factors, including the volume of contrast material injected, the degree of surrounding soft tissue injury, the presence of scar tissue from previous injuries, and the length of time from injury to arthrography.[264] Arthrography performed after considerable delay may not reveal the presence of ligamentous injury; arthrography performed after appropriate conservative or operative therapy may not demonstrate previously evident abnormalities.[265]

Ankle arthrography is a reliable method of delineating these ligamentous injuries. Its reported accuracy is 75 to 90 per cent.[268, 269] Some observers report less success, particularly in diagnosing double injuries of the lateral ligaments.[266, 775] In these cases, massive extravasation related to one injury may obscure extravasation related to a second injury. A combination of ankle arthrography and tenography may provide more reliable information in these instances.[775]

Any of these ankle injuries may be associated with abnormalities on plain films, including soft tissue swelling and avulsion fractures at the osseous sites of attachment of the specific ligament. Furthermore, stress radiography may indicate ligament weakening by revealing abnormal widen-

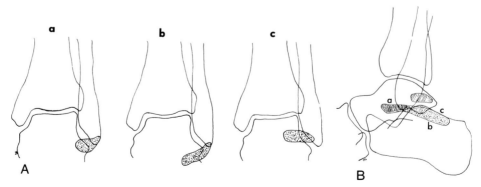

**FIGURE 13–120.** Ankle arthrography: Normal ligamentous anatomy.
**A, B** Diagrammatic representation of the major lateral ligaments of the ankle. On anteroposterior **(A)** and lateral **(B)** views, these ligaments include the anterior talofibular ligament (a), calcaneofibular ligament (b), and posterior talofibular ligament (c). Note that they nearly are horizontal in course, arising from the lateral malleolus and surrounding the lateral aspect of the ankle.

*Illustration continued on opposite page*

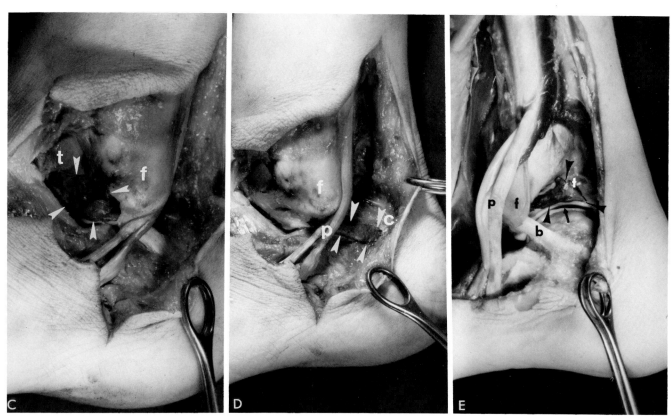

**FIGURE 13-120** *Continued*

**C–E** Dissection identifying the major lateral ligaments of the ankle (ligaments are painted with tantalum). The anterior talofibular ligament **(C)** (arrowheads) extends from the distal end of the fibula (f) to the talus (t). The calcaneofibular ligament **(D)** (arrowheads) originates from the posterior aspect of the distal fibula (f) and inserts on the superior aspect of the calcaneus (c). It is intimate with the tendons of the peroneal muscles (p). The posterior talofibular ligament **(E)** (arrowheads) extends from the fibula (f) to the talus (t). Note its relationship to the calcaneofibular ligament (b), peroneal tendons (p), and posterior subtalar joint (arrow).

*Illustration continued on following page*

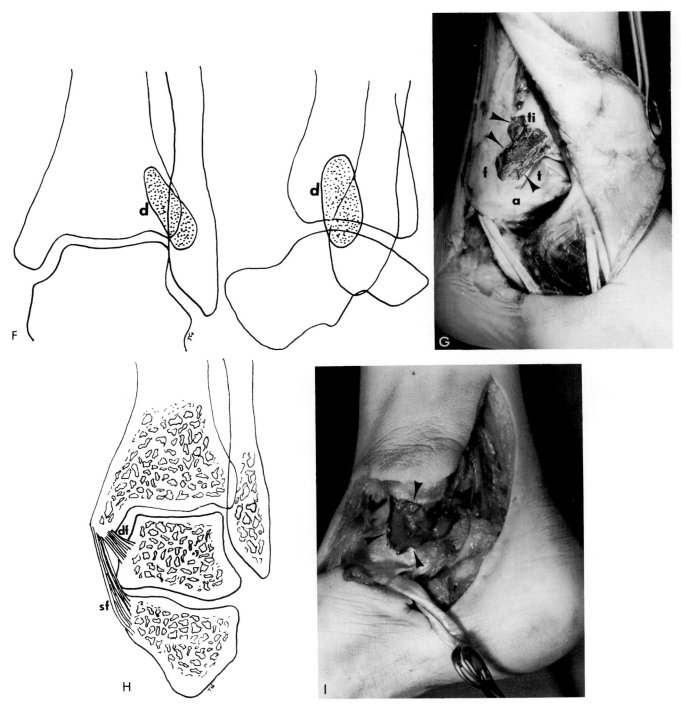

**FIGURE 13–120** *Continued*

**F** Diagrammatic representation of the distal anterior tibiofibular ligament (d) on anteroposterior and lateral views. This ligament extends from the anterior and lateral aspects of the distal end of the tibia to the anterior portion of the distal fibula.

**G** Dissection of ankle to reveal the distal anterior tibiofibular ligament (arrowheads). In this anterior oblique view, the ligament can be traced from its origin on the tibia (ti) to its insertion on the fibula (f). It is located above the dome of the talus (t) and the anterior talofibular ligament (a).

**H** Diagrammatic representation of a coronal section through the deltoid ligament. Superficial (sf) and deep (df) fibers are evident.

**I** Dissection of ankle to reveal the deltoid ligament. On this lateral view, the tantalum-coated deep fibers of the ligament (arrowheads) are seen. The posterior tibial tendon and long flexor tendons are held by the clamp.

(**A, B, F, H,** Courtesy of T. Goergen, M.D., Escondido, California; **C–E, G, I,** from Kaye JJ, Bohne WH: *Radiology 125*:659, 1977.)

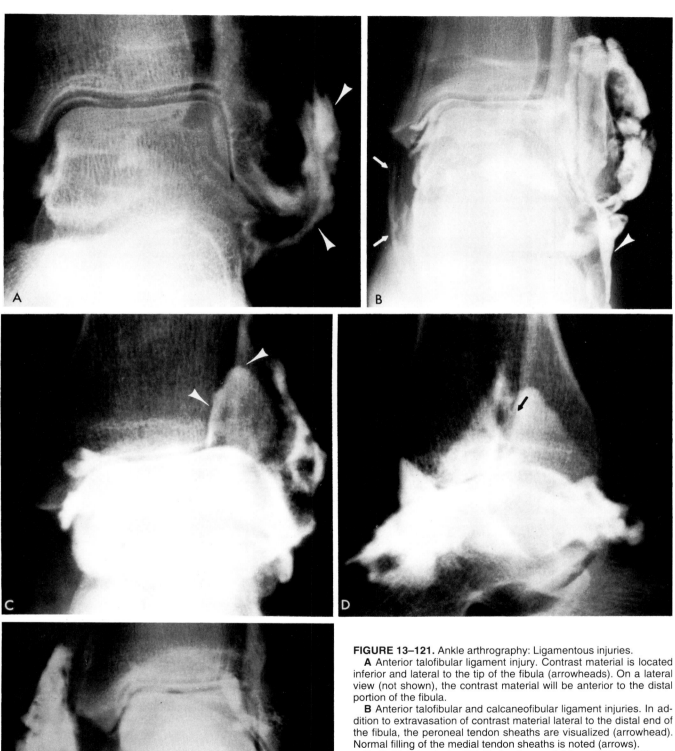

**FIGURE 13–121.** Ankle arthrography: Ligamentous injuries.

**A** Anterior talofibular ligament injury. Contrast material is located inferior and lateral to the tip of the fibula (arrowheads). On a lateral view (not shown), the contrast material will be anterior to the distal portion of the fibula.

**B** Anterior talofibular and calcaneofibular ligament injuries. In addition to extravasation of contrast material lateral to the distal end of the fibula, the peroneal tendon sheaths are visualized (arrowhead). Normal filling of the medial tendon sheaths is noted (arrows).

**C, D** Distal anterior tibiofibular ligament injury. Oblique **(C)** and lateral **(D)** views reveal extravasation between the distal tibia and fibula (arrowheads). The normal clear zone anterior to the distal fibula has been obliterated (arrow).

**E** Deltoid ligament injury. Contrast material has extravasated beneath and medial to the medial malleolus (arrowhead).

ing of the joint.[366, 608] Evidence also indicates a potential role for MR imaging in the identification of sites of ligamentous (and tendinous) injury about the ankle (see Chapter 70).

### Other Traumatic Disorders

**Transchondral Fracture.** Osteochondral fractures (osteochondritis dissecans) of the talar dome are not infrequent.[276, 277] Arthrography in this situation will outline the integrity of the overlying cartilage and the presence of intra-articular cartilaginous bodies. The arthrographic technique should be modified so that air alone or air with 1 to 2 ml of radiopaque contrast material is utilized.

**Soft Tissue and Bony Intra-articular Debris** (Fig. 13–122). As noted earlier, arthrography alone or in combination with conventional tomography or CT scanning may outline pieces of cartilage or both cartilage and bone within the joint cavity after ankle trauma. In addition, a mass consisting of hyalinized connective tissue may lodge between fibula and talus after an inversion sprain,[278] leading to persistent or intermittent pain over the lateral aspect of the ankle. Arthrography can delineate the abnormal tissue in this condition.

**Adhesive Capsulitis** (Fig. 13–123). Posttraumatic adhesive capsulitis in the ankle has been described.[79, 355, 469] This condition, which classically has been recognized as a com-

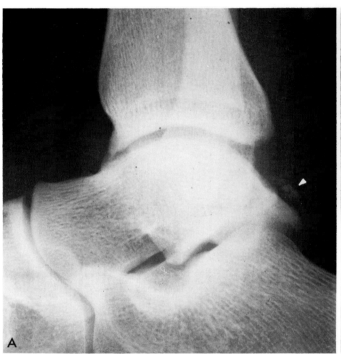

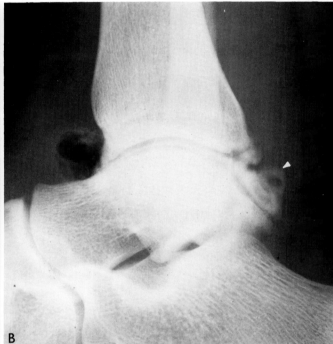

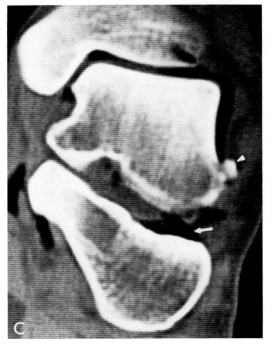

**FIGURE 13–122.** Ankle arthrography: Intra-articular osseous body.

**A** An initial radiograph demonstrates an osseous dense area (arrowhead) adjacent to the talus.

**B** Arthrography confirms its intra-articular location, the dense region producing a filling defect (arrowhead) in the contrast-filled joint cavity. (Courtesy of M. K. Dalinka, M.D., Philadelphia, Pennsylvania.)

**C** Computed arthrotomography using air alone in a different patient shows an osseous fragment (arrowhead) in the lateral recess of the joint on a direct coronal scan. Note the air in the posterior subtalar joint (arrow).

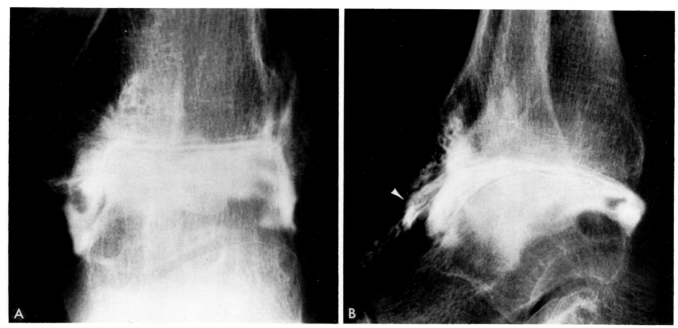

**FIGURE 13–123.** Ankle arthrography: Adhesive capsulitis. The oblique view **(A)** reveals decreased joint volume and irregularities of capsular attachment. On the lateral view **(B),** no filling of normal anterior and posterior recesses has occurred, and extravasation of contrast material is seen along the needle track (arrowhead).

plication of trauma about the shoulder, is not confined to the shoulder joint but may occur elsewhere. In the ankle, patients develop restricted motion after trauma to bone or soft tissue. Arthrography delineates a decrease in the articular capacity, with resistance to injection of contrast material, obliteration of normal anterior and posterior recesses or tibiofibular syndesmosis, opacification of lymphatic vessels,[661] and extravasation of contrast material along the needle track.

### Rheumatoid Arthritis

As in other joints, rheumatoid arthritis of the ankle may be delineated with arthrography.[22, 615] A nodular, corrugated synovial pattern, diminished cartilaginous surface, and lymphatic filling (a nonspecific finding)[616] may be apparent. On rare occasions, synovial cysts may be delineated.

## Peroneal Tenography

Contrast opacification of the peroneal tendons (peroneal tenography) may provide useful information in patients with articular or traumatic disorders.[279, 280, 356, 357, 617, 618, 696]

### Technique

After administration of a local anesthetic, a 22 gauge, 1.5 inch needle is inserted into the common peroneal sheath above the lateral malleolus. The tendon can be palpated easily in this region, and the needle is advanced in an inferior direction until firm resistance is met. Under fluoroscopic control, 10 to 20 ml of Renografin is administered and traced as the material flows in an inferior and superior direction along the sheath. Radiographs are taken in anteroposterior, lateral, and oblique projections. An anteroposterior tunnel view also is obtained with forefoot inversion and the radiographic beam angled 45 degrees toward the

head.[279] Contrast material then can be aspirated and lidocaine is injected.

### Normal Peroneal Tenogram (Fig. 13–124)

The peroneus longus and peroneus brevis muscles occupy the lateral aspects of the leg and foot. The peroneus longus extends from the lateral condyle of the tibia, the head and upper two thirds of the lateral aspect of the fibula, and the intermuscular septa and fasciae around the lateral malleolus obliquely across the sole of the foot to attach to the medial cuneiform and base of the first metatarsal. The peroneus brevis shares a common sheath with the peroneus longus as the two tendons pass around the lateral malleolus. This tendon originates from the lower two thirds of the lateral surface of the fibula and adjacent intermuscular septa and inserts into the base of the fifth metatarsal.

The normal peroneal tenogram outlines the common sheath of the peroneus longus and peroneus brevis muscles and the point of bifurcation of this sheath into separate sheaths enclosing either tendon. These sheaths can be traced for variable distances in the foot, appearing smooth in outline and containing a radiolucent tendon, without displacement.

### Peroneal Tenography After Local Trauma
### (Figs. 13–125 and 13–126)

Painful disability after calcaneal fractures may result from one of four major factors[281]: posttraumatic arthritis of the subtalar or talocalcaneonavicular joints; stenosing tenosynovitis of the peroneal tendons[282, 283, 618]; excessive bone formation on the plantar aspect of the heel; and injury to the septa of the heel pad. In most instances, peroneal dysfunction may be suspected by deformity and widening of the lateral aspect of the calcaneus beneath the fibula. In

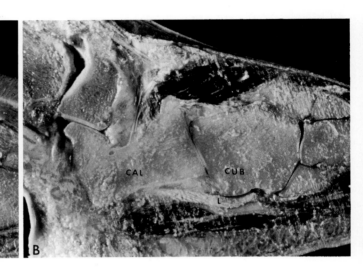

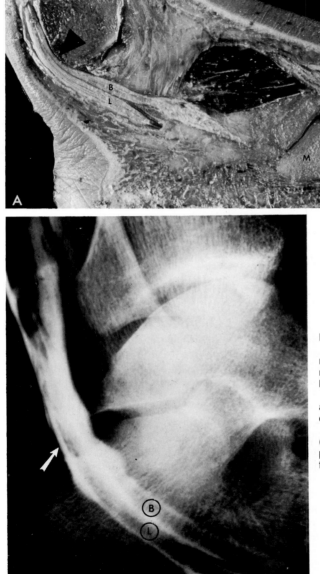

**FIGURE 13–124.** Peroneal tenography: Anatomy and normal tenogram.

**A** A lateral sagittal section of the foot and ankle demonstrates the peroneus brevis **(B)** and peroneus longus (L) tendons passing around the lateral malleolus (arrowhead). The peroneus brevis can be followed close to the base of the fifth metatarsal (M).

**B** A slightly more medial sagittal section through the calcaneus (CAL) and cuboid (CUB) bone outlines the peroneus longus (L) tendon as it crosses underneath the foot.

**C** The normal peroneal tenogram reveals a smooth synovial sheath (arrow) separating into sheaths enclosing the peroneus brevis (B) and peroneus longus (L) tendons. No impingement or deviation of the contrast-filled sheaths can be seen.

(From Resnick D, Goergen TG: Radiology *115*:211, 1975.)

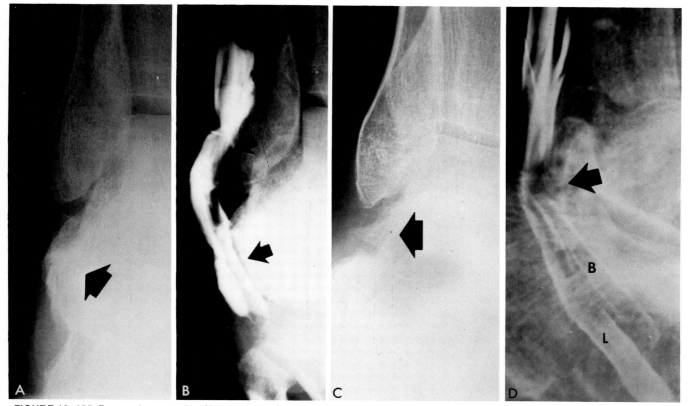

**FIGURE 13–125.** Peroneal tenography: Abnormalities after trauma.

**A, B** Patient with previous calcaneal fracture. Initial radiograph **(A)** reveals deformity of the lateral surface of the calcaneus (arrow). The peroneal tenogram **(B)** indicates lateral displacement (upper arrow) and compression (lower arrow) of the peroneal tendons and sheath.

**C, D** A second patient with previous calcaneal fracture. The plain film **(C)** reveals a lateral calcaneal spicule (arrow) beneath the fibula. The peroneal tenogram **(D)** outlines impingement and compression of the sheath as it passes around the lateral malleolus (arrow) associated with incomplete filling of the peroneus brevis (B) and peroneus longus (L) sheaths.

**(B, D,** From Resnick D, Goergen TG: Radiology *115*:211, 1975.)

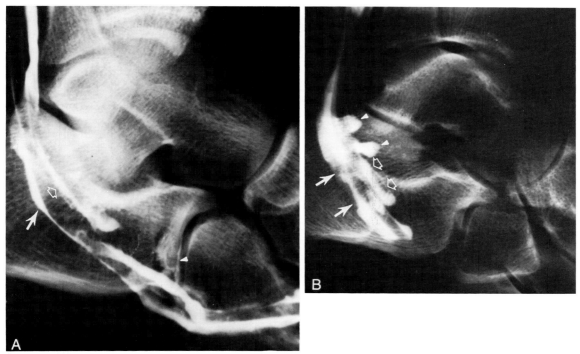

**FIGURE 13–126.** Peroneal tenography: Stenosing and nodular tenosynovitis.

**A** A lateral view after injection of the peroneal tendon sheaths shows filling of the peroneus longus (solid arrow) and peroneus brevis (open arrow) sheaths. Contrast material enters the calcaneocuboid joint (arrowhead), indicative of a capsular tear or defect in the tendon sheath. There is nonfilling of the superior margin of the peroneus brevis, consistent with fibrosis.

**B** In a second patient, the margins of the peroneus longus (solid arrows) and peroneus brevis (open arrows) tendon sheaths are markedly irregular, with pseudodiverticula (arrowheads) of the peroneus brevis tendon sheath.

(From Gilula LA, et al: Radiology *151*:581, 1984.)

some patients, however, the source of pain may be more obscure. In these patients, peroneal tenography is useful.

The tenogram may show several abnormal findings: (1) extrinsic compression and irregularity of the sheath; (2) lateral or anterior displacement of the tendons and sheath; (3) complete obstruction of contrast flow; and (4) tendon rupture.

Peroneal tenography and subtalar arthrography can be accompanied by lidocaine injection to localize the source of obscure pain in patients with previous calcaneal fractures.[280] This distinction may aid the surgeon; stenosing peroneal tenosynovitis may require only excision of a protruding calcaneal spicule, whereas subtalar arthritis may necessitate an extensive arthrodesis.

Acute peroneal tendon dislocation is an infrequent injury that usually results from skiing accidents.[284, 285] After extreme dorsiflexion of the foot, strong contraction of the peroneal tendons may occur. This contraction tears the fibular periosteum and superior peroneal retinaculum and may dislodge a small fragment of fibular cortex. Initial radiographs will reveal soft tissue swelling and an osseous fragment in this clinical setting. Peroneal tenography might be useful in delineating the position of the displaced peroneal tendons.

A report has appeared of a recurrent ganglion about the lateral aspect of an ankle that was injected with contrast material.[286] Opacification of the peroneus longus tendon sheath was observed, which led to appropriate surgery.

## Additional Tenography and Retrocalcaneal Bursography (Figs. 13–127 and 13–128)

Contrast opacification of additional tendon sheaths about the ankle and the retrocalcaneal bursa has been undertaken.[287–298, 617–619, 700, 776, 777] Opacification of the tendon sheaths is not difficult, particularly in patients with rheumatoid arthritis, and consists of introducing a 22 gauge, 1.5 inch needle directly into the distended structure and injecting several milliliters of contrast material. The retrocalcaneal bursa can be punctured with a 22 gauge, 1.5 inch needle introduced adjacent to the Achilles tendon. The needle is advanced until it contacts the upper posterior surface of the calcaneus. Up to 1 ml of contrast material then is injected. In rheumatoid arthritis, irregularity and nodularity of the synovial lining of the sheath and bursa are observed. Tenographic findings accompanying stenosing tenosynovitis are similar to those seen with peroneal tendon sheath opacification.[618]

Although MR imaging currently is used as a diagnostic technique preferable to tenography in the assessment of the tendons about the ankle (see Chapter 70), tenography remains important in the treatment of tenosynovitis.[700] Injection of local anesthetic agents and corticosteroid preparations directly into the affected tendon sheath may have therapeutic benefit.

## Arthrography of Talocalcaneal Joints

Arthrographic evaluation of either or both talocalcaneal joints has been employed to investigate congenital, traumatic, and articular disorders. Injection of the talocalcaneonavicular joint is relatively easy; injection of the posterior subtalar joint is more difficult.[290]

## Technique

Injection of the talocalcaneonavicular joint is accomplished under fluoroscopy using a 22 gauge, 1.5 inch needle and 60 per cent Renografin. The needle is introduced from a dorsal approach and is aimed directly downward into the talonavicular space, approximately 1 cm medial to the dorsalis pedis artery. Upon entrance into the joint, 3 to 4 ml of contrast material is injected. Films are taken in anteroposterior, lateral, oblique, and axial projections.

Injection into the posterior subtalar joint can be made from a medial, posterior, or lateral approach.[290, 778] Using the medial approach, a 22 gauge, 3.5 inch needle is introduced behind the medial malleolus, 1 cm posterior and inferior to the posterior tibial artery. The needle is advanced under fluoroscopic control in an anterosuperior direction into the space between the posterior aspects of the talus and calcaneus. Taking care not to introduce the needle through the interosseous ligament into the talocalcaneonavicular space, inject 1.5 to 2.5 ml of Renografin. Anteroposterior, oblique, lateral, and axial radiographs are obtained.

The point of needle insertion for the more easily accomplished lateral approach to the posterior subtalar joint is adjacent to the fibula. With fluoroscopic guidance the needle is advanced vertically into the joint while the medial aspect of the patient's foot is against the radiographic table. The remainder of the examination is similar to that using the medial approach.

## Normal Arthrography of Talocalcaneonavicular and Posterior Subtalar Joints (Fig. 13–129)

The normal arthrogram of the talocalcaneonavicular joint demonstrates a smooth synovial cavity extending in a gradual curve, which is concave posteriorly, about the anterior aspect of the talus. The cavity extends dorsally to the talar neck and ventrally along the plantar aspect of the talus. It covers the sustentaculum tali. There is no communication with the calcaneocuboid, posterior subtalar, or cuneonavicular joints.

The contrast-filled posterior subtalar joint appears as a linear dense area between the posterior halves of talus and calcaneus along the lateral aspect of the foot. A recess appears as a sausage-shaped collection of contrast material at the posterior margin of the joint.[291] Medial and lateral recesses also are evident. No contrast material flows into the region of the sinus tarsi.[778] In 10 to 20 per cent of arthrograms, communication is present between the posterior subtalar joint and the ankle. Rarely is communication observed between the posterior subtalar joint and talocalcaneonavicular cavity.

## Trauma (Fig. 13–130)

Trauma may lead to abnormalities of the talocalcaneal joints. After calcaneal fractures, posttraumatic arthritis of the neighboring joints may cause significant disability. Selective injection of contrast material with lidocaine into each of the neighboring joints will lead to accurate appraisal as to the source of the symptoms.[280] Injections are made into one joint—the ankle, subtalar, or talocalcaneonavicular joint—and the patient then is asked to walk for approximately 30 minutes to determine if the lidocaine has relieved the pain. If the first injection is unsuccessful, another joint is injected, and the procedure is repeated until

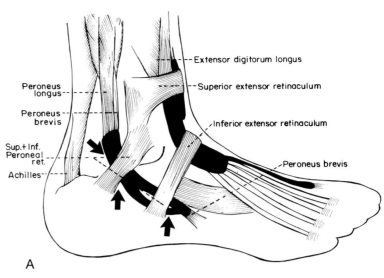

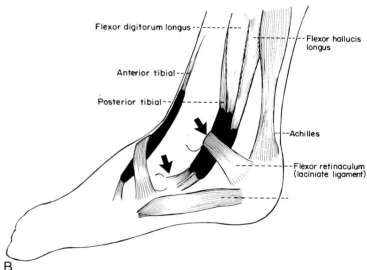

**FIGURE 13–127.** Tenography of the ankle and foot. Normal anatomy. The lateral **(A)** and medial **(B)** tendons and sheaths are indicated. (From Gilula LA, et al: Radiology *151*:581, 1984.)

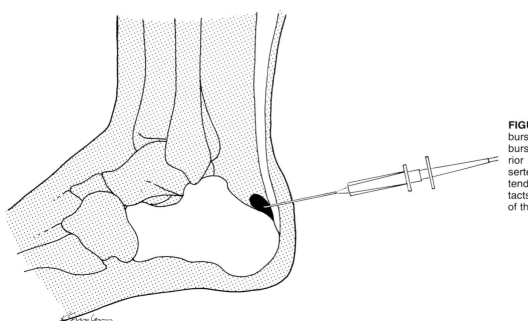

**FIGURE 13–128.** Retrocalcaneal bursography: Technique. The bursa is punctured from a posterior approach. The needle is inserted adjacent to the Achilles tendon and advanced until it contacts the upper posterior surface of the calcaneus.

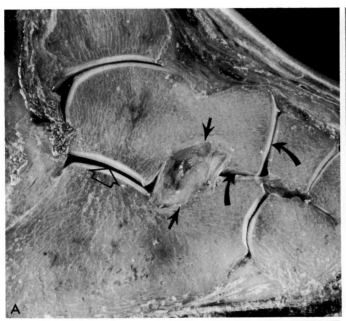

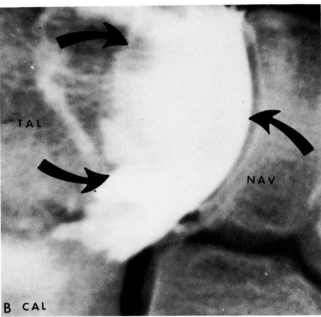

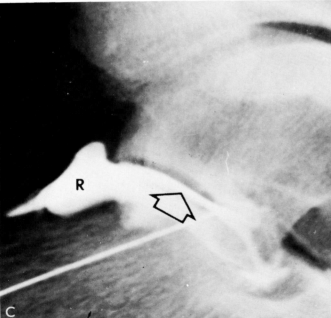

**FIGURE 13–129.** Arthrography of the talocalcaneonavicular and posterior subtalar joints: Anatomy and normal arthrograms.

**A** Sagittal section of the ankle and foot. Observe the talocalcaneonavicular joint (curved arrows) between talus, navicular, and calcaneus, and the posterior subtalar joint (open arrow) between posterior facets of the calcaneus and talus. Interosseous ligaments (straight arrows) separate the two cavities.

**B** An oblique projection during arthrography of the talocalcaneonavicular joint. Note the partially filled articular cavity (arrows) between the talus (TAL), navicular (NAV), and calcaneus (CAL).

**C** A lateral projection during arthrography of the posterior subtalar joint reveals filling of the articular cavity (arrow) with visualization of a normal posterior recess (R). The talocalcaneonavicular joint does not opacify.

(From Resnick D: Radiology *111*:581, 1974.)

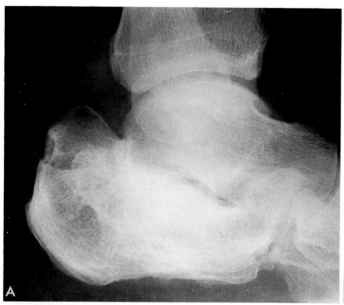

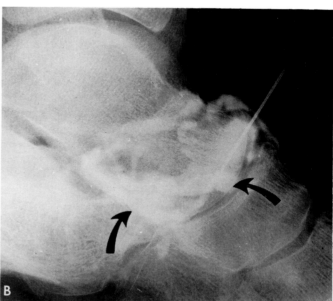

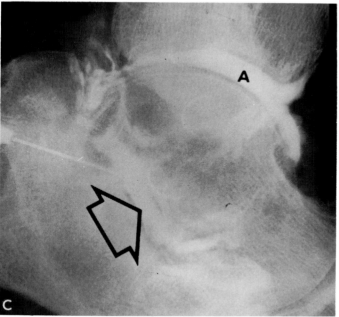

**FIGURE 13-130.** Arthrography of the talocalcaneonavicular and posterior subtalar joints: Abnormalities after trauma. A patient with a previous calcaneal fracture and persistent heel pain. The initial film **(A)** indicates narrowing, sclerosis, and deformity of the posterior subtalar joint and flattening of the superior surface of the calcaneus. Injection of the talocalcaneonavicular joint **(B)** with a mixture of lidocaine and contrast material reveals irregularity of the articular cavity (arrows) and gave some temporary relief of pain. Similarly, injection of the posterior subtalar joint **(C)** (arrow) provided additional relief of pain, demonstrating posterior extravasation of contrast material as well. The ankle joint (A) has opacified. These findings indicated that the patient's symptoms were originating from both the talocalcaneonavicular and posterior subtalar joints. A triple arthrodesis might be the most appropriate therapy.

the painful articulation is identified. In some instances, incomplete contrast opacification of a specific articulation indicates posttraumatic fibrous ankylosis of the joint. On the basis of findings related to contrast and lidocaine arthrography, the surgeon can plan the most effective therapy for the patient.

Talocalcaneal joint arthrography also may be useful in studying patients with posttraumatic sinus tarsi syndrome.[292, 293, 778, 779] These patients develop pain in the midtarsal area over the lateral aspect of the sinus tarsi. It has been suggested that, in this condition, normal synovial folds of the posterior subtalar joint about the interosseous ligament are obliterated. These findings can be revealed by posterior subtalar arthrography, in which the normal recesses about the ligament are not opacified.[293] These changes are related to synovial hyperplasia and do not develop immediately after trauma. The arthrogram should be delayed for some time until the joint effusion diminishes and synovial hypertrophy has occurred. Additional arthrographic findings of the sinus tarsi syndrome are a smooth and round appearance to the anterior margin of the posterior subtalar joint and, in some cases, extravasation of contrast material into the sinus tarsi region.[778] An associated rupture of the calcaneofibular ligament is common.

### Arthritis

In rheumatoid arthritis, abnormalities include distention of the posterior portion of the joint capsule, limited or irregular opacification of the anterior recess, and filling defects caused by hypertrophic synovitis.[620] Direct corticosteroid injection into the articulation may be beneficial.

### Developmental Disorders

**Tarsal Coalition.** Talocalcaneonavicular arthrography has been employed in patients with tarsal coalition.[294] Coalitions between the talus and sustentaculum tali of the calcaneus frequently are difficult to detect on initial radiographs. A tangential view of the area has been recommended (the Harris-Beath view).[295] On occasion, multiple tangential views with varying degrees of angulation of the incident beam and conventional tomography or CT scanning are necessary. Osseous, fibrous, or cartilaginous sustentacular-talar coalitions can be diagnosed with arthrography of the talocalcaneonavicular joint. After introduction of contrast material, routine anteroposterior, lateral, and oblique views are supplemented by axial views taken with varying degrees of beam angulation (35 degrees, 45 degrees, 55 degrees). The normal sustentacular-talar articulation (middle facets of the talocalcaneonavicular joint) will be filled with contrast material. In the presence of a coalition, this space will not be opacified.

**Clubfeet.** Simultaneous arthrography of the ankle and talocalcaneonavicular joint has been advocated in studying children with clubfeet.[296–299] The degree of talar deformity is not determined readily on plain films because of the small size of the ossification centers in the infant's foot. By opacification of these two articular cavities, measurements of the length and width of the talus, the orientation of the talocalcaneonavicular joint, the trochlear curvature, and the talocrural recesses can be made.[299] These measurements may allow selection of a more appropriate treatment in refractory or recurrent clubfeet.[367, 368]

### Arthrography of the Midfoot and Forefoot

Opacification of the joints of the midfoot and forefoot (Fig. 13–131) has been described in normal persons[17, 22, 300, 301] and in patients with rheumatoid arthritis.[22, 287] In general, arthrography is accomplished easily by introducing a 22 gauge or 25 gauge needle directly into the joint under fluoroscopic control. In rheumatoid arthritis, a typical corrugated synovial pattern may be seen, and saccular enlargement of the joint cavity, particularly on the plantar aspects of the metatarsophalangeal joints, can be observed. On rare occasions, a sinus tract between an involved metatarsophalangeal joint and the skin is delineated.

## MISCELLANEOUS AREAS

### Apophyseal Joints

The injection of contrast material, anesthetic agent, corticosteroid preparation, or any combination of the three, into the apophyseal joints of the lumbar spine has been advocated in the diagnosis and treatment of the facet syndrome.[302–304, 621–629, 780] This term was introduced in 1933 by Ghormley,[630] who emphasized that aches and pains in the back were analogous to those accompanying articular disorders in the appendicular skeleton. The apophyseal joints subsequently were identified as a source of such pain by Badgley in 1941[631] and Pedersen and collaborators in 1956,[632] and reproduction of the clinical manifestations during the injection of hypertonic saline in the region of the facet joints was documented by Hirsch and coworkers in 1963.[633]

The fact that abnormalities of the apophyseal joint can lead to significant symptoms and signs is consistent with its anatomy. The apophyseal joint, a synovium-lined space existing between the inferior articular process of one vertebra and the superior articular process of the subjacent vertebra, contains small meniscoid structures composed of synovial villi, fat, and fibrous tissue that may become inflamed or trapped between the apposing osseous surfaces.[634] The capsule of the facet joint is richly innervated by the dorsal ramus of the lumbar spinal nerve, with each joint having a bisegmental innervation.[621]

The facet syndrome leads to pain, which is exacerbated with rotary motion, in the lower back, thighs, buttocks, and legs and to focal tenderness over the affected joint. Its manifestations are not entirely specific and are simulated by other abnormalities of the vertebral column; conversely, the facet syndrome can be misinterpreted as evidence of a herniated intervertebral disc. This diagnostic dilemma underscores the continuing controversy regarding the existence and importance of the facet syndrome in clinical practice.[625] The results of direct injection of the lumbar apophyseal joints with anesthetic, corticosteroids, and contrast material do not entirely resolve this controversy but lend support to the pioneering investigations of Ghormley, Badgley, and Pedersen and others,[630–632] who emphasized the contribution of the apophyseal joints to low back pain.

The intrinsically curved lumbar apophyseal joints are less accessible to direct puncture than many of the articulations of the body; however, the puncture technique is not difficult and can be accomplished with fluoroscopy and, occasionally, CT. The patient first is placed prone on the table and,

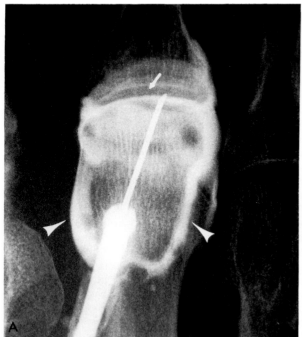

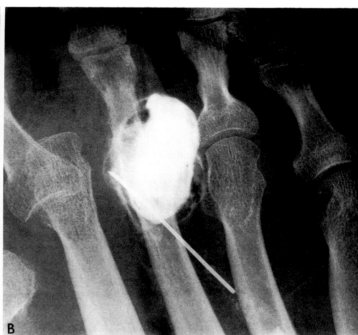

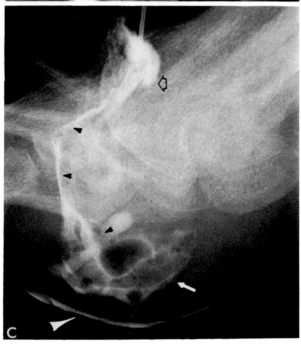

**FIGURE 13–131.** Arthrography of the forefoot: Normal and abnormal arthrograms.

**A** A normal arthrogram of the metatarsophalangeal joint reveals large proximal recesses (arrowheads) and smooth articular cartilage (arrow).

**B** Metatarsophalangeal joint arthrography in rheumatoid arthritis. Observe cystic dilation of the articular cavity, which, on lateral films, was located primarily on the plantar aspect of the joint. Typical rheumatoid erosions and subluxations are evident.

**C** Metatarsophalangeal joint arthrography in rheumatoid arthritis. A lateral view indicates the presence of a sinus with contrast opacification of the articular cavity (open arrow), sinus tract (small arrowheads), plantar cyst (solid arrow), and skin surface (large arrowhead).

in this position or with only slight rotation of the body into an oblique attitude, the posterior portion of the joint surface is brought into profile. Although the degree of rotation that is necessary will vary according to the spinal level being examined and the precise orientation of the articular facets, it must be emphasized that minimal rotation of the patient's body generally is adequate. Increasing obliquity, even as great as 45 degrees, will profile the anterior portion of the apophyseal joint, which will be misinterpreted by an inexperienced examiner as evidence that the patient is in the correct position to accomplish the injection. As only the posterior aspect of the joint is accessible to puncture, acceptance of this exaggerated oblique position will result in technical failure. CT is best reserved for those patients who have significant degenerative abnormalities in the apophyseal joints, in whom posteriorly located osteophytes may block the entrance of the needle.

Under fluoroscopic control, a 20 or 22 gauge spinal needle is directed vertically into the joint space until bone or cartilage is reached (Fig. 13–132). The position of the needle tip can be checked by having the patient turn from one side to the other; it should remain in close alignment with the apophyseal joint during this maneuver.

The choice of injection level is based primarily on clinical evidence, especially focal tenderness over a joint.[621] Injection of multiple levels on one or both sides of the body sometimes is required, although it is advisable to examine only one spinal level at a time so that the results of the injection can be analyzed more precisely.

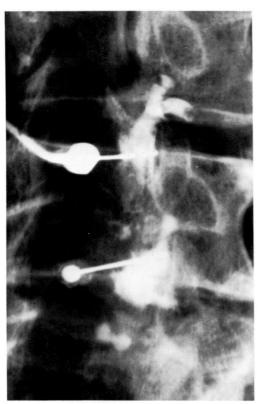

**FIGURE 13–132.** Arthrography of the lumbar apophyseal joints. Observe the needle placement in two consecutive apophyseal joints. Some extravasation of contrast material is evident at the lower level, whereas in the upper joint all of the contrast agent is within the joint.

There is no uniform agreement regarding the amount and the constituency of the solution that should be instilled. It is common practice to inject initially a small amount of radiopaque contrast material (0.5 to 1.5 ml) to confirm the proper placement of the needle, followed by the instillation of approximately 1.0 ml of 0.25 per cent bupivacaine hydrochloride (Marcaine) and 40 mg of methylprednisolone acetate (Depo-Medrol).[621]

When a large volume of material is injected its extravasation, especially in the epidural space, commonly is seen. The diffusion of the anesthetic agent as well as the corticoid medication into the periarticular tissues as a result of capsular rupture may allow these substances to contact other structures, including the branches of the sinuvertebral nerve. In such instances, any relief of back pain cannot reliably be attributed to abnormalities of an apophyseal joint. The use of a smaller injection volume (0.5 ml of radiopaque contrast material and 0.5 to 0.7 ml of a more concentrated anesthetic agent) has been recommended by some investigators as a more suitable solution for injection when the purpose is principally diagnostic rather than therapeutic.[626]

The arthrogram itself is used mainly to confirm the intracapsular position of the needle tip, revealing a smooth, oval joint capsule in the frontal projection and an S-shaped configuration in the oblique projection. Arthrographic abnormalities occasionally are seen, including an irregular or nodular appearance in the presence of synovial proliferation or synechiae, and a constricted joint (adhesive capsulitis) in some instances of osteoarthritis.[621] Although visualization of lymphatics may indicate synovial inflammation, it is not a specific finding, resulting also from overdistention of a normal joint. Similarly, extravasation of the contrast agent from the superior or inferior recess of the joint more frequently is a manifestation of capsular distention and rupture due to a large injection volume than a result of inherent weakness of the capsule itself. Capsular changes, however, including distortion and irregularity, are observed in patients with previous laminectomy or spinal fusion, or both.[621]

In the presence of spondylolysis, opacification of one lumbar facet joint will outline an abnormal communication with the adjacent facet joint via a tract or channel.[303, 635, 636] Rarely, communication with contralateral facet joints also is observed in cases of spondylolysis.[635] Such patterns of abnormal joint connections are consistent with tearing of the articular capsule due to the separation of the edges of the bone. Contrast material also may insinuate itself between an articular process and an anomalous ossicle at its tip.[637]

Reports of the therapeutic effects after the intra-articular injection of an anesthetic agent and a corticosteroid preparation have varied. Destouet and coworkers[621] observed immediate improvement in 20 of 41 patients who had no previous surgery after one spinal level was injected. Recurrent symptoms developed in 15 of these 20 patients. Of the 21 patients whose symptoms did not respond to the intitial injection, 13 were injected at a second level, and four of these demonstrated improvement and have remained free of symptoms. Of 13 patients who had had previous surgery, five improved after one level was injected, although only one of these remained free of pain. In summary, these investigators reported that 54 per cent of 54 patients showed a favorable response to facet block, which was temporary in the majority of cases.

Carrera[628] observed a beneficial therapeutic response to injection of the lumbar facet joints in 13 of 20 patients (65 per cent), of whom six patients remained free of symptoms for more than 6 months. Lippitt[623] classified his results in 99 patients receiving a total of 117 facet joint injections as excellent in 17 per cent, good in 25 per cent, fair in 9 per cent, mediocre in 4 per cent, and unchanged in 44 per cent. Fairbank and collaborators,[624] in an investigation of 25 patients who received local anesthetic injection into a maximally tender lumbar apophyseal joint, indicated that 14 patients (54 per cent) had immediate relief from pain, which, in approximately one half of the patients, was permanent. Raymond and Dumas[626] observed an overall response rate of 16 per cent for temporary relief in 25 patients when a smaller amount of injection solution was used; although their reported success rate was lower than that of most other series, and a long-term therapeutic benefit was not apparent, these authors concluded that a larger volume of solution and the addition of corticosteroids are indicated only when the study is being performed for a therapeutic rather than a diagnostic purpose. Lynch and Taylor[679] reported partial or complete relief of back pain 6 months after the procedure in 56 per cent of 50 patients and emphasized the importance of intra-articular injection without tissue extravasation. Murtagh[780] reported long-term relief of clinical manifestations after such injection in over 50 per cent of cases, whereas Jackson and coworkers[782] indicated less favorable results regarding the diagnostic and therapeutic benefits of injection into the lumbar facet joints.

Arthrography of the facet joints in the cervical spine has received less attention.[638, 639, 783, 784] The study is performed with the patient in the prone position and the neck flexed as far as possible to keep the joint interspace vertical. Fluoroscopic guidance allows the accurate placement of a 22 gauge spinal needle into the joint from a posterior or lateral approach. Care must be exercised so that the needle is not advanced too deeply, reaching the intervertebral foramen and injuring the vertebral artery or nerve root. A combination of radiopaque contrast material, anesthetic agent, and corticosteroid preparation can be used to produce relief from pain attributable to abnormalities of the facet joints. The relief of symptoms commonly is not permanent, however.[783, 784]

Although synovial cysts may arise from a facet joint, especially at the fourth and fifth lumbar levels, and may lead to significant neurologic manifestations, their demonstration usually is provided by myelography, CT, or MR imaging, rather than by arthrography (see Chapter 40).[640–643, 680, 681] Myelography reveals a nonspecific, posteriorly located extradural mass, whereas CT and MR imaging show somewhat more diagnostic findings consisting of a cystic lesion that is adjacent to a degenerated facet joint with calcification of its wall and, occasionally, gas in its center. Direct percutaneous puncture with opacification of a synovial cyst is possible and allows instillation of corticosteroids.[697] Similarly, corticosteroid preparations can reach the synovial cyst during injection and overdistention of the adjacent apophyseal articulation. Such injections can provide symptomatic relief.[781]

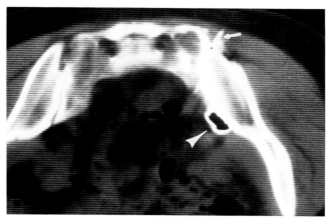

**FIGURE 13–133.** Arthrography of the sacroiliac joint. The needle has been placed in the sacroiliac joint (arrow). Contrast agent, air, lidocaine, and a corticosteroid preparation have been injected; observe anterior extravasation of the material (arrowhead) on this transaxial CT image.

## Sacroiliac Joints

Arthrography of the sacroiliac joints is indicated only as a sequel to aspiration in cases of suspected infection or crystal deposition disease. Although fluoroscopy can be used to monitor needle placement,[644] the author prefers to use CT for this purpose (Fig. 13–133). The patient is placed prone on the table, and, after initial transaxial scans of the joint, the site of skin puncture and the angle of needle insertion can be determined. Owing to the obliquity of the juxta-articular osseous surfaces, the lower portion of the sacroiliac joint should be entered. The needle usually is directed in a posteromedial to anterolateral direction and should be advanced beyond the interosseous ligaments to reach the joint cavity. CT scans can be used to monitor needle advancement. Once an aspirate is recovered, opacification of the joint with radiopaque contrast material documents the precise location of the needle tip.

## Interspinous Ligaments

Radiographic examination of the lumbar interspinous ligaments using contrast material has been described.[305] The material is injected bilaterally. In normal situations, the ligament appears as a flat, spindle-shaped filling defect surrounded by contrast material; in abnormal cases, the contrast material penetrates the ligament itself.

## Craniocervical Joints

Arthrography of the normal joints between the occiput, atlas, and axis has been performed.[306] No clinical application has yet been documented for this procedure, but use of this technique in patients with rheumatoid arthritis may be helpful in their management.

## Costovertebral Joints

Arthrographic opacification of the lower costovertebral joints has been described.[785] The procedure may have diagnostic and, when combined with corticosteroid injection, therapeutic benefit.

## SUMMARY

This chapter has stressed the many indications for contrast opacification of joint cavities, tendon sheaths, and bursae. These procedures generally are simple to perform, and the information they provide may be essential for proper diagnosis and treatment. The introduction and refinement of MR imaging, however, has led to major modifications with regard to the manner in which arthrography, tenography, and bursography are employed. Indeed, MR imaging has invaded the territory once held firm by these other diagnostic methods and, at many institutions, has become the imaging technique of choice in the assessment of internal derangements of the knee, glenohumeral and temporomandibular joints, ankle, and other articulations.

## References

1. Ranawat CS, Freiberger RH, Jordan LR, et al: Arthrography in the rheumatoid wrist joint. A preliminary report. J Bone Joint Surg [Am] 51:1269, 1969.
2. Harrison MO, Freiberger RH, Ranawat CS: Arthrography of the rheumatoid wrist joint. AJR 112:480, 1971.
3. Kessler I, Silberman Z: Experimental study of the radiocarpal joint by arthrography. Surg Gynecol Obstet 112:33, 1961.
4. Ranawat CS, Harrison MO, Jordan LR: Arthrography of the wrist joint. Clin Orthop 83:6, 1972.
5. Resnick D: Arthrography in the evaluation of arthritic disorders of the wrist. Radiology 113:331, 1974.
6. Trentham CE, Hamm RL, Masi AT: Wrist arthrography: Review and comparison of normal, rheumatoid arthritis and gout patients. Semin Arthritis Rheum 5:105, 1975.
7. Resnick D: Early abnormalities of the pisiform and triquetrum in rheumatoid arthritis. Ann Rheum Dis 35:46, 1976.
8. Resnick D: Rheumatoid arthritis of the wrist. The compartmental approach. Med Radiogr Photogr 52:50, 1976.
9. Resnick D: Rheumatoid arthritis of the wrist: Why the ulnar styloid? Radiology 112:29, 1974.
10. Stenström R, Wegelius O: Clearance of ¹²⁵I-labelled urographin from knee joints in rheumatoid arthritis. Acta Rheum Scand 16:151, 1970.
11. Wiljasalo M, Julkunen H, Salven I: Lymphography in rheumatic diseases. Ann Med Intern Fenn 55:125, 1966.
12. Lewin JR, Mulhern LM: Lymphatic visualization during contrast arthrography of the knee. Radiology 103:577, 1972.
13. Weston WJ: Lymphatic filling during positive contrast arthrography in rheumatoid arthritis. Australas Radiol 13:368, 1969.
14. Rieunau G, Gay R, Martinez C, et al: Lesions de l'articulation radio-cubitale inférieure dans les traumatismes de l'avant-bras et du poignet. Intérêt de l'arthrographie. Rev Chir Orthop 57 (Suppl 1):253, 1971.
15. Andrén L, Eiken O: Arthrographic studies of wrist ganglions. J Bone Joint Surg [Am] 53:299, 1971.
16. Gerber NJ, Dixon AS: Synovial cysts and juxta-articular bone cysts (geodes). Semin Arthritis Rheum 3:323, 1974.
17. Weston WJ: The normal arthrograms of the metacarpophalangeal, metatarsophalangeal and interphalangeal joints. Australas Radiol 13:211, 1969.
18. Resnick D, Danzig LA: Arthrographic evaluation of injuries of the first metacarpophalangeal joint: Gamekeeper's thumb. AJR 126:1046, 1976.
19. Bowers WH, Hurst LC: Gamekeeper's thumb. Evaluation by arthrography and stress roentgenography. J Bone Joint Surg [Am] 59:519, 1977.
20. Linscheid RL: Arthrography of the metacarpophalangeal joint. Clin Orthop 103:91, 1974.
21. Glogowski A, Laval-Jeantet M, Stora P: Arthrographie des doigts et du carpe dans les rhumatismes inflammatoires. J Radiol Electrol Med Nucl 57:873, 1976.
22. Weston WJ, Palmer DG: Soft Tissues of the Extremities. A Radiologic Study of Rheumatic Disease. New York, Springer-Verlag, 1977.
23. Moberg E, Stener B: Injuries to the ligaments of the thumb and fingers. Diagnosis, treatment and prognosis. Acta Chir Scand 106:166, 1954.
24. Neviaser RJ, Wilson JN, Lievano A: Rupture of the ulnar collateral ligament of the thumb (gamekeeper's thumb). Correction by dynamic repair. J Bone Joint Surg [Am] 53:1357, 1971.
25. Stener B: Displacement of the ruptured ulnar collateral ligament of the metacarpophalangeal joint of the thumb. A clinical and anatomical study. J Bone Joint Surg [Br] 44:869, 1962.
26. Schultz RJ, Fox JM: Gamekeeper's thumb. Result of skiing injuries. NY State J Med 73:2329, 1973.
27. Brewerton DA: Tenography in the rheumatoid hand. Hand 2:46, 1970.
28. Brewerton DA: Radiographic studies in the rheumatoid hand. Br J Radiol 42:487, 1969.
29. Palmer DG: Dynamics of joint disruption. NZ Med J 78:166, 1973.
30. Resnick D: Roentgenographic anatomy of the tendon sheaths of the hand and wrist: Tenography. AJR 124:44, 1975.
31. Resnick D: Osteomyelitis and septic arthritis complicating hand injuries and infections: Pathogenesis of roentgenographic abnormalities. J Can Assoc Radiol 27:21, 1976.
32. Weston WJ: The ulnar bursa. Australas Radiol 17:216, 1973.
33. Weston WJ: The digital sheaths of the hand. Australas Radiol 13:360, 1969.
34. Kaplan E: Functional and Surgical Anatomy of the Hand. 2nd Ed. Philadelphia, JB Lippincott Co, 1965.
35. Lampe E: Surgical anatomy of the hand with special reference to infections and trauma. Clin Symp 21:66, 1969.
36. Scheldrup E: Tendon sheath patterns in hand. Surg Gynecol Obstet 93:161, 1951.
37. Kanavel A: Infections of the Hand: A Guide to the Surgical Treatment of Acute and Chronic Suppurative Processes in the Fingers, Hand and Forearm. 7th Ed. Philadelphia, Lea & Febiger, 1939.
38. Gad P: Anatomy of the volar part of the capsules of the finger joints. J Bone Joint Surg [Br] 49:362, 1967.
39. Leach R, Odom J Jr: Systemic causes of carpal tunnel syndrome. Postgrad Med 44:127, 1968.
40. Phalen G: Carpal tunnel syndrome: Seventeen years' experience in diagnosis and treatment of six hundred fifty-four hands. J Bone Joint Surg [Am] 48:211, 1966.
41. Eto RT, Anderson PW, Harley JD: Elbow arthrography with the application of tomography. Radiology 115:283, 1975.
42. Arvidsson H, Johansson O: Arthrography of the elbow joint. Acta Radiol 43:445, 1955.
43. Chirls M: Arthrography in the diagnosis of joint disease. J Med Soc NJ 63:61, 1966.
44. Del Buono MS, Solarino GB: Arthrography of the elbow with double contrast media. Ital Clin Orthop 14:223, 1962.
45. Mouterde P, Massare C, Deburge A: Luxation traumatique du coude de l'adulte étude arthrographique. Aspect clinique d'une série de 100 cas. Ann Chir 29:743, 1975.
46. Haage H: Röntgendiagnostik der Gelenkschwellung des Ellenbogens. ROFO 118:45, 1973.
47. Weston WJ: The synovial changes at the elbow in rheumatoid arthritis. Australas Radiol 15:170, 1971.
48. Goode JD: Synovial rupture of the elbow joint. Ann Rheum Dis 27:604, 1968.
49. Ehrlich GE, Guttmann GG: Valvular mechanisms in antecubital cysts of rheumatoid arthritis. Arthritis Rheum 16:259, 1973.
50. Erhlich GE: Antecubital cysts in rheumatoid arthritis—a corollary to popliteal (Baker's) cysts. J Bone Joint Surg [Am] 54:165, 1972.
51. Bäckdahl M: The caput ulnae syndrome in rheumatoid arthritis. A study of the morphology, abnormal anatomy and clinical picture. Acta Rheumatol Scand Suppl 5:5, 1963.
52. Weston WJ: The lead arthrogram—plumbography. Skel Radiol 2:169, 1978.
53. Weston WJ: The olecranon bursa. Australas Radiol 14:323, 1970.
54. Killoran PJ, Marcove RC, Freiberger RH: Shoulder arthrography. AJR 103:658, 1968.
55. Kernwein GA, Roseberg B, Sneed WR Jr: Arthrographic studies of shoulder joint. J Bone Joint Surg [Am] 39:1267, 1957.
56. Lindblom K: Arthrography and roentgenography in ruptures of the tendons of the shoulder joint. Acta Radiol 20:548, 1939.
57. Nelson DH: Arthrography of the shoulder. Br J Radiol 25:134, 1952.
58. Neviaser JS: Arthrography of shoulder joint: Study of findings in adhesive capsulitis of shoulder. J Bone Joint Surg [Am] 44:1321, 1962.
59. Samilson R, Raphael RL, Post L, et al: Arthrography of shoulder joint. Clin Orthop 20:21, 1961.
60. Reeves B: Arthrography of shoulder. J Bone Joint Surg [Br] 48:424, 1966.
61. Den Herder BA: Clinical significance of arthrography of humeroscapular joint. Radiol Clin Biol 46:185, 1977.
62. Nelson CL: The use of arthrography in athletic injuries of the shoulder. Orthop Clin North Am 4:775, 1973.
63. Nelson CL, Burton RI: Upper extremity arthrography. Clin Orthop 107:62, 1975.
64. Preston BJ, Jackson JP: Investigation of shoulder disability by arthrography. Clin Radiol 28:259, 1977.
65. Schneider R, Ghelman B, Kaye JJ: A simplified injection technique for shoulder arthrography. Radiology 114:738, 1975.
66. Dalinka MK: A simple aid to the performance of shoulder arthrography. AJR 129:942, 1977.
67. Ghelman B, Goldman AB: The double contrast shoulder arthrogram: Evaluation of rotator cuff tears. Radiology 124:251, 1977.
68. Goldman AB, Ghelman B: The double-contrast shoulder arthrogram. A review of 158 studies. Radiology 127:655, 1978.
69. Debeyre J, Patte D, Elmelik E: Repair of ruptures of the rotator cuff of the shoulder with a note on advancement of the supraspinatus muscle. J Bone Joint Surg [Br] 47:36, 1965.
70. Wolfgang GL: Surgical repair of tears of the rotator cuff of the shoulder. Factors influencing the result. J Bone Joint Surg [Am] 56:14, 1974.
71. McLaughlin HL: Rupture of the rotator cuff. J Bone Joint Surg [Am] 44:979, 1962.

72. Neviaser JS: Ruptures of rotator cuff. Clin Orthop 3:92, 1954.
73. Weber J, Kecskés S: Arthrografie bei Periarthritis humeroscapularis. ROFO 124:573, 1976.
74. Andrén L, Lundberg BJ: Treatment of rigid shoulders by joint distention during arthrography. Acta Orthop Scand 36:45, 1965.
75. Neviaser JS: Adhesive capsulitis of the shoulder. A study of the pathological findings in periarthritis of the shoulder. J Bone Joint Surg 27:211, 1945.
76. Lippmann RK: Frozen shoulder; periarthritis; bicipital tenosynovitis. Arch Surg 47:283, 1943.
77. Lidström A: Den ''frusna'' skuldran. Nord Med 69:125, 1963.
78. Lundberg BJ: The frozen shoulder. Clinical and radiographical observations. The effect of manipulation under general anesthesia. Structure and glycosaminoglycan content of the joint capsule. Local bone metabolism. Acta Orthop Scand (Suppl) 119:5, 1969.
79. Goldman AB, Katz MC, Freiberger RH: Post-traumatic adhesive capsulitis of the ankle: Arthrographic diagnosis. AJR 127:585, 1976.
80. Ennevaara K: Painful shoulder joint in rheumatoid arthritis: A clinical and radiologic study of 200 cases, with special reference to arthrography of the glenohumeral joint. Acta Rheum Scand Suppl 11:1, 1967.
81. Bankart ASB: The pathology and treatment of recurrent dislocation of the shoulder joint. Br J Surg 26:23, 1938.
82. DeSmet AA, Ting YM, Weiss JJ: Shoulder arthrography in rheumatoid arthritis. Radiology 116:601, 1975.
83. Weiss JJ, Thompson GR, Doust V, et al: Rotator cuff tears in rheumatoid arthritis. Arch Intern Med 135:521, 1975.
84. Burgener FA, Weiss JJ, Doust V: Die Schulterarthrographie bei primär chronischer Polyarthritis. ROFO 116:490, 1972.
85. Weston WJ: Enlarged axillary glands in rheumatoid arthritis. Australas Radiol 15:55, 1971.
86. Armbuster TG, Slivka J, Resnick D, et al. Extraarticular manifestations of septic arthritis of the glenohumeral joint. AJR 129:667, 1977.
87. Weston WJ: The intrasynovial fatty masses in chronic rheumatoid arthritis. Br J Radiol 46:213, 1974.
88. DeSeze S, Hubault A, Rampon S: Senile haemorrhagic shoulder. Ann Rheum Dis 27:292, 1968.
89. Weston WJ: Arthrography of the acromio-clavicular joint. Australas Radiol 18:213, 1974.
90. Heubelin GW, Greene GS, Conforti VP: Hip joint arthrography. AJR 68:736, 1952.
91. Katz JF: Arthrography in Legg-Calvé-Perthes disease. J Bone Joint Surg [Am] 50:467, 1968.
92. Severin E: Arthrography in congenital dislocation of the hip. J Bone Joint Surg 21:304, 1939.
93. Kenin A, Levine J: A technique for arthrography of the hip. AJR 68:107, 1952.
94. Mitchell GP: Arthrography in congenital displacement of the hip. J Bone Joint Surg [Br] 45:88, 1963.
95. Astley R: Arthrography in congenital dislocation of the hip. Clin Radiol 18:253, 1967.
96. Ozonoff MB: Controlled arthrography of the hip: A technic of fluoroscopic monitoring and recording. Clin Orthop 93:260, 1973.
97. Salvati EA, Ghelman B, McLaren T, et al: Subtraction technique in arthrography for loosening of total hip replacement fixed with radiopaque cement. Clin Orthop 101:105, 1974.
98. Guerra J Jr, Armbuster TG, Resnick D, et al: The adult hip: An anatomic study. Part II. The soft tissue landmarks. Radiology 128:11, 1978.
99. Razzano CD, Nelson CL, Wilde AH: Arthrography of the adult hip. Clin Orthop 99:86, 1974.
100. Freiberger RH: Congenital dislocation of the hip. Hip diseases of infancy and childhood. Curr Prob Radiol 3:4, 1973.
101. Grech P: Video-arthrography in hip dysplasia. Clin Radiol 23:202, 1972.
102. Patel D: Arthroscopy of the plicae-synovial folds and their significance. Am J Sports Med 6:217, 1978.
103. Pipkin G: Knee injuries: The role of the suprapatellar plica and suprapatellar bursa in simulating internal derangements. Clin Orthop 74:161, 1971.
104. Harty M, Joyce JJ III: Synovial folds in the knee joint. Orthop Rev 7:91, 1977.
105. Kaye JJ, Winchester PH, Freiberger RH: Neonatal septic ''dislocation'' of the hip: True dislocation or pathological epiphyseal separation? Radiology 114:671, 1975.
106. Glassberg GB, Ozonoff MB: Arthrographic findings in septic arthritis of the hip in infants. Radiology 128:151, 1978.
107. Lachman RS, Rimoin DL, Hollister DW: Arthrography of the hip. A clue to the pathogenesis of the epiphyseal dysplasias. Radiology 108:317, 1973.
108. Hardaker WT Jr, Whipple TL, Bassett FM III: Diagnosis and treatment of the plica syndrome of the knee. J Bone Joint Surg [Am] 62:221, 1980.
109. Axer A, Schiller MG: The pathogenesis of the early deformity of the capital femoral epiphysis in Legg-Calvé-Perthes syndrome (LCPS). An arthrographic study. Clin Orthop 84:106, 1972.
110. Gershuni DH, Axer A, Hendel D: Arthrographic findings in Legg-Calvé-Perthes disease and transient synovitis of the hip. J Bone Joint Surg [Am] 60:457, 1978.
111. Jonsäter S: Coxa plana, a histo-pathologic and arthrographic study. Acta Orthop Scand Suppl 12:5, 1953.
112. Murphy WA, Siegel MJ, Gilula LA: Arthrography in the diagnosis of unexplained chronic hip pain with regional osteopenia. AJR 129:283, 1977.
113. Armstrong P, Saxton H: Ilio-psoas bursa. Br J Radiol 45:493, 1972.
114. Warren R, Kaye JJ, Salvati EA: Arthrographic demonstration of an enlarged iliopsoas bursa complicating osteoarthritis of the hip—a case report. J Bone Joint Surg [Am] 57:413, 1975.
115. O'Connor DS: Early recognition of iliopectineal bursitis. Surg Gynecol Obstet 57:674, 1933.
116. Dalinka MK, Cohen GS, Wershba M: Knee arthrography. CRC Crit Rev Radiol Sci 4:1, 1973.
117. Keats TE, Staatz DS, Bailey RW: Pneumoarthrography of the knee. Surg Gynecol Obstet 94:361, 1952.
118. Lindblom K: The arthrographic appearance of the ligaments of the knee joint. Acta Radiol 19:582, 1938.
119. Lindblom K: Arthrography of the knee, a roentgenographic and anatomical study. Acta Radiol Suppl 74:7, 1948.
120. Andrén L, Wehlin L: Double contrast arthrography of the knee with horizontal roentgen ray beam. Acta Orthop Scand 29:307, 1960.
121. Freiberger RH, Killoran PJ, Cardona G: Arthrography of the knee by double contrast method. AJR 97:736, 1966.
122. Butt WP, McIntyre JL: Double contrast arthrography of the knee. Radiology 92:487, 1969.
123. Angell FL: Fluoroscopic technique of double contrast arthrography of the knee. Radiol Clin North Am 9:85, 1971.
124. Angell FL: A restraint device for arthrography of the knee. Radiology 98:186, 1971.
125. Gelmon MI, Riding LJ: Arthrography of the knee. Appl Radiol 4:19, 1975.
126. Gilula LA: A simplified stress device for knee arthrography. Radiology 122:828, 1977.
127. Levinsohn EM: A new simple restraining device for fluoroscopically monitored knee arthrography. Radiology 122:827, 1977.
128. Nicks AJ, Mihalko M: A simple device to open the knee joint space during double contrast arthrography. Radiology 122:827, 1977.
129. Lee KR, Sanders WF: A practical stress device for knee arthrography. Radiology 127:542, 1978.
130. O'Malley BP: Value of delayed films in knee arthrography. J Can Assoc Radiol 25:144, 1974.
131. Ricklin P, Rüttimann A, Del Buono MS: Meniscus Lesions—Practical Problems of Clinical Diagnosis, Arthrography and Therapy. New York, Grune & Stratton, 1971.
132. Montgomery CE: Synovial recesses in knee arthrography. AJR 121:86, 1974.
133. Russell E, Hamm R, LePage JR, et al. Some normal variations of knee arthrograms and their anatomical significance. J Bone Joint Surg [Am] 60:66, 1978.
134. Nicholas JA, Freiberger RH, Killoran PJ: Double contrast arthrography of the knee. Its value in the management of 225 knee derangements. J Bone Joint Surg [Am] 52:203, 1970.
135. Heiser S, LaBriola JH, Meyers MH: Arthrography of the knee. Radiology 79:822, 1962.
136. McIntyre JL: Arthrography of the lateral meniscus. Radiology 105:531, 1972.
137. Jelaso DV: The fascicles of the lateral meniscus: An anatomic-arthrographic correlation. Radiology 114:335, 1975.
138. Wickstrom KT, Spitzer RM, Olsson HE: Roentgen anatomy of the posterior horn of the lateral meniscus. Radiology 116:617, 1975.
139. Fetto JF, Marshall JL, Ghelman B: An anomalous attachment of the popliteus tendon to the lateral meniscus. Case report. J Bone Joint Surg [Am] 59:548, 1977.
140. Ringertz HG: Arthrography of the knee. I. Localization of lesions. Acta Radiol Diagn 14:138, 1973.
141. Ringertz HG: Arthrography of the knee. II. Isolated and combined lesions. Acta Radiol Diagn 17:235, 1976.
142. Hall FM: Buckled meniscus. Radiology 126:89, 1978.
143. Bramson RT, Staple TW: Double contrast knee arthrography in children. AJR 123:838, 1975.
144. Stenström R: Diagnostic arthrography of traumatic lesions of the knee joint in children. Ann Radiol 18:391, 1975.
145. Saddawi ND, Hoffman BK: Tear of the attachment of a normal medial meniscus of the knee in a four year old child. J Bone Joint Surg [Am] 52:809, 1970.
146. Noble J, Hamblen, DL: The pathology of the degenerate meniscus lesion. J Bone Joint Surg [Br] 57:180, 1975.
147. Noble J: Lesions of the menisci. Autopsy incidence in adults less than fifty-five years old. J Bone Joint Surg [Am] 59:480, 1977.
148. Hernandez FJ: Cysts of the semilunar cartilage of the knee. A light and electron microscopic study. Acta Orthop Scand 47:436, 1976.
149. Burgan DW: Arthrographic findings in meniscal cysts. Radiology 101:579, 1971.
150. Wroblewski M: Trauma and the cystic meniscus: Review of 500 cases. Injury 4:319, 1971.
151. Raine GET, Gonet LCL: Cysts of the menisci of the knee. Postgrad Med J 48:49, 1972.
152. Hall FM: Arthrography of the discoid lateral meniscus. AJR 128:993, 1977.
153. Haveson SB, Rein BI: Lateral discoid meniscus of the knee: Arthrographic diagnosis. AJR 109:581, 1970.
154. Smillie IS: The congenital discoid meniscus. J Bone Joint Surg [Br] 30:671, 1948.
155. Kaplan EB: Discoid lateral meniscus of the knee joint. Nature, mechanism and operative treatment. J Bone Joint Surg [Am] 39:77, 1957.
156. Fisher AGT: The disk-shaped external semilunar cartilage. Br Med J 1:688, 1936.
157. Cave EF, Staples OS: Congenital discoid meniscus. A cause of internal derangement of the knee. Am J Surg 54:371, 1941.

158. Jeannopoulos CL: Observations on discoid menisci. J Bone Joint Surg [Am] 32:649, 1950.

159. Murdoch G: Congenital discoid medial semilunar cartilage. J Bone Joint Surg [Br] 38:564, 1956.

160. Riachi E, Phares A: An unusual deformity of the medial semilunar cartilage. J Bone Joint Surg [Br] 45:146, 1963.

161. Richmond DA: Two cases of discoid medial cartilage. J Bone Joint Surg [Br] 40:268, 1958.

162. Ross JA, Tough ICK, English TA: Congenital discoid cartilage. Report of a case of discoid medial cartilage with an embryological note. J Bone Joint Surg [Br] 40:262, 1958.

163. Weiner B, Rosenberg N: Discoid medial meniscus: Association with bone changes in the tibia. A case report. J Bone Joint Surg [Am] 56:171, 1974.

164. Resnick D, Goergen TG, Kaye JJ, et al: Discoid medial meniscus. Radiology 121:575, 1976.

165. Philippon J: Étude des malformations congénitales méniscales par arthropneumographie. J Radiol Electrol Med Nucl 40:1, 1959.

166. Moes CAF, Munn JD: The value of knee arthrography in children. J Can Assoc Radiol 16:226, 1965.

167. Nathan PA, Cole SC: Discoid meniscus—a clinical and pathological study. Clin Orthop 64:107, 1969.

168. Dashefsky JH: Discoid lateral meniscus in three members of a family. J Bone Joint Surg [Am] 53:1208, 1971.

169. Symeonides PP, Ioannides G: Ossicles in the knee menisci. Report of three cases. J Bone Joint Surg [Am] 54:1288, 1972.

170. Weaver JB: Calcification and ossification of the menisci. J Bone Joint Surg 24:873, 1942.

171. Rosen IE: Unusual intrameniscal lunulae. Three case reports. J Bone Joint Surg [Am] 40:925, 1958.

172. Glass RS, Barnes WM, Kells DU, et al: Ossicles of knee menisci. Report of seven cases. Clin Orthop 111:163, 1975.

173. Bernstein RM, Olsson HE, Spitzer RM, et al: Ossicle of the meniscus. AJR 127:785, 1976.

174. Pederson HE: The ossicles of the semilunar cartilages of rodents. Anat Rec 105:1, 1949.

175. Suzuki K, Izawa T, Eguro H: Ossification of semilunar cartilage. Report of a case. J Jpn Orthop Assoc 44:467, 1970.

176. Doyle JR, Eisenberg JH, Orth MW: Regeneration of knee menisci: A preliminary report. J Trauma 6:50, 1966.

177. Smillie IS: Observations on the regeneration of the semilunar cartilages in man. Br J Surg 31:398, 1944.

178. Goldenberg RR: Refracture of a regenerated internal semilunar cartilage. J Bone Joint Surg 17:1054, 1935.

179. Massare C, Bard M, Tristant H: Intérêt de l'arthrographie du genou dans les gonalgies après méniscectomie. Revue de 200 dossiers personnels. J Radiol Electrol Med Nucl 55:401, 1974.

180. Debnam JW, Staple TW: Arthrography of the knee after meniscectomy. Radiology 113:67, 1974.

181. Laasonen EM, Wilppula E: Why a meniscectomy fails. Acta Orthop Scand 47:672, 1976.

182. Dandy DJ, Jackson RW: The diagnosis of problems after meniscectomy. J Bone Joint Surg [Br] 57:349, 1975.

183. Jackson JP: Degenerative changes in the knee after meniscectomy. Br Med J 2:525, 1968.

184. Appel H: Late results after meniscectomy in the knee joint. A clinical and roentgenologic follow-up investigation. Acta Orthop Scand (Suppl 133):6, 1970.

185. Tapper EM, Hoover NW: Late results after meniscectomy. J Bone Joint Surg [Am] 51:517, 1969.

186. Gear MWL: The late results of meniscectomy. Br J Surg 54:270, 1967.

187. Huckell JR: Is meniscectomy a benign procedure? A long term follow-up study. Can J Surg 8:254, 1965.

188. McGinty JB, Geuss LF, Marvin RA: Partial or total meniscectomy. A comparative analysis. J Bone Joint Surg [Am] 59:763, 1977.

189. Mittler S, Freiberger RH, Harrison-Stubbs M: A method of improving cruciate ligament visualization in double contrast arthrography. Radiology 102:441, 1972.

190. Dalinka MK, Gohel VK, Rancier L: Tomography in the evaluation of the anterior cruciate ligament. Radiology 108:31, 1973.

191. Pavlov H, Torg JS: Double contrast arthrographic evaluation of the anterior cruciate ligament. Radiology 126:661, 1978.

192. Pavlov H, Freiberger RH: An easy method to demonstrate the cruciate ligaments by double contrast arthrography. Radiology 126:817, 1978.

193. Dalinka MK, Garofola J: The infrapatellar synovial fold: A cause for confusion in the evaluation of the anterior cruciate ligament. AJR 127:589, 1976.

194. Anderson PW, Maslin P: Tomography applied to knee arthrography. Radiology 110:271, 1974.

195. Wershba M, Dalinka MK, Coren GS, et al: Double contrast knee arthrography in the evaluation of osteochondritis dissecans. Clin Orthop 107:81, 1975.

196. Horns JW: Single contrast knee arthrography in abnormalities of the articular cartilage. Radiology 105:537, 1972.

197. Thomas RH, Resnick D, Alazraki NP, et al: Compartmental evaluation of osteoarthritis of the knee. A comparative study of available diagnostic modalities. Radiology 116:585, 1975.

198. Horns JW: The diagnosis of chondromalacia by double contrast arthrography of the knee. J Bone Joint Surg [Am] 59:119, 1977.

199. Thijn CJP: Double contrast arthrography in meniscal lesions and patellar chondropathy. Radiol Clin Biol 45:345, 1976.

200. Newberg A, Wales L: Radiographic diagnosis of quadriceps tendon rupture. Radiology 125:367, 1977.

201. Smason JB: Post-traumatic fistula connecting prepatellar bursa with knee joint. Report of a case. J Bone Joint Surg [Am] 54:1553, 1972.

202. Jelaso DV, Morris GA: Rupture of the quadriceps tendon: Diagnosis by arthrography. Radiology 116:621, 1975.

203. Duncan AM: Arthrography in rupture of the suprapatellar bursa with pseudocyst formation. AJR 121:89, 1974.

204. Anderson PW, Harley JD, Maslin PU: Arthrographic evaluation of problems with united tibial plateau fractures. Radiology 119:75, 1976.

205. Taylor AR: Arthrography of the knee in rheumatoid arthritis. Br J Radiol 42:493, 1969.

206. Taylor AR, Ansell BM: Arthrography of the knee before and after synovectomy for rheumatoid arthritis. J Bone Joint Surg [Br] 54:110, 1972.

207. Hall AP, Scott JT: Synovial cysts and rupture of the knee joint in rheumatoid arthritis; an arthrographic study. Ann Rheum Dis 25:32, 1966.

208. Pinder IM: Treatment of the popliteal cyst in the rheumatoid knee. J Bone Joint Surg [Br] 55:119, 1973.

209. Wolfe RD, Giuliano VJ: Double-contrast arthrography in the diagnosis of pigmented villonodular synovitis of the knee. AJR 110:793, 1970.

210. Greenfield MM, Wallace KM: Pigmented villonodular synovitis. Radiology 54:350, 1950.

211. Sanderud A: Pigmented villonodular synovitis. Acta Orthop Scand 24:155, 1955.

212. Goergen TG, Resnick D, Niwayama G: Localized nodular synovitis of the knee: A report of two cases with abnormal arthrograms. AJR 126:647, 1976.

213. Granowitz SP, Mankin HJ: Localized pigmented villonodular synovitis of knee. J Bone Joint Surg [Am] 49:122, 1967.

214. Hoffa A: Über Röntgenbilder nach Sauerstoffeinblasung in das Kniegelenk. Berl Klin Wschr 43:940, 1906.

215. Muckle DS, Monahan P: Intra-articular ganglion of the knee. Report of two cases. J Bone Joint Surg [Br] 54:520, 1972.

216. Crittenden JJ, Jones DM, Santarelli AG: Knee arthrogram in synovial chondromatosis. Radiology 94:133, 1970.

217. Prager RJ, Mall JC: Arthrographic diagnosis of synovial chondromatosis. AJR 127:344, 1976.

218. Weitzman G: Lipoma arborescens of the knee. Report of a case. J Bone Joint Surg [Am] 47:1030, 1965.

219. Burgan DW: Lipoma arborescens of the knee: Another cause of filling defects on a knee arthrogram. Radiology 101:583, 1971.

220. Brodsky AE: Synovial hemangioma of the knee joint. Bull Hosp Joint Dis 17:58, 1956.

221. Coventry MB, Harrison EG Jr, Martin JF: Benign synovial tumors of the knee: A diagnostic problem. J Bone Joint Surg [Am] 48:1350, 1966.

222. Moon NF: Synovial hemangioma of the knee joint. A review of previously reported cases and inclusion of two new cases. Clin Orthop 90:183, 1973.

223. Resnick D, Oliphant M: Hemophilia-like arthropathy of the knee associated with cutaneous and synovial hemangiomas. Report of 3 cases and review of the literature. Radiology 114:323, 1975.

224. Forrest J, Staple TW: Synovial hemangioma of the knee. Demonstration by arthrography and arteriography. AJR 112:512, 1971.

225. Thomas ML, Andress MR: Angioma of the knee demonstrated by angiography and arthrography—report of a case. Acta Radiol Diagn 12:217, 1972.

226. Salerno NR, Menges JF, Borns PF: Arthrograms in hemophilia. Radiology 102:135, 1972.

227. Dalinka MK, Coren G, Hensinger R, et al: Arthrography in Blount's disease. Radiology 113:161, 1974.

228. Siffert RS, Katz JF: The intra-articular deformity in osteochondrosis deformans tibiae. J Bone Joint Surg [Am] 52:800, 1970.

229. Lindgren PG, Willen R: Gastrocnemio-semimembranosus bursa and its relation to the knee joint. I. Anatomy and histology. Acta Radiol Diagn 18:497, 1977.

230. Doppman JL: Baker's cyst and the normal gastrocnemio-semimembranosus bursa. AJR 94:646, 1965.

231. Wilson PD, Eyre-Brook AL, Francis JD: Clinical and anatomical study of semimembranosus bursa in relation to popliteal cyst. J Bone Joint Surg 20:963, 1938.

232. Burleson RJ, Bickel WH, Dahlin DC: Popliteal cyst: Clinico-pathologic survey. J Bone Joint Surg [Am] 38:1265, 1956.

233. Baker WM: Formation of synovial cysts in leg in connection with disease of knee joint. St Bartholomew's Hosp Rep 13:245, 1877.

234. Gristina AG, Wilson PD: Popliteal cysts in adults and children: Review of 90 cases. Arch Surg 88:357, 1964.

235. Hoffman BK: Cystic lesions of popliteal space. Surg Gynecol Obstet 116:551, 1963.

236. Jayson MIV, Dixon AS: Intra-articular pressure in rheumatoid arthritis of the knee. III. Pressure changes during joint use. Ann Rheum Dis 29:401, 1970.

237. Taylor AR, Rana NA: A valve. An explanation of the formation of popliteal cysts. Ann Rheum Dis 32:419, 1973.

238. Palmer DG: Anteromedial synovial cysts at the knee joint in rheumatoid disease. Australas Radiol 16:79, 1972.

239. Schmidt MC, Workman JB, Barth WF: Dissection or rupture of a popliteal cyst. A syndrome mimicking thrombophlebitis in rheumatic diseases. Arch Intern Med *134*:694, 1974.
240. Swett HA, Jaffe RB, McIff EB: Popliteal cysts: Presentation as thrombophlebitis. Radiology *115*:613, 1975.
241. Solomon L, Berman L: Synovial rupture of knee joint. J Bone Joint Surg [Br] *54*:460, 1972.
242. Iacano V, Gauvin G, Zimbler S: Giant synovial cyst of the calf and thigh in a patient with granulomatous synovitis. Clin Orthop *115*:220, 1976.
243. Pallardy G, Fabre P, Ledoux-Lebard G, et al: L'arthrographie due genou dans l'étude des bursites et des kystes synoviaux. J Radiol Electrol Med Nucl 50:481, 1969.
244. Shapiro RF, Resnick D, Castles JJ, et al: Fistulization of rheumatoid joints. Spectrum of identifiable syndromes. Ann Rheum Dis *34*:489, 1975.
245. Perri JA, Rodnan GP, Mankin HJ: Giant synovial cysts of the calf in patients with rheumatoid arthritis. J Bone Joint Surg [Am] 50:709, 1968.
246. Lapayowker MS, Cliff MM, Tourtellotte CD: Arthrography in the diagnosis of calf pain. Radiology 95:319, 1970.
247. Pastershank SP, Mitchell DM: Knee joint bursal abnormalities in rheumatoid arthritis. J Can Assoc Radiol 28:199, 1977.
248. Wolfe RD, Colloff B: Popliteal cysts. An arthrographic study and review of the literature. J Bone Joint Surg [Am] *54*:1057, 1972.
249. Bryan RS, DiMichele JD, Ford GL Jr: Popliteal cysts. Arthrography as an aid to diagnosis and treatment. Clin Orthop 50:203, 1967.
250. Grepl J: Beitrag zur positiven Arthrographie bei pathologischen Veränderungen der Bursae popliteae. ROFO *119*:84, 1973.
251. Clark JM: Arthrography diagnosis of synovial cysts of the knee. Radiology *115*:480, 1975.
252. Cooperberg PL, Tsang I, Truelove L, et al: Grey scale ultrasound in the evaluation of rheumatoid arthritis of the knee. Radiology *126*:759, 1978.
253. Ambanelli U, Manganelli P, Nervetti A, et al: Demonstration of articular effusions and popliteal cysts with ultrasound. J Rheumatol *3*:134, 1976.
254. Carpenter JR, Hattery RR, Hunder GG, et al: Ultrasound evaluation of the popliteal space. Comparison with arthrography and physical examination. Mayo Clin Proc *51*:498, 1976.
255. Rudikoff JC, Lynch JJ, Philipps E, et al: Ultrasound diagnosis of Baker cyst. JAMA *235*:1054, 1976.
256. Moore CP, Sarti DA, Lovie JS: Ultrasonographic demonstration of popliteal cysts in rheumatoid arthritis. A noninvasive technique. Arthritis Rheum *18*:577, 1975.
257. Meire HB, Lindsay DJ, Swinson DR, et al: Comparison of ultrasound and positive contrast arthrography in the diagnosis of popliteal and calf swellings. Ann Rheum Dis *33*:221, 1974.
258. Levin MH, Nordyke RA, Ball JJ: Demonstration of dissecting popliteal cysts by joint scans after intra-articular isotope injections. Arthritis Rheum *14*:591, 1971.
259. Cooper RA: Computerized tomography (body scan) of Baker's cyst. J Rheumatol *5*:184, 1978.
260. Dixon AS, Grast C: Acute synovial rupture in rheumatoid arthritis: Clinical and experimental observations. Lancet *1*:742, 1964.
261. Tait GBW, Bach F, Dixon AS: Acute synovial rupture: Further observations. Ann Rheum Dis *24*:273, 1965.
262. Barbaric ZL, Young LW: Synovial cyst in juvenile rheumatoid arthritis. AJR *116*:655, 1972.
263. Toyama WM: Familial popliteal cysts in children. Am J Dis Child *124*:586, 1972.
264. Olson RW: Arthrography of the ankle: Its use in the evaluation of ankle sprains. Radiology *92*:1439, 1969.
265. Broström L, Liljedahl SO, Lindvall N: Sprained ankles. II. Arthrographic diagnosis of recent ligament ruptures. Acta Chir Scand *129*:485, 1965.
266. Spiegel PK, Staples OS: Arthrography of the ankle joint: Problems in diagnosis of acute lateral ligament injuries. Radiology *114*:587, 1975.
267. Arner O, Ekengren K, Hulting B, et al: Arthrography of the talocrural joint: Anatomic, roentgenographic and clinical aspects. Acta Chir Scand *113*:253, 1957.
268. Fordyce AJW, Horn CV: Arthrography in recent injuries of the ligament of the ankle. J Bone Joint Surg [Br] *54*:116, 1972.
269. Ala-Ketola L, Puranen J, Koivisto E, et al: Arthrography in the diagnosis of ligament injuries and classification of ankle injuries. Radiology *125*:63, 1977.
270. Mehrez M, El Geneidy S: Arthrography of the ankle. J Bone Joint Surg [Br] *52*:308, 1970.
271. Fussell ME, Godley DR: Ankle arthrography in acute sprains. Clin Orthop *93*:278, 1973.
272. Sanders HWA: Ankle arthrography and ankle distortion. Radiol Clin Biol *46*:1, 1977.
273. Gordon RB: Arthrography of the ankle joint. Experience in 107 studies. J Bone Joint Surg [Am] *52*:1623, 1970.
274. Percy EC, Hill RO, Callaghan JE: The "sprained" ankle. J Trauma *9*:972, 1969.
275. Kaye JJ, Bohne WHO: A radiographic study of the ligamentous anatomy of the ankle. Radiology *125*:659, 1977.
276. Smith GR, Winquist RA, Allan NK, et al: Subtle transchondral fractures of the talar dome: A radiological perspective. Radiology *124*:667, 1977.
277. Berndt AL, Harty M: Transchondral fractures (osteochondritis dissecans) of the talus. J Bone Joint Surg [Am] *41*:988, 1959.
278. Wolin I, Glassman F, Sideman S, et al: Internal derangement of the talofibular component of the ankle. Surg Gynecol Obstet *91*:193, 1950.
279. Deyerle WM: Long term follow-up of fractures of the os calcis. Diagnostic peroneal synoviagram. Orthop Clin North Am *4*:213, 1973.
280. Resnick D, Goergen TG: Peroneal tenography in previous calcaneal fractures. Radiology *115*:211, 1975.
281. Garcia A, Parkes J: Fractures of the foot. *In* N Giannestras (Ed): Foot Disorders. Medical and Surgical Management. Philadelphia, Lea & Febiger, 1973.
282. Burman M: Stenosing tendovaginitis of the foot and ankle; studies with special reference to the stenosing tendovaginitis of the peroneal tendons at the peroneal tubercle. Arch Surg *67*:686, 1953.
283. Webster FS: Peroneal tenosynovitis with pseudotumor. J Bone Joint Surg [Am] *50*:153, 1968.
284. Earle AS, Moritz JR, Tapper EM: Dislocation of the peroneal tendons at the ankle: An analysis of 25 ski injuries. Northwest Med *71*:108, 1972.
285. Church CC: Radiographic diagnosis of acute peroneal tendon dislocation. AJR *129*:1065, 1977.
286. Daffner RH, Whitfield PW: Recurrent ganglion cyst: The value of preoperative ganglionography. AJR *129*:345, 1977.
287. Palmer DG: Tendon sheaths and bursae involved by rheumatoid disease at the foot and ankle. Australas Radiol *14*:419, 1970.
288. Resnick D, Feingold ML, Curd J, et al: Calcaneal abnormalities in articular disorders. Rheumatoid arthritis, ankylosing spondylitis, psoriatic arthritis and Reiter syndrome. Radiology *125*:355, 1977.
289. Weston WJ: The bursa deep to tendo Achillis. Australas Radiol *14*:327, 1970.
290. Resnick D: Radiology of the talocalcaneal articulations. Anatomic considerations and arthrography. Radiology *111*:581, 1974.
291. Weston WJ: Traumatic effusions of the ankle and posterior subtaloid joints. Br J Radiol *31*:445, 1958.
292. Meyer JM: L'arthrographie de l'articulation sous-astragalienne postérieure et de l'articulation de Chopart. Thèse Méd Genève, No 3318, 1973.
293. Meyer JM, Lagier R: Post-traumatic sinus tarsi syndrome. An anatomical and radiological study. Acta Orthop Scand *48*:121, 1977.
294. Kaye JJ, Ghelman B, Schneider R: Talocalcaneonavicular joint arthrography for sustentacular-talar tarsal coalitions. Radiology *115*:730, 1975.
295. Harris RI, Beath T: Etiology of peroneal spastic flat foot. J Bone Joint Surg [Br] *30*:624, 1948.
296. Sahlstedt B: Simultaneous arthrography of the talocrural and talonavicular joints in children. I. Technique. Acta Radiol Diagn *17*:545, 1976.
297. Hjelmstedt A, Sahlstedt B: Simultaneous arthrography of the talocrural and talonavicular joints in children. II. Comparison between anatomic and arthrographic measurements. Acta Radiol Diagn *17*:557, 1976.
298. Hjelmstedt A, Sahlstedt B: Simultaneous arthrography of the talocrural and talonavicular joints in children. II. Measurements on normal feet. Acta Radiol Diagn *18*:513, 1977.
299. Hjelmstedt A, Sahlstedt B: Simultaneous arthrography of the talocrural and talonavicular joints in children. IV. Measurements on congenital club feet. Acta Radiol Diagn *19*:223, 1978.
300. Weston WJ: Positive contrast arthrography of the normal midtarsal joints. Australas Radiol *13*:365, 1969.
301. Resnick D: Roentgen features of the rheumatoid mid and hindfoot. J Can Assoc Radiol *27*:99, 1976.
302. Glover JR: Arthrography of the joints of the lumbar vertebral arches. Orthop Clin North Am *8*:37, 1977.
303. Ghelman B, Doherty JH: Demonstration of spondylolysis by arthrography of the apophyseal joint. AJR *130*:986, 1978.
304. Mooney V, Robertson J: The facet syndrome. Clin Orthop *115*:149, 1976.
305. Köhler R: Contrast examination of the lumbar interspinous ligaments. Preliminary report. Acta Radiol *52*:21, 1959.
306. Dirheimer Y, Ramsheyi A, Reolon M: Positive arthrography of the craniocervical joint. Neuroradiology *12*:257, 1977.
307. McGaw WH, Weckesser EC: Pneumarthrograms of the knee. A diagnostic aid in internal derangements. J Bone Joint Surg *27*:432, 1945.
308. Meschan I, McGraw WH: Newer methods of pneumoarthrography of the knee with an evaluation of the procedure in 315 operated cases. Radiology *49*:675, 1947.
309. Kleinberg S: Pulmonary embolism following oxygen injection of a knee. JAMA *89*:172, 1927.
310. Pavlov H, Ghelman B, Warren RF: Double-contrast arthrography of the elbow. Radiology *130*:87, 1979.
311. Roback DL: Elbow arthrography: Brief technical considerations. Clin Radiol *30*:311, 1979.
312. Gilula LA, Schoenecker PL, Murphy WA: Shoulder arthrography as a treatment modality. AJR *131*:1047, 1978.
313. Slätis P, Aalto K: Medial dislocation of the tendon of the long head of the biceps brachii. Acta Orthop Scand *50*:73, 1979.
314. El-Khoury GY, Albright JP, Abu Yousef MM, et al: Arthrotomography of the glenoid labrum. Radiology *131*:333, 1979.
315. Zachrisson BE, Ejeskär A: Arthrography in dislocation of the acromioclavicular joint. Acta Radiol Diagn *20*:81, 1979.
316. Schwartz AM, Goldberg MJ: The medial adductor approach to arthrography of the hip in children. Radiology *132*:483, 1979.
317. Tegtmeyer CJ, McCue FC III, Higgins SM, et al: Arthrography of the knee: A comparative study of the accuracy of single and double contrast techniques. Radiology *132*:37, 1979.

318. Hall FM: Further pitfalls in knee arthrography. J Can Assoc Radiol 29:179, 1978.
319. Barrie HJ: The pathogenesis and significance of meniscal cysts. J Bone Joint Surg [Br] 61:184, 1979.
320. Buckwalter JA, Dryer RF, Mickelson MR: Arthrography in juxtaarticular cysts of the knee. Two cases diagnosed by delayed roentgenograms. J Bone Joint Surg [Am] 61:465, 1979.
321. Enis JE, Ghandur-Mnaymneh L: Cyst of the lateral meniscus causing erosion of the tibial plateau. A case report. J Bone Joint Surg [Am] 61:441, 1979.
322. Berson BL, Hermann G: Torn discoid menisci of the knee in adults. Four case reports. J Bone Joint Surg [Am] 61:303, 1979.
323. Kossoff J, Naimark A, Corbett M: Case report 85. Skel Radiol 4:45, 1979.
324. Pavlov H, Hirschy JC, Torg JS: Computed tomography of the cruciate ligaments. Radiology 132:389, 1979.
325. Rau WS, Kauffmann G: Röntgendiagnostik des Knorpelschadens am Kniegelenk. Radiologe 18:451, 1978.
326. Kormano M, Mäkelä P: Lymphatics filled at knee arthrography. Acta Radiol Diagn 19:853, 1978.
327. Pudlowski RM, Gilula LA, Kyriakos M: Intra-articular lipoma with osseous metaplasia: Radiographic-pathologic correlation. AJR 132:471, 1979.
328. Gordon GV, Edell S, Brogadir SP, et al: Baker's cysts and true thrombophlebitis. Report of two cases and review of the literature. Arch Intern Med 139:40, 1979.
329. Gillies H, Seligson D: Precision in the diagnosis of meniscal lesions: A comparison of clinical evaluation, arthrography, and arthroscopy. J Bone Joint Surg [Am] 61:343, 1979.
330. Hallel T, Salvati EA: Osteochondritis dissecans following Legg-Calvé-Perthes disease. Report of three cases. J Bone Joint Surg [Am] 58:708, 1976.
331. Dalinka MK, Lally JF, Gohel VK: Arthrography of the lateral meniscus. AJR 121:79, 1974.
332. Harley JD: An anatomic-arthrographic study of the relationships of the lateral meniscus and the popliteus tendon. AJR 128:181, 1977.
333. Weiner B, Rosenberg N: Discoid medial meniscus: Association with bone changes in the tibia. A case report. J Bone Joint Surg [Am] 56:171, 1974.
334. Fairbank TJ: Knee joint changes after meniscectomy. J Bone Joint Surg [Br] 30:664, 1948.
335. Ganel A, Engel J, Ditzian R, et al: Arthrography as a method of diagnosing soft-tissue injuries of the wrist. J Trauma 19:376, 1979.
336. Hall FM: Elbow arthrography. Radiology 132:775, 1979.
337. Mink JH, Richardson A, Grant TT: Evaluation of glenoid labrum by double-contrast shoulder arthrography. AJR 133:883, 1979.
338. Mikasa M: Subacromial bursography. J Jpn Orthop Assoc 53:225, 1979.
339. Rosenthal DI, Murray WT, Jauernek RR, et al: Stressing the knee joint for arthrography. Radiology 134:250, 1980.
340. Bowen AD III: Have you tried this knee arthrography stress device? AJR 134:197, 1980.
341. Foote GA: Delayed films in double contrast knee arthrography. Australas Radiol 22:273, 1978.
342. Pavlov H, Goldman AB: The popliteus bursa: An indicator of subtle pathology. AJR 134:313, 1980.
343. Schuldt DR, Wolfe RD: Clinical and arthrographic findings in meniscal cysts. Radiology 134:49, 1980.
344. Conforty B, Lotem M: Ossicles in human menisci: Report of two cases. Clin Orthop 144:272, 1979.
345. Vahvanen V, Aalto K: Meniscectomy in children. Acta Orthop Scand 50:791, 1979.
346. Noble J, Erat K: In defense of the meniscus. A prospective study of 200 meniscectomy patients. J Bone Joint Surg [Br] 62:7, 1980.
347. Seidl G, Scherak O, Hofner W: Antefemoral dissecting cysts in rheumatoid arthritis. Radiology 133:343, 1979.
348. Eyanson S, Macfarlane JD, Brandt KD: Popliteal cyst mimicking thrombophlebitis as the first indication of knee disease. Clin Orthop 144:215, 1979.
349. Rauschning W, Lindgren PG: Popliteal cysts (Baker's cysts) in adults. I. Clinical and roentgenological results of operative excision. Acta Orthop Scand 50:583, 1979.
350. Lindgren PG, Rauschning W: Clinical and arthrographic studies on the valve mechanism in communicating popliteal cysts. Arch Orthop Traum Surg 95:245, 1979.
351. Ireland J, Trickey EL, Stoker DJ: Arthroscopy and arthrography of the knee. A critical review. J Bone Joint Surg [Br] 62:3, 1980.
352. Levinsohn EM, Baker BE: Prearthrotomy diagnostic evaluation of the knee: Review of 100 cases diagnosed by arthrography and arthroscopy. AJR 134:107, 1980.
353. Korn MW, Spitzer RM, Robinson KE: Correlations of arthrography with arthroscopy. Orthop Clin North Am 10:535, 1979.
354. Lindholmer E, Foged N, Jensen JT: Arthrography of the ankle. Value in diagnosis of rupture of the lateral ligaments. Acta Radiol Diagn 19:585, 1978.
355. Moppes PI, Hoogenband CR, Greep JM: Adhesive capsulitis of the ankle (frozen ankle). Arch Orthop Traum Surg 94:313, 1979.
356. Abraham E, Stirnaman JE: Neglected rupture of the peroneal tendons causing recurrent sprains of the ankle. Case report. J Bone Joint Surg [Am] 61:1247, 1979.
357. Evans GA, Frenyo SK: The stress-tenogram in the diagnosis of ruptures of the lateral ligament of the ankle. J Bone Joint Surg [Br] 61:347, 1979.
358. Neviaser TJ: Arthrography of the shoulder. Orthop Clin North Am 11:205, 1980.
359. Gershuni DH, Axer A, Hendel D: Arthrography as an aid to diagnosis, prognosis, and therapy in Legg-Calvé-Perthes' disease. Acta Orthop Scand 51:505, 1980.
360. Ferrer-Roca O, Vilalta C: Lesions of the meniscus. Part I: Macroscopic and histologic findings. Clin Orthop 146:289, 1980.
361. Ferrer-Roca O, Vilalta C: Lesions of the meniscus. Part II: Horizontal cleavages and lateral cysts. Clin Orthop 146:301, 1980.
362. Reichelt A, Hehne HJ, Rau WS, Schlageter M: Die doppel Kontrastarthrographie bei der Chondropathia patellae—klinische und experimentelle Studie zur Pathogenese und Diagnostik. Z Orthop 117:746, 1979.
363. Beyer D, Fiedler V, Schütt H, et al: Hypertrophie des hoffaschen fettkörperseine arthrographische diagnose? Röntgen-Bl 32:429, 1979.
364. Rauschning W, Lindgren PG: The clinical significance of the valve mechanism in communicating popliteal cysts. Arch Orthop Traum Surg 95:251, 1979.
365. Hermann G, Hochberg F: Lipoma arborescens: Arthrographic findings. Orthopedics 3:19, 1980.
366. Van Moppes FI, VanEngelshoven JMH, Van de Hoogenband CR: Comparison between talar tilt, anterior drawer sign and ankle arthrography in ankle ligament lesions. J Belge Radiol 62:441, 1979.
367. Hjelmstedt EA, Sahlstedt B: Arthrography as a guide in the treatment of congenital clubfoot. Acta Orthop Scand 51:321, 1980.
368. Hjelmstedt A, Sahlstedt B: Talo-calcaneal osteotomy and soft tissue procedures in the treatment of clubfoot. Parts I, II. Acta Orthop Scand 51:335, 349, 1980.
369. Mink JH, Dickerson R: Air or CO₂ for knee arthrography? AJR 134:991, 1980.
370. Sedgwick WG, Gilula LA, Lesker PA, et al: Wear particles: Their value in knee arthrography. Radiology 136:11, 1980.
371. Dalinka MK: Arthrography. New York, Springer-Verlag, 1980.
372. Freiberger RH, Kaye JJ: Arthrography. New York, Appleton-Century-Crofts, 1979.
373. Anderson TM Jr: Arthrography. Radiol Clin North Am 19:215, 1981.
374. Goldman AB, Dines DM, Warren RF: Shoulder Arthrography. Technique, Diagnosis, and Clinical Correlation. Boston, Little, Brown, 1982.
375. Arndt R-D, Horns JW, Gold RH, et al: Clinical Arthrography. Baltimore, Williams & Wilkins, 1981.
376. Guerra J Jr, Resnick D: Practical aspects of arthrography. Part 1. Examination techniques. Appl Radiol, Mar-April, 1984, p 83.
377. Apple JS, Martinez S, Khoury MB, et al: A comparison of Hexabrix and Renografin-60 in knee arthrography. AJR 145:139, 1985.
378. Guerra J Jr, Resnick D, Haghighi P, et al: Investigation of a new arthrographic contrast agent: Iotrol. Invest Radiol 19:228, 1984.
379. Enzmannn DR, Young S: Arthrography using perfluorocarbon compounds. Invest Radiol 16:46, 1981.
380. Pastershank SP, Resnick D, Niwayama G, et al: The effect of water-soluble contrast media on the synovial membrane. Radiology 143:331, 1982.
381. Murray RC, Forrai E: Transitory eosinophilia localised in the knee joint after pneumarthrography. J Bone Joint Surg [Br] 32:74, 1950.
382. Hasselbacher P, Schumacher HR: Synovial fluid eosinophilia following arthrography. J Rheumatol 5:173, 1978.
383. Hall FM, Rosenthal DI, Goldberg RP, et al: Morbidity from shoulder arthrography: Etiology, incidence, and prevention. AJR 136:59, 1981.
384. Hall FM, Goldberg RP, Wyshak G, et al: Shoulder arthrography: Comparison of morbidity after use of various contrast media. Radiology 154:339, 1985.
385. Goldberg RP, Hall FM, Wyshak G: Pain in knee arthrography: Comparison of air vs. CO₂ and respiration vs. no respiration. AJR 136:377, 1981.
386. Goldberg RP, Hall FM: Pain and pH. AJR 135:875, 1980.
387. Kim KS, Lachman R: In vitro effects of iodinated contrast media on the growth of staphylococci. Invest Radiol 17:305, 1982.
388. Dawson P, Becker A, Holton JM: The effect of contrast media on the growth of bacteria. Br J Radiol 56:809, 1983.
389. Dory MA, Wautelet MJ: Arthrography in septic arthritis. Lidocaine- and iodine-containing contrast media are bacteriostatic. Arthritis Rheum 28:198, 1985.
390. Resnick D, Kerr R, André M, et al: Digital arthrography in the evaluation of painful joint prostheses. Invest Radiol 19:432, 1984.
391. Resnick D, André M, Kerr R, et al: Digital arthrography of the wrist: A radiographic and pathologic investigation. AJR 142:1187, 1984.
392. Resnik CS, Fronek J, Frey C, et al: Intra-articular pressure determination during glenohumeral joint arthrography. Preliminary investigation. Invest Radiol 19:45, 1984.
393. Cone RO, Yaru N, Resnick D, et al: Intracapsular pressure monitoring during arthrographic evaluation of painful hip prostheses. AJR 141:885, 1983.
394. Newberg AH, Muhn CS, Robbins AH: Complications of arthrography. Radiology 155:605, 1985.
395. Greenberger PA, Patterson R, Simon R, et al: Pretreatment of high risk patients requiring radiographic contrast media studies. J Allerg Clin Immun 67:185, 1981.
396. Totty WG, Murphy WA: Pneumoarthrography: Reemphasis of a neglected technique. J Can Assoc Radiol 35:264, 1984.
397. Dalinka MK, Osterman AL, Albert AS, et al: Arthrography of the wrist and shoulder. Orthop Clin North Am 14:193, 1983.
398. Kricun ME: Wrist arthrography. Clin Orthop 187:65, 1984.
399. Gilula LA, Totty WG, Weeks PM: Wrist arthrography. The value of fluoroscopic spot viewing. Radiology 146:555, 1983.
400. Schwartz AM, Ruby LK: Wrist arthrography revisited. Orthopedics 5:883, 1982.
401. Braunstein EM, Louis DS, Green TL, et al: Fluoroscopic and arthrographic evaluation of carpal instability. AJR 144:1259, 1985.

402. Berger RA, Blair WF, El-Khoury GY: Arthrotomography of the wrist. The triangular fibrocartilage complex. Clin Orthop *172*:257, 1983.
403. Blair WF, Berger RA, El-Khoury GY: Arthrotomography of the wrist: An experimental and preliminary clinical study. J Hand Surg [Am] *10*:350, 1985.
404. Tirman RM, Weber ER, Snyder LL, et al: Midcarpal wrist arthrography for detection of tears of the scapholunate and lunotriquetral ligaments. AJR *144*:107, 1985.
405. Mikic ZDJ: Arthrography of the wrist joint. An experimental study. J Bone Joint Surg [Am] *66*:371, 1984.
406. Wu G, Whitehouse GH, Littler TR: The demonstration of lymphatic channels on wrist arthrography with particular reference to associated lymphoedema. Rheumatol Rehabil *21*:65, 1982.
407. Palmer AK, Levinsohn EM, Kuzma GR: Arthrography of the wrist. J Hand Surg *8*:15, 1983.
408. Levinsohn EM, Palmer AK: Arthrography of the traumatized wrist. Correlation with radiography and the carpal instability series. Radiology *146*:647, 1983.
409. Berger RA, Blair WF, El-Khoury GY: Arthrotomography of the wrist. The palmar radiocarpal ligaments. Clin Orthop *186*:224, 1984.
410. Tehranzadeh J, Labosky DA: Detection of intraarticular loose osteochondral fragments by double-contrast wrist arthrography. A case report of a basketball injury. Am J Sports Med *12*:77, 1984.
411. Meyer VE, Winter P: Osteochondrosis dissecans des distalen radioulnaren Gelenkes. Orthopäde *10*:66, 1981.
412. Mohanti RC, Kar N: Study of triangular fibrocartilage of the wrist joint in Colles' fracture. Injury *11*:321, 1980.
413. Moneim MS, Omer GE Jr: Wrist arthrography in acute carpal injuries. Orthopedics *6*:299, 1983.
414. Tehranzadeh J, Labosky DA, Gabrielle OF: Ganglion cysts and tear of triangular fibrocartilages of both wrists in a cheerleader. Am J Sports Med *11*:357, 1983.
415. Rosenthal DI, Murray WT, Smith RJ: Finger arthrography. Radiology *137*:357, 1983.
416. Engel J, Luboshitz S, Israeli A, et al: Tenography in De Quervain's disease. Hand *13*:142, 1981.
417. Teng MM, Murphy WA, Gilula LA, et al: Elbow arthrography: A reassessment of the technique. Radiology *153*:611, 1984.
418. Mink JH, Eckardt JJ, Grant TT: Arthrography in recurrent dislocation of the elbow. AJR *136*:1242, 1981.
419. Josefsson PO, Andren L, Gentz CF, et al: Arthrography of the dislocated elbow joint. Acta Radiol Diagn *25*:143, 1984.
420. Blane CE, Kling TF Jr, Andrews JC, et al: Arthrography in the post-traumatic elbow in children. AJR *143*:17, 1984.
421. Pirani M, Lange-Mechlen I, Cockshott WP: Rupture of a posterior synovial cyst of the elbow. J Rheumatol *9*:94, 1982.
422. Burt TB, MacCarter DK, Gelman MI, et al: Clinical manifestations of synovial cysts. West J Med *133*:99, 1980.
423. Villers P, Moitrel C, Chemin JJ: L'arthrographie de l'épaule en double contraste. Ann Radiol *23*:599, 1980.
424. De Smet AA: Arthrographic demonstration of the subcoracoid bursa. Skel Radiol *7*:275, 1982.
425. Bretzke CA, Crass JR, Craig EV, et al: Ultrasonography of the rotator cuff. Normal and pathologic anatomy. Invest Radiol *20*:311, 1985.
426. Middleton WD, Edelstein G, Reinus WR, et al: Sonographic detection of rotator cuff tears. AJR *144*:349, 1985.
427. Craig EV: The geyser sign and torn rotator cuff: Clinical significance and pathomechanics. Clin Orthop *191*:213, 1984.
428. Ahovuo J, Paavolainen P, Slatis P: The diagnostic value of arthrography and plain radiography in rotator cuff tears. Acta Orthop Scand *55*:220, 1984.
429. Garcia JF: Arthrographic visualization of rotator cuff tears. Optimal application of stress to the shoulder. Radiology *150*:595, 1984.
430. Kilcoyne RF, Matsen FA III: Rotator cuff tear measured by arthropneumotomography. AJR *140*:315, 1983.
431. Rizk TE, Pinals RS: Frozen shoulder. Semin Arthritis Rheum *11*:440, 1982.
432. Binder AI, Bulgen DY, Hazleman BL, et al: Frozen shoulder: An arthrographic and radionuclear scan assessment. Ann Rheum Dis *43*:365, 1984.
433. Dines D, Warren RF, Inglis AE: Surgical treatment of lesions of the long head of the biceps. Clin Orthop *164*:164, 1982.
434. Braunstein EM, O'Connor G: Double-contrast arthrotomography of the shoulder. J Bone Joint Surg [Am] *64*:192, 1982.
435. Kleinman PK, Kanzaria PK, Goss TP, et al: Axillary arthrotomography of the glenoid labrum. AJR *141*:993, 1984.
436. Pappas AM, Goss TP, Kleinman PK: Symptomatic shoulder instability due to lesions of the glenoid labrum. Am J Sports Med *11*:279, 1983.
437. McGlynn FJ, El-Khoury G, Albright JP: Arthrography of the glenoid labrum in shoulder instability. J Bone Joint Surg [Am] *64*:506, 1982.
438. Kinnard P, Tricoire J-L, Levesque R-Y, et al: Assessment of the unstable shoulder by computed arthrography. A preliminary report. Am J Sports Med *11*:157, 1983.
439. Shuman WP, Kilcoyne RF, Matsen FA, et al: Double-contrast computed tomography of the glenoid labrum. AJR *141*:581, 1983.
440. Deutsch AL, Resnick D, Mink JH, et al: Computed and conventional arthrotomography of the glenohumeral joint: Normal anatomy and clinical experience. Radiology *143*:603, 1984.
441. Resnik CS, Deutsch AL, Resnick D, et al: Arthrotomography of the shoulder. Radiographics *4*:963, 1984.
442. Caspari RB: Shoulder arthroscopy: A review of the present state of the art. Contemp Orthop *4*:523, 1980.
443. Johnson LL: Arthoscopy of the shoulder. Orthop Clin North Am *11*:197, 1980.
444. Lombardo SJ: Arthroscopy of the shoulder. Clin Sports Med *2*:309, 1983.
445. Cone RO, Danzig L, Resnick D, et al: The bicipital groove: Radiographic, anatomic, and pathologic study. AJR *141*:781, 1983.
446. DePalma AF: Surgery of the Shoulder. 3rd Ed. Philadelphia, JB Lippincott Co, 1983, pp 55–60, 512–558.
447. Warwick R, Williams PL (Eds): Gray's Anatomy. 35th Br Ed. Philadelphia, WB Saunders Co, 1973, pp 407–471.
448. Uhthoff HK, Piscopo M: Anterior capsular redundancy of the shoulder: Congenital or traumatic. An embryological study. J Bone Joint Surg [Br] *67*:363, 1985.
449. Townley CO: The capsular mechanism in recurrent dislocation of the shoulder. J Bone Joint Surg [Am] *32*:370, 1950.
450. DePalma AF, Cooke AJ, Prabhakar M: The role of the subscapularis in recurrent anterior dislocations of the shoulder. Clin Orthop *54*: 35, 1967.
451. Symeonides PP: The significance of the subscapularis muscle in the pathogenesis of recurrent anterior dislocation of the shoulder. J Bone Joint Surg [Br] *54*:476, 1972.
452. Turkel SJ, Panio MW, Marshall JL, et al: Stabilizing mechanisms preventing anterior dislocation of the glenohumeral joint. J Bone Joint Surg [Am] *63*:1208, 1981.
453. Freeland AE, Higgins RW: Anterior shoulder dislocation with posterior displacement of the long head of the biceps tendon. Arthrographic findings. A case report. Orthopedics *8*:468, 1985.
454. Nance EP Jr, Jones TB, Kaye JJ: Dissecting synovial cysts of the shoulder: A complication of chronic rotator cuff tears. AJR *138*:739, 1982.
455. Sanders TR, Staple TW: Percutaneous catheter drainage of septic shoulder joint. Radiology *147*:270, 1983.
456. Neer CS: Anterior acromioplasty for the chronic impingement syndrome in the shoulder. J Bone Joint Surg [Am] *54*:41, 1972.
457. Cone RO III, Resnick D, Danzig L: Shoulder impingement syndrome: Radiographic evaluation. Radiology *150*:29, 1984.
458. Penny JN, Welsh RP: Shoulder impingement syndromes in athletes and their surgical management. Am J Sports Med *9*:11, 1981.
459. Ha'eri GB, Wiley AM: Shoulder impingement syndrome. Results of operative release. Clin Orthop *168*:128, 1982.
460. Strizak AM, Danzig L, Jackson DW, et al: Subacromial bursography. An anatomical and clinical study. J Bone Joint Surg [Am] *64*:196, 1982.
461. Strife JL, Towbin R, Crawford A: Hip arthrography in infants and children: The inferomedial approach. Radiology *152*:536, 1984.
462. Crawford AH, Carothers TA: Hip arthrography in the skeletally immature. Clin Orthop *162*:54, 1982.
463. Newberg AH, Wetzner SM: Digital subtraction arthrography. Radiology *154*:238, 1985.
464. Hendrix RW, Wixson RL, Rana NA, et al: Arthrography after total hip arthroplasty: A modified technique used in the diagnosis of pain. Radiology *148*:647, 1983.
465. Azouz EM: Apparent or true neonatal hip dislocation? Radiologic differential diagnosis. Can Med Assoc J *129*:595, 1983.
466. Ogden JA, Lee KE, Rudicel SA, et al: Proximal femoral epiphysiolysis in the neonate. J Pediatr Orthop *4*:285, 1984.
467. Guyer B, Levinsohn EM: Recurrent anterior dislocation of the hip: Case report with arthrographic findings. Skel Radiol *10*:262, 1983.
468. Klein A, Sumner TE, Volberg FM, et al: Combined CT-arthrography in recurrent traumatic hip dislocation. AJR *138*:963, 1982.
469. Griffiths HJ, Utz R, Burke J, et al: Adhesive capsulitis of the hip and ankle. AJR *144*:101, 1985.
470. Lequesne M, Becker J, Bard M, et al: Capsular constriction of the hip: Arthrographic and clinical considerations. Skel Radiol *6*:1, 1981.
471. Kaelin A: Une cause rare de blocage traumatique de la hanche chez l'enfant. Int Orthop (SICOT) *8*:9, 1984.
472. Ueo T, Hamabuchi M: Hip pain caused by cystic deformation of the labrum acetabulare. Arthritis Rheum *27*:947, 1984.
473. Steinbach LS, Schneider R, Goldman AB, et al: Bursae and abscess cavities communicating with the hip. Diagnosis using arthrography and CT. Radiology *156*:303, 1985.
474. Chaiamnuay P, Davis P: An unusual case of inguinal swelling. Arthritis Rheum *27*:239, 1984.
475. Weinreb JC, Cohen JM, Maravilla KR: Iliopsoas muscles: MR study of normal anatomy and disease. Radiology *156*:435, 1985.
476. Penkava RR: Iliopsoas bursitis demonstrated by computed tomography. AJR *135*:175, 1980.
477. Peters JC, Coleman BG, Turner ML, et al: CT evaluation of enlarged iliopsoas bursa. AJR *135*:392, 1980.
478. Carrera GF, Papadakes N, Imray TJ: Retropsoas extension of ruptured hip capsule: Arthrographic demonstration. AJR *135*:1293, 1980.
479. Janus CL, Hermann G: Enlargement of the iliopsoas bursa: Unusual cause of cystic mass on pelvic sonogram. J Clin Ultrasound *10*:133, 1982.
480. Lyons JC, Peterson LFA: The snapping iliopsoas tendon. Mayo Clin Proc *59*:327, 1984.
481. Nunziata A, Blumenfeld I: Cadeva a resorte. A proposito de una variedad. Prensa Med Argent *38*:1997, 1951.
482. House AJG: Orthopaedists and ballet. Clin Orthop *89*:52, 1972.

483. Schaberg JE, Harper MC, Allen WC: The snapping hip syndrome. Am J Sports Med 12:361, 1984.
484. Gerber AM, Resnick D: Knee joint puncture after patellectomy. Clin Orthop 154:337, 1981.
485. Martin IR, Stoner P: An efficient apparatus for liver arthrography. Br J Radiol 58:483, 1985.
486. Salazar JE, Sebes JI, Scott RL: The supine view in double-contrast knee arthrography. AJR 141:585, 1983.
487. Hammond DI, Liver JA: Prone and supine views in double-contrast knee arthrography. J Can Assoc Radiol 35:262, 1984.
488. Weaver JW: Stereoscopic spot filming in arthrography. AJR 138:172, 1982.
489. Hotchkiss RN, Tew WP, Hungerford DS: Cartilaginous debris in the injured human knee. Correlation with arthroscopic findings. Clin Orthop 168:144, 1982.
490. Evans CH, Mears DC, Stanitski CL: Ferrographic analysis of wear in human joints. Evaluation by comparison with arthroscopic examination of symptomatic knees. J Bone Joint Surg [Br] 4:572, 1982.
491. Shakespeare DT, Rigby HS: The bucket-handle tear of the meniscus. A clinical and arthrographic study. J Bone Joint Surg [Br] 65:383, 1983.
492. Schafer H: Das Meniskusganglion. Früherkennung durch Ausmessung standardisierter Arthrogramme. ROFO 136:505, 1982.
493. Segal P, Perringerard I, Raguet M, et al: Etude étiopathogénique des kystes du ménisque externe. Rev Chir Orthop 69:55, 1983.
494. Dickhaut SC, DeLee JC: The discoid lateral-meniscus syndrome. J Bone Joint Surg [Am] 64:1068, 1982.
495. Dickason JM, Del Pizzo W, Blazina ME, et al: A series of ten discoid medial menisci. Clin Orthop 168:75, 1982.
496. Johnson RG, Simmons EH: Discoid medial meniscus. Clin Orthop 167:176, 1982.
497. Hermann G, Berson BL: Discoid medial meniscus: Two cases of tears presenting as locked knee due to athletic trauma. Am J Sports Med 12:74, 1984.
498. Clark CR, Ogden JA: Development of the menisci of the human knee joint. Morphological changes and their potential role in childhood meniscal injury. J Bone Joint Surg [Am] 65:538, 1983.
499. Engber WD, Mickelson MR: Cupping of the lateral tibial plateau associated with a discoid meniscus. Orthopedics 4:904, 1981.
500. Mariani PP, Puddo G: Meniscal ossicle. A case report. Am J Sports Med 9:392, 1981.
501. Radin EL, de Lamotte F, Maquet P: Role of the menisci in the distribution of stress in the knee. Clin Orthop 185:290, 1984.
502. Kurosawa H, Fukubayashi T, Nakajima H: Load-bearing mode of the knee joint: Physical behavior of the knee joint with or without menisci. Clin Orthop 149:283, 1980.
503. Korkala O, Karaharju E, Gronblad M, et al: Articular cartilage after meniscectomy. Rabbit knees studied with the scanning electron microscope. Acta Orthop Scand 55:273, 1984.
504. Shapiro F, Glimcher MJ: Induction of osteoarthrosis in the rabbit knee joint: Histologic changes following meniscectomy and meniscal lesions. Clin Orthop 147:287, 1980.
505. Northmore-Ball MD, Dandy DJ, Jackson RW: Arthroscopic, open partial, and total meniscectomy. J Bone Joint Surg [Br] 65:400, 1983.
506. Tregonning RJA: Closed partial meniscectomy. Early results for single tears with meniscal symptoms. J Bone Joint Surg [Br] 65:378, 1983.
507. Goodfellow JW: Closed meniscectomy. J Bone Joint Surg [Br] 65:373, 1983.
508. Heatley FW: The meniscus—can it be repaired? J Bone Joint Surg [Br] 62:397, 1980.
509. Cabaud HE, Rodkey WG, Fitzwater JE: Medial meniscus repairs. An experimental and morphologic study. Am J Sports Med 9:129, 1981.
510. Arnoczky SP, Warren RF: Microvasculature of the human meniscus. Am J Sports Med 10:90, 1982.
511. Danzig L, Resnick D, Gonsalves M, et al: Blood supply to the normal and abnormal menisci of the human knee. Clin Orthop 172:271, 1983.
512. Arnoczky SP, Warren RF: The microvasculature of the meniscus and its response to injury. An experimental study in the dog. Am J Sports Med 11:131, 1983.
513. El-Khoury GY, Usta HY, Berger RA: Meniscotibial (coronary) ligament tears. Skel Radiol 11:191, 1984.
514. Henry JH, Craven RP Jr: Traumatic meniscal lesions in children. South Med J 74:1336, 1981.
515. King AG: Meniscal lesions in children and adolescents: A review of the pathology and clinical presentation. Injury 15:105, 1983.
516. Arcomano JP, Anetrella LJ: Visualizing the interior cruciate ligament. AJR 138:1189, 1982.
517. Reider B, Clancy W, Langer LO: Diagnosis of cruciate ligament injury using single contrast arthrography. Am J Sports Med 12:451, 1984.
518. Pavlov H, Warren RF, Sherman MF, et al: The accuracy of double-contrast arthrographic evaluation of the anterior cruciate ligament. A retrospective review of one hundred and sixty-three knees with surgical confirmation. J Bone Joint Surg [Am] 65:175, 1983.
519. Pavlov H: The radiographic diagnosis of the anterior cruciate ligament deficient knee. Clin Orthop 172:57, 1983.
520. Brody GA, Pavlov H, Warren RF, et al: Plica synovialis infrapatellaris: Arthrographic sign of anterior cruciate ligament disruption. AJR 140:767, 1983.
521. Braunstein EM: Anterior cruciate ligament injuries: A comparison of arthrographic and physical diagnosis. AJR 138:423, 1982.

522. Warren RF, Levy IM: Meniscal lesions associated with anterior cruciate ligament injury. Clin Orthop 192:32, 1983.
523. Passariello R, Trecco F, De Paulis F, et al: Computed tomography of the knee joint: Technique of study and normal anatomy. J Comput Assist Tomogr 7:1035, 1983.
524. Passariello R, Trecco F, De Paulis F, et al: Computed tomography of the knee joint: Clinical results. J Comput Assist Tomogr 7:1043, 1983.
525. Reiser M, Rupp N, Karpf PM, et al: Erfahrungen mit der CT-arthrographie der Kreuzbänder des Kniegelenkes. ROFO 137:327, 1982.
526. Rickards D, Chapman JA: Computed tomography of the anterior cruciate ligament. Clin Radiol 35:327, 1984.
527. Golimbu C, Firooznia H, Rafii M, et al: Computerized tomography of the posterior cruciate ligaments. Comput Radiol 6:233, 1982.
528. Deramos RK: CT diagnosis of torn meniscus. Comput Radiol 6:263, 1982.
529. Jurik AG, Jorgensen J, Helmig O, et al: Computed tomography of the knee with reference to meniscal tears. A preliminary report. Acta Radiol Diagn 25:433, 1984.
530. Li KC, Henkelman M, Poon PY, et al: MR imaging of the normal knee. J Comput Assist Tomogr 8:1147, 1984.
531. Turner DA, Prodromos CC, Petasnick JP, et al: Acute injury of the ligaments of the knee: Magnetic resonance evaluation. Radiology 154:717, 1985.
532. Sartoris DJ, Kursunoglu S, Pineda C, et al: Detection of intra-articular bodies in the knee using computed arthrotomography. Radiology 155:447, 1985.
533. Kaufmann J, Langlotz M: Ist die idiopathische Chondropathia patellae mit radiologischen methoden Diagnostizierbar? ROFO 141:422, 1984.
534. Reiser M, Karpf P-M, Bernett P: Diagnosis of chondromalacia patellae using CT arthrography. Eur J Radiol 2:181, 1982.
535. Boven F, Bellemans M-A, Geurts J, et al: A comparative study of the patello-femoral joint on axial roentgenogram, axial arthrogram, and computed tomography following arthrography. Skel Radiol 8:179, 1982.
536. Boven F, Bellemans M-A, Geurts J, et al: The value of computed tomography scanning in chondromalacia patellae. Skel Radiol 8:183, 1982.
537. Aprin H, Broukhim B: Early diagnosis of acute rupture of the quadriceps tendon by arthrography. Clin Orthop 195:185, 1985.
538. Deutsch AL, Resnick D, Dalinka MK, et al: Synovial plicae of the knee. Radiology 141:627, 1981.
539. Apple JS, Martinez S, Hardaker WT, et al: Synovial plicae of the knee. Skel Radiol 7:251, 1982.
540. Jackson RW: The sneaky plicae. J Rheumatol 7:437, 1980.
541. Jouanin T, Dupont JY, Halimi P, et al: The synovial folds of the knee joint: Anatomical study based on the dissection of 200 knee joints. Anat Clin 4:47, 1982.
542. Kinnard P, Levesque RY: The plica syndrome. A syndrome of controversy. Clin Orthop 183:141, 1984.
543. Dorfmann H, Orengo P, Amarenco G: Pathology of the synovial folds in the knee. The value of arthroscopy. Rev Rhum Mal Osteoartic 50:324, 1983.
544. Harrewyn JM, Algnan M, Renoux M, et al: Pathological synovial folds in the knee joint (synovial plica). Arthroscopic treatment. Rev Rhum Mal Osteoartic 49:3, 1982.
545. Gray DJ, Gardner E: Prenatal development of the human knee and superior tibiofibular joints. Am J Anat 86:235, 1950.
546. Pipkin G: Lesions of the suprapatellar plica. J Bone Joint Surg [Am] 32:363, 1950.
547. Aprin H, Shapiro J, Gershwind M: Arthrography (plica views). A noninvasive method for diagnosis and prognosis of plica syndrome. Clin Orthop 183:90, 1984.
548. Frija G, Halimi P, Dupont JY, et al: Expression radiologique des plicae du genou. Ann Radiol 25:375, 1982.
549. Boven F, De Boeck M, Potvliege R: Synovial plicae of the knee on computed tomography. Radiology 147:805, 1983.
550. Dory MA: Arthrographic recognition of the mediopatellar plica of the knee. Radiology 150:608, 1984.
551. Thijn CJP, Hillen B: Arthrography and the medial compartment of the patello-femoral joint. Skel Radiol 11:183, 1984.
552. Klein W: The medial shelf of the knee. A follow-up study. Arch Orthop Traum Surg 102:67, 1983.
553. Schulitz KP, Hille E, Kochs W: The importance of the mediopatellar synovial plica for chondromalacia patellae. Arch Orthop Traum Surg 102:37, 1983.
554. Richmond JC, McGinty JB: Segmental arthroscopic resection of the hypertrophic mediopatellar plica. Clin Orthop 178:185, 1983.
555. Nottage WM, Sprague NF III, Auerbach BJ, et al: The medial patellar plica syndrome. Am J Sports Med 11:211, 1983.
556. Vaughan-Lane T, Dandy DJ: The synovial shelf syndrome. J Bone Joint Surg [Br] 64:475, 1982.
557. Jackson RW, Marshall DJ, Fujisawa Y: The pathologic medial shelf. Orthop Clin North Am 13:307, 1982.
558. Moller H: Incarcerating mediopatellar synovial plica syndrome. Acta Orthop Scand 52:357, 1981.
559. Reid GD, Glasgow M, Gordon DA, et al: Pathological plicae of the knee mistaken for arthritis. J Rheumatol 7:573, 1980.
560. Cooke TD, Wyllie J: Anatomic separation of the suprapatellar pouch spares its involvement by rheumatoid synovitis in the knee. Rheumatol Int 1:99, 1981.
561. San Dretto MA, Wartinbee DR, Carrerra GF, et al: Suprapatellar plica synovialis: A common arthrographic finding. J Can Assoc Radiol 33:163, 1982.
562. Darlington D, Hawkins CF: Nail-patella syndrome with iliac horns and heredi-

tary nephropathy. Necropsy report and anatomical dissection. J Bone Joint Surg [Br] *49*:164, 1967.

563. Reider B, Marshall JL, Warren RF: Persistent vertical septum in the human knee joint. J Bone Joint Surg [Am] *63*:1185, 1981.

564. Fujikawa K: Arthrographic study of the rheumatoid knee. Part I. Synovial proliferation. Ann Rheum Dis *40*:332, 1981.

565. Fujikawa K, Tanaka Y, Matsubayashi T, et al: Arthrographic study of the rheumatoid knee. Part 2. Articular cartilage and menisci. Ann Rheum Dis *40*:344, 1981.

566. Guerra J Jr, Newell JD, Resnick D, et al: Gastrocnemio-semimembranosus bursal region of the knee. AJR *136*:593, 1981.

567. Rauschning W: Anatomy and function of the communication between knee joint and popliteal bursae. Ann Rheum Dis *39*:354, 1980.

568. Rauschning W, Fredriksson BA, Wilander E: Histomorphology of idiopathic and symptomatic popliteal cysts. Clin Orthop *164*:306, 1982.

569. Wigley RD: Popliteal cysts: Variations on a theme of Baker. Semin Arthritis Rheum *12*:1, 1982.

570. Shepherd JR, Helms CA: Atypical popliteal cyst due to lateral synovial herniation. Radiology *140*:66, 1981.

571. O'Dell JR, Andersen PA, Hollister JR, et al: Anterior tibial mass: An unusual complication of popliteal cysts. Arthritis Rheum *27*:113, 1984.

572. Corbetti F, Schiavon F, Fiocco U, et al: Unusual antefemoral dissecting cyst. Br J Radiol *58*:675, 1985.

573. Thevenon A, Hardouin P, Duquesnoy B: Popliteal cyst presenting as an anterior tibial mass. Arthritis Rheum *28*:477, 1985.

574. Fedullo LM, Bonakdarpour A, Moyer RA, et al: Giant synovial cysts. Skel Radiol *12*:90, 1984.

575. Hertzanu Y, Mendelsohn DB, Firer P: Calcified bodies in a giant Baker's cyst. S Afr Med J *65*:973, 1984.

576. Rosenthal DI, Schwartz AN, Schiller AL: Case report 179. Skel Radiol *7*:142, 1981.

577. Kattapuram SV: Case report 181. Skel Radiol *7*:279, 1982.

578. McLeod BC, Charters JR, Straus AK, et al: Gas-like radiolucencies in a popliteal cyst. Rheumatol Int *3*:143, 1983.

579. Fam AG, Wilson SR, Holmberg S: Ultrasound evaluation of popliteal cysts in osteoarthritis of the knee. J Rheumatol *9*:428, 1982.

580. Lukes PJ, Herberts P, Zachrisson BE: Ultrasound in the diagnosis of popliteal cysts. Acta Radiol Diagn *21*:663, 1980.

581. Gompels BM, Darlington LG: Evaluation of popliteal cysts and painful calves with ultrasonography: Comparison with arthrography. Ann Rheum Dis *41*:355, 1982.

582. Harper J, Schubert F, Benson MD, et al: Ultrasound and arthrography in the detection of ruptured Baker's cysts. Australas Radiol *26*:281, 1982.

583. Hermann G, Yeh H-C, Lehr-Janus C, et al: Diagnosis of popliteal cyst: Double-contrast arthrography and sonography. AJR *137*:369, 1981.

584. Abdel-Dayem HM, Barodawala YK, Papademetriou T: Scintigraphic arthrography. Comparison with contrast arthrography and future applications. Clin Nucl Med *7*:516, 1982.

585. Lamki L: Baker's cyst. Radionuclide arthrographic findings. Clin Nucl Med *10*:147, 1985.

586. Wallner RJ, Dadparvar S, Croll MN, et al: Demonstration of an infected popliteal (Baker's) cyst with three-phase skeletal scintigraphy. Clin Nucl Med *10*:153, 1985.

587. Schwimmer M, Edelstein G, Heiken JP, et al: Synovial cysts of the knee: CT evaluation. Radiology *154*:175, 1985.

588. Lee KR, Tines SC, Price HI, et al: The computed tomographic findings of popliteal cysts. Skel Radiol *10*:26, 1983.

589. Lee KR, Tines SC, Yoon JW: CT findings of suprapatellar synovial cysts. J Comput Assist Tomogr *8*:296, 1984.

590. Hull RG, Rennie JAN, Eastmond CJ, et al: Nuclear magnetic resonance (NMR) tomographic imaging for popliteal cysts in rheumatoid arthritis. Ann Rheum Dis *43*:56, 1984.

591. Smith DL, Bennett RM: Popliteal cyst rupture in SLE—superior rupture and an infected calf cyst. J Rheumatol *8*:518, 1981.

592. Ruiz EP, Eguren TT, Palop MJ, et al: Fistule cutanée d'un kyste poplite chez une patiente atteinte de polyarthrite rhumatoide. Rev Rhum Mal Osteoartic *52*:115, 1985.

593. Grepl J: Wert der positiven Arthrographie zur Diagnostik und Pathogenese retrofemoraler Bakerzysten. Z Orthop *120*:1, 1982.

594. Patrone NA, Ramsdell GM: Baker's cyst and venous thrombosis. South Med J *74*:768, 1981.

595. DeSmet AA, Neff JR: Knee arthrography for the preoperative evaluation of juxta-articular masses. Radiology *143*:633, 1982.

596. Griffiths HT, Elston CW, Colton CL, et al: Popliteal masses masquerading as popliteal cysts. Ann Rheum Dis *43*:60, 1984.

597. Bogumill GP, Bruno PD, Barrick EF: Malignant lesions masquerading as popliteal cysts. A report of three cases. J Bone Joint Surg [Am] *63*:474, 1981.

598. Littlejohn GO, Brand CA, Ada A, et al: Popliteal cysts and deep venous thrombosis: Tc-99m red blood cell venography. Radiology *155*:237, 1985.

599. Giyanani VL, Grozinger KT, Gerlock AJ Jr, et al: Calf hematoma mimicking thrombophlebitis: Sonographic and computed tomographic appearance. Radiology *154*:779, 1985.

600. Robb D: Obstruction of the popliteal artery by synovial cyst. Br J Surg *48*:221, 1960.

601. Haid SP, Conn J, Bergan JJ: Cystic adventitial disease of the popliteal artery. Arch Surg *101*:765, 1970.

602. Shute K, Rothnie NG: The aetiology of cystic arterial disease. Br J Surg *60*:397, 1973.

603. St Pierre RK, Jones PJ, Fleming LL: Arthroscopy and arthrography of the knee: A comparative study. South Med J *74*:1322, 1981.

604. Stoker DJ, Renton P, Fulton A: The value of arthrography in the management of internal derangements of the knee: The first 1000 are the worst. Clin Radiol *32*:557, 1981.

605. Thijn CJP: Accuracy of double-contrast arthrography and arthroscopy of the knee joint. Skel Radiol *8*:187, 1982.

606. Daniel D, Daniels E, Aronson D: The diagnosis of meniscus pathology. Clin Orthop *163*:218, 1982.

607. Marymont JV, Lynch MA, Henning CE: Evaluation of meniscus tears of the knee by radionuclide imaging. Am J Sports Med *11*:432, 1983.

608. Sauser DD, Nelson RC, Lavine MH, et al: Acute injuries of the lateral ligaments of the ankle: Comparison of stress radiography and arthrography. Radiology *148*:653, 1983.

609. van Moppes FI, van den Hoogenband CR, van Engelshoven JMA, et al: Arthrography, talar tilt and surgical findings after inversion trauma of the ankle. ROFO *134*:413, 1981.

610. van Moppes FI, van den Hoogenband CR: The significance of the peroneus tendon sheath in ankle arthrography. ROFO *132*:573, 1980.

611. Vuust M: Arthrographic diagnosis of ruptured calcaneofibular ligament. I. A new projection tested on experimental injury post mortem. Acta Radiol Diagn *21*:123, 1980.

612. Vuust M, Niedermann B: Arthrographic diagnosis of ruptured calcaneofibular ligament. II. Clinical evaluation of a new method. Acta Radiol Diagn *21*:231, 1980.

613. Lindholmer E, Andersen A, Andersen SB, et al: Arthrography of the ankle. Value in diagnosis of rupture of the calcaneofibular ligament. Acta Radiol Diagn *24*:217, 1983.

614. van Moppes FI, Meijer F, van den Hoogenband CR: Arthrographic differential diagnosis between ruptures of the anterior talofibular ligament, the joint capsule and the anterior tibiofibular ligament. Diagn Imag *49*:171, 1980.

615. Dirheimer Y, Ludig J-J, Meyer P: L'arthrographie de la cheville dans la polyarthrite rhumatoide. Rhumatologie *25*:343, 1973.

616. van Moppes FI, van den Hoogenband CR, Betts-Brown A: Filling of lymphatic vessels in ankle arthrography. Diagn Imag *49*:171, 1980.

617. Teng MMH, Destouet JM, Gilula LA, et al: Ankle tenography: A key to unexplained symptomatology. Part I. Normal tenographic anatomy. Radiology *151*:575, 1984.

618. Gilula LA, Oloff L, Caputi R, et al: Ankle tenography: A key to unexplained symptomatology. Part II. Diagnosis of chronic tendon disabilities. Radiology *151*:581, 1984.

619. Canoso JJ, Wohlgethan JR, Newberg AH, et al: Aspiration of the retrocalcaneal bursa. Ann Rheum Dis *43*:308, 1984.

620. Beaudet F, Dixon AS: Posterior subtalar joint synoviography and corticosteroid injection in rheumatoid arthritis. Ann Rheum Dis *40*:132, 1981.

621. Destouet JM, Gilula LA, Murphy WA, et al: Lumbar facet joint injection: Indication, technique, clinical correlation, and preliminary results. Radiology *145*:321, 1982.

622. Destouet JM, Murphy WA: Lumbar facet block. Indications and technique. Orthop Rev *14*:57, 1985.

623. Lippitt AB: The facet joint and its role in spine pain. Management with facet joint injections. Spine *9*:746, 1984.

624. Fairbank JCT, Park WM, McCall IW, et al: Apophyseal injection of local anesthetic as a diagnostic aid in primary low-back pain syndromes. Spine *6*:598, 1981.

625. Murphy WA: The facet syndrome. Radiology *151*:533, 1984.

626. Raymond J, Dumas J-M: Intraarticular facet block: Diagnostic test or therapeutic procedure? Radiology *151*:333, 1984.

627. Carrera GF: Lumbar facet joint injection in low back pain and sciatica. Description of technique. Radiology *137*:661, 1980.

628. Carrera GF: Lumbar facet joint injection in low back pain and sciatica. Preliminary results. Radiology *37*:665, 1980.

629. Dory MA: Arthrography of the lumbar facet joints. Radiology *140*:23, 1981.

630. Ghormley RK: Low back pain with special reference to the articular facets with presentation of an operative procedure. JAMA *101*:1773, 1933.

631. Badgley CE: The articular facets in relation to low-back pain and sciatic radiation. J Bone Joint Surg [Am] *23*:481, 1941.

632. Pedersen HE, Blunck CFJ, Garner E: The anatomy of lumbosacral posterior rami and meningeal branches of spinal nerves (sinuvertebral nerves): With an experimental study of their functions. J Bone Joint Surg [Am] *38*:377, 1956.

633. Hirsch C, Ingelmark BE, Miller M: The anatomical basis for low back pain: Studies on the presence of sensory nerve endings in ligamentous, capsular and intervertebral disc structures in the human lumbar spine. Acta Orthop Scand *33*:1, 1963.

634. Hadley LA: Anatomico-roentgenographic studies of the posterior spinal articulations. AJR *86*:270, 1961.

635. Maldague B, Mathurin P, Malghem J: Facet joint arthrography in lumbar spondylolysis. Radiology *140*:29, 1981.

636. Park WM, McCall IW, Benson D, et al: Spondylarthrography: The demonstration of spondylolysis by apophyseal joint arthrography. Clin Radiol *36*:427, 1985.

637. Raymond J, Dumas J-M: Anomalous ossicle of the articular process: Arthrography and facet block. AJR *141*:1233, 1983.

638. Dory MA: Arthrography of the cervical facet joints. Radiology *148*:379, 1983.

639. Dussault RG, Nicolet V: Cervical facet joint arthrography. J Can Assoc Radiol 36:79, 1985.
640. Hemminghytt S, Daniels DL, Williams VM: Intraspinal synovial cysts: Natural history and diagnosis by CT. Radiology 145:375, 1982.
641. Schulz EE, West WL, Hinshaw DB, et al: Gas in a lumbar extradural juxtaarticular cyst. Sign of synovial origin. AJR 143:875, 1984.
642. Spencer RR, Jahnke RW, Hardy TL: Dissection of gas into an intraspinal synovial cyst from contiguous vacuum facet. J Comput Assist Tomogr 7:886, 1983.
643. Kurz LT, Garfin SR, Unger AS, et al: Intraspinal synovial cyst causing sciatica. J Bone Joint Surg [Am] 67:865, 1985.
644. Hendrix RW, Lin P-JP, Kane WJ: Simplified aspiration or injection technique for the sacro-iliac joint. J Bone Joint Surg [Am] 64:1249, 1982.
645. Kaplan P, Tu H, Lydiatt D, et al: Temporomandibular joint arthrography of normal subjects: Prevalence of pain with ionic versus nonionic contrast agents. Radiology 156:825, 1985.
646. Roy C, Godin C, Dussault RG: Complementary role of wrist arthrography in non-union of scaphoid fractures. J Can Assoc Radiol 36:194, 1985.
647. Mack LA, Matsen FA III, Kilcoyne RF, et al: US evaluation of the rotator cuff. Radiology 157:205, 1985.
648. Mink JH, Harris E, Rappaport M: Rotator cuff tears: Evaluation using double-contrast shoulder arthrography. Radiology 157:621, 1985.
649. Resnick D: Frozen shoulder. Ann Rheum Dis 44:805, 1985.
650. Hoilund-Carlsen PF, Meinicke J, Christiansen B, et al: Joint distention arthrography for disabling hip pain. A controlled clinical trial. Scand J Rheumatol 14:179, 1985.
651. Middleton WD, Reinus WR, Totty WG, et al: US of the biceps tendon apparatus. Radiology 157:211, 1985.
652. Kaye JJ: Knee arthrography today. Radiology 157:265, 1985.
653. Passariello R, Trecco F, de Paulis F, et al: Meniscal lesions of the knee joint: CT diagnosis. Radiology 157:29, 1985.
654. Ghelman B: Meniscal tears of the knee: Evaluation by high-resolution CT combined with arthrography. Radiology 157:23, 1985.
655. Reicher MA, Rauschning W, Gold RH, et al: High-resolution magnetic resonance imaging of the knee joint: Normal anatomy. AJR 145:895, 1985.
656. Reicher MA, Bassett LW, Gold RH: High-resolution magnetic resonance imaging of the knee joint: Pathologic correlations. AJR 145:903, 1985.
657. Kay SP, Gold RH, Bassett LW: Meniscal pneumatocele. A case report of spontaneous, persistent intra-articular and juxta-articular gas. J Bone Joint Surg [Am] 67:1117, 1985.
658. Comba D, Quaglia F, Magliano GE: Massive discoid medial meniscus. A case report. Acta Orthop Scand 56:340, 1985.
659. Wolfe RD, Dieden JD: Cruciate ligament injury: Diagnostic difficulties in the presence of meniscal injury. Radiology 157:19, 1985.
660. Rovere GD, Adair DM: Medial synovial shelf plica syndrome. Treatment by intraplical steroid injection. Am J Sports Med 13:382, 1985.
661. van Moppes FI, Meijer F, van den Hoogenband CR: Lymphatic filling in ankle arthrography. AJR 145:651, 1985.
662. Ingram C, Stoker DJ: Contrast media in double-contrast arthrography of the knee: A comparison of ioxaglate and iothalamate preparations. Br J Radiol 59:143, 1986.
663. Gilula LA, Reinus WR, Totty WG: Midcarpal wrist arthrography. AJR 146:645, 1986.
664. Middleton WD, Reinus WR, Totty WG, et al: Ultrasonographic evaluation of the rotator cuff and biceps tendon. J Bone Joint Surg [Am] 68:440, 1986.
665. Crass JR, Craig EV, Feinberg SB: Sonography of the postoperative rotator cuff. AJR 146:561, 1986.
666. Middleton WD, Reinus WR, Melson GL, et al: Pitfalls of rotator cuff sonography. AJR 146:555, 1986.
667. Craig EV: The acromioclavicular joint cyst. An unusual presentation of a rotator cuff tear. Clin Orthop 202:189, 1986.
668. Calvert PT, Packer NP, Stoker DJ, et al: Arthrography of the shoulder after operative repair of the torn rotator cuff. J Bone Joint Surg [Br] 68:147, 1986.
669. Ahovuo J, Paavolainen P, Slatis P: Diagnostic value of sonography in lesions of the biceps tendon. Clin Orthop 202:184, 1986.
670. Rafii M, Firooznia H, Golimbu C, et al: CT arthrography of the capsular structures of the shoulder. AJR 146:361, 1986.
671. de Carvalho A, Jurik AG: Joint fluid after aspiration. A disturbing factor in knee arthrography. Acta Radiol Diagn 26:715, 1985.
672. Manco LG, Kavanaugh JH, Fay JJ, et al: Meniscus tears of the knee: Prospective evaluation with CT. Radiology 159:147, 1986.
673. Beltran J, Noto AM, Mosure JC, et al: Meniscal tears: MR demonstration of experimentally produced injuries. Radiology 158:691, 1986.
674. Beltran J, Noto AM, Herman LJ, et al: Joint effusions: MR imaging. Radiology 158:133, 1986.
675. Selby B, Richardson ML, Montana MA, et al: High resolution sonography of the menisci of the knee. Invest Radiol 21:332, 1986.
676. Salazar JE, Duke RA, Winer-Muram HT: Locking and unlocking of the knee: arthrographic demonstration. AJR 146:575, 1986.
677. Soren A: On the etiology of congenital malformation of the meniscus. Arch Orthop Trauma Surg 104:283, 1985.
678. Podgorski M, Edmonds J: Bidirectional knee joint rupture. J Rheumatol 12:1180, 1985.
679. Lynch MC, Taylor JF: Facet joint injection for low back pain. A clinical study. J Bone Joint Surg [Br] 68:138, 1986.

680. Mercader J, Gomez JM, Cardenal C: Intraspinal synovial cyst: Diagnosis by CT. Follow-up and spontaneous remission. Neuroradiology 27:346, 1985.
681. Bland JH, Schmidek HH: Symptomatic intraspinal cynovial cyst in a 66-year-old marathon runner. J Rheumatol 12:1006, 1985.
682. Corbetti F, Malatesta V, Camposampiero A, et al: Knee arthrography: Effects of various contrast media and epinephrine on synovial fluid. Radiology 161:195, 1986.
683. Warner JJ, Becker GJ, Robb JA, et al: Digital subtraction arthrography following hip arthroplasty. Appl Radiol 15:59, 1986.
684. Manaster BJ: Digital wrist arthrography: Precision in determining the site of radiocarpal-midcarpal communication. AJR 147:563, 1986.
685. Singson RD, Feldman F, Rosenberg ZS: Elbow joint: Assessment with double-contrast CT arthrography. Radiology 160:167, 1986.
686. Akbarnia BA, Silberstein ML, Rende RJ, et al: Arthrography in the diagnosis of fractures of the distal end of the humerus in infants. J Bone Joint Surg [Am] 68:599, 1986.
687. Beltran J, Gray L, Bools JC, et al: Rotator cuff lesions of the shoulder: Evaluation by direct sagittal CT arthrography. Radiology 160:161, 1986.
688. El-Khoury GY, Kathol MH, Chandler JB, et al: Shoulder instability: Impact of glenohumeral arthrotomography on treatment. Radiology 160:669, 1986.
689. Dorrell JH, Catterall A: The torn acetabular labrum. J Bone Joint Surg [Br] 68:400, 1986.
690. Burk DL Jr, Kanal E, Brunberg JA, et al: 1.5-T surface-coil MRI of the knee. AJR 147:293, 1986.
691. Gallimore GW Jr, Harms SE: Knee injuries: High-resolution MR imaging. Radiology 160:457, 1986.
692. Reicher MA, Hartzman S, Duckwiler GR, et al: Meniscal injuries: Detection using MR imaging. Radiology 159:753, 1986.
693. Spence KF Jr, Robertson RJ: Medial meniscal cysts. Orthopedics 9:1093, 1986.
694. Dumas J-M, Eddé DJ: Meniscal abnormalities: Prospective correlation of double-contrast arthrography and arthroscopy. Radiology 160:453, 1986.
695. Dory MA: Arthrography of the ankle joint in chronic instability. Skel Radiol 15:291, 1986.
696. Blanshard KS, Finlay DBL, Scott DJA, et al: A radiological analysis of lateral ligament injuries of the ankle. Clin Radiol 37:247, 1986.
697. Jacob JR, Weisman MH, Mink JH, et al: Reversible cause of back pain in rheumatoid arthritis: An apophyseal joint cyst. Arthritis Rheum 29:431, 1986.
698. McGinty JB, Johnson LL, Jackson RW, et al: Uses and abuses of arthroscopy: A symposium. J Bone Joint Surg [Am] 74:1563, 1992.
699. Hall FM: Arthrography: Past, present, and future. AJR 149:561, 1987.
700. Baker KS, Gilula LA: The current role of tenography and bursography. AJR 154:129, 1990.
701. Obermann WR, Kieft GJ: Knee arthrography: A comparison of iohexol, ioxaglate sodium meglumine, and metrizoate. Radiology 162:729, 1987.
702. Obermann WR, Bloem JL, Hermans J: Knee arthrography: Comparison of iotrolan and ioxaglate sodium meglumine. Radiology 173:197, 1989.
703. Mrose HE, Rosenthal DI: Arthrography of the hand and wrist. Hand Clin 7:201, 1991.
704. Quinn SF, Belsole RS, Greene TL, et al: Work in progress: Postarthrography computed tomography of the wrist: Evaluation of the triangular fibrocartilage complex. Skel Radiol 17:565, 1989.
705. Gilula LA, Hardy DC, Totty WG, et al: Fluoroscopic identification of torn intercarpal ligaments after injection of contrast material. AJR 149:761, 1987.
706. Pittman CC, Quinn SF, Belsole R, et al: Digital subtraction wrist arthrography: Use of double contrast technique as a supplement to single contrast arthrography. Skel Radiol 17:119, 1988.
707. Quinn SF, Pittman CC, Belsole R, et al: Digital subtraction wrist arthrography: Evaluation of the multiple-compartment technique. AJR 151:1173, 1988.
708. Belsole RJ, Quinn SF, Greene TL, et al: Digital subtraction arthrography of the wrist. J Bone Joint Surg [Am] 72:846, 1990.
709. Levinsohn EM, Palmer AK, Coren AB, et al: Wrist arthrography: The value of the three compartment injection technique. Skel Radiol 16:539, 1987.
710. Zinberg EM, Palmer AK, Coren AB, et al: The triple-injection wrist arthrogram. J Hand Surg [Am] 13:803, 1988.
711. Levinsohn EM, Rosen ID, Palmer AK: Wrist arthrography: Value of the three-compartment injection method. Radiology 179:231, 1991.
712. Manaster BJ: The clinical efficacy of triple-injection wrist arthrography. Radiology 178:267, 1991.
713. Wilson AJ, Gilula LA, Mann FA: Unidirectional joint communications in wrist arthrography: An evaluation of 250 cases. AJR 157:105, 1991.
714. Herbert TJ, Faithfull RG, McCann DJ, et al: Bilateral arthrography of the wrist. J Hand Surg [Br] 15:233, 1990.
715. Manaster BJ, Mann RJ, Rubenstein S: Wrist pain: Correlation of clinical and plain film findings with arthrographic results. J Hand Surg [Am] 14:466, 1989.
716. Gilula LA, Hardy DC, Totty WG: Distal radioulnar joint arthrography. AJR 150:864, 1988.
717. Hardy DC, Totty WG, Carnes KM, et al: Arthrographic surface anatomy of the carpal triangular fibrocartilage complex. J Hand Surg [Am] 13:823, 1988.
718. Viegas SF, Ballantyne G: Attritional lesions of the wrist joint. J Hand Surg [Am] 12:1025, 1987.
719. Maloney MD, Sauser DD, Hanson EC, et al: Adhesive capsulitis of the wrist: Arthrographic diagnosis. Radiology 167:187, 1988.
720. Hanson EC, Wood VE, Thiel AE, et al: Adhesive capsulitis of the wrist. Diagnosis and treatment. Clin Orthop 234:51, 1988.
721. Yates C, Sullivan JA: Arthrographic diagnosis of elbow injuries in children. J Pediatr Orthop 7:54, 1987.

722. Gundry CR, Schils JP, Resnick D, et al: Arthrography of the post-traumatic knee, shoulder, and wrist. Current status and future trends. Radiol Clin North Am 27:957, 1989.

723. Naimark A, Baum A: Pitfall to avoid. Injection of the subcoracoid bursa: A cause of technical failure in shoulder arthrography. J Can Assoc Radiol 40:170, 1989.

724. Sholkoff SD, Cook J: Arthrography for acromioclavicular joint cysts. AJR 151:838, 1988.

725. Crass JR: Current concepts in the radiographic evaluation of the rotator cuff. CRC Crit Rev Diagn Radiol 28:23, 1988.

726. Bjorkenheim J-M, Paavolainen P, Ahovuo J, et al: The intraarticular pressure during shoulder arthrography. A diagnostic aid in rotator cuff tear. Acta Orthop Scand 58:128, 1987.

727. Stiles RG, Resnick D, Sartoris DJ, et al: Rotator cuff disruption: Diagnosis with digital arthrography. Radiology 168:705, 1988.

728. Nelson MC, Leather GP, Nirschl RP, et al: Evaluation of the painful shoulder. A prospective comparison of magnetic resonance imaging, computerized tomographic arthrography, ultrasonography, and operative findings. J Bone Joint Surg [Am] 73:707, 1991.

729. Misamore GW, Woodward C: Evaluation of degenerative lesions of the rotator cuff. A comparison of arthrography and ultrasonography. J Bone Joint Surg [Am] 73:704, 1991.

730. Wasilewski SA, Frankl U: Rotator cuff pathology. Arthroscopic assessment and treatment. Clin Orthop 267:65, 1991.

731. Burk DL Jr, Karajick D, Kurtz AB, et al: Rotator cuff tears: Prospective comparison of MR imaging with arthrography, sonography, and surgery. AJR 153:87, 1989.

732. Fukuda H, Mikasa M, Yamanaka K: Incomplete thickness rotator cuff tears diagnosed by subacromial bursography. Clin Orthop 223:51, 1987.

733. Neviaser TJ: Adhesive capsulitis. Orthop Clin North Am 18:439, 1987.

734. Neviaser RJ, Neviaser TJ: The frozen shoulder. Diagnosis and management. Clin Orthop 223:59, 1987.

735. Keating JF, Kelly IG: Frozen shoulder: A retrospective analysis of 56 patients. J Orthop Rheumatol 3:11, 1990.

736. Parker RD, Froimson AI, Winsberg DD, et al: Frozen shoulder. I. Chronology, pathogenesis, clinical picture, and treatment. Orthopedics 12:868, 1989.

737. Morency G, Dussault RG, Robillard P, et al: Arthrographie distensive dans le traitement de la capsulite adhésive de l'épaule. J Can Assoc Radiol 40:84, 1989.

738. Corbeil V, Dussault RG, Leduc BE, et al: Capsulite rétractile de l'épaule: Étude comparative de l'arthrographie avec corticothérapie intra-articulaire avec ou sans distension capsulaire. J Can Assoc Radiol 43:127, 1992.

739. Ozaki J, Nakagawa Y, Sakurai G, et al: Recalcitrant chronic adhesive capsulitis of the shoulder. Role of contracture of the coracohumeral ligament and rotator interval in pathogenesis and treatment. J Bone Joint Surg [Am] 71:1511, 1989.

740. Rakofsky M, Arias C, Wagner JJ: Case report 633. Skel Radiol 19:532, 1990.

741. Ribbans WJ, Mitchell R, Taylor GJ: Computerized arthrotomography of primary anterior dislocation of the shoulder. J Bone Joint Surg [Br] 72:181, 1990.

742. Pennes DR, Jonsson K, Buckwalter K, et al: Computed arthrotomography of the shoulder: Comparison of examinations made with internal and external rotation of the humerus. AJR 153:1017, 1989.

743. Wilson AJ, Totty WG, Murphy WA, et al: Shoulder joint: Arthrographic CT and long-term follow-up, with surgical correlation. Radiology 173:329, 1989.

744. Habibian A, Stauffer A, Resnick D, et al: Comparison of conventional and computed arthrotomography with MR imaging in the evaluation of the shoulder. J Comput Assist Tomogr 13:968, 1989.

745. Singson RD, Feldman F, Bigliani LU, et al: Recurrent shoulder dislocation after surgical repair: Double-contrast CT arthrography. Work in progress. Radiology 164:425, 1987.

746. Pennes DR: Shoulder joint: Arthrographic CT appearance. Radiology 175:878, 1990.

747. Renner JB, Agee MW: Treatment of suppurative arthritis by percutaneous catheter drainage. AJR 154:135, 1990.

748. Kilcoyne RF, Kaplan P: The lateral approach for hip arthrography. Skel Radiol 21:239, 1992.

749. Walker CW, FitzRandolph RL, Collins DN, et al: Arthrography of painful hips following arthroplasty: Digital versus plain film subtraction. Skel Radiol 20:403, 1991.

750. Kelcz F, Peppler WW, Mistretta CA, et al: K-edge digital subtraction arthrography of the painful hip prosthesis: A feasibility study. AJR 155:1053, 1990.

751. Swan JS, Braunstein EM, Capello W: Aspiration of the hip in patients treated with Girdlestone arthroplasty. AJR 156:545, 1991.

752. Glynn TP Jr, Kreipke DL, DeRosa GP: Computed tomography arthrography in traumatic hip dislocation. Intra-articular and capsular findings. Skel Radiol 18:29, 1989.

753. Matsui M, Ohzono K, Saito S: Painful cystic degeneration of the limbus in the hip. J Bone Joint Surg [Am] 70:448, 1988.

754. Fritz P, Mariette X, Clerc D, et al: Rectus femoris sheath: A new localization of hip synovial cyst. J Rheumatol 16:1575, 1989.

755. Yasuda M, Ono M, Naono T, et al: Multiple rheumatoid bursal cysts. J Rheumatol 16:986, 1989.

756. Berquist TH, Bender CE, Maus TP, et al: Pseudobursae: A useful finding in patients with painful hip arthroplasty. AJR 148:103, 1987.

757. Silver SF, Connell DG, Duncan CP: Case report 550. Skel Radiol 18:327, 1989.

758. Staple TW, Mork A: Snapping tendon syndrome: Hip tenography with fluoroscopic monitoring. Radiology 166:873, 1988.

759. Harper MC, Schaberg JE, Allen WC: Primary iliopsoas bursography in the diagnosis of disorders of the hip. Clin Orthop 221:238, 1987.

760. Freiberger RH, Pavlov H: Knee arthrography. Radiology 166:489, 1988.

761. Langer JE, Meyer SJF, Dalinka MK: Imaging of the knee. Radiol Clin North Am 28:975, 1990.

762. Manco LG, Berlow ME: Meniscal tears—comparison of arthrography, CT, and MRI. CRC Crit Rev Diagn Imag 29:151, 1989.

763. Lantz B, Singer KM: Meniscal cysts. Clin Sports Med 9:707, 1990.

764. Woods GW, Whelan JM: Discoid meniscus. Clin Sports Med 9:695, 1990.

765. McCabe JP, Gilmore MFX: Spontaneous rupture of the suprapatellar bursa. J Bone Joint Surg [Br] 72:927, 1990.

766. Schäfer H: Synovialfalten des Kniegelenkes. Die Plica parapatellaris medialis. ROFO 147:640, 1987.

767. Hodge JC, Ghelman B, O'Brien SJ, et al: Synovial plicae and chondromalacia patellae: Correlation of results of CT arthrography with results of arthroscopy. Radiology 186:827, 1993.

768. Martinez D, Millner PA, Coral A, et al: Case report 745. Skel Radiol 21:393, 1992.

769. Armstrong SJ, Watt I: Lipoma arborescens of the knee. Br J Radiol 62:178, 1989.

770. Kirkham B, Churchill M, Dasgupta B, et al: Anterolateral rupture of popliteal cysts in rheumatoid arthritis. Ann Rheum Dis 50:187, 1991.

771. Petros DP, Hanley JF, Gilbreath P, et al: Posterior compartment syndrome following ruptured Baker's cyst. Ann Rheum Dis 49:944, 1990.

772. Haller J, Resnick D, Sartoris D, et al: Arthrography, tenography, and bursography of the ankle and foot. Clin Podiatr Med Surg 5:893, 1988.

773. Raatikainen T, Putkonen M, Puranen J: Arthrography, clinical examination, and stress radiograph in the diagnosis of acute injury to the lateral ligaments of the ankle. Am J Sports Med 20:2, 1992.

774. Wrazidlo W, Karl E-L, Koch K: Die arthrographische Diagnostik der vorderen Syndesmosenruptur am oberen Sprunggelenk. ROFO 148:492, 1988.

775. Bleichrodt RP, Kingma LM, Binnendijk B, et al: Injuries of the lateral ankle ligaments: Classification with tenography and arthrography. Radiology 173:347, 1989.

776. Reinus WR, Gilula LA, Lesiak LF, et al: Tenography in unresolved ankle tenosynovitis. Orthopedics 10:497, 1987.

777. Cheung Y, Rosenberg ZS, Magee T, et al: Normal anatomy and pathologic conditions of ankle tendons: Current imaging techniques. RadioGraphics 12:429, 1992.

778. Goossens M, De Stoop N, Claessens H, et al: Posterior subtalar joint arthrography. A useful tool in the diagnosis of hindfoot disorders. Clin Orthop 249:248, 1989.

779. Meyer J-M, Garcia J, Hoffmeyer P, et al: The subtalar sprain. A roentgenographic study. Clin Orthop 226:169, 1988.

780. Murtagh FR: Computed tomography and fluoroscopy guided anesthesia and steroid injection in facet syndrome. Spine 13:686, 1988.

781. Bjorkengren AG, Kurz LT, Resnick D, et al: Symptomatic intraspinal synovial cysts: Opacification and treatment by percutaneous injection. AJR 149:105, 1987.

782. Jackson RP, Jacobs RR, Montesano PX: Facet joint injection in low-back pain. A prospective statistical study. Spine 13:966, 1988.

783. Roy DF, Fleury J, Fontaine SB, et al: Clinical evaluation of cervical facet joint infiltration. J Can Assoc Radiol 39:118, 1988.

784. Hove B, Gyldensted C: Cervical analgesic facet joint arthrography. Neuroradiology 32:456, 1990.

785. Benhamou CL, Roux Ch, Gervais T, et al: Costo-vertebral arthropathy. Diagnositic and therapeutic value of arthrography. Clin Rheumatol 7:220, 1988.

786. Zobel MS, Borrello JA, Siegel MJ, et al: Pediatric knee MR imaging: Pattern of injuries in the immature skeleton. Radiology 190:397, 1994.

787. Richards RD, Sartoris DJ, Pathria MN, et al: Hill-Sachs lesion and normal humeral groove: MR imaging features allowing their differentiation. Radiology 190:665, 1994.

788. Ogden JA, Ganey TM, Arrington JA, et al: Meniscal ossification. I. Human. Skeletal Radiol 23:167, 1994.

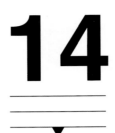

# 14

# Angiography

*Joseph J. Bookstein, M.D.*

Angiography fulfills a legitimate role in the imaging armamentarium of skeletal disease. Although the technique ordinarily is unnecessary, a broad variety of skeletal diseases constitute occasional indications for angiography. Vascular injury often coexists with musculoskeletal trauma and, if suspected, specific arteriographic diagnosis of the nature and extent of arterial injury usually is required. Active bleeding at sites not readily amenable to surgical control may be treated effectively by transcatheter hemostasis. In patients with bone tumors, arteriography sometimes is indicated for evaluation of tumor extent and nature, and also to assess any direct invasion or involvement of major arteries. Clinical manifestations of bone tumors can be palliated by intra-arterial chemotherapeutic infusions or by embolization. Articular disorders and vascular diseases may be confused: for example, a popliteal aneurysm or venous thrombosis may produce symptoms and signs that resemble those of arthritis or a synovial cyst. Angiomatous malformations may be diagnosed and treated through angio-

graphic techniques. Angiographic demonstration of arterial anatomy often is requested prior to the use of bone or soft tissue grafts. Thus, although each of the foregoing indications occurs infrequently, the large variety of indications results in reasonably frequent application of angiographic techniques in patients with skeletal disorders.

This chapter considers in some detail the role of arteriography in the assessment of musculoskeletal disease. Additional information related to this assessment can be found in many other chapters in this book.

## TRAUMA

Blunt or penetrating skeletal trauma is one of the most frequent indications for skeletal angiography.[1-3] Arteriography may demonstrate traumatic aneurysms, intimal dissections, transections, thromboses, and arteriovenous communications (Figs. 14–1 to 14–4). Even minor arterial injuries may lead to arterial thrombosis or embolization. Arteriography and vascular therapy, therefore, should be applied liberally and early, before the development of overt sequelae. Specific indications include the following:

1. Direct signs of vascular injury, such as pallor and decreased temperature of the injured extremity, loss of distal pulses, or vascular bruit.
2. Fracture with absent or diminished distal pulses.
3. Penetrating trauma proximate to a major artery, regardless of the presence or absence of direct signs of arterial injury.
4. Major pelvic hemorrhage after pelvic trauma, in which case transcatheter embolization is a particularly effective form of treatment.
5. Massive, disproportionate, or progressive limb swelling compatible with arterial or venous hemorrhage or venous thrombosis.

Although trauma often produces venous injury and venous hemorrhage, such injuries usually are of little additional clinical significance, and the veins are studied infrequently by venography.

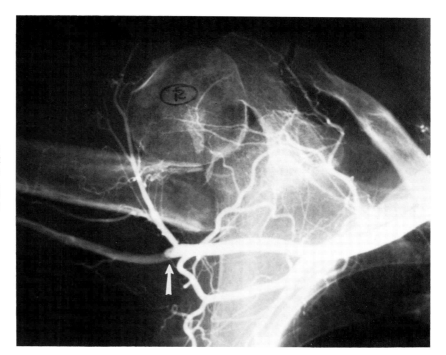

**FIGURE 14–1.** Arterial injury associated with blunt trauma to the shoulder. After the patient suffered this displaced humeral neck fracture, the entire upper extremity became pulseless, pale, and cool. The angiogram demonstrates an intimal tear and partial obstruction of the high brachial artery (arrow).

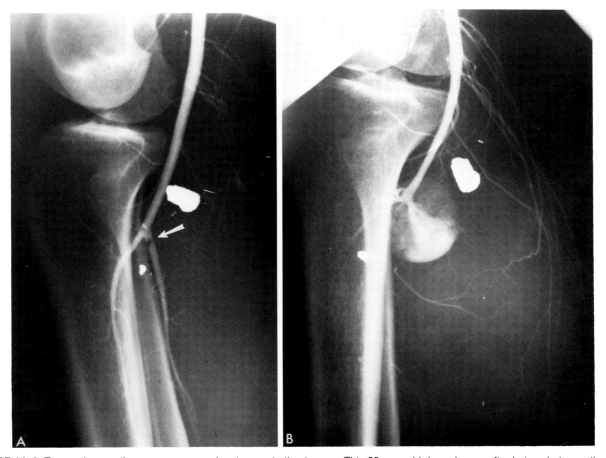

**FIGURE 14–2.** Traumatic mycotic aneurysm secondary to penetrating trauma. This 29 year old drug abuser, after being shot near the knee, had marked joint swelling and tenderness and a cool foot. After the initial arteriogram **(A)**, he developed a clostridial infection that was treated with hyperbaric oxygen. After institution of heparin therapy a month after injury, he developed a sudden painful, pulsatile swelling in the right popliteal fossa, clinically thought to represent an abscess or aneurysm.

　**A** Initial arteriogram demonstrates an intimal tear at the origin of the tibioperoneal trunk (arrow) and downstream compression of this artery by a hematoma. Also, several bullet fragments are evident.

　**B** Arteriogram obtained 1 month later, after sudden development of popliteal swelling, shows a mycotic aneurysm.

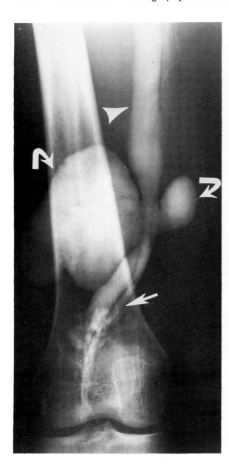

**FIGURE 14–3.** Pulsatile venous aneurysm and arteriovenous fistula after penetrating injury from an ice pick several years earlier. The arteriogram demonstrates two venous aneurysms at the site of fistula (curved arrows), early venous opacification of a somewhat dilated superficial femoral vein (arrowhead), and delayed flow in the small postfistulous popliteal artery (straight arrow).

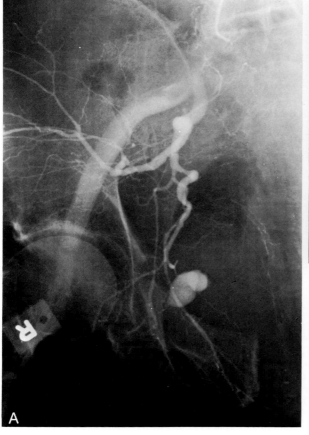

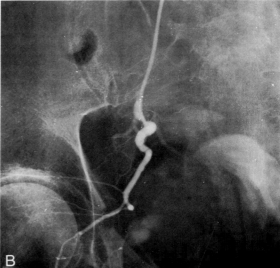

**FIGURE 14–4.** Pelvic fracture with massive hematoma. The patient had received 12 units of transfused blood. The hemorrhage was treated by embolization.

**A** The initial arteriogram demonstrates extravasation from the obturator artery.

**B** After transcatheter placement of two Gelfoam fragments, the bleeding artery has been obstructed, and the bleeding was controlled permanently.

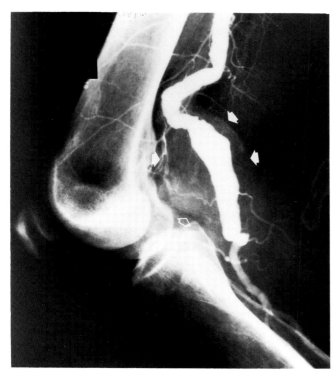

**FIGURE 14–5.** Ordinary atherosclerotic aneurysm in a patient with a cool left foot and barely pulsatile mass in left popliteal fossa. Note that much of the aneurysm is filled with nonopacified clot. The margin is demarcated by minimal intimal calcification (open and solid arrows). (Courtesy of L. Wexler, M.D., Stanford, California.)

## TRANSCATHETER HEMOSTASIS

Hemorrhage may occur in and around bones and joints, most frequently after trauma. Usually the hemorrhage is self-limited or is controlled surgically. Occasionally, however, control of the hemorrhage via transcatheter embolization may be an attractive alternative. For example, pelvic fractures, particularly those involving the pubic rami, may produce life-threatening hemorrhage. Selective catheterization and embolization of the appropriate internal iliac branches can be a simple life-saving measure[1, 4–6] (Fig. 14–4). Postoperative hemorrhage after orthopedic procedures, with or without associated infection, has been treated in the same manner.[7] Transcatheter therapy of hemophilic hemarthrosis also may be feasible.

## ANEURYSMS AND OTHER PRIMARY ARTERIAL DISEASES

### Aneurysms

Aneurysms not infrequently involve the popliteal artery (Fig. 14–5) and produce a mass in the popliteal space that simulates superficially joint disease or a soft tissue tumor. Clinical examination almost always reveals intrinsic pulsation, however, and the aneurysm will not expand the suprapatellar bursa, as would a knee joint effusion. Popliteal aneurysms rarely rupture but are prone to thrombose or produce downstream embolization. Although diagnosis is readily confirmed with ultrasonography or MR imaging, arteriography of the aneurysm and adjacent vessels is indicated in planning surgery.

Several articles report the development of arterial aneurysms in association with osteochondromas about the knee joint[8, 9] (see Chapter 83). The usual proximity of the popliteal artery to the rough aspect of the osteochondroma and the mechanical trauma secondary to motion of the knee joint combine to produce chronic arterial injury and eventual aneurysm. In the case illustrated in Figure 14–6, rapid expansion of the aneurysm simulated malignant transformation of the osteochondroma.

### Cystic Mucinous Degeneration

Cystic mucinous degeneration may involve the popliteal artery. The usual manifestations are ischemic, often of abrupt onset in young men, secondary to arterial obstruction by the cyst; rarely the mass is palpable, simulating a primary articular lesion. Hemorrhage into the cyst may occur, producing an intramural hematoma. The cause is unknown; a congenital origin is postulated by some investigators because the condition may affect relatively young patients.[10, 11]

### Popliteal Entrapment Syndrome

The popliteal entrapment syndrome is produced by compression of the popliteal artery by the medial head of the gastrocnemius muscle (Fig. 14–7). It generally is manifested as intermittent claudication in a young, otherwise normal patient. The compression may be due to either (1) abnormal position of the popliteal artery medial to the medial head of the gastrocnemius muscle, or (2) compression of a normally situated popliteal artery by an anomalous laterally inserting slip from the medial head of the gastrocnemius.[12, 13]

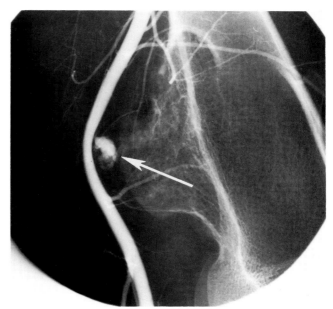

**FIGURE 14–6.** Aneurysm secondary to femoral exostosis. This patient with multiple exostoses developed pain, tenderness, and enlargement over an exostosis near the knee, and malignant degeneration was suspected.

Magnification arteriogram in the lateral view shows no pathologic vessels in the region of the exostosis to suggest malignancy. Instead, a pseudoaneurysm is beginning to opacify (arrow) at the site of chronic arterial injury from the exostosis.

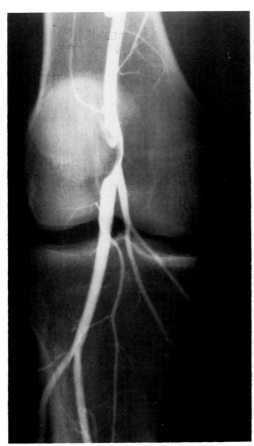

**FIGURE 14–7.** Popliteal entrapment syndrome. Compression of the popliteal artery by the medial head of the gastrocnemius muscle in a 20 year old man who developed claudication while at work. The artery appears to be smoothly compressed from its lateral aspect. The normal course of the artery suggests that compression is due to an aberrant slip of the medial head of the gastrocnemius muscle, not to an anomalous course of the popliteal artery medial to a normal gastrocnemius muscle. Some associated intimal changes were noted at operation. (Although this was not mentioned, the possibility of some mural thickening due to cyst or hemorrhage also is suspected.) Operative release of the head of the gastrocnemius muscle and endarterectomy resulted in relief of symptoms. (Courtesy of A. B. Crummy, M.D., Milwaukee, Wisconsin.)

### Hypothenar Hammer Syndrome

The hypothenar hammer syndrome is characterized by thrombosis, spasm, or aneurysm of the ulnar artery secondary to repetitive minor, usually occupational, trauma.[14] Because of the variability of the arterial supply to the fingers and the associated collateral circulation, any one finger or combination of fingers may show signs of ischemia. Arteriography demonstrates narrowing, occlusion, or aneurysm of the ulnar artery, usually adjacent to the hook of the hamate.[15] Most symptomatic patients will have multiple occlusions involving digital arteries, metacarpal arteries, and palmar arches. The distal occlusions apparently are secondary to emboli that have arisen within the ulnar artery (Fig. 14–8).

### TUMORS AND OTHER MASSES

Arteriography has been advocated in evaluating the type, extent, and behavioral characteristics of bone tumors.[16–21] In the author's opinion, this advocacy should be tempered somewhat. Biopsy is much more reliable in evaluating behavioral characteristics; plain films, CT scans, and MR images generally are adequate in determining extent (see Chapter 83).

Giant cell tumor usually involves para-articular bone, most frequently the femoral condyles. The tumor usually is hypervascular and has been studied angiographically with some frequency.[19, 22] An example is shown in Figure 14–9. Angiography may be relatively helpful in cases with an important soft tissue component.[19]

Angiography also has been used in tumor therapy.[23] Transcatheter embolization has been advocated in the palliative management of pain or hemorrhage of bone tumors[8, 24] (Fig. 14–9). Regression of arteriographic features of a bone tumor can play a useful role in evaluating response after chemotherapy.[25] Angiography may assume wider future application when effective chemotherapeutic agents are developed that are optimally administered intra-arterially, or when transcatheter embolization becomes more generally accepted.

Arteriography has assumed a larger role in evaluating the nature and extent of soft tissue masses.[16, 18, 21, 26–28] In the author's experience, the procedure is reliable only in the evaluation of arteriovenous malformations or hemangiomas, and even here reliability is incomplete (see Chapter 95). Examples of vascular malformations are shown in Figures 14–10 to 14–12. In some of these vascular masses, extent cannot be well evaluated angiographically because all or portions of the lesion may not opacify, even after pharmacoangiography.[16, 26] Although histologic-arteriographic correlates of malignancy or benignancy have been described, their accuracy may be insufficient for clinical application.

Transcatheter therapy is being applied increasingly in the management of peripheral vascular malformations.[28–31] Temporary control of pain, swelling, or hemorrhage usually can be achieved by obstructing major vessels leading to the malformation, but symptoms usually recur after a variable period of time owing to development of collateral circulation (Fig. 14–11). Efforts currently are being directed toward embolic obliteration of the small vessels within the lesion, rather than the large feeding vessels outside the lesion, in an attempt to prevent recurrences.

### AUTOIMMUNE DISEASES

A considerable number of arterial diseases have been described that are loosely characterized by inflammation, proliferation, or destruction of components of the arterial wall. Many are associated with symptoms and signs of arthritis. Polyarteritis nodosa, Takayasu's arteritis, and giant cell arteritis are examples of such diseases. These diseases generally are believed to have an autoimmune basis and to be a response to intravascular deposition of immune complexes or to attachment of autoimmune antibodies to arterial and other tissues. These diseases have been classified by a variety of schema[32–34] (see Chapter 36): by histologic appearance (polyarteritis nodosa, giant cell arteritis, necrotizing arteritis, leukocytoclastic angiitis); by areas of involvement (temporal arteritis, polymyalgia rheumatica); by pathogenesis (allergic arteritis); by acuteness of disease (Churg-Strauss arteritis); by size of vessel involved (aorti-

*Text continued on page 419*

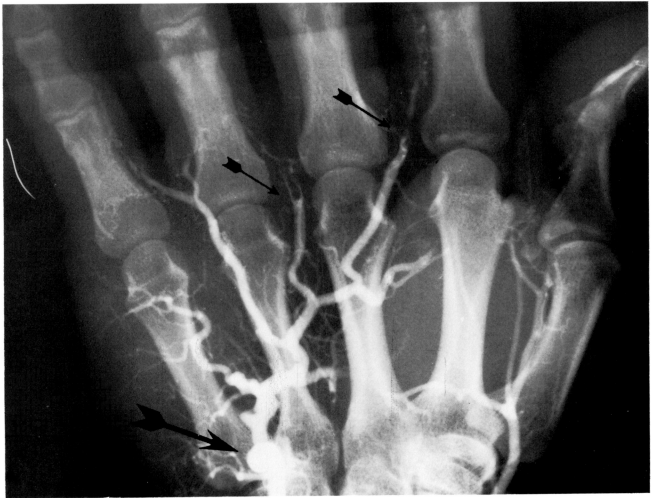

**FIGURE 14–8.** Hypothenar hammer syndrome. This 30 year old tool and dye worker had symptoms of Raynaud's phenomenon. His occupation involved repeated minor trauma to the ulnar aspect of his hand. The arteriogram demonstrates minor irregularity and dilation of the distal ulnar artery (large arrow). Multiple small emboli have originated in the ulnar artery and lodged in the proper digital arteries (small arrows).

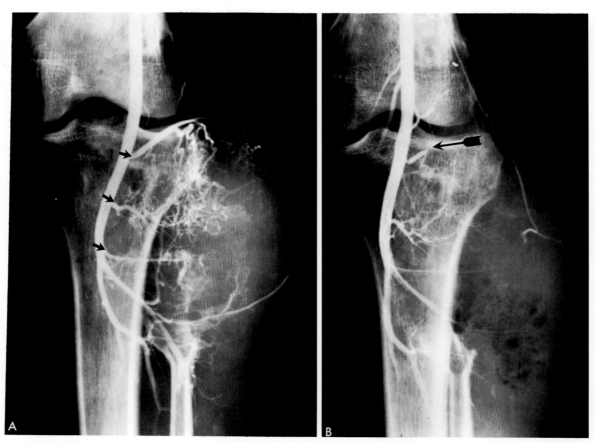

**FIGURE 14–9.** Diagnostic and therapeutic arteriography of a giant cell tumor. Thirty-five year old man with giant cell tumor of the fibula. The patient already had had two other giant cell tumors removed from other sites, and had another tumor in the opposite leg. Bleeding had been severe and difficult to control after prearteriographic biopsy. Arteriography was performed as part of a plan to resect the multiple, histologically benign giant cell lesions while trying to avoid amputation and maintain locomotive ability.

   **A** Arteriogram demonstrates abundant tumor vessels of the fibular lesion (arrows). There also appears to be tumor vascularity within the tibia (subsequently confirmed by additional biopsy).

   **B** Arteriogram after embolization demonstrates effective devascularization of the tumor. Gas in the soft tissues is secondary to an intervening biopsy. Arrow indicates the site of occlusion of the lateral inferior geniculate artery.

   (From Feldman F, et al: AJR *123*:130, 1975. Copyright 1975, American Roentgen Ray Society.)

**FIGURE 14–10.** Angiography of a para-artic- ular soft tissue hemangioma. Thirty year old man with limited ability to extend the elbow. Minor soft tissue fullness was present on clinical examination. Prior operations had re- vealed infiltrating hemangioma.

**A** Arterial phase shows no definite abnor- mality.

**B** Parenchymal phase 15 minutes after intra-arterial injection of tolazoline (Prisco- line) shows faint accumulations of contrast medium in the hemangioma. The striated pattern of accumulation indicates diffuse in- filtration of muscle by the lesion, confirmed at exploratory operation.

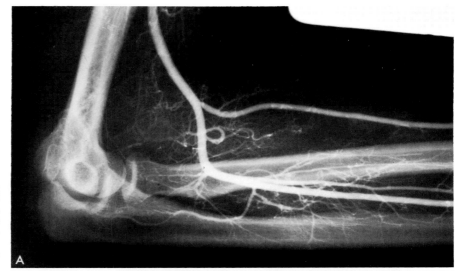

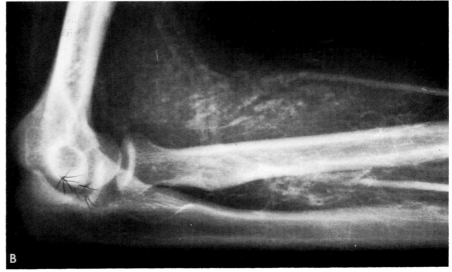

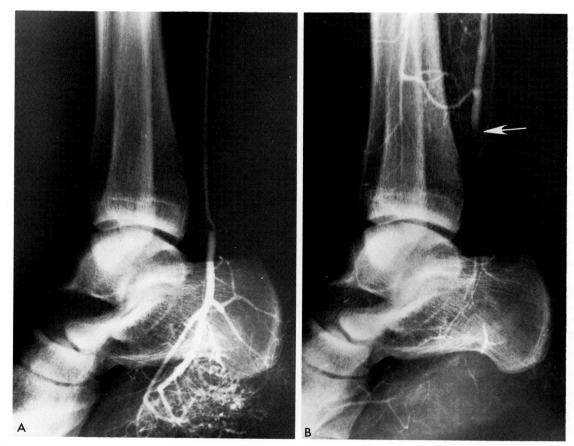

**FIGURE 14–11.** Transcatheter therapy of a subcalcaneal hemangioma. This 16 year old boy had severe pain on walking due to this hemangioma. Three previous operations had not provided permanent relief, and amputation was being considered.

**A** Posterior tibial arteriogram prior to embolization shows most of the hypervascular lesion.

**B** After embolization with both small and large particles of Ivalon (Unipoint, Inc., High Point, North Carolina), the hemangioma is poorly perfused. The posterior tibial artery became occluded (arrow) after the smaller emboli had been delivered into the lesion.

Clinical status improved greatly, and the patient was relatively asymptomatic for 1 year, when pain again returned. Repeat arteriography demonstrated persistent occlusion of the embolized arteries, but additional collateral vessels to the lesion had developed, which were reembolized. Three separate embolic therapeutic sessions eventually were held, with clinical improvement after each one. Each time, smaller Ivalon fragments were being used, in an effort to obliterate the lesion from within.

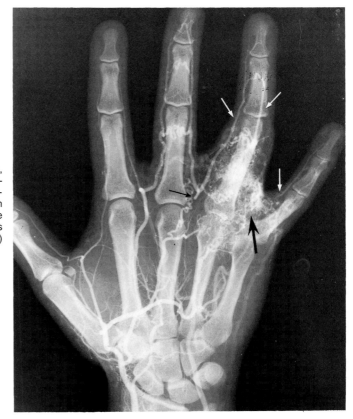

**FIGURE 14–12.** Angiography of typical arteriovenous malformation, which persisted after ligation of several feeding arteries. Arteriography again was performed in preparation for another attempt at removal of this para-articular mass, which limited mobility at the fourth metacarpophalangeal joint, and which bled intermittently. Despite prior surgical occlusion of all of the regional proper digital arteries (small arrows), these arteries as well as the lesion (large arrow) continue to opacify via collateral routes.

tis, polyarteritis nodosa of medium-sized vessels); by constellation of involved organs or tissues (small vessels of lung and kidney—Wegener's disease; capillaries of lung and kidney—Goodpasture's syndrome; medium-sized arteries, synovial membranes, muscle tenderness—polymyalgia arteritica[31, 35]). Because of the lack of general agreement regarding classification as well as the tremendous overlap among diseases, and for want of a system based on fundamental objective criteria, it may be advisable to characterize the arteritides by specifying all the aforementioned features: acuteness; vessels, organs, and tissues involved; histologic evidence of necrosis, giant cells, aneurysms, or intimal proliferation; and angiographic evidence of aneurysms or intimal proliferation.

### Rheumatoid Arthritis

Rheumatoid arthritis is expressed predominantly as a disease of synovial membranes, but in a significant percentage of cases vascular disease also is present, which occasionally becomes of clinical significance. Muscle biopsies have revealed arteritis in 8.8 per cent of cases of rheumatoid arthritis,[36] and active vasculitis has been noted in 25 per cent of an autopsied series.[37] Histologic features of rheumatoid vasculitis include mild perivascular or adventitial inflammation, intimal thickening with little or no cellular reaction,[38, 39] arterial thromboses, and necrotizing arteriolar panarteritis.[40] Corticosteroid therapy has been implicated as a possible etiologic factor in those cases with necrotizing arteritis. Aortitis or aortic valvulitis also is an associated finding,[41] and spontaneous aortic rupture has been reported

after steroid therapy for rheumatoid arthritis.[42] Arteriographic studies have been infrequent. Laws and colleagues[39] demonstrated arterial stenoses of the digital arteries in 26 of 38 patients with rheumatoid arthritis, with frequent collateral circulation. Nonspecific hyperemia was present in 22 of 37 patients, particularly near bony erosions or regions of synovial proliferation in joints or tendon sheaths.

### Giant Cell Arteritis

Giant cell arteritis (also called temporal, cranial, or granulomatous arteritis) is a form of vasculitis characterized histologically by necrosis of the arterial wall and granulomatous vascular reaction with giant cells. Medium-sized arteries, such as the temporal, subclavian, or popliteal arteries, are involved most frequently, but virtually any artery, including the aorta, may be affected. Many extravascular manifestations are associated, including fatigue, fever, anorexia, weight loss, synovitis, and visual disturbances.[9]

### Polymyalgia Rheumatica

Polymyalgia rheumatica (also called polymyalgia arteritica) is characterized by recurrent rheumatic discomfort involving muscles and joints, particularly of the shoulder and hip girdles, systemic manifestations of fever and malaise, elevated sedimentation rate, and, usually, associated arteritis of medium-sized vessels.[11, 29] Two thirds of patients will have palpable synovial thickening or effusion at some point during their illness. Hands and sternoclavicular, acromioclavicular, sacroiliac, and pubic joints are predisposed to

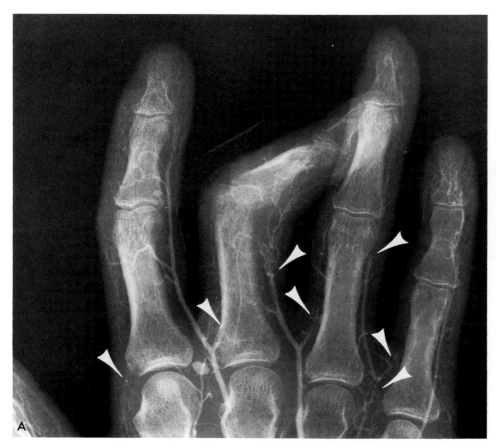

**FIGURE 14–13.** Examples of digital involvement in several arteritides.
**A** Scleroderma. Note multiple proper digital arterial occlusions (arrowheads) and marked ulnar deviation of the middle phalanx of the third finger due to scleroderma. Minor irregularities of the proper digital artery of the index finger also are present.

*Illustration continued on opposite page*

involvement. Joint biopsy will demonstrate nonspecific synovitis and capsulitis. Arterial biopsy will show arteritis in about 50 per cent of cases; usually giant cells are prominent, and the appearance and distribution of disease generally are indistinguishable from those of giant cell arteritis. The marked overlap between polymyalgia rheumatica and giant cell arteritis suggests that both are manifestations of the same disease process.[43]

### Scleroderma

Scleroderma (Figs. 14–13 and 14–14) is expressed primarily as a disease of small arteries, but joint involvement, often resembling rheumatoid arthritis, is not infrequent.[44, 45] In a series of 24 patients with scleroderma who had arthritic symptoms, one or more skeletal abnormalities were present in the hands or wrists of each; in seven patients, features resembled rheumatoid arthritis.[44] Histologic examination of digital arteries from patients with scleroderma consistently has revealed uniquely extensive arterial disease.[39] Intimal arteriolar thickening is the most frequent manifestation, but panarteritis also may occur. Small arteries throughout the body may be involved. The kidneys are particularly predisposed, and small renal vessels, usually at the interlobular level, are involved in 90 per cent of persons dying with the disease.[46]

Angiography reflects the severe arterial disease noted histologically. In a review of 31 digital arteriograms of patients with scleroderma,[47] severe stenoses or occlusions,

usually multiple, were present in 29. Most commonly the proper digital arteries were involved in their middle or distal portions. The vascular beds of the terminal digits often were obliterated. In patients with clinical evidence of renal disease, renal arteriography usually demonstrates extensive obstructive and occlusive disease of interlobular arteries and innumerable renal cortical microinfarcts and scars (Fig. 14–14).

### Systemic Lupus Erythematosus

Systemic lupus erythematosus (SLE) (Fig. 14–13) is the most frequent of the collagen vascular disorders. Its features reveal significant overlap with those of rheumatoid arthritis. Approximately one third of patients with rheumatoid arthritis will show positive LE cell preparations, and an equal number of patients with SLE will have a positive test for rheumatoid factor.[48, 49] Most patients will have arthritic symptoms at some point in the course of disease, and radiographic signs of soft tissue or bony abnormalities also are frequent.[24, 50] For example, hand radiographs in 59 patients with SLE demonstrated abnormalities in 34, most commonly periarticular calcification or swelling, acral sclerosis, malalignment, or soft tissue calcification.[24]

Vascular manifestations of SLE generally are confined to the very small arteries, such as interlobular arteries of the kidney, or to renal glomerular capillaries. Histologic changes may vary widely; mild abnormalities are characterized by deposition of fibrinoid material within the intima,

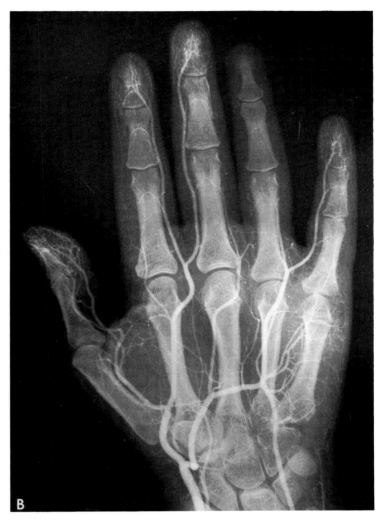

**FIGURE 14–13** *Continued*

**B** Systemic lupus erythematosus. Ordinarily such large arteries are not involved in systemic lupus erythematosus, but in this patient the proper digital arteries of the second through fifth digits show occlusions indistinguishable from those in scleroderma.

*Illustration continued on following page*

generally accompanied by fibroblast proliferation. Progressive deposition of material leads to luminal compromise and destruction of wall muscle and elastic elements. In advanced disease, necrotizing arteritis can develop.[51] Digital arteriograms in some patients with SLE show arterial occlusions that may be indistinguishable from those occurring in scleroderma (Fig. 14–13B). Renal arteriograms in SLE reaffirm the predominantly small-vessel distribution of disease; most abnormality occurs within renal glomeruli, with loss of glomerular granularity on magnification renal arteriograms. Interlobular arteries commonly are narrowed but are not occluded.

### Polyarteritis Nodosa

Polyarteritis nodosa (Figs. 14–13 and 14–14), along with the other collagen vascular diseases that already have been mentioned, frequently produces mild arthralgias and myalgias, but actual joint effusion is unusual. The predominant manifestation is a necrotizing arteritis that may affect arteries anywhere in the body. Arteriography of involved areas may demonstrate small aneurysms, a feature virtually pathognomonic of necrotizing arteritis. Aneurysms may not develop, or at least are not visible, in many cases. Once

formed, they also may disappear, apparently as a result of healing.[52] Other features include arterial stenoses, occlusions, collateral circulation, marginal irregularities, and evidence of tissue infarction. Arteries in and around joints may be affected (Fig. 14–13C) but rarely are studied angiographically. Renal arteries are involved in a high percentage of cases, usually in patients with hypertension or hematuria, and renal arteriography may be the most effective method for reaching a diagnosis (Fig. 14–14B).

### VENOUS DISEASES

The swelling and tenderness of thrombophlebitis sometimes may simulate joint disease clinically. Venography is the most definitive diagnostic procedure. In the presence of thrombosis of lower extremity veins, intraluminal defects due to thrombi almost always are visualized (Fig. 14–15). Fresh thrombi largely fill the obstructed venous lumen, and commonly they demonstrate convex proximal and distal margins. A thin rim of contrast medium may be insinuated between the thrombus and the venous wall.

A popliteal cyst of the knee joint may simulate the swelling of thrombophlebitis.[53] Contrast arthrography, as well as MR imaging and venography, will permit specific diagno-

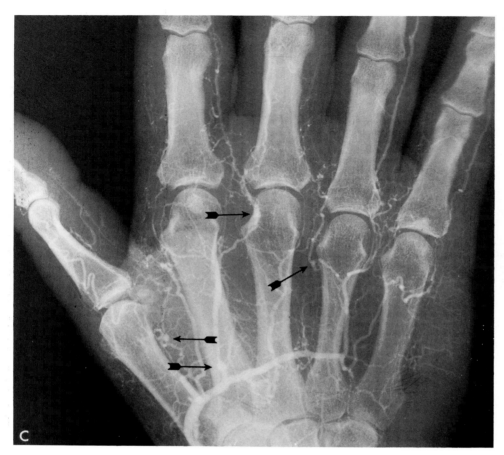

**FIGURE 14–13** *Continued*
**C** Polyarteritis nodosa. Multiple proper digital arteries and the ulnar artery are occluded, a distribution similar to that of scleroderma. The presence of a number of small aneurysms (arrows), however, suggests the possibility of a necrotizing arteritis.

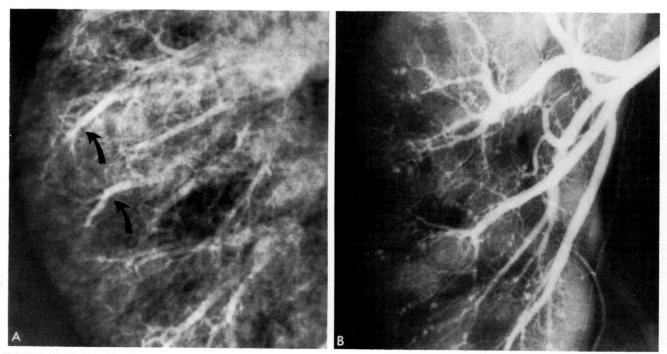

**FIGURE 14–14.** Renal involvement in various arteritides.
  **A** Scleroderma (3 ×). Arteries visualized (arrows) are the distal interlobar arteries. Interlobular arteries of the cortex are not seen, because they are either occluded or markedly narrowed. The coarse mottling of the nephrogram reflects multiple tiny scars due to microinfarcts.
  **B** Polyarteritis nodosa (nonmagnified angiography). The disease tends to involve arteries of larger caliber than does scleroderma. Note multiple occlusions of distal interlobar arteries, with multiple associated aneurysms reflecting the presence of a necrotizing process.

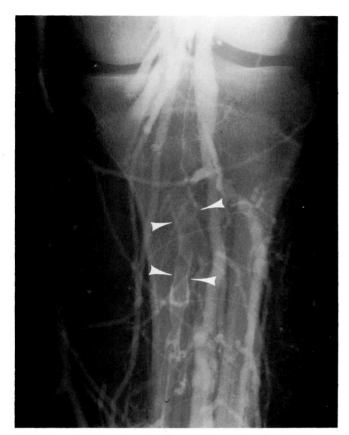

**FIGURE 14–15.** Thrombophlebitis producing pain and swelling about the knee joint. Note the thin accumulation of contrast medium between the intraluminal thrombus and the vein wall, confirming the presence of thrombus (arrowheads).

sis. Indeed, a popliteal cyst may coexist with venous obstruction, in view of the propensity of these cysts to obstruct the popliteal vein.

## Klippel-Trenaunay Syndrome

A triad consisting of cutaneous hemangiomas, bone and soft tissue hypertrophy, and venous varices has been termed the Klippel-Trenaunay syndrome (see Chapter 63). A broad spectrum of expressions is reported: involvement of one lower extremity; involvement of multiple limbs; diffuse skeletal and facial involvement; vascular malformations (sometimes bleeding); hypertrophy of the pelvis and viscera; arteriovenous malformations (Parke-Weber syndrome); lymphatic malformations.[54, 55] In the author's experience, most patients have had involvement of only one lower extremity by port-wine cutaneous hemangioma, bone and soft tissue hypertrophy, and varices. Angiography ordinarily was requested to evaluate the possibility of arteriovenous malformation, but in none of the author's cases was such malformation present, and the arteries appeared normal. Instead, a venous abnormality of the deep system was present in each of these cases. Usually the venous abnormality was characterized by total absence of all or part of the deep system (Fig. 14–16). In one or two cases, only a localized stenosis of the deep system was present.

## MISCELLANEOUS DISORDERS

### Occupational Acro-osteolysis

Occupational acro-osteolysis was described in 1967 by Wilson and coworkers.[56] The syndrome (see Chapter 94) is characterized primarily by resorption of portions of distal phalangeal tufts, some digital tenderness, and Raynaud's phenomenon. It was observed in 31 of 3000 workers involved in the manufacture of polyvinylchloride.[50] Arteriography in one patient demonstrated mild hypervascularity adjacent to areas of bone resorption (Fig. 14–17) and distal occlusion of the princeps pollicis artery.

### Frostbite

The importance of vascular injury in the pathogenesis of frostbite is well recognized.[57, 58] Experimental studies have demonstrated that within minutes of thawing, capillaries and venules become occluded with thrombi. Several hours later, most of the blood flow is via peripheral precapillary shunts. Arteriography will demonstrate marked slowing of blood flow in sizeable branches, probably due to spasm and more distal obstruction (Fig. 14–18). As the condition improves, arterial flow improves, but residual occlusions may persist.

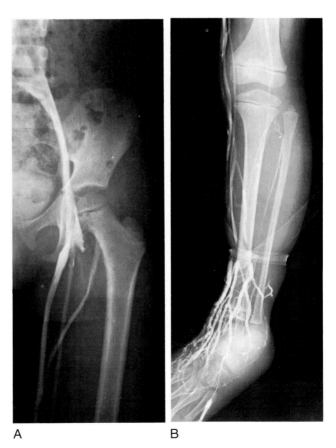

A         B

**FIGURE 14–16.** Klippel-Trenaunay syndrome in an 8 year old girl. This patient had relatively increased length and thickness of the left lower extremity, a port-wine malformation over the thigh and buttock, and varices. The venogram demonstrates complete absence of a deep venous system in the leg and thigh. The iliac vein is smaller than usual but otherwise normal.

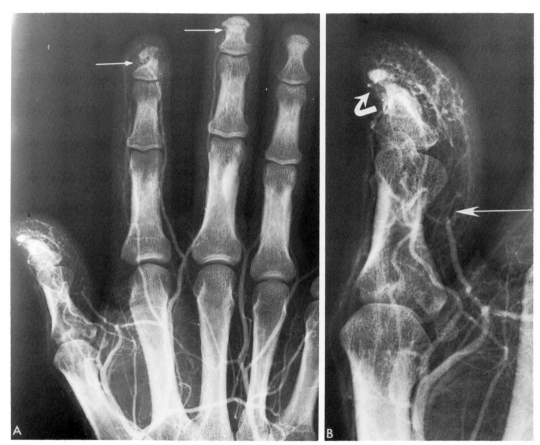

**FIGURE 14–17.** Occupational acro-osteolysis. A 28 year old man with a history of 2½ years of exposure to polyvinylchloride complained of tingling and pallor of the hands on exposure to cold. The hands had swollen intermittently in response to cold in the past but now were swollen permanently.

**A** Conventional arteriogram of the hand shows no major arterial occlusions, except in the thumb. There has been resorption of the distal phalanges, producing transverse defects (arrows).

**B** Arteriogram of the thumb, performed on cardboard. Note the excellent detail that can be obtained with this technique. Straight arrow indicates the site of occlusion of the princeps pollicis artery. Curved arrow indicates the transverse line of bone resorption. (From Bookstein JJ: *In* AK Poznanski [Ed]: The Hand in Radiologic Diagnosis. Philadelphia, WB Saunders Co, 1974.)

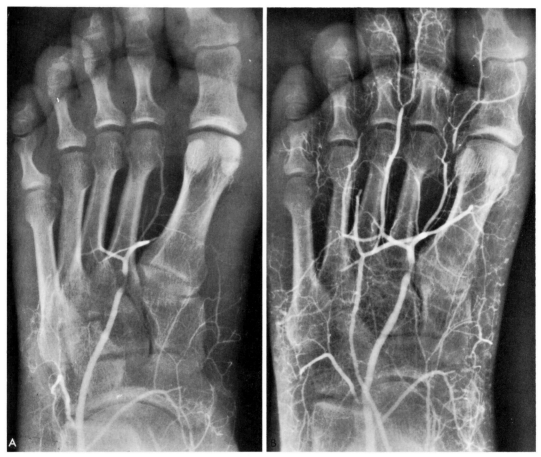

**FIGURE 14–18.** Frostbite. A 30 year old man suffered pedal frostbite after becoming lost and walking in the snow for 36 hours.

**A** Angiography of the left foot 3 days after cold exposure showed slow flow with concentric tubular narrowing of the distal dorsalis pedis artery, severe spasm of the metatarsal arch, and lack of opacification of the digital arteries of the first, third, fourth, and fifth toes. Reserpine (0.5 mg) was injected into the left superficial femoral artery.

**B** Repeat angiography after 2 days demonstrates much less spasm. Portions of all toes now are perfused. The patient was discharged a few weeks later, after losing only a small amount of tissue from the large toe.

(From Gralino BJ, et al: Radiology *119*:301, 1976.)

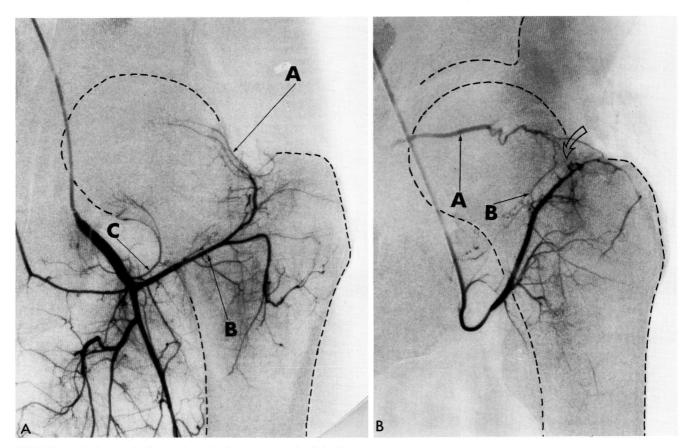

**FIGURE 14–19.** Superselective angiography in osteonecrosis of the hip.

**A** Normal left hip for comparison. Superselective injection of the medial circumflex artery. A, Superior capsular branches; B, superior branch of the medial circumflex artery, which surrounds the femoral neck posteriorly; C, inferior capsular branch.

**B** Necrosis of the left femoral head. Mild depression of the femoral head was evident on plain lateral projection. Superselective injection of the superior branch of the medial circumflex artery shows obvious interruption of the superior capsular arteries and their stumps (open arrow). Reflux of contrast material from a hypertrophied posterior branch of the femoral neck (B) into the inferior gluteal artery is seen (A).

(Modified after Théron J: Radiology *124*:649, 1977.)

## Osteonecrosis of the Femoral Head

The ischemic origin of osteonecrosis of the femoral head has been assumed for many years. Théron[59] has demonstrated occlusion of the superior capsular arteries in such patients using superselective arteriography of the medial and lateral circumflex, obturator, and superior and inferior gluteal arteries (Fig. 14–19). Normally, the femoral head is supplied primarily by arteries arising from the medial femoral circumflex artery. In patients with idiopathic osteonecrosis of the femoral head, occlusion of branches may be evident in the early phases. Later the branches may recanalize. It remains to be determined, however, whether the arterial occlusion is the cause or the effect of the necrosis.

Phlebography and manometry of the diaphysis or metaphysis of tubular bones have been performed in ischemic necrosis and other affections of the hip. Findings frequently have been interpreted as reflecting partial venous obstruction or inadequacy.[60–62] Several authors[60, 62] have implied that venography holds a place in clinical management or in earlier diagnosis. In the author's opinion, the range of normal phlebograms still is inadequately defined, the interpretations are difficult and subjective, and the images seem partially dependent on technical factors.

## Reflex Sympathetic Dystrophy

Reflex sympathetic dystrophy syndrome currently is the accepted term for a constellation of symptoms that may follow trauma to the upper or lower extremity (see Chapter 51). The symptoms generally are out of proportion to the severity of injury and are manifested by several of the following characteristics: (1) intense or unduly prolonged pain that may persist long after obvious skin or bone injuries have healed, (2) vasomotor disturbances, particularly erythema, (3) delayed functional recovery, and (4) various trophic changes of bone and skin. Synonyms of reflex sympathetic dystrophy include painful posttraumatic osteoporosis, Sudeck's atrophy, causalgia, and the shoulder-hand syndrome.[63–65] This syndrome also may develop after bypass vascular surgery for peripheral vascular insufficiency.

The most tenable explanation for the syndrome is that trauma produces a self-sustaining disturbance of autonomic regulation. No consensus has yet been reached regarding the exact mechanism of nerve injury, nerve feedback, and amplification. Clinical features include extreme sensitivity of the skin in the involved region; skin erythema, warmth, and swelling; unwillingness to use the extremity; and radiographic evidence of osteoporosis.

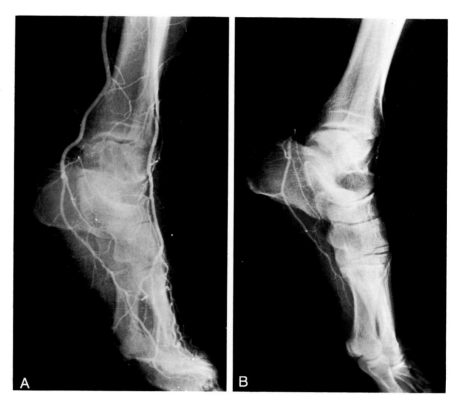

**FIGURE 14–20.** Reflex sympathetic dystrophy. Two months earlier, this 50 year old man had had a ligamentous injury of the knee after sliding into second base in a baseball game. Pain subsequently had been constant and somewhat progressive. The leg was slightly swollen and had a bluish discoloration suggesting thrombophlebitis. A venogram had been normal. The arteriogram was obtained to evaluate arteriovenous shunting.

**A** The initial study demonstrates enlarged anterior and posterior tibial vessels. All of the small arteries of the foot were dilated, and the veins opacified densely and early. Contrast material reached the foot about 10 seconds earlier on the involved leg than on the normal contralateral leg.

**B** The second arteriogram was obtained after intra-arterial infusion of 6 mg of the beta-adrenergic blocker propranolol (Inderal). The pain had disappeared, and remained in abeyance for 20 days. The arteries have resumed normal caliber, and arteriovenous shunting has disappeared.

Various features of this syndrome have suggested the possibility of vascular disease. The angiographic features in reflex sympathetic dystrophy may be somewhat unusual (Fig. 14–20). Blood flow is markedly accelerated on the involved side, with dilation of small veins (particularly of the heel pad) and early venous opacification. These features suggest opening of precapillary arteriovenous shunts. After placing a tourniquet on the leg, the arteries may constrict disproportionately and the signs of increased flow may disappear promptly, but temporarily.

A variety of treatments have been advocated, including acupuncture, physical therapy, corticosteroids, and sympathectomy. Marked clinical benefit has been described after intravenous injection of the beta-adrenergic antagonist propranolol.[63, 64] Immediately after such therapy, arteriography may show disappearance of the hypervascularity and a normal rate of flow (Fig. 14–20).

### Fibrous Dysplasia

The bony lesions of fibrous dysplasia may be quite hypervascular, although the degree of vascularity probably is variable.[66–68] Hypervascular lesions may assume clinical significance through spontaneous hemorrhage; isolated reports of spontaneous scalp or nasal hemorrhage may be found.[66, 68] When bony lesions are very extensive, high output cardiac failure can occur.

The author has encountered a 13 year old girl with the McCune-Albright syndrome (fibrous dysplasia, sexual precocity, and café-au-lait spots). Her osseous fibrodysplastic lesions were extensive and involved all four extremities, the shoulder and pelvic girdles, and the skull and spine. Some of her most distressing symptoms were the result of high output cardiac failure. Cardiac catheterization indicated output of 22 liters/min. Bruits were present over the thighs, and superimposed arteriovenous malformations had been suspected. Arteriography, however, indicated that the fibrous dysplastic lesions themselves explained the arteriovenous shunting. Each lesion demonstrated marked hypervascularity (Fig. 14–21), with enlarged arterial feeders and early opacification of large draining medullary veins.

### Massive Osteolysis of Gorham

This rare syndrome is characterized by rapidly progressive osteolysis of one or several bones (see Chapter 94). The process may lead to complete disappearance of the affected bones, but prognosis for life is good.[69] The major long bones and pelvic or shoulder girdles are involved most frequently. Young adults are affected most often, and a history of preceding trauma is common. The pathologic tissue is characterized by proliferating capillaries. The cause is unknown, although some physicians consider the disease to be a form of hemangiomatosis.

Arteriograms have been described as demonstrating hypervascularity with arteriovenous shunting.[70] The vascular pattern is not suggestive of neoplasm, and, in this regard, arteriography may be of differential diagnostic value.

### SUMMARY

The role of angiography in the diagnosis and treatment of a variety of musculoskeletal problems is described in this chapter. This role includes the documentation of vascular injury after trauma, the control of hemorrhage, the visualization of a variety of primary arterial diseases that are

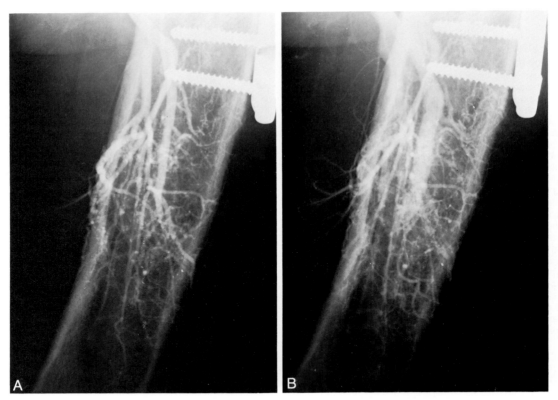

**FIGURE 14–21.** McCune-Albright syndrome. This 13 year old girl had extensive lesions of fibrous dysplasia throughout her body, café-au-lait spots, and precocious puberty. Numerous pathologic fractures had occurred in the past. Arteriography was performed to demonstrate the location of some of the major arteriovenous shunts and to evaluate the efficacy of transcatheter embolization. The magnification arteriograms of a femoral lesion demonstrate the typical hypervascularity and arteriovenous shunting that were observed in many other lesions as well. In **A**, note the increased numbers of medullary vessels. In **B**, early dense opacification of a large vein is present.

associated with or may resemble joint disease, the evaluation of the nature and extent of soft tissue masses, the visualization of arteritis complicating collagen vascular disorders, and the detection of peripheral venous abnormalities, which may simulate articular or periarticular disease.

## References

1. Ben-Menachem Y, Coldwell DM, Young JW, et al: Hemorrhage associated with pelvic fractures: Causes, diagnosis, and emergent management. AJR *157*:1005, 1991.
2. Damron T, McBeath A: Diagnosis and management of vascular injuries associated with skeletal trauma. Orthop Rev *19*:1063, 1990.
3. Odland MD, Gisbert VL, Gustilo RB, et al: Combined orthopedic and vascular injury in the lower extremities: Indications for amputation. Surgery *108*:660, 1990.
4. Ring EJ, Athanasoulis C, Waltman AC, et al: Arteriographic management of hemorrhage following pelvic fracture. Radiology *109*:65, 1973.
5. Ring EJ, Waltman AC, Athanasoulis C, et al: Angiography in pelvic trauma. Surg Gynecol Obstet *139*:375, 1974.
6. van Urk H, Perlberger RR, Muller H: Selective arterial embolization for control of traumatic pelvic hemorrhage. Surgery *83*:133, 1978.
7. Rubin BE, Fortune WP, May MM: Therapeutic embolization for postoperative hemorrhage about the hip of a patient with Pseudomonas infection. J Bone Joint Surg [Am] *60*:988, 1978.
8. Rouanet JP, Chalut J, Bacourt F, et al: Rare cause of arterial aneurysm: Exostosis. J Radiol Electrol Med Nucl *57*:171, 1976.
9. Greenway G, Resnick D, Bookstein JJ: Popliteal pseudoaneurysm as a complication of adjacent osteochondroma: Angiographic diagnosis. AJR *132*:294, 1979.
10. DeLaurentis DA, Wolferth CC, Wolf FM, et al: Mucinous adventitial cysts of the popliteal artery in an 11 year old girl. Surgery *74*:456, 1973.
11. Schlesinger A, Gottesman L: Cystic degeneration of the popliteal artery. AJR *127*:1043, 1976.
12. Inada K, Hirose M, Iwashima Y, et al: Popliteal artery entrapment syndrome: A case report. Br J Surg *65*:613, 1978.
13. Insua JA, Young JR, Humphries AW: Popliteal artery entrapment syndrome. Arch Surg *101*:771, 1970.
14. Conn J, Bergan JJ, Bell JL: Hypothenar hammer syndrome: Post-traumatic digital ischemia. Surgery *68*:1122, 1970.
15. Bookstein JJ: Arteriography. *In* AK Poznanski (Ed): The Hand in Radiologic Diagnosis. 2nd Ed. Philadelphia, WB Saunders Co, 1984, pp 97–112.
16. Hudson TM, Haas G, Enneking WF, et al: Angiography in management of musculoskeletal tumors. Surg Gynecol Obstet *141*:11, 1975.
17. Kindblom L-G, Merck C, Svendsen P: Myxofibrosarcoma: A pathologico-anatomical, microangiographic and angiographic correlative study of eight cases. Br J Radiol *50*:876, 1977.
18. Levin DC, Gordon DH, McSweeney J: Arteriography of peripheral hemangiomas. Radiology *121*:625, 1976.
19. Prando A, deSantos LA, Wallace S, et al: Angiography in giant-cell bone tumors. Radiology *130*:323, 1979.
20. Yaghmai I: Angiographic features of osteosarcoma. AJR *129*:1073, 1977.
21. Yaghmai I: Angiographic manifestations of soft-tissue and osseous hemangiopericytomas. Radiology *126*:653, 1978.
22. Feldman F, Casarella WJ, Dick HM, et al: Selective intraarterial embolization of bone tumors. AJR *123*:130, 1975.
23. Mitty HA, Hermann G, Abdelwahab IF, et al: Role of angiography in limb-tumor surgery. RadioGraphics *11*:1029, 1991.
24. Weissman BN, Rappoport AD, Sosman JL, et al: Radiographic findings in the hands in patients with systemic lupus erythematosus. Radiology *126*:313, 1978.
25. Chuang VP, Benjamin R, Jaffe N, et al: Radiographic and angiographic changes in osteosarcoma after intraarterial chemotherapy. AJR *139*:1065, 1982.
26. Ekelund L, Laurin S, Lunderquist A: Comparison of a vasoconstrictor and a vasodilator in pharmacoangiography of bone and soft tissue tumors. Radiology *122*:95, 1977.
27. Hutcheson J, Klatte EC, Kremp R: The angiographic appearance of myositis ossificans circumscripta. Radiology *102*:57, 1972.
28. Levin DC, Watson RC, Baltaxe HA: Arteriography in diagnosis and management of acquired peripheral soft-tissue masses. Radiology *104*:53, 1972.
29. Natali J, Merland JJ: Superselective arteriography and therapeutic embolization for vascular malformations (angiodysplasias). J Cardiovasc Surg *17*:465, 1976.
30. Olcott C, Newton TH, Stoney RJ, et al: Inter-arterial embolization in the management of arteriovenous malformations. Surgery *79*:3, 1976.

31. Svendler C-A, Sonderlundh S: Angiographic diagnosis in polymyalgia arteritica. Acta Radiol (Diagn) *18*:333, 1977.
32. Zvaifler NJ: Vasculitides: Classification and pathogenesis. Aust NZ J Med *8* (Suppl 1):134, 1978.
33. Hunder GG, Allen GL: Giant cell arteritis: A review. Bull Rheum Dis *29*:980, 1978.
34. deShazo RD: The spectrum of systemic vasculitis. Postgrad Med *58*:78, 1975.
35. Ostberg G: On arteritis with special reference to polymyalgia arteritica. Acta Pathol Microbiol Scand (Suppl) *237*:1, 1973.
36. Sokoloff J, Wilens SL, Bunim JJ: Arteritis of striated muscle in rheumatoid arthritis. Am J Pathol *27*:157, 1951.
37. Cruickshank B: The arteritis of rheumatoid arthritis. Ann Rheum Dis *13*:136, 1954.
38. Laws JW, Lillie JG, Scott JT: Arteriographic appearances in rheumatoid arthritis and other disorders. Br J Radiol *36*:477, 1963.
39. Laws JW, Sallab RA, Scott JT: An arteriographic and histologic study of digital arteries. Br J Radiol *40*:740, 1967.
40. Williams RC Jr: Rheumatoid Arthritis as a Systemic Disease. Philadelphia, WB Saunders Co, 1974, p 56.
41. Clark WS, Kulka JP, Bauer W: Rheumatoid aortitis with aortic regurgitation. Am J Med *22*:580, 1957.
42. Smith DC, Hirst AE: Spontaneous aortic rupture associated with chronic steroid therapy for rheumatoid arthritis in two cases. AJR *132*:271, 1979.
43. Bruk MI: Articular and vascular manifestations of polymyalgia rheumatica. Ann Rheum Dis *26*:103, 1967.
44. Rabinowitz JG, Twersky J, Guttadauria M: Similar bone manifestations of scleroderma and rheumatoid arthritis. AJR *121*:35, 1974.
45. Resnick D, Greenway G, Vint VC, et al: Selective involvement of the first carpometacarpal joint in scleroderma. AJR *131*:283, 1978.
46. Cannon PJ, Hassar M, Case DB, et al: The relationship of hypertension and renal failure in scleroderma (progressive systemic sclerosis) to structural and functional abnormalities of the renal cortical circulation. Medicine *53*:1, 1974.
47. Dabich L, Bookstein JJ, Zweifler A, et al: Digital arteries in patients with scleroderma: Arteriographic and plethysmographic study. Arch Intern Med *130*:708, 1972.
48. Freidman IA, Sickley JF, Poske RM, et al: The LE phenomenon in rheumatoid arthritis. Ann Intern Med *46*:1113, 1957.
49. Ziff M: The agglutination reaction in rheumatoid arthritis. J Chronic Dis *5*:644, 1957.
50. Budin J, Feldman F: Soft tissue calcifications in systemic lupus erythematosus. AJR *124*:358, 1975.
51. Talbott JH: Collagen Vascular Diseases. New York, Grune & Stratton, 1974, p 1.
52. Robins J, Bookstein JJ: Regressing aneurysms in periarteritis nodosa. Radiology *104*:39, 1972.
53. Doppman JL: Baker's cyst and normal gastrocnemiosemimembranosus bursa. AJR *94*:646, 1965.
54. Azouz EM: Hematuria, rectal bleeding and pelvic phleboliths in children with the Klippel-Trenaunay syndrome. Pediatr Radiol *13*:82, 1983.
55. Macpherson RI, Letts RM: Skeletal diseases associated with angiomatosis. J Can Assoc Radiol *29*:90, 1978.
56. Wilson R, McCormick W, Tatum C, et al: Occupational acroosteolysis. JAMA *201*:577, 1967.
57. Gralino BJ, Porter JM, Rösch J: Angiography in the diagnosis and therapy of frostbite. Radiology *119*:301, 1976.
58. Quintanilla R, Krusen FH, Esser HE: Studies on frostbite with special reference to treatment and the effect on minute blood vessels. Am J Physiol *149*:149, 1947.
59. Théron J: Superselective angiography of the hip. Radiology *124*:649, 1977.
60. Green NE, Griffin PP: Intra-osseous venous pressure in Legg-Perthes disease. J Bone Joint Surg [Am] *64*:666, 1982.
61. Iwasaki K, Okasaki T, Ikeda S, et al: The haemodynamics of Perthes disease. Int Orthop (SICOT) *6*:142, 1982.
62. Manninger J, Bird T, Zolczer L, et al: The diagnostic role of intraosseous phlebography in the affections of the hip in childhood. Arch Orthop Trauma Surg *96*:203, 1980.
63. Schutzer SF, Gossling HR: The treatment of reflex sympathetic dystrophy syndrome. J Bone Joint Surg [Am] *66*:625, 1984.
64. Simon G: Letter to the Editor. JAMA *227*:327, 1974.
65. Visitsunthron U, Prete P: Reflex sympathetic dystrophy of the lower extremity. West J Med *135*:62, 1981.
66. Graf CJ, Perret GE: Spontaneous recurrent hemorrhage as an unusual complication of fibrous dysplasia of the skull. J Neurosurg *52*:570, 1980.
67. Jelsma F: Primary Tumors of the Calvaria, with Special Consideration of the Clinical Problems. Springfield, Ill, Charles C. Thomas, 1959, p 66.
68. Matson DD: Neurosurgery of Infancy and Childhood. Springfield, Ill, Charles C. Thomas, 1969, p 617.
69. Gorham LW, Stoup AP: Massive osteolysis. J Bone Joint Surg [Am] *37*:985, 1955.
70. Kolar J, Zidkovd H, Matejovsky Z, et al: Radiology of massive osteolysis syndrome. Radiol Diagn *22*:369, 1981.

# 15

# Radionuclide Techniques

*Naomi Alazraki, M.D.*

The dynamic nature of bone provides the basic theme for interpretation of bone scans. The integrity of bone as a living tissue in constant activity is displayed by the scintillation camera or scanner on x-ray or Polaroid film images. In addition to its role as the structural support of the body, bone is important in the regulation of many elements in the body, including calcium, phosphate, and hydrogen ion, and therefore is an important indicator of many disease processes. Until the emergence of the bone scan as a clinical procedure in 1961, only radiography was available for imaging the skeletal system. As demonstrated by various investigations,[1] osseous destruction may not be seen on a radiograph until as much as 50 per cent or more of the bone in a vertebral body has been destroyed. With this recogni-

tion that radiography was a relatively insensitive technique for evaluating abnormalities of the bone, enthusiasm for a more sensitive imaging approach developed. In 1961, Fleming and coworkers[2] demonstrated localization of strontium-85 in normal bone with increased uptake of the radionuclide at sites of osseous abnormalities. Since that time, the high sensitivity of the bone scan, particularly following advances in radiopharmaceutical preparations and in imaging instruments, has been well established by many investigators.[3–8]

## HISTORICAL ASPECTS AND TECHNIQUES

The use of radionuclides for evaluating the skeletal system has a history that long predates the advent of the $^{85}$Sr bone scan. Bone necrosis, osteomyelitis, and bone neoplasms were described in radium dial workers between 1917 and 1925.[9, 10] Chronic ingestion of the radium by these workers resulted in deposition of the radioactive material in the bone. In 1935, Chiewitz and Hevesy[11] studied phosphorus metabolism in rats and noted that $^{32}$P was deposited in the bones of adult rats. In studying the metabolism of neoplasms of bone, Treadwell and associates[12] in 1942 used $^{89}$Sr, a beta ray emitter, as a tracer, and with autoradioactive studies identified deposition of the radioactive strontium in the osteogenic productive regions in normal bone as well as in osteosarcomas. After these observations, in 1958 Bauer and Ray[13] noted that strontium behaved biologically similarly to calcium. Between 1958 and 1961, several investigators,[14, 15] using $^{85}$Sr and a point-dash counting technique, studied patients with bone metastases, and finally the technique of the bone scan emerged in 1961.[16] Unfortunately, there is no isotope of calcium that emits gamma rays in energy ranges suitable for imaging with the instruments that are available today. Thus, strontium was utilized as the next best imitator of calcium.

In addition to the bone scan, other radioactive techniques that can be used to evaluate bone or mineral metabolism have included autoradiography, mineral absorption or photon densitometry, and neutron activation analysis for the determination of whole body calcium levels. Autoradiography generally is used as a research tool and involves the administration of a beta-emitting radionuclide to an animal. After an appropriate time during which incorporation of the radionuclide into the tissue to be studied (i.e., the bone) takes place, the animal is killed. The tissue is sectioned, and a photographic emulsion is applied over the section. The tissue remains in contact with the emulsion for a sufficient length of time to allow exposure of the emulsion from the beta emissions of the radionuclide in the sectioned tissue. When the film is developed, the degree of darkening of the emulsion will be proportional to the number of beta emissions from the radionuclide in the tissue. The autoradiograph, therefore, serves as a way of visualizing the site of uptake of the radioisotope on a cellular level. In the case of radioactive $^{32}$P or an isotope of calcium, quantitation of the amount of radionuclide in the section provides a basis for determining major mineral and organic metabolic patterns in bone and rates of bone turnover.[17]

Heightened awareness of the prevalence of osteoporosis, particularly among postmenopausal women, and the high cost and morbidity of this disease have spurred interest in effective and practical methods for early detection of osteoporosis to help prevent the significant consequences of this disease. A number of methods for determining bone mineral content, including single photon absorptiometry, dual photon absorptiometry, and CT using single energy and dual energy methods, are being used clinically (see Chapter 52). Tied to the selection of a technique for osteoporosis screening is the choice of bone(s) to be examined. The lumbar spine, although consisting of both trabecular and cortical bone, is predominantly trabecular in composition; the middle portion of the radius consists of approximately 95 per cent cortical bone; the distal portion of the radius is composed of 75 per cent cortical and 25 per cent trabecular bone; and the calcaneus is all trabecular bone.[133, 134] Because of this heterogeneous nature of the skeleton, each method of bone mineral analysis (dual photon absorptiometry, single photon absorptiometry, CT) has unique advantages and limitations. Precision, reliability, radiation exposure, and cost of each technique also must be considered.

Single photon absorptiometry, as originally described, involves scanning of a patient's wrist that is placed between an $^{125}$I source and a sodium iodide detector.[18] The greater the mineral content of the bone, the fewer the number of photons that penetrate the bone to be detected by the sodium iodide crystal. Quantitation of bone density of the distal portion of the radius (or some other accessible defined point) can be accomplished at different intervals, allowing estimation of the patient's response to therapy and of the progression of various diseases, such as secondary hyperparathyroidism,[19] osteoporosis,[20] and other conditions that alter bone mineral content.[21] Dual photon absorptiometry (see Chapter 52) is used as a method of detecting osteoporosis by determining the bone mineral content in the lumbar spine.[135] A gadolinium-153 ($^{153}$Gd) source emits photons of 44 (Europium k x-rays at 42 and 48 keV) and 100 keV (x-rays at 97 and 103 keV), which are transmitted through the lumbar spine. The instrument that is used for dual photon absorptiometry is a smaller version of a rectilinear scanning device with a sodium iodide detector in the upper probe that detects the transmitted photons from the source, which is housed in the lower probe. The total integrated mineral in the path of the beam is measured, and

uniform soft tissue thickness, which is critical for the successful application of single photon absorptiometry, is not required. Mathematically, the use of a softer (44 keV) photon in concert with a harder photon (100 keV) allows differentiation between soft tissue and bone so that bone mineral density alone can be measured accurately; bone mineral in grams per cubic centimeter is calculated by the simultaneous solution of two equations describing the intensity of the transmitted radiation beam for the 44 and 100 keV energies, respectively.[205] The separate contributions of cortical and trabecular bone cannot be determined by this technique, however. As the lumbar spine is a mixture of cortical and trabecular bone, some centers also obtain measurements (using single or dual photon absorptiometry) derived from the calcaneus or the radius, or both.[136–141] In addition, as the hip is a common site of fracture in osteoporosis, dual photon measurements of this region also are made.

In vivo neutron activation analysis has been used in some centers to determine total body calcium content. This procedure involves bombarding the subject with neutrons from a nuclear reactor or a particle accelerator. The neutrons are absorbed by the atomic nuclei in the tissue, producing isotopes of the bombarded elements. The radioactive isotopes can be measured and the amount of the stable element originally present in the subject then can be calculated, as for a given number of neutrons entering a sample, the quantity of the radioactive isotope that is produced will be closely proportional to the amount of the stable element originally present. In humans, small doses of neutrons are used to measure large quantities of material. For a few minutes, the patient is exposed to a uniform neutron flux and then is transferred to a whole body counter, in which gamma rays emitted by the produced radioactive isotopes can be measured. With a neutron dose of about 1 roentgen equivalent— man (rem), sodium, chlorine, and calcium can be determined within a few percentage points.[22–25] This procedure, however, is not used clinically for a number of reasons, including the limited availability of neutron fluxes and whole body counters, as well as the potentially high radiation exposure resulting from the production of radioactive isotopes in vivo that have varying physical half-lives. These radioisotopes continue to expose the patient to radiation long after the neutron flux bombardment has ceased. Despite these limitations in the procedure, various investigators have reported the feasibility of determining total body calcium by in vivo neutron activation analysis. As more than 99 per cent of the body's calcium is located within the skeleton, the measurement of total body calcium reflects the state of bone mineralization.

In clinical practice, radionuclide imaging is the technique that is used most widely in the detection of some bone abnormalities. As in most procedures in nuclear medicine, the bone scan is an extremely sensitive but relatively nonspecific method. Any process that disturbs the normal balance of bone production and resorption can produce an abnormality on the bone scan. These abnormalities may be manifested as regions of increased or decreased activity. The great majority of lesions appear as focal areas of increased activity, as the usual response to an insult is osteogenesis. In normal images, the skeleton has clear areas that show greater and lesser concentration of the radionuclide. These differences in the degree of radionuclide concentration throughout the normal skeleton usually correspond to differences in bone turnover; for example, in children the epiphyses and physeal (growth) plates (sites at which bone turnover is most rapid and active) appear as foci of intense tracer activity. In adults, metaphyses of tubular bones may show more activity than diaphyses.

The amount of radiopharmaceutical agent accumulated in any region of bone depends on two major factors: the rate of bone turnover and the integrity of the blood supply. Of these two factors, the intactness of the vascular supply appears to have a more important influence on the bone scan; if there is an absence of blood perfusion to a localized region of bone, the radiopharmaceutical agent cannot be delivered to this area, and a photon-deficient, or "cold," region may be visualized on the scan.[26] Genant and associates[27] studied the rates of both blood flow and osteogenesis in experimental animal models and confirmed that the rate of blood flow in bone is the most important factor in determining the degree of radiopharmaceutical uptake on the bone scan. Studies that were performed earlier using fluorine-18[28] also established the importance of bone perfusion in the production of the bone scan.[29] Siegel and coworkers[30] reported experimental data using technetium-99m hydroxyethylene diphosphonate ($^{99m}$Tc-HEDP), which also suggested that bone blood flow is the major factor in determining the distribution of the radiopharmaceutical; after femoral artery ligation, a decrease in $^{99m}$Tc-diphosphonate uptake in the bones of the affected limb was seen, even in the presence of healing fractures. Studies by Sagar and associates[132] in animals have uncovered a nonproportional relationship between increments in bone blood flow and augmentation of $^{99m}$Tc-methylene diphosphonate ($^{99m}$Tc-MDP) uptake. These investigators suggested a "diffusion-limited" phenomenon governing the bone uptake of $^{99m}$Tc-MDP in response to increased bone blood flow. They found that a fourfold increase in tibial blood flow produced only a 33 per cent augmentation of $^{99m}$Tc-MDP tibial uptake. After sectioning of the tibial sympathetic nerve supply, the diffusion-limitation effect of enhanced $^{99m}$Tc-MDP uptake in response to increased blood supply persisted, but at a higher flow rate level.

## RADIOPHARMACEUTICALS

Over the years, a number of radiopharmaceutical agents have been used for bone scanning. Strontium-85 was the first imageable radionuclide that was successful in allowing identification of abnormalities within bone. The basis for its behavior is its ability to substitute biologically for calcium and be incorporated into the hydroxyapatite crystal of bone as a strontium-hydroxyapatite structure.[31] After the strontium has reached the bone via the blood stream, it is believed to diffuse freely across the capillary membrane. Strontium is incorporated rapidly into the bones; approximately 30 to 50 per cent of the administered dose is labeled to the bones within 1 hour after its administration. The remainder of the $^{85}$Sr is excreted by the kidneys and the gastrointestinal tract. Superimposed activity in the gastrointestinal tract may interfere with bone imaging, which makes it advisable to perform the scan several days after injection of the strontium (usually 7 days).[16] Strontium-85 is a very poor radionuclide for clinical use because of its 65 day physical half-life and unfavorable gamma energy emission of 513 keV. To minimize the patient's radiation exposure,

only small doses of 100 microcuries ($\mu$Ci) can be used. At this dose level, and with the added disadvantage of the sodium iodide crystal's inefficiency for detecting the high energy gamma emission of the $^{85}$Sr, a bone scan takes several hours to perform and results in images of relatively poor quality compared with the images that can be obtained with other agents. Strontium-87m is a more effective radiopharmaceutical than $^{85}$Sr, as it has a 388 keV gamma ray emission and only a 2.8 hour physical half-life. Its disadvantages are that it is extremely expensive, as an yttrium generator produced agent ($^{85}$Y$\rightarrow$ $^{85m}$Sr), and its short physical half-life requires that imaging be performed 2 to 3 hours after injection, at a time when plasma levels of $^{87m}$Sr still are elevated enough to cause an unfavorable bone-to-blood background count ratio.

Fluorine-18 has a 1.9 hour physical half-life and therefore is not widely available; its use is limited to centers with rapid access to a cyclotron or reactor that produces radioisotopes for medical use. Fluorine-18 is a positron emitter; the resulting 511 keV annihilation x-rays can be imaged by the conventional scintillation imaging systems that are available in most institutions. However, a 511 keV photon requires heavy collimation and is imaged inefficiently by the scintillation camera.

Nonetheless, some authors have obtained good imaging results using the scintillation camera, a high energy collimator, and fluorine-18 as $^{18}$F-fluorodeoxyglucose ($^{18}$FDG) to simulate positron emission tomography (PET) imaging of myocardial metabolism[214] and potentially for bone imaging. Indeed, in the early 1970s, $^{18}$F bone scanning was performed using two opposed scintillation camera detectors without collimators and coincidence detection circuitry. Although $^{18}$F has physical limitations when used as a bone imaging agent, it has superior biologic characteristics. Approximately 50 per cent of the administered dose is incorporated into the $Ca_{10}(PO_4)_6(OH)_2$ (calcium hydroxyapatite) crystal, probably by exchange for hydroxyl radicals, which are of similar physical size to the fluorine atom.[32, 33] The remaining 50 per cent of the injected $^{18}$F is excreted rapidly by the kidneys so that blood clearance is faster for $^{18}$F than it is for the other bone-seeking radiopharmaceuticals that have been used. Even when imaging is performed at 2 to 3 hours after intravenous or oral administration of $^{18}$F, the bone-to-blood and bone-to-soft tissue background count ratios are very favorable.

In 1971, Subramanian and McAfee introduced $^{99m}$Tc-polyphosphate as a bone imaging agent.[34] Subsequent work resulted in the discovery of other $^{99m}$Tc-labeled phosphate compounds, such as HEDP, PPi (pyrophosphate), and MDP,[35, 36] compounds that have improved the resolution of bone imaging dramatically, allowing definition of small osseous anatomic structures. Technetium-99m has a physical half-life of 6 hours and emits a 140 keV gamma ray, which is ideal for imaging with the available scintillation cameras and scanners. The low radiation exposure resulting from this agent permits the use of doses of 15 to 20 mCi for each bone scan. Thus, a whole body, head-to-toe image in an anterior or a posterior projection may be obtained in 20 to 35 min, and approximately 1 hour is required to produce both posterior and anterior total body images of exceptionally high quality, depending on instruments and biologic variables.

The $^{99m}$Tc-phosphate compounds that currently are used

for bone imaging can be categorized as condensed phosphates (inorganic compounds) and phosphonates (organic compounds). The first of the phosphate radiopharmaceuticals introduced for clinical imaging was polyphosphate as $^{99m}$Tc-tripolyphosphate, an inorganic compound composed of chains of three phosphate residues. This compound rapidly was replaced by a longer chain polyphosphate containing approximately 46 phosphate residues.[37] Pyrophosphate, which contains only two phosphate residues, subsequently replaced the polyphosphates. The diphosphonates, which are organic analogues of pyrophosphate and are more stable clinically than the polyphosphates in that they are not susceptible to enzymatic hydrolysis in vivo, also gained clinical confidence. Agents in this category that are used widely today are HEDP, MDP, and HDP (hydroxymethylene diphosphonate). Imidodiphosphonate, which contains a P-N-P bond,[38] is another category of polyphosphate compound that can be labeled with $^{99m}$Tc and used for bone imaging. Other potential phosphate-containing bone imaging compounds include phosphonate analogues of chelating agents (DTPA, EDTA) and other variations on the methylene phosphonic acid structure.

Technetium-99m is the most widely used radioisotope in clinical nuclear medicine. After binding to various pharmaceuticals, it is used for brain, liver, and lung scans, radionuclide angiographic studies, cardiac ejection fraction and gated cardiac blood pool wall motion studies, as well as bone and bone marrow scans. It is eluted from a molybdenum-99 generator in the form of pertechnetate ion ($^{99m}$TcO$_4^-$), which is a +7 valence state. Technetium-99 pertechnetate is used in its ionic sodium pertechnetate form for radionuclide angiographic studies, and thyroid, salivary gland, gastric mucosal, or Meckel's diverticulum imaging. After intravenous injection of $^{99m}$Tc-pertechnetate, it localizes throughout the extracellular fluids in the body. If $^{99m}$Tc-pertechnetate is mixed with a solution of one of the phosphate or phosphonate compounds and then is injected intravenously, the distribution in vivo remains the same as for technetium pertechnetate alone, indicating a failure of the technetium to be bound to the phosphate or phosphonate. Technetium-99m must be in a chemically reduced form for binding or chelation to occur. Reduction of technetium from a +7 valence state (TcO$_4^-$) to a +4 valence state is accomplished easily by mixing the $^{99m}$Tc-pertechnetate after its elution from the generator with tin (Sn$^{+2}$) in the form of stannous chloride. Mixing the $^{99m}$Tc-pertechnetate, stannous chloride, and one of the phosphate compounds in a solution results in a technetium-tin-phosphate complex that preferentially localizes within bone when injected intravenously.[31]

Bone uptake localization half-times have been measured as 15 to 30 min, which is much more rapid than the half-time disappearance from the blood, which has been measured at about 1 hour. The technetium-phosphate complex that is not localized within bone is excreted into the urine by means of glomerular filtration. Slight variations occur among the various phosphate compounds in the proportion of the administered dose that localizes in the bone and in the rate of excretion of the compound by the kidneys. At 1 hour after intravenous administration, 58 per cent of the administered MDP, 48 per cent of administered HEDP, and 47 per cent of administered PPi were found in the bones.[37] In a comparison of skeletal uptakes of three diphosphonates

(HEDP, MDP, and HDP) by whole body retention at 24 hours after injection, Fogelman and associates[142] reported values of 18.3, 30.3, and 36.6 per cent, respectively. These results appear to indicate that slight alterations in diphosphonate molecular structure may have significant effects on bone uptake. In a study of $^{99m}$Tc-HDP and $^{99m}$Tc-MDP, based on imaging at 2 and 4 hours after injection, both agents revealed the same number of skeletal lesions, but the retention of tracer in bone compared with that in soft tissue was greater, and image quality was better with $^{99m}$Tc-HDP than with $^{99m}$Tc-MDP.[143] Studies of blood clearance and urinary excretion of the technetium-phosphate complexes[37, 39] have shown that diphosphonate compounds are cleared more rapidly from the blood than either pyrophosphate or polyphosphate. MDP appears to be cleared from the blood more rapidly than HEDP, which enhances MDP's slight advantage in bone deposition and, therefore, its role as a radiopharmaceutical for bone imaging.

The phosphate compounds are bound to protein after intravenous injection. The degree of protein binding may influence the blood clearance and urinary excretion rates of these compounds. Another factor that contributes to differences in rates of blood clearance is the variable nature of the binding of the compounds to red blood cells. For example, 10 to 30 per cent of the whole blood $^{99m}$Tc-pyrophosphate is bound to red cells at 1 to 3 hours after injection.[40] Conversely, only a negligible amount of $^{99m}$Tc-HEDP or $^{99m}$Tc-MDP is bound to these cells. Six hour urine collections show that about 68 per cent of the administered technetium-labeled diphosphonate compounds is excreted, compared with 50 per cent of the technetium-labeled pyrophosphate compounds and 46 per cent of the technetium-labeled polyphosphate compounds.

All of these phosphate compounds can inhibit both formation and dissolution of hydroxyapatite crystals in vitro and in vivo. In fact, these agents, particularly the diphosphonates, have been used in the management of patients with Paget's disease of bone[41] and of some patients with idiopathic calcinosis universalis. Pharmacologic doses of diphosphonate may retard bone growth and ectopic calcification in these patients. The mechanism of this action has been postulated to be the accretion of the diphosphonate onto the mineral surfaces of bone, resulting in a retardation of further buildup or loss of mineral ion. Inhibition of the conversion of noncrystalline calcium phosphate to hydroxyapatite crystal by diphosphonate also has been proposed.

The mechanism by which the $^{99m}$Tc-labeled phosphate compounds are incorporated into bone is not understood entirely. Because the technetium-phosphate compounds do not carry significant ionic charge, they may be able to diffuse relatively freely across the bone capillary wall, similarly to the behavior of strontium and fluorine. Having arrived at the bone site, therefore, the phosphate compound may chemisorb (chemical and physical processes leading to adsorption) at kink and dislocation sites on the surface of the hydroxyapatite, resulting in a release of tin and $^{99m}$Tc, which are hydrolyzed and deposited either separately or together as hydrated tin oxide and technetium dioxide.[30] Sites of rapid bone turnover, such as growth centers and reactive bone lesions, are associated with a large mineral surface that is available for exchange and chemisorption by the $^{99m}$Tc-tin-phosphate complex. Although the hypothesis that the $^{99m}$Tc-phosphate compounds bind at the bone crystal surface is the current dominant theory, it also has been proposed that such binding predominates at the organic matrix, particularly the immature collagen.[42, 43]

## INSTRUMENTS

The most widely used instrument for imaging skeletal distribution of radionuclides is the scintillation camera, which may be equipped with a scanning mode for displaying the whole body distribution of the radiopharmaceutical on a single x-ray film. Scintillation cameras detect the distribution of radiopharmaceutical in vivo by recording externally the interactions of gamma rays emitted from the body with a sodium iodide crystal in the camera head. The scintillation camera detection system involves an array of photomultiplier tubes ranging in number from 37 to 61 in current models (one manufacturer marketed a 91 tube camera), which process the scintillations that result from interactions of the gamma rays in the sodium iodide crystal such that each gamma ray interaction of the appropriate energy level is displayed on an XY axis corresponding in position to its origin in the body. This results in an image of the distribution of the radionuclide in vivo. The images are recorded on Polaroid film with a radioactive scintillation displayed as a white dot, or on x-ray film with a radioactive scintillation displayed as a black dot. The scintillation camera may be equipped with a 10 inch diameter sodium iodide crystal, a 15 inch diameter sodium iodide crystal, or a 20 inch diameter sodium iodide crystal. The detector heads may be round or rectangular.

Lead collimators are needed in front of the sodium iodide crystal to minimize the number of scattered photons that can interact with the crystal. For $^{99m}$Tc bone and joint imaging, either high resolution or all-purpose low energy collimators are used. If stationary spot imaging is performed, 100,000 to 500,000 counts are obtained per image, the greater count rate resulting in a higher quality image, which of course takes longer to obtain. For spot images, it is advisable to use a pinhole or low energy converging collimator to magnify small regions of interest and maximize the resolution of the image.

Equipping the scintillation camera with a scanning mode option consisting of either a moving table or a moving detector head will permit the obtaining of total body images, which can be displayed on a single 8 × 10 inch x-ray film. A total body radionuclide bone image in the anterior or posterior projection obtained 2 hours after intravenous injection of 15 mCi of $^{99m}$Tc-labeled phosphate compounds generally will take about 30 min. If 25 mCi is used with a dual head imaging system, anterior and posterior whole body images can be obtained simultaneously in about 15 min. The time obviously is dependent on the collimator used, the degree of uptake of the radiopharmaceutical in the bones, the amount of renal excretion, the size and build of the patient, the number of millicuries injected, the time elapsed between injection and imaging, and the width of the window setting around the 140 keV photon energy peak of $^{99m}$Tc. In most institutions, at least anterior and posterior total body views are obtained, supplemented with spot images of questionably abnormal regions. A 20 per cent window usually is used, limiting the recording of counts to those photons that fall within 20 per cent of the 140 keV peak of activity.

The rectilinear scanner is an older imaging instrument that has been phased out of production. It only has one photomultiplier tube behind a single sodium iodide crystal of either 3 inch, 5 inch, or 8 inch diameter that moves across and down the body, recording the radiation that is detected beneath it. The counts are displayed by blackening of an x-ray film on a point-by-point basis. These instruments are tomographic in that they use focusing collimators and preferentially record counts from a plane at a particular depth in the body.

The current state of the art is the single photon emission computed tomography (SPECT) camera, which generates tomographic images, displaying multiple planes of selective activity from a single scan of the body. The camera rotates 360 degrees around the patient, acquiring multiple (usually 60 to 64) planar image projections from which tomographic slice images are generated. These can be viewed in coronal, sagittal, and transaxial projections. These instruments offer a potential similar to that of CT imaging devices. This approach can provide more detailed information, both qualitative and quantitative, on the localization of radiopharmaceuticals in bones and joints. Indeed, several reports indicate the superior ability of SPECT over planar bone imaging in the detection of bone lesions.[144–146]

Manufacturers have introduced dual and triple head scintillation camera systems that provide higher count SPECT imaging capability, or, alternatively, can be used to decrease patient scan time without sacrificing counts. Bone scans generally are done using the 180 degree opposed large crystal dual head systems.

## CLINICAL APPLICATIONS

Since the emergence of bone scanning in 1961, the clinical utility of this technique has continued to grow. Originally, the bone scan methodology gained clinical attention because of its ability to provide more sensitive detection than routine radiography in the evaluation of metastatic disease. Certainly, radionuclide bone imaging is widely used in the detection of osseous metastasis in patients with primary neoplasms that frequently spread to the bone (e.g., carcinoma of the prostate or breast). In addition to neoplasm, the bone scan is valuable in the early diagnosis of osteomyelitis and in evaluating the response of the infection to therapy. Radionuclide bone imaging has not yet achieved wide clinical use in metabolic diseases. Potentially, however, the bone imaging may be a sensitive indicator of metabolic alterations. It also may prove valuable in following the therapeutic responses in particular metabolic disorders. Vascular diseases such as ischemic necrosis lend themselves well to examination by bone scan, because radionuclide bone imaging is so sensitive to blood flow and to the reparative osteogenic processes that usually accompany vascular diseases of the bone. After traumatic insults to bone, the radionuclide study may be particularly helpful clinically in processes in which the radiograph is not so sensitive—for example, stress fractures. Articular diseases also can be well evaluated with scintigraphy. Thus, a partial list of indications for radionuclide bone imaging would include the following:

1. To screen for bone metastases.
2. To localize metastases for diagnostic biopsies and to

evaluate for suitability of bone radionuclide therapy (strontium-89) to relieve bone pain from metastatic disease.

3. To diagnose osteomyelitis before radiographic changes are evident; to aid in differentiating cellulitis from osteomyelitis; and to aid in evaluating painful prostheses for infection and for loosening.

4. To detect and evaluate the extent of articular involvement in various forms of arthritis, including osteoarthritis, rheumatoid arthritis, and rheumatoid variant disorders.

5. To aid in the workup and characterization of benign bone lesions, particularly those that are sometimes difficult to visualize by radiographic techniques because of their nature or location.

6. To aid in the diagnosis of stress fractures and other traumatic injuries not evident on plain radiographs.

7. To aid in the workup of compression fractures, particularly when there is a question of the age of the compression fracture, as may occur in medicolegal cases.

8. To evaluate bone pain of any cause in the presence of normal radiographs.

9. To aid in diagnosis and management of ischemic necrosis of bone.

10. To aid in management of myositis ossificans.

11. To aid in the prognostic evaluation of microvascular competence required to support healing of soft tissue ulcerations in patients with peripheral vascular disease; and to aid in the selection of amputation site or level.

In recent years, however, the clinical applications of radionuclide bone imaging have been influenced dramatically by the introduction and refinement of MR imaging, a diagnostic method that generally is equally sensitive and often more specific than bone scintigraphy. MR imaging, however, is more expensive than radionuclide bone imaging and does not provide whole body images of the skeleton.

### Neoplasm

**Skeletal Metastasis.** The axial skeleton is a major site of metastases; of all skeletal metastases, approximately 80 per cent localize in the axial skeleton, 10 per cent in the skull, and 10 per cent in the long bones.[44] Various studies have documented that approximately 10 to 40 per cent of patients with skeletal metastases have normal radiographs at a time when the bone scan is abnormal, and fewer than 5 per cent of bone scans are normal when radiographs show localized abnormalities.[16] It is not uncommon for the bone scan of a patient who is free of any bone pain and whose radiographs are entirely normal to show multiple foci of metastatic disease. Occasionally, a region may be painful and yet normal on radionuclide bone images. In these latter cases, evaluation by radiography may show a lytic lesion that apparently has not caused sufficient reactive bone formation on a histologic level to result in increased radiopharmaceutical accumulation on the bone scan. Anaplastic tumors and multiple myeloma are two major categories of malignant disease that characteristically may not stimulate sufficient osteoblastic reaction for an abnormal focus to be imaged on scan. Nonetheless, if the bone scan demonstrates regions of abnormal increased uptake, successful bone pain relief in this disease can be achieved with strontium-89 ther-

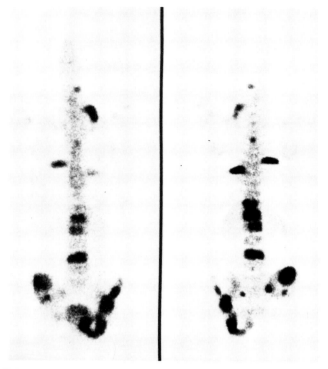

**FIGURE 15–1.** Metastatic bone disease: Anterior and posterior views from a $^{99m}$Tc-pyrophosphate bone scan in a patient with primary cancer of the prostate. Multiple hot foci of increased uptake of the radiopharmaceutical agent are seen involving the spine, pelvis, and ribs. The lesions are concentrating the radiopharmaceutical agent so avidly that the blood background, kidneys, and normal bones are hardly visible.

apy.[218, 219] Figure 15–1 demonstrates a radionuclide bone image in a patient with metastatic bone disease.

Lesions that are osteolytic radiographically are not necessarily purely osteolytic histologically. At a cellular level, both osteoblastic and osteoclastic activity may be increased. The lytic nature of a lesion evident radiographically simply reflects the fact that the resorption process is occurring at a more rapid rate than the osteogenic process. In these cases, the bone scan usually is positive because it reflects osteogenic activity in the lesion, which usually is increased above that in the normal adjacent bone. In approximately 5 per cent of metastases, the bone scan indeed is negative in the presence of a radiographically evident destructive lesion, indicating that the osteogenesis within the lesion or its blood supply is not greater than that in the normal surrounding bone.

The bone scan frequently is used to follow the response of neoplasm to irradiation, chemotherapy, or hormone therapy in patients with cancer and bone metastases. It is not uncommon to see dramatic changes in the bone scan after therapy, with resolution of previously abnormal areas throughout the skeleton, findings that usually are interpreted as a favorable therapeutic response. This response cannot necessarily be interpreted to mean that no viable tumor cells remain in a region that has converted to normal on the radionuclide images, however (Fig. 15–2). An individual lesion also may show apparent worsening on a bone scan obtained after completion of therapy. In some cases,

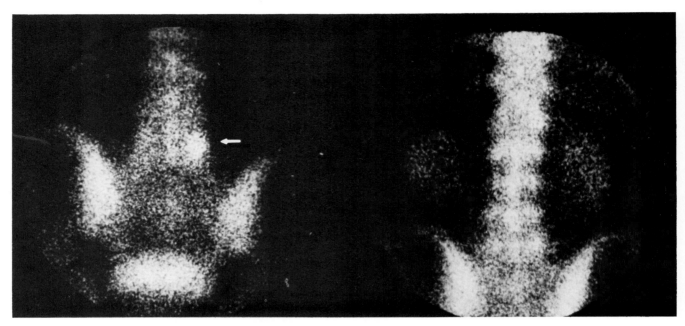

**FIGURE 15–2.** Metastatic disease with response to chemotherapy: Scintillation camera views of the patient's lower spine after $^{99m}$Tc-pyrophosphate scans obtained approximately 1 year apart in a patient with primary cancer of the prostate. On the image at left, a focus of increased activity is noted in the right side of the L5 vertebral body (arrow). One year later, the abnormal focus in L5 no longer is apparent. The patient had been treated with chemotherapy for prostate cancer and responded well.

this response has been identified as a transient process, which may represent repair and healing of the bone rather than progression of disease. This "flare" phenomenon has been estimated to occur in 10 to 15 per cent of breast cancer patients with bone metastases who are treated with chemotherapy[147] and in about 6 per cent of prostate cancer patients who are treated with chemotherapeutic regimens for stage D$_2$ disease.[148]

Another scintigraphic pattern that may be associated with widespread metastatic bone disease is the "superscan" seen on whole body imaging. When metastatic bone disease is far advanced, the skeletal system may avidly extract the radiopharmaceutical from the blood, resulting in greater than 50 per cent bone concentration of the radiopharmaceutical and leaving less available radionuclide for excretion by the kidneys. Consequently, on the image, the kidneys may not be visualized and the blood background may be markedly free of radioactivity, with the generalized bone-to-background ratio of counts being unusually high (Figs. 15–3 and 15–4). Conversely, one or more photon-deficient or cold areas can represent the scintigraphic response to skeletal metastases (Fig. 15–5).

In about 6 to 8 per cent of patients with skeletal metastases, only a single focal lesion may be seen on the scan. The significance of solitary abnormalities on bone scans in patients with known extraosseous malignant lesions was addressed in a report of 1129 consecutive patients.[215] Solitary abnormalities in bone were identified in 172 patients (15 per cent). In 90 of the 172 patients, the cause of the abnormality on the scan was established. Sixty-four per cent of these abnormalities were related to metastases and 36 per cent were related to benign processes.[216]

In another study of scintigraphically evident bone lesions in 246 patients with cancer but no known metastases, 14 per cent of newly detected lesions were proved to be malig-

nant, and 38 per cent were proved to be benign.[216] Seventy-four per cent of the patients in this study had breast cancer. Of those bone scan abnormalities for which the accompanying radiographs were normal, 17 per cent were related to skeletal metastases. Overall, more than 50 per cent of the bone metastases in this study were not evident on radiographs. These data suggest that newly discovered abnormal foci detected on a bone scan require further radiographic or other imaging correlation or biopsy.

Solitary rib lesions present unique diagnostic difficulties. A review of 2851 bone scans done at a cancer center documented that only 1.4 per cent of cancer patients had solitary rib lesions, and 90 per cent of these were associated with a benign cause, such as trauma or postoperative radiation therapy.[153] Whereas the frequency of solitary rib lesions may be very low, Harbert and coworkers[154] found that 22 per cent of 471 cancer patients studied had one or more rib lesions. They described broad scintigraphic characteristics of rib lesions on the basis of their intensity and appearance in serial studies. Fractures often were focal rather than linear, with decreasing intensities over a period of 3 to 6 months, and aligned so that two or more ribs in the same location were involved (Figs. 15–6 and 15–7). In one study of one or two abnormalities detected on bone scans in cancer patients, the ribs were the single most common site for scan-positive and radiograph-negative abnormalities, but only 8 per cent of the scintigraphically positive areas were related to skeletal metastases.[216]

In contrast to radiographic characteristics that aid in the differentiation between benign and malignant processes, scintigraphic abnormalities can give only a very general indication of the aggressiveness of the lesion. When a single lesion is found on the radiographs, the scan is helpful in confirming the solitary nature of the lesion, in identifying the presence of other bone lesions, and in characterizing the

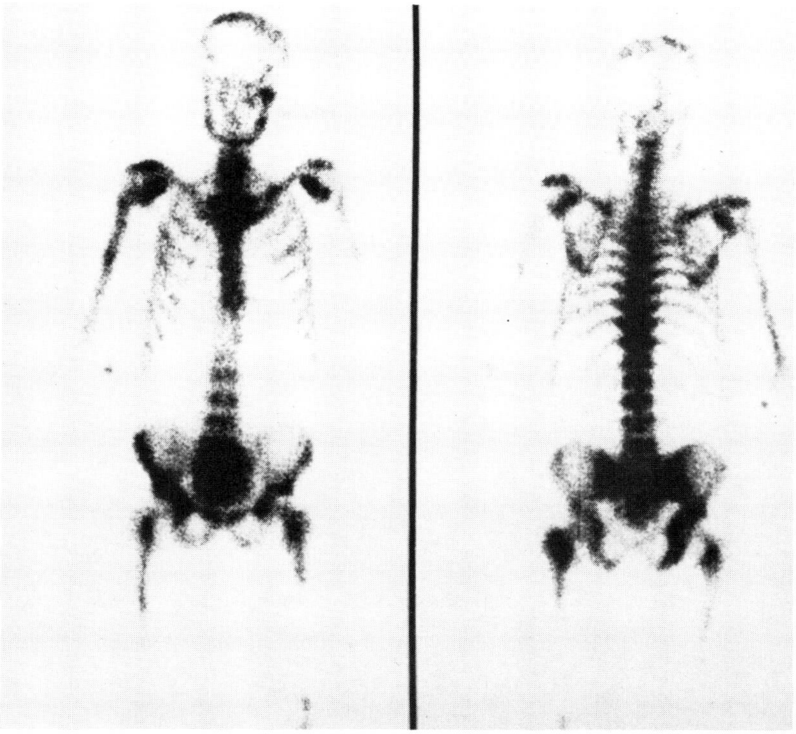

**FIGURE 15–3.** "Superscan" in metastatic disease: Anterior and posterior whole body images from a $^{99m}$Tc-pyrophosphate scan in a patient with primary cancer of the prostate. The superscan pattern shows absence of activity in the kidneys, low blood background activity, and generalized, uniformly increased uptake by all the bones in the body. Some areas of greater and lesser uptake can be identified on closer examination, particularly in the right humerus, the left distal end of the femur, the right posterior pelvis and iliac bone, the left mandible, the skull, and the ribs.

lesion as "high grade" or "low grade" in radiopharmaceutical concentration. In general, malignant lesions are hyperemic and, therefore, "hotter" on the scintigraphic image than benign lesions (Fig. 15–8). There are many reported exceptions to this general rule.[155–159] Additionally, a radionuclide angiogram can be performed with the scintillation camera centered over the radiographically identified abnormality at the time of intravenous injection of the radiopharmaceutical; the degree of vascularity of the lesion can be surmised on sequential frames by comparing the vascularity at the site of abnormality with that of surrounding normal bone.

Attempts to define the best approach to the detection of skeletal metastases by combining radiography and nuclear imaging, with an eye to cost effectiveness, have been considered. In one study,[45] an analysis of examinations requested by clinicians without radiologic guidance in 141 patients being evaluated for tumor staging indicated that excessive studies were performed in 18 per cent of these patients and that inadequate or inappropriate studies were performed in 27 per cent. In actuality, the necessary data for arriving at the optimum combined radiographic and nuclear imaging approach to determine the presence of skeletal metastasis in various neoplasms still are in the process of being gathered. McNeil[44] has approached the problem by first examining the frequency of bone metastases at autopsy in several malignant diseases. A decision-making analysis for the use of bone scans in primary and secondary tumors then is based on data currently available on the yield of the abnormal bone scan in that disease relative to autopsy results, the assumed health benefits associated with information gained from the scan, and the financial costs. These analyses have been applied to breast cancer, lung cancer, prostate cancer, and primary malignant bone tumors.

***Breast Cancer.*** A large disparity exists between the frequency of bone metastases from breast cancer found at autopsy and that detected at the time of initial therapy and follow-up. Indications are that many persons have occult bone metastases, undetected at the time of surgery and early follow-up. The frequency of bone metastases at autopsy in patients with primary breast cancer ranges from 50 to 85 per cent. The reported frequency of bone metastases in patients with primary breast cancer at the time of surgery and thereafter has varied considerably.[46–48] Bone pain is an unreliable indicator of the presence or absence of bone metastases from breast cancer; indeed, a report has indicated that 60 per cent of patients with such cancer and bone pain had no evidence of metastases, whereas 44 per cent of patients without pain had bone metastases.[160] The occurrence rate of positive bone scans for metastatic disease in patients with breast cancer at the stage 1 or 2 level has ranged from 2 to 38 per cent. Most studies indicate that the frequency of a true-positive bone scan in stage 1 or 2 disease is in the neighborhood of 2 per cent, whereas in stage 3 disease the frequency of true-positive bone scans increases to about 28 per cent. Investigators have found that bone metastasis becomes apparent on follow-up scans 3 to 4 years after surgery in about 20 to 30 per cent of patients who had negative bone scans and no evidence of bone metastases at the time of surgery.[46–48] Fifty per cent of the patients in whom bone metastases were seen at 3 years after treatment actually had manifested their disease by 12 months after therapy and 75 per cent by 18 months after therapy. The increased sensitivity of the scan compared with the radiograph appears to give the scan a 6 to 18

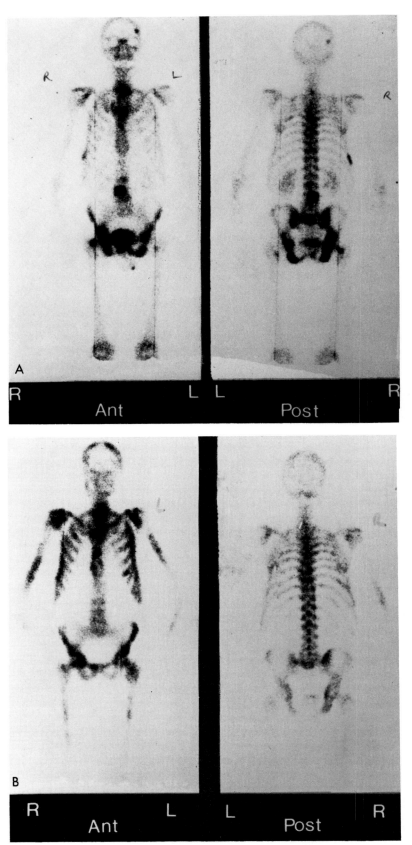

**FIGURE 15–4.** Progression of metastatic bone disease: Anterior and posterior $^{99m}$Tc-methylene diphosphonate (MDP) whole body images in a patient with primary cancer of the prostate.

**A** Observe multiple focal regions of increased activity in the pelvic bones, lumbar spine, ribs, and skull. The findings are suggestive of metastatic disease.

**B** The same patient was reimaged approximately 1 year later. The patient's metastatic bone disease has progressed to the pattern of a superscan, reflecting generalized involvement of almost every bone in the body. The pattern consists of poor visualization of the kidneys, very low blood background activity, and generalized increased bone activity with some irregularities noted on careful inspection, particularly in the humeri, femora, skull, and ribs.

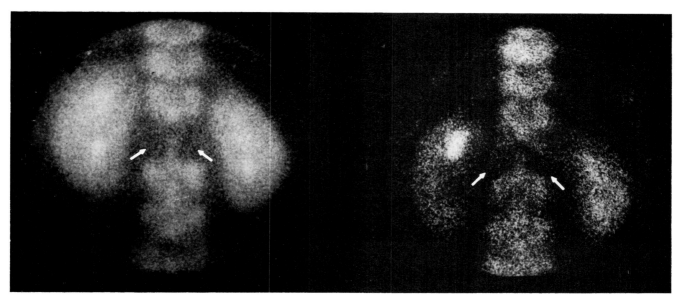

**FIGURE 15–5.** Cold focus in metastatic disease: Single scintillation camera views of the upper lumbar spine in two patients; the patient on the left has primary lung cancer, whereas the patient on the right has primary breast cancer. Both patients have metastatic disease involving the bones. The photon-deficient or "cold" region shown in each of these scans is a reflection of metastatic disease in the lumbar vertebral bodies (arrows). Note that the spinous processes of the lumbar vertebrae in both cases appear to be intact. The cold region seen on the scan is postulated to be a secondary effect either of total interruption of blood supply to the vertebral body because of the presence of necrotic tumor that has outgrown its blood supply or of total replacement of the bony structure by tumor, leaving no viable osteoblasts to produce bone that can accrete the radiopharmaceutical agent. Incidentally noted is a dilated calyx in the upper pole of the left kidney in the patient with breast cancer.

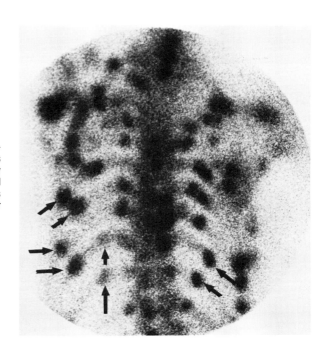

**FIGURE 15–6.** Rib fractures. Focal and rounded regions of increased uptake in the ribs correspond to sites of fractures in this patient. Arrows indicate fractures that line up from one rib to the next, indicating that they probably occurred at the same time. As the degree of intensity of abnormal radionuclide is influenced by the age of the fracture (younger fractures taking up more radionuclide than older ones), the fractures in the left lower rib cage (vertical arrows) probably are older than most of the others.

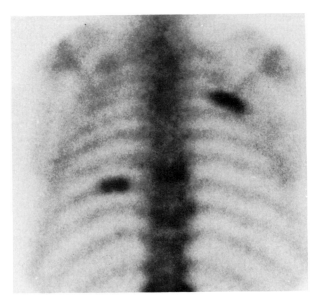

**FIGURE 15–7.** Rib metastases. Two abnormal areas of increased radiopharmaceutical uptake in ribs are aligned with the longitudinal axis of the ribs, a pattern more consistent with bone metastases than fractures.

month lead over the radiograph in converting to abnormal results. McNeil has concluded from these data that patients with clinical stage 3 breast carcinoma should have preoperative bone scans.[44] Patients with stage 1 and stage 2 disease should have baseline evaluations at the time of therapy and follow-up scans at 6, 12, 18, and 24 months to detect those who may have had occult metastatic disease, undetected at the time of initial therapy. McNeil's rationale is not accepted universally, with opinions varying from those that question the value of including bone scans in the routine evaluation of patients with early breast carcinoma to those that indicate that such scans are fundamental to this evaluation and clearly superior to routine radiography.[160, 201–203]

Although most patients with bone metastases from breast cancer have multiple focal regions of increased uptake of the radionuclide distributed throughout the skeleton, localized uptake in the sternum, probably related to spread of tumor from the internal mammary chain nodes, is a characteristic pattern. The sternal abnormality often is asymmetric, with more uptake on the side of the primary breast tumor.[217]

***Lung Cancer.*** Two to 35 per cent of patients with stage 1 or 2 adenocarcinoma, epidermoid carcinoma, or large cell carcinoma of the lung reveal a true-positive yield for bone metastases on bone scan.[49, 50] At autopsy, the frequency of such metastases in patients with primary lung cancer ranges from 30 to 50 per cent. Comparative studies of the bone scan and radiograph in the detection of skeletal metastases in this neoplasm have not yet been accomplished. Because adequate data are lacking, it is difficult to conclude that preoperative bone scans are or are not warranted in the workup of patients with lung cancer, although McNeil has suggested that even if the yield is low, the operative mortality rate in this disease may justify a preoperative bone scan.[44]

Bone scan abnormalities seen in patients with lung can-

cer and bony metastases include the following patterns: (1) diffuse bone involvement, particularly of the distal small bones; (2) photopenic lesions; (3) chest wall involvement, which may reflect pleural disease; (4) symmetric tubular bone involvement related to hypertrophic osteoarthropathy, which is seen in about 10 per cent of patients with lung cancer.

***Prostate Cancer.*** The frequency of bone metastases at autopsy in patients with primary prostate carcinoma ranges from 50 to 70 per cent. A Veterans Administration cooperative study has shown that patients with stage 1 or 2 disease (stages A and B) had a 7 per cent yield of positive bone scans, whereas in patients with more advanced, stage 3 disease, 18 per cent had positive bone scans.[44] It is apparent that a large number of patients with primary prostate carcinoma develop positive bone scans on follow-up examinations. Characteristically, only 54 per cent of patients with bone metastases have pain at the time of their scan conversion from normal to abnormal, whereas 12 per cent of those without detectable bone metastases may have pain.[51] Thus, pain apparently is a symptom that is difficult to interpret as an indicator of the presence or absence of bone metastases. The high frequency of bone metastases detected in this disease even during early stages strongly supports the routine use of the bone scan in staging of the disease and follow-up of these patients.[160–162, 164]

Of available tests for detecting spread of prostate cancer to bone, the bone scan is highly sensitive[44] and quite specific, even compared to the prostate specific antigen (PSA) blood test, which does not distinguish between bone and soft tissue metastases. The economic advantage of the PSA

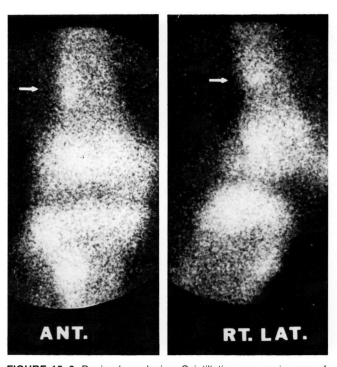

**FIGURE 15–8.** Benign bone lesion: Scintillation camera images of the right knee from a $^{99m}$Tc-pyrophosphate bone scan. In both views, the distal diaphysis of the femur shows a focus of increased activity, which corresponds to a benign fibrous cortical defect (arrows). The degree of increased activity is much less than the normal activity in the metaphyses of this young adult.

test over the bone scan has led to its routine use as a screening method, however. Current practice uses a PSA value greater than 8 units to indicate a need for a bone scan to allow identification of bone metastases. If the PSA value is normal or less than 8 units, bone metastases are highly unlikely.

Strontium-89 has been demonstrated to be an effective therapy for bone pain resulting from osteoblastic metastases. Most of the reported studies have been based on patients with prostate or breast cancers in whom conventional therapies have failed. Significant relief from bone pain is achieved in about 80 per cent of cases and total relief in about 25 per cent. Reports have indicated that strontium-89 may delay progression of disease.[218, 219] Investigative trials to determine if therapeutic benefit can be obtained from earlier use of strontium-89 in patients with documented bone metastases, but prior to development of bone pain, are being planned. The mechanism by which strontium-89 relieves pain is not understood. Clearly, its beta emissions result in radiation to sites of skeletal metastasis. Its major toxicity is hematologic, requiring careful monitoring of the platelet count. Other bone localizing agents that diminish pain related to skeletal metastasis (e.g., rhenium and sumarium) are being evaluated in clinical trials. These agents possess a shorter life than strontium-89, therefore delivering their radiation more rapidly and resulting in more rapid pain relief. The pain relief afforded by these agents, however, is not of long duration.

***Thyroid Cancer.*** Generally, the bone scan is recognized as the most sensitive imaging method for the detection of bone metastases. However, in the case of thyroid cancer metastatic to bone, iodine-131 imaging using high scanning doses (5 to 10 mCi) or thallium-201 may be more sensitive than conventional bone scan for the detection of differentiated bone metastases of thyroid tumor.[220, 221] In one report of eight patients with metastatic thyroid cancer, conventional bone scan missed 60 per cent of bone metastases that were seen on [131]I images.[220] More recently, thallium SPECT imaging has been reported as a significant improvement over other approaches.[221]

After therapy of thyroid cancer with 100 mCi or greater of [131]I, whole body imaging at 7 to 10 days probably provides an excellent opportunity of optimized sensitivity for detection of bone and other metastases from thyroid cancer. Such imaging also provides evidence of the achievement of [131]I localization and hence radiation delivery to tumor foci in bones and other tissues.

***Primary Malignant Bone Tumors.*** The frequency of skeletal metastases at autopsy in patients with primary osteosarcoma is about 25 per cent. Although pulmonary metastases also are frequent in these patients, Goldstein and coworkers[52] reported that about 15 per cent of patients developed bone metastases in the absence of or prior to lung metastases. These investigators also noted that approximately 25 per cent of all bone lesions were seen by 7 months, 50 per cent by 14 months, and 75 per cent by 24 months after clinical presentation. Thus, it seems reasonable that children with osteosarcoma should have a bone scan as a baseline study to verify the presence or absence of distant metastases. On the other hand, the question of whether or not the bone scan is more accurate than the radiograph in delineating the local extent of the primary tumor (in osteosarcoma as well as in other primary bone sarcomas) is

unanswered, as general hyperperfusion of the involved extremity may account for a larger abnormality on the scan than on the radiograph without necessarily being indicative of tumor extension.[149–152]

Rees and colleagues[222] reported on 27 children with localized osteosarcoma, of whom 18 subsequently developed lung metastases and three developed bone metastases. Seven of the 18 patients with lung metastases showed abnormal pulmonary uptake of the bone-seeking radionuclide in sites of metastasis. Detection of the bone metastases in three patients did not alter therapy. These authors concluded that the bone scan is useful in the initial assessment of metastases and subsequent follow-up evaluation in selected cases, but not in cases in which no suspicion of bone metastases exists. An important function of bone scans in primary bone tumors is to identify polyostotic involvement.[223] The bone scan, because it is more sensitive than radiography, should be the preferred method.

In Ewing's sarcoma, about 60 per cent of patients have bone metastases at autopsy.[44] At the time of clinical presentation, bone metastases were diagnosed in 12 per cent of children with Ewing's sarcoma, whereas 33 per cent of patients showed bone metastases on follow-up examinations.[53, 54] These skeletal metastases occurred prior to or in the absence of pulmonary metastases in more than half the patients who were studied. Such metastases have been reported to be more frequent when the primary neoplasm is located in the axial skeleton.[165] On the basis of available data, it would seem reasonable that children with Ewing's sarcoma should have a bone scan at the time of initial presentation and during follow-up periods of at least 2 years.

***Neuroblastoma.*** Bone scanning has been recommended as the screening procedure of choice in children suspected of having skeletal metastases in neuroblastoma.[55] Gilday and associates found no false-negative bone scans in 30 cases of neuroblastoma and recommended that radiographs be obtained only if a lesion was evident on the nuclear image.[55] Other investigators[56, 163, 166] have reported false-negative bone scans in neuroblastoma. In one series,[56] a total of 18 lesions were detected in six patients, of which 14 were demonstrated by radiography and only four were positive by radiography and scintigraphy. Skeletal foci of neuroblastoma show predilection for the metaphyseal regions of long bones, at which sites the scintigraphic abnormalities may be obscured by the avid uptake of radiopharmaceutical in adjacent physes. This fact, coupled with the small size and lytic nature of the lesion, is cited as an explanation for the false-negative radionuclide examinations in patients with neuroblastoma.[56] Abnormal accumulation of the bone-seeking radionuclide at the site of the primary tumor represents, however, an additional benefit of the bone scan in patients with neuroblastoma.[160, 166]

Despite some inconsistencies in scintigraphic findings, the bone scan clearly is superior to radiography in cases of skeletal metastases related to neuroblastoma, with a sensitivity of 90 per cent versus 69 per cent for radiography in one series[223] and 74 per cent for radiography in another series.[224] Reports comparing bone scan and metaiodobenzyl-guanidine (MIBG) labeled to [123]I have revealed mixed results. In one study[225] of 44 children with neuroblastoma, [123]I-MIBG scanning showed more skeletal involvement (161 sites) than did bone scanning (100 sites). Five patients with abnormal foci on bone scan had normal MIBG scans, however. Thus, the $^{99m}$Tc-MDP bone scan is recommended as the primary screening method for the detection of skeletal metastases in neuroblastoma, although $^{123}$I-MIBG is believed to be the best whole body imaging method for soft tissue involvement in neuroblastoma.[226] Therapy using $^{131}$I-MIBG has been tried with mixed results. Using 100 to 250 mCi of $^{131}$I-MIBG, partial remissions were seen in four of eight patients.[227]

**Benign Bone Tumors and Tumor-Like Lesions.** In the evaluation of benign bone lesions, the scan may be valuable clinically, particularly in patients with pain in whom radiographs fail to reveal a bone lesion. Not uncommonly, small lesions that are difficult to see on the radiograph because of their location may be quite apparent on the bone scan. An osteoid osteoma is a lesion that characteristically is quite "hot" on the bone scan and yet may be difficult to detect on a radiograph[57] (Fig. 15–9). Closer inspection documents that a "double density" characterizes the region of increased activity on the bone scan in patients with an osteoid osteoma.[167] Autoradiography confirms that the central nidus of the tumor accumulates greater amounts of the radiopharmaceutical than the surrounding sclerotic bone, accounting for the double density appearance.[168] Radionuclide techniques also have been used to localize the nidus while the patient is in the operating room. Sterilized radiation probes are used for this purpose at the time of surgery in a patient who has received an intravenous injection of the bone-seeking radionuclide approximately 3 hours prior to the operation. After surgical exposure of the bone, the head of the probe is moved along the surface of the bone until the point of highest gamma emission is identified.[169] Autoradiography of the excised specimen can be done to confirm that the nidus has been removed.[168]

Several other benign bone lesions frequently are "hot" on the bone scan, including Paget's disease and fibrous dysplasia. The extent of radiopharmaceutical concentration in these lesions reflects the degree of hyperemia and osteogenesis.

Bone cysts show normal or slightly increased radiopharmaceutical concentration, and a central area of decreased counts may be present. When a fracture complicates a bone cyst, the scan will be "hot." In the absence of such a fracture, the radionuclide appearance may be useful in distinguishing between a benign cyst and a malignant bone lesion.

In the skull, a mild degree of increased uptake in the frontal or parasagittal region usually will reflect the presence of hyperostosis frontalis internis. The mild nature of the augmented radionuclide activity and its characteristic anatomic distribution allow accurate diagnosis in these cases. In children, sutural sites may show increased activity, which regresses to normal after closure of the sutures. In infants, the bone scan may be of clinical value in examining patients with potential premature closure of sutures and in determining the need for surgical intervention.[58, 59]

Bone islands have a variable appearance on the bone scan. When larger than 3 cm in size, they may be manifested as focal regions of increased activity on the bone scan. Generally, bone islands that are less than 3 cm in size show normal uptake of the radiopharmaceutical. The bone scan, when accompanied by a radionuclide angiogram performed at the time of intravenous injection of the radiopharmaceutical, may be helpful in differentiating a bone island from a more aggressive lesion, as an element of increased vascularity would make the diagnosis of bone island unlikely.

Other benign bone tumors and tumor-like lesions, including eosinophilic granuloma, fibrous cortical defect, enchondroma, aneurysmal bone cyst,[170] and osteochondroma, frequently will show increased radiopharmaceutical uptake on the nuclear images. The scan may be clinically helpful in identifying multiple lesions in these diseases, as well as in their follow-up, particularly if malignant transformation is suspected.

## Infection

The diagnosis of bone infection remains a major clinical problem, particularly as the radiograph is relatively insensitive to the early changes of osteomyelitis and frequently may not become positive until 10 to 14 days after the onset of the disease. The sensitivity of the bone scan is such that as early as 24 hours after the onset of symptoms, the scan may be positive and usually will remain positive until the lesion is healed completely.[60] The role of the radionuclide study in the evaluation of osseous inflammatory disease includes (1) early detection, (2) differentiation of osteomyelitis from cellulitis, and (3) identification of renewed activity in cases of chronic osteomyelitis. Regarding the first, the high degree of sensitivity of the bone scan for identifying and localizing the abnormality in the presence of normal radiographs makes the scan important clinically in the workup of patients with possible osteomyelitis. Occasionally, very early in the course of osteomyelitis, the lesion will appear on the scan as a "cold" or photon-deficient focus.[26, 61] This appearance probably can be explained by the pathophysiology of early osteomyelitis, specifically an interruption of bone blood supply secondary to sludging and thrombosis induced by the inflammatory infiltration of cells, which may originate in the marrow. Several such

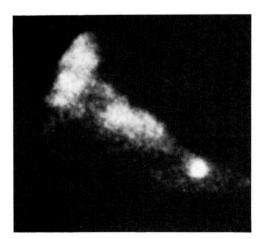

**FIGURE 15–9.** Osteoid osteoma: A lateral view of the left foot from a $^{99m}$Tc-MDP bone scan in a patient complaining of pain in the left foot. A focal region of markedly increased uptake in the forefoot is identified and is consistent with the diagnosis of osteoid osteoma.

cases have been reported, particularly in neonates or young children. With time, the pattern of a focally increased region of activity will replace the photon-deficient area as bone repair occurs and an infarctive process is replaced by a hyperemic response. Thus, the spectrum of the radionuclide pattern in osteomyelitis varies from areas that are photon-deficient to those that have augmented radionuclide activity (Fig. 15–10). Between these two points, of course, lies the range for a normal degree of uptake. If the patient is imaged during the transient normal period on this spectrum, a false-negative scan will result.

As a consequence of false-negative results ranging in frequency from 5 per cent to as high as 60 per cent early in the course of osteomyelitis, particularly in infants and small children, $^{67}$Ga bone imaging has been used as an adjunct to technetium imaging. Gallium-67 citrate images are obtained 6 and 24 hours after the injection of 5 mCi for the diagnosis of osteomyelitis. Reports on the use of $^{67}$Ga for imaging active osteomyelitis uniformly have revealed correct identification of infection in nearly all cases. In many patients, particularly children, the gallium images are more accurate in identifying focal lesions adjacent to growth plates that were masked by adjacent high-intensity uptake on bone scans. Figure 15–11A shows the bone scan and Figure 15–11B the gallium scan from a 21 year old man complaining of right hip pain. The bone scan failed to show a definite abnormality, and only in retrospect, after visualization of the abnormality in the right sacroiliac joint on the gallium

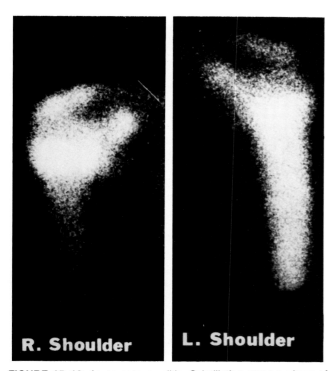

**FIGURE 15–10.** Acute osteomyelitis: Scintillation camera views of the shoulders in a patient with osteomyelitis. The left shoulder view shows a markedly increased uptake involving the proximal portion of the humerus and extending to the level of the midshaft. At a later time, radiographs of this region showed periosteal elevation and other findings consistent with the diagnosis of acute osteomyelitis. The right shoulder is normal.

study, was a faint degree of increased uptake identified on the technetium study. Osteomyelitis subsequently was confirmed by blood cultures and radiography.

The differentiation between osteomyelitis and cellulitis may be a very difficult clinical problem in which sequential $^{99m}$Tc-MDP and $^{67}$Ga imaging may be helpful,[62, 63] both for diagnosis and for monitoring the response to therapy. The three phase or four phase bone scan is widely used for these purposes. At the time of intravenous injection of $^{99m}$Tc-MDP, sequential imaging with the scintillation camera centered over the bone in question produces a radionuclide angiogram (phase one) that is followed by an immediate blood pool image (also, phase one), disclosing the degree of vascular abnormality of the involved bone. Generally, in either osteomyelitis or cellulitis, increased vascularity will be seen. Routinely, delayed images are obtained in several projections at about 2 hours after injection (phase two). In either osteomyelitis or cellulitis, focal increased activity may be seen on these images in the region in question. If a second set of delayed images is made at about 5 hours after injection (phase three), the ratio of counts in the region being examined relative to the surrounding normal bone will have increased compared with the ratio at 2 hours in patients with osteomyelitis. The fourth phase is a 24 hour image that further accentuates the increasing count accumulation in regions of osteomyelitis relative to normal bone. In cellulitis, however, just the opposite would be expected: The ratio of counts would decrease slowly over this time period, as most of the activity within the region is due to the hypervascular characteristics of the soft tissue inflammation. Although both $^{67}$Ga- and $^{111}$In-labeled leukocytes are highly sensitive detectors of osteomyelitis, it may be difficult to determine if the activity is the result of bone or soft tissue infection, or both. The approach of combined radionuclide angiography, blood pool imaging, and conventional and delayed nuclear bone imaging (the four phase bone scan), supplemented by $^{67}$Ga- or $^{111}$In-labeled leukocyte imaging, or both, is demonstrated in Figures 15–12 to 15–15.

Although $^{67}$Ga-citrate and $^{111}$In-labeled leukocytes are widely used in the diagnosis of acute and chronic osteomyelitis, most knowledgeable physicians probably would prefer the three or four phase technetium phosphate bone scan as the initial nuclear imaging procedure, especially in the evaluation of acute osteomyelitis. The reports of false-negative results on $^{99m}$Tc-phosphate scans, particularly in neonates and young children, were based on conventional 2 or 3 hour static imaging, not three or four phase studies. The radiation dose from indium in particular, and, to a lesser extent, from gallium is high for a neonate; therefore, such studies usually are accomplished after a normal $^{99m}$Tc-phosphate bone scan in neonates or young children when clinical suspicion persists. In adults the sensitivity of the three phase bone scan in the detection of osteomyelitis has been reported as 90 to 100 per cent and its specificity as 73 to 89 per cent.[166, 171, 228–230] In one study of adults with peripheral vascular disease and suspected osteomyelitis, the four phase bone scan showed a sensitivity of 80 per cent and a specificity of 87 per cent,[212] results that were slightly better than those of the three phase study in the same patient group.

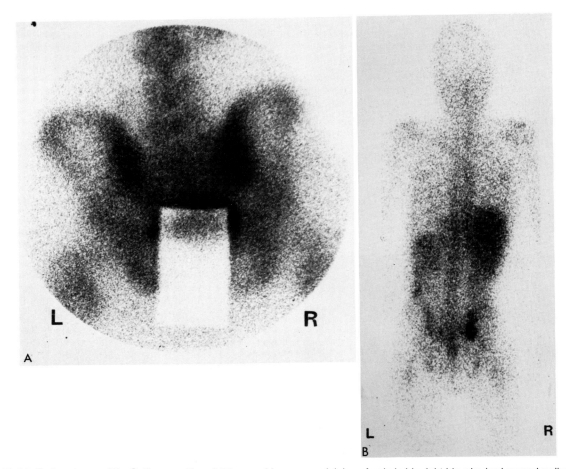

**FIGURE 15–11.** Early osteomyelitis: Gallium positive. A 21 year old man complaining of pain in his right hip who had normal radiographs was referred from the emergency room for a bone scan to determine if a focus of osteomyelitis was present.

   **A** On the $^{99m}$Tc-MDP image, an area of equivocal abnormality in the right sacroiliac joint is seen.

   **B** A $^{67}$Ga scan was performed because of the suspicion of osteomyelitis. The right sacroiliac region is highly positive on the gallium scan, confirming the probable diagnosis of osteomyelitis. Blood cultures eventually revealed *Staphylococcus aureus*, and radiographs became positive approximately 1 week later.

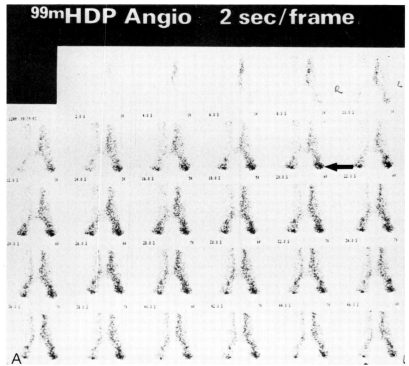

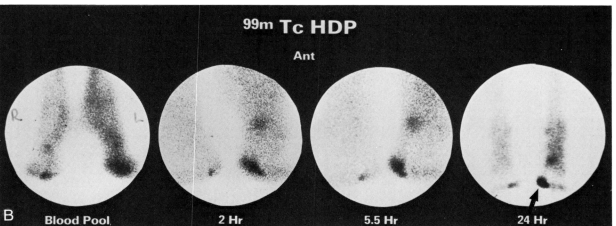

**FIGURE 15–12.** Four phase bone scan: Osteomyelitis versus cellulitis.

**A** Radionuclide angiogram of the feet in a patient with a diabetic ulcer over the left great toe. The sequential 2 sec images (left to right) show generalized hypervascularity in the left foot in comparison to the right, with a focus of more intense activity over the left great toe (arrow).

**B** Blood pool and delayed images of the ⁹⁹ᵐTc-HDP bone scan of the feet show that the region of abnormal activity in the left first toe persists (arrow) in comparison to the normal right foot. This pattern of abnormal, persistent uptake of the radionuclide, even at 24 hours, is consistent with the diagnosis of osteomyelitis. Note also that the other bones of the involved foot show generalized increased uptake as well, probably reflecting hypervascularity due to inflammation.

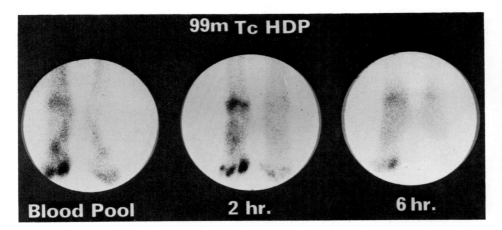

**FIGURE 15–13.** Osteomyelitis versus soft tissue infection. Three phase bone scan in a patient with persistent ulcerations of the toes. Although there is increased uptake of the radionuclide in the blood pool and 2 hour images, the significantly diminished bone activity at 6 hours makes the diagnosis of osteomyelitis unlikely.

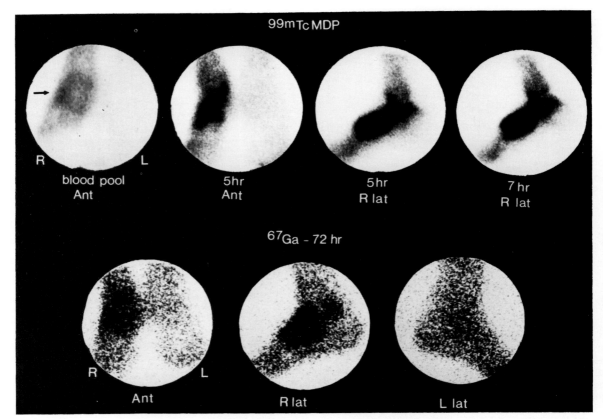

**FIGURE 15–14.** Osteomyelitis versus cellulitis: Bone and gallium scans. $^{99m}$Tc-MDP immediate blood pool image, delayed $^{99m}$Tc-MDP images, and $^{67}$Ga scan images of the feet in a diabetic patient are shown. Note that the blood pool image shows markedly increased activity involving the right foot, particularly the region of the tarsal bones (arrow). Delayed images show persistence of increased activity in the region of the tarsal bones, with an increasing ratio of counts in the tarsal bone area relative to other bones at 7 hours. The $^{67}$Ga scan confirms a high probability of osteomyelitis involving the tarsal bones because of the markedly increased uptake seen in the abnormal foot relative to the normal left side. Later radiographic studies confirmed the presence of osteomyelitis involving several of the tarsal bones.

**FIGURE 15–15.** Active osteomyelitis around metallic plates and screws in the femur and tibia. Bone scan images (left column), including left lateral and anterior views, show abnormal, increased uptake in the regions of bone infection involving the metal plate and screws in the tibia (double arrows) and femur. The $^{67}$Ga images (middle column) show a matching pattern of abnormal, increased uptake in the regions of bone infection (arrows). The $^{111}$In leukocyte images (right column) show the same areas of abnormal, increased uptake as on the bone and gallium images (black arrows) in the tibia but, in addition, these images reveal abnormal increased uptake in the suprapatellar bursa and knee joint (single black arrow above and single white arrow below). In addition to osteomyelitis, the $^{111}$In leukocyte images have documented septic arthritis.

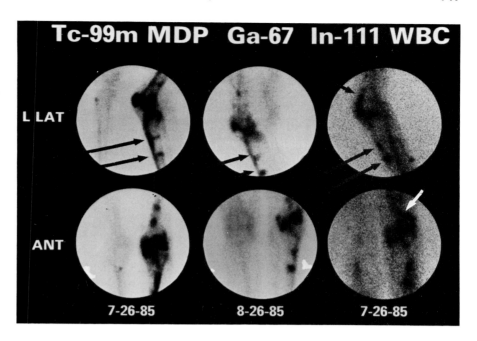

A more recent report by Schauwecker[231] indicates that the sensitivity for $^{111}$In leukocyte imaging in acute osteomyelitis is 90 to 95 per cent for all bones, but for chronic osteomyelitis sensitivity varies by location (i.e., 94 per cent for peripheral bones and 53 per cent for central bones).

For combined bone and gallium scans, several patterns have been described,[232] but only the pattern in which abnormal gallium uptake exceeds the abnormal bone scan uptake indicates active bone infection reliably. Unfortunately, this scan pattern is seen in only 25 to 28 per cent of patients with bone infection.[231, 232] Gallium is excellent in excluding osteomyelitis, if results are normal, and confirming osteomyelitis when the criterion of discordant or increased gallium accumulation exceeding bone scan accumulation is met.

The high false-negative results of the technetium bone scans in cases of acute osteomyelitis in pediatric patients perhaps are related to a masking effect produced by the normal activity characteristic of the regions of rapid growth in the metaphyses and epiphyses and diminished blood flow that is characteristic in the very early stages of osteomyelitis. In fact, a spectrum in the pattern of radiopharmaceutical uptake in bone lesions is observed, ranging from regions of photon deficiency (cold areas) to regions of augmented activity (hot areas). If the lesion is cold or hot scintigraphically, it is identified easily on the scan, but if its pattern of activity lies between these two points, it is missed easily. Despite these drawbacks, scintigraphic imaging of bone is considered the optimal diagnostic technique for the assessment of acute osteomyelitis, although an argument can be presented for using $^{111}$In leukocyte scanning first in adults who reveal chronic degenerative or traumatic bone changes on radiographs.

In chronic osteomyelitis, comparisons of $^{99m}$Tc-phosphate bone imaging and $^{67}$Ga-citrate imaging suggest higher accuracy of the gallium scan in detecting the response or lack of response of the infection to therapy.[63] One limitation of the $^{99m}$Tc-phosphate bone scan in following the response of

therapy in cases of chronic osteomyelitis is its sensitivity to bone remodeling and proliferation. Gallium uptake, however, truly may be more indicative of the presence of infection because it is not as sensitive to bone remodeling. It has been suggested that the clinically important pattern in evaluating this response to therapy is the general direction of the changing scintigraphic findings on serial gallium scans (i.e., toward more normal or more abnormal findings). The clinical utility of the gallium scan has been found to be most significant in patients whose clinical assessment was uncertain.[63] In one study, 14 patients with chronic osteomyelitis were followed over a 2 year period by clinical, radiographic, and bone and gallium scans, which were obtained approximately every 6 months.[63] The results indicated that although radiographic findings did not change substantially over the course of therapy, both the bone scan and the gallium scan revealed changes that reflected the response to therapy accurately. When there was poor response or no response, little or no change was seen in the scans. Bone scans tended to remain positive for longer periods of time than did the gallium scans, probably because of continued bone remodeling and osteogenesis, even after the infectious process had subsided. The gallium scan, on the other hand, tended to remain positive only as long as an active infectious process continued.[63] Figure 15–16 demonstrates follow-up studies of a patient with chronic osteomyelitis using bone and gallium scans over a 2 year period.

With regard to $^{111}$In leukocyte imaging, comparative studies of this technique and $^{99m}$Tc-phosphate bone imaging in animals with acute osteomyelitis indicate that white blood cell scans can detect the disease earlier than technetium phosphate bone scans or conventional radiographs.[172] In patients, $^{111}$In leukocyte scanning has been judged effective in the evaluation of patients with pain after hip arthroplasty,[173] although gallium and technetium phosphate scanning also has been used for this purpose (see later discussion). In the detection of renewed activity of infection

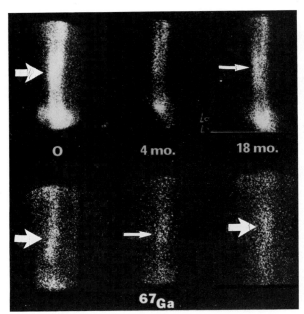

**FIGURE 15–16.** Chronic osteomyelitis: Clinical failure. A patient with chronic osteomyelitis was treated with antibiotic therapy without clinical improvement. The $^{99m}$Tc-phosphate images (above) and the gallium images (below) both show persistence of an abnormal focus of increased uptake (arrows).

in patients with chronic osteomyelitis, $^{111}$In appears to represent a superior radionuclide agent.[174, 175]

Patients with septic arthritis also have been studied by $^{99m}$Tc-MDP, $^{67}$Ga, and $^{111}$In leukocyte imaging. All of these radionuclide examinations can reveal abnormalities, although factors such as the age of the process may modify the findings. Lisbona and Rosenthall[64] documented in their series that changing activity of $^{67}$Ga uptake paralleled the patient's clinical course more closely than did the $^{99m}$Tc-MDP image in septic arthritis.

In acute osteomyelitis, bone and gallium scans have been used to follow the response to therapy and as a potential guide for determining when intravenous antibiotics should be discontinued.[65] Scans improved markedly within the first 2 or 4 weeks of treatment, but abnormalities persisted at 6 weeks in over 50 per cent of cases, despite clinical resolution of disease.

Pain after joint replacement may be caused by loosening of the prosthesis, infection, or both. Evaluation of $^{67}$Ga or $^{99m}$Tc-phosphate bone imaging has been performed for diagnosis of infection or loosening of prostheses. In one series of 26 patients with hip or knee prostheses who had bone and gallium scans and who underwent subsequent surgery, correlation of the scintigraphic and surgical results revealed a 75 per cent sensitivity for the diagnosis of infection by both gallium and bone scans, with a specificity of 73 per cent.[66] Scan evidence for presence or absence of loosening was in agreement with the surgical findings in 16 patients with loosening and in two patients without loosening. The sensitivity for detecting loosening by scan was 100 per cent, whereas the specificity was 40 per cent. The overall results of the radionuclide study in classifying the prosthesis correctly as diseased or nondiseased (loosening with or without infection) was 80 per cent. This study reported

a 75 per cent sensitivity and 73 per cent specificity for the scan diagnosis of infection. There were several false-positive scans, most of which had been obtained in patients with rheumatoid arthritis. The radionuclide criteria that were used for the diagnosis of infection were moderate to severe focal increased uptake on both bone and gallium images. The diagnosis of loosening was based on an abnormal bone scan, which varied in severity from very mild to severe alterations, and a gallium scan that was only mildly abnormal or even normal. Figures 15–17 to 15–19 demonstrate the bone and gallium scan results in patients with painful prostheses. Additional studies[67-71] have revealed a high degree of accuracy in correlating implant loosening with scan results, whereas other authors[66] have reported a somewhat poorer ability of the scans to distinguish infection from loosening. Nonetheless, a normal bone scan would appear to weigh heavily against the need for surgical intervention for loosening or infection of prostheses.

The radionuclide study also can be used in the assessment of osteomyelitis involving the stump of an amputated limb. Frequently, because of constant irritation to the bone produced by weight-bearing on the prosthesis, the radiograph will show osseous irregularities that make the diagnosis of early osteomyelitis very difficult. Likewise, the bone scan may show increased radionuclide uptake secondary to the continual trauma to the distal part of the stump. Markedly increased uptake, however, exceeded by abnormal activity on a gallium image, should alert the physician to a high probability of osteomyelitis (Fig. 15–20). Gallium activity that is equal to or less than that on the bone scan is not specific for osteomyelitis, although it does not exclude that possibility.

A cadre of new agents are under investigation for imaging infection. To some extent a sense of urgency is connected to bringing these new products to market because of the hazards associated with $^{111}$In leukocyte scanning, which requires handling of blood and blood products. Human polyclonal (nonspecific) immunoglobulin G (IgG) shows promise as an agent to image infection if labeled to indium-111 or technetium-99m.[235] This type of new agent for imaging of infection is being received enthusiastically because it appears to be effective clinically and consists of a simple kit preparation that does not require withdrawal of blood from patients. This labeled immunoglobulin is thought to bind to Fc receptors expressed by cells involved in the inflammatory response (macrophages, polymorphonuclear leukocytes, lymphocytes).[236] In one study of 84 patients whose suspected infections were evaluated with $^{111}$In-labeled polyclonal IgG, the images had a sensitivity of 92 per cent and a specificity of 95 per cent.[237] This study demonstrated that this radiopharmaceutical is useful in the assessment of infections related to a variety of organisms and in a variety of osseous and extraosseous sites.

Work from Austria showed that imaging with a $^{99m}$Tc-labeled monoclonal antigranulocyte antibody (BW 250/183) in 34 patients who had suspected inflammation of soft tissue and bone was 95 per cent sensitive.[238] The specificity (85%) was somewhat lower, reflecting the difficulty of distinguishing between infection and inflammation without infection, both of which lead to accumulation of leukocytes. The monoclonal antibody BW 250/183 reacts with an epitope of a nonspecific cross-reacting antigen on the surface of granulocytes.

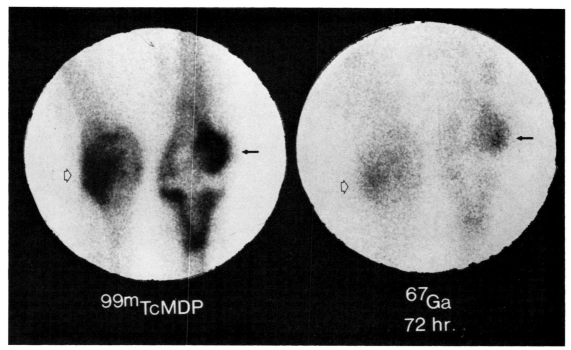

**FIGURE 15–17.** Painful prosthesis: Loosening versus infection. The ⁹⁹ᵐTc-MDP bone image and ⁶⁷Ga image of the knees in a patient with underlying rheumatoid arthritis and a painful left knee prosthesis are shown. The ⁹⁹ᵐTc-MDP study shows increased uptake around the tibial portion of the prosthesis and a focus of increased uptake in the lateral femoral portion, which is matched by markedly increased uptake on the gallium image in the same regions (solid arrows). The findings are consistent with osteomyelitis, which was confirmed at surgery. Increased uptake is seen on bone and gallium images in the opposite knee affected by rheumatoid arthritis (open arrows).

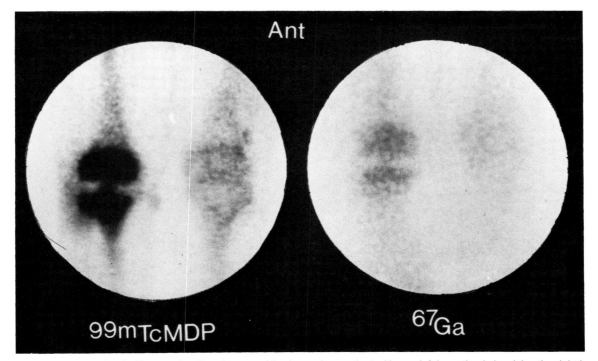

**FIGURE 15–18.** Painful prosthesis: Bone and gallium images of the knees in a patient with a painful prosthesis involving the right knee. Both bone and gallium studies show markedly increased uptake about both femoral and tibial components. These scan results are not diagnostic of infection. At surgery, presence of infection was confirmed.

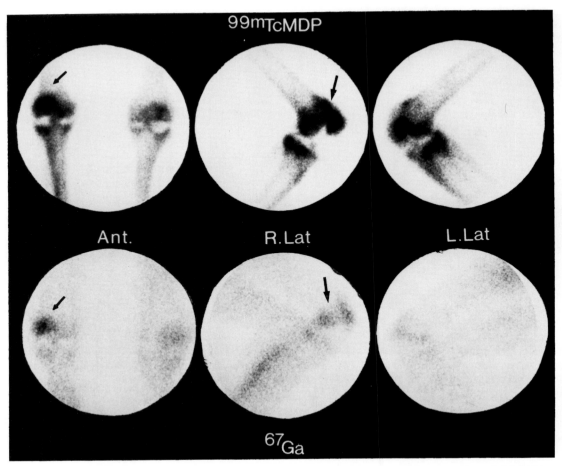

**FIGURE 15–19.** Painful prosthesis: Bone and gallium images in a patient with bilateral knee prostheses and a painful right knee. The right knee shows markedly increased uptake in the femoral component on both bone and gallium studies (arrows). At surgery, no infection was found; however, abundant granulation tissue and loosening of the prosthesis were noted.

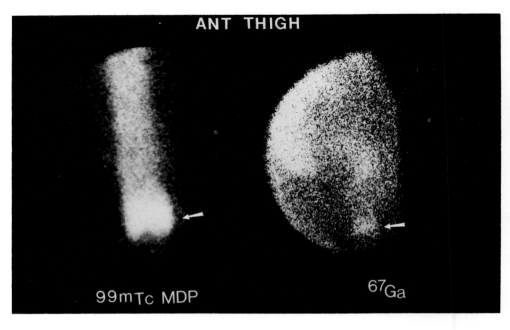

**FIGURE 15–20.** Amputation: Evaluation of stump for infection. $^{99m}$Tc-MDP bone and $^{67}$Ga images of the distal stump of an above-the-knee amputation being evaluated for possible osteomyelitis. Note that markedly increased uptake is seen at the distal stump on the $^{99m}$Tc-MDP image, with a focus of increased uptake on the gallium image (arrows). The patient was treated for osteomyelitis.

A potential complication of $^{99m}$Tc-labeled monoclonal antibody imaging is the precipitation of an immunologic response to the antibody and possible reactions to a second administration. Human anti-mouse antigens, which are able to bind to the monoclonal antibody at its variable region (anti-idiotype antibodies), were detected at low levels in only 1 of 20 patients studied, indicating relative safety.[238]

A major deficiency of the $^{111}$In-labeled leukocyte study and techniques using some of the newer agents is that imaging is delayed for 24 hours. $^{99m}$Tc-HMPAO-labeled leukocytes have been studied as a potential alternative for $^{111}$In-labeled white blood cells; reports on the accuracy of this technique for early imaging have been mixed. Mountfield and coworkers[239] reported that compared to $^{111}$In-labeled leukocyte scanning, $^{99m}$Tc-HMPAO leukocyte imaging performed 4 hours after administration of radiopharmaceutical agent is highly sensitive (100 per cent) for detecting infections but has a very low specificity. After 24 hours, $^{99m}$Tc-HMPAO-labeled leukocyte images remained sensitive (100 per cent), as did $^{111}$In-labeled leukocyte images after 24 hours, but specificity for $^{99m}$Tc-HMPAO (62 per cent) still was significantly lower than that of $^{111}$In-labeled leukocytes (86 per cent).

Although results with $^{99m}$Tc-HMPAO-labeled leukocyte imaging are encouraging, the handling of blood for labeling leukocytes detracts from its appeal. It is much more likely that $^{111}$In-labeled immunoglobulin G or the $^{111}$In- or $^{99m}$Tc-labeled antigranulocyte antibody agents will replace $^{111}$In-labeled leukocytes as the preferred imaging agent for infection after the favorable review by the Food and Drug Administration of the new drug application.

MR imaging studies in patients with suspected osteomyelitis indicate similar problems as described for radionuclide studies. Specificity for osteomyelitis is reduced because traumatic changes or tumors of bone can mimic osteomyelitis on the MR image. Although bone infection usually is associated with increased signal intensity on T2-weighted spin echo MR images, some culture-proved cases of osteomyelitis show low signal intensity on both T1- and T2-weighted images, which also is characteristic of fibrous dysplasia and other conditions. Metallic implants diminish the utility of MR imaging because of the presence of artifacts. Nonetheless, MR imaging clearly has advantages over CT,[233] and reported sensitivity and specificity are comparable to those of nuclear imaging.[234]

## Trauma

**Stress Injuries.** Conventional radiography has proved to be an extremely sensitive tool for detecting fractures and for following the healing response. Some fractures, however, are not detected readily by conventional radiography. A good example of such a fracture is the stress fracture. Stress fractures result from repetitive prolonged muscular action on a bone that is unaccustomed to such stress. *Fatigue fractures* and *insufficiency fractures* are two types of stress fractures. The fatigue fracture most commonly affects military recruits and athletes who impose repetitive, perhaps abnormal, muscular stress or torque on normal bones. The insufficiency fracture occurs as a result of normal physiologic stresses on abnormal bones having deficient elastic resistance. Conditions that predispose to insufficiency fractures include osteoporosis, osteomalacia, Paget's disease,

osteopetrosis, rheumatoid arthritis, fibrous dysplasia, hyperparathyroidism, and irradiation.

The bone scan may be helpful in imaging either fatigue or insufficiency fractures, especially when radiographs are unrevealing. The high degree of sensitivity of the bone scan surpasses that of radiography in detecting stress fractures and other forms of periosteal injury without fracture. Wilcox and coworkers[72] reported an evaluation of bone scintigraphy in 34 patients with physical findings and histories suggestive of stress fracture in the lower extremity. Of the 34 persons, 21 had abnormal studies, 11 involving the femoral neck, nine involving the tibia, and one involving the femur. All the abnormal radionuclide studies were apparent prior to or at the time of appearance of radiographic changes. Of the nine with abnormal tibial studies, radiographic changes never evolved in three. No false-negative results were found among the 13 patients with normal scintigrams. Other studies have confirmed that the bone scan is an effective technique for the early diagnosis of a stress fracture[73, 176–180] (Figs. 15–21 and 15–22).

Another stress injury is the shin splint. This term is applied to tightness and aching in the lower legs on exercise, commonly encountered in athletes. Tendinitis, myositis, and periostitis of the anterior or posterior muscle groups of the leg all are probably involved. On bone scan, shin splint pain is associated with periosteal deposition of the radiopharmaceutical, with the appearance of a "double stripe" sign, similar to that reported in hypertrophic

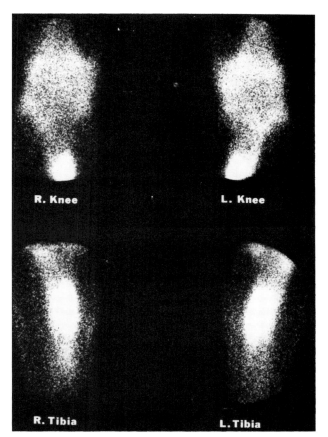

**FIGURE 15–21.** Stress fractures. $^{99m}$Tc-Pyrophosphate bone images of both lower legs in a 21 year old military recruit complaining of pain in the shins. Marked increased uptake is noted over the proximal ends of both tibia. The findings are consistent with stress fractures.

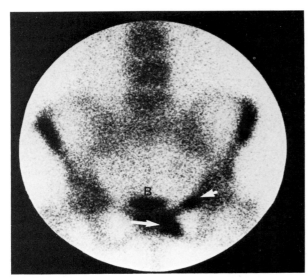

**FIGURE 15–22.** Stress fractures. This abnormal bone scan from a 30 year old female athlete indicates stress fractures in the superior pubic ramus and parasymphyseal bone (arrows). A small amount of radiopharmaceutical excretion is seen in the bladder (B). A radiograph (not shown) revealed a mild degree of bone sclerosis in the region of the symphysis pubis but no findings to correspond to the pubic ramus lesion.

osteoarthropathy.[181, 182] In these cases, the scan reflects periosteal injury rather than a true stress fracture of bone (Fig. 15–23); in a true stress fracture, the bone scan shows abnormally increased radionuclide uptake that traverses horizontally across the shaft of the long bone (see Chapter 67).

Matin[76] has described five stages of stress fractures ranging from minimal periosteal reaction (stage I) to a full-thickness stress fracture (stage V). The importance in distinguishing these stages is the time requirement for satisfactory treatment. A periosteal reaction can require as little as 1 or 2 weeks of rest, whereas a stage V stress fracture may require at least 6 weeks of rest and possibly immobilization.

**Athletic Injuries.** Sports medicine specialists know the desirability of providing objective evidence to dedicated athletes of the need to refrain from training to allow an

injury to heal.[240] The bone scan often provides such evidence, even when radiographs do not, and it provides information regarding the severity of the injury. The most commonly encountered such injury is a stress fracture. Other occult fractures include injury to the hook of the hamate, usually acquired from playing tennis, baseball, or golf. Enthesopathies are subtle injuries that may be difficult to diagnose but may be apparent on the bone scan. Bursitis may be associated with sports activities and may be apparent on SPECT bone scans, even though not seen on routine radiographs, MR images, or even planar bone scans.[241]

Abnormal increased activity in the patella has many causes, including fracture, osteoarthritis, and chondromalacia.[242] Furthermore, the finding of a "hot" patella on bone scan often is not associated with significant symptoms.

**Fracture Healing.** Studies of the pathophysiology of fracture healing show that repair at the fracture site usually begins within 24 hours after the event. Bone scans may show focal abnormalities, perhaps as early as 24 hours after injury, but usually by 3 days.[74] The degree of uptake on the bone scan increases, reaching a maximum within several weeks.[75] This phase then is followed by a decrease in uptake, eventually approaching normal levels (Fig. 15–24). Matin[76] reported that 80 per cent of 204 patients with fractures had abnormal bone scans at 24 hours after injury, and 95 per cent had abnormal scans by 72 hours. Several investigators[76–78] have found that fractures can appear abnormal on scans obtained within a few hours of injury, although differences in the scintigraphic time pattern have been noted in older patients compared with persons under 65 years of age. Older patients reveal a lag in the appearance of augmented activity at the fracture site on the scan and in the rapidity with which the scan returns to normal.

Although there is some variability in the time of appearance of fractures on scan, even greater variability exists in the time periods necessary for return of the scan to normal. It is not uncommon to identify abnormal increased focal uptake at a fracture site that is several years old, even as much as 20 years old. Nonetheless, it may be possible to identify the approximate age of a fracture on the scan by the degree of increased uptake (Fig. 15–25). Generally, recent fractures show intense increased uptake, whereas

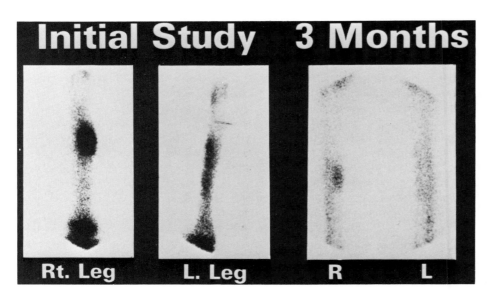

**FIGURE 15–23.** Stress fractures and periosteal injury. A 16 year old female runner complaining of shin splints has a true stress fracture (stage V) in the right tibia and periosteal reaction (stage II) in the left tibia. A subsequent examination 3 months later shows rapid resolution of the periosteal reaction on the left with mild residual abnormality at the site of the true stress fracture on the right. (Courtesy of P. Matin, M.D., Roseville, California.)

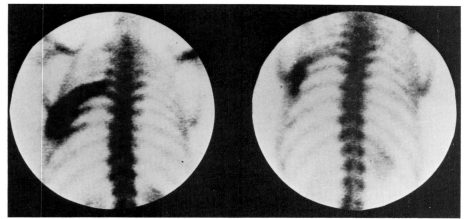

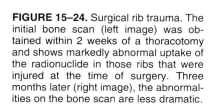

**FIGURE 15–24.** Surgical rib trauma. The initial bone scan (left image) was obtained within 2 weeks of a thoracotomy and shows markedly abnormal uptake of the radionuclide in those ribs that were injured at the time of surgery. Three months later (right image), the abnormalities on the bone scan are less dramatic.

older fractures show normal or mild increased uptake. Because the radiograph may not be helpful in distinguishing between an acute compression fracture and one that has been present for years (if there are no prior radiographs for comparison), the bone scan may have a medicolegal impact in some cases.

Reported studies have examined the potential contribution of the bone scan in assessing the course of fracture healing and nonunion and in predicting which fractures might respond favorably to percutaneous electrical stimulation.[79, 80] In a study of patients with fibrous union, bone scans showed two patterns of radionuclide concentration: (1) intense activity at the fracture site, which appeared quite homogeneous, and (2) a line of decreased activity (negative defect) at the fracture site surrounded by increased uptake on both sides.[80] Of 66 patients with intense radionuclide activity at the fracture site, 62 showed evidence of a good healing response with electrical stimulation. In nine patients with a negative radionuclide defect at the fracture site, eight did not respond to percutaneous electrical stimulation (Fig. 15–26).

Similarly, persistent radionuclide activity can be noted at sites of surgical trauma. This is not infrequent after craniotomy or prosthetic joint surgery. Typically, within 6 to 9 months after surgery, the bone scan should return to a relatively normal baseline level of uptake around a prosthesis (Fig. 15–27). Not infrequently, heterotopic ossification can appear about a joint prosthesis; radiopharmaceutical uptake in the heterotopic bone must not be mistaken for another process, such as infection or loosening (Fig. 15–28).

**Child Abuse.** In the evaluation of children suspected of being abused, published studies comparing radionuclide bone scans and skeletal radiographic surveys have arrived at conflicting conclusions. Some investigators[196–198] present data to support the superiority of bone scanning over radiography in detecting skeletal lesions of child abuse, whereas other authors[199] indicate that the bone scan should be a secondary test after complete radiographic skeletal survey when occult fractures are suspected clinically. Haase and colleagues[196] reported on 44 child abuse patients who had both bone scan and radiographs. Twenty-six had negative scans and negative radiographs. In two cases, radiographically evident skull fractures were undetected by scan; in five of seven cases with positive scans, normal radiographs were obtained initially, but later radiographs showed evidence of osseous lesions. Thus, these investigators concluded that a bone scan and skull radiographs should be obtained initially to evaluate child abuse victims.

The bone scan has certain limitations in evaluating child abuse: Healed fractures may not be evident; epiphyseal and metaphyseal fractures may be difficult to detect because of the normally augmented uptake of the radiopharmaceutical in these regions; and technical details such as the use of pinhole collimation and careful positioning of the patient are critical to accurate analysis. False-negative results of bone scanning are most likely to be obtained in the neonate and young child. Thus, the specific age of the patient may be an important consideration in selecting an imaging approach to evaluating child abuse.

**Iatrogenic Trauma and Steroid Effect.** Joint aspiration and bone or bone marrow biopsy are frequently performed diagnostic procedures. When a bone scan follows one of these procedures, the question of the effect of the iatrogenic trauma on the bone scan often is raised. Several studies

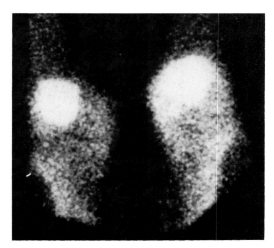

**FIGURE 15–25.** Patellar fractures. $^{99m}$Tc-MDP knee image shows bilateral "hot" patellae. The differential diagnosis for hot patellae includes chondromalacia, degenerative joint disease, fractures, and other conditions. In this case, radiographs (not shown) confirmed the presence of bilateral patellar fractures.

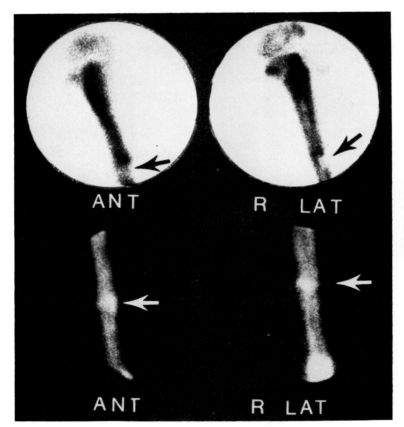

**FIGURE 15–26.** Fracture nonunion: $^{99m}$Tc-MDP bone images of a patient with nonunion of a fracture site in the tibia at the time when the upper row of images was obtained (black arrows). Several months later, follow-up $^{99m}$Tc-MDP images show activity bridging the gap of the previously photon-deficient fracture site (white arrows). This indicates successful healing.

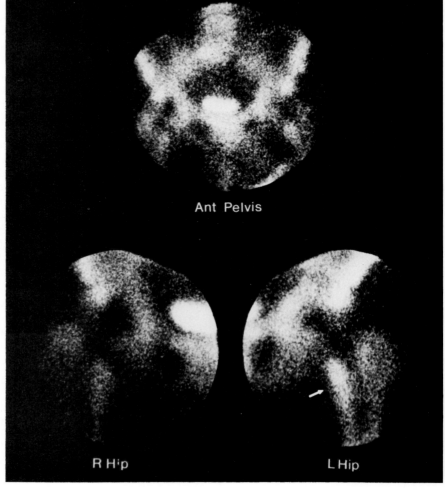

**FIGURE 15–27.** Hip prostheses: $^{99m}$Tc-Pyrophosphate bone images of the pelvis and both hips in a patient with bilateral hip prostheses that had been implanted more than 9 months previously. The right hip is normal and the left hip shows very mildly increased uptake over a medial portion of the femoral part of the prosthesis (arrow). The scan is considered to be normal.

454

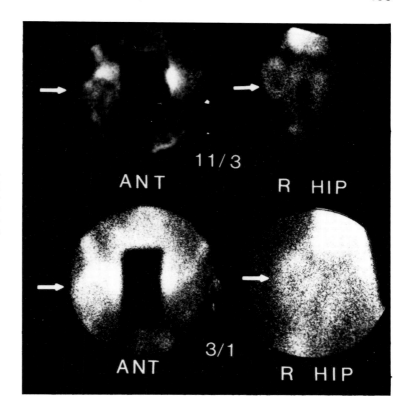

**FIGURE 15–28.** Hip prosthesis with heterotopic ossification: 99mTc-Pyrophosphate bone images of the pelvis and right hip in a patient with a right hip prosthesis and complicating heterotopic ossification. Uptake of the radiopharmaceutical agent can be seen extending around the prosthesis into the soft tissues, indicating heterotopic bone formation (arrows).

have addressed these issues[207–209] and their authors have concluded that in adult patients or animals, the aspiration or biopsy usually does not alter the bone scan.[207] It appears, however, that skeletal maturity and anatomic sites in the bone must be considered in the evaluation of the effect of biopsy or aspiration procedures on subsequently performed bone scans. In a study performed to assess the effect of injury by needle aspiration or drilling of metaphyseal and diaphyseal areas in immature and mature bones, Alazraki and colleagues[208] showed that in 12 immature rabbits, such trauma to metaphyseal regions had no effect on the subsequent 99mTc-phosphate bone images. Diaphyseal trauma always resulted in definitely abnormal bone scan images in mature and immature rabbits, but metaphyseal trauma in mature animals was accompanied by variable results. In an analysis of joint needle aspiration and contrast arthrography in mature dogs, Traughber and coworkers[209] found no effect on the bone scans that were done at 24 and 96 hours after the procedure.

Although osseous trauma is detected sensitively by the bone scan, reported experience in patients receiving corticosteroid therapy indicates that bone scanning may fail to detect fractures.[210] In a study in rabbits, Scott and colleagues[211] found that detection of bone trauma by the scan definitely was impaired in animals being given high doses of corticosteroids. The sensitivity of the bone scan was markedly diminished in the first week after the trauma and only mildly decreased 3 weeks after the injury. Similar, but less dramatic, results were related to low doses of corticosteroids.

### Metabolic Bone Disease

A balance between the two continuous processes of cancellous and cortical bone resorption and production is nec-

essary for maintaining normal calcium homeostasis and normal skeletal structural integrity. Specific imbalances in osseous resorption and production exist in many metabolic diseases, imbalances which, if sufficiently severe, become apparent on radionuclide studies. Generally, metabolic diseases affect all parts of the skeleton. In some specific entities, however, particular bones may be affected more than others, and it is the characteristic distribution of disease throughout the skeleton that provides the basis for accurate scintigraphic as well as radiographic diagnosis.

Until recently, the use of nuclear imaging in metabolic bone disease was extremely limited. Gradually, an increasing number of reports have addressed the role of bone imaging and quantitative radionuclide and photon densitometry studies in the evaluation of such disease. The sensitivity of bone scintigraphy in detecting focal abnormalities of bone has been documented in metabolic disorders.[81–83] For example, the insufficiency type of stress fracture (pseudofracture) that may appear in osteomalacia can be identified as a focal area of increased uptake on bone scans even when radiologic surveys are normal, although subsequent coned-down radiographs of areas of radionuclide abnormalities may confirm the presence of these fractures.[81] Studies have indicated that the appearance of the bone scan in some patients with osteomalacia is sufficiently different from that in normal persons that the presence of a metabolic disorder can be identified. Generally the mean bone-to-soft tissue uptake ratio of counts in the osteomalacia group has been significantly higher than in the control group. Fogelman and coworkers[81] reported a mean 24 hour 99mTc-HEDP retention of 41 per cent in osteomalacia patients, compared with about 20 per cent in normal persons. In osteomalacia, the most consistent subjective abnormality on bone imaging was an increased uptake of tracer in the long bones, the wrists, the calvarium, and the mandible.[183, 184] These findings also have been noted in other metabolic disorders, such as hyperparathyroidism. Increased activity in the costochondral junctions and the appearance of a "tie sternum" have been cited as additional radionuclide characteristics of some metabolic disorders, as have focal regions of increased uptake at sites of pseudofractures and brown tumors in hyperparathyroidism.

The radiograph is a relatively insensitive tool for detecting the presence and the extent of bone disease in patients with primary hyperparathyroidism. Quantitative analysis of the radionuclide distribution has been examined as a means of diagnosing and evaluating the extent of this disease. Measurement of rates of disappearance from blood and urinary excretion of $^{99m}$Tc-labeled phosphate was performed in normal persons and in patients with primary hyperparathyroidism, pseudohypoparathyroidism, and postsurgical untreated hypoparathyroidism.[82] The blood disappearance curves of the labeled phosphate were identical in these three groups. Significantly increased urinary excretion of labeled tracer, however, was recorded in those persons with hyperparathyroidism and pseudohypoparathyroidism. The bone scans were abnormal in 58 per cent of the hyperparathyroid patients, with focal abnormalities being evident in the distal extremities, the skull, and the mandible. About half of these patients showed radiographic abnormalities, including subperiosteal resorption and osteopenia. In other studies of patients with primary hyperparathyroidism, investigators have documented increased whole body retention of $^{99m}$Tc-labeled phosphate.[83–86] Their findings suggest that monitoring of excretion and retention of labeled phosphate might be a more sensitive means of determining abnormalities that accompany certain metabolic bone diseases than is whole body imaging.

In renal osteodystrophy[85] bone scans usually reveal absence of renal images, reflecting poor renal function. Furthermore, focal abnormalities similar to those that occasionally are seen in scans of patients with primary hyperparathyroidism may be identified. Increased activity has been reported in the ends of the long bones and at the costochondral junctions in as many as 80 per cent of these patients when radiographic abnormalities were identified in only 48 per cent.[85] Quantitative monitoring shows markedly increased 24 hour retention of the labeled phosphate as well as increased skeletal tracer accumulation relative to that in soft tissue.

In patients with osteomalacia, whole body monitoring also shows an increase in the 24 hour retention of the labeled phosphate. The images demonstrate increased bone-to-soft tissue activity ratios of varying degrees, sometimes identifiable as a "superscan." The scans also may show focal areas of increased uptake in the axial skeleton, long bones, wrists, costochondral junctions, sternum, calvarium, mandible, and sites of pseudofractures.

Scintigraphic patterns in patients with osteoporosis apparently are quite variable; studies may be normal or reveal areas of increased or decreased radiopharmaceutical localization in bones. Whole body retention of labeled phosphates usually is normal.[84] Disuse bone atrophy results in osteoporosis, which by experimental and clinical studies has been found to be associated with a high rate of bone formation. Scans have shown increased radiopharmaceutical concentration in bones affected by disuse osteoporosis.[87]

Increased regional bone blood flow has been postulated to explain the augmented concentration of radiopharmaceutical in bones of paralyzed limbs. Patients with paraplegia of longer than 9 years' duration, however, may not have increased technetium-phosphate localization in the paralyzed limbs. Radiocalcium balance and kinetic studies in disuse osteoporosis have shown that during the first several years of disuse, bone formation is increased up to twice normal and bone resorption is increased even more; the results of radionuclide studies in patients with long-standing paralysis are consistent with their having decreased osteogenesis as well as decreased bone resorption in the paralyzed limbs.[88]

Other entities that have been evaluated by bone scintigraphy include regional migratory osteoporosis and reflex sympathetic dystrophy or Sudeck's atrophy. In regional migratory osteoporosis, focal abnormalities on bone scan may be seen even before radiographic changes become evident. In addition, the scan may remain positive even after clinical recovery. One report[89] describing the bone scan in this entity concluded that the diagnosis can be strongly suggested by the correlation of history, laboratory findings, physical examination, radiography, and bone scan, thereby sparing patients multiple invasive procedures, such as biopsy and angiography. In migratory osteoporosis, severe joint pain may be accompanied by scan findings of "migrating" increased periarticular uptake.[90] Increased osseous blood flow to the involved, osteoporotic areas also has been demonstrated by dynamic radionuclide angiographic studies.

## Paget's Disease

In 1877, Sir James Paget described osteitis deformans in a patient whom he had followed for 20 years.[91] As radiography became established, the frequency of Paget's disease became increasingly evident as asymptomatic cases were detected. Autopsy studies show a frequency of Paget's disease of 3 per cent in persons older than 40 years.[92] The occurrence of the disease increases with age and it is most prevalent during the seventh decade of life, with men being affected more frequently than women. The pathophysiology of Paget's disease is characterized by increased bone resorption and increased formation of abnormal bone that is highly cellular, containing numerous vascular spaces and a disorganized trabecular pattern. The abnormal bone that is produced is subject to deformity from normal weight-bearing. Pain is a common clinical complaint in pagetic patients. Complications include pathologic fracture, secondary degenerative joint disease, and sarcomatous degeneration to osteosarcoma, chondrosarcoma, or fibrosarcoma. These complications occur in fewer than 3 per cent of patients with Paget's disease.[93]

Polyostotic involvement predominates in this disease. The bones that are involved most often include the pelvis, thoracolumbar vertebrae, femur, skull, scapula, tibia, and humerus in approximate order of descending frequency. Bone blood flow and osteogenesis are increased markedly, and therefore the bone scan shows characteristic intense increased activity in the affected areas. The deformity and the enlargement of the bones that are seen on radiographs are equally characteristic on the radionuclide images.

The markedly increased blood flow in affected bones suggests the possibility that arteriovenous fistulas are

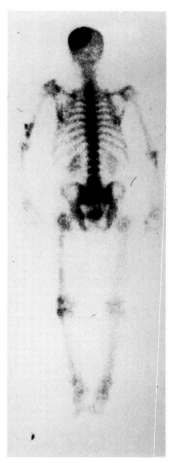

**FIGURE 15–29.** Paget's disease: Osteoporosis circumscripta. Total body $^{99m}$Tc-MDP bone image in a patient with early Paget's disease involving the skull.

formed within the osseous tissue as part of the disease process. However, the presence of arteriovenous fistulas has not been documented by histology, arteriography, or radiolabeled microsphere techniques. In patients with as much as 35 per cent of the skeleton involved by Paget's disease, high cardiac outputs have been reported owing to the markedly increased blood flow to the affected bones.[94]

Radiographically, Paget's disease may become manifest as lytic or sclerotic foci. During the early osteoporotic or lytic phase, most typically seen in the cranial vault as osteoporosis circumscripta, the bone scan shows markedly increased activity, with greater activity at the advancing margins of the lesion and less increased activity in its central portion[95] (Fig. 15–29). As the disease progresses and the osteolytic and osteoblastic activities become equalized, the radiographs may show a mixed sclerotic and lytic pattern, which then may be followed by a predominantly osteoblastic radiologic appearance. In the later sclerotic phase of the disease, increased osteoblastic and osteoclastic activity may have ceased, and the healed lesions, which still are apparent radiographically, may appear normal on the scan. Thus, the bone scan may be useful in determining true activity of the disease process,[96, 97] as the radiograph will remain static in the sclerotic phase. In assessing response of pagetic bone to therapy with calcitonin, diphosphonate, or mithramycin, the bone scan may be particularly helpful, and the changing

radionuclide pattern even may be quantitated with computer techniques (Fig. 15–30).

## Vascular Disease

**Ischemic Necrosis of Bone.** The diagnosis and prognosis of ischemic necrosis of bone are major clinical problems that have not yet been characterized well enough by any available diagnostic technique to guide clinical management accurately. Interruption of blood supply to a bone may result from many pathologic processes, including trauma, hematologic problems, vasculitis, metabolic disorders, fat embolization, and corticosteroid therapy. Radiographically, detection of ischemic necrosis is very difficult, as the affected bone has a degree of radiodensity that is similar to that of normal bone. A true increase in the bone radiodensity follows, due to compression of dead bone and revascularization with an accompanying production of new bone. These changes, however, may not become apparent radiographically for several weeks or even months after the acute process. Despite the recent emphases on the role of MR imaging in the assessment of osteonecrosis (see Chapter 80), bone scintigraphy remains an effective diagnostic technique. Initially, on the bone scan, if there has been a substantial interruption of blood supply, the radiopharmaceutical cannot reach the involved area and there may be decreased activity on the scan. As the bone reacts to the insult and attempts to repair the damage with revascularization and reossification, scintigraphy may show increased activity in the involved area. Later, secondary degenerative joint disease may appear, with a concomitant increase in radionuclide uptake about the joint.[98]

Thus, foci of ischemic necrosis of bone may appear on scintillation images as areas of either decreased or increased radiopharmaceutical uptake. Presumably, as the radionuclide pattern changes between these two states, there may be a period in which normal uptake is evident. Therefore, it is important to obtain high resolution images of the affected regions. Either converging or pinhole collimation will be helpful in the recognition of focal "cold" defects, especially if adjacent reactive changes with increased radiopharmaceutical uptake already are present. Figure 15–31 demonstrates the findings of increased uptake about a recent femoral neck fracture, accompanied by osteonecrosis of the femoral head, which has resulted in a "cold" area on the image. The pinhole collimator markedly improves the interpreter's ability to identify the two distinct abnormalities.

Orthopedic surgeons who deal with problems of ischemic necrosis, particularly of the femoral heads, need to consider at an early disease stage, before radiographic flattening of the femoral head is evident, whether or not arthroplasty is necessary. If osteonecrosis of the femoral head has resulted in nonviable bone that has lost its ability to recover, it may be advisable to perform a femoral head replacement prior to the development of secondary degenerative changes of the hip. If the affected femoral head will revascularize and recover, however, such extensive surgery may not be required. Attempts to use the bone scan as a prognostic indicator in this clinical setting have not met with uniform success.[185, 186]

Ischemic necrosis of bone occurs in as many as 17 per cent of patients after renal transplantation.[187] In 85 per cent of these cases, ischemic necrosis is evident within 2 years

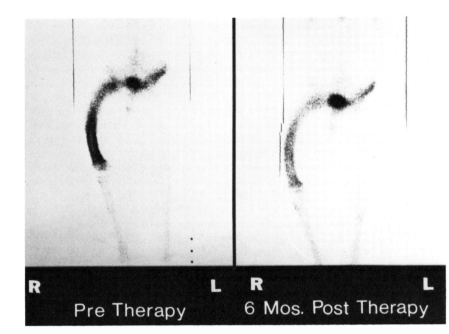

**FIGURE 15–30.** Paget's disease: Response to therapy—two anterior view total body bone images obtained 6 months apart after calcitonir therapy in a patient with Paget's disease. The images show a typical pagetic femoral deformity with markedly increased uptake and apparent enlargement and bowing of the osseous structure. After therapy, the degree of increased uptake in the pagetic bone is greatly lessened.

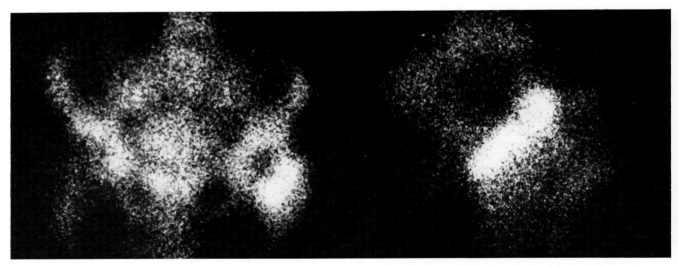

**FIGURE 15–31.** Ischemic necrosis: $^{99m}$Tc-Pyrophosphate bone images of the pelvis (left) and left hip (right) with pinhole collimator view in a patient with an acute fracture through the femoral neck and secondary ischemic necrosis of the left femoral head. The pinhole view shows that the femoral head is cold and that the linear fracture through the femoral neck is hot.

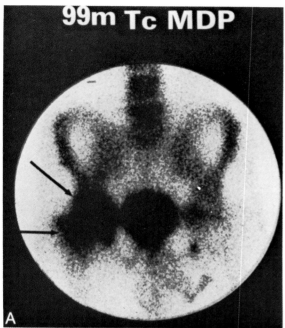

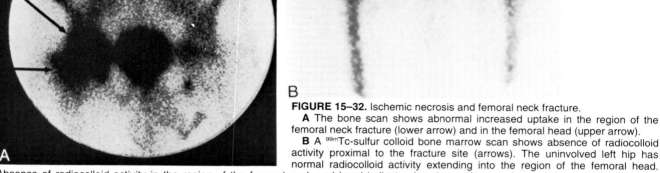

**FIGURE 15–32.** Ischemic necrosis and femoral neck fracture.
    **A** The bone scan shows abnormal increased uptake in the region of the femoral neck fracture (lower arrow) and in the femoral head (upper arrow).
    **B** A [99m]Tc-sulfur colloid bone marrow scan shows absence of radiocolloid activity proximal to the fracture site (arrows). The uninvolved left hip has normal radiocolloid activity extending into the region of the femoral head. Absence of radiocolloid activity in the region of the femoral neck and head indicates impairment in vascularity, consistent with ischemic necrosis.

after the transplantation. In a prospective study describing the use of [99m]Tc-MDP bone scans for the early detection of ischemic necrosis in patients with a renal transplant, Spencer and Maisey[187] noted a 12 per cent frequency of minor fractures, many of which would not have been detected if not for the bone scan. The bone scan has been found effective in the diagnosis of ischemic bone necrosis accompanying other disorders, such as systemic lupus erythematosus.[188] This effectiveness may be increased using single photon emission CT (SPECT).[189]

Another imaging approach, bone marrow imaging, has been used to predict the viability of bone in patients with ischemic necrosis.[99] In general, the absence of radiocolloid uptake in the femoral head and neck on the bone marrow scan indicates vascular impairment, whereas the presence of radiocolloid uptake indicates an intact vascular supply through the femoral marrow space (Fig. 15–32). Initial studies were accomplished using [99m]Tc-sulfur colloid, a particle of about 200 to 500 nm in size. The major problem encountered with this agent was that no scintigraphic activity was detected in the bone marrow of femoral heads in about 50 per cent of normal patients. Turner,[193] however, showed that when [99m]Tc-antimony colloid, with a smaller particle size of about 10 nm, was used, marrow activity could be detected in the femoral heads in 28 of 30 normal patients. These same investigators, using the antimony radiopharmaceutical experimentally in rabbits, found diminished marrow activity after surgical interruption of the blood supply to the femoral head. They also applied this technique successfully to the diagnosis of ischemic necrosis of the femoral head in patients who had had a subcapital fracture of the femoral neck.

In patients with sickle cell anemia, both bone and bone marrow imaging may be helpful in the diagnosis of infarction, revealing focal regions of decreased activity in acute bone infarcts.[100] With healing, the bone scan converts from a pattern of decreased focal activity to one of increased focal activity in the affected region, whereas the bone marrow scan may show the return of radiocolloid concentration in the affected area.[101] Differentiation between bone infarction and osteomyelitis in patients with sickle cell anemia whose first manifestation is pain is difficult even with the use of bone, bone marrow, and gallium imaging, however. Although increased activity of gallium occurs in regions of osteomyelitis, this agent also may accumulate in regions of infarction. A bone marrow scan may show abnormal regions of decreased uptake in osteomyelitis, whereas the bone marrow scan may remain normal in septic arthritis. Thus, in the differentiation between osteomyelitis and septic arthritis, the bone marrow scan may be helpful.[102]

**Legg-Calvé-Perthes Disease.** In the evaluation of Legg-Calvé-Perthes disease, the bone scan has been cited for its superior sensitivity in comparison to radiography.[190, 191] The necrosis of the femoral capital epiphyses that affects children 4 to 8 years of age, more frequently boys, is believed to be of vascular origin. Characteristically, early in the course of this disease, radionuclide imaging shows a focal region of decreased radiopharmaceutical uptake in the anterolateral aspect of the proximal femoral epiphysis, although the entire epiphysis may be involved in some cases. Revascularization and healing subsequently are demonstrated on the scan as areas of increased activity in the femoral head and adjacent femoral neck.[103] In clinical practice, the problem of differentiation between Legg-Calvé-Perthes disease and synovitis may arise. In the latter situation, the scan shows increased periarticular activity but no epiphyseal defect. In addition, the gallium scan may be helpful in the diagnosis of septic arthritis. The prognosis in Legg-Calvé-Perthes disease has been related to the degree of epiphyseal involvement.[104] A more accurate assessment of the extent of epiphyseal involvement can be obtained if pinhole imaging techniques are used to optimize the image details of small areas within hips of pediatric patients (Fig. 15–33).

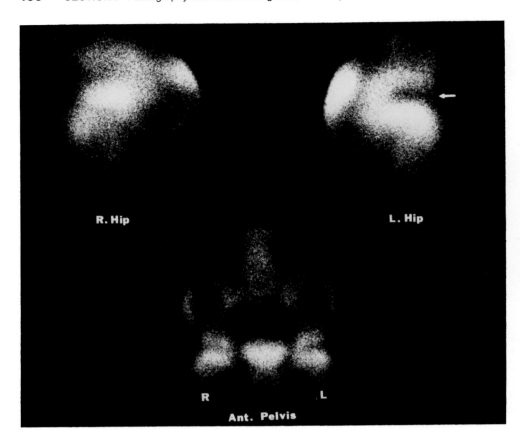

**FIGURE 15–33.** Legg-Calvé-Perthes disease: $^{99m}$Tc-Pyrophosphate bone images in a 6 year old child. The left hip view shows a larger area of decreased counts in the region of the femoral growth plate (arrow), consistent with the diagnosis of Legg-Calvé-Perthes disease. The finding could easily be missed on the anterior pelvis view but is seen on the pinhole collimator view.

**Slipped Capital Femoral Epiphysis.** Compromise of the blood supply to the femoral head is a known sequela of slipped capital femoral epiphyses. $^{99m}$Tc-diphosphonate bone scans usually show increased uptake in the physis and adjacent metaphysis of the femur in cases of epiphyseal slippage, probably reflecting an increase in metabolic bone activity associated with repair at the site of physeal fracture. Decreased uptake in the femoral head on the side of the slipped epiphysis also may be seen, indicating compromise of the blood supply[192] and, perhaps, impending ischemic necrosis, although the correlation between decreased radiopharmaceutical uptake in the affected femoral head and the development of ischemic necrosis probably needs further documentation.

**Caisson Disease.** In experimental bone necrosis, the radionuclide bone scan shows abnormalities of increased uptake, probably reflecting new bone formation during a reactive or reparative process, within 3 weeks of the causative insult and many weeks prior to any detectable abnormality on radiographs.[194] Thus, it has been suggested that bone scans are a better technique for early diagnosis of caisson disease than radiography.

### Articular Disease

The first radionuclide joint images were obtained in 1965 with $^{131}$I-labeled albumin,[105] with the rationale that joints involved in inflammatory disease would show increased tracer accumulation due to increased synovial blood flow and abnormal synovial capillary permeability. $^{131}$I-labeled albumin, an intravascular label, therefore, seemed to be the appropriate agent. In 1967, $^{99m}$Tc-pertechnetate, which lo-

calizes in the blood pool and the extracellular fluid compartments, was used for joint imaging.[106] These joint images were far superior to the $^{131}$I-labeled albumin images because of the preferred physical characteristics of $^{99m}$Tc for imaging with the scintillation camera or scanner compared with the 365 keV gamma emission of $^{131}$I. Soon after the introduction of $^{99m}$Tc-labeled phosphate compounds for bone imaging in 1971,[8] these agents were applied to joint imaging as well.[107] Because diseases affecting the joints also stimulate osteogenesis in the periarticular bone, it was thought that joints affected by arthritis would have abnormal uptake of the phosphate-labeled agents in the adjacent bone. Furthermore, there is an increase in synovial vascularity secondary to the joint disease, which also causes increased vascularity in the adjacent bone. The result on imaging, therefore, is focally increased tracer accumulation in the periarticular osseous structures. Comparisons of the $^{99m}$Tc-labeled phosphate images with $^{99m}$Tc-pertechnetate images have indicated that the phosphate-labeled compounds are far more sensitive in detecting abnormal joints than the pertechnetate.[108]

In the presence of a joint effusion with increased synovial capillary permeability, these agents diffuse across the synovial membrane into the effusion. These tracers also may bind to proteins within the joint capsule or in the joint fluid. Additionally, with $^{99m}$Tc-labeled phosphate compounds, the same principles that govern its uptake within bone also apply to its accumulation in articular diseases (i.e., chemical and physical processes resulting in adsorption onto hydroxyapatite crystals at bone surfaces, with close correlation to bone blood flow and bone surface-to-volume ratios). Epiphyseal and metaphyseal bone typically has a higher bone surface-to-volume ratio and higher local blood flow than other areas of bone.[109] In degenerative arthritis, destruction of articular cartilage also results in abnormal stress on the bone adjacent to the chondral surface. Thus, remodeling and sclerosis of bone occur and are accompanied by increased blood supply to the region.

In most institutions, [99m]Tc-labeled phosphate compounds for joint imaging are used in doses similar to those used for bone imaging (i.e., 15 to 20 mCi), with scintigraphy performed approximately 2 hours after the intravenous injection of the material. The patient is encouraged to drink fluids so as to optimize the renal excretion of the tracer from the blood background. Generally, a total body image will be obtained in anterior and posterior projections unless the examination is limited to specific joints. Alternatively, in a joint survey, scintillation camera images with a converging collimator may be used to evaluate each individual joint, accumulating approximately 250,000 counts per image for peripheral joints. If a whole body scan is performed, spot images using the converging or pinhole collimator for abnormal joints may be performed selectively. For careful evaluation of any one joint, frontal and lateral views should be obtained, particularly in the knees, because increased activity related to the overlying patella and patellofemoral compartment may be misinterpreted as lateral femorotibial compartment disease on a frontal view. For the hips, anterior and posterior views are important and are obtained routinely. In children, frog-leg and straight anteroposterior views of the hips may be helpful.

**Normal Joints.** Normal joints show symmetric activity, although the shoulder joint on the side of dominant handedness occasionally shows more activity than that in the opposite shoulder. Greatest activity normally is seen in the periarticular regions, with predictable variations in the degree of activity for different joints. For example, in the hand, activity around joints normally is greatest in the wrist and in the metacarpophalangeal joints, with uniform diminishing activity, which progresses from the first to the fifth digit. For each individual digit, the activity is greatest in the proximal joints and diminishes distally. The degree of activity in epiphyseal regions in children is much greater than the activity seen in periarticular structures in adults. For example, around the knee joint in an adult, the degree of increased activity is proportional to the mass of bony structures (e.g., the medial femoral condyle has slightly more activity than the lateral femoral condyle), and the normal degree of periarticular activity is elevated only minimally compared with that in other bony structures.

**Degenerative Joint Disease.** In the evaluation of osteoarthritis of the knee, Thomas and coworkers[110] demonstrated a practical application for radionuclide joint imaging in guiding the orthopedic surgeon in deciding on the need for surgery and in selecting a surgical approach. Fifty-six osteoarthritic knees in 52 men and 1 woman being considered for surgery were evaluated by history, physical examination, assessment of knee function, radiography with and without weight-bearing, double-contrast arthrography, and [99m]Tc-polyphosphate bone imaging. All methods were correlated finally with direct inspection by either arthroscopy or surgery. The radionuclide joint imaging correlated more closely than any of the other techniques with direct inspection. The results of the bone scan indicated the extent and the severity of the joint disease and affected the choice of

surgery. High tibial valgus osteotomy generally is more successful in patients with varus deformity in whom the lateral femorotibial compartment has been preserved; if lateral compartmental disease is present, a high tibial valgus osteotomy probably will be unsuccessful, leaving unicompartmental replacement of the involved medial femorotibial compartment and total knee replacement as the surgical alternatives. On the basis of clinical examination and radiography with and without weight-bearing, 28 knees in this series had absent or mild lateral femorotibial compartmental disease. The radionuclide images in 15 knees and the arthrogram in five knees detected a higher level of disease in the lateral femorotibial compartment than was suspected otherwise. The radionuclide study confirmed absence of lateral tibial and femoral disease in 10 of the 28 cases and presence of mild disease in three cases. The surgical management plan was altered because of the detection of moderate lateral compartment abnormalities in seven of the 28 patients. Long-term evaluation of these patients will be needed to establish the validity of this approach (Fig. 15–34).

**Rheumatoid Arthritis and Rheumatoid Variant Diseases.** Documentation of the sensitivity of the bone scan in detecting and estimating the extent of joint involvement in patients with rheumatoid arthritis or a rheumatoid variant disease, such as psoriatic arthritis, ankylosing spondylitis, and Reiter's syndrome, has been reported in several studies.[111–114] The bone scan is considered the most sensitive imaging indicator of active disease in these arthritides. The

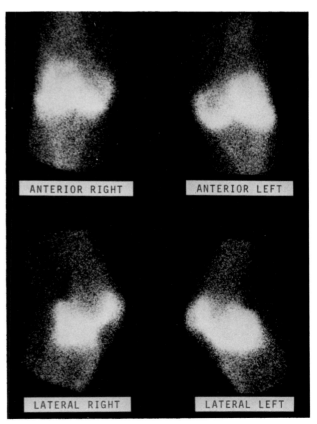

**FIGURE 15–34.** Degenerative knee disease: [99m]Tc-Polyphosphate bone images of the knees in a patient with severe osteoarthritis showing marked tricompartment abnormalities on both sides.

pattern of abnormal radionuclide activity in rheumatoid arthritis, consisting of symmetric peripheral joint abnormalities, may be distinguishable from that in the rheumatoid variant diseases, which tend to have more central skeletal involvement and asymmetric peripheral joint abnormalities. Compared with the radiograph, however, the bone scan is less specific in its ability to distinguish among the clinical entities. Nonetheless, the scintigraphic abnormalities often appear before radiographic or clinical abnormalities. The bone scan shows greatest sensitivity in detecting abnormalities in the smaller peripheral joints. For the shoulder, hip, and knee joints, the frequency of clinical abnormality is equal to or slightly greater than the frequency of focal increased activity on the bone scan. In the axial skeleton of patients with rheumatoid arthritis, the results are less conclusive. Abnormalities of the sacroiliac joints as measured by increased radionuclide activity are found to be more common than abnormalities noted by clinical and radiographic examinations. Other studies using computer profiles of the distribution of radioactivity on images of the sacroiliac joints also have indicated more frequent detection of increased activity than could be correlated with clinical or radiographic abnormalities.[114] These findings have supported a broad variation in the normal degree of radiopharmaceutical uptake in the sacroiliac joints. On radionuclide images of the spine, it may be difficult to distinguish between active and inactive disease and the presence or absence of coincident disorders, such as degenerative disease.

Studies of quantitative images of the sacroiliac joints using computer-generated ratios of activity over the sacroiliac regions versus that in the central portion of the sacrum, or profile curves of the changes in uptake across the sacroiliac region, have suggested that separate ratios should be obtained for each sacroiliac joint and, perhaps, for the superior, middle, and inferior regions of each joint as well.[113, 114] This would indicate that disease can be so localized within the sacroiliac joint as to affect only one joint or only one region of the articulation. The application of quantitative sacroiliac joint radionuclide examination may prove to be useful in following the course of patients with ankylosing spondylitis or sacroiliitis of psoriatic arthritis or Reiter's syndrome, and in many HLA-B27–positive persons without back pain or radiographic evidence of sacroiliac joint disease. Lentle and colleagues[113] observed an association between sacroiliitis and increased sacroiliac-to-sacrum count ratios in patients who were suspected clinically of having ankylosing spondylitis or Reiter's syndrome and who had the histocompatibility antigen HLA-B27. They also detected scan evidence of sacroiliitis in patients with psoriasis, uveitis, or Crohn's disease, some of whom had normal radiographs.

Weissberg and colleagues[112] reported that 23 joints of 640 joints examined in patients with rheumatoid variant disorders were noted to have radiographic changes of osteoarthritis, and 21 of these manifested no increased activity by bone scan. In addition, 10 of 14 patients with rheumatoid arthritis who had degenerative changes in the spine had normal radionuclide uptake in the spine on scan. Several reports have shown that patients with classic ankylosing spondylitis in whom ankylosis of the sacroiliac joints was noted on radiography showed normal or slightly decreased radionuclide activity in the sacroiliac joints on scintigraphy. This probably reflected the inactivity of disease at the time

of the scan.[112–114, 116] Thus, it would appear that the radionuclide examination may offer a means of differentiating inflammatory from degenerative joint alterations and active from "burned-out" disease. Correlation of the radionuclide study with the radiograph is necessary for fuller understanding of the disease processes that are present.

In patients with rheumatoid arthritis, the characteristic pattern that is seen on bone scan consists of symmetric involvement of joints.[115] In the knees, usually symmetric medial and lateral femorotibial compartmental uptake occurs with or without increased radionuclide accumulation in the patellofemoral compartment. In a few patients with classic rheumatoid arthritis, asymmetric involvement has been seen. This finding, which is more frequent in the initial stages of the disease, possibly reflects the localized distribution of stress forces and remodeling that can be seen very early in the inflammatory process. A pattern consisting of a dense band of increased activity at the epiphyseal-metaphyseal area about the small joints of the hands and the feet, which often is seen normally in young patients, has been noted in older patients with rheumatoid arthritis.

Follow-up bone scans in patients being treated for rheumatoid arthritis do not always correlate with the clinical course of the disease. Some investigators have noted that joints actually may show increased radionuclide activity in the face of clinical improvement. Nonetheless, the bone scan is considered to be an extremely sensitive indicator of activity in rheumatoid arthritis and rheumatoid variant dis-

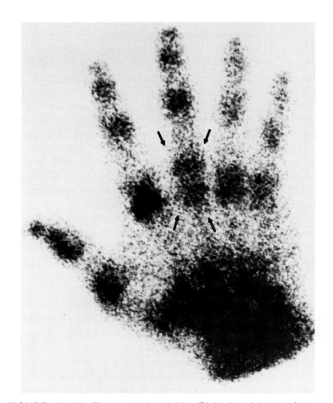

**FIGURE 15–35.** Rheumatoid arthritis: Right hand image from a ⁹⁹ᵐTc-pyrophosphate bone study in a patient with rheumatoid arthritis. Bands of activity at epiphyseal-metaphyseal areas (arrows) normally may be seen in young patients. In middle-aged persons, they are abnormal. Multiple joints of the hand and wrist are involved in this patient. (From Weissberg DL, et al: AJR *131*:665, 1978. Copyright 1978, American Roentgen Ray Society.)

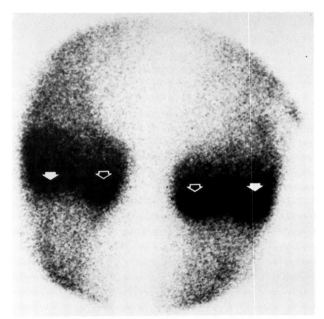

**FIGURE 15–36.** Rheumatoid arthritis: Radionuclide bone images of both knees in a patient with rheumatoid arthritis. Images show symmetric distribution of abnormal activity in all femorotibial compartments, medially (open arrows) and laterally (solid arrows). (From Weissberg DL, et al: AJR *131*:665, 1978. Copyright 1978, American Roentgen Ray Society.)

eases. Weissberg and associates[112] reported on a comparison between nuclear imaging using $^{99m}$Tc-pyrophosphate and clinical or radiologic evaluation in over 1000 joints of patients with various articular disorders, especially arthritis. The results indicated agreement between the scan and the radiograph in 67 per cent of examined joints. Abnormal scan activity was seen in 20 per cent of the joints that had no radiographic abnormalities, whereas 13 per cent of the joints examined showed radiographic abnormality in the absence of bone scan abnormality (Figs. 15–35 to 15–41).

In addition to the arthritides that were discussed previously, the bone scan and the gallium scan are positive in septic arthritis (Fig. 15–42).

**Subtalar Coalition.** Subtalar coalition may occur as a congenital condition in the form of a fibrous, cartilaginous, or osseous bridge. As discussed in Chapter 90, the bone scan represents an effective screening examination.[195]

**Radionuclide Arthrography.** Radionuclide arthrography has been used clinically to aid in the identification of loosening of the femoral component of a total hip arthroplasty, although the radionuclide technique is reported not to be useful for evaluating the acetabular component. With regard to the femoral component, comparative studies of standard and radionuclide arthrography have reported superior accuracy of the radionuclide technique when correlated with surgery.[205, 206] One method employs the intraarticular injection of 10 to 15 ml of 60 per cent diatrizoate

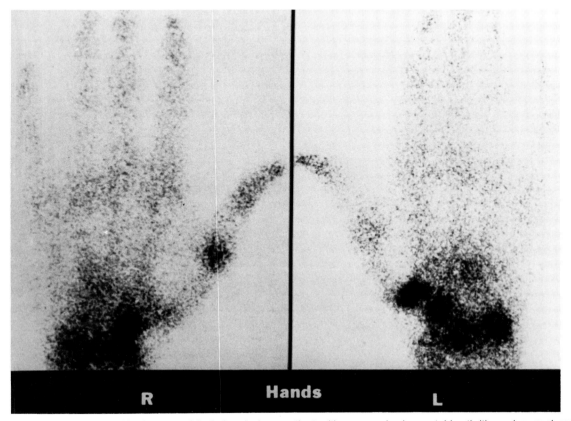

R    **Hands**    L

**FIGURE 15–37.** Rheumatoid arthritis: Images of both hands in a patient with very early rheumatoid arthritis and normal radiographs. Abnormalities are identified in both wrists and in the metacarpophalangeal joint of the right thumb.

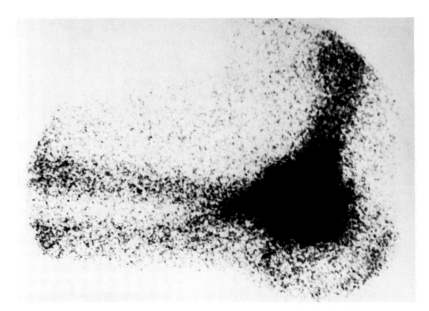

**FIGURE 15–38.** Rheumatoid arthritis: The right elbow of a patient with rheumatoid arthritis and with effusion of this joint. Increased activity in the joint and surrounding soft tissue confirms the presence of active disease.

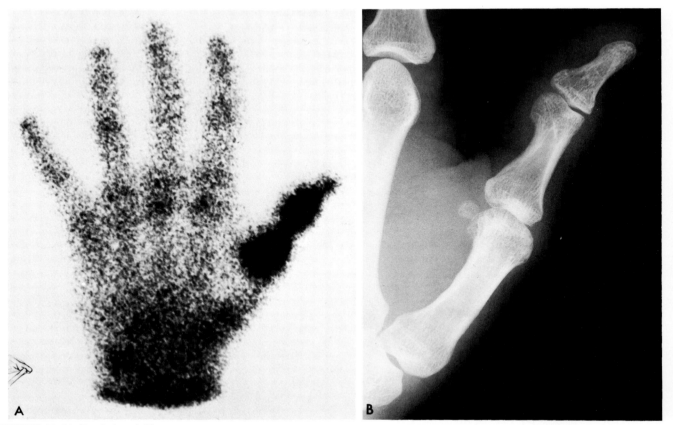

**FIGURE 15–39.** Psoriatic arthritis.
  **A** Radionuclide bone image shows foci of increased uptake in the interphalangeal and metacarpophalangeal joints of the thumb. Other joints are normal.
  **B** Radiograph shows only minimal periarticular soft tissue swelling. Later radiographic and clinical abnormalities developed in these joints.
  (From Weissberg DL, et al: AJR *131*:665, 1978. Copyright 1978, American Roentgen Ray Society.)

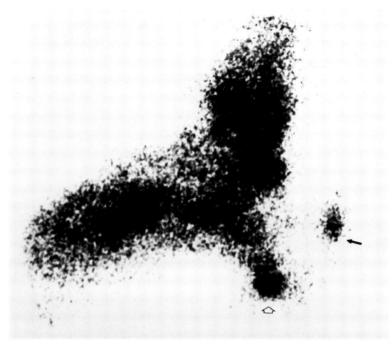

**FIGURE 15–40.** Ankylosing spondylitis: Left foot and ankle on a $^{99m}$Tc-pyrophosphate bone study in a patient with ankylosing spondylitis. The focus at the inferior aspect of the calcaneus (open arrow) corresponds to a site of small cortical erosion and bone production seen on the radiograph, whereas the focus of increased activity in the superoposterior aspect of the calcaneus (solid arrow) corresponds to inflammatory changes in the retrocalcaneal bursa.

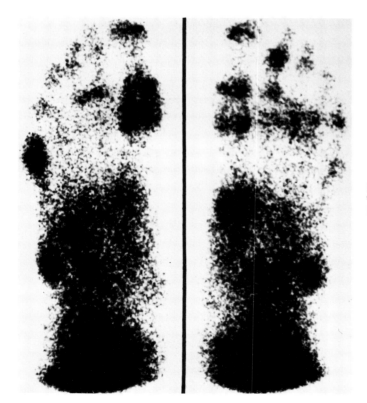

**FIGURE 15–41.** Psoriatic arthritis: Images of both feet from a $^{99m}$Tc-pyrophosphate bone study in a patient with psoriatic arthritis. Note the asymmetric involvement of distal joints.

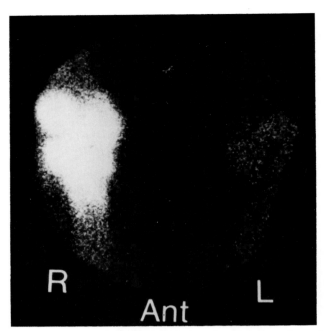

**FIGURE 15–42.** Septic arthritis: $^{99m}$Tc-Pyrophosphate knee images in a patient with septic arthritis involving the right knee.

meglumine, followed by 1 mCi of $^{99m}$Tc-sulfur colloid in a volume of 1 ml through the same needle. After radiographs are obtained, imaging with the scintillation camera follows. Other methods also have been used (Fig. 15–43).

### Diseases of Soft Tissue

A multitude of soft tissue lesions have been reported to concentrate bone-seeking radiopharmaceuticals[117–125] (Table 15–1) (Figs. 15–44 and 15–45). In identifying a cause for uptake of these agents by soft tissue, it is important to correlate the scan with a radiograph of the affected region, as soft tissue calcification or heterotopic ossification may be evident. Even in the absence of any soft tissue densities on the radiograph, however, the presence of microscopic foci of calcification or heterotopic bone formation below the limits of resolution of the radiograph cannot be excluded. Bone- and calcium-forming tumors such as osteosarcoma, neuroblastoma, and colonic carcinoma metastases, myositis ossificans, dermatomyositis, diffuse interstitial pulmonary calcification associated with hyperparathyroidism or mitral stenosis, metastatic soft tissue calcification, and cardiac valvular calcifications are examples of lesions with foci of calcification or ossification that may be positive on bone scans. In addition, certain lesions that typically do not show calcification may concentrate the bone-seeking radiopharmaceuticals, including various benign or malignant soft tissue tumors, myocardial and cerebral infarction, pyogenic and fungal soft tissue infections, noninfectious inflammatory diseases of the heart and skeletal muscle, amyloidosis, healing soft tissue wounds, intramuscular injection sites, and normal and diseased breast tissue.[12]

The factors that determine the localization of the $^{99m}$Tc-labeled phosphate compounds in noncalcified or nonossified soft tissue tumors are not well understood. Increased vascularity, altered capillary permeability or cellular calcium metabolism, presence of immature collagen, and

atypical binding of the $^{99m}$Tc-phosphate compound to phosphatase enzymes are among the factors that have been considered in attempts to explain the localization of the bone-seeking radiopharmaceuticals in the soft tissue lesions.[31, 124] In the cases in which calcification or ossification is present in the soft tissue lesion, the mechanism of $^{99m}$Tc-phosphate compound uptake is presumed to be adsorption to the calcific focus similar to the adsorption of $^{99m}$Tc-phosphate compound that occurs onto the hydroxyapatite crystal in normal bone. In fact, the composition of the pathologic calcifications in many of these lesions has been shown to be similar to that of calcium deposits found in normal bone on x-ray diffraction studies.

In cases of damaged muscle (e.g., myocardial infarcts, inflammatory myopathies, or ischemic injuries of skeletal muscle), the mechanism for concentration of the $^{99m}$Tc-phosphate compounds is thought to be related to the abnormal movement of calcium from plasma into the damaged muscle cell. These compounds are able to move into the damaged cells through abnormally permeable sarcolemma and then to adsorb onto the intracellular calcium deposits.[124] Use of $^{99m}$Tc-phosphate compounds for imaging acute myocardial infarcts has become common in clinical practice and is quite sensitive for detecting myocardial infarction between 24 hours and 7 days after the acute injury.[126] Prior to 24 hours and later than 7 days after the infarct, the sensitivity of concentration of the $^{99m}$Tc-phosphate compounds within the infarcted myocardial muscle falls off precipitously, for reasons that are not well understood.

Paraosteoarthropathy, or ectopic ossification associated with neuromuscular disorders, develops in approximately 20 to 30 per cent of patients after spinal cord injury and in some series in as many as 50 per cent of such patients.[127, 128] It also is associated with other forms of paraplegia and quadriplegia; because it may lead to joint ankylosis, it is a serious complication. The cause of such ossification is not known. Ectopic ossification associated with spinal cord injury most often begins 4 to 10 weeks after the injury and progresses for approximately 6 to 14 months, with the eventual formation of hard, bony masses that may be pal-

*Text continued on page 471*

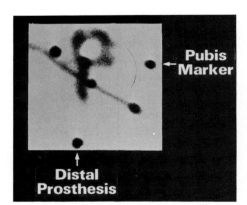

**FIGURE 15–43.** Radionuclide arthrography. In this patient, a femoral prosthesis was being evaluated for possible loosening. After injection into the joint space of 1 mCi of $^{99m}$Tc-sulfur colloid, imaging was performed to ascertain whether the radionuclide activity extends down the shaft of the prosthesis. In the absence of loosening, the activity should remain at the injection site. This scan shows abnormal radionuclide activity along the femoral component of the prosthesis, indicating loosening.

**TABLE 15–1. Lesions That Have Been Associated With Soft Tissue Uptake of
$^{99m}$Tc-Phosphate Compounds**

**Breast**
Lactation
Fat necrosis
Mazoplasia
Gynecomastia
Postmastectomy
Breast prosthesis
Fibrocystic disease and
  mammary dysplasia
Primary breast cancer
Metastatic breast carcinoma

**Cardiovascular System**
Acute or chronic myocardial
  infarction
Unstable angina
Left ventricular aneurysm
Aortic aneurysm
Myocardial contusion
Mönckeberg's sclerosis
Calcified valves
Calcified coronary arteries
Prosthetic valves
Chemotherapy
Radiotherapy
Amyloidosis
Pericarditis and endocarditis
Chagas' disease
Metastatic calcification
Malignant pericardial effusions
Metastases to heart
Hemangiopericytoma

**Gastrointestinal System**
Milk-alkali syndrome
Intestinal infarction
Abdominal aneurysm
Gastric calcification
Necrotizing enterocolitis
Trauma from nasogastric tube
Metastatic calcification
Metastases from rectal
  adenocarcinoma
Mucinous adenocarcinoma of
  the stomach
Malignant ascites
Colorectal metastases

**Genitourinary System**
Acute tubular necrosis
Chemotherapy
Radiotherapy
Kidney (after radiographic
  contrast)
Iron excess
Thalassemia major
Nephrocalcinosis
Phimosis
Orchitis
Wolman's disease
Leiomyoma of uterus
Chronic renal failure
Kidney in sickle cell anemia
Hypernephroma
Transplant ischemia
Erythroleukemia
Metastatic calcification
Urinoma
Primary renal tumors
Lymphatic lymphosarcoma
Ovarian carcinoma
Metastatic seminoma

**Head, Neck, and Neurologic
System**
Cerebrovascular accident
Brain abscess
Thyroid nodule
Arteriovenous malformation
Cerebritis
Chronic subdural hematoma
Cerebral infarction
Metastatic calcification (thyroid)
Cerebral tumors
Calcified thyroid carcinoma
Brain metastases
Medullary carcinoma
Schwannoma
Neurilemoma
Primary neuroblastoma

**Liver**
Amyloidosis
Postarteriography status
Necrosis
Aluminum excess
Cholangiocarcinoma
Metastases from colon
  carcinoma
Malignant melanoma
Metastases from oat cell
  carcinoma of lung
Neuroblastoma, soft tissue
  uptake
Metastases from osteosarcoma

**Lung**
Radiotherapy
Fibrothorax
Sarcoidosis
Interstitial pulmonary
  calcification
Berylliosis
Lung nodules in chronic
  hemodialysis
Metastatic calcification
Bronchogenic carcinoma
Metastases from osteogenic
  sarcoma
Malignant pleural effusion

**Muscle and Periarticular
Tissues**
Iron dextran injection
Rhabdomyolysis
Polymyositis
Muscle trauma
Overexertion
McArdle's syndrome and
  disorders of glycogenolysis
Muscular dystrophy
Postrevascularization
Myositis ossificans
Precordial electrostimulation
Electric burns
Sickle cell disease
Ischemia
Chemoperfusion
Radiotherapy
Amyloidosis
Synovitis
Calcific tendinitis
Gouty tophi
Calcified myoma
Ipsilateral uptake after lumbar
  sympathectomy
Fibromatosis
Cartilaginous exostosis
Migratory osteolysis
Calcinosis universalis
Dystrophic calcifications
Extravasated calcium gluconate
Rhabdomyosarcoma
Synovioma

**Skin and Subcutaneous
Tissues**
Electrical burns
Precordial electrostimulation
Filariasis
Inflamed breast implant
Pseudoxanthoma elasticum
Amyloidosis
Calcinosis universalis
Tumoral calcinosis
Infiltrated calcium solution
Soft tissue inflammation
Abscess
Surgical incision
Radiotherapy
Hyperhidrosis
Fat necrosis
Spinal cord injury
Drug injection
Urinary contamination
Dermatomyositis
Soft tissue abscess
Healing wound
Chemoperfusion
Soft tissue irradiation
Folds of fat
Neurofibroma
Metastatic calcification
Angiolipoma
Lipoma
Hematoma
Fibromatosis
Soft tissue sarcoma
Liposarcoma
Malignant fibrous histiocytoma
Ewing's sarcoma of soft parts
Osteosarcoma

**Spleen and Hematologic
System**
G6PD deficiency
Hemosiderosis
Infarction (sickle cell anemia)
Thalassemia major
Uptake in SS disease
Splenic lymphoma
Reticulum cell sarcoma
Lymphosarcoma

**Other**
Filarial infestation
Christmas disease
Lymphoma
Uterine fibroid
Neuroblastoma
Ganglioneuroblastoma

From Alazraki N: *In* JC Harbert, AFG da Rocha (Eds): Textbook of Nuclear Medicine. Vol. 2, Clinical Applications. Philadelphia, Lea & Febiger, 1984.

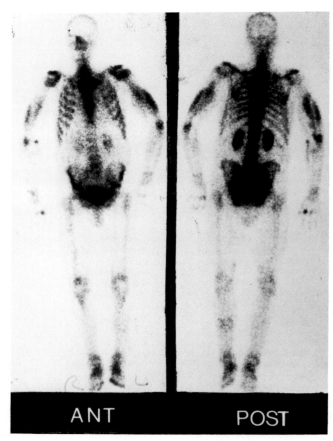

**FIGURE 15–44.** Soft tissue disease: Anterior and posterior $^{99m}$Tc-pyrophosphate bone images in a patient with an inflammatory polymyositis. The bone-seeking radiopharmaceutical agent has accumulated in the skeletal muscles, particularly in the upper arms.

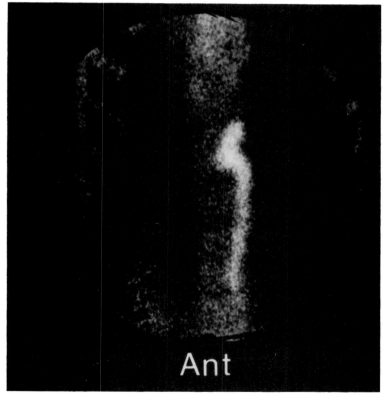

**FIGURE 15–45.** Soft tissue scar: Scintillation camera image shows increased uptake in a linear pattern over the abdomen in a patient 2 weeks after abdominal surgery. The radionuclide uptake corresponds in location to the patient's abdominal scar.

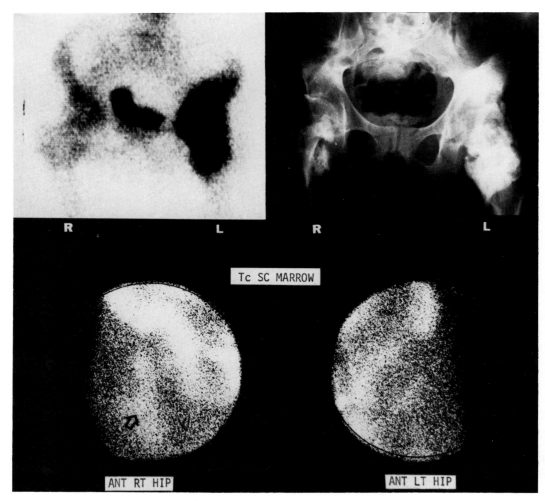

**FIGURE 15–46.** Heterotopic ossification: Radionuclide bone image and radiograph (above) in a patient with spinal cord injury and heterotopic bone formation surrounding both hip joints. $^{99m}$Tc-Sulfur colloid bone marrow images (below) show uptake of radiopharmaceutical agent in the region of the heterotopic bone (arrow), particularly in the right hip. This indicates the presence of bone marrow formation in the maturing heterotopic bone.

pable in the soft tissues. Radiographs often are normal in the early stages or may show soft tissue swelling within the first 3 weeks. By 2 or 3 months, bone may become apparent, after which a trabecular pattern may become evident. By 12 to 18 months, the mass of new bone becomes stable radiographically. The bone scan in these patients commonly is abnormal before radiographic changes are evident, and it shows an early increase in accumulation of $^{99m}$Tc-phosphate in the involved region.[129, 130] Furthermore, bone and bone marrow scanning is effective in assessing the maturity of the ectopic bone. If surgical resection is planned to relieve flexion-extension deformity or limitation of motion, it is advisable to be certain that the ectopic bone has matured at the time of surgical intervention, as the likelihood of recurrence then will be minimized. Other laboratory tests, such as the measurement of serum alkaline phosphatase levels or urinary hydroxyproline excretion, have not been reliable predictors of the maturity of the ectopic bone. Serial bone scans show that the activity within the ectopic bone tends to decline, reaching a plateau level as the ossification reaches maturity. Bone marrow scanning using $^{99m}$Tc-labeled sulfur colloid, which is trapped in the reticuloendothelial cells of the marrow, reveals uptake in the ectopic bone only when bone marrow has been formed. Thus, the presence of bone marrow activity is another indicator of the maturity of the ectopic bone (Fig. 15–46).

## Irradiation Injury

After irradiation, the bone scan usually shows decreased osseous uptake of the radiopharmaceutical relative to the level of uptake in the bone outside the therapy port. Occasionally, very shortly after radiation therapy, the bone scan will show increased uptake. These radionuclide changes can be explained by available histologic data. Initially there is an increase in the remodeling of cortical bone, which peaks between 3 and 6 months after irradiation. Changes in bone vascularity accompany the bone remodeling,[131] and there is increased regional skeletal blood flow, presumably because of an inflammatory response to radiation. Subsequently the hyperemia subsides, as does the increased tracer accumulation. Microvascular injury affecting the osteoblasts adds to a reduction in new bone formation, resulting in eventual decreased uptake on the bone scan. Because irradiation of normal bone is associated with extensive changes on the bone scan, the use of the radionuclide study to monitor the therapeutic response of a bone lesion to radiation therapy is questionable.

## SUMMARY

During approximately 30 years of experience with bone scanning, broad expansions in the clinical impact of radionuclide imaging on disorders of bones, joints, and soft tissues have occurred. This increased impact had its groundwork laid by advances in radiopharmaceuticals and instruments that are used for bone imaging. The progression from $^{85}$Sr- to $^{99m}$Tc-labeled phosphate and phosphonate compounds, coupled with the advance from crude rectilinear scanning techniques to whole body scintillation imaging with large crystal cameras and sophisticated electronics, has encouraged use of radionuclide techniques in the evaluation of musculoskeletal diseases. Many clinical studies have

documented the high degree of sensitivity of the bone scan compared with that of the radiograph in detecting osseous and articular abnormalities. Currently, the relative diagnostic roles of bone scintigraphy and MR imaging are being investigated.

## References

1. Schmorl G, Junghanns H: The Human Spine in Health and Disease. 2nd American Ed. New York, Grune & Stratton, 1971, pp 2, 158.
2. Fleming WH, McIlraith JD, King ER: Photoscanning of bone lesions utilizing strontium-85. Radiology 77:635, 1961.
3. Charkes ND, Sklaroff DM: Early diagnosis of metastatic bone cancer by photoscanning with strontium-85. J Nucl Med 5:168, 1964.
4. DeNardo GL, Volpe JA: Detection of bone lesions with the strontium-85 scintiscan. J Nucl Med 7:219, 1966.
5. Harmer CL, Burns JE, Sams A, et al: The value of fluorine-18 for scanning bone tumors. Clin Radiol 20:204, 1969.
6. Galasko CSB: Detection of skeletal metastases from carcinoma of the breast. Surg Gynecol Obstet 132:1019, 1971.
7. Blau M, Nagler W, Bender MA: Fluorine-18: A new isotope for bone scanning. J Nucl Med 3:332, 1962.
8. Subramanian G, McAfee JG, O'Mara RE, et al: $^{99m}$Tc-polyphosphate PP46: A new radiopharmaceutical for skeletal imaging (Abstr). J Nucl Med 12:399, 1971.
9. Blum T: Osteomyelitis of the mandible and maxilla. J Am Dent Assoc 11:802, 1924.
10. Looney WB: The initial medical and industrial use of radioactive materials (1915–1940). AJR 72:838, 1954.
11. Chiewitz O, Hevesy G: Radioactive indicators in the study of phosphorus metabolism in rats. Nature (London) 136:754, 1935.
12. Treadwell A de G, Low-Beer BV, Friedell HL, et al: Metabolic studies on neoplasm of bone with the aid of radioactive strontium. Am J Med Sci 204:521, 1942.
13. Bauer GCH, Ray RD: Kinetics of strontium metabolism in man. J Bone Joint Surg [Am] 40:171, 1958.
14. Bauer, GCH, Wendeberg B: External counting of $^{47}$Ca and $^{85}$Sr in studies of localized skeletal lesions in man. J Bone Joint Surg [Br] 41:558, 1959.
15. Gynning I, Langeland P, Lindberg S, et al: Localization with $^{85}$Sr of spinal metastases in mammary cancer and changes in uptake after hormone and roentgen therapy. Acta Radiol 55:119, 1961.
16. DeNardo GL, Jacobson SJ, Raventos A: $^{85}$Sr bone scan in neoplastic disease. Semin Nucl Med 2:18, 1972.
17. Jowsey J, Riggs BL: Assessment of bone turnover by microradiography and autoradiography. Semin Nucl Med 2:3, 1972.
18. Cameron JR, Sorenson J: Measurement of bone mineral in vivo: An improved method. Science 142:230, 1963.
19. Griffiths HJL, Zimmerman RE, Bailey G, et al: The use of photon absorptiometry in the diagnosis of renal osteodystrophy. Radiology 109:277, 1973.
20. Goldsmith NF, Johnston JO, Ury H, et al: Bone mineral estimation in normal and osteoporotic women. J Bone Joint Surg [Am] 53:83, 1971.
21. Mazess RB (Ed): Third International Conference on Bone Mineral Measurement. AJR 126:1266, 1976.
22. Fremlin JH: Determination of whole-body calcium by neutron activation analysis in vivo. Semin Nucl Med 2:86, 1972.
23. Cohn SH, Dombrowski CS: Measurement of total-body calcium, sodium, chlorine, nitrogen, and phosphorus in man by in vivo neutron activation analysis. J Nucl Med 12:499, 1971.
24. Nelp WB, Palmer HE, Murano R, et al: Measurement of total body calcium (bone mass) in vivo with the use of total body neutron activation analysis. J Lab Clin Med 76:151, 1971.
25. Chamberlain MJ, Fremlin JH, Peters DK, et al: Total-body calcium by whole body neutron activation: A new technique for study of bone disease. Br Med J 2:581, 1968.
26. Goergen TG, Alazraki NP, Halpern SE, et al: "Cold" bone lesions: A newly recognized phenomenon of bone imaging. J Nucl Med 15:1120, 1973.
27. Genant HK, Bautovich GJ, Singh M, et al: Bone-seeking radionuclides: An in vivo study of factors affecting skeletal uptake. Radiology 113:373, 1974.
28. Van Dyke D, Anger HO, Yano Y, et al: Bone blood flow shown with $^{18}$F and the positron camera. Am J Physiol 209:65, 1965.
29. Charkes ND, Makler PT, Philips C: Studies of skeletal tracer kinetics. I. Digital-computer solution of a five compartment model of ($^{18}$F) fluoride kinetics in humans. J Nucl Med 19:1301, 1978.
30. Siegel BA, Donovan RL, Alderson PO, et al: Skeletal uptake of $^{99m}$Tc-diphosphonate in relation to local bone blood flow. Radiology 120:121, 1976.
31. Jones AG, Francis MD, Davis MA: Bone scanning: Radionuclide reaction mechanisms. Semin Nucl Med 6:3, 1976.
32. Blau M, Ganatra R, Bender MA: $^{18}$F-fluoride for bone imaging. Semin Nucl Med 2:31, 1972.
33. O'Mara RE, Subramanian G: Experimental agents for skeletal imaging. Semin Nucl Med 2:38, 1972.
34. Subramanian G, McAfee JG: A new complex of $^{99m}$Tc for skeletal imaging. Radiology 99:192, 1971.

35. Thrall JH: Technetium-99m labeled agents for skeletal imaging. CRC Crit Rev Clin Radiol Nucl Med 8:1, 1976.
36. Merrick MV: Bone scanning. Br J Radiol 48:327, 1975.
37. Davis MA, Jones AG: Comparison of 99mTc-labeled phosphate and phosphonate agents for skeletal imaging. Semin Nucl Med 6:19, 1976.
38. Subramanian G, McAfee JG, Blair RJ, et al: Technetium-99m labeled stannous imidodiphosphate, a new radiodiagnostic agent for bone scanning: Comparison with other 99mTc complexes. J Nucl Med 16:1137, 1975.
39. Krishnamurthy GT, Tubis M, Endow JS, et al: Clinical comparison of the kinetics of 99mTc labeled polyphosphate and diphosphonate. J Nucl Med 15:848, 1974.
40. Subramanian G, McAfee JG, Blair RJ, et al: Technetium-99m methylene diphosphonate—a superior agent for skeletal imaging: Comparison with other technetium complexes. J Nucl Med 16:744, 1975.
41. Khairi MRA, Altman RD, DeRosa GP, et al: Sodium etidronate in the treatment of Paget's disease of bone. A study of long-term results. Ann Intern Med 87:656, 1977.
42. Rosenthall L, Kaye M: Observations in the mechanism of 99mTc-labeled phosphate complex uptake in metabolic bone disease. Semin Nucl Med 6:59, 1976.
43. Kaye M, Silverton S, Rosenthall L: Technetium-99m-pyrophosphate: Studies in vivo and in vitro. J Nucl Med 16:40, 1975.
44. McNeil BJ: Rationale for the use of bone scans in selected metastatic and primary bone tumors. Semin Nucl Med 8:336, 1978.
45. Mall JC, Bekerman C, Hoffer PB, et al: A unified radiological approach to the detection of skeletal metastases. Radiology 118:323, 1976.
46. Citrin DL, Furnival CM, Bessent RG, et al: Radioactive technetium phosphate bone scanning in preoperative assessment and follow-up study of patients with primary cancer of the breast. Surg Gynecol Obstet 143:360, 1976.
47. Gerber FH, Goodreau JJ, Kirchner PT: Tc-99m EHDP bone scanning in breast cancer. J Nucl Med 16:529, 1975.
48. McNeil BJ, Pace PD, Gray EB, et al: Preoperative and follow-up bone scans in patients with primary carcinoma of the breast. Surg Gynecol Obstet 147:745, 1978.
49. Ramsdell JW, Peters RM, Taylor AT, et al: Multiorgan scans for staging lung cancer: Correlation with clinical evaluation. J Thorac Cardiovasc Surg 73:653, 1977.
50. Gutierrez AC, Vincent RG, Bakshi S, et al: Radioisotope scans in the evaluation of metastatic bronchogenic carcinoma. J Thorac Cardiovasc Surg 69:934, 1975.
51. Schaffer DL, Pendergrass HP: Comparison of enzyme, clinical, radiographic, and radionuclide methods of detecting bone metastases from carcinoma of the prostate. Radiology 121:431, 1976.
52. Goldstein H, McNeil BJ, Zufalle E, et al: Changing indications for bone scintigraphy in patients with osteosarcoma. Radiology 135:177, 1980.
53. Goldstein H, McNeil BJ, Zufalle E, et al: Is there still a place for bone scanning in Ewing's sarcoma? J Nucl Med 21:10, 1980.
54. McNeil BJ, Cassady JR, Geiser CF, et al: Fluorine-18 bone scintigraphy in children with osteosarcoma or Ewing's sarcoma. Radiology 109:627, 1973.
55. Gilday DL, Ash JM, Reilly BJ: Radionuclide skeletal survey for pediatric neoplasms. Radiology 123:399, 1977.
56. Kaufman RA, Thrall JH, Keyes JW Jr, et al: False-negative bone scans in neuroblastoma metastatic to the ends of long bones. AJR 130:131, 1978.
57. Gilday DL, Ash JM: Benign bone tumors. Semin Nucl Med 6:33, 1976.
58. Gates GF, Dore EK: Detection of craniosynostosis by bone scanning. Radiology 115:665, 1976.
59. Sty JR, Boedecker RA, Babbitt DP: Skull scintigraphy in infantile hypophosphatasia. J Nucl Med 20:305, 1979.
60. Handmaker H, Leonards R: The bone scan in inflammatory osseous disease. Semin Nucl Med 6:95, 1976.
61. Teates CD, Williamson BRJ: "Hot and cold" bone lesion in acute osteomyelitis. AJR 129:517, 1977.
62. Gilday DL, Paul DJ, Paterson J: Diagnosis of osteomyelitis in children by combined blood pool and bone imaging. Radiology 117:331, 1975.
63. Alazraki NP, Fierer J, Resnick D: Chronic osteomyelitis: Monitoring by 99mTc-phosphate and 67Ga-citrate imaging. AJR 145:767, 1985.
64. Lisbona R, Rosenthall L: Observations on the sequential use of 99mTc-phosphate complex and 67Ga imaging in osteomyelitis, cellulitis, and septic arthritis. Radiology 123:123, 1977.
65. Kolyvas E, Rosenthall L, Ahronheim GA, et al: Serial 67Ga-citrate imaging during treatment of acute osteomyelitis in childhood. Clin Nucl Med 3:461, 1978.
66. Alazraki NP, Minteer-Convery M, Convery FR: Accuracy of bone and gallium scanning in patients with painful prosthetic replacement. Proceedings of the Society for Nuclear Medicine, 4th Annual Western Regional Meeting, Monterey, California. 1979 (Abstr).
67. Williamson BRJ, McLaughlin RE, Wang GJ, et al: Radionuclide bone imaging as a means of differentiating loosening and infection in patients with a painful total hip prosthesis. Radiology 133:723, 1979.
68. Rosenthall L, Lisbona R, Hernandez M, et al: 99mTc-pp and 67Ga imaging following insertion of orthopedic devices. Radiology 133:717, 1979.
69. Reing CM, Richin PF, Kenmore PI: Differential bone scanning in the evaluation of a painful total joint replacement. J Bone Joint Surg [Am] 61:933, 1979.
70. Sakimura IT, Dorr L, Montgomery J, et al: Bone and gallium scan following total hip replacement to differentiate loosening from infection. Proceedings of the Society for Nuclear Medicine, 4th Annual Western Regional Meeting, 1979 (Abstr).
71. Hattner RS, Hunter J, Genant HK, et al: Utility of skeletal scintigraphy in the detection of failed total knee arthroplasty. Proceeding Society for Nuclear Medicine, 4th Annual Western Regional Meeting, Monterey, California, 1979 (Abstr).
72. Wilcox JR Jr, Moniot AL, Green JP: Bone scanning in evaluation of exercise related stress injuries. Radiology 123:699, 1977.
73. Geslien GE, Thrall JH, Espinosa JL, et al: Early detection of stress fractures using 99mTc-polyphosphate. Radiology 121:683, 1976.
74. Marty R, Denney J, McKamey MR, et al: Bone trauma and related benign disease: Assessment by bone scanning. Semin Nucl Med 6:107, 1976.
75. Wendeberg B: Mineral metabolism of fractures of the tibia in man studied with external counting of Sr85. Acta Orthop Scand (Suppl) 52:1, 1961.
76. Matin P: The appearance of bone scans following fractures, including immediate and long-term studies. J Nucl Med 20:1227, 1979.
77. Rosenthall L, Hill RO, Chuang S: Observation on use of 99mTc-phosphate imaging in peripheral bone trauma. Radiology 119:637, 1976.
78. Fordham EW, Ramachandran PC: Radionuclide imaging of osseous trauma. Semin Nucl Med 4:411, 1974.
79. Stevenson JS, Bright RW, Dunson GL, et al: Technetium-99m phosphate bone imaging: A method for assessing bone graft healing. Radiology 110:391, 1974.
80. Alavi A, Desai A, Esterhai J, et al: Bone scanning in the evaluation of non-united fractures. J Nucl Med 20:647, 1979.
81. Fogelman I, McKillop JH, Bessent RG, et al: The role of bone scanning in osteomalacia. J Nucl Med 19:245–248, 1978.
82. Krishnamurthy GT, Brickman AS, Blahd WH: Technetium-99m-Sn-pyrophosphate pharmacokinetics and bone image changes in parathyroid disease. J Nucl Med 18:236, 1977.
83. Sy WM: Bone scan in primary hyperparathyroidism. J Nucl Med 15:1089, 1974.
84. Fogelman I, Bessent RG, Turner JG, et al: The use of whole-body retention of Tc-99m diphosphonate in the diagnosis of metabolic bone disease. J Nucl Med 19:270, 1978.
85. Sy WM, Mittal AK: Bone scan in chronic dialysis patients with evidence of secondary hyperparathyroidism and renal osteodystrophy. Br J Radiol 48:878, 1975.
86. Wiegmann T, Rosenthall L, Kaye M: Technetium-99m pyrophosphate bone scans in hyperparathyroidism. J Nucl Med 18:231, 1977.
87. Prakash V, Kamel NJ, Lin MS, et al: Increased skeletal localization of 99mTc diphosphonate in paralyzed limbs. Clin Nucl Med 1:48, 1976.
88. Rasmussen H, Bordier P: The Physiological and Cellular Basis of Metabolic Bone Disease. Baltimore, Williams & Wilkins Co., 1974.
89. Bray ST, Partain CL, Teates CD, et al: The value of the bone scan in idiopathic regional migratory osteoporosis. J Nucl Med 20:1268, 1979.
90. Strashun A, Chayes Z: Migratory osteolysis. J Nucl Med 20:129, 1979.
91. Paget J: On a form of chronic inflammation of bones (osteitis deformans). Med Chir Trans 60:37, 1877.
92. Schmorl G: Uber Ostitis deformans Paget. Virchows Arch Pathol Anat Physiol 283:694, 1932.
93. Serafini AN: Paget's disease of bone. Semin Nucl Med 6:47, 1976.
94. Rhodes BA, Greyson ND, Hamilton CR Jr, et al: Absence of arteriovenous shunts in Paget's disease of bone. N Engl J Med 287:686, 1972.
95. Rausch JM, Resnick D, Goergen TG, et al: Bone scanning in osteolytic Paget's disease: Case report. J Nucl Med 18:699, 1976.
96. Wellman HN, Schauwecker D, Robb JA, et al: Skeletal scinti-imaging and radiography in the diagnosis and management of Paget's disease. Clin Orthop 127:55, 1977.
97. Shirazi PH, Ryan WG, Fordham EW: Bone scanning in evaluation of Paget's disease of bone. CRC Crit Rev Clin Radiol Nucl Med 5:523, 1974.
98. Alazraki NP: Aseptic necrosis discussion. In BA Siegel (Ed): Nuclear Radiology Syllabus. Chicago, American College of Radiology, 1978.
99. Meyers MH, Telfer N, Moore TM: Determination of the vascularity of the femoral head with technetium-99m sulphur colloid. J Bone Joint Surg [Am] 59:658, 1977.
100. Lutzker LG, Alavi A: Bone and marrow imaging in sickle cell disease: Diagnosis of infarction. Semin Nucl Med 6:83, 1976.
101. Alavi A, Bond JP, Kuhl DE, et al: Scan detection of bone marrow infarcts in sickle cell disorders. J Nucl Med 15:1003, 1974.
102. Feigin DS, Strauss HW, James AE Jr: The bone marrow scan in experimental osteomyelitis. Skel Radiol 1:103, 1976.
103. Danigelis JA: Pinhole imaging in Legg-Perthes' disease: Further observations. Semin Nucl Med 6:69, 1976.
104. Catterall A: The natural history of Perthes' disease. J Bone Joint Surg [Br] 53:37, 1971.
105. Weiss TE, Maxfield WS, Murison PJ, et al: Iodinated human serum albumin (I-131) localization studies of rheumatoid arthritis joints by scintillation scanning. Arthritis Rheum 8:976, 1965.
106. Alarcón-Segovia D, Trujegue M, Tovaz E, et al: Scintillation scanning of the joints with technetium-99m. Proceedings of the Annual Meeting of the American Rheumatism Association, New York, 1967.
107. Desaulniers M, Fuks A, Hawkins D, et al: Radiotechnetium polyphosphate joint imaging. J Nucl Med 15:417, 1974.
108. Bekerman C, Genant HK, Hoffer PB, et al: Radionuclide imaging of the bones and joints of the hand: A definition of normal and comparison of sensitivity using 99mTc-pertechnetate and 99mTc-diphosphonate. Radiology 118:653, 1975.
109. Holfer PB, Genant HK: Radionuclide joint imaging. Semin Nucl Med 6:121, 1976.

110. Thomas RH, Resnick D, Alazraki NP, et al: Compartmental evaluation of osteoarthritis of the knee: A comparative study of available diagnostic modalities. Radiology *116*:585, 1975.
111. McCarty DJ, Polcyn RE, Collins PA: <sup>99m</sup>Technetium scintiphotography in arthritis. II. Its nonspecificity and clinical and roentgenographic correlations in rheumatoid arthritis. Arthritis Rheum *13*:21, 1970.
112. Weissberg DL, Resnick D, Taylor A, et al: Rheumatoid arthritis and its variants: Analysis of scintiphotographic, radiographic, and clinical examinations. AJR *131*:665, 1978.
113. Lentle BC, Russell AS, Percy JS, et al: The scintigraphic investigation of sacroiliac disease. J Nucl Med *18*:529, 1977.
114. Goldberg RP, Genant HK, Shimshak R, et al: Applications and limitations of quantitative sacroiliac joint scintigraphy. Radiology *128*:683, 1978.
115. Sy WM, Bay R, Camera A: Hand images: Normal and abnormal. J Nucl Med *18*:419, 1977.
116. Russell AS, Lentle BC, Percy JS: Investigation of sacroiliac disease: Comparative evaluation of radiological and radionuclide techniques. J Rheumatol *2*:45, 1975.
117. Brown M, Swift TR, Spies SM: Radioisotope scanning in inflammatory muscle disease. Neurology *26*:517, 1976.
118. Rosenthal DI, Chandler HC, Azizi F: Uptake of bone imaging agents by diffuse pulmonary metastatic calcification. AJR *129*:871, 1977.
119. Buja LM, Tofe AJ, Kulkarni PV, et al: Sites and mechanisms of localization of technetium-99m phosphorus radiopharmaceuticals in acute myocardial infarcts and other tissues. J Clin Invest *60*:724, 1977.
120. Byun HH, Rodman SG, Chung KE: Soft tissue concentration of <sup>99m</sup>Tc-phosphates associated with injections of iron dextran complex. J Nucl Med *17*:374, 1976.
121. Garcia AC, Yeh SDJ, Benua RS: Accumulation of bone-seeking radionuclides in liver metastasis from colon carcinoma. Clin Nucl Med *2*:265, 1977.
122. Rosenfield N, Treves S: Osseous and extraosseous uptake of fluorine-18 and technetium-99m polyphosphate in children with neuroblastoma. Radiology *111*:127, 1974.
123. Alazraki NP: Soft tissue localization of bone imaging radiopharmaceuticals. *In* BA Siegel (Ed): Nuclear Radiology Syllabus. Chicago, American College of Radiology, 1978.
124. Siegel BA, Engel WK, Derrer EC: Localization of technetium-99m diphosphonate in acutely injured muscle. Relationship to muscle calcium deposition. Neurology *27*:230, 1977.
125. Poulouse KP, Reha RC, Eckelman WC: Extra-osseous localization of Tc-99m-pyrophosphate. Br J Radiol *48*:724, 1975.
126. Berman DS, Amsterdam EA, Hines HH, et al: New approach to interpretation of technetium-99m pyrophosphate scintigraphy in detection of acute myocardial infarction. Clinical assessment of diagnostic accuracy. Am J Cardiol *39*:341, 1977.
127. Silver JR: Heterotopic ossification: A clinical study of its possible relationship to trauma. Paraplegia *7*:220, 1969.
128. Alazraki NP: Myositis ossificans associated with spinal cord injury. *In* BA Siegel (Ed): Nuclear Radiology Syllabus. Chicago, American College of Radiology, 1978.
129. Tanaka T, Rossier AB, Hussey RW, et al: Quantitative assessment of para-osteo-arthropathy and its maturation on serial radionuclide bone images. Radiology *123*:217, 1977.
130. Suzuki Y, Hisada K, Takeda M: Demonstration of myositis ossificans by <sup>99m</sup>Tc-pyrophosphate bone scanning. Radiology *111*:663, 1974.
131. King MA, Casarett GW, Weber DA: A study of irradiated bone. I. Histopathologic and physiologic changes. J Nucl Med *20*:1142, 1979.
132. Sagar VV, Piccone JM, Charkes ND: Studies of skeletal tracer kinetics. III. Tc-99m (Sn) methylenediphosphonate uptake in the canine tibia as a function of blood flow. J Nucl Med *20*:1257, 1979.
133. Wahner HW, Dunn WL, Riggs BL: Assessment of bone mineral. Part I. J Nucl Med *25*:1134, 1984.
134. Wahner HW, Riggs BL, Beabout JW: Diagnosis of osteoporosis: Usefulness of photon absorptiometry at the radius. J Nucl Med *18*:432, 1977.
135. Jensen GF, Christiansen C, Boesen J, et al: Relationship between bone mineral content and frequency of postmenopausal fractures. Acta Med Scand *213*:61, 1983.
136. Health and Public Policy Committee, American College of Physicians, Philadelphia, PA: Radiologic methods to evaluate bone mineral content. Ann Intern Med *100*:908, 1984.
137. Riggs BL, Wahner HW, Seeman E, et al: Changes in bone mineral density of the proximal femur and spine with aging. J Clin Invest *7*:716, 1982.
138. Mazess RB, Peppler WW, Chesney RW, et al: Does bone measurement on the radius indicate skeletal status? Concise Communication. J Nucl Med *25*:281, 1984.
139. Yano K, Wasnich RD, Vogel JM, et al: Bone mineral measurements among middle-aged and elderly Japanese residents in Hawaii. Am J Epidemiol *119*:751, 1984.
140. Wahner HW, Dunn WL, Riggs BL: Assessment of bone mineral. Part 2. J Nucl Med *25*:1241, 1984.
141. Krolner B, Nielsen SP, Lund B, et al: Measurement of bone mineral content (BMC) of the lumbar spine, II. Correlation between forearm BMC and lumbar spine BMC. Scand J Clin Lab Invest *40*:665, 1980.
142. Fogelman I, Pearson DW, Bessent RG, et al: A comparison of skeletal uptakes of three diphosphonates by whole-body retention: Concise communication. J Nucl Med *22*:880, 1981.
143. Van Duzee BF, Schaefer JA, Ball JD, et al: Relative lesion detection ability of Tc-99m HMDP and Tc-99m MDP: Concise communication. J Nucl Med *25*:166, 1984.
144. Collier BD, Johnson RP, Carrera GF, et al: Painful spondylolysis or spondylolisthesis studied by radiography and single-photon emission computed tomography. Radiology *154*:207, 1985.
145. Collier BD, Carrera GF, Johnson RP, et al: Detection of femoral head avascular necrosis in adults by SPECT. J Nucl Med *26*:979, 1985.
146. Stromqvist B, Brismar J, Hansson LI: Emission tomography in femoral neck fracture for evaluation of avascular necrosis. Acta Orthop Scand *54*:872, 1983.
147. Rossleigh MA, Lovegrove FTA, Reynolds PM, et al: The assessment of response to therapy of bone metastases in breast cancer. Aust NZ J Med *14*:19, 1984.
148. Pollen JJ, Witzum KC, Ashburn WL: The flare phenomenon in radionuclide bone scan in metastatic prostate cancer. AJR *142*:773, 1984.
149. Hudson TM, Chew FS, Manaster BJ: Radionuclide bone scanning of medullary chondrosarcoma. AJR *139*:1071, 1982.
150. Thrall JH, Geslien GE, Corcoron RJ, et al: Abnormal radionuclide deposition patterns adjacent to focal skeletal lesions. Radiology *115*:659, 1975.
151. Simon MA, Kirchner PT: Scintigraphic evaluation of primary bone tumors. J Bone Joint Surg [Am] *62*:758, 1980.
152. Dahlin DC: Bone Tumors. 3d Ed. Springfield, Ill, Charles C Thomas, 1978.
153. Tumeh SS, Beadle G, Kaplan WD: Clinical significance of solitary rib lesions in patients with extraskeletal malignancy. J Nucl Med *26*:1140, 1985.
154. Harbert JC, George FH, Kerner ML: Differentiation of rib fractures from metastases by bone scanning. Clin Nucl Med *6*:359, 1981.
155. Bushnell D, Shirazi P, Khedkar N, et al: Ewing's sarcoma seen as a "cold" lesion on bone scans. Clin Nucl Med *8*:173, 1983.
156. Siddiqui AR, Ellis JH: "Cold spot" on bone scan at the site of primary osteosarcoma. Eur J Nucl Med *7*:480, 1982.
157. Veluvolu P, Collier BD, Isitman AT, et al: Scintigraphic skeletal "doughnut" sign due to giant cell tumor of the fibula. Clin Nucl Med *9*:631, 1984.
158. Novetsky GJ, Berlin L: The solitary hand lesion: Bone scintigraphy of monostotic fibrous dysplasia. Clin Nucl Med *9*:590, 1984.
159. Humphry A, Gilday DL, Brown RG: Bone scintigraphy in chondroblastoma. Radiology *137*:497, 1980.
160. McNeil BJ: Value of bone scanning in neoplastic disease. Semin Nucl Med *14*:277, 1984.
161. Schaffer DL, Pendergrass HP: Comparison of enzyme, clinical radiographic and radionuclide methods of detecting bone metastases from carcinoma of the prostate. Radiology *121*:431, 1976.
162. Shafer RB, Reinke DB: Contribution of the bone scan, serum acid and alkaline phosphatase, and the radiographic bone survey to the management of newly-diagnosed carcinoma of the prostate. Clin Nucl Med *2*:200, 1977.
163. Howman-Giles RB, Gilday DL, Ash JM: Radionuclide skeletal survey in neuroblastoma. Radiology *131*:497, 1979.
164. Pollen JJ, Gerber K, Ashburn WL, et al: Nuclear bone imaging in metastatic cancer of the prostate. Cancer *47*:2585, 1981.
165. Nair N: Bone scanning in Ewing's sarcoma. J Nucl Med *26*:349, 1985.
166. Podrasky AE, Stark DD, Hattner RS, et al: Radionuclide bone scanning in neuroblastoma: Skeletal metastases and primary tumor localization of 99m Tc-MDP. AJR *141*:469, 1983.
167. Helms CA, Hattner RS, Vogler JB: Osteoid osteoma: Radionuclide diagnosis. Radiology *151*:779, 1984.
168. Ghelman B, Vigorita VJ: Postoperative radionuclide evaluation of osteoid osteomas. Radiology *146*:509, 1983.
169. Colton CL, Hardy JG: Evaluation of a sterilizable radiation probe as an aid to the surgical treatment of osteoid-osteoma. Technical note. J Bone Joint Surg [Am] *65*:1019, 1983.
170. Hudson TM: Scintigraphy of aneurysmal bone cysts. AJR *142*:761, 1984.
171. Maurer AH, Chan DPC, Camargo EE, et al: Utility of three-phase skeletal scintigraphy in suspected osteomyelitis: Concise Communication. J Nucl Med *22*:941, 1981.
172. Raptopoulos V, Doherty PW, Goss TP, et al: Acute osteomyelitis: Advantage of white cell scans in early detection. AJR *139*:1077, 1982.
173. Mulamba L, Ferrant A, Leners N, et al: Indium-111 leukocyte scanning in the evaluation of painful hip arthroplasty. Acta Orthop Scand *54*:695, 1983.
174. Shauwecker DS, Park HM, Mock BH, et al: Evaluation of complicating osteomyelitis with Tc-99m MDP, In-111 granulocytes, and Ga-67 citrate. J Nucl Med *25*:849, 1984.
175. Merkel KD, Brown ML, Dewanjee MK, et al: Comparison of indium-labeled-leukocyte imaging with sequential technetium-gallium scanning in the diagnosis of low-grade musculoskeletal sepsis. J Bone Joint Surg [Am] *67*:465, 1985.
176. Devereaux MD, Parr GR, Lachman SM, et al: The diagnosis of stress fractures in athletes. JAMA *252*:531, 1984.
177. Noakes TD, Smith JA, Lindenberg G, et al: Pelvic stress fractures in long distance runners. Am J Sports Med *13*:120, 1985.
178. Koch RA, Jackson DW: Pubic symphysitis in runners. A report of two cases. Am J Sports Med *9*:62, 1981.
179. Jackson DW, Wiltse LL, Dingeman RD, et al: Stress reactions involving the pars interarticularis in young athletes. Am J Sports Med *9*:304, 1981.
180. Fink-Bennett DM, Benson MT: Unusual exercise-related stress fractures. Clin Nucl Med *9*:430, 1984.
181. Lieberman CM, Hemingway DL: Scintigraphy of shin splints. Clin Nucl Med *5*:31, 1980.

182. Terry DW Jr, Isitman AT, Holmes RA: Radionuclide bone images in hypertrophic pulmonary osteoarthropathy. AJR *124*:571, 1975.

183. Rai GS, Webster SGP, Wraight EP: Isotopic scanning of bone in the diagnosis of osteomalacia. Am Geriatr Soc *29*:45, 1981.

184. Wilkins WE, Chalmers A, Sanerkin NG, et al: Osteomalacia in the elderly: The value of radio-isotope bone scanning in patients with equivocal biochemistry. Age Aging *12*:195, 1983.

185. Drane WE, Rudd TG: Femoral head viability following hip fracture prognostic role of radionuclide bone imaging. Clin Nucl Med *10*:141, 1984.

186. Greiff J, Lanng S, Hoilund-Carlsen PF, et al: Early detection by Tc-99m Sn-pyrophosphate scintigraphy of femoral head necrosis. Acta Orthop Scand *51*:119, 1980.

187. Spencer JD, Maisey M: A prospective scintigraphic study of avascular necrosis of bone in renal transplant patients. Clin Orthop *194*:125, 1985.

188. Conklin JJ, Alderson PO, Zizic TM, et al: Comparison of bone scan and radiograph sensitivity in the detection of steroid-induced ischemic necrosis of bone. Radiology *147*:221, 1983.

189. Collier BD, Carrera GF, Johnson RP, et al: Detection of femoral head avascular necrosis in adults by SPECT. J Nucl Med *26*:979, 1985.

190. Sutherland AD, Savage JP, Paterson DC, et al: The nuclide bone-scan in the diagnosis and management of Perthes' disease. J Bone Joint Surg [Br] *62*:3, 1980.

191. Cavailloles F, Bok B, Bensahel H: Bone scintigraphy in the diagnosis and follow up of Perthes' disease. Eur J Nucl Med *7*:327, 1982.

192. Gelfand MJ, Strife JL, Braham EJ, et al: Bone scintigraphy in slipped capital femoral epiphysis. Clin Nucl Med *8*:613, 1983.

193. Turner JH: Post-traumatic avascular necrosis of the femoral head predicted by preoperative technetium-99m antimony-colloid scan. J Bone Joint Surg [Am] *65*:786, 1983.

194. Gregg PJ, Walder DN: Scintigraphy versus radiography in the early diagnosis of experimental bone necrosis. J Bone Joint Surg [Br] *62*:214, 1980.

195. Goldman AB, Pavlov H, Schneider R: Radionuclide bone scanning in subtalar coalitions: Differential considerations. AJR *138*:427, 1982.

196. Haase GM, Ortiz VN, Sfakianakis GN, et al: The value of radionuclide bone scanning in the early recognition of deliberate child abuse. J Trauma *20*:10, 1980.

197. Smith FW, Gilday DL, Ash JM, et al: Unsuspected costo-vertebral fractures demonstrated by bone scanning in the child abuse syndrome. Pediatr Radiol *10*:103, 1980.

198. Sty JR, Starshak RJ: The role of bone scintigraphy in the evaluation of the suspected abused child. Radiology *146*:369, 1983.

199. Merten DF, Radkowski MA, Leonidas JC: The abused child: A radiological reappraisal. Radiology *146*:377, 1983.

200. Amundsen TR, Siegel MJ, Siegel BA: Osteomyelitis and infarction in sickle cell hemoglobinopathies: Differentiation by combined technetium and gallium scintigraphy. Radiology *153*:807, 1984.

201. Lee Y-TN: Bone scanning in patients with early breast carcinoma: Should it be a routine staging procedure? Cancer *47*:486, 1981.

202. Citrin DL, Hougen C, Zwiebel W, et al: The use of serial bone scans in assessing response of bone metastases to systemic treatment. Cancer *47*:680, 1981.

203. Front D, Schneck SO, Frankel A, et al: Bone metastases and bone pain in breast cancer: Are they closely associated? JAMA *242*:1747, 1979.

204. Pollen JJ, Gerber K, Ashburn WL, et al: Nuclear bone imaging in metastatic cancer of the prostate. Cancer *47*:2585, 1981.

205. Uri G, Wellman H, Capello W, et al: Scintigraphic and x-ray arthrographic diagnosis of femoral prosthesis loosening: Concise Communication. J Nucl Med *25*:661, 1984.

206. Rosenthall L, Aldis AE, Hill RO: Combined radionuclide and radiocontrast arthrography for evaluating hip arthroplasty. Eur J Nucl Med *10*:531, 1985.

207. Tyler JL, Powers TA: Bone scanning after marrow biopsy: Concise Communication. J Nucl Med *23*:1085, 1982.

208. Alazraki N, Moitoza J, Heaphy J, et al: The effect of iatrogenic trauma on the bone scintigram—an animal study: Concise Communication. J Nucl Med *25*:978, 1984.

209. Traughber PD, Manaster BJ, Murphy K, et al: Bone scanning of joints after needle aspiration and/or contrast arthrography. AJR *146*:87, 1986.

210. Scott S, Alazraki N, Manaster B: Failure of bone scanning to detect fractures in a woman on chronic steroid therapy. Skel Radiol *12*:204, 1984.

211. Scott S, Alazraki N, Manaster B, et al: Effect of steroid intake on radionuclide bone scan accuracy for detecting bone trauma. In preparation.

212. Alazraki N, Dries D, Datz F, et al: The value of a 24-hour image (four phase bone scan) in assessing osteomyelitis in patients with peripheral vascular disease. J Nucl Med *26*:711, 1985.

213. Alazraki N: The musculoskeletal system. *In* JC Harbert, AFG da Rocha (Eds.)

214. Bax JJ, Visser FC, van Lingen A, et al: 18F-fluorodeoxyglucose and SPECT to detect viable myocardium after recent infarction. Eur J Nucl Med *200*:841, 1993.

215. Corcoran RJ, Thrall JH, Kyle RW, et al: Solitary abnormalities in bone scans of patients with extraosseous malignancies. Nucl Med *121*:663, 1976.

216. Jacobson AF, Stomper PC, Cronin EB, et al: Bone scans with one or two new abnormalities in cancer patients with no known metastases: Reliability of interpretation of initial correlative radiographs. Radiology *174*:503, 1990.

217. Fordham EW, Ali A: Skeletal imaging in malignant disease. Bone, Golden's Diagn Nucl Med *67*:1011, 1979.

218. Robinson RG, Preston DF, Baxter KG, et al: Clinical experience with strontium-89 in prostatic and breast cancer patients. Semin Oncol *20*:44, 1993.

219. Porter AT, McEwan AJB: Strontium-89 as an adjuvant to external beam radiation improves pain relief and delays disease progression in advanced prostate cancer: Results of a randomized controlled trial. Semin Oncol *20*(Suppl 2):38, 1993.

220. Castillo LA, Yeh SDJ, Leeper RD: Bone scans in bone metastases from functioning thyroid carcinoma. Clin Nucl Med *5*:200, 1980.

221. Charkes ND, Vitti RA, Brooks K: Thallium-201 SPECT increases detectability of thyroid cancer metastases. J Nucl Med *31*:147, 1990.

222. Rees CR, Siddiqui AR, duCret R: The role of bone scinitgraphy in osteogenic sarcoma. Skel Radiol *15*:365, 1986.

223. Podrasky AE, Stark DD, Hattner RS, et al: Radionuclide bone scanning in neuroblastoma: Skeletal metastases and primary tumor localization of $^{99m}$ Tc-MDP. AJR *141*:469, 1983.

224. Baker M, Siddiqui AR, Provisor A, et al: Radiographic and scintigraphic skeletal imaging in patients with neuroblastoma: Concise communication. J Nucl Med *24*:467, 1983.

225. Gordon I, Peters AM, Gutman A, et al: Skeletal assessment in neuroblastoma—the pitfalls of iodine-123-MIBG scans. J Nucl Med *31*:129, 1990.

226. Gilday DL, Greenberg M: The controversy about the nuclear medicine investigation of neuroblastoma. J Nucl Med *31*:135, 1990.

227. Sisson JC, Shapiro B, Hutchinson RJ, et al: Locating and treating adrenergic tumors with a presynaptic radiopharmaceutical: In vivo imaging of neurotransmitter function in brain, heart and tumors (abstract). ACNP Nuclear Medicine Symposium, University of Michigan, Ann Arbor, 1990.

228. Alazraki N, Dries DJ, Datz F, et al: Value of a 24 hour image four phase bone scan in assessing osteomyelitis in patients with peripheral vascular disease. J Nucl Med *26*:711, 1985.

229. Maurer AH, Chen CDP, Camargo EE, et al: Utility of three-phase skeletal scintigraphy in suspected osteomyelitis. J Nucl Med *22*:941, 1981.

230. Seldin DW, Heiken JP, Feldman F, et al: Effect of soft-tissue pathology on detection of pedal osteomyelitis in diabetes. J Nucl Med *26*:988, 1985.

231. Schauwecker DS: Osteomyelitis: Diagnosis with In-111 labeled leukocytes. Radiology *171*:141, 1989.

232. Tumeh SS, Aliabadi P, Weissman NB, et al: Chronic osteomyelitis: Bone and gallium scan patterns associated with active disease. Radiology *158*:685, 1986.

233. Chandnani VP, Beltran J, Morris CS, et al: Acute experimental osteomyelitis and abscesses: Detection with MR imaging versus CT. Radiology *174*:233, 1990.

234. Erdman WA, Tamburro F, Jayson HT, et al: Osteomyelitis: Characteristics and pitfalls of diagnosis with MR imaging. Radiology *180*:533, 1991.

235. Rubin RH, Fischman AJ, Callahan RJ, et al: $^{111}$In-labeled nonspecific immunoglobulin scanning in the detection of focal infection. N Engl J Med *321*:935, 1989.

236. Fishman AJ, Rubin RH, White JA, et al: Localization of Fc and Fab fragments of nonspecific polyclonal IgG at focal sites of inflammation. J Nucl Med *31*:1199, 1990.

237. Fishman AJ, Rubin RH, Khaw BA, et al: Detection of acute inflammation with $^{111}$In-labeled nonspecific polyclonal IgG. Semin Nucl Med *18*:335, 1988.

238. Lind P, Langsteger W, Koltringer P, et al: Immunoscintigraphy of inflammatory processes with a technetium-99m-labeled monoclonal antigranulocyte antibody (MAb BW 250/183). J Nucl Med *31*:417, 1990.

239. Mountfield PJ, Kettle AG, O'Doherty MJ, et al: Comparison of technetium-99m-HMPAO leukocytes with indium-111 oxine leukocytes for localizing intraabdominal sepsis. Radiology *31*:311, 1990.

240. Matire JR: The role of nuclear medicine bone scans in evaluating pain in athletic injuries. Clin Sports Med *6*:713, 1987.

241. Alazraki N: Musculoskeletal imaging. *In* A Taylor, F Datz (Eds): Clinical Practice of Nuclear Medicine. New York, Churchill Livingstone, 1991, p 379.

242. Kipper MS, Alazraki N, Feiglin DH: The "hot" patella. Clin Nucl Med *4*:411, 1974.

Textbook of Nuclear Medicine. Volume 2. Clinical Applications. 2nd Ed. Philadelphia, Lea & Febiger, 1984, p 157.

# 16

# Needle Biopsy of Bone

*Donald Resnick, M.D.*

Open biopsy is an accepted surgical procedure in the diagnosis of a variety of skeletal disorders, including neoplastic, inflammatory, and metabolic conditions. Because this procedure requires considerable time and expense, operating room space, and personnel, as well as use of general anesthesia in most cases, repeated attempts have been made in the past to devise special instruments for percutaneous needle biopsy of bone.[1-13] More recently, advances in radiology, including image intensification, biplane videofluoroscopy, CT, and high resolution radionuclide bone scanning, have emphasized that radiologists are in a unique position to perform such closed needle biopsies.[14-16]

The bone specimen can be obtained in one of two ways: an aspiration by needle or a core by trephine. Tissue obtained by needle aspiration is small in quantity and distorted, with loss of cellular configuration; tissue obtained by trephine biopsy is greater in quantity and intact, although this technique requires larger needle size. Needle aspiration is most useful for tissue culture to exclude infection, although some investigators report the value of needle aspiration in establishing a wide variety of clinical diagnoses[17, 18, 28]; trephine biopsy is a better technique for histologic diagnosis.[19, 29, 30]

## ADVANTAGES AND DISADVANTAGES

Some of the advantages of closed needle biopsy of bone over open biopsy are obvious:

1. The method is relatively simple and the instruments are not technically complicated. The physician can gain expertise in the procedure in a short period of time. Closed needle biopsy can be accomplished quickly, usually within 45 minutes.

2. The patient is not submitted to any great risk. General anesthesia is not required and, in fact, the technique can be applied as an outpatient procedure, although we recommend that the patient be observed in the hospital for 24 hours after biopsy. Local complications such as infection are infrequent, and damage to internal organs does not occur if the procedure is accomplished carefully. The patient is not subjected to a major operative procedure even if a deep area of the skeleton must be biopsied.

3. Use of modern fluoroscopic equipment facilitates accurate needle placement, and the site of such needle placement can be permanently recorded with spot film or overhead radiographs prior to biopsy. CT scanning and scintigraphy can be used to further facilitate the procedure.

The major disadvantages of closed needle biopsy are the following:

1. A relatively small amount of material is withdrawn. This is particularly true with fine needle biopsies in which meager cytologic material may not be representative of the entire lesion, leading to an inaccurate pathologic diagnosis. This disadvantage is not so apparent with trephine biopsy, as a larger quantity of tissue is removed. In certain situations, repeat closed or open biopsy is necessary.

2. The biopsy procedure is relatively ''blind'' so that the ideal area of the lesion may not be biopsied. Use of high quality fluoroscopic control and CT minimizes this disadvantage.

3. The success of this procedure requires an experienced

pathologist who cooperates closely with the radiologist. For open biopsies, however, a similar situation exists, in which cooperation among a capable orthopedic surgeon, radiologist, and pathologist is required.

4. Although theoretically it is possible that closed biopsy of a tumor could lead to its dissemination in neighboring and distant tissues, this is not a realistic complication of the procedure.

## INDICATIONS AND CONTRAINDICATIONS

Although the indications for needle biopsy of bone will vary from one institution to another, certain guidelines do exist. General indications for this procedure follow.

### Neoplastic Disease

With regard to patients with suspected or proved *skeletal metastasis*, potential indications for closed bone biopsy include the following[34, 35]:

1. Patients with a known primary tumor who have a solitary bone lesion detected by conventional radiography, CT, MR imaging, or scintigraphy, or any combination of the four, in whom verification of the nature of the lesion will influence treatment. In many such persons the osseous abnormality will indeed represent a site of metastasis, but such documentation may be necessary for appropriate therapy planning. When the radiographic characteristics of the bone lesion are not typical of metastases from the known primary tumor (e.g., a purely osteolytic lesion in a patient with prostatic carcinoma or a purely osteosclerotic lesion in a patient with adenocarcinoma of the lung), the need for biopsy is more obvious, serving either to eliminate the diagnosis of skeletal metastasis or to uncover a second primary neoplasm. Furthermore, when the radionuclide bone scan alone is positive, the nonspecific nature of this examination must be understood; positive bone scans are encountered at sites of benign neoplasms and nontumorous conditions.

2. Patients without a known primary tumor who have solitary or multiple osteolytic or osteoblastic lesions in whom the most probable diagnosis is metastatic disease. In such persons, bone biopsy represents a direct means to establish quickly the cellular characteristics of the metastatic focus and, depending upon these characteristics, govern subsequent decisions regarding the need for and type of further diagnostic evaluation (see Chapter 85). This indication could be expanded to include tumors, such as lymphomas, for which the anticipated modes of treatment would be chemotherapy or radiation therapy rather than surgery. The diagnosis of multiple myeloma should be documented by appropriate laboratory examination rather than by closed bone biopsy. After this diagnosis has been established, sternal or iliac crest marrow aspiration is a more appropriate examination. Occasionally closed biopsy techniques are useful in a patient with a solitary plasmacytoma.

The closed biopsy technique also is indicated in evaluating debilitated patients with bone lesions that are not readily accessible to open biopsy, in whom a long surgical procedure would not be well tolerated.

3. Patients with known multiple primary tumors who

have one or more bone lesions. Percutaneous bone biopsy helps determine the type of tumor causing the bone lesion, thereby allowing the initiation of appropriate therapy.

4. Patients with a primary tumor in whom there is need to determine whether viable tumor cells are present in a radiographically stable metastatic bone lesion (or lesions).

5. Patients with a known primary tumor that is in clinical remission who have developed a new bone lesion (or lesions). A closed biopsy of the lesion may document the presence of metastasis from the known neoplasm or from a new primary tumor, or the presence of a nontumorous condition.

6. Patients who have received radiation therapy for a primary tumor or metastatic bone lesion, or both, who develop osseous abnormalities in the irradiated skeleton whose nature is not clear. Such changes may relate to radiation-induced osteopenia, necrosis or sarcoma (see Chapter 73), osteomyelitis, or new or recurrent metastasis from the known primary tumor or a new neoplasm.

7. Patients with a non-neoplastic skeletal problem (e.g., Paget's disease, osteomyelitis) that may predispose to metastatic seeding, who develop a new aggressive lesion at the site of bone involvement whose nature is not clear.

With regard to *primary tumors of bone or soft tissue*, the advantages of closed biopsy over surgical intervention and open biopsy are less clear.[80–82, 98] Although adequate sampling of tissue is fundamental to the success of any closed biopsy procedure, it is especially important in patients with primary osseous or soft tissue neoplasms. Failure to obtain adequate tissue is more prevalent in bone tumors that are mainly or purely osteosclerotic. The chances of successful diagnosis are increased if biopsy specimens of osteoblastic tumors are obtained from their soft tissue components or osteolytic areas, or both.[36] The Tru-Cut biopsy needle is well suited to the evaluation of primary soft tissue tumors or the nonosseous component of primary malignant bone tumors. Although fine needle aspiration of primary soft tissue neoplasms has met with some success,[37–39, 73] the technique is not widely used.

### Metabolic Disease

To accurately establish the presence and type of metabolic disease, open wedge resection or percutaneous biopsy of the iliac crest should be accomplished, as it is necessary to obtain a full-thickness bone sample with both cortices and medulla.[20] Large-core biopsy needles are used for this procedure, providing adequate material for qualitative and quantitative histologic evaluation (see Chapter 20).[32, 40, 41, 74] Despite the large size of the needles, this type of biopsy procedure is safe and can be performed on an outpatient basis.[74]

### Infectious Disease

Closed needle biopsy or aspiration can be useful in establishing a diagnosis of osteomyelitis and septic arthritis.[83] Material should be obtained for both histologic diagnosis and appropriate tissue culture.

Aspiration of superficial joints is accomplished easily, even in the absence of radiographic equipment. Aspiration of the hip, glenohumeral joint, discovertebral junction,[42, 84] and sacroiliac joint[43, 44] is best attempted with fluoroscopic or CT guidance.[33]

## Articular Disease

Although closed bone biopsy usually is not necessary in the diagnosis of articular disorders, it may be used to evaluate patients with subchondral cystic lesions in whom the exact diagnosis is in doubt. In this fashion, the presence of osteonecrosis, infection, degenerative disease, rheumatoid arthritis, or intraosseous ganglia may be substantiated. Percutaneous biopsy of the synovial membrane can provide useful data in patients with a variety of articular disorders.[85]

## Miscellaneous Diseases

Closed bone biopsies can provide information in numerous additional diseases, including Paget's disease, fibrous dysplasia, eosinophilic granuloma, and sarcoidosis.

Caution should be employed in obtaining biopsy material from a vertebral lesion with extensive destruction because of the possibility of causing considerable hemorrhage and spinal instability. Furthermore, a right-sided approach to vertebral lesions should be used whenever possible because of the presence of the aorta on the left side.

Metastatic deposits from certain primary neoplasms, such as thyroid and renal carcinoma, may be extremely vascular. It is not uncommon to note excessive bleeding during closed biopsy of these lesions, although the hemorrhage generally is controlled.

## BIOPSY SITES

Use of radionuclide studies in the localization of appropriate biopsy sites should be emphasized. Scintigraphy may allow identification of additional lesions that are more accessible to closed needle biopsy than the initially detected abnormality. Closed needle biopsy of radiographically and scintigraphically positive lesions is more successful than biopsy of lesions that are apparent only on radionuclide scans, although definite diagnoses may be established in the latter situation as well.[16, 31]

Scintigraphy also can be used to determine the precise entrance point prior to closed (or open) biopsy of lesions that are difficult to visualize fluoroscopically. This is particularly useful for abnormalities in the ribs,[45–49, 86] although some investigators suggest that solitary lesions of the ribs that are demonstrable by radionuclide examination but not by radiographic examination should not be biopsied.[19]

The preferred biopsy site is a prominent area of a non–weight-bearing bone. Additional accessible areas for biopsy are the pelvis and extremities. Biopsy of the lumbar spine is performed more easily than biopsy of the thoracic spine.[50, 51] Biopsy of the cranial vault and ribs should be undertaken with appropriate caution to ensure that the needle is not inserted too deeply.

## NEEDLES: TYPES AND TECHNIQUES

A variety of needles are available for both trephine and aspiration biopsy. Trephine needles are of two basic types[19]

(Fig. 16–1): some needles such as the Vim-Silverman (Fig. 16–1A) and Westerman-Jensen needles contain narrow, paired cutting blades that engage the tissue[21, 22]; other needles, such as the Kormed (Fig. 16–1B), Craig (Fig. 16–1C), Turkel, Ackermann, and Meunier (Fig. 16–1D, E) needles, consist of round tubes with serrated edges that cut the tissue.[10, 23] Modifications of these basic types of needles have been suggested.[52, 53, 93–95, 97]

In the author's experience, the Kormed, Ackermann, and Craig[23] needles have been used most extensively (Figs. 16–2 and 16–3). The procedure for using the Craig needle is simple. After administration of local anesthetic into the skin, subcutaneous tissue, and periosteum, a blunt guide is inserted through the skin down to the biopsy site and its position is checked with fluoroscopy. A cannula is placed over the guide and held firmly against the bone. The guide is removed, and the cutting needle then is inserted through the cannula. This needle is approximately 2.5 cm longer than the cannula, this distance representing the depth of the biopsy specimen to be taken. With a to-and-fro twisting motion using a variable amount of pressure, the cutting needle is driven into the bone and its position is again checked with fluoroscopy. A radiograph is obtained for documentation of accurate needle placement. While at its full depth, the needle is moved back and forth to dislodge the specimen from surrounding osseous tissue. The cutting needle then is removed, and the cannula is left in place. The cannula subsequently can be moved to a different location if a second biopsy specimen is required. The tissue is removed from the cutting needle with a long, thin probe and placed in an appropriate specimen container.

Modifications of this technique occasionally are required. CT, rather than fluoroscopy, may be used for procedural monitoring (see later discussion). A syringe can be attached to the end of the cutting needle, providing suction as the needle is removed. When the tissue required for biopsy is very friable, the cutting needle may be replaced with the ''worm,'' a component of the Craig trephine biopsy set that has two sharp tines, or hooks, designed to grasp friable tissue.[54] The worm is rotated carefully in a clockwise direction as the tines engage the tissue; it then is withdrawn through the cannula. Contrast material can be introduced into a cystic lesion of bone through the biopsy needle to delineate any solid component of the lesion that should be biopsied.[72]

Minor differences exist between the Craig and both the Turkel and Ackermann needles.[19] With these latter instruments, the guide and cannula are inserted together. The cutting and removing of the specimen are accomplished in a fashion similar to that employed with the Craig needle. Of these three needles, the Ackermann needle is preferred for obtaining biopsy specimens of vascular lesions. The Turkel needle is more useful for evaluating sclerotic lesions because it contains stronger teeth on its cutting surface.

The Westerman-Jensen and Vim-Silverman needles are particularly useful for biopsies of soft tissues and weakened bone. These needles contain three basic parts: an outer needle, an obturator, and inner blades. Initially, the obturator and outer needle are inserted through the skin into the bone or soft tissue. The obturator then is removed and the inner needle with its engaging blades is inserted beyond the tip of the outer needle, grasping the osseous or soft tissues.

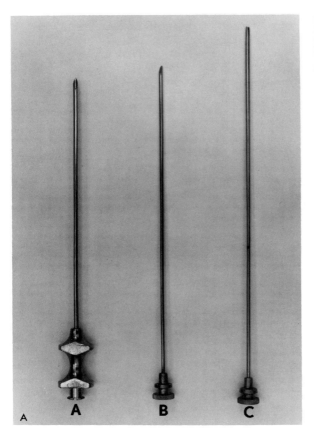

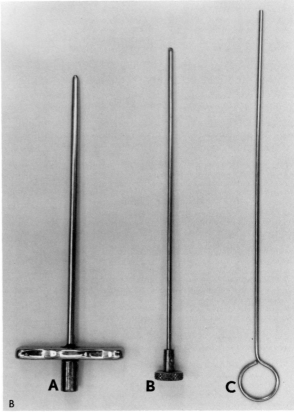

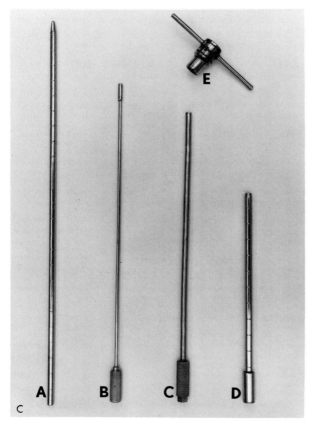

**FIGURE 16–1.** Types of trephine needles.

**A** Vim-Silverman needle: Parts consist of an outer needle (A), obturator (B), and inner blades (C). The outer needle and obturator are inserted together. The obturator then is removed and the inner needle is inserted beyond the tip of the outer needle, engaging the biopsy tissue.

**B** Kormed needle: Parts consist of an outer needle (A), obturator (B), and probe (C). The outer needle and obturator are inserted together. The obturator is removed and the needle is advanced into the bone with a to-and-fro motion. After the needle is removed, the probe can be used to remove the biopsy tissue.

**C** Craig needle: Parts consist of a guide (A), probe (B), cutting needle (C), cannula (D), and handle (E). The guide is inserted into the biopsy site and the cannula is placed over the guide and held firmly against the bone. After the guide is removed, the cutting needle is inserted through the cannula. The handle is placed on the needle and the needle is advanced, using a to-and-fro motion. After the needle is removed, the probe can be used to dislodge the specimen.

*Illustration continued on opposite page*

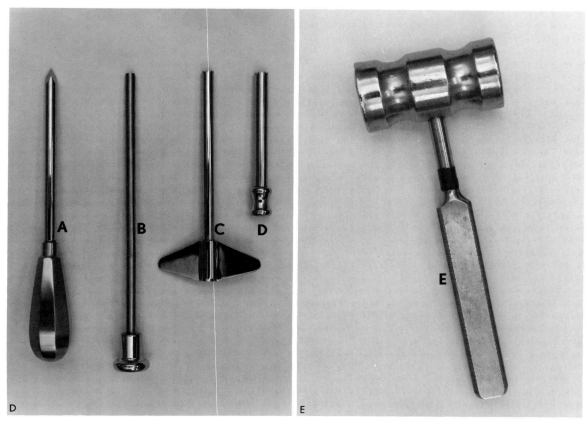

**FIGURE 16–1** *Continued*

**D, E,** Meunier needle: Pertinent parts are guides (A, B), inner needle (C), outer needle (D), and hammer (E). Prior to biopsy, local anesthetic should be administered. A spinal needle is inserted through the skin and directed against the bone. A tap with the hammer (E) allows the needle to enter the bone marrow. A small amount of lidocaine can be administered directly into the marrow. The guide (B) and outer needle (D) can be inserted down to the biopsy site. The guide is removed and the outer needle is advanced into the bone. The inner needle (C) is inserted through the outer needle and extended into the bone with a twisting motion. The caliber of this needle allows a large specimen to be removed.

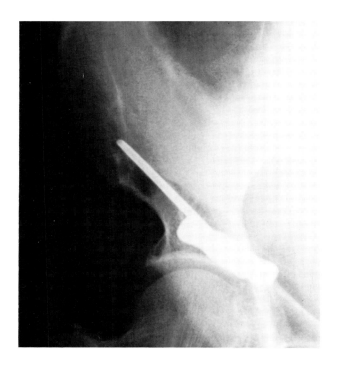

**FIGURE 16–2.** Iliac biopsy with Kormed needle: Skeletal metastasis. Observe that the outer needle has engaged a segment of abnormal bone.

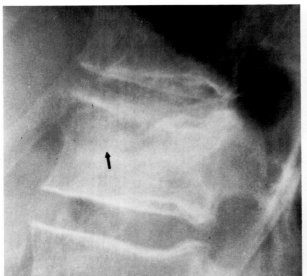
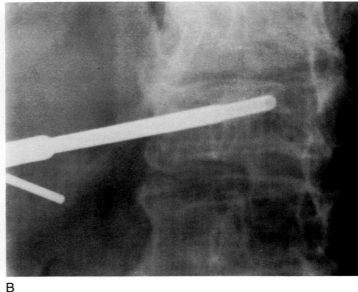

A          B

**FIGURE 16–3.** Lumbar vertebral body biopsy with Craig needle: Healing fracture. An initial radiograph revealed no abnormalities. One year later, collapse of the superior aspect of the lumbar vertebral body with adjacent lysis and sclerosis is apparent (arrow) **(A)**. The patient denied trauma. The cutting needle is anchored into the vertebral body **(B)**. Biopsy revealed a healing fracture without tumor.

The outer needle then is advanced further, enclosing the inner needle, and both needles are removed together.

With any of the trephine needles, biopsy of a purely osteosclerotic lesion or one surrounded by a thickened cortical surface can require intense physical exertion. This problem is accentuated if the bone being biopsied has an acutely curved surface, a situation that is encountered in the long tubular bones. In this instance, the biopsy instrument has a tendency to slip. Use of a hand drill, either to provide a cortical defect in which the biopsy needle can be secured firmly or to form a cortical tunnel to the underlying abnormal medullary canal through which the needle can be inserted, facilitates the procedure in such difficult cases.[55, 56] Newer types of biopsy needles have incorporated power drills[99] that, in some instances, may be affixed to two concentric telescoping stainless steel tubes containing sawteeth that face in opposite directions (Fig. 16–4). When the tubes are rotated in opposing directions, the passing teeth act like blades of scissors,[57] providing an adequate core of soft and hard tissues.[58]

Aspiration needles of different sizes are available.[7, 12, 14, 17, 18, 24, 25] For evaluating many lesions, an 18 or 20 gauge needle may be sufficient. The needle with stylet is guided into the lesion with gentle pressure under fluoroscopic control. The stylet is removed and a syringe is used for tissue aspiration. It has been suggested that rotation of the syringe will allow more adequate biopsy samples. The material is placed on appropriate slides for cytologic examination and, if required, in laboratory containers for culture and bacteriologic identification.

In some situations, aspiration-type cutting needles, such as the Westcott, Chiba, and Tru-Cut needles, are employed. Such needles, particularly the Tru-Cut, are most useful for biopsy of primary soft tissue neoplasms, providing a large specimen free of maceration.[89] The Tru-Cut needle also is beneficial in obtaining material from osteolytic lesions and

the bone marrow, although in the latter instance, a cortical window must be made first.[89]

Aspiration probes recently have been designed for performing percutaneous discectomy,[59, 60, 87] although the clinical feasibility of this procedure is not yet documented fully.

## ADDITIONAL TECHNIQUES OF NEEDLE BIOPSY

Before biopsy, patients should be evaluated for coagulopathy.[89] In some instances, such evaluation will require an appropriate protocol for selected clotting studies, such as platelet count, prothrombin time, and partial thromboplastin time. The patient should not eat on the morning of the examination and is given both a mild sedative and pain medication (e.g., 50 to 75 mg of intramuscularly injected meperidine hydrochloride with or without 10 mg of diazepam by mouth).[61] An intravenous catheter is placed in the arm and saline solution is administered to keep the line open. All pertinent radiographs and radionuclide examinations are reviewed prior to the study. The examination is performed using single plane or biplane fluoroscopy.[62, 63, 88] The latter method is particularly useful when a vertebral body is being biopsied. Ample local anesthetic is infiltrated into the skin, subcutaneous tissue, and periosteum at the biopsy site. Fluoroscopic guidance is employed during the procedure. Bed rest and a mild analgesic agent may be required for 24 hours afterward. Following rib biopsy, chest radiographs should be obtained to exclude the presence of a pneumothorax.

Although CT, with its cross-sectional display and excellent density resolution, has been employed successfully to monitor closed biopsy procedures of the musculoskeletal system,[50, 64, 65, 75, 84, 90, 91] it is not needed in the vast majority of cases. In most patients, it makes little difference in the

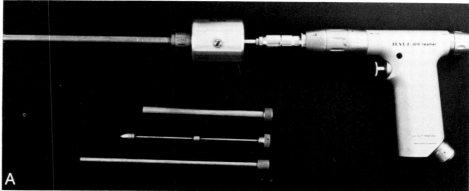

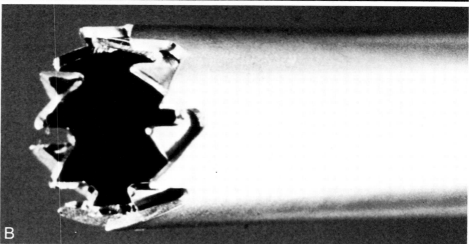

**FIGURE 16–4.** CORB counterrotating biopsy needle.

**A** The power supply is connected to the gear box from which extend the cutting tubes.

**B** Two thin-walled concentric telescoping stainless steel tubes contain sawteeth that are oriented in different directions. One tube rotates clockwise and the other rotates counterclockwise.

(Courtesy of M. Dalrymple, San Diego, California, and of Zimmer Corporation, Warsaw, Indiana.)

length or cost of the procedure whether fluoroscopy or CT is used for monitoring. Some reports indicate superiority of CT guidance of closed biopsy in certain locations such as the spine[50, 91]; in the author's experience, lumbar vertebral biopsy is easier, more convenient, and equally safe when monitored with fluoroscopy, especially when the advancing biopsy needle is inserted at an angle, as is commonly necessary when obtaining tissue from the fifth lumbar vertebral body or lumbosacral disc. For this lumbar vertebral body or the lumbosacral disc, finding the precise location of the end of the needle may require multiple transaxial CT scans, prolonging the examination time. CT is best reserved for biopsy of the thoracic or cervical spine and for those cases in which biopsy of a primary soft tissue neoplasm, infectious site, or a soft tissue component of a primary osseous process is attempted (Fig. 16–5). Occasionally, CT will delineate modifications of the cortex of a tubular bone that will influence the success of the biopsy procedure.[65]

Biopsy techniques for vertebral bodies using fluoroscopic or CT guidance have been well outlined.[13, 77, 92, 100] These techniques vary, depending on the level of the vertebral lesion. If possible, a right-sided approach should be employed.

### Biopsy of the Tenth Through Twelfth Thoracic Vertebrae and the Lumbar Vertebrae (Fig. 16–6A)

The patient is placed in the prone position on the table. The point of needle entrance is 6.5 cm from the spinous process of the vertebra to be biopsied. A 20 gauge spinal needle is inserted at an angle of 145 degrees to the horizontal and is passed slowly down to the bone. Inserting the needle at a greater angle may allow the dura to be entered; inserting the needle at a lesser angle may result in failure to encounter the vertebral body. The angle of 145 degrees is ideal for biopsy of the vertebral body; it must be altered slightly if the posterior elements are to be biopsied. After checking the needle position under fluoroscopy and administering appropriate anesthetic, the physician inserts the biopsy needle in the same fashion.

When the fifth lumbar vertebra is to be biopsied, frequently it is necessary to insert the needle lateral to the vertebra above and to angle it in an inferior direction (Fig. 16–7).

### Biopsy of the First Through Ninth Thoracic Vertebrae (Fig. 16–6B)

The patient is placed prone on the table. The point of entrance of the spinal needle is about 4 cm from the spinous process of the vertebra to be biopsied. The needle is inserted at an angle of 120 to 125 degrees from the horizontal, passing over the superior aspect of the adjacent rib. The needle position is monitored several times with fluoroscopy or CT as the needle is passed down to the bone. Appropriate anesthetic is administered, and the biopsy needle is inserted in the same fashion. Penetration of either needle should not exceed 7 cm.

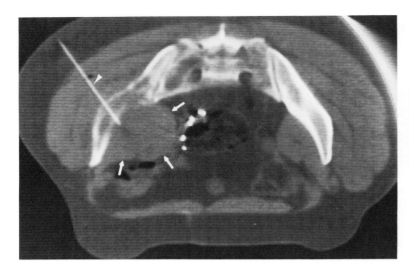

**FIGURE 16–5.** Biopsy with CT guidance. In this 64 year old patient with adenocarcinoma of the colon, a large osteolytic lesion of the ilium extended to the acetabulum. Monitoring of the aspiration biopsy procedure (done with the patient in a prone position) with CT allows accurate placement of the needle (arrowhead) within a large soft tissue component (arrows) of the lesion.

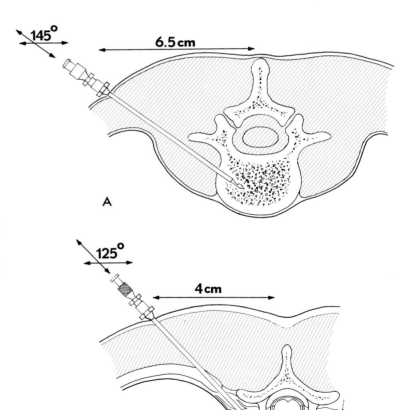

**FIGURE 16–6.** Technique of spinal biopsy.

**A** Lower thoracic and lumbar vertebrae: The needle is inserted 6.5 cm from the spinous process at an angle of 145 degrees from the horizontal.

**B** Upper thoracic vertebrae: The needle is inserted approximately 4 cm from the midline, over the rib at an angle of 125 degrees from the horizontal.

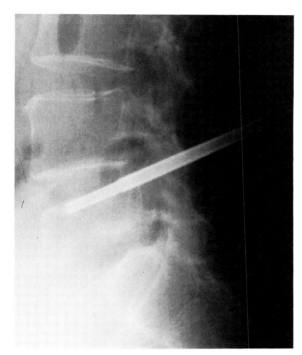

**FIGURE 16–7.** Technique of spinal biopsy for the fifth lumbar vertebral body. Observe that the Craig needle has been advanced in an inferior direction, owing to the presence of the iliac crest at a lower level. In this case a biopsy of the upper portion of the vertebral body documented that the cause of an osteolytic area was a cartilaginous node.

## PROCESSING OF THE BIOPSY SPECIMEN

Although it always is advisable to contact the pathology department prior to performing the biopsy, thereby ensuring correct handling of the specimen, certain guidelines for handling specimens are summarized here. It should be obvious that no matter how carefully the procedure is planned and how meticulous the biopsy technique is, improper processing of the removed fluid or tissue will result in a nondiagnostic study.

Fluid aspirates should be transferred immediately to culture tubes or delivered rapidly to the laboratory for plating.[63] In cases of suspected articular infection in which no fluid is recovered spontaneously, the instillation of nonbacteriostatic, sterile saline solution should be followed by reaspiration of the joint contents.

Blood that is aspirated from the osseous lesion should not be discarded, as it frequently will provide an accurate diagnosis.[66] The blood is allowed to clot in a syringe or plastic cap, and then it is sent as a tissue specimen in formalin to the laboratory and processed separately from the removed tissue. Smears also can be made from small drops of blood.

Tissue aspirates may be handled in several ways.[63, 67] They can be embedded in paraffin for routine histologic analysis or processed for cytologic examination. Trephine cores generally are placed in formalin, decalcified, embedded in paraffin, sectioned, and stained. Crush artifacts in the tissue can be avoided if the specimen is removed from the cutting needle with gentle pressure.

If electron microscopy is being considered as an adjunct to the routine histologic analysis, a portion of the tissue should be placed in glutaraldehyde, not formaldehyde.[39, 68] Less commonly employed tissue examinations include cytologic studies, tissue imprints, and immunofluorescence.[68]

## RESULTS OF NEEDLE BIOPSY

Most observers believe that trephine biopsy is superior to aspiration biopsy in establishing a histologic diagnosis because of the larger sample of tissue obtained. The accuracy of trephine biopsy, however, depends in large part on the expertise of the pathologist as well as on the adequacy of the specimen. Debnam and Staple reported that an accurate diagnosis was made or disease was excluded in 81 per cent of patients or 74 per cent of biopsy sites,[19] which was a higher accuracy rate than had been recorded previously.[11, 26, 27] They attributed their relative success to careful selection of patients and biopsy sites, the use of bone scanning, detailed radiographic study of involved sites, and careful biopsy technique under fluoroscopic control. More recently, Murphy and associates[63] reported an overall accuracy of 94 per cent in 169 skeletal biopsy procedures; the accuracy for confirmation or exclusion of cancer was 95 per cent, and that for confirmation or exclusion of inflammation was 97 per cent. In an analysis of the results of 120 percutaneous bone biopsies, Tehranzadeh and collaborators[61] found a 72 per cent concurrence of biopsy findings with the patients' other clinical abnormalities and subsequent course, a poor success rate (44 per cent) in the diagnosis of primary bone tumors, and better success in diagnosing skeletal metastasis, especially in the spine. Stoker and Kissin[76] reported an overall accuracy rate of 89 per cent in a review of 135 vertebral biopsies. Fraser-Hill and Renfrew,[80] upon reviewing their experience with 102 percutaneous needle biopsies, reported an accuracy of 82 per cent in patients with skeletal metastasis, 90 per cent in those with suspected musculoskeletal infections, and 83 per cent in those with primary musculoskeletal tumors. Stoker and associates,[96] in a review of 208 biopsy procedures, reported an overall accuracy rate of 97 per cent. Although there is apparent variability in the success rate of this procedure, needle biopsy of bone, when performed and interpreted carefully, can be an accurate procedure.[78]

## COMPLICATIONS

The procedure usually is performed without significant complication. Mild pain and discomfort are common. Hemorrhage can result when biopsy specimens are obtained from patients with vascular tumors or when a venous or arterial structure is injured, particularly in biopsies of the spine. Acute paraplegia has been reported occasionally after spinal biopsy.[27] Paresis related to anesthetizing major motor nerves occurs, but it usually resolves in several hours.[89] Pneumothorax may complicate spine[63, 69] or rib biopsy, and sinus tracts infrequently may appear after biopsy of a superficial infectious lesion. Additional reported complications include footdrop, pneumonia, pneumoretroperitoneum, meningitis, and even death, but these are extremely rare.[61, 79] The potential for local or systemic spread of tumor during or after the biopsy procedure has been studied in animals.[70, 71] Although it appears to be of little practical importance in humans, when biopsy of a primary tumor is done, the biopsy should be accomplished in such a way that the needle tract can be resected along with the specimen.[89, 101] Therefore, the shortest needle path to the lesion is not always the most desirable. In selected patients, needle biopsy of bone is a safe procedure, which can be readily accomplished in the Radiology Department.

## References

1. Siffert R, Arkin AM: Trephine biopsy of bone with special reference to lumbar vertebral bodies. J Bone Joint Surg [Am] 31:146, 1949.
2. Ackermann W: Vertebral trephine biopsy. Ann Surg 143:373, 1956.
3. Kendall PH: Needle biopsy of vertebral bodies. Ann Phys Med 5:236, 1960.
4. Valls J, Ottolenghi CE, Schajowicz F: Aspiration biopsy in the diagnosis of lesions of vertebral bodies. JAMA 136:376, 1948.
5. Martin HE, Stewart FW: Advantages and limitations of aspiration biopsy. AJR 35:245, 1936.
6. Hyman G: Comparison of bone-marrow aspiration and skeletal roentgenograms in diagnosis of metastatic carcinoma. Cancer 8:576, 1955.
7. Ottolenghi CE: Diagnosis of orthopedic lesions by aspiration biopsy. Results of 1061 punctures. J Bone Joint Surg [Am] 37:443, 1955.
8. Hoffman WJ: New technique and instruments for obtaining biopsy specimens. Am J Cancer 15:212, 1931.
9. Robertson RC, Ball RP: Destructive spine lesions: Diagnosis by needle biopsy. J Bone Joint Surg 17:749, 1935.
10. Turkel H, Bethell FH: Biopsy of bone marrow performed by new and simple instrument. J Lab Clin Med 28:1246, 1943.
11. Ackermann W: Application of the trephine for bone biopsy. Results in 635 cases. JAMA 184:11, 1963.
12. Schajowicz F, Derqui JC: Puncture biopsy in lesions of the locomotor system. Review of results in 4050 cases, including 941 vertebral punctures. Cancer 21:531, 1968.
13. Ottolenghi CE: Aspiration biopsy of the spine. J Bone Joint Surg [Am] 51:1531, 1969.
14. Lalli AF: Roentgen-guided aspiration biopsies of skeletal lesions. J Can Assoc Radiol 21:71, 1970.
15. Rabinov K, Goldman H, Rosbash H, et al: The role of aspiration biopsy of focal lesions in lung and bone by simple needle and fluoroscopy. AJR 101:932, 1967.
16. Debnam JW, Staple TW: Needle biopsy of bone. Radiol Clin North Am 13:157, 1975.
17. Thommesen P, Frederiksen P: Fine needle aspiration biopsy of bone lesions: Clinical value. Arch Orthop Scand 47:137, 1976.
18. Akerman M, Berg NO, Persson BM: Fine needle aspiration biopsy in the evaluation of tumor-like lesions of bone. Acta Orthop Scand 47:129, 1976.
19. Debnam JW, Staple TW: Trephine bone biopsy by radiologists. Results of 73 procedures. Radiology 116:607, 1975.
20. Johnson KA, Kelly PJ, Jowsey J: Percutaneous biopsy of the iliac crest. Clin Orthop 123:34, 1977.
21. Tenopyr J, Silverman I: The importance of biopsy in tumor diagnosis. Radiology 36:57, 1941.
22. Ellis LD, Jensen WN, Westerman MP: Needle biopsy of bone and marrow. Arch Intern Med 114:213, 1964.
23. Craig FS: Vertebral body biopsy. J Bone Joint Surg [Am] 38:93, 1956.
24. Hajdu SI, Melamed MR: Needle biopsy of primary malignant bone tumors. Surg Gynecol Obstet 133:829, 1971.
25. Schajowicz F: Aspiration biopsy in bone lesions. J Bone Joint Surg [Am] 37:465, 1955.
26. Cramer LE, Kuhn C III, Stein AH Jr: Needle biopsy of bone. Surg Gynecol Obstet 118:1253, 1964.
27. Stahl DC, Jacobs B: Diagnosis of obscure lesions of the skeleton. Evaluation of biopsy methods. JAMA 201:229, 1967.
28. Adler O, Rosenberger A: Fine needle aspiration biopsy of osteolytic metastatic lesions. AJR 133:15, 1979.
29. Moore TM, Meyers MH, Patzakis MJ, et al: Closed biopsy of musculoskeletal lesions. J Bone Joint Surg [Am] 61:375, 1979.
30. DeSantos LA, Murray JA, Ayala AG: The value of percutaneous needle biopsy in the management of primary bone tumors. Cancer 43:735, 1979.
31. Collins JD, Bassett L, Main GD, et al: Percutaneous biopsy following positive bone scans. Radiology 132:439, 1979.
32. Meunier P, Courpron P, Giroux JM, et al: Bone histomorphometry as applied to research on osteoporosis and to the diagnosis of hyperosteoidosis states. In SP Nielsen, E Hjorting-Hansen (Eds): Calcified Tissues 1975: Proceedings of the Eleventh European Symposium on Calcified Tissues. Copenhagen, Denmark, FADL Publishing Co, 1976, p 354.
33. Hardy DC, Murphy WA, Gilula LA: Computed tomography in planning percutaneous bone biopsy. Radiology 134:447, 1980.
34. Zornoza J: Needle biopsy of metastases. Radiol Clin North Am 20:569, 1982.
35. Edeiken B, de Santos LA: Percutaneous needle biopsy of the irradiated skeleton. Radiology 146:653, 1983.
36. Ayala AG, Zornoza J: Primary bone tumors: Percutaneous needle biopsy. Radiologic-pathologic study of 222 biopsies. Radiology 149:675, 1983.
37. Akerman M, Idvall I, Rydholm A: Cytodiagnosis of soft tissue tumors and tumor-like conditions by means of fine needle aspiration biopsy. Arch Orthop Traum Surg 96:61, 1980.
38. Rydholm A, Akerman M, Idvall I, et al: Aspiration cytology of soft tissue tumors. A prospective study of its influence on choice of surgical procedure. Int Orthop (SICOT) 6:209, 1982.
39. Kindblom L-G: Light and electron microscopic examination of embedded fine-needle biopsy specimens in the preoperative diagnosis of soft tissue and bone tumors. Cancer 51:2264, 1982.
40. Faugere M-C, Malluche HH: Comparison of different bone-biopsy techniques for qualitative and quantitative diagnosis of metabolic bone diseases. J Bone Joint Surg [Am] 65:1314, 1983.
41. Nilsson BE, Wiklund P-E: Iliac crest biopsy in the diagnosis of metabolic bone disease. A method study. Acta Med Scand 213:151, 1983.
42. Joshi KB, Brinker RA: Fine needle diagnosis in lumbar osteomyelitis. Skel Radiol 10:173, 1983.
43. Vinceneux PH, Lasserre PP, Grossin M: Technique de ponction-biopsie percutanée au trocart de l'articulation sacro-iliaque pour le diagnostic bactériologique et histologique des sacro-iliites. Rev Rhum Mal Osteoartic 48:93, 1981.
44. Hendrix RW, Lin P-JP, Kane WJ: Simplified aspiration or injection technique for the sacro-iliac joint. J Bone Joint Surg [Am] 64:1249, 1982.
45. Little AG, DeMeester TR, Kirchner PT, et al: Guided biopsies of abnormalities on nuclear bone scans. Technique and indications. J Thorac Cardiovasc Surg 85:396, 1983.
46. Froelich JW, McKusick KA, Strauss HW, et al: Localization of bone lesions for open biopsy. Radiology 146:549, 1983.
47. Burkhalter JL, Patel BR, Harrison RB: Radionuclide bone scan as an aid in localizing lesions for bone biopsy. Skel Radiol 9:246, 1983.
48. Shih W-J, DeLand FH, Domstad PA, et al: Open rib biopsy guided by radionuclide technique. Ann Thorac Surg 38:59, 1984.
49. Zegel HG, Turner M, Velchik MG, et al: Percutaneous osseous needle aspiration biopsy with nuclear medicine guidance. Clin Nucl Med 9:89, 1984.
50. Adapon BD, Legada BD Jr, Lim EVA, et al: CT-guided closed biopsy of the spine. J Comput Assist Tomogr 5:73, 1981.
51. Fyfe IS, Henry APJ, Mulholland RC: Closed vertebral biopsy. J Bone Joint Surg [Br] 65:140, 1983.
52. Jacobson H: Percutaneous bone biopsy with a simple punch instrument. Indications, results and complications. Acta Radiol Diagn 23:415, 1982.
53. Pais MJ, Lightfoote JB, Burnett K, et al: Trephine bone biopsy system: A refined needle for radiologists. Radiology 153:253, 1984.
54. Gilula LA, Destouet JM, Murphy WA: Valuable "worm" of the Craig skeletal biopsy set. Radiology 142:787, 1982.
55. Cohen MA, Zornoza J, Finkelstein JB: Percutaneous needle biopsy of long-bone lesions facilitated by the use of a hand drill. Radiology 139:750, 1981.
56. Kattapuram SV, Rosenthal DI, Phillips WC: Trephine biopsy of the skeleton with the aid of a hand drill. Radiology 152:231, 1984.
57. Manual, CORB biopsy needle. Zimmer Corporation, Warsaw, Indiana.
58. Matthews LS, Braunstein EM: A counter rotating power drill for needle biopsy. Clin Orthop 184:217, 1984.
59. Onik G, Helms CA, Ginsberg L, et al: Percutaneous lumbar discectomy using a new aspiration probe: Porcine and cadaver model. Radiology 155:251, 1985.
60. Onik G, Helms CA, Ginsberg L, et al: Percutaneous lumbar disckectomy using a new aspiration probe. AJR 144:1137, 1985.
61. Tehranzadeh J, Freiberger RH, Ghelman B: Closed skeletal needle biopsy: Review of 120 cases. AJR 140:113, 1983.
62. Carrera GF, Gonyo JE, Barthelemy CR: Fluoroscopically guided percutaneous bone biopsy. JAMA 246:884, 1981.
63. Murphy WA, Destouet JM, Gilula LA: Percutaneous skeletal biopsy 1981: A procedure for radiologists—results, review, and recommendations. Radiology 139:545, 1981.
64. Murphy WA: Radiologically guided percutaneous musculoskeletal biopsy. Orthop Clin North Am 14:233, 1983.
65. Gatenby RA, Mulhern CB Jr, Moldofsky PJ: Computed tomography guided thin needle biopsy of small lytic bone lesions. Skel Radiol 11:289, 1984.
66. Hewes RC, Vigorita VJ, Freiberger RH: Percutaneous bone biopsy: The importance of aspirated osseous bood. Radiology 148:69, 1983.
67. Frable WJ: Fine-needle aspiration biopsy: A review. Hum Pathol 14:9, 1983.
68. Simon MA: Biopsy of musculoskeletal tumors. J Bone Joint Surg [Am] 64:1253, 1982.
69. El-Khoury GY, Terepka RH, Mickelson MR, et al: Fine-needle aspiration biopsy of bone. J Bone Joint Surg [Am] 65:522, 1983.
70. Robertson WW Jr, Janssen HF: Hematoma formation after bone biopsy: A canine model. South Med J 76:966, 1983.
71. Robertson WW Jr, Janssen HF, Pugh JL: The spread of tumor-cell-sized particles after bone biopsy. J Bone Joint Surg [Am] 66:1243, 1984.
72. de Santos LA, Edeiken BS: Intralesional injection of contrast media for percutaneous needle biopsy of bone. Radiology 143:789, 1982.
73. Akerman M, Rydholm A, Persson BM: Aspiration cytology of soft tissue tumors. The 10-year experience at an Orthopedic Oncology Center. Acta Orthop Scand 56:407, 1985.

74. Hodgson SF, Johnson KA, Muhs JM, et al: Outpatient percutaneous biopsy of the iliac crest: Methods, morbidity, and patient acceptance. Mayo Clin Proc 61:28, 1986.

75. Mick CA, Zinreich J: Percutaneous trephine bone biopsy of the thoracic spine. Spine 10:737, 1985.

76. Stoker DJ, Kissin CM: Percutaneous vertebral biopsy: A review of 135 cases. Clin Radiol 36:569, 1985.

77. Larédo J-D, Bard M: Thoracic spine: percutaneous trephine biopsy. Radiology 160:485, 1986.

78. Mink J: Percutaneous bone biopsy in the patient with known or suspected osseous metastases. Radiology 161:191, 1986.

79. Williams MP, Ford GA: Pneumoretroperitoneum following iliac crest trephine. Br J Radiol 59:935, 1986.

80. Fraser-Hill MA, Renfrew DL: Percutaneous needle biopsy of musculoskeletal lesions. 1. Effective accuracy and diagnostic utility. AJR 158:809, 1992.

81. Fraser-Hill MA, Renfrew DL, Hilsenrath PE: Percutaneous needle biopsy of musculoskeletal lesions. 2. Cost effectiveness. AJR 158:813, 1992.

82. Dollahite HA, Tatum L, Moinuddin SM, et al: Aspiration biopsy of primary neoplasms of bone. J Bone Joint Surg [Am] 71:1166, 1989.

83. Cotty PH, Fouquet B, Pleskof L, et al: Spondylodiscitis: Intérêt de la biopsie radioguidée. A propos de 30 cas. J Neuroradiol 15:13, 1988.

84. Hoffer FA, Strand RD, Gebhardt MC: Percutaneous biopsy of pyogenic infection of the spine in children. J Pediatr Orthop 8:442, 1988.

85. Beaulé V, Larédo J-D, Cywiner C, et al: Synovial membrane: Percutaneous biopsy. Radiology 177:581, 1990.

86. Prasad R, Olson WH: Bone marking for biopsy using radionuclide bone imaging. Cancer 60:2205, 1987.

87. Sakou T, Masuda A: Percutaneous diskectomy for lumbar disk herniation. A preliminary report. Clin Orthop 286:174, 1993.

88. Hayt DB: Use of light localizer in fluoroscopically guided percutaneous procedures. AJR 149:623, 1987.

89. Kattapuram SV, Rosenthal DI: Percutaneous biopsy of skeletal lesions. AJR 157:935, 1991.

90. Frager DH, Goldman MJ, Seimon LP, et al: Computed tomography guidance for skeletal biopsy. Skel Radiol 16:644, 1987.

91. Kattapuram SV, Rosenthal DI: Percutaneous biopsy of the cervical spine using CT guidance. AJR 149:539, 1987.

92. Dufauverrier R, Morcet N, Méadeb J, et al: Interventional radiology of the spine. Medicamundi 37:84, 1992.

93. Hauenstein KH, Wimmer B, Beck A, et al: Knochenbiopsie unklarer knochenläsionen mit einer neuen 1,4 mm messenden Biapsiekanüle. Radiologe 28:251, 1988.

94. Quinn SF, Demlow T, Dunkley B: Temno biopsy needle: Evaluation of efficacy and safety in 165 biopsy procedures. AJR 158:641, 1992.

95. Fornage BD: Fine-needle aspiration biopsy with a vacuum test tube. Radiology 169:553, 1988.

96. Stoker DJ, Cobb JP, Pringle JAS: Needle biopsy of musculoskeletal lesions. A review of 208 procedures. J Bone Joint Surg [Br] 73:498, 1991.

97. Iaccarino V, Sadile F, Vetrani A, et al: Percutaneous intralesional brushing of cystic lesions of bone: a technical improvement of diagnostic cytology. Skel Radiol 19:187, 1990.

98. Simon MA, Biermann JS: Biopsy of bone and soft-tissue lesions. J Bone Joint Surg [Am] 75:616, 1993.

99. Ahlström KH, Aström KG: CT-guided bone biopsy performed by means of a coaxial biopsy system with an eccentric drill. Radiology 188:549, 1993.

100. Renfrew DL, Whitten CG, Wiese JA, et al: CT-guided percutaneous transpedicular biopsy of the spine. Radiology 180:574, 1991.

101. Davies NM, Livesley PJ, Cannon SR: Recurrence of an osteosarcoma in a needle biopsy track. J Bone Joint Surg [Br] 75:977, 1993.

# SECTION

# II

# Imaging of the Postoperative Patient

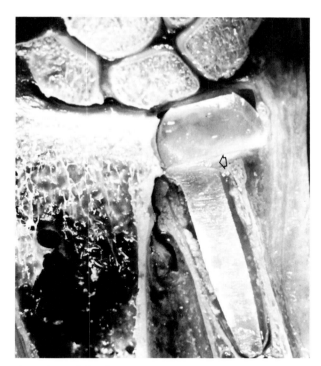

**Imaging of the Postoperative Patient:** Silicone ulnar head prosthesis in rheumatoid arthritis: Note the fracture of the prosthesis (arrow).

# 17

# Imaging After Surgery in Extraspinal Sites

*Barbara N. Weissman, M.D.*

This chapter is concerned with a description of some of the more commonly encountered orthopedic devices and techniques. In each instance, essential principles that are fundamental to the correct interpretation of pertinent imaging studies are provided, but, owing to the complexity of the subject, the interested reader also may wish to consult additional sources.

## FRACTURE FIXATION

Fixation refers to the maintenance of the position of fracture fragments during healing. Hardware may be placed directly across the fracture site (internal fixation), or the area may be immobilized by casts or by appliances fixed to the adjacent bone (external fixation).

### Internal Fixation Devices

Internal fixation devices usually are inserted after open reduction of the fracture fragments. In some cases, however, percutaneous placement of internal fixation devices may follow closed fracture reduction.

**Pins.** Wires, pins, nails, and rods generally are distinguished on the basis of size. Wires are the thinnest. Kirschner wires have spatulate ends and are thin (0.028 to 0.062 inch) in an attempt to decrease the frequency of pin tract infection. The soft tissue end of the wire may be cut off beneath the skin or its protruding end bent or capped to prevent injury. Steinmann pins are thicker than Kirschner wires. Kirschner wires and Steinmann pins may be smooth or threaded; threaded varieties usually require general anesthesia at the time of their removal.[1,2] Kirschner wires are used for percutaneous or open fixation of fractures involving the small bones of the hands and feet.[2] They should be inserted obliquely in relation to the fracture line. Because they are thin and smooth, they may be placed across a physeal plate without causing significant injury.[178] Kirschner wires also may serve as guides over which cannulated screws are placed.

**Intramedullary Nails and Rods.**[3-7] Nails are thicker than pins, and rods generally are thicker than nails. Clinically, however, these terms often are used interchangeably.[178] Intramedullary rods are used primarily for the treatment of closed transverse or short oblique midshaft fractures of the long bones. Rods should be strong enough to resist angular deformity, but their ability to resist rotation

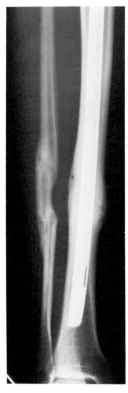

**FIGURE 17–1.** Healing tibial fracture. An intramedullary rod has maintained essentially anatomic alignment of the tibia during healing. Because endosteal blood supply is damaged, healing is due largely to periosteal callus formation.

(torque) is limited unless an interlocking mechanism is incorporated into the nail design. Similarly, compression can occur at the fracture site with telescoping along the rod unless proximal and distal interlocking screws are used.

Insertion of an intramedullary rod damages the blood supply to the endosteum; therefore, healing occurs exclusively by periosteal new bone formation and organization of the hematoma formed around the fracture site (Fig. 17–1). Fluted rods may allow earlier revascularization to occur. Once healing occurs (i.e., about 18 months after lower limb fractures), the rods usually are removed.

Rush pins are round in cross section and have a sled-runner point; a hooked opposite end aids in extraction and helps prevent distal pin migration[5, 6] (Fig. 17–2).

Various types of nails have been developed. The *Kuntscher nail* is rigid, cloverleaf-shaped in cross section, and split longitudinally for part of its length so that it can expand when bone resorption occurs around it.[7]

*Ender nails* are slightly curved, round in cross section, and semi-elastic. When multiple Ender nails are used, rotational stability is improved[8, 9] (Fig. 17–3). These nails may be used for the treatment of femoral, humeral, or tibial fractures. In cases of intertrochanteric fractures, three to five nails are inserted in a retrograde fashion proximal to the medial femoral condyle after the fracture has been reduced.

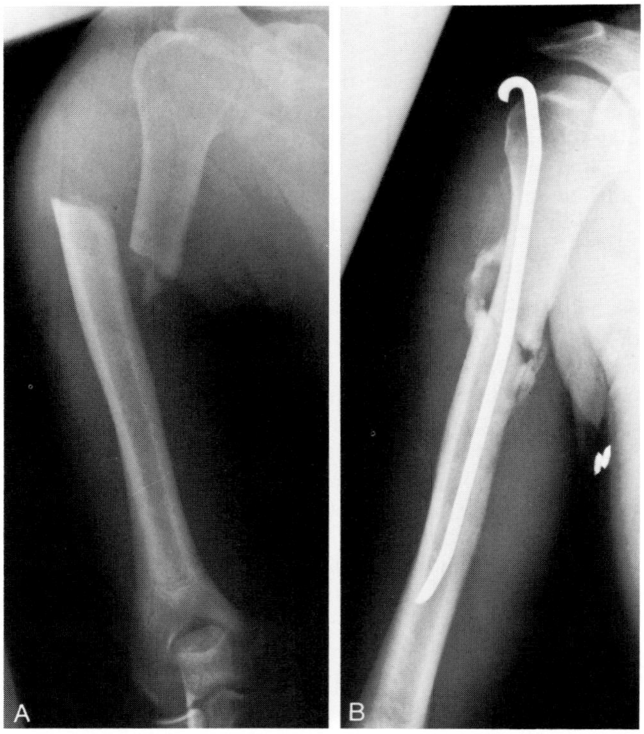

**FIGURE 17–2.** Rush pin.

**A** Anteroposterior view immediately after injury shows a humeral shaft fracture with angular deformity, displacement, and overriding.

**B** After closed reduction, a Rush pin stabilizes the fracture. A moderate amount of callus is present.

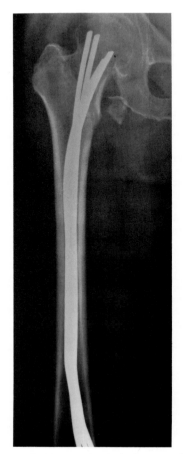

**FIGURE 17–3.** Healing intertrochanteric fracture after insertion of Ender nails. Four Ender nails have been threaded across the intertrochanteric fracture site. The nails fill the medullary canal and their proximal tips fan out in the femoral head.

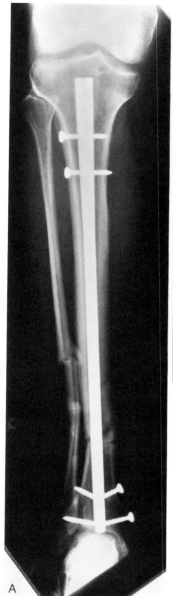

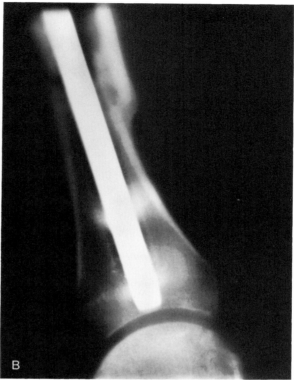

**FIGURE 17–4.** Disruption of intramedullary fixation.

**A** An anteroposterior radiograph shows that shortening has occurred at the tibial fracture site with disruption of the distal transfixing screws and migration of the rod distally.

**B** Conventional tomography confirms the integrity of the subchondral bone of the tibia.

Complications of intramedullary pins, rods, and nails include splitting of the shaft of the bone; inability to advance or withdraw the nail; separation of fracture fragments; penetration of the nail into an adjacent joint; pain from a prominent end of the fixation device; inadequate immobilization of the fracture (leading to nonunion); fracture, bending, or loosening of the rod; migration of the rod; fracture at the site of Ender nail insertion; fat embolization; rod corrosion; and spread of infection along the shaft of the bone. Some of these complications are illustrated in Figures 17–4 to 17–6.

When loosening of an intramedullary nail occurs, periosteal callus formation is abundant and may extend along the entire length of the diaphysis.[1] It is thought that such periosteal reaction results from motion of the fracture fragments in relation to the nail, forcing fluid through Volkmann's canals, with elevation of the periosteum. When no motion of the fracture fragments occurs and fixation is rigid, periosteal callus is limited to the area near the fracture site.

Fractures treated by intramedullary fixation usually are diaphyseal in location and transverse or short oblique in contour. This form of fixation usually is contraindicated in open or compound wounds.[1] Locking intramedullary nails have holes in them that allow screws (transfixation screws) to be inserted to fix the rod within the bone. Interlocking screws placed both proximal and distal to the fracture site will inhibit compression and rotation and are used primarily for treatment of comminuted diaphyseal femoral and tibial fractures.[179, 180]

Insertion of screws into only one end of the intramedullary nail provides "dynamic" fixation in which compression at the fracture site may occur but rotation of the nail in the medullary canal is controlled by the transfixation screw. Second generation femoral locking nails allow placement of a large diameter sliding proximal lag screw

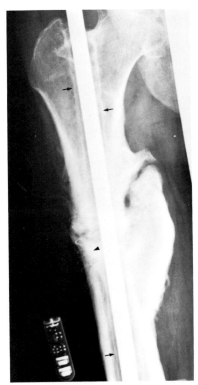

**FIGURE 17–5.** Hypertrophic nonunion. Motion of the rod is documented by the radiolucent zones around it (arrows). The fracture has not healed despite the large amount of periosteal reaction medially. An electrical stimulation device with a helical cathode (arrowhead) is present. (From Weissman BN, Sledge CB: Orthopedic Radiology. Philadelphia, WB Saunders Co, 1986.)

and distal transfixation screws for treatment of ipsilateral femoral neck or intertrochanteric fractures and comminuted fractures of the femoral shaft[180] (Fig. 17–7).

The Gamma nail (Howmedica, Rutherford, New Jersey) is a sliding hip screw with a short intramedullary rod, which can accommodate interlocking screws. The theoretical advantages of this implant over conventional sliding hip screws are more efficient load transfer through the femoral calcar because of the relatively medial location of the femoral stem in comparison to a sideplate; the shorter lever arm, which reduces the risk of implant failure; the maintenance of the compression screw feature to allow controlled impaction of the fracture site; and the closed nature of the procedure for insertion of the Gamma nail.

**Wires.** Wires may be placed around the fracture fragments (cerclage) for compression. The surgical exposure necessary for the placement of cerclage wires may interfere with periosteal circulation and fracture healing.[3] Fracture of the wire, bone resorption under the wire, and irritation of adjacent soft tissues by the twisted ends of the wire may complicate the procedure.

Tension band wiring is based on a concept developed by Pauwels in which tensile forces on a bone are neutralized so that compression alone occurs at the fracture site. The underlying principle is that an eccentrically loaded bone is subjected to bending (tensile) forces on its convex side and to compression forces on its concave side. A plate or wire along the convex side is used to absorb the tensile forces, allowing compression forces alone to act on the fracture

site.[10] Steinmann pins may be used to hold the tension band and to provide rotational stability (Figs. 17–8 and 17–9).

**Screws.** Cortical screws are threaded over their length. They are used primarily to secure plates or nail-plate devices to bone, and they should penetrate both the near and the far cortices (Fig. 17–10).

Cancellous lag screws are threaded distally and have smooth proximal shafts (Figs. 17–10 and 17–11). The threads are wider than those of cortical screws so that they hold better in cancellous bone. When cancellous screws are used to produce compression across a fracture, the threaded portion of the screw should be completely within the distal fracture fragment, and the screw threads should not cross the fracture line. Cortical screws also may function as lag screws by overdrilling the proximal cortex so that only the distal threads engage the bone. Cannulated screws have a central channel so that they may be inserted over a wire or pin for accurate placement. The pin is positioned and repositioned if necessary. When appropriate position is achieved, the cannulated screw is inserted and the pin is removed (Fig. 17–12).

The Herbert screw is a cannulated screw that is threaded proximally and distally but not centrally.[11] The pitch of the threads differs proximally and distally, so that as the screw is tightened, the fracture fragments are drawn together.[179] This type of screw is used primarily in the treatment of nonunion of the scaphoid bone, serving to hold the bone graft between the fracture fragments (Fig. 17–13).

Interference screws are short, fully threaded screws with a cancellous thread pattern and a recessed head.[181] They are

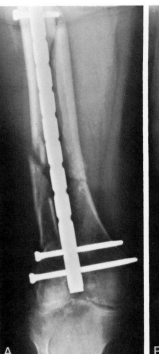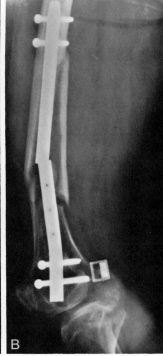

**FIGURE 17–6.** Nonunion of fracture with broken intramedullary rod. These radiographs were obtained 10 months after multiple trauma.

**A** The anteroposterior view shows an intramedullary rod with proximal and distal interlocking screws. The fracture has not united. The discontinuity in the rod is difficult to see on this view.

**B** The fracture of the rod now is obvious. It occurred through one of the screw holes.

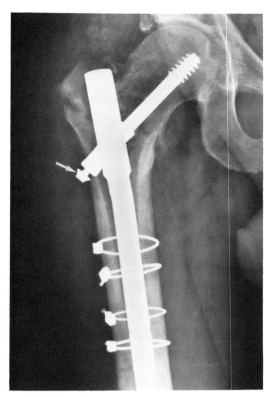

**FIGURE 17–7.** Intramedullary nail and dynamic hip screw for fixation of comminuted intertrochanteric fracture. This patient suffered multiple injuries in a high-speed motor vehicle accident. An intramedullary nail with a dynamic hip screw has been used for internal fixation of the intertrochanteric fracture. The compression screw can be seen (arrow). Cerclage wires were used to hold a nondisplaced longitudinal fracture of the midshaft of the femur.

used in cruciate ligament reconstructions, in which they wedge the bone of a bone-tendon-bone graft against the wall of the tunnel[178] (Fig. 17–14).

The sliding screw plate[12–15] (dynamic compression screw, dynamic hip screw) is used primarily in the treatment of intertrochanteric fractures, but it also is used in cases of femoral neck and subtrochanteric fractures. This device provides fixation while allowing impaction to occur at the fracture during healing and weight-bearing. The key feature in the use of the sliding screw plate apparatus is the achievement of a stable reduction (by anatomic restoration in stable fractures or by displacement techniques in comminuted, unstable fractures). The ultimate stability of the fracture depends on the reduction, rather than on the screw and plate absorbing the stress.

The sliding screw plate apparatus consists of a lag screw and a side plate with a barrel (Fig. 17–15). The threaded portion of the screw is placed in the femoral head, and its shaft is inserted into the barrel of the side plate. Rotation between the barrel and side plate is prevented in some designs by flattening of one side of the screw and barrel. A small compression screw also may be used, which, when inserted into the shaft of the lag screw and tightened, provides additional impaction at the fracture site.

The tip of the lag screw should be located centrally within the femoral head. In a review of frontal and lateral radiographs of patients who underwent sliding screw plate fixation of intertrochanteric fractures, Mulholland and Gunn[13] classified the location of the screw tip as being approximately central (position 1) or eccentric (positions 2 and 3). In position 2, the tip of the screw was between one half a screw diameter and one screw diameter from the center of the head, and in position 3, the center of the screw tip was more than one screw diameter from the center line of the femoral head. A screw in position 3 on both radiographic views invariably moved within the femoral head. Screws in positions 1 and 2, with the tip within one half inch from the articular surface, were never associated with movement. Slight inferior and posterior screw placement may be used to decrease the possibility of "cutting out" of the screw.

The threads of the lag screw should be in the subchondral bone, with the screw tip optimally about one half inch from the articular surface (Fig. 17–16). The side plate should lie flush with the femoral shaft, and the screws attaching it to

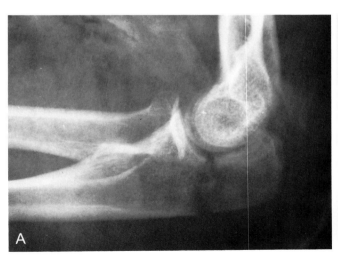
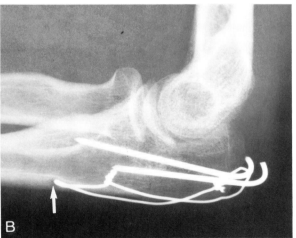

**FIGURE 17–8.** Tension band wiring.
  **A** The initial lateral view shows an olecranon fracture with a few millimeters of separation at the fracture margins.
  **B** A lateral radiograph after surgery shows a tension band wire extending through a drill hole in the ulna distally (arrow) and around Kirschner wires proximally. The prominent ends of the Kirschner wires produced symptoms, and the hardware subsequently was removed.

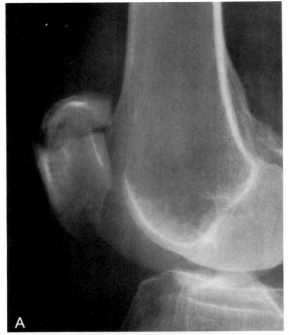

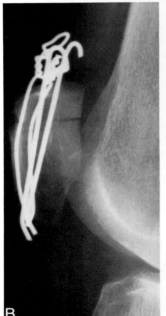

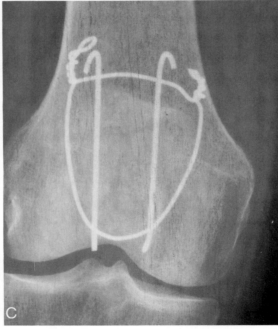

**FIGURE 17–9.** Tension band wiring.

**A** The lateral view shows a displaced transverse fracture of the superior pole of the patella. A nondisplaced fracture involves the inferior pole.

**B, C** Lateral **(B)** and anteroposterior **(C)** views show tension band wiring resulting in marked improvement in alignment.

**FIGURE 17–10.** Cortical and cancellous screws.

**A** The cortical screw often is used to secure plates to bone.

**B** Cortical screws may function as lag screws by overdrilling the proximal cortex so that only the distal threads engage bone.

**C** The cancellous (lag) screw has distal threads and a smooth proximal shaft. The threads are more widely spaced than those of a cortical screw.

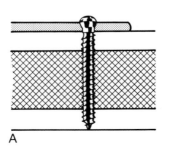

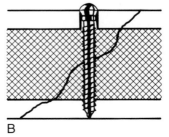

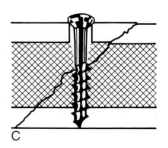

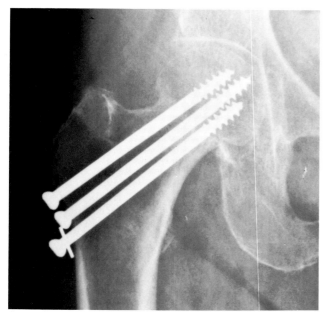

**FIGURE 17–11.** Cancellous screws. These Knowles' pins provide compression at the subcapital fracture site.

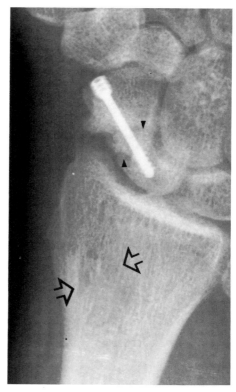

**FIGURE 17–13.** Bone grafting for nonunion of a scaphoid fracture. A bone graft (arrowheads) is held in place by the Herbert screw. The radial donor graft site is faintly visible (open arrows).

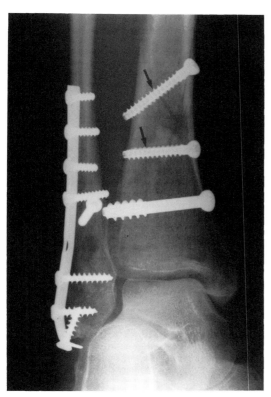

**FIGURE 17–12.** Cannulated screws. Cannulated screws (arrows) were used for interfragmentary compression.

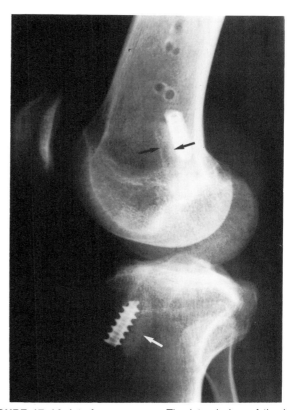

**FIGURE 17–14.** Interference screw. The lateral view of the knee after anterior cruciate ligament reconstruction shows the interference screws holding the bone graft (arrows) of a bone-tendon-bone graft preparation in the surgically created tunnels. (Courtesy of A. Newberg, M.D., Boston, Massachusetts.)

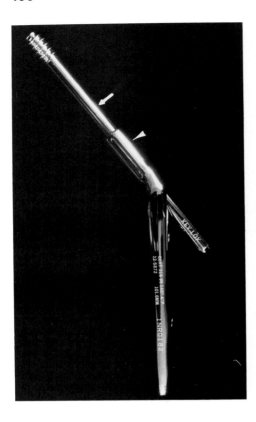

**FIGURE 17–15.** Sliding screw plate. The lag screw (arrow) can telescope through the barrel (arrowhead) of the side plate as bone resorption occurs at the fracture site.

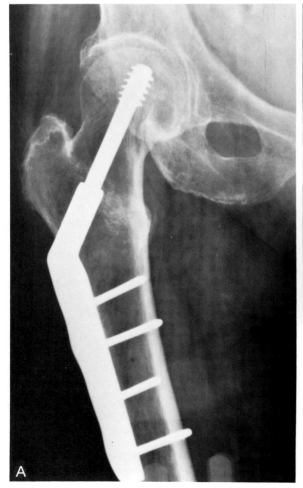

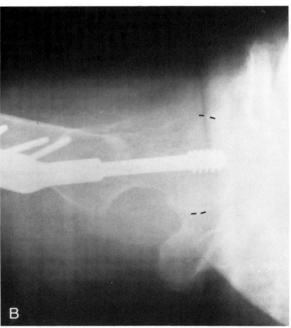

**FIGURE 17–16.** Compression screw plate. Anteroposterior **(A)** and lateral **(B)** views show a well-positioned compression screw with the tip of the screw located centrally in the femoral head on both views. The intertrochanteric fracture has healed. A portion of the surface of the femoral head is indicated by interrupted lines in **B**.

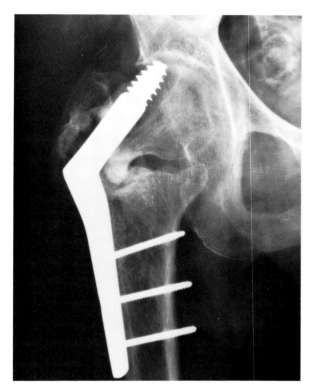

**FIGURE 17–17.** Nonunion of intertrochanteric fracture with "cutting out" of compression screw. The compression screw tip was positioned in the lateral half of the femoral head. No compression of the screw could occur because the screw threads are already abutting on the barrel. The cortical screws holding the side plate are unnecessarily long and could cause soft tissue injury. Collapse of the fracture into a varus position and nonunion have occurred, causing the tip of the screw to "cut out" laterally.

caused by nonunion of the fracture, producing increased stress on the hardware. Occasionally the screw will become disengaged from the barrel (Fig. 17–19) and even may protrude into the pelvis.[12] Stress fracture of the femur proximal to the screw, bending or breaking of the side plate, and rotation of the femoral head on the lag screw are additional complications of sliding screw plate fixation.

**Plates.**[1, 10, 19–20] A plate can be used to provide one or more of the following functions: static or dynamic compression, neutralization, and buttressing[10] (Fig. 17–20).

Static compression refers to the production of axial compression along fractures, with the potential advantages of more rigid fixation, a smaller fracture gap to be bridged, and reduction in the external immobilization required. Compression can be achieved either by attaching a tension device to a plate at the time of internal fixation or by using a particular type of plate, the dynamic compression plate (see next paragraph). When a tension device is used, the compression plate is screwed to one side of the fracture and the tension device then is screwed to the bone near the opposite end of the plate. This device is hooked to the plate and tightened, producing compression along the fracture site. When the appropriate degree of compression is achieved, the plate is secured to the bone with multiple screws, and the tension device is removed, its site of attachment to bone being recorded by the screw hole that is visible on subsequent radiographs. Disadvantages of compression plating include the longer surgical incision that is necessary when a tension device is used and the possibility of refracture after the plate is removed, owing to the bone atrophy that occurs beneath it.

The dynamic compression plate has screw holes with sloped sides that correspond to the slope of the undersur-

the cortex should just penetrate the far cortex. The barrel of the side plate should not contact the proximal fracture fragment to allow impaction of bone at the fracture site.[12] The degree of telescoping of the sliding screw is measured by noting the change in the distance from the end of the barrel to the first screw thread on the initial radiographs in comparison to the most current examination. Correction factors that account for changes in patient positioning may be applied to this measurement, although in clinical practice this correction usually is unnecessary.[16] Telescoping usually averages 7 mm.[12]

Several complications of sliding screw plate fixation occur. "Cutting out" of the nail can be limited by correct placement of the screw (Fig. 17–17). It should be noted, however, that the location of the screw tip may not be assessed accurately by frontal and lateral views owing to the inability to see the screw tip and the adjacent cortex in an exactly tangential projection. This is particularly true when the screw tip is located peripherally in the femoral head.[17] Penetration of the screw into the joint may occur owing to failure of the device to telescope (Fig. 17–18). If the lag screw is too short, telescoping may be limited by contact between the threaded portion of the screw and the barrel. This essentially converts the sliding screw plate into a one piece unit. Other causes of failure to telescope include excessive friction between the barrel and the nail or contact between the proximal fracture fragment and the barrel of the side plate.[12] Bending or breaking of the nail usually is

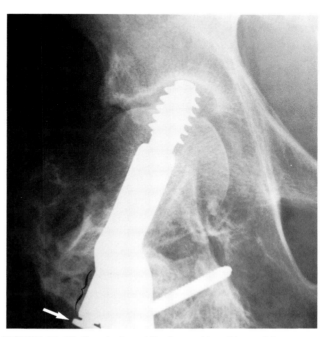

**FIGURE 17–18.** Penetration of the femoral head by a sliding screw. Some impaction at the fracture site in the femoral neck has occurred, as evidenced by the sliding screw protruding from the barrel (bracket). The fracture has collapsed into a varus position, and the screw has penetrated the femoral head and eroded the acetabulum. The small compression screw (arrow) is visible.

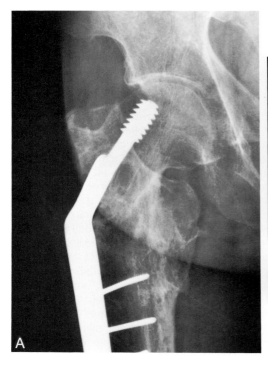

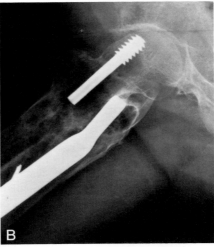

**FIGURE 17–19.** Disengaged compression screw.

**A** The anteroposterior view shows the screw to overlie the lateral portion of the femoral head. An intertrochanteric fracture has healed, with a large amount of periosteal reaction and varus deformity.

**B** The frog-leg lateral view shows that the compression screw had actually disengaged from the barrel (a finding not very obvious in **A**).

face of the screw. As the screws are tightened, the screw head glides down the incline of the screw hole, toward the center of the plate. The bone fragment in which that screw is inserted is shifted toward the center of the plate, thus producing compression at the fracture line. The dynamic compression plate allows compression of a fracture line between adjacent screw holes and, therefore, may be used for the treatment of comminuted and segmental fractures as well as for the treatment of simple fractures.

A plate that is used for neutralization bridges a comminuted fracture and transmits bending or torsional forces from the proximal to the distal fragment, protecting the intervening fracture fragments from these forces. When applied to a cortical surface that is concave, the plate is bent slightly so that its central portion is not in contact with the bone. Before the plate is applied, the fracture fragments are reduced and held by lag screws. The ends of the plate initially are fixed to the bone and then the central screws are inserted, producing impaction or compression at the fracture site.[1]

Plates used for buttressing support an area of thin cortex or cancellous bone graft, preventing collapse. These plates are under compression (rather than tension) and are used near joints, such as in the tibial metaphysis, to prevent deformity after fracture fixation and grafting.

Plates are categorized into straight plates and plates with special shapes.[178] Straight plates include those with round holes, dynamic compression plates, tubular plates, and reconstruction plates. Dynamic compression plates are recognizable on radiographs by their oval holes. Tubular plates have a concave inner surface to conform to the curvature of the underlying bone. Reconstruction plates can be bent to conform to the shape of the underlying bone (Fig. 17–21). A condylar blade plate has a U-shaped blade fixed to a side plate. It is used primarily for fixation of fractures of the proximal or distal portion of the femur. A dynamic condylar screw may be used in place of the 95 degree condylar blade plate (Fig. 17–22). It has the same 95 degree angle between the screw and side plate (to allow valgus alignment) and AO dynamic compression screw holes in the side plate. The screw is the same as the AO dynamic hip screw. One advantage of the dynamic condylar screw over the blade plate is its easier positioning as the screw is positioned over a guidewire so that adjustments can be made. Once the screw is positioned it may be turned to facilitate placement of the side plate along the femoral shaft. This apparatus is used for fixation of high subtrochanteric femoral fractures, peritrochanteric fractures with subtrochanteric extension, and distal femoral fractures.

Fracture may occur after compression plating. It has several causes. The bone under the plate may atrophy, predisposing to fracture and necessitating protection of the extremity after the plate is removed. Differences between the rigidity of the plate and that of the bone predispose to fracture near the end of the plate, and this propensity is reduced by inserting the end screws through only one cortex (Fig. 17–23). After removal of plates, fractures may occur through the screw holes, although these usually become filled with woven bone at about 6 weeks. Additional complications of plating also are encountered (Figs. 17–24 and 17–25).

## External Fixation Devices[21–26]

External fixation of fractures was introduced in the 1930s and 1940s to provide immobilization of fractures while maintaining the potential for adjusting fracture position. In addition, external fixators may be used for compression at sites of attempted fusion (Fig. 17–26) and for distraction during attempted limb lengthening. Several devices are

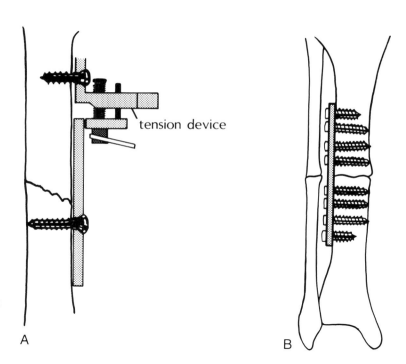

**FIGURE 17–20.** Functions of plates.
   **A** Static compression.
   **B** Dynamic compression after correction of nonunion with varus deformity.
   **C** Buttressing.
   **D** Neutralization.
   (Redrawn after Muller ME, et al: Manual of Internal Fixation, Technique Recommended by the AO Group. J Schatzker, et al, Transl. New York, Springer-Verlag, 1979.)

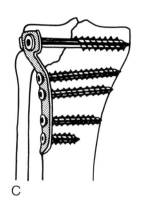

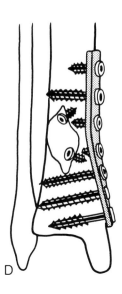

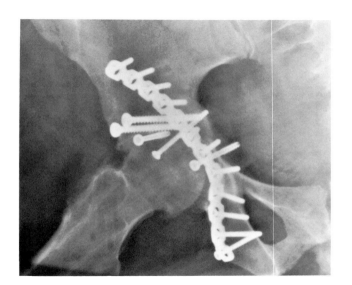

**FIGURE 17–21.** Reconstruction plate. This patient suffered transverse and posterior acetabular rim fractures. The reconstruction plate has been contoured to fit the posterior column of the acetabulum.

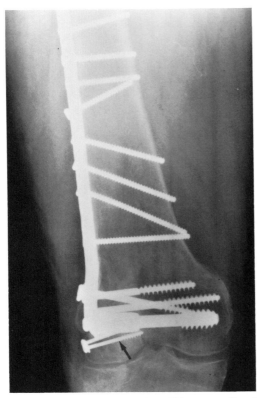

**FIGURE 17–22.** Condylar screw (DCS). This man suffered a comminuted intra-articular supracondylar femoral fracture. The 6 month postoperative radiograph shows cancellous screws holding the lateral condylar fragment (arrow), interfragmentary cortical screws placed in a lag fashion, and a condylar screw plate. The fracture lines are largely obliterated.

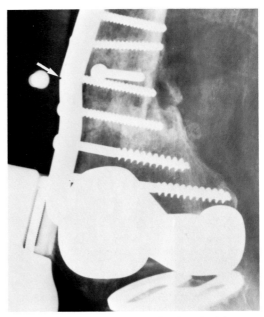

**FIGURE 17–24.** Broken plate. A blade plate had been used for fracture fixation. An anteroposterior view of the knee after reinjury had shown angulation of the plate. This oblique view confirms the presence of a fracture of the plate (arrow). A total knee prosthesis and ligamentous laxity also are present.

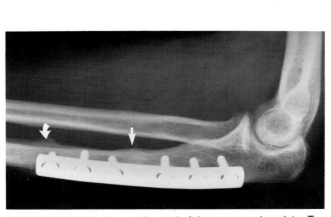

**FIGURE 17–23.** Fracture at the end of the compression plate. Ten months after compression plating and 1 month after a new injury, the original ulnar fracture has healed (straight arrow). A new fracture has occurred near the end of the plate (curved arrow). (From Weissman BN, Sledge CB: Orthopedic Radiology. Philadelphia, WB Saunders Co, 1986.)

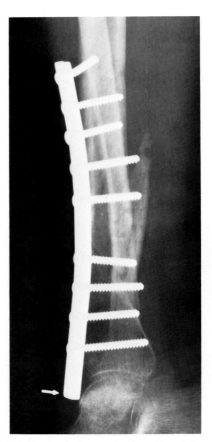

**FIGURE 17–25.** Mechanical complication after plating. This plate was inserted at the time of bone grafting of a tibial fracture that had failed to unite. The end of the plate (arrow) impinges on the talus.

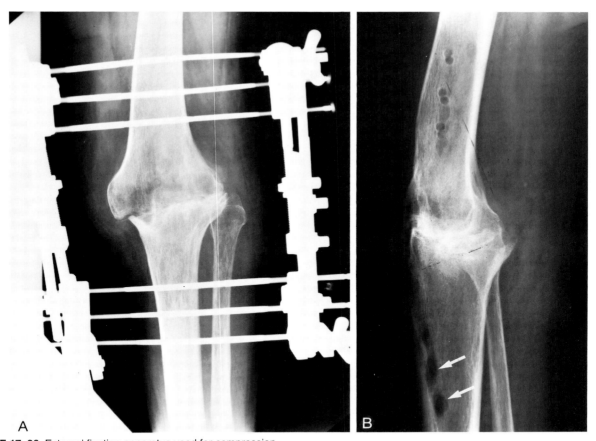

**FIGURE 17–26.** External fixation apparatus used for compression.

**A** An infected prosthesis has been removed. The external fixation (Hoffman) apparatus maintains compression at the site of attempted fusion.

**B** A lateral view after healing of the fusion shows the areas of radiolucency around the tibial pin tracts (arrows), indicating infection. The noninfected femoral pin tract sites are sharply defined.

available that consist of one or more frames anchored to the bone with pins.

Some indications for external fixation of fractures include open fractures in which comminution is present, especially in cases of segmental bone loss and soft tissue damage; the presence of major vascular damage requiring repair; severe osteoporosis; and extensive epiphyseal and metaphyseal comminution. External fixators also are used in the treatment of infected, nonunited fractures and during healing of free vascularized bone grafts.

Advantages of external fixation are greater ease in nursing and skin care and the possibility of patient mobility while the device is being used. When used for the treatment of pelvic fractures, relief of pain and reduced hemorrhage have been noted[22, 25, 26] (Fig. 17–27).

Several complications are associated with the use of ex-

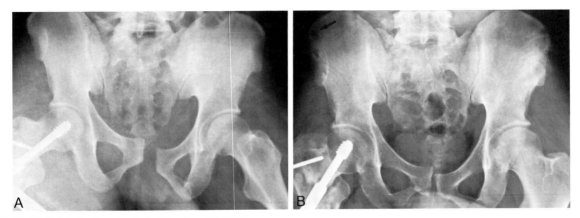

**FIGURE 17–27.** Pelvic fracture treated with external fixation.

**A** A vertical right sacral fracture is present, with disruption of the right neural foramina. Separation of the pubic symphysis is seen.

**B** External fixation was applied, with improvement in alignment. The defects from the iliac pins can be seen. Resorption of bone has occurred around at least one of these (arrow) due to infection.

ternal fixation. Pin tract infections are most frequent when large amounts of soft tissue are traversed by the pins. The use of stronger pins and better fixation at the bone-pin interface decrease the frequency of these infections,[21] although they have been observed in 4 per cent of tibial fractures treated by external fixation in one series.[21] Radiographic evidence of pin tract infection includes bone resorption around pin tracts, ring sequestra, and adjacent periosteal reaction. Soft tissue damage may lead to pain and contracture. Delayed union or nonunion may result from distraction of fracture fragments and long periods without weight-bearing while the external fixation apparatus is being employed. It has been suggested that the duration of external fixation therefore should be relatively short (5 to 10 weeks for tibial fractures), after which gradual weight-bearing in a cast is advisable.[21]

The Ilizarov frame recently has been introduced in the United States.[182, 183] This frame consists of circular rings that surround the limb and are connected by a series of longitudinal bars with adjustable thread and nut distraction points. Traction wires provide fixation to bone. The system is both strong and adaptable. It is used most often for limb lengthening or for treatment of limb deformities associated with malunion or nonunion or congenital disorders. A "corticotomy" procedure in which a metaphyseal osteotomy is performed is used to divide the bone without disturbing the nutrient vessels in the marrow.[183] Radiographic examination plays a critical role in assessing treatment results. Young and coworkers emphasized the need to obtain radiographs of the entire bone to evaluate alignment and often additional views centered on the distraction site to evaluate healing.[182] Bone formation develops at the distraction site within 15 weeks, appearing early as hazy opacity within the gap. Sonography may be useful for detecting bone formation in the gap earlier than on radiographs[184] and for detecting the cystlike collections that develop occasionally.

### Polymethylmethacrylate[27–33]

Polymethylmethacrylate (PMMA) came into widespread use in orthopedic surgery in the 1960s with the introduction by Charnley of a metal-to-plastic total hip prosthesis bonded to bone with PMMA cement.[34] Additional uses of PMMA have since been developed. In patients with metastatic disease of the long bones or pelvis, PMMA has been used as an adjunct to internal fixation so that prompt weight-bearing and pain relief are achieved (Fig. 17–28). Harrington and collaborators[30] reviewed their experience with 375 cases of impending or actual pathologic fracture treated by local tumor resection, internal fixation (or a prosthesis), and intramedullary PMMA. Criteria used for prophylactic fixation were a well-defined osteolytic lesion greater than 3 cm in diameter, an osteolytic lesion that destroyed 50 per cent or more of the cortex, or persistent pain in the area of an osteolytic focus. Eighty-five per cent of patients so treated had excellent or good pain relief and 94 per cent regained the ability to walk.

PMMA instilled into an area of cortical destruction increases the strength of that bone (Fig. 17–29). Ryan and Begeman[33] created 2.5 cm cortical defects in cadaveric femora and compared the strengths of intact femora, femora containing these defects, and femora containing defects filled with PMMA. An approximately 50 per cent increase

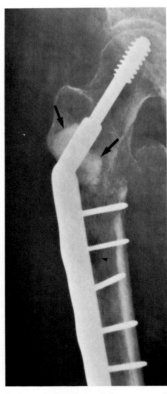

**FIGURE 17–28.** Polymethylmethacrylate as an adjunct in the treatment of pathologic fracture. This patient suffered a pathologic fracture through a metastatic focus arising from renal carcinoma. A sliding screw plate device was inserted, with PMMA instilled into the medullary canal (arrows). Several areas of lytic bone destruction remain (one indicated by an arrowhead).

in axial load strength was noted in the PMMA treated femora over that in the bones with unfilled defects. The intact femora were 44 per cent stronger than those specimens with filled defects. Improved strength in torque also was demonstrated in the femora with filled as compared to unfilled lesions.

Investigations of the effects of PMMA on fracture healing have shown conflicting results. Harrington and coworkers noted that the presence of PMMA cement in the medullary canal did not interfere with healing.[30] Even in cases in which large cortical gaps were filled with cement, healing by periosteal new bone occurred. An experimental investigation of fracture healing in dogs after intramedullary fixation with PMMA in the medullary canal or plate fixation with PMMA along the periosteum has shown deficient healing in six of eight animals, however.[28]

Radiation therapy often is used in conjunction with curettage and internal fixation for the treatment of pathologic fracture. The presence of PMMA apparently does not interfere with local radiation therapy.[30]

In addition to using PMMA for the treatment of pathologic fractures, cement also has been used to improve fracture fixation in osteoporotic patients. Thus, Bartucci and collaborators[27] noted a lower rate of complications of fixation in unstable, comminuted intertrochanteric fractures that were reduced approximately anatomically and in which PMMA was instilled into the femoral head and neck than in those cases in which PMMA was omitted. In patients with initially stable intertrochanteric fractures, the rates of

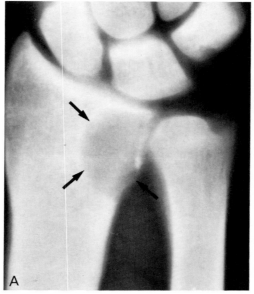
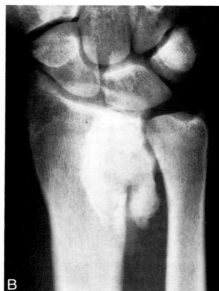

**FIGURE 17–29.** Polymethylmethacrylate filling a defect created by removal of tumor.

**A** A frontal conventional tomogram shows an osteolytic lesion in the distal end of the radius (arrows) that proved to be a giant cell tumor.

**B** Curettage was performed, and the lesion was filled with PMMA.

(Courtesy of P. Cochran, M.D., West Roxbury, Massachusetts.)

complications of fixation were equivalent whether or not PMMA was used. These investigators believed that the cement within the proximal fragment distributed varus forces over a greater area in the proximal fragment and improved screw fixation. Extrusion of cement into the fracture site was kept to a minimum.

Antibiotics in powder form may be added to the powdered polymer before it is mixed with the liquid monomer at the time of surgery[185] (Fig. 17–30). The cement will elute antibiotics at greater concentration than can be achieved by systemic administration, and this form of treatment is without hazard when appropriate amounts of antibiotics are administered.[185, 186]

## ELECTRICAL STIMULATION[37–45]

Application of electrical currents of 5 to 20 microamperes has been shown to stimulate bone formation at the cathode. In general, two methods of electrical stimulation of bone formation currently are available: direct current stimulation and pulsing electromagnetic fields.

Direct current stimulation requires placement of the cathode into the fracture or nonunion site. Brighton and collaborators have used stainless steel Kirschner wires that are insulated except at their tips and are inserted percutaneously into the site of nonunion.[39] The anode is placed on the skin. Paterson and coworkers have used a surgically implanted apparatus with a helical titanium cathode to achieve electrical stimulation[42, 43] (Fig. 17–31).

Pulsing electromagnetic fields are used by applying an external apparatus over the fracture site (Fig. 17–32). The apparatus is connected to household current for 10 to 12 hours per day. No surgical procedures are necessary, and the treatment has no known risk.

Fracture healing after electrical stimulation occurs in about 80 per cent of cases, a rate of healing that is similar to that of bone graft surgery. Contraindications to electrical stimulation include the presence of a pseudarthrosis with a fluid-filled cavity, a large gap at the fracture site, or active infection.

## BONE GRAFTS[46–74]

### Terminology

Bone grafts are described according to their origins, the type of bone used for grafting, and the method of graft placement.

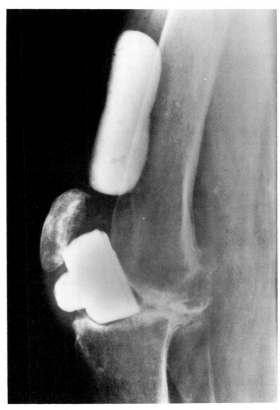

**FIGURE 17–30.** Antibiotic spacers. In this patient a septic total knee replacement was removed. Antibiotic-impregnated PMMA spacers were inserted. The tibiofemoral spacer has migrated from its original position, keeping the tibia subluxed anteriorly and allowing the posterior soft tissues to tighten.

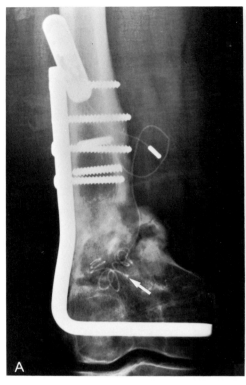 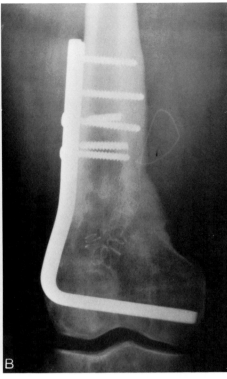

**FIGURE 17–31.** Fracture healing after electrical stimulation.

**A** Nonunion occurred after femoral osteotomy. Electrical stimulation with a helical cathode (arrow) was begun.

**B** Healing is complete. The apparatus, except for the cathode, has been removed.

(From Weissman BN, Sledge CB: Orthopedic Radiology. Philadelphia, WB Saunders Co, 1986.)

The following terms are used to identify origins of bone grafts:

*Autografts:* The transplanted bone is derived from the same person receiving it.

*Allografts* (homografts): The transplanted material is derived from another person of the same species.

*Xenografts* (heterografts): The transplanted material is derived from a member of a different species.

The types of bone used for grafting include cortical bone, cancellous bone, or both cortical and cancellous bone. Cancellous bone grafts are used primarily to promote osteogenesis, whereas cortical bone grafts are used to provide structural stability. When corticocancellous bone grafts are used, they are positioned so that the cancellous surface abuts on the soft tissues to facilitate vascular ingrowth.[55]

Grafts also may be described according to their composition, position, and shape. Onlay grafts consist of cortical bone that is placed across a bony defect (such as a nonunion) and held by screws to a surgically denuded or drilled surface of the host bone. The sliding inlay graft consists of bone cut from the proximal fragment and slid distally across a bony defect. The dowel graft consists of a core of cancellous bone that is inserted into a surgically created channel to stimulate osteogenesis. Muscle pedicle grafts are used primarily in the treatment of femoral neck fractures and fractures associated with nonunion.[75, 76] A segment of bone that includes the insertion of the quadratus femoris muscle is detached from the intertrochanteric region of the femur and moved into a prepared site bridging the fracture. Screws are used to hold the graft in place. Strut grafts, often composed of a rib or fibula, provide stability and stimulate osteogenesis; these are used most often in the spine (Fig. 17–33). H-grafts are shaped so that they may be wedged between spinous processes.

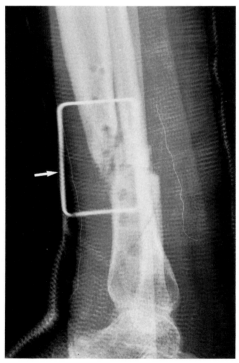

**FIGURE 17–32.** Pulsing electromagnetic fields. This patient had a nonunion of a tibial fracture. The lateral view shows that the tibial hardware has been removed and a fibular osteotomy has been performed. The locator block (arrow) used to center the electrical stimulation device is seen to overlie the fracture site.

## Indications

Bone grafts generally are used to promote healing or provide stability, or both. Possible situations in which bone

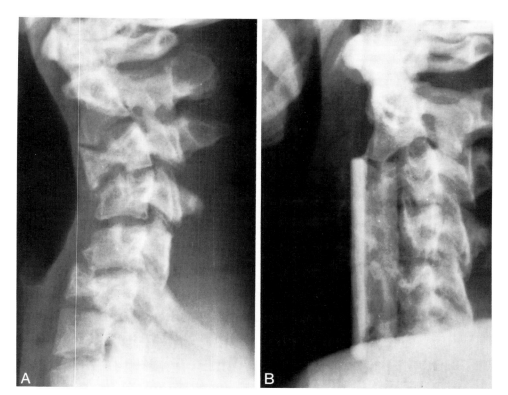

**FIGURE 17–33.** Strut graft.

**A** This patient had marked kyphosis as a consequence of injury, with multiple vertebral body fractures. Posterior decompression had been done (note the absence of the C5 spinous process and laminae and a portion of the spinous process of C4).

**B** An anterior fusion was done with insertion of a cadaveric fibula allograft. The vertebral alignment is improved.

(Courtesy of T. Cochran, M.D., West Roxbury, Massachusetts.)

grafting may be used include filling of bony defects or cavities (Figs. 17–34 and 17–35); bridging of joints for arthrodesis; bridging of large defects in a long bone[66]; promoting healing in cases of nonunion; and promoting union or filling defects in cases of delayed union, malunion, fresh fracture, or osteotomy.[4]

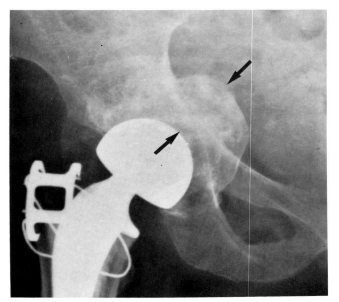

**FIGURE 17–34.** Acetabular bone grafting. This patient had severe bilateral protrusio acetabuli deformity. A bipolar endoprosthesis was inserted, and the acetabular defect was filled with bone graft (arrows).

## Bone Formation After Grafting[49]

Cancellous bone grafts have greater capacity to induce new bone formation than do cortical grafts. If the cancellous graft is immobile, a process of ''creeping substitution'' takes place, in which new bone is deposited on the scaffold of dead trabeculae. The origin of this new bone is controversial and includes the graft itself or the differentiation of host osteoprogenitor cells. Bone induction refers to the process by which tissue that normally is non–bone-forming is stimulated to produce bone. As summarized by Brown and Cruess,[49] three factors are necessary for bone induction to occur: a stimulus (such as the presence of decalcified bone matrix),[63] a potentially osteogenic cell, and a favorable environment.[49] One stimulus to new bone formation may be a diffusible ''bone morphogenetic protein'' that is found in bone matrix and that stimulates mesenchymal cells to differentiate into bone-forming cells.[60]

Allografts generally are less satisfactory than autografts in that new bone formation is slower, vascular penetration is slower and less dense, and bone replacement tends to be superficial. Rejection of allografts because of sensitization of the host by antigens in the graft is a major reason for considering them inferior to autografts. Freezing or freeze-drying of allograft material may decrease its antigenicity, but in addition freeze-drying appears to diminish the torsional and bending strength of the graft.[67] Allografts do not contribute new bone-forming cells but do induce new bone formation in the host. After transplantation of fresh allografts in animals, two phases of bone production have been seen: an early phase of bone formation by the graft that ends in the death of the new bone and a second phase of bone formation by the host.

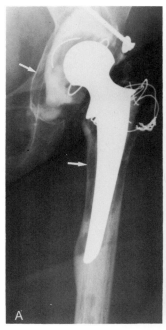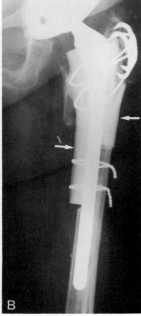

**FIGURE 17–35.** Massive allograft for reconstruction after failure of a total hip replacement.

**A** Marked resorption has occurred around the cemented acetabular and femoral components (arrows).

**B** A cadaver allograft (arrows) has been used to replace the proximal portion of the femur. A new prosthesis has been inserted.

The histologic sequence of repair is similar initially for both cortical and cancellous grafts.[55] All but the most superficial cells of the graft die, owing to a lack of adequate blood supply. Necrosis occurs within the marrow and the haversian canals and leads to a macrophage response. Ingrowth of granulation tissue consisting of small capillaries and primitive mesenchymal tissue occurs. In cancellous grafts, new bone is deposited along the surfaces of dead trabeculae (Table 17–1). The central areas of necrotic bone are resorbed. Finally, marrow spaces are refilled by active bone marrow. Cortical grafts undergo a more prolonged period in which bone resorption occurs along the haversian canals. The resorption process then is followed by the laying down of new bone. Both the bone resorption and the

### TABLE 17–1. Some Comparisons Between Cancellous and Cortical Bone Grafts

| Cancellous Graft | Cortical Graft |
| --- | --- |
| Better survival of osteogenic cells because the structure allows diffusion and early microvascular anastomoses | Dense bone is a barrier to diffusion |
| Large endosteal surface supplies osteoprogenitor cells | Small endosteal surface |
| Abundant red marrow supplies many osteoprogenitor cells | Fewer osteoprogenitor cells |
| Healing by creeping substitution; new bone is deposited on dead trabeculae followed by removal of necrotic matrix | Removal of necrotic matrix from around the central canals of osteons occurs first followed by new bone formation |
| Relatively weak | Relatively strong |

bone production phases predominate peripherally and are limited or nonexistent in the deeper cortex.

Cortical grafts undergo resorption of bone around the central canals of the osteon, which is followed by the laying down of appositional new bone. During the phase of bone removal, porosity and weakening of a cortical graft may lead to fracture or loss of fixation.[50, 51] Enneking and collaborators[53] noted in dogs that cortical bone grafts were substantially weakened by internal porosity at 6 weeks and remained weak for 6 months, regaining nearly normal strength at 1 year. At that time, slightly more than half of the transplant had been replaced by new bone. Similar studies in humans have shown that grafts are repaired in the same fashion, but the sequence takes approximately twice as long as it does in the dog.[52]

### Vascularized Bone Grafts[46, 58, 73]

In the 1970s, microsurgical techniques were developed that allowed bone grafts and their associated vasculature to be transplanted so that the grafts remained viable. Currently, the success rate of this procedure is greater than 90 per cent.[72] Although union and hypertrophy of transplanted bone occur early (Fig. 17–36), the frequency of union has been reported to be no different from that of conventional grafts performed in dogs.[50] Another comparison of various types of grafts in dogs has shown revascularized autografts

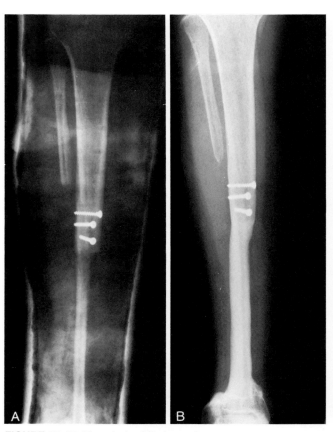

**FIGURE 17–36.** Vascularized fibular graft.

**A** After removal of a long segment of the distal portion of the tibia for tumor, a vascularized segment of fibula was used to bridge the defect.

**B** Bony union occurred proximally and distally between the graft and the tibia; subsequently, hypertrophy of the graft has occurred.

to be superior in terms of early incorporation, hypertrophy, and greatest mechanical strength.[74]

Vascularized bone grafting takes hours to perform and requires highly skilled personnel. This procedure, therefore, usually is reserved for cases of massive bone loss (e.g., greater than 12 cm), those in which more conventional techniques have failed,[49] or those in which an inadequate soft tissue bed is present.[50]

### Massive Cadaver Allografts[187–192]

Massive cadaver allografts are used for limb salvage in the treatment of primary bone tumors and for reconstruction in patients with severe bone loss after failed joint replacement (Fig. 17–35B). In selected cases, such as after resection of aggressive benign bone tumors or bone sarcomas, reconstruction is performed by insertion of massive bone graft consisting of bone, articular cartilage, and accompanying tendons or ligaments. Bone formation (by creeping substitution) occurs at the host-graft junction and is presumed to require many years before remodeling of the entire graft occurs. The graft, therefore, functions largely as a spacer. The fate of the articular cartilage is unknown. It is thought that the cartilage surface eventually is replaced by fibrocartilage and secondary osteoarthritis supervenes.[190]

Mnaymneh and coworkers evaluated 70 osteoarticular grafts performed to reconstruct extremities after tumor resection.[190] Satisfactory results occurred in 85 per cent of patients who were free of tumor recurrence. Mankin and colleagues, however, noted that, of 62 patients with osteoarticular allograft implantation followed 2 years or more, only 65 per cent had good or excellent functional results.[189] This was not as good as was noted in patients with intercalary grafts (a bone graft between two segments of host bone).

Failure of massive allografts most often is due to infection or fracture.[188] In the series of Mankin and associates (62 osteoarticular grafts, 19 intercalary grafts, and seven allografts with prostheses), a high complication rate was noted, including infection in 13 per cent, allograft fracture in 16.5 per cent, and nonunion in 11 per cent.[189] Infection occurred in 4.3 per cent of cases collected by Mnaymneh and coworkers and in 11.7 per cent of cases reviewed by Lord and colleagues, and it was responsible for 82 per cent of failures in one series.[188, 190] Fractures of massive allografts occurred in almost 16 per cent of 274 bone tumor patients studied by Berrey and coworkers.[187] Three types of fracture were identified: (1) fractures characterized by rapid destruction of the graft in the absence of tumor recurrence or infection, (2) fractures occurring through the shaft of the allograft, and (3) fractures involving the articular surface. Type 1 fractures were uncommon, type 2 were more common in men, and type 3 were more common in women and were thought to be caused by osteonecrosis. Fractures occurred from 6 to 100 months after surgery.

### Donor Sites

The most frequently used donor sites for bone grafting are the iliac crest, tibia, fibula, greater trochanter, distal portion of the radius, and the posterior elements of the spine.

The ilium is a good source of cancellous bone grafts. When the patient is supine, cancellous bone is removed from the area below the anterior superior iliac spine. The inner table of bone is left intact to avoid the development of a muscular hernia. If more cancellous bone is needed, dissection is extended posteriorly, taking care not to injure the sciatic nerve or the sacroiliac joint.

Fibular grafts are obtained from the middle one third to one half of the bone because this area may be excised without adverse effects. The distal one quarter as well as the proximal segment of the fibula should remain intact to ensure stability at the ankle and knee.[55, 72]

Complications at donor graft sites appear to be few. McGrath and Watson[62] reviewed donor sites in the distal portion of the radius, proximal portion of the ulna, and metacarpus, carpus, and phalanges and found no complications after a 22 month period. Nonetheless, fracture may occur after cortical graft removal (e.g., from the tibia), and intraoperative bleeding and postoperative pain may follow iliac crest biopsy. Laurie and collaborators[59] assessed patients after graft removal from the ilium (60 cases) or the thoracic cage (44 cases). Nine per cent of patients had pleural lacerations after removal of more than one rib, and 6.8 per cent had persistent chest pain 2 years after surgery. Early morbidity related to iliac donor sites was greater than that associated with rib resection and included intraoperative and postoperative blood loss, delayed healing of incisions directly over the iliac crest, and pain. Later, painful scars and abnormalities of bone contour were noted. Ten per cent of patients had pain 2 years after removal of bone from the iliac crest, but the pain was not so severe as that occurring after rib resection. Stress fractures, hernias through an iliac donor site, and gait problems have been noted in other reports.[59]

### Radiologic Examination

At follow-up examinations, healing of iliac donor sites is seen to occur with sclerosis at the margins of the osseous defects. Bone excrescences from the donor site may occur and be accompanied by pain.[193] Radiographic evaluation of 18 rib and eight iliac bone graft donor sites showed complete regeneration occurring in children and in adults under the age of 30 years. Regeneration failed to occur in those over 30 years of age.[68]

Graft healing generally is documented by loss of the sharp margins between the graft and the host bone, eventually leading to osseous union with bone continuity across the graft-host junction. Conventional tomography may be helpful in this evaluation. Fibrous union is suggested by the persistence of a thin residual radiolucent area between the graft and the host bone.[48]

The time required to achieve union depends on the size and the type of graft, the local conditions, and the site of the surgery. Grafts used in the treatment of nonunion of tibial fractures require 3 to 6 months for union to occur.[48] Similarly, incorporation of vascularized grafts usually is accomplished by 6 months.[73] Vascularized grafts in the mandible generally heal within 4 to 6 weeks, those in the forearm within 8 to 12 weeks, and those in the leg within 4 to 6 months.[72]

Sequential radiographic examinations of cortical grafts have shown changes in graft density and size. Autogenous cortical grafts decrease in radiodensity during the first 6 to 10 months after surgery and then increase in radiodensity.

Hypertrophy of these autografts has been reported in 32 per cent, atrophy in 9 per cent, and no change in 58 per cent of cases.[52]

### Scintigraphic Examination

Histologic and scintigraphic evaluation of conventional autogenous bone grafts in dogs has shown that periosteal new bone formation can result in a positive bone scan despite the nonviability of the graft.[47] With regard to vascularized bone grafts, the accumulation of the bone scanning agent in the area of the graft within the first week after transplantation indicates both an intact vasculature and metabolically viable bone; conversely, the absence of such uptake of the bone scanning agent on serial radionuclide examinations suggests segmental nonviability[47, 61] (Fig. 17–37). Accumulation of the bone-seeking radionuclide after this 1 week period, however, may be due to the laying down of new bone on the surface of dead trabeculae and does not indicate either vascular patency or the presence of viable graft. Blood perfusion and blood pool scans are helpful in confirming vascular patency in the first 2 weeks after surgery. Marrow scintigraphy[194] has been used successfully to study the viability of vascularized iliac crest grafts to the femoral neck.[195] Tracer uptake corresponding to the region of the graft indicates viability.

### Magnetic Resonance Imaging

Manaster and coworkers have used MR imaging to evaluate the vessels of the leg prior to grafting using vascularized fibular grafts.[196] The arterial anatomy was shown to be defined correctly by the preoperative MR images in all cases. Follow-up assessment with MR imaging was believed to be unnecessary.

### Complications

Enneking and colleagues[52] defined delayed union in cortical grafts as the absence of healing 12 months after surgery (Fig. 17–38). Graft failure may be associated with progressive bone resorption, leading to a decrease in the size and density of the graft and ultimately to its disappearance[48] (Fig. 17–39). Similar graft resorption may be due to

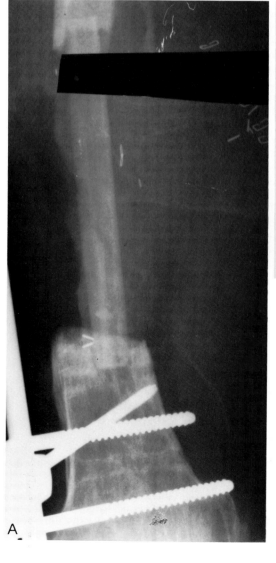

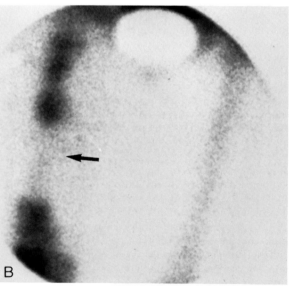

**FIGURE 17–37.** Absent blood flow to vascularized graft.
**A** A vascularized bone graft was used to bridge a defect created by the removal of a long segment of bone affected with chronic osteomyelitis.
**B** A bone scan shows absent isotope uptake in the graft (arrow), suggesting nonviability.

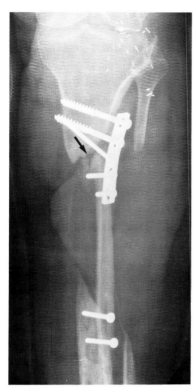

**FIGURE 17–38.** Failure of bone grafting. A vascularized fibular graft was used to bridge a tibial defect caused by removal of an infected, nonunited fracture. Prior vascular injury and repair had occurred. Despite multiple attempts at supplemental grafting, union never occurred proximally (arrow) and the patient eventually underwent amputation.

recurrent tumor or infection (Fig. 17–40). Infection often is evident clinically and is suggested radiographically by the presence of soft tissue swelling, erosion, and osteoporosis of adjacent host bone.

Stress fractures within cortical grafts are not uncommon and have been observed in six of 22 vascularized grafts greater than 10 cm in length in the lower extremities in one series.[72] Callus formation was demonstrated about these fractures within 4 weeks. Stress fractures also have been noted in patients with autogenous cortical bone grafts.[52] Stress fractures usually occur only after union of the graft to the host bone is seen, and they may fail to heal without operative treatment.

## RESECTION ARTHROPLASTY

Resection arthroplasties consist of the removal of one or both articular surfaces of a joint. Currently these techniques are used primarily as salvage procedures after failed total joint replacement surgery.

### Girdlestone Arthroplasty[77–91]

In the preantibiotic era (1921) G.R. Girdlestone developed a resection arthroplasty for secondarily infected tuberculous hips that allowed debridement of infected tissues and adequate drainage.[83] In 1943, the technique was reported in detail for the treatment of acute pyogenic infection of the hip unresponsive to the available antibiotics (sulfanilamides and penicillin), drainage, and immobiliza-

tion.[83] Currently, however, the operation is thought of primarily as a salvage procedure, performed when an infected total hip prosthesis is removed. It also is used in some instances of infectious arthritis in preference to hip fusion.[91]

As described by Girdlestone, the operation leaves "no cartilage, no diseased bone, no dead tissues and no dead spaces."[83] Through a lateral approach perpendicular to the muscular planes, the gluteal muscles, greater trochanter, lateral acetabulum, acetabular cartilage, femoral head and neck, and joint capsule are removed. As performed by Girdlestone, the acetabular floor was removed if an intrapelvic abscess was found. The resulting large funnel-shaped cavity was packed with gauze and drains, with healing occurring over the subsequent few months. Splinting or traction was used to prevent proximal displacement of the femur, which might close the wound. In subsequent descriptions of the procedure, the wounds have been closed and femoral osteotomy has been performed to improve stability in patients undergoing resection for noninfectious arthritis.[81, 85, 87] The term "Girdlestone arthroplasty" currently is applied in a general sense to any hip joint resection.

A Girdlestone arthroplasty may be used in the treatment of an infection after total hip replacement. Deep infection occurs in 1 to 2 per cent of such replacements.[79] In selected cases, antibiotic therapy has been combined with a single stage revision to a new total hip prosthesis.[88] In other cases, a Girdlestone arthroplasty (sometimes combined with subsequent reinsertion of a total hip replacement) is necessary.

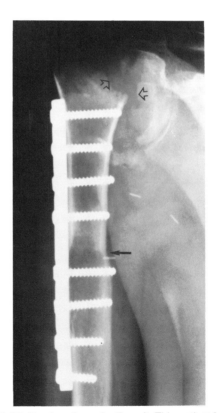

**FIGURE 17–39.** Fracture through allograft. This patient had had an allograft 3 years previously after resection of a chondrosarcoma. The graft has united to the host bone (arrow). A fracture of the graft has occurred (open arrows). This was thought to have begun at an area of revascularization from adjacent soft tissue attachments. Pathologic examination of the removed allograft showed necrotic bone.

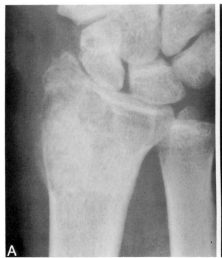
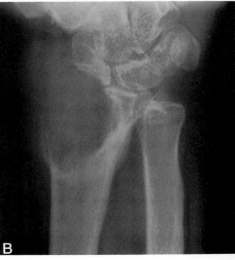
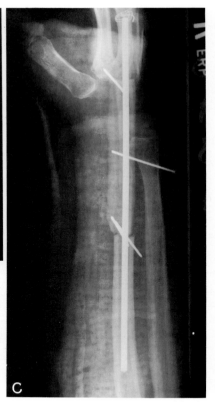

**FIGURE 17–40.** Recurrent tumor destroying bone graft.
   **A** A giant cell tumor of the radius had been removed by curettage and the defect packed with bone graft.
   **B** Recurrent tumor has destroyed the graft, the distal portion of the radius, and a portion of the scaphoid.
   **C** The distal end of the radius and carpus have been resected and the defect bridged by a fibular graft. An intramedullary rod and several pins are noted.

The presence of any of the following has been reported to be an indication for Girdlestone arthroplasty after total hip replacement: virulent, resistant organisms; gram-negative organisms; two or more concomitant strains of organisms; unhealthy and edematous soft tissues; a draining sinus; radiographic evidence of well-established osteomyelitis with bone erosion; and severe loss of bone substance.[88] The results of Girdlestone arthroplasty after removal of an infected hip prosthesis have not been as dismal as might be expected. Pain relief and control of infection occur in over 80 per cent of patients.[79, 80, 86, 90] Shortening of the affected extremity, a Trendelenburg gait, and joint instability are invariable sequelae that make walking difficult and tiring.[79] Radiographs confirm complete removal of the femoral neck, acetabular rim, and PMMA cement (Fig. 17–41). Although optimally all cement is removed, residual cement does not necessarily result in continued infection.[77, 79, 80] Thus, Bourne and coworkers noted residual cement in 11 cases, and only one of these required reoperation to control infection.[79] The position at which the femur lies in relation to the acetabulum should be noted.

The technique for performing aspiration arthrography after Girdlestone arthroplasty has been described by Swan and coworkers.[197]

## ARTHRODESIS (JOINT FUSION)

Arthrodesis refers to the surgical stiffening of a joint (derived from the Greek *arthron,* meaning ''joint,'' and *desis,* ''a binding together'').[92] Such surgery usually is performed to provide stability or to relieve pain resulting from joint damage owing to prior infection, injury, or failed joint replacement surgery. The bony fusion performed may be intra-articular, extra-articular, or a combination of the two.

### Ankle[93–110]

Even in the current era of total joint replacement surgery, ankle arthrodesis remains a valuable procedure for the alleviation of pain due to arthritis, the treatment of paralytic instability, and salvage after a failed total ankle replacement. Results after ankle fusion are surprisingly good.[102–104] The adequacy of function after ankle fusion is believed to be attributable to compensatory motion of the small joints of the ipsilateral foot, altered motion of the ankle of the contralateral limb, making gait symmetric, and the use of footwear with an appropriate heel height.[102] Although compensatory motion of the midtarsal joints has been considered to be an important factor in maintaining function after ankle fusion, Jackson and Glasgow[98] found that the normal range of dorsiflexion and plantar flexion of the foot after fusion actually was decreased by an average of 75 per cent in comparison to the opposite (normal) side. Stewart and collaborators[109] noted that only 17 per cent of patients had increased midtarsal mobility postoperatively, 53 per cent had decreased midtarsal motion, and 30 per cent had no change in motion in comparison to the contralateral foot. The presence of a flexible midfoot apparently is not essential for achieving an acceptable result after ankle fusion.

Since the introduction of ankle fusion in 1878, more than 20 techniques for achieving tibiotalar fusion have been developed.[96] Significant surgical advances have included posterior displacement of the foot to increase stability, the addition of bone graft, and compression across the fusion

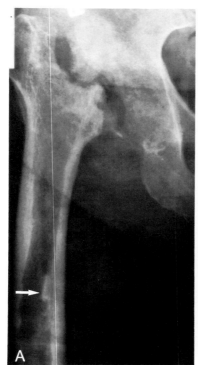
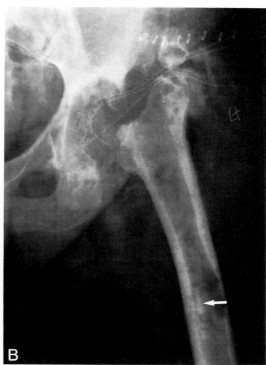

**FIGURE 17–41.** Girdlestone arthroplasties. This patient had infected total hip prostheses bilaterally, necessitating bilateral Girdlestone arthroplasties. Some cement remains in each femoral canal (arrows). In the right femur **(A)** infection recurred at the area of retained cement, whereas in the left hip **(B)** infection did not recur.

site.[95] The Charnley compression arthrodesis consists of resection of the articular surfaces of the tibia and talus and compression of these surfaces to eliminate shear and maintain bony apposition (Fig. 17–42). Steinmann pins are inserted in the distal portion of the tibia and in the talus anterior to its axis so that compression will hold the anterior

portion of the arthrodesis together and the pull of the Achilles tendon will keep the posterior edges apposed.[95]

Optimal foot position for ankle arthrodesis has been debated, but current studies imply that fusion should be done with the foot in the neutral position in both men and women,[97] although Boobbyer noted that up to 5 degrees of plantar flexion of the foot is satisfactory in women.[94] Greater than 10 degrees of plantar flexion has been found to be the foot position most likely to be associated with postoperative pain.[104] The degree of flexion of the foot can be evaluated on radiographs by measuring the angle between the long axis of the tibia and the long axis of the talus (drawn through the midportion of the talar head) (Fig. 17–43). Optimally, no varus or valgus angulation of the foot should be present.[94, 103, 104] Although radiographic measurement of varus and valgus angulation may be difficult and even unreliable,[103] some authors use the angle between the long axis of the tibia and the lateral margin of the talus on the anteroposterior view for this assessment.[104] The talus may be shifted posteriorly. Fusion of the ankle in 5 to 10 degrees of external rotation has been suggested as an important feature so that pushoff can be accomplished by pronating the foot. The degree of external rotation generally is evaluated clinically.

Radiographically identifiable complications occurring after ankle arthrodesis include pseudarthrosis, malunion, infection, and osteoarthritis of the small joints of the foot. Pseudarthrosis has been reported in up to 30 per cent of cases. In general, union occurs clinically at an average of 18.6 weeks after surgery[105] but is slower when fusion is done as a salvage rather than as a primary procedure. Abnormal peripheral sensation in the limb may predispose to nonunion. Morrey and Wiedeman[104] define delayed union as the clinical presence of motion at the operative site or the obvious lack of bony union on radiographic examina-

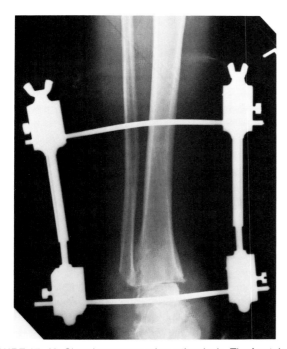

**FIGURE 17–42.** Charnley compression arthrodesis. The frontal view shows the resected margins of the tibia and talus held in apposition by the Charnley compression device. The bowing of the pins attests to the compression. The malleoli have been resected.

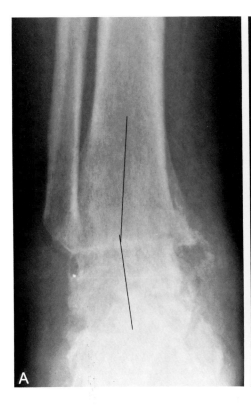
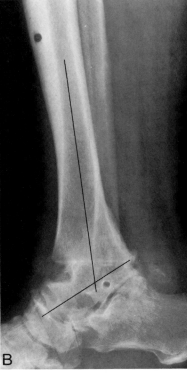

**FIGURE 17–43.** Ankle fusion.

**A** The anteroposterior view shows no remaining radiolucency along the tibiotalar surface, indicating healing. Varus alignment is present between the long axis of the tibia and that of the talus.

**B** This lateral view does not include the bottom of the foot. The angle between the long axis of the tibia and the long axis of the talus (through its midportion) has been used to determine the degree of plantar flexion.

tion at 6 months after surgery. Nonunion is said to have occurred when the same findings are present 12 months after surgery. Malposition after fusion was noted in 12 per cent of patients in one series[104] (Fig. 17–44). Postopera-

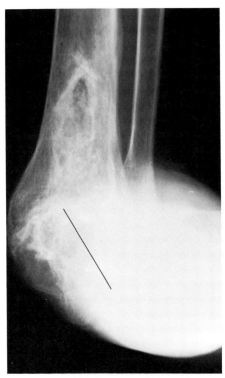

**FIGURE 17–44.** Ankle fusion with valgus deformity. Ankle fusion was attempted after a failed total ankle prosthesis was removed. The ankle is fused in a valgus position. The fibula impinged on the lateral aspect of the foot and revision surgery was necessary. The line indicates the approximate axis of the talus.

tively, careful evaluation of foot position and apposition at the fusion site is necessary to ensure that correct position is maintained. Infections may occur along the tracts of the pins that are used for compression or at the site of attempted fusion. Morrey and Wiedeman found infection in 23 per cent of patients evaluated; in six of 14 cases, infection occurred at the tibial pin site and in 10 of 14 cases, it occurred at the fusion site.[104] In four patients, nonunion resulted. Pain after ankle fusion has been attributed in some cases to the development of osteoarthritis in the joints of the foot. Despite the radiographic demonstration of osteoarthritis, however, several studies have shown no correlation between the development or progression of midtarsal arthritis and the clinical result.[102, 104, 108] Mazur and colleagues[102] noted more severe osteoarthritic changes in the subtalar and midtarsal joints of patients with marked plantar flexion after fusion.

## Hip[111–121]

The startling success of total hip replacement and the availability of treatment for tuberculous arthritis have severely curtailed the use of hip fusion. Reports indicating a high rate of failure after total hip replacement in young persons, however, have sparked renewed interest in hip fusion as a primary procedure and as a salvage procedure after failed total hip replacement.[122] Successful hip arthrodesis results in a painless, stable hip and the ability to engage in strenuous activity. Therefore, it is a procedure to be considered in young patients with incapacitating pain from unilateral hip damage. The procedure can "buy time" and later be revised to a total hip replacement.

Hip arthrodesis was introduced in the United States by Albee in 1908.[119] Since then, a large number of techniques have been introduced to achieve intra-articular, combined intra- and extra-articular, or purely extra-articular fusion.

Intra-articular arthrodesis includes removing the surface of the femoral head and acetabulum and, then, maintaining the femoral head in contact with the acetabulum by means of external or internal fixation, or both. Graft material also may be used.

The degree of hip abduction occurring after fusion may be documented on radiographs using a horizontal reference line (along the bottom of the sacroiliac joints or the ischia) and a line drawn along the femoral shaft[119]; similarly, the position of hip flexion may be evaluated on lateral radiographs.[113] An investigation has indicated that hip flexion of about 30 degrees results in the greatest patient comfort; greater flexion may improve the patient's ability to sit but makes walking more difficult, whereas less hip flexion makes walking easier and sitting more difficult.[113, 121] The appropriate degree of hip abduction depends on the amount of shortening of the leg that is present; when there is no shortening, slight adduction of the fused hip has been shown by Stinchfield and Cavallaro[121] to produce the most normal gait. In adults, the leg usually is fused in a position of 5 to 15 degrees of external rotation.[120]

The results of hip fusion generally are good. Stinchfield and Cavallaro observed that all patients in whom solid fusion developed were free of hip pain.[121] Sponseller and colleagues[119] reviewed 53 patients who underwent surgical fusion prior to the age of 35 years and who were followed for more than 20 years; 78 per cent of the patients were satisfied with the surgical outcome, and most were able to carry out normal activities.

The major complications of hip arthrodesis relate to the inability to achieve solid fusion and the long-term effect of such surgery on other joints. Several large series have revealed a relatively high frequency of pseudarthrosis (Fig. 17–45). Thus, Lipscomb and McCaslin[116] studied 347 patients and noted a 22 per cent frequency of pseudarthrosis and Stinchfield and Cavallaro[121] found a 23 per cent frequency of pseudarthrosis, although more than half of affected patients were not incapacitated. Malposition, defined as the presence of greater than 15 degrees of adduction or abduction or 60 degrees or more of flexion, also may occur. Back pain may be prominent and was noted in all patients in one series[114] who were followed for longer than 10 years. The pain often is relieved after total hip replacement.[117] Ipsilateral knee pain has been noted in 45 per cent and contralateral knee pain in 26 per cent of patients[119] (Fig. 17–46). In addition, contralateral hip pain occurs and is not always alleviated by total hip replacement on the fused side.

## OSTEOTOMY

The term "osteotomy" refers to the surgical cutting of bone. Osteotomies usually are performed to correct or reduce deformity. A closing wedge osteotomy refers to the removal of a triangular bony wedge from one side and approximation of the resection margins; an example is the intertrochanteric varus osteotomy. An opening wedge osteotomy is performed by cutting the bone at an angle, causing one side to open. The defect then is filled with bone graft. A rotational osteotomy consists of rotating the distal fragment on its long axis. A displacement osteotomy involves a shift in the position of the distal fragment with relation to the proximal one (e.g., the McMurray medial displacement intertrochanteric osteotomy). Shish kebob osteotomies are used to correct severe bowing deformities of the long bones, such as may occur in osteogenesis imperfecta. The shaft is cut in several places, and the fragments are threaded on an intramedullary rod.[141]

### High Tibial Osteotomy[142–152]

Normally, 60 per cent of weight-bearing forces on the knee are transmitted through the medial femorotibial compartment and 40 per cent are transmitted through the lateral femorotibial compartment.[143] Increased weight-bearing stresses in one of these compartments related to varus or valgus alignment abnormalities may result in osteoarthritis with progressive cartilage loss. This cartilage loss further shifts stress to the involved compartment. The rationale for high tibial osteotomy is to correct this abnormal angulation and to shift stress (in a more normal amount) to the other compartment.[143] Results of osteotomy generally are better when varus deformity, rather than valgus deformity, is present initially.[145]

High tibial osteotomy usually is employed in active patients under 65 years of age with pain in the knee caused by osteoarthritis. In older patients, total knee replacement is performed more often. Osteotomy allows patients to continue vigorous activities, including sports, and may be used as an interim procedure before total knee replacement is necessary. The knee should have good mobility and stability, and pain should be localized to the radiographically narrowed femorotibial compartment. Clinical results are improved when less than 10 degrees of varus deformity is present on radiographs obtained with the patient erect.[145]

Standing views using 36 inch films that include the leg from hip to ankle are recommended for preoperative evaluation. Under normal circumstances, when points are drawn

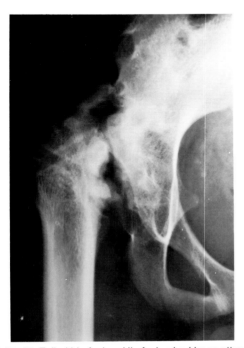

**FIGURE 17–45.** Failed hip fusion. Hip fusion had been attempted in childhood. The osseous defects relate to prior attempts at internal fixation. Osteolyis in the femoral head, bone sclerosis, a shallow acetabulum, and a small ilium are present. No bony union has occurred.

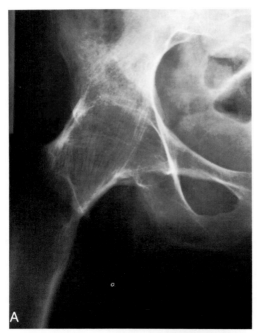

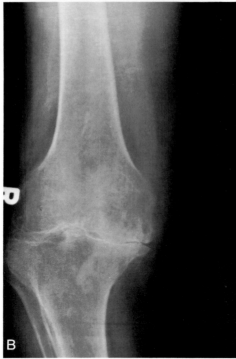

**FIGURE 17–46.** Hip fusion with ipsilateral osteoarthritis.
   **A** The frontal view shows the solid right hip fusion. Osteopenia and muscular atrophy are evident.
   **B** The frontal view of the ipsilateral knee shows severe osteoarthritis. The patient required total hip and total knee replacements.

at the centers of the femoral head, the knee, and the ankle, they all fall on a straight line (the mechanical axis) (Fig. 17–47). This axis is altered in patients with genu varum or genu valgum (Fig. 17–48). Surgical correction of the angular deformity using a high tibial osteotomy is aimed at restoration of the normal mechanical axis with overcorrection of about 3 to 5 degrees.[146]

   If standing views that do not include the hip and ankle

are obtained, they should contain enough of the femoral and tibial shafts to allow measurement of the varus or valgus deformity that is present. Such measurements facilitate surgical correction that attempts to achieve about 10 degrees of valgus alignment.

   The Coventry high tibial osteotomy involves resection of a wedge of bone from the tibial metaphysis between the joint and the tibial tubercle. Usually, a closing wedge osteotomy is done. The thicker part of the wedge to be removed is located laterally (valgus osteotomy) in a patient with genu varum, so that when the bone margins are brought together, an overall valgus alignment of the knee is achieved. The degree of correction and the amount of bone to be removed are determined from the preoperative radiographs[143] (Fig. 17–49). Because shortening of the leg is produced by the tibial osteotomy, an osteotomy of the fibular shaft, fibular head excision, or division of the proximal tibiofibular joint (allowing the fibular head to slide proximally) is necessary.

   Maquet advocates a barrel vault osteotomy for the treatment of osteoarthritis with varus deformity of the knee.[146] With this procedure, greater degrees of varus deformity can be corrected. The technique involves a curved osteotomy performed proximal to the tibial tubercle. The fragments then are rotated to obtain the desired correction, and the distal fragment is displaced anteriorly.

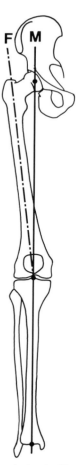

**FIGURE 17–47.** The mechanical axis. Normally, a straight line can be drawn from the center of the femoral head through the center of the knee to the center of the ankle. This is the mechanical axis (M). The femoral shaft axis (F) normally deviates from the mechanical axis.

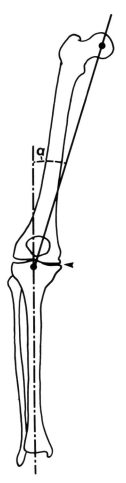

**FIGURE 17–48.** Deformity in osteoarthritis. The deformity resulting from osteoarthritis can be determined on radiographs that include the hip, knee, and ankle, obtained with the patient erect. The angle (a) between lines drawn connecting the center of the femoral head, the knee, and the tibial plafond is a measure of the deformity that is present. Medial cartilage space narrowing (arrowhead) with varus deformity is shown. (Redrawn after Maquet P: Treatment of osteoarthritis of the knee by osteotomy. In UH Weil [Ed]: Progress in Orthopedic Surgery, Vol 4. New York, Springer-Verlag, 1980.)

Distal femoral supracondylar osteotomy is used when osteoarthritis is accompanied by a valgus deformity.[146] One pair of Steinmann pins is inserted through the femoral condyles and another is inserted through the femoral shaft, creating an angle that is required for correction of the deformity and 1 to 2 degrees of overcorrection. After osteotomy, the proximal fragment is impacted into the distal one until the pins are parallel. A compression device then is applied.

Good or excellent results have been observed in 97 per cent of patients who were examined 2 years after high tibial osteotomy,[145] although the frequency of a successful outcome appears to deteriorate progressively after that time. The specific postoperative alignment has not been shown statistically to correlate with a successful final result, and recurrent varus deformity is not necessarily associated with an unsatisfactory surgical outcome. The average time required for healing of a high tibial osteotomy is 9 weeks.

Complications occurring after this procedure are infrequent. Fracture or ischemic necrosis of the proximal tibial fragment may occur, but infection[143] and non-union (Fig. 17–50) are rare.

## Proximal Femoral Osteotomy[153–172]

In 1925, Lorenz introduced high femoral osteotomy for the treatment of osteoarthritis of the hip.[165] McMurray[163, 164] subsequently described medial femoral displacement osteotomy for this disease and, in the 1950s, Pauwels popularized angulation osteotomy.[163, 164] Angulation osteotomies now are performed in relatively young patients with osteoarthritis of the hip due to increased unit loading.

Many theories have been proposed to explain the beneficial effects of osteotomy in patients with osteoarthritis of the hip. Compressive force of three to four times body weight normally is generated across the hip joint during monopedal stance.[170] This force is the vectorial sum of body weight acting through the distance from the center of the sacrum to the center of the femoral head and of the hip abductors acting through a distance from the greater trochanter to the center of the femoral head (Fig. 17–51). When the articular surfaces of the joint are congruent, this force is distributed over a larger surface area than when the surfaces are incongruent. Excessive unit loading is a cause of osteoarthritis and may occur, for example, from increased body weight or from incongruent joint surfaces (when only portions of the articular surface are available to transmit load). Pauwels noted that in patients with incongruent joint surfaces, pressure on the joint can be reduced by increasing the weight-bearing area by means of adduction (varus) or abduction (valgus) osteotomy.[169] In addition to increasing surface area, relaxation of the adjacent musculature is produced at the time of osteotomy with a consequent decrease in the compressive forces on the hip.

Candidates for proximal femoral osteotomy have pain due to osteoarthritis of the hip and generally are younger than candidates for total hip replacement.[170] Obese persons and those engaged in heavy labor are not ideal subjects for this osteotomy. Hip flexion of at least 80 degrees and adduction or abduction of 15 degrees or more should be present.

**Medial Displacement Osteotomy.** Oblique intertrochanteric osteotomy with maximum medial displacement of the distal fragment (Lorenz osteotomy) was introduced for the treatment of osteoarthritis by McMurray.[163, 164] It was believed that the body weight would be transmitted directly from the pelvis to the distal femoral fragment. Rotation of the proximal fragment occurs inadvertently in some cases and produces better clinical results than those that are observed when displacement is unaccompanied by rotation. The displacement osteotomy with inadvertent rotation of the proximal fragment is similar to the varus osteotomy with medial displacement of the distal fragment (see following discussion).

**Adduction (Varus) and Abduction (Valgus) Osteotomy** (Fig. 17–52). The varus osteotomy is performed when the femoral head is essentially hemispherical, cartilage loss is evident in the superior and lateral portions of the joint, and the articulation is more congruent with the hip in abduction.[170] In this procedure, a carefully measured wedge of bone, wider medially, is removed and the femoral head is rotated medially (15 to 40 degrees) until the articular surfaces are congruent. The adductor muscles are released

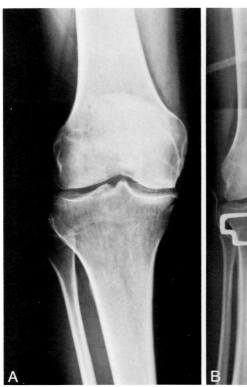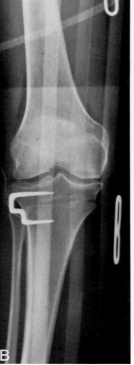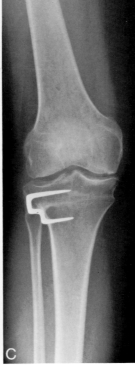

**FIGURE 17–49.** High tibial osteotomy.

**A** Osteoarthritis with cartilage loss in the medial femorotibial space, osteophytosis, and varus deformity are present. Pain was localized to the medial compartment.

**B** Immediately after high tibial osteotomy, valgus alignment is noted.

**C** A follow-up examination 4 years later shows the healed osteotomy site. The valgus angulation is maintained.

and the abductors and iliopsoas muscles are relaxed by the change in position of the trochanters. The distal femoral fragment is displaced medially so that it is aligned with the mechanical axis of the leg. Without this shift, excessive

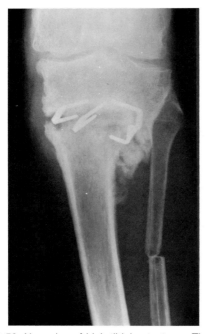

**FIGURE 17–50.** Nonunion of high tibial osteotomy. The osteotomy had been performed in a more distal location than usual. Hypertrophic nonunion at the osteotomy site has developed, with marked bone sclerosis and periosteal reaction. A fibular shaft osteotomy had also been done.

load would be placed on the medial femorotibial compartment of the knee.[159]

Valgus osteotomy is considered when the femoral head is not hemispherical and when adduction improves congruency.[170] A wedge of bone is removed that is wider laterally. The lower margin of the removed segment is at the level of the lesser trochanter and perpendicular to the femoral shaft. The femoral head is rotated laterally with some overcorrection so that the cartilage space is about 2 mm wider at the lateral acetabular margin than centrally.[169] The distal fragment is displaced laterally. Bombelli and associates[154] noted that the rotation of the femoral head should be enough that capsular structures are placed under tension and osteophytes that increase the surface area of the joint are induced to form.

In patients with insufficient acetabular coverage of the femoral head, correction in more than one plane may be done (i.e., valgus extension osteotomy). Extension and flexion refer to rotation of the femoral head posteriorly (extension) or anteriorly (flexion).

**Radiologic Examination.** The trabecular pattern and the appearance of the subchondral bone plate reflect the magnitude and the distribution of forces placed on the joint. In the acetabulum, the subchondral bone plate (the ''sourcil'') normally is uniform in thickness, and a corresponding uniform distribution of force occurs on that portion of the joint.[169] In patients with eccentric loading (such as those with acetabular dysplasia), focal areas of subchondral sclerosis develop (Fig. 17–53). With marked increase in stress, bone resorption and cyst formation occur. Thus, radiographs document uneven stress distribution, and if loading is improved postoperatively, these abnormal findings should regress.

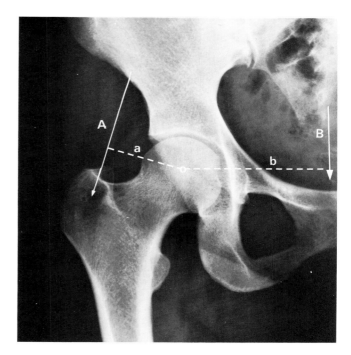

**FIGURE 17–51.** Forces on the hip in monopedal stance. Normally a balance exists between the abduction muscular forces (A) acting through distance a and the body weight (B) (less the weight of the stance limb) acting through distance b. o, Center of femoral head.

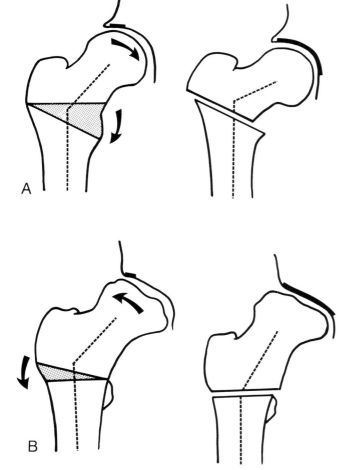

**FIGURE 17–52.** Femoral osteotomy.
  **A** Varus osteotomy.
  **B** Valgus osteotomy.
  (From Weissman BN, Sledge CB: Orthopedic Radiology. Philadelphia, WB Saunders Co, 1986.)

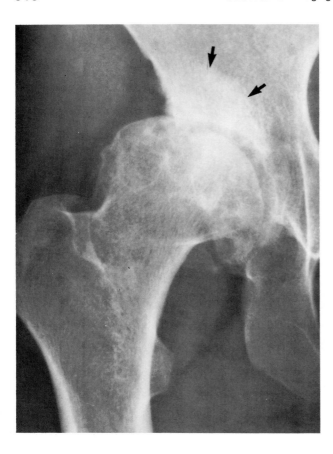

**FIGURE 17–53.** Acetabular dysplasia with secondary osteoarthritis. Severe cartilage loss is accompanied by hypertrophic lipping. The abnormal stress on the acetabulum is reflected by the zone of bone sclerosis (arrows).

Preoperative radiography is used not only to document abnormal unit loading but also to determine the degree of surgical correction that is necessary. Fluoroscopy with the leg in various degrees of adduction, abduction, and flexion documents the degree of rotation that most improves the cartilage space. Lateral views or CT scanning with reformatted images will demonstrate anterior acetabular deficiency.

Postoperative radiographs document the degree of correction provided by the osteotomy, the healing of the osteotomy site, and any regression of the preoperative osteoarthritic changes (Fig. 17–54).[153, 167] The osteotomy site heals gradually, with trabecular continuity normally achieved at about 4 months after surgery.[171]

Evidence of bone resorption adjacent to the orthopedic appliances may be due to abnormal motion or infection (Fig. 17–55). Nonunion is indicated by the development of bone sclerosis and irregular bone resorption along the osteotomy surfaces.

**Results.** Relief of pain after proximal femoral osteotomy often is immediate and may be long-lasting. Evaluation of 50 hips with displacement osteotomies performed at least 9.3 years previously showed the procedure to be of lasting benefit in 87 per cent of cases.[166] After 10 years, 74 per cent of hips were pain-free at rest, and 96 per cent had improvement in pain on weight-bearing. Regression of subchondral cysts and bone sclerosis has been observed in 46 per cent of cases and often is accompanied by dramatic relief of pain.[166] Widening of the cartilage space may occur, presumably related to proliferation of fibrocartilage.

In contrast to the long-term benefits already noted, Reigstad and Gronmark[171] reviewed 103 consecutive medial dis-

placement femoral osteotomies and noted good results in only 70 per cent at 1 year after surgery, in 51 per cent at 5 years after surgery, and in 30 per cent at 10 years after surgery. Thus, "the clinical effect of osteotomy is unpredictable and not as long-lasting as was previously believed."[171] Miegel and Harris[165] found that 12 to 15 years after medial displacement osteotomy, 66 per cent of patients had required cup or total joint arthroplasties.

## PROCEDURES FOR ISCHEMIC NECROSIS OF THE FEMORAL HEAD

Ischemic necrosis of the femoral head typically occurs in young adults. In approximately 75 per cent of cases, a predisposing factor is identified. Although symptoms begin unilaterally, the opposite hip becomes involved in more than one half of cases, almost always within 2 years after the diagnosis has been established in the initially affected hip.[173] Without treatment, progressive collapse of the femoral head is almost inevitable. Treatment strategies used prior to osseous collapse include core decompression, bone grafting, rotational osteotomy, and angular osteotomy.[174]

Core decompression is a procedure in which a core of bone is removed beginning in the lateral cortex of the femur just distal to the greater trochanter and terminating in the anterolateral segment of the femoral head (Fig. 17–56). Partial weight-bearing on crutches is maintained for at least 6 weeks after the procedure. The rationale for core decompression is the finding of elevated bone marrow pressures in patients suspected of having ischemic necrosis, even when radiographs are normal. Such elevations in pressure may be related, for example, to infection or to neoplas-

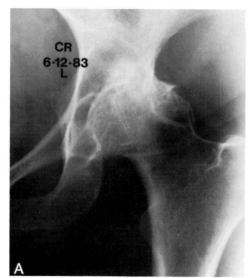

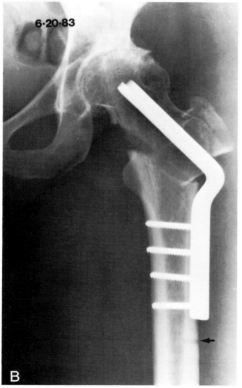

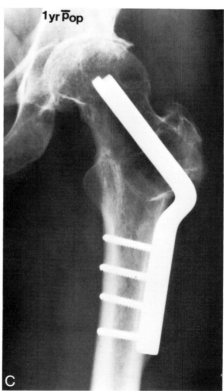

**FIGURE 17–54.** Successful intertrochanteric osteotomy.

**A** Preoperative radiograph shows severe osteoarthritis with cartilage loss, sclerosis, and osteophytes.

**B** Radiograph immediately after varus osteotomy. Note the screw defect from the tension device (arrow).

**C** One year later, a thin cartilage space has developed. The patient's pain was relieved.

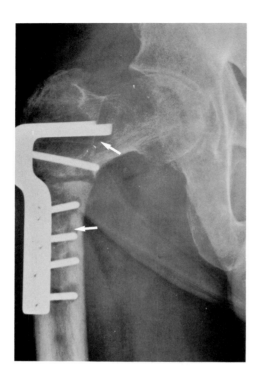

**FIGURE 17–55.** Delayed union of intertrochanteric osteotomy. Following intertrochanteric osteotomy, loosening of the hardware occurred with areas of bone resorption evident (arrows). No infection was found and healing occurred after reoperation and immobilization.

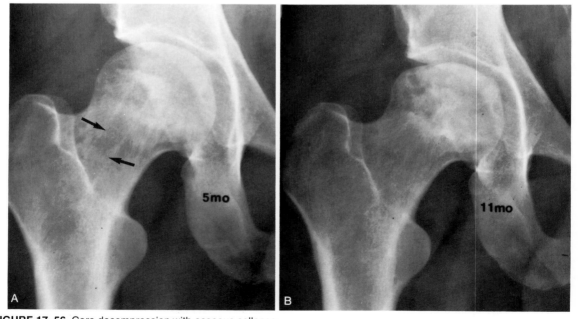

**FIGURE 17–56.** Core decompression with osseous collapse.
**A** Five months after core decompression (arrows) for ischemic necrosis of the femoral head, no osseous collapse is evident.
**B** Six months after **A,** the femoral head has collapsed.

tic or Gaucher's cells that exist in the marrow and lead to compression of intraosseous capillaries, reducing intramedullary circulation.[175] Removal of a core of bone from the femoral head and neck lowers the bone marrow pressure. This treatment is thought to have lasting benefit in early (stages I and II) disease.

MR imaging has been used to gauge the results of core decompression.[198–201] Evaluation of patients with the bone marrow edema pattern (possibly an early stage of osteonecrosis) has shown return to normal marrow signal after core decompression.[199, 200] In a series of 32 hips with osteonecrosis examined with MR imaging before and after core decompression, the size of the lesion appeared to be the most important factor in predicting femoral head collapse.[199] Thus, four of nine large lesions demonstrated progressive collapse, whereas none of the smaller or moderate-sized lesions collapsed. Signal characteristics remained unchanged in most cases. Similarly, Saito and colleagues confirmed a relationship between the size of lesion and surgical outcome in cases of stages II and III osteonecrosis.[198]

Bone grafting represents a procedure in which a core of bone is removed (as in the core decompression procedure), after which the defect is filled with bone graft.[174] Vascularized fibular grafts may be used in an attempt to revascularize a necrotic femoral head.[196] The femoral head is reamed out and packed with cancellous bone graft. A fibular graft is then placed as far as possible into a tunnel drilled in the femoral head and neck for decompression and curettage. The vascularized fibular graft, its vascular supply, and a surrounding muscle cuff are positioned within the tunnel; thus, the graft alone does not entirely fill the tunnel. Follow-up radiographs should show incorporation of the proximal fibular graft as evidenced by blurring of its margins, occurring in an average of 6 months after surgery. Healing of the femoral head graft usually is not visible but the contour of the femoral head should be evaluated. It was noted by Manaster and coworkers[181] that graft incorporation and femoral head collapse appeared to be related such that graft incorporation and maintenance of a normal contour of the femoral head tend to occur together.

The Sugioka osteotomy is a rotational osteotomy in which the femoral head is rotated anteriorly and inferiorly so that the area of osseous involvement is shifted into a non–weight-bearing position.[176, 177] Angulation osteotomy may be done with rotation of the femoral head medially (varus) and posteriorly (extension) to shift the affected area of bone to a non–weight-bearing position.

## SUMMARY

Knowledge of orthopedic devices and techniques is a prerequisite to accurate interpretation of postoperative radiographs. A variety of internal fixation devices, including pins, nails, rods, screws, and plates, in addition to external fixation devices and PMMA cement, are used in fracture fixation. Electrical stimulation may be used to promote fracture healing, and numerous techniques of bone grafting are advocated in the treatment of many skeletal processes. Resection arthroplasty, arthrodesis, and osteotomy represent additional orthopedic methods.

## References

1. Sisk TD: Fractures. In AS Edmonson, AH Crenshaw (Eds): Campbell's Operative Orthopedics. St Louis, CV Mosby, 1980, p 509.
2. Meals RA, Meuli HC: Carpenter's nails, phonograph needles, piano wires, and safety pins: The history of operative fixation of metacarpal and phalangeal fractures. J Hand Surg [Am] 10:144, 1985.
3. Johnson KD, Johnston DWC, Parker B: Comminuted femoral-shaft fractures: Treatment by roller traction, cerclage wires and an intramedullary nail, or an interlocking intramedullary nail. J Bone Joint Surg [Am] 66:1222, 1984.
4. Edmonson AS: Surgical techniques. In AS Edmonson, AH Crenshaw (Eds): Campbell's Operative Orthopedics. St Louis, CV Mosby, 1980, p 19.
5. Rush LV, Rush HL: Evolution of medullary fixation of fractures by the longitudinal pin. Am J Surg 78:324, 1949.
6. Rush LV, Rush HL: Intramedullary fixation of fractures of the humerus by the longitudinal pin. Surgery 27:268, 1950.
7. Kuntscher GBG: The Kuntscher method of intramedullary fixation. J Bone Joint Surg [Am] 40:17, 1958.
8. Ender GH: Treatment of pertrochanteric and subtrochanteric fractures of the femur with Ender pins. In The Hip: 6th Open Scientific Meeting of the Hip Society. Proceedings, Vol 6. St Louis, CV Mosby, 1978, p 187.
9. Harris LJ: Condylocephalic nailing of proximal femoral fractures. In CM Evarts (Ed): AAOS Instructional Course Lectures. St Louis, CV Mosby, 1983, p 292.
10. Müller ME, Allgower M, Schneider R, et al: Manual of Internal Fixation: Technique Recommended by the AO Group. J Schatzker et al, Transl. New York, Springer-Verlag, 1979.
11. Faithfull DK, Herbert TJ: Small joint fusions of the hand using the Herbert bone screw. J Hand Surg [Br] 9:167, 1984.
12. Sartoris DJ, Kerr R, Georgen T, et al: Sliding-screw plate fixation of proximal femoral fractures: Radiographic assessment. Skel Radiol 14:104, 1985.
13. Mulholland RC, Gunn DR: Sliding screw plate fixation of intertrochanteric femoral fractures. J Trauma 12:581, 1972.
14. Ecker ML, Joyce JJ III, Kohl EJ: The treatment of trochanteric hip fractures using a compression screw. J Bone Joint Surg [Am] 57:23, 1975.
15. Laros GS, Moore JF: Complications of fixation in intertrochanteric fractures. Clin Orthop 101:110, 1974.
16. Doppelt SH: The sliding compression screw—today's best answers for stabilization of intertrochanteric hip fractures. Orthop Clin North Am 11:507, 1980.
17. Walters R, Simon SR: Joint destruction, a sequel of unrecognized pin penetration in patients with slipped capital femoral epiphyses. In The Hip: 8th Open Scientific Meeting of the Hip Society. Proceedings, Vol 8. St Louis, CV Mosby, 1980, 416.
18. Sarmiento A, Mullis DL, Lata LL, et al: A quantitative comparative analysis of fracture healing under the influence of compression plating vs. closed weight-bearing treatment. Clin Orthop 149:232, 1980.
19. Terjesen T, Benum P: Mechanical effects of metal plate fixation. In vitro investigation of intact and osteotomized human and rabbit tibiae. Acta Orthop Scand 54:256, 1983.
20. Terjesen T: Bone healing after metal plate fixation and external fixation of the osteotomized rabbit tibia. Acta Orthop Scand 55:69, 1984.
21. Mears DC: External Skeletal Fixation. Baltimore, Williams & Wilkins, 1983.
22. Seligson D, Pope M: Concepts in External Fixation. New York, Grune & Stratton, 1982.
23. Slatis P, Karaharjo EO: External fixation of unstable pelvic fractures: Experiences in 22 patients treated with a trapezoid compression frame. Clin Orthop 151:73, 1980.
24. Wild JJ Jr, Hanson GW, Tullos HS: Unstable fractures of the pelvis treated by external fixation. J Bone Joint Surg [Am] 64:1010, 1982.
25. Aho AJ, Nieminen SJ, Nylamo DI: External fixation by Hoffman-Vidal-Adrey. Osteotaxis for severe tibial fractures. Treatment scheme and technical criticism. Clin Orthop 181:154, 1983.
26. Mears DC, Fu GH: Modern concepts of external skeletal fixation of the pelvis. Clin Orthop 151:65, 1980.
27. Bartucci EJ, Gonzalez MH, Cooperman DR, et al: The effect of adjunctive methylmethacrylate on failures of fixation and function in patients with intertrochanteric fractures and osteoporosis. J Bone Joint Surg [Am] 67:1094, 1985.
28. Enis JE, McCollough NC III, Cooper JS: Effects of methylmethacrylate in osteosynthesis. Clin Orthop 105:283, 1974.
29. Harrington KD, Johnston JO, Turner RH, et al: The use of methylmethacrylate as an adjunct in the internal fixation of malignant neoplastic fractures. J Bone Joint Surg [Am] 54:1665, 1972.
30. Harrington KD, Sim FH, Enis JE, et al: Methylmethacrylate as an adjunct in internal fixation of pathological fractures. J Bone Joint Surg [Am] 58:1047, 1976.
31. Lewallen RP, Pritchard DJ, Sim FH: Treatment of pathologic fractures or impending fractures of the humerus with Rush rods and methylmethacrylate. Experience with 55 cases in 54 patients; 1968–1977. Clin Orthop 166:193, 1982.
32. Ohashi T, Inoue S, Kajikawa K: External skeletal fixation using methylmethacrylate. Current technique, clinical results, and indications. Clin Orthop 178:121, 1983.
33. Ryan JR, Begeman PC: The effects of filling experimental large cortical defects with methylmethacrylate. Clin Orthop 185:306, 1984.

34. Owen R, Goodfellow J, Bullough P: Scientific Foundation of Orthopaedics and Traumatology. Philadelphia, WB Saunders Co, 1980.

35. Clark CR, Keggi KJ, Penjabi MM: Methylmethacrylate stabilization of the cervical spine. J Bone Joint Surg [Am] 66:40, 1984.

36. Asnis SE, Lesniewski P, Dowling T Jr: Anterior decompression and stabilization with methylmethacrylate and a bone bolt for treatment of pathologic fractures of the cervical spine. A report of two cases. Clin Orthop 187:139, 1984.

37. Bassett CAL: The development and application of pulsed electromagnetic fields (PEMFs) for ununited fractures and arthrodeses. Orthop Clin North Am 15:61, 1984.

38. Bassett CAL, Mitchell SN, Gaston SR: Pulsing electromagnetic field treatment in ununited fractures and failed arthrodeses. JAMA 247:623, 1982.

39. Brighton CT, Black J, Friedenberg ZB, et al: A multicenter study of the treatment of non-union with constant direct current. J Bone Joint Surg [Am] 63:2, 1981.

40. Day L: Electrical stimulation in the treatment of ununited fractures. Clin Orthop 161:54, 1981.

41. Esterhai JL Jr, Brighton CT, Heppenstall RB, et al: Detection of synovial pseudarthrosis by 99mTc scintigraphy: Application to treatment of traumatic nonunion with constant direct current. Clin Orthop 161:15, 1981.

42. Paterson DC, Lewis GN, Cass CA: Treatment of delayed union and nonunion with implanted direct current stimulator. Clin Orthop 148:117, 1980.

43. Paterson DC, Lewis GN, Cass CA: Treatment of congenital pseudarthrosis of the tibia with direct current stimulation. Clin Orthop 148:129, 1980.

44. Steinberg ME, Brighton CT, Steinberg BR, et al: Treatment of avascular necrosis of the femoral head by a combination of bone grafting, decompression, and electrical stimulation. Clin Orthop 186:137, 1984.

45. Weber BG, Brunner C: The treatment of nonunions without electrical stimulation. Clin Orthop 161:24, 1981.

46. Berggren A, Weiland AJ, Dorfman H: Free vascularized bone grafts: Factors affecting their survival and ability to heal to recipient bone defects. Plast Reconstr Surg 69:19, 1982.

47. Berggren A, Weiland AJ, Ostrup LT: Bone scintigraphy in evaluating the viability of composite bone grafts revascularized by microvascular anastomoses, conventional autogenous bone grafts, and free non-revascularized periosteal grafts. J Bone Joint Surg [Am] 64:799, 1982.

48. Bowerman JW, Hughes JL: Radiology of bone grafts. Radiol Clin North Am 13:467, 1975.

49. Brown KLB, Cruess RL: Bone and cartilage transplantation in orthopaedic surgery. J Bone Joint Surg [Am] 64:270, 1982.

50. Dell PC, Burchardt H, Glowczewskie FP Jr: A roentgenographic, biomechanical, and histologic evaluation of vascularized and non-vascularized segmental fibular canine autografts. J Bone Joint Surg [Am] 67:105, 1985.

51. Enneking WF, Burchardt H, Puhl JJ, et al: Physical and biological aspects of repair in dog cortical-bone transplants. J Bone Joint Surg [Am] 57:237, 1975.

52. Enneking WF, Eady JL, Burchardt H: Autogenous cortical bone grafts in the reconstruction of segmental skeletal defects. J Bone Joint Surg [Am] 62:1039, 1980.

53. Frame JW, Browne RM, Brady CL: Biologic basis for interpositional autogenous bone grafts to the mandible. J Oral Maxillofac Surg 40:407, 1982.

54. Frame JW, Edmondson HD, O'Kane MM: A radio-isotope study of the healing of mandibular bone grafts in patients. Br J Oral Surg 21:277, 1983.

55. Heppenstall RB: Bone grafting. In RB Heppenstall: Fracture Treatment and Healing. Philadelphia, WB Saunders Co, 1980, p 89.

56. Heppenstall RB: The present role of bone graft surgery in treating nonunion. Orthop Clin North Am 15:113, 1984.

57. Kandel RA, Pritzker KPH, Langer F, et al: The pathologic features of massive osseous grafts, Hum Pathol 15:141, 1984.

58. Lau RSF, Leung PC: Bone graft viability in vascularized bone graft transfer. Br J Radiol 55:325, 1982.

59. Laurie SWS, Kaban LB, Mulliken JB, et al: Donor-site morbidity after harvesting rib and iliac bone. Plast Reconstr Surg 73:933, 1984.

60. Lindholm TS, Urist MR: A quantitative analysis of new bone formation by induction in composite grafts of bone marrow and bone matrix. Clin Orthop 150:288, 1980.

61. Lisbona R, Rennie WRJ, Daniel RK: Radionuclide evaluation of free vascularized bone graft viability. AJR 134:387, 1980.

62. McGrath MH, Watson HK: Late results with local bone graft donor sites in hand surgery. J Hand Surg [Am] 6:234, 1981.

63. Mellonig JT, Bowers GM, Cotton WR: Comparison of bone graft materials. Part II. New bone formation with autografts and allografts: A histological evaluation. J Periodontol 52:297, 1981.

64. Mendes DG, Roffman M, Silbermann M: Reconstruction of the acetabular wall with bone graft in arthroplasty of the hip. Clin Orthop 186:29, 1984.

65. Mullikan JB, Kaban LB, Glowacki J: Induced osteogenesis—the biological principle and clinical applications. J Surg Res 37:487, 1984.

66. Noellert RC, Louis DS: Long-term follow-up of nonvascularized fibular autografts for distal radial reconstruction. J Hand Surg [Am] 10:335, 1984.

67. Pelker RR, Friedlaender GE, Markham TC: Biomechanical properties of bone allografts. Clin Orthop 174:54, 1983.

68. Psilakis JM, Woisky R: A study of regeneration of donor areas of bone grafts. Ann Plast Surg 10:391, 1983.

69. Roffman M, Silbermann M, Mendes DG: Incorporation of bone graft covered with methylmethacrylate onto acetabular wall. An experimental study. Acta Orthop Scand 54:580, 1983.

70. Salama R: Xenogeneic bone grafting in humans. Clin Orthop 174:113, 1983.

71. Smith TF: Bone graft physiology. Survival and incorporation of the graft. J Am Podiatry Assoc 73:70, 1983.

72. Taylor GI: The current status of free vascularized bone grafts. Clin Plast Surg 10:185, 1983.

73. Weiland AJ: Vascularized free bone transplants. J Bone Joint Surg [Am] 63:166, 1981.

74. Weiland AJ, Phillips TW, Randolph MA: Bone grafts: A radiologic, histologic and biomechanical model comparing autografts, allografts, and free vascularized bone grafts. Plast Reconstr Surg 74:368, 1984.

75. Meyers MH, Harvey JP Jr, Moore TM: Delayed treatment of subcapital and transcervical fractures of the neck of the femur with internal fixation and a muscle pedicle bone graft. Orthop Clin North Am 5:743, 1974.

76. Meyers MH, Harvey JP Jr, Moore TM: The muscle pedical bone graft in the treatment of displaced fractures of the femoral neck: Indications, operative technique, and results. Orthop Clin North Am 5:779, 1974.

77. Ahlgren S-A, Gudmundsson G, Bartholdsson E: Function after removal of a septic total hip prosthesis. Acta Orthop Scand 51:541, 1980.

78. Bittar ES, Petty W: Girdlestone arthroplasty for infected total hip arthroplasty. Clin Orthop 170:83, 1982.

79. Bourne RB, Hunter GA, Rorabeck CH, et al: A six-year follow-up of infected total hip replacements managed by Girdlestone's arthroplasty. J Bone Joint Surg [Br] 66:340, 1984.

80. Canner GC, Steinberg ME, Heppenstall RB, et al: The infected hip after total hip arthroplasty. J Bone Joint Surg [Am] 66:1393, 1984.

81. Batchelor JS: Excision of the femoral head and neck in cases of ankylosis and osteoarthritis of the hips. Proc R Soc Med 38:689, 1945.

82. Fenelon GCC, Von Foerster G, Engelbrecht E: Disarticulation of the hip as a result of failed arthroplasty. A series of 11 cases. J Bone Joint Surg [Br] 62:441, 1980.

83. Girdlestone GR: Acute pyogenic arthritis of the hip. An operation giving free access and effective drainage. Lancet 1:419, 1943.

84. Girdlestone GR: Acute pyogenic arthritis of the hip. An operation giving free access and effective drainage. Clin Orthop 170:4, 1982.

85. Gruca A: The treatment of quiescent tuberculosis of the hip joint by excision and "dynamic" osteotomy. J Bone Joint Surg [Br] 32:174, 1950.

86. McElwaine JP, Colville J: Excision arthroplasty for infected total hip replacements. J Bone Joint Surg [Br] 66:168, 1984.

87. Milch H: Resection-angulation operation for arthritis of hip. Bull Hosp Joint Dis 9:187, 1948.

88. Miley GB, Scheller AD Jr, Turner RH: Medical and surgical treatment of the septic hip with one-stage revision arthroplasty. Clin Orthop 170:76, 1982.

89. Murray WR, Lucas DB, Inman VT: Femoral head and neck resection. J Bone Joint Surg [Am] 46:1184, 1964.

90. Parr PL, Croft C, Enneking WF: Resection of the head and neck of the femur with and without angulation osteotomy. A follow-up of thirty-eight patients. J Bone Joint Surg [Am] 53:935, 1971.

91. Tuli SM, Mukherjee SK: Excision arthroplasty for tuberculous and pyogenic arthritis of the hip. J Bone Joint Surg [Br] 63:29, 1981.

92. Stedman's Medical Dictionary, 22nd Ed. Baltimore, Williams & Wilkins, 1972.

93. Barr JS, Record EE: Arthrodesis of the ankle joint. Indications, operative technic and clinical experience. N Engl J Med 248:53, 1953.

94. Boobbyer GN: The long-term results of ankle arthrodesis. Acta Orthop Scand 52:107, 1981.

95. Charnley J: Compression arthrodesis of the ankle and shoulder. J Bone Joint Surg [Br] 33:180, 1951.

96. Davis RJ, Millis MB: Ankle arthrodesis in the management of traumatic ankle arthrodesis: A long-term retrospective study. J Trauma 20:674, 1980.

97. Hefti FL, Baumann JU, Morscher EW: Ankle joint fusion—determination of optimal position by gait analysis. Acta Orthop Trauma Surg 96:187, 1980.

98. Jackson A, Glasgow M: Tarsal hypermobility after ankle fusion—fact or fiction? J Bone Joint Surg [Br] 61:470, 1979.

99. Kennedy JC: Arthrodesis of the ankle with particular reference to the Gallie procedure. A review of fifty cases. J Bone Joint Surg [Am] 42:1308, 1960.

100. King HS, Watkins TB Jr, Samuelson KM: Analysis of foot position in ankle arthrodesis and its influence on gait. Orthop Trans 3:347, 1979.

101. Lance EM, Paval A, Fries I, et al: Arthrodesis of the ankle joint: A follow-up study. Clin Orthop 142:146, 1979.

102. Mazur JM, Schwartz E, Simon SR: Ankle arthrodesis. Long-term follow-up with gait analysis. J Bone Joint Surg [Am] 61:964, 1979.

103. Morgan CD, Henke JA, Bailey RW, et al: Long-term results of tibiotalar arthrodesis. J Bone Joint Surg [Am] 67:546, 1985.

104. Morrey BF, Wiedeman GP Jr: Complications and long-term results of ankle arthrodesis following trauma. J Bone Joint Surg [Am] 62:777, 1980.

105. Rothacker GW Jr, Cabanela ME: External fixation for arthrodesis of the knee and ankle. Clin Orthop 180:101, 1983.

106. Scranton PE, Fu FH, Brown TD: Ankle arthrodesis: A comparative clinical and biomechanical evaluation. Clin Orthop 151:234, 1980.

107. Scranton PE Jr: Use of internal compression in arthrodesis of the ankle. J Bone Joint Surg [Am] 67:550, 1985.

108. Stewart M: Arthrodesis. In AS Edmonson, AH Crenshaw (Eds): Campbell's Operative Orthopedics. St Louis, CV Mosby, 1980, p 1100.

109. Stewart MJ, Beeler, TC, McConnell JC: Compression arthrodesis of the ankle. Evaluation of a cosmetic modification. J Bone Joint Surg [Am] 65:219, 1983.

110. Verhelst MP, Mulier JC, Hoogmartens MJ, et al: Arthrodesis of the ankle joint

with complete removal of the distal part of the fibula. Experience with the transfibular approach and three different types of fixation. Clin Orthop *118:*93, 1976.

111. Brewster RC, Coventry MB, Johnson EW Jr: Conversion of the arthrodesed hip to a total hip arthroplasty. J Bone Joint Surg [Am] *57:*27, 1975.
112. Fulkerson JP: Arthrodesis for disabling hip pain in children and adolescents. Clin Orthop *128:*296, 1977.
113. Core DR, Murray MP, Sepic SB, et al: Walking patterns of men with unilateral surgical hip fusion. J Bone Joint Surg [Am] *57:*759, 1975.
114. Greiss ME, Thomas RJ, Freeman MAR: Sequelae of arthrodesis of the hip. J R Soc Med *73:*497, 1980.
115. Kostuik J, Alexander D: Arthrodesis for failed arthroplasty of the hip. Clin Orthop *188:*173, 1984.
116. Lipscomb PR, McCaslin FE Jr: Arthrodesis of the hip. Review of 371 cases. J Bone Joint Surg [Am] *43:*923, 1961.
117. Lubahn JD, McCollister K, Evarts C, et al: Conversion of ankylosed hips to total hip arthroplasty. Clin Orthop *153:*146, 1980.
118. Price CT, Lovell WW: Thompson arthrodesis of the hip in children. J Bone Joint Surg [Am] *62:*1118, 1980.
119. Sponseller PD, McBeath AA, Perpich M: Hip arthrodesis in young patients. A long-term follow-up study. J Bone Joint Surg [Am] *66:*853, 1984.
120. Stewart M: Arthrodesis. *In* AS Edmonson, AH Crenshaw (Eds): Campbell's Operative Orthopedics. St Louis, CV Mosby, 1980, p 1113.
121. Stinchfield FE, Cavallaro WU: Arthrodesis of the hip joint. J Bone Joint Surg [Am] *32:*48, 1950.
122. Chandler HP, Reineck FT, Wixson RL, et al: Total hip replacement in patients younger than thirty years. J Bone Joint Surg [Am] *63:*1426, 1981.
123. Brown MD: Lumbar spine fusion. *In* BE Finneson (Ed): Low Back Pain. Philadelphia, JB Lippincott, 1980.
124. Calabrese AS, Freiberger RH: Acquired spondylolysis after spinal fusion. Radiology *81:*492, 1963.
125. Calenoff L, Hendrix RW, Schafer MF: Surgical fusion of the posttraumatic spine: A radiologic assessment. CRC Crit Rev Diagn Imaging *23:*269, 1985.
126. Dawson EG, Clader TJ, Bassett LW: A comparison of different methods used to diagnose pseudarthrosis following posterior spinal fusion for scoliosis. J Bone Joint Surg [Am] *67:*1153, 1985.
127. DePalma AF, Marone PJ: Spondylosis following spinal fusion. Report of a case. Clin Orthop *15:*208, 1959.
128. Dwyer AF: Experience of anterior correction of scoliosis. Clin Orthop *93:*191, 1973.
129. Eismont FJ, Simeone FA: Bone overgrowth (hypertrophy) as a cause of late paraparesis after scoliosis fusion. A case report. J Bone Joint Surg [Am] *63:*1016, 1981.
130. Foley MJ, Lee C, Calenoff L, et al: Radiologic evaluation of surgical cervical spine fusion. AJR *138:*79, 1982.
131. Foley MJ, Calenoff L, Hendrix RW, et al: Thoracic and lumbar spine fusion: Postoperative radiologic evaluation. AJR *141:*373, 1983.
132. Hall JE: Current concepts review. Dwyer instrumentation in anterior fusion of the spine. J Bone Joint Surg [Am] *63:*1188, 1981.
133. Harrington PR, Dickson JH: An eleven-year clinical investigation of Harrington instrumentation. A preliminary report of 578 cases. Clin Orthop *93:*113, 1973.
134. Kestler OC: Overgrowth (hypertrophy) of lumbosacral grafts, causing a complete block. Bull Hosp Joint Dis *27:*51, 1966.
135. Macnab I, Dall D: The blood supply of the lumbar spine and its application to the technique of intertransverse lumbar fusion. J Bone Joint Surg [Br] *53:*628, 1971.
136. Simmons JW: Posterior lumbar interbody fusion with posterior elements as chip grafts. Clin Orthop *193:*85, 1985.
137. Swank S, Lonstein JE, Moe JH, et al: Surgical treatment of adult scoliosis. J Bone Joint Surg [Am] *63:*268, 1981.
138. Vanden Brink KD, Edmonson AS: *In* AS Edmonson, AH Crenshaw (Eds): Campbell's Operative Orthopedics. St Louis, CV Mosby, 1980, p 1939.
139. Wang GJ, Reger SI, Shao ZH, et al: Comparative strength of anterior spinal fixation with bone graft or polymethylmethacrylate. Experimental operations and observations on dogs. Clin Orthop *188:*303, 1984.
140. Wilkinson RH, Willi UV, Gilsanz V, et al: Radiographic evaluation of the spine after surgical correction of scoliosis. AJR *133:*703, 1979.
141. Ford LT: Osteotomies. Nomenclature and uses. Radiol Clin North Am *13:*79, 1975.
142. Coventry MB: Osteotomy about the knee for degenerative and rheumatoid arthritis. Indications, operative technique, and results. J Bone Joint Surg [Am] *55:*23, 1973.
143. Coventry MB: Current concepts review. Upper tibial osteotomy for osteoarthritis. J Bone Joint Surg [Am] *67:*1136, 1985.
144. Coventry MB, Bowman PW: Long-term results of upper tibial osteotomy for degenerative arthritis of the knee. Acta Orthop Belg *48:*139, 1982.
145. Insall JN, Joseph DM, Msika C: High tibial osteotomy for varus gonarthrosis. A long-term follow-up study. J Bone Joint Surg [Am] *66:*1040, 1984.
146. Maquet P: Treatment of osteoarthritis of the knee by osteotomy. *In* UH Weil (Ed): Progress in Orthopedic Surgery, Vol 4. Joint Preserving Procedures of the Lower Extremities. New York, Springer-Verlag, 1980, p 57.
147. Myrnerts R: Optimal correction in high tibial osteotomy for varus deformity. Acta Orthop Scand *51:*689, 1980.
148. Schatzker J, Burgess RC, Glynn MK: The management of nonunions following high tibial osteotomies. Clin Orthop *193:*230, 1985.
149. Tjornstrand B, Svensson K, Thorngren KG: Prediction of long-term outcome

150. Tjornstrand B, Selvik G, Egund N, et al: Roentgen stereophotogrammetry in high tibial osteotomy for gonarthrosis. Arch Orthop Trauma Surg *99:*73, 1981.
151. Vainionpää S, Läike E, Kirves P, et al: Tibial osteotomy for osteoarthritis of the knee. A five to ten-year follow-up study. J Bone Joint Surg [Am] *63:*938, 1981.
152. Wagner H: Principles of corrective osteotomies in osteoarthrosis of the knee. *In* UH Weil (Ed): Progress in Orthopedic Surgery, Vol 4. Joint Preserving Procedures of the Lower Extremities. New York, Springer-Verlag, 1980, p 75.
153. Adam A, Spence AJ: Intertrochanteric osteotomy for osteoarthritis of the hip. A review of fifty-eight operations. J Bone Joint Surg [Br] *40:*219, 1958.
154. Bombelli R, Gerundini M, Aronson J: The biomechanical basis for osteotomy in the treatment of osteoarthritis of the hip: Results in younger patients. *In* The Hip: 12th Open Scientific Meeting of the Hip Society. St Louis, CV Mosby, 1984, p 18.
155. Brand RA, Pedersen DR: Computer modeling of surgery and a consideration of the mechanical effects of proximal femoral osteotomies. *In* The Hip: 12th Open Scientific Meeting of the Hip Society. St Louis, CV Mosby, 1984, p 193.
156. Conforty B: Femoral osteotomy for correction of sequelae of conservative treatment of congenital dislocation of the hip. Isr J Med Sci *16:*284, 1980.
157. Day B, Shim SS, Leung G: Effect of the high femoral osteotomy upon the vascularity and blood supply of the hip joint. Surg Gynecol Obstet *158:*443, 1984.
158. Ferguson AB Jr: High intertrochanteric osteotomy for osteoarthritis of the hip. J Bone Joint Surg [Am] *46:*1159, 1964.
159. Fidler M: Planning an intertrochanteric femoral osteotomy. Acta Orthop Scand *55:*501, 1984.
160. Harris NH, Kirwan E: The results of osteotomy for early primary osteoarthritis of the hip. J Bone Joint Surg [Br] *46:*447, 1964.
161. Malkin SAS: Femoral osteotomy in treatment of osteoarthritis of the hip. Br Med J *1:*304, 1936.
162. Maquet P, Radin EL: Osteotomy as an alternative to total hip replacement in young adults. Clin Orthop *123:*138, 1977.
163. McMurray TP: Osteo-arthritis of the hip joint. Br J Surg *22:*716, 1935.
164. McMurray TP: Osteo-arthritis of the hip joint. J Bone Joint Surg *21:*1, 1939.
165. Miegel RE, Harris WH: Medial-displacement intertrochanteric osteotomy in the treatment of osteoarthritis of the hip. A long-term follow-up study. J Bone Joint Surg [Am] *66:*878, 1984.
166. Mogensen A, Zoega H, Marinko P: Late results of intertrochanteric osteotomy for advanced osteoarthritis of the hip. Acta Orthop Scand *51:*85, 1980.
167. Osborne GV, Fahrni WH: Oblique displacement osteotomy for osteoarthritis of the hip joint. J Bone Joint Surg [Br] *32:*148, 1950.
168. Parr PL, Croft C, Enneking WF: Resection of the head and neck of the femur with and without angulation osteotomy. A follow-up study of thirty-eight patients. J Bone Joint Surg [Am] *53:*935, 1971.
169. Pauwels F: Biomechanics of the Normal and Diseased Hip. Theoretical Foundation, Technique and Result of Treatment. An Atlas. New York, Springer-Verlag, 1976, p 146.
170. Poss R: Current concepts review. The role of osteotomy in the treatment of osteoarthritis of the hip. J Bone Joint Surg [Am] *66:*144, 1984.
171. Reigstad A, Gronmark T: Osteoarthritis of the hip treated by intertrochanteric osteotomy. A long-term follow-up. J Bone Joint Surg [Am] *66:*1, 1984.
172. Wardle EN: Displacement osteotomy of the upper end of the femur. J Bone Joint Surg [Br] *37:*568, 1955.
173. Lotke PA, Steinberg ME: Osteonecrosis of the hip and knee. Bull Rheum Dis *35:*1, 1985.
174. Enneking WF: The choice of surgical procedures in idiopathic aseptic necrosis. *In* The Hip: 7th Open Scientific Meeting of the Hip Society. St Louis, CV Mosby, 1979, p 238.
175. Hungerford DS, Zizic TM: Pathogenesis of ischemic necrosis of the femoral head. Hip, p 249, 1983.
176. Sugioka Y: Transtrochanteric anterior rotational osteotomy of the femoral head in the treatment of osteonecrosis affecting the hip: A new osteotomy operation. Clin Orthop *130:*191, 1978.
177. Sugioka Y: Transtrochanteric rotational osteotomy in the treatment of idiopathic and steroid-induced femoral head necrosis, Perthes' disease, slipped capital femoral epiphysis and osteoarthritis of the hip. Indications and results. Clin Orthop *184:*12, 1984.
178. Slone RM, Heare MM, Vander Griend RA, et al: Orthopedic fixation devices. RadioGraphics *11:*823, 1991.
179. Weissman BN, Reilly DT: Diagnostic imaging evaluation of the postoperative patient following musculoskeletal trauma. Radiol Clin North Am *27:*1035, 1989.
180. Browner BD, Mast J, Mendes M: Principles of internal fixation. *In* BD Browner, et al (Eds): Skeletal Trauma. Philadelphia, WB Saunders Co, 1992, p 243.
181. Manaster BJ: Imaging knee ligament reconstructions. *In* Syllabus: A Categorical Course in Musculoskeletal Radiology. Advanced Imaging of Joints: Theory and Practice. Presented at the 79th Scientific Assembly and Annual Meeting of the Radiological Society of North America, 1993.
182. Young JWR, Kovelman H, Resnik CS, et al: Radiologic assessment of bones after Ilizarov procedures. Radiology *177:*89, 1990.
183. Green S: The Ilizarov method. *In* BD Browner, et al (Eds): Skeletal Trauma. Philadelphia, WB Saunders Co, 1992, p 543.
184. Young JWR, Kostrubiak IS, Resnik CS, et al: Sonographic evaluation of bone

production in the distraction site for Ilizarov limb lengthening procedures. AJR *154:*125, 1990.

185. Buchholz HW, Elson RA, Heiner K: Antibiotic-loaded acrylic cement: Current concepts. Clin Orthop *190:*96, 1984.
186. Murray WR: Use of antibiotic-containing bone cement. Clin Orthop *190:*89, 1984.
187. Berrey BH, Lord CF, Gebhardt MC, et al: Fractures of allografts. Frequency, treatment and end results. J Bone Joint Surg [Am] *72:*825, 1990.
188. Lord CF, Gebhardt MC, Tomford WW, et al: Infection in bone allografts. J Bone Joint Surg [Am] *70:*369, 1988
189. Mankin HJ, Doppelt S, Tomford W: Clinical experience with allograft implantation. The first ten years. Clin Orthop *174:*69, 1983.
190. Mnaymneh W, Malinin TI, Makley JT, et al: Massive osteoarticular allografts in the reconstruction of extremities following resection of tumors not requiring chemotherapy and radiation. Clin Orthop *197:*76, 1985.
191. Musculo DL, Petracchi LJ, Ayerza MA, et al: Massive femoral allografts followed for 22 to 36 years. J Bone Joint Surg [Br] *74:*887, 1992.
192. Parrish FF: Allograft replacement of all or part of the end of a long bone following excision of a tumor. J Bone Joint Surg [Am] *55:*1, 1973.
193. Fern ED, Saleh M: Bone spurs: A symptomatic complication of iliac crest bone harvesting. J Orthop Rheumatol *6:*103, 1993.
194. Itoh K, Minami A, Sakuma T, et al: The use of three-phase bone imaging in vascularized fibular and iliac bone grafts. Clin Nuc Med *14:*494, 1989.
195. Cheung HS, Steward IET, Ho KC, et al: Vascularized iliac crest grafts: Evaluation of viability status with marrow scintigraphy. Radiology *186:*241, 1993.
196. Manaster BJ, Coleman DA, Bell DA: Pre- and postoperative imaging of vascularized fibular grafts. Radiology *176:*161, 1990
197. Swan JS, Braunstein EM, Capello W: Aspiration of the hip in patients treated with Girdlestone arthroplasty. AJR *156:*545, 1991.
198. Saito S, Ohzono K, Ono K: Joint-preserving operations for idiopathic avascular necrosis of the femoral head. Results of core decompression, grafting and osteotomy. J Bone Joint Surg [Br] *70:*78, 1988.
199. Chan TW, Dalinka MK, Steinberg ME, et al: MRI appearance of femoral head osteonecrosis following core decompression and bone grafting. Skel Radiol *20:*103, 1991.
200. Hofmann S, Engel A, Neuhold A, et al: Bone-marrow oedema syndrome and transient osteoporosis of the hip. J Bone Joint Surg [Br] 75:210, 1993.
201. Neuhold A, Hofmann S, Engel A, et al: Bone marrow edema of the hip: MR findings after core decompression. J Comp Assist Tomogr *16:*951, 1992.

# 18

# Imaging After Spine Surgery

*Mini N. Pathria, M.D., and Steven R. Garfin, M.D.*

The surgical treatment of low back pain has followed three major trends in the past century.[1] Originally, degenerative or herniated discs were considered the most important cause of low back pain, leading to the development of laminectomy and diskectomy. The next major trend was the addition of spinal fusion because spinal instability was considered to be the cause when the patient continued to have back pain after disc excision.[1] The latest trend is directed to the treatment of radiculopathy, rather than back pain, deformity, or instability alone. Currently, numerous surgical techniques are employed, including percutaneous interventional procedures, osseous resection or decompression, realignment, and fusion. A vast array of spinal hardware systems has been developed to address the full spectrum of spinal disorders.[2, 3] In this chapter, the major indications, methods, instrument systems, and complications related to spinal surgery are reviewed. For a more comprehensive discussion of this complicated topic, the interested reader is referred to the references indicated.

## INTERVENTIONAL SPINAL PROCEDURES

A variety of nonoperative percutaneous interventional procedures have been devised for the treatment of back pain with or without leg pain, particularly in the lumbar region. These include radiofrequency coagulation or injections of local anesthetic agents or corticosteroids, or both, into the facet joints for back pain, epidural injections for leg pain, and percutaneous diskectomy or chymopapain chemonucleolysis for disc herniation.[4–9] Many of these techniques remain controversial and their role in the treatment of back or leg pain still has not been established clearly.

Injection of corticosteroids and anesthetic agents into the facet joints is used primarily to treat patients with a poorly defined clinical symptom complex referred to as the "facet syndrome."[4, 5, 10] The "facet syndrome" was named by Ghormley in 1933 and its importance as a cause of back pain became widely known through the work of Mooney and Robertson in 1976.[5, 10] The symptoms of the facet syndrome are nonspecific, consisting of pain in the low back, buttock, and thigh in the absence of sensory or motor neurologic deficit. Mooney and Robertson showed that this entire syndrome could be produced in normal volunteers by the injection of hypertonic saline solution into the facet joints.[5] The mechanism by which the facet joint causes pain is poorly understood, making specific diagnosis of the facet syndrome difficult. Postulated mechanisms include synovitis, mechanical entrapment of synovial fringes, joint distention with adjacent neural compression, adhesive capsulitis, segmental instability, and degenerative arthritis.[4–6, 8, 9, 11] In most cases, the facet syndrome is a diagnosis of exclusion. Radiologists generally have agreed that the radiographic appearance of the facet joints and the presence of degenerative osteoarthropathy are poorly correlated with the existence of facet joint pain. Part of the difficulty in assessing the role of facet joint arthrosis is the inability to evaluate these articulations reliably solely on the basis of plain films. The sensitivity of conventional radiographs for facet osteoarthrosis is low, particularly for mild or moderate disease.[12] Oblique radiographs, which are most sensitive for facet arthrosis, have a sensitivity of only 23 per cent for mild osteoarthrosis and underestimate significantly the degree of disease in moderate or severe degeneration of this joint.[12] Because clinical and radiographic findings are poor indicators of the exact site of facet arthropathy, typically multiple joints are injected at one sitting.

The specific explanation for the efficacy of facet joint

injection remains unknown.[4–6, 13] Most studies documenting successful response have used injection volumes of 3 to 6 ml into the facet joint, thereby producing sufficient capsular distention to cause rupture of the joint and produce extravasation.[4, 5, 9, 14] The normal capacity of the facet joint is only 1 to 2 ml.[4, 6] Injection of small volumes, less than 2 ml, prevents capsular rupture and subsequent extravasation into the epidural and periarticular spaces. Raymond and Dumas injected the facet joints in 25 patients with only 1 ml per joint and noted a dramatic reduction in therapeutic efficacy compared to the results of other investigators using larger volumes.[6] They suggested that capsular rupture, with subsequent epidural and periarticular diffusion, is a necessary component of a successful facet block.[6] Their data imply that a successful facet block after injection of a large volume does not constitute an indication for facet joint fusion because relief of discomfort may be due to extra-articular sources of pain in many patients.

The facet syndrome has remained a controversial entity because many of the early studies that showed improvement after facet joint injection were poorly designed and unblinded.[4, 13] Difficulty in establishing a precise diagnosis also makes it harder to interpret the success of facet injection therapy. Early studies suggested that short-term relief could be obtained in 59 to 94 per cent of patients and long-term benefits persisted in 20 to 54 per cent of patients injected.[4, 5, 9] More recent studies, including a large prospective randomized controlled trial comparing saline solution versus intra-articular anesthetic agents and steroids versus extra-articular anesthetic agents and steroids, have shown that a significant placebo effect exists and that many complex psychosocial factors are correlated with obtaining pain relief.[4, 13] Lilius and coauthors have shown that 36 per cent of patients receive long-term pain relief after facet joint injection, regardless of whether saline solution or medication is injected and irrespective of the exact site of injection.[13]

Facet joint injection is not limited to treatment of the facet syndrome. Injection of corticosteroids also has been used for the percutaneous treatment of symptomatic intraspinal synovial cysts.[15] These cysts or ganglia typically develop adjacent to a degenerated lumbar facet joint and communicate with the diseased joint, allowing simultaneous delivery of the pharmaceutical agent to the joint and cyst by facet injection.[11, 15] Bjorkengren and colleagues reported successful treatment of three patients with lumbar synovial cysts with this method, obtaining complete resolution of symptoms in two patients and partial resolution in the other.[15] Although one patient's cyst did decrease in size after the procedure, symptomatic relief was obtained even without significant change in the appearance or size of the cystic cavity.[15]

Epidural injection of saline solution, anesthetic agents, corticosteroids, or combinations of these agents also has been used to provide short-term, and sometimes permanent, relief of sciatica.[4, 16, 17] This technique, like facet block, remains controversial with highly variable success rates, ranging from 23 to 84 per cent, reported in the literature.[4, 6, 17] Most studies suggesting benefit from this technique have been poorly designed, lacking patient randomization, blinding, adequate control groups, and objective criteria for response.[17] Cuckler and associates evaluated epidural injec-

tion of steroids versus saline solution in a well-designed prospective, randomized double-blind trial and found no difference in efficacy between the two groups.[16, 17] The therapeutic effect noted in the group injected with saline solution may be related to distention due to the volume effect of the injection rather than to the delivery of any specific agent.

Epidural injection, unlike facet joint injection, has been associated with an array of serious complications. Epidural anesthesia has been implicated as a cause for intraspinal inflammatory lesions (such as arachnoiditis), subarachnoid cysts, and spinal cord abnormalities (such as surface irregularity, intramedullary cysts, and myelomalacia).[18] These complications presumably are due to inadvertent intradural injection, flow from the epidural into the intradural space, or a reaction to the preservative agents in the vials of anesthetic.[18] Hypercortisolism, aseptic meningitis, pyogenic and tuberculous meningitis, adhesive arachnoiditis, and sclerosing spinal pachymeningitis all have been related to the use of epidural steroids, presumably as a consequence of intradural steroid extravasation.[17, 19] To minimize these complications, epidural injection may be performed under fluoroscopic guidance.

The role of chemonucleolysis in the management of leg pain related to disc herniation also is controversial. Chemonucleolysis, also known as intradiscal nucleolysis, is performed by injecting a proteolytic or chondrolytic enzyme, such as chymopapain or collagenase, into the substance of a herniated disc.[7, 20] The technique was first used in humans in 1964 with chymopapain, derived from papain, an extract of papaya latex.[7] Collagenase was first used in clinical trials in 1981 and never achieved the widespread initial acceptance of chymopapain. Success rates for chymopapain chemonucleolysis initially were encouraging, typically ranging from 75 to 85 per cent.[20–23] These early high success rates were obtained in patients with radiculopathy due to a documented disc herniation. Much of the benefit from chemonucleolysis has been thought to result from the natural history of disc herniation, with symptomatic improvement in the majority of patients regardless of therapy. Decrease in the extent of disc herniation after the procedure has been documented, but similar findings of diminution in size of the herniated fragment also are seen in patients treated conservatively, without any specific chemolytic intervention.[24] More recently, randomized trials comparing chemonucleolysis with diskectomy in patients not responding to nonoperative therapy show that the failure rate at 1 year is significantly lower with the operative technique.[16]

Serious complications such as anaphylaxis, transverse myelitis with paraplegia, and subarachnoid hemorrhage, as well as a mortality rate of 0.02 per cent (identical to that of surgical diskectomy) have been reported with the use of chymopapain.[7, 20, 21] Sensitivity reactions to chymopapain develop in 1 to 5 per cent of patients; of these, approximately one quarter result in systemic anaphylaxis.[7, 8, 20, 21] Chymopapain chemonucleolysis is contraindicated in patients allergic to the enzyme or papaya, in patients who previously had been injected with chymopapain, in pregnant women, and in those with spinal stenosis or cauda equina syndrome.[21] The technique is not suitable for patients with nonspecific back pain or patients with disc herniation with sequestered fragments. The high complication rate has led to a marked reduction in the use of enzymatic chemonucleolysis.[23, 25]

Percutaneous diskectomy (PCD) has gained popularity as a nonsurgical treatment for herniated lumbar nucleus pulposus. Manual PCD, performed via a posterolateral lumbar approach using elongated rongeurs passed through a cannula, was first developed by Hijikata in 1975.[26] Initially most manual PCDs were performed through a cannula 4 mm or larger; common complications associated with a cannula this size were soft tissue bleeding and hematoma formation.[23] More serious complications associated with the manual PCD technique are discitis, occurring in approximately 1 per cent of patients, direct trauma to adjacent vascular structures, and neurologic injury, the last two particularly when general anesthesia is employed.[23]

Automated techniques also are available, which are easier technically and perhaps safer. Onik and coworkers are credited as the first authors to describe a fully automated percutaneous diskectomy system to remove disc material.[25, 27] The system they described used a 2.8 mm cannula through which a 2 mm cutting probe, known as the Nucleotome, is passed.[25, 27] The cutting probe uses a reciprocating suction cutter under continuous irrigation to remove disc fragments. Automated PCD appears to have a low complication rate, probably owing to the relatively small size of the cannula and the blunt tip of the distal end of the device, which prevents passage through the anterior annulus.[23] The most common serious complication associated with automated PCD appears to be discitis, but the prevalence of this complication is less than 1 per cent.[23]

Both manual and automated PCDs have acceptably low morbidity and mortality rates. One disadvantage of both techniques is the difficulty encountered in cannulating at L5-S1 owing to the steep angle necessary to clear the iliac crest.[23] Sequestered disc fragments are a contraindication for both techniques.[23, 25, 26] Success rates for PCD range from 53 to 87 per cent, compared to a successful outcome in over 90 per cent of properly selected patients undergoing microdiskectomy or limited surgical diskectomy.[23, 25, 26] The reason for the success of PCD is unclear; no laboratory data have been obtained that explain the pathophysiologic basis of the therapeutic response to PCD.[23] There does not appear to be any correlation between the quantity of disc removed and the therapeutic result.[25]

## DISKECTOMY AND DECOMPRESSION

Resection of bone is performed most commonly for decompression of spinal stenosis, for decompression of traumatic lesions, and to provide access to the disc for diskectomy. The extent of decompression or bone removal varies, depending on the clinical indication. Very small amounts of bone need to be removed to perform diskectomy in patients without central or foraminal stenosis. Extensive resection may be necessary in the patient with severe spinal canal impingement at multiple levels, which typically results from extensive degenerative spinal stenosis. Both anterior and posterior approaches are used. Decompression may be performed alone or combined with spinal fusion or spinal instrumentation (or with both) if immobilization is deemed necessary.

## Thoracic and Lumbar Spine

Laminotomy and laminectomy are resectional techniques typically employed for the removal of a herniated disc in the lumbar spine. The resection for access to a herniated disc often is unilateral because the majority of disc herniations are posterolateral and disc material can be removed easily through a unilateral defect, known as a laminotomy or hemilaminectomy. In a laminotomy, resection often is limited to the margins of the laminae (cephalic, caudal, or both), whereas the entire lamina from its cephalic to its caudal margin is resected during laminectomy.[28] Inadequate visualization, particularly through a very small or ''keyhole'' laminotomy, may result in inadequate decompression or intraoperative injury to the nerve root at the surgical site.[29–33] A laminotomy defect usually can be recognized on the anteroposterior radiograph by noting unilateral widening of the interlaminar space but often is difficult to identify on transaxial CT scans and MR images owing to the limited nature of the bone resection.[28] Even if the osseous defect is not apparent on cross-sectional imaging, loss of portions of the ligamentum flavum underlying the resection and distortion of the overlying soft tissues may be recognized.[34, 35] Hemilaminectomy is apparent readily on conventional radiography, CT scanning, and MR imaging due to the presence of a unilateral defect in the laminar bone. The major advantage of laminotomy versus laminectomy is less bone removal and, therefore, presumably a lower likelihood of postoperative instability.[29, 36, 37] Most surgeons agree that only the amount of bone necessary for adequate visualization should be resected for simple disc herniation.

Total laminectomy with foraminotomy or facetectomy is a more extensive resection than that required for simple disc excision. This procedure commonly is employed for the treatment of symptomatic lumbar stenosis. Unlike laminotomy and laminectomy for disc removal, the resection often is bilateral and includes resection of the spinous process, resulting in an unroofing of the spinal canal.[28] Foraminotomies typically involve removal of the medial half of the facet, preserving the interfacet joint and the pars interarticularis.[29] Foraminotomy results in loss of the normal width and obliquity of the inner margin of the facet, producing instead a narrowed facet with a straight medial border. The inferior tip of the facet may be truncated or the facet may be completely absent (facetectomy) when extensive resection has been performed (Fig. 18–1).

The facet joints and posterior intervertebral ligaments are the spine's principal posterior stabilizers; resection of the complete facet leads to increased likelihood of instability if an arthrodesis is not carried out simultaneously.[38, 39] A few authors have suggested that the extent of decompression does not correlate with the presence of postoperative slippage but most surgeons consider facetectomy to be a destabilizing procedure.[40] Patients with underlying degenerative spondylolisthesis appear to be at highest risk for progressive instability after decompressive surgery.[40] Wide fenestration, consisting of removal of only the medial parts of the inferior facets and adjoining ligamenta flava, has been advocated as an alternative method of decompression for spinal stenosis.[39] In a wide fenestration, the interlaminar bone is removed only when the central spinal canal is narrow. Many patients with symptoms of stenosis of the spinal canal are relieved of symptoms even if the laminae

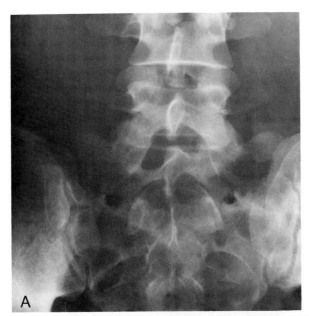

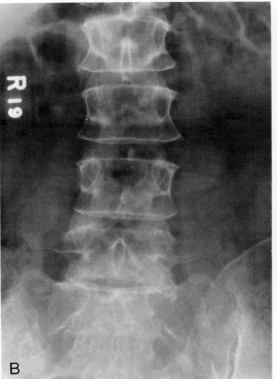

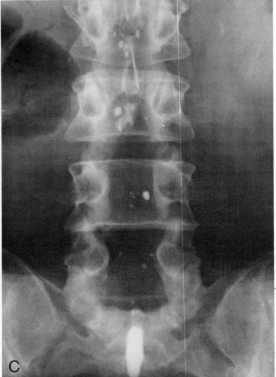

**FIGURE 18–1.** Resection and decompression procedures.

**A** A hemilaminotomy defect is seen at the cranial aspect of the right lamina of a transitional L5 vertebra.

**B** The inferior facet of L3 has been resected on the left side and the tip of the superior facet of L4 has become truncated after foraminotomy of the left L3-L4 neural foramen for stenosis.

**C** Extensive resection of the posterior elements with uproofing of the spinal canal for spinal stenosis is seen. Note the absence of the spinous processes, laminae (laminectomy), and large portions of the facets in the lower lumbar spine.

are not resected completely.[39] This operation is not used in patients who already have degenerative spondylolisthesis but may prevent instability in patients with focal spinal stenosis and normal alignment.

Thinning of the inferior articular facet at the site of facetectomy predisposes this structure to the development of a postoperative stress fracture. Typical symptoms include new pain, local tenderness, pain on rotational movements, and relief with recumbency.[41] The most common locations for postfacetectomy fractures are the pars interarticularis and the inferior tip of the facet; less common locations include the lamina and spinous process.[42] Zinreich and collaborators found postoperative fractures in over 15 per cent of patients with postsurgical failed back syndrome; the majority in their series involved the pars interarticularis.[42] Rothman and coworkers, using reformatted CT in patients with prior lumbar surgery, found the pars to be intact in their patients but noted the presence of a horizontal fracture at the base of the inferior facet in 6 per cent of patients[41] (Fig. 18–2). Both fractures are difficult to visualize radiographically and may be confused with each other on CT scans unless careful attention is paid to the exact site and orientation of the fracture line. With CT, both pars and facet fractures are difficult to detect on transaxial images alone so these areas should be carefully assessed on sagittal and coronal reconstructions.[41]

The extent of decompression necessary for the successful management of spinal stenosis is highly variable and depends on the extent of disease. Imaging plays a key role in detecting, defining the extent and cause of, and localizing areas of stenosis. Lumbar spinal stenosis is produced by osseous or soft tissue-induced narrowing of the spinal canal, lateral recess, or intervertebral foramen.[29, 37, 43] Experimental data based on an animal model of lumbar stenosis suggest that constriction of the spinal canal of more than 50 per cent is the critical point that results in neurologic deficits and histologic abnormalities.[44] Classification of lumbar stenosis into congenital or acquired groups as well as categorization by level, location, and underlying pathologic condition is based on a combination of clinical, electromyographic, and radiographic parameters.[29, 43, 44]

In a patient with single-level stenosis, adequate surgical treatment includes removal of sufficient portions of the laminae, and often of the medial aspects of the facet joints, to cause decompression. Laminotomies of the superior and inferior vertebrae may be adequate; in selected cases a complete laminectomy may be avoided.[29] Multilevel stenosis necessitates more extensive surgery, with resection of all laminar and facet bone in the areas of stenosis.[29] The majority of patients with lumbar stenosis severe enough to warrant surgery require multilevel decompression. In Hall and colleagues' series of 68 patients undergoing decompressive laminectomy, only 19 had decompression of two or fewer levels.[43]

Postoperative vertebral subluxation is the most common complication encountered in patients after extensive decompressive surgery of the posterior thoracic or lumbar region.[29, 38, 40] Spinal deformities occurring after multiple laminectomies are most likely to develop in the growing child. The skeletally immature person has a 50 per cent rate of occurrence of cervicothoracic or thoracic kyphosis after posterior decompressive surgery.[38] In the adult, risk factors for postoperative instability include underlying degenerative spondylolisthesis, advanced age, primary neural disorder, rheumatoid arthritis, or recurrent trauma.[29, 30] Underlying degenerative spondylolisthesis appears to be the most significant risk factor. The prevalence of postoperative instability in patients with preexisting anterolisthesis approaches 65 per cent.[29] Most patients with preexisting spondylolisthesis are elderly women, in whom malalignment is approximately twice as frequent as in men.[40]

Patients deemed to be at high risk for instability after decompressive lumbar laminectomy typically undergo fusion with posterolateral or intertransverse bone grafting at the time of operation.[29, 37, 39] Numerous internal fixation devices have become available that are designed to prevent further subluxation while the bone fusion is consolidating.[29] Herkowitz and Kurz evaluated the postoperative results in 50 patients with single-level spinal stenosis associated with degenerative lumbar spondylolisthesis.[36] Half of the patients underwent decompression and intertransverse fusion with cortical and corticocancellous iliac crest graft; the others had an identical decompression but no fusion. Herkowitz and Kurz noted a 36 per cent rate of pseudarthrosis in their patients undergoing intertransverse fusion after decompression of single-level lumbar spinal stenosis.[36] Despite this high pseudarthrosis rate, long-term follow-up showed significantly better overall results, with less leg pain and less progression of anterolisthesis, in the 25 patients undergoing fusion.[36]

On the basis of a review of all studies of operative intervention for lumbar stenosis published in the previous decade, Katz and associates reported that success rates ranged from 64 to 95 per cent.[37] Many studies, however, were based on short follow-up periods, inexplicit criteria,

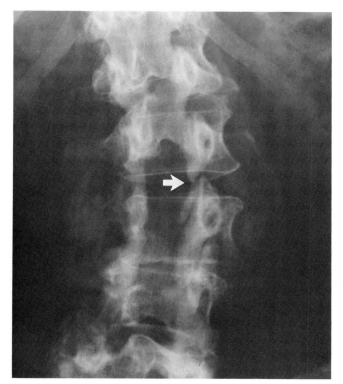

**FIGURE 18–2.** Facet fracture. A horizontal fracture of the caudal tip of the left L2 inferior facet (arrow) has occurred after foraminotomy. The defect developed several years after foraminotomy.

and physician rather than patient assessments.[37] From the results of a long-term study, Katz and coauthors concluded that the benefits of operation deteriorate over time, particularly in patients with coexisting morbid conditions, such as rheumatoid arthritis, osteoarthritis, cardiovascular disease, and chronic pulmonary disease.[37] The advanced age of most patients undergoing decompressive surgery for spinal stenosis results in a high rate of postoperative complications, particularly if an arthrodesis is performed.[45]

Tears of the dura are not uncommon during resectional surgery. Failure to recognize normal anatomic variants, such as spina bifida occulta or the normal wide interlaminar space between L5 and S1, can lead to inadvertent tearing of the dura and entry into the spinal canal.[46] Dural tears generally are detected and repaired at the time of operation; small undetected dural leaks typically heal spontaneously, but large leaks may persist and form large paraspinal fluid collections[1, 30, 34, 47, 48] (Fig. 18–3). Postoperative pseudomeningocele is an uncommon complication resulting from a chronic unrecognized or incompletely repaired dural tear.[31, 49, 50] The prevalence of postoperative pseudomeningocele (also known as extradural pseudocyst, iatrogenic meningocele, and postoperative diverticulum) is difficult to establish. Reported prevalence rates range from 0.07 to 2 per cent.[1, 49]

There are no specific plain film or tomographic findings of a postoperative pseudomeningocele. Prior to the introduction of CT and MR imaging, the diagnosis was established by myelography on noting filling of a cavity with contrast material posterior to the surgical laminectomy site. Currently, the diagnosis is established with CT or MR imaging. With CT the pseudomeningocele appears as a rounded mass of low attenuation posterior to the thecal sac; the margin typically consists of a well-defined rim of higher attenuation due to pseudocapsule formation.[49] This appearance must be distinguished from the normal anteroposterior elongation and minimal outpouching of an intact thecal sac through a bilateral laminectomy defect.[28, 34, 49] With MR imaging, the signal intensity of the collection corresponds

to that of cerebrospinal fluid, although increased signal intensity may be seen in cases complicated by hemorrhage.[35] In the majority of cases, communication between the collection and the thecal sac can be established by noting passage of myelographic contrast material from the thecal sac into the collection, although the passage may be delayed or absent in some cases owing to healing of the dural tear.[34, 49]

Major vascular injury may occur during lumbar diskectomy if the anterior longitudinal ligament is disrupted, allowing passage of surgical instruments into the retroperitoneal space.[32, 51, 52] Intraoperative lateral radiographs may underestimate the risk of annular rupture because of the curvature of the anterior disc margin and the presence of magnification.[53] Up to 75 per cent of cases of vascular damage involve a major artery; 10 to 20 per cent of cases develop an arteriovenous fistula, typically between the common iliac artery and vein.[51, 52]

Decompression also is used occasionally for the management of fractures and dislocations leading to spinal canal compromise. Realignment alone may obviate the need for decompressive surgery in the majority of cases. Considerable controversy exists over the relative merits of anterior versus posterior approaches and over the benefits of concomitant fusion and instrumentation if decompression is necessary. Nowhere is this controversy more evident than in the debate over the optimal management of the burst fracture with neurologic deficit caused by retropulsed bone. Decompression by simple laminectomy, posterolateral decompression with removal of bone fragments, distraction rodding, anterior decompression, and anterior decompression with instrumentation all have been used for the management of this common injury.[54–57] Decompression by laminectomy is associated with a high risk of kyphosis and instability and is not recommended.[54, 58] Some decompression is accomplished by posterior distraction alone, presumably because of an intact posterior longitudinal ligament realigning the retropulsed fracture fragments.[57, 59] However, distraction rodding alone often does not provide adequate osseous decompression or realignment of these injuries.[56, 57, 60–62] Posterior and posterolateral decompression of retropulsed bone fragments, combined with application of hardware, may be necessary.[50, 55, 57, 61] The major advantage of posterior decompression is that it can be performed at the same time as posterior stabilization and instrumentation.

Some authors advocate anterior decompression for burst fractures as the direct visualization of both the anterior and the middle spinal columns facilitates adequate decompression.[58, 63–65] Anterior grafting, anterior hardware application, or use of posterior instruments may be employed to provide stability after the anterior decompression. Anterior strut grafting or some other form of stabilization typically is necessary after adequate anterior decompression as the vertebral body is so comminuted that it acts as a "vacant space," providing no support for the anterior column.[59] The major disadvantage of anterior decompression combined with posterior hardware application is the longer operating time and the frequent need to perform two separate operations, even though they may be performed successively, without delay, in selected cases.

The anterior approach for thoracic and lumbar spinal decompression was described first in 1934 but did not become popular until the 1950s, when it was employed for

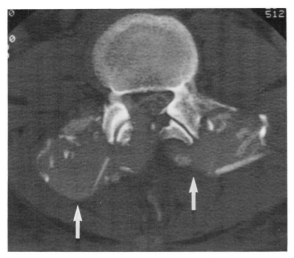

**FIGURE 18–3.** Dural tear. A transaxial CT scan obtained after the administration of intrathecal contrast agent demonstrates a leak of cerebrospinal fluid into the paraspinal soft tissues (arrows). Immature bone graft is present from the recent laminectomy and fusion procedure.

decompression of tuberculous spondylitis producing paraplegia.[63] Anterior decompression now is employed for fractures, infection, and rigid kyphosis, and for debridement of neoplasm.[63] Decompression of degenerative spondylosis in the thoracic and lumbar regions is performed via the posterior approach as previously discussed. In the thoracolumbar and lumbar regions, anterior decompression is destabilizing and requires some type of fusion to achieve stability. Single-level upper thoracic surgery, such as decompression of a herniated thoracic disc, may not require arthrodesis because of the stability afforded by the rib cage and the limited resection that typically is required.[66]

### Cervical Spine

Unlike the lumbar region, access to herniated cervical discs via the posterior approach is limited significantly because of the presence of the spinal cord. The anterior approach is preferred for management of cervical disc disease when concomitant diskectomy and fusion are performed. Laminectomy typically is reserved for patients requiring decompression for cervical spinal stenosis and usually is performed at multiple levels. Cervical spondylitic myelopathy is multifactional, being due to a combination of progressive degenerative cervical spondylosis, direct spinal cord compression, cord ischemia, and, often, an underlying congenitally narrow spinal canal.[67] The functional diameter of the canal is narrowed in both flexion and extension; this dynamic compression, in conjunction with abnormal exaggerated motion at the spondylitic level, has been employed to support the use of routine fusion in conjunction with decompression in the management of patients with severe spondylitic myelopathy.[67]

Extensive cervical laminectomy for decompression of myelopathy without adequate fusion can lead to progressive subluxation and kyphosis, producing a ''swan-neck'' deformity[68] (Fig. 18–4). This deformity rarely is seen after a single-level laminectomy or after multiple unilateral hemilaminectomies. Presumably it is the result of loss of posterior ligamentous and osseous stability, aggravated by con-

comitant muscle weakness.[68] Anterior fusion typically is necessary for correction, although this may be technically difficult when the deformity is severe. Laminoplasty was developed to prevent this postoperative complication; this technique widens the canal and theoretically maintains stability.

Anterior cervical decompression with fusion is advocated for the management of patients with neurologic deficit after traumatic injury to the cervical region resulting in spinal cord compression by anteriorly located bone or disc fragments.[69–71] Improvement in neurologic function has been documented in 81 per cent of patients with incomplete quadriplegia, and functional return of at least one motor root has been observed in 54 per cent of those with complete quadriplegia after adequate anterior surgery.[70, 71]

## SPINAL FUSION WITHOUT INSTRUMENTATION

Intervertebral fusion of the spine using bone graft first was attempted in 1911, after a few unsuccessful attempts to stabilize the spine with silk, silver wire, celluloid bars, and steel bars.[72–75] The first successful spinal fusions with bone graft were reported independently by Albee[74] and Hibbs.[75] Both authors described the use of autologous bone graft applied to the posterior thoracolumbar spine for the treatment of tuberculous gibbus deformity.[74, 75] Since that time, numerous reports have been published on the use of bone graft and other materials, placed anteriorly, posteriorly, or at both sites, at all spinal levels to achieve spinal fusion. Cotler and associates have summarized the four general reasons for performing an arthrodesis of the spine. These include (1) prevention of progressive spinal deformity; (2) maintenance of corrected deformity; (3) reestablishment of spinal stability; and (4) elimination of pain caused by motion between spinal segments.[3] Spinal fusion may be carried out alone or combined with decompressive surgery or application of spinal hardware, or both.

### Graft Materials

The graft material used most commonly for achieving spinal fusion is bone, whether it be autograft or allograft.[76] Autograft may be obtained from numerous anatomic regions, with the iliac crest being the site used most widely. The ilium offers a variety of osseous contours and is a source for cortical, corticocancellous, and cancellous graft harvest. The main advantages of autograft are histocompatibility, availability, and high osteogenic potential owing to the presence of viable osteoprogenitor cells.[3, 77] Banked allograft bone is used when the patient's own bone stock is of limited quantity or of poor quality, usually as a consequence of metabolic bone disease or previous surgical harvesting. The use of allograft decreases operative time and eliminates the risk of donor site complications, particularly hemorrhage in patients with cardiovascular compromise or graft collapse in patients with severe osteoporosis.[45, 77–79] The major disadvantages of allografts are potential for transmission of disease, a slower rate of vascularization, failure of incorporation (nonunion), and higher rates of collapse.[78] Anterior fusions with allografts tend to have a better incorporation rate than posterior fusions with this material. Higher fusion rates are achieved with autogenous

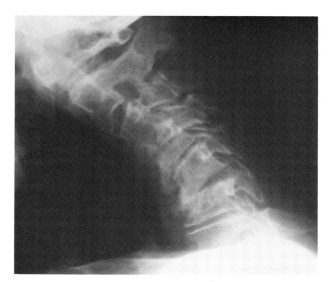

**FIGURE 18–4.** Postlaminectomy kyphosis. Severe cervical kyphosis has occurred after laminectomies at C5 and C6 for degenerative spondylosis. Disc space loss is seen at multiple cervical levels.

bone than with allograft; xenografts have the lowest fusion rate.[76] Kiel bone (bovine source), the most widely studied xenograft, rarely undergoes osseous union but does serve as a scaffold for dense fibrous tissue.[80]

The initial bone grafts that were used consisted of cortical or corticocancellous strips derived from autologous spinous processes removed at the time of operation. In 1933, Ghormley developed the technique of using autogenous iliac crest cancellous bone for use in lumbosacral fusion.[72] Porous cancellous grafts are revascularized rapidly by osteoblastic laying down of new bone on preexisting trabeculae. Incorporation of cancellous grafts typically is complete by 6 months.[81] In 1933, Burns described the use of an autologous cortical tibial strut graft employing an anterior approach for the reduction and fusion of a high grade spondylolisthesis at L5-S1 in an adolescent boy.[82] The use of strong cortical strut grafts to obtain immediate stability continues but iliac crest, rib, or fibular constructs have replaced the tibia as the major graft source. The use of vascularized strut grafts derived from autologous rib also has been reported.[76, 80]

Cortical grafts, although they are stronger mechanically, are revascularized more slowly than cancellous bone. Revascularization takes place via the existing haversian system and bone exterior.[77] Long strut grafts have a slower incorporation rate than short segment fusions. Solid union of cortical grafts may take up to 2 years to develop and nonunion rates for rib or fibular strut grafts range from 8 to 37 per cent.[76, 77] Fibular grafts are the slowest grafts to incorporate and are quite weak at their distal ends approximately 6 months after insertion, when revascularization is beginning.[63, 81] After the ends have incorporated, the central region is relatively weakened and more prone to fracture.

Major complications related to harvest sites for autologous graft include fracture of the underlying bone when a large amount of bone has been harvested, infection, and damage of overlying soft tissue structures. Removal of large bicortical bone graft, particularly when associated with splitting of the inner and outer tables of the ilium, predisposes the bone to fracture.[79, 83] Infection at the graft site may be associated with infection at the site of spinal fusion, presumably due to simultaneous contamination of both sites.[79, 84] Anterior iliac crest harvesting can produce cosmetic deformity and damage the lateral femoral cutaneous nerve or the lateral branch of the hypogastric nerve, producing anterolateral thigh numbness and pain.[79, 85] Posterior iliac crest graft harvest can produce gait disturbance from gluteal weakness and sacroiliac joint instability. Other complications associated with iliac crest harvest include hematoma formation and persistent local pain.[3, 79] Fibular graft harvest is associated commonly with leg pain, which may persist for a long time, and less frequently with damage to the overlying soft tissue structures.[85] Ankle and knee joint dysfunction can be avoided by using only the middle third of the fibular diaphysis for the graft.

Nonosseous sources of graft material include polymethylmethacrylate (PMMA), which is used widely for reconstruction after debridement or resection of spinal neoplasms, bioactive ceramic spacers, and manufactured hydroxyapatite bone graft substitutes.[76, 86–89] Other substances under investigation as bone graft substitutes include tricalcium phosphate, demineralized bone matrix, and bone morphogenetic protein.[3]

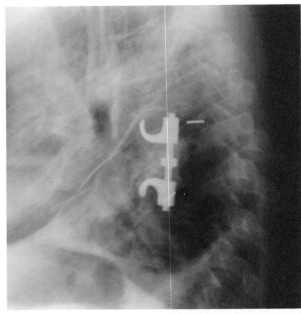

**FIGURE 18–5.** Methylmethacrylate fixation. A lateral view of the midthoracic spine demonstrates placement of methylmethacrylate after corpectomy. A distraction Knodt rod also has been placed to augment the construct. Note the characteristic central nut on the Knodt rod.

PMMA is a resinous acrylic material formed by mixing its liquid and powder components at the time of operation.[90] PMMA is used most widely after corpectomy and debridement of spinal neoplasms, particularly metastatic disease.[76, 88] It is strongest in compression but does not resist tension so that this material frequently is used in the anterior spinal regions. PMMA can be molded to any desired shape, and its material properties are unaffected by radiation and chemotherapy, both of which are known to inhibit bone healing.[76] Use of PMMA alone or, more typically, PMMA in conjunction with metallic internal fixation and bone grafting, facilitates early mobilization of the patient with a malignant lesion[76, 88] (Fig. 18–5). This substance also has been used for fixation after trauma and to fill osseous defects created by severe osteoporosis or rheumatoid arthritis or defects caused by previous instrument insertion or loosening prior to reinstrumentation.[80, 91–94]

The major disadvantages of PMMA include increased rates of infection and mechanical loosening. Mechanical loosening is common because the material interdigitates only with native bone and never undergoes incorporation. Gradual resorption at the bone-cement interface, leading to loss of fixation and subsequent extrusion of the construct, is the most frequent complication, accounting for over 80 per cent of cases of PMMA failure.[76, 88] Resorption at the bone-acrylic interface with subsequent loosening typically occurs within 1 year; therefore, PMMA fixation is recommended only as a salvage technique in patients with a short life expectancy.[88, 92] Infection of PMMA is common because of its suppression of leukocyte function and, unlike infection of bone graft or metallic hardware, requires extensive debridement and removal of the material, which is considerably more difficult to remove in toto than metal constructs.[92, 95] The substance appears homogeneous and has a density similar to that of soft tissue on conventional radiographs. Radiopaque material, typically barium, is added to the PMMA during manufacture to render it more easy to visualize radiographically. Loosening prior to shifting or extrusion often is difficult to detect because of the irregular, undulating margins of the construct. PMMA exhibits inhomogeneity on CT scans, in which entrapped air bubbles also may be apparent in intact noninfected graft; in MR images, PMMA exhibits signal void with all sequences.[90]

Synthetic or manufactured hydroxyapatite grafts have been developed for use as bone graft substitutes. Bone graft substitutes derived from the calcium carbonate exoskeleton of certain varieties of sea coral, which has been converted into porous hydroxyapatite, have become available commercially.[86, 87] Although these implants lack the osteoprogenitor cells and bone-producing factors found in viable autologous bone, they do serve as an effective nonantigenic scaffolding for bone ingrowth and incorporation.[87] Some of these constructs have little inherent mechanical stability, which precludes their use in situations in which they must bear large structural loads.[86] Once incorporated, however, their structural strength is stronger than that of bone.[86] On initial radiographs, the implants appear much denser than normal bone and do not exhibit the organized, linear trabecular pattern of bone-based graft materials (Fig. 18–6). As the graft is incorporated, loss of its homogeneous architecture and marginal irregularities are seen.[86]

## Thoracic and Lumbar Spine

Hibbs performed the first spinal arthrodesis in the United States in 1911, when he used strips of autologous spinous process bone placed over posterior elements denuded of cartilage to fuse the posterior thoracic and lumbar vertebral joints.[75] In the same year, Albee reported the use of cortical tibial graft laid into sagittal clefts created in the thoracolumbar spinous processes.[74] Albee's procedure was popular for some time but was soon replaced by the more successful Hibbs fusion.[72] Hibbs midline fusion technique and its subsequent modifications remained the standard spinal fusion operation for over half a century.[72] The posterior approach still remains the standard method of obtaining fusion in the thoracic and lumbar regions, but the site of fusion has been modified. Currently, most lumbar arthrodeses are performed posterolaterally, adjacent to the posterior elements rather than in the midline. Midline posterior fusion does not allow decompression, has a symptomatic pseudarthrosis rate of 20 to 30 per cent and now is rarely used as an isolated procedure.[32] Posterolateral fusions are performed either posterior to the transverse processes (intertransverse fusion) or overlying the posterolateral surfaces of the facet joint and lamina (interlaminar fusion), or both fusions are done.

Anterior interbody fusions are performed much less frequently than the standard posterolateral arthrodesis. Interbody fusions at the level of the lumbar intervertebral disc can be performed using either an anterior or a posterior approach. Interbody grafting of the lumbar spine via a posterior approach, known as a posterior lumbar interbody fusion (PLIF), was developed to provide more stable fixation than could be achieved by posterior graft alone. In 1944, Briggs and Milligan reported the use of a round bone peg derived from the spinous process to perform a PLIF after decompression and diskectomy for degenerative disc

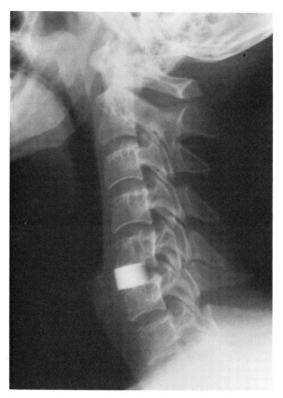

**FIGURE 18–6.** Hydroxyapatite graft. An interbody coralline-based hydroxyapatite graft is seen at C5-C6. Anterior distraction is present at the surgical level in this patient, producing hyperlordosis and narrowing of the interlaminar distance.

disease.[96] They performed a combined interbody and posterior fusion and were able to obtain osseous union in most cases. In the late 1940s, similar techniques were reported by numerous authors, particularly by Cloward, and PLIFs became widely used in the lower lumbar spine.[51, 72, 97]

A variety of materials have been used for PLIF fusions, the most common being autologous bone in the form of tricortical or cortical cylindrical dowels, usually cut from the ilium.[98] Large iliac strut grafts also may be used to obtain more stable immediate fixation. Fibular strut grafts similarly have been inserted using a posterior approach for spondyloptosis and offer superior strength in comparison to the standard iliac corticocancellous grafts.[99–101] More recently, PLIFs using metallic fixation devices placed at the level of the disc space have been described[98] (Fig. 18–7). These devices currently are experimental and their role in obtaining spinal fusion has not yet been established. PLIF can be combined with rigid posterior hardware, such as pedicle screw fixation.[97]

Anterior interbody fusions are used when anterior decompression is necessary or when the posterior elements are grossly insufficient and to augment inadequate or incomplete posterior fusions. Anterior surgical approaches to the thoracic and lumbar spine initially were developed for the treatment of tuberculous abscesses.[72] The primary purpose of these early anterior operations was decompression and debridement, not fusion. In the 1930s, reports began to appear describing anterior interbody grafting of the lumbar spine for fusion of isthmic spondylolisthesis.[72, 82] Several reports outlining the use of cortical and cancellous grafting

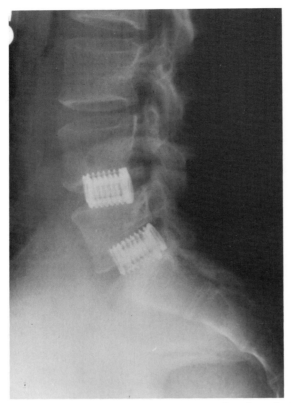

**FIGURE 18–7.** Posterior lumbar interbody fusion. Ray Cage fixation devices are seen at L4-L5 and L5-S1. These cylindrical devices are embedded in the vertebral bodies and allow for bone ingrowth.

necessary for successful incorporation.[83] The interbody graft should appear rectangular, as wedge-shaped grafts that are taller anteriorly tend to extrude owing to spinal hyperextension[83] (Fig. 18–8). Minor degrees of graft protrusion anterior to the vertebral margin tend to resorb spontaneously and do not cause any major problems. Cortical strut grafts are used when multilevel vertebral body resection is performed. Because of the high mechanical stresses in this region, all types of strut grafts used in the thoracic and lumbar regions have been reported to fracture or collapse.[76] Rib grafts, particularly when they span long segments, are considerably weaker than fibular grafts, but both can fracture when exposed to the forces generated, particularly at the thoracolumbar and lumbar regions.[76, 80]

Anterior thoracic and lumbar approaches are associated with a variety of complications. Along with failure of the graft itself, complications related to the adjacent vascular, neural, and visceral structures may be encountered.[85, 102, 103] Vascular complications are rare but are most likely to occur in patients with preexisting vascular abnormalities such as aneurysm, pseudoaneurysm, other underlying anomalies, or extensive calcific atherosclerosis.[85] Injury to the thoracic duct with resultant chylothorax also is rare but has a 50 per cent mortality rate unless recognized and managed appropriately[104] (Fig. 18–9). Neural injury is uncommon but may lead to dysfunction, often temporary, of the lumbosacral plexus, parasympathetic paraspinous lumbar chain, sympathetic plexus, or, rarely, cauda equina owing to direct penetration of the spinal canal.[85, 103] Visceral injuries to the pleura, diaphragm, peritoneum, ureter, and intrathoracic and intra-abdominal organs, also can occur during the anterior lumbar approach.[83, 85, 102]

anteriorly in the thoracic and lumbar regions appeared before any similar methods were developed in the cervical region.[72] Single-level intervertebral fusions typically are performed by the placement of a cancellous or corticocancellous interbody graft. Anterior interbody grafts tend to show some settling prior to fusion; this settling may be

## Cervical Spine

The objectives of surgical fusion of the cervical spine are to obtain and maintain physiologic alignment, eliminate excessive motion, correct or prevent instability, and avoid the development of kyphotic deformity.[3, 105] Anterior, pos-

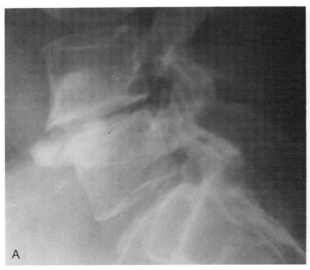

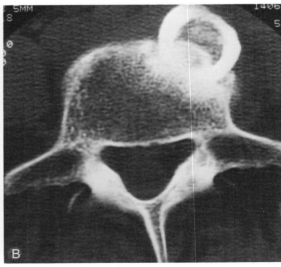

**FIGURE 18–8.** Graft extrusion.
**A** Anterior extrusion of an L4-L5 interbody graft is present.
**B** The transaxial CT scan demonstrates the extruded graft extending anterolaterally to the vertebral margin. This graft was left in situ and developed resorption of the extruded region, followed by fusion.

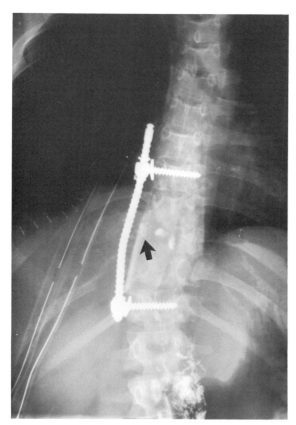

**FIGURE 18–9.** Thoracic duct tear. Anterior strut graft and Edwards universal rod (older version) with Kostuik screws were placed for a fracture-dislocation at T10-T11. The patient developed a chylothorax postoperatively. A lymphangiogram demonstrates extravasation at the surgical site (arrow) due to an iatrogenic tear of the thoracic duct.

terior or combined approaches all are used. In contrast to the lumbar region, simple bone grafting is employed more commonly using an anterior interbody approach rather than a posterior one. Grafting alone rarely is sufficient for posterior stabilization, so posterior grafting typically is combined with use of some form of metallic hardware to provide stability until the graft incorporates.

Anterior operative approaches to the cervical spine, as for the thoracic and lumbar regions, initially were developed for debridement of granulomatous abscess and for biopsy and resection of neoplasms.[71] Anterior interbody fusions subsequently were devised primarily for the treatment of cervical spondylosis and degenerative disc disease. The first major series of anterior fusions was described by Robinson and Smith in 1955, who performed anterior removal of the degenerated intervertebral cervical disc, followed by anterior bone grafting to obtain interbody fusion.[106] In 1958, the anterior approach for removal of degenerated discs and interbody fusion was further popularized by Cloward, who emphasized the concomitant removal of symptomatic osteophytes using this approach.[107] Since that time, anterior fusions have undergone only minor modifications but their indications have broadened to include traumatic lesions, cervical stenosis, inflammatory arthropathies, ligamentous ossification, and many other pathologic cervical conditions requiring an anterior decompression.

Some controversy exists over whether single-level diskectomy requires interbody fusion, although many surgeons routinely graft such cases. Anterior intervertebral grafting is considered essential after anterior multilevel decompression to restore spinal stability and function.[76] In patients with multiple levels of disc degeneration, interbody grafts can be used at all operated levels, or strut grafting may be employed. Anterior cervical fusion typically is performed by placing corticocancellous autologous bone grafts in the region of the intervertebral disc after removal of a degenerated disc and any significant osteophytes. The graft functions as a mechanical spacer that maintains or increases disc height and also distracts the neural foramina, decreasing the compressive effect of foraminal osteophytes.[81] The most commonly used anterior methods of placing bone grafts are the Smith-Robinson, keystone (Simmons, Bailey-Badgley), and Cloward techniques. The most widely used is the tricortical Smith-Robinson graft that is obtained from the iliac crest. The graft is horseshoe shaped and is placed with the cortices directed anteriorly and laterally. The Smith-Robinson graft can be seen easily on the lateral radiograph as a rectangular wedge of corticocancellous bone that fits snugly between the intact endplates.[105] Fracture, collapse, and extrusion of the Smith-Robinson graft are minimized by making it at least 6 mm (preferably 8 to 9 mm) high, 2 mm higher than the degenerated disc, preparing the endplates parallel to each other, and countersinking the graft 2 mm posterior to the anterior vertebral body cortex.[76, 80, 103] The Cloward graft is larger, consisting of a circular dowel that is of cortical bone on the outside and of cancellous bone centrally, which projects into the vertebral body through indistinct endplates.[105, 107] The cortical ends are directed anteriorly and posteriorly so that the circular cortical contour of the graft and the slightly larger defect in the adjacent vertebral endplates and bodies are most apparent on the anteroposterior projection. The Cloward procedure allows the surgeon to perform a more extensive resection of the vertebral body and associated osteophytosis than the standard Smith-Robinson procedure.[105] The Bailey-Badgley graft is a rectangular corticocancellous graft that is inlaid into a trough fashioned in the anterior portion of the vertebral bodies.[108] It also allows for resection of vertebral endplates and osteophytes. In vitro testing suggests that the horseshoe configured Smith-Robinson graft is stronger and exhibits more initial stability than the strut or dowel graft.[109] The strength of the Smith-Robinson method is due to the configuration of the graft and, more importantly, the preservation of intact vertebral endplates.[109] The Cloward graft is the weakest and also the most likely to become extruded.[80, 109] Cervical strut grafts are used after corpectomy and allow for replacement of one or multiple vertebral bodies. Anterior strut grafting or augmentation with posterior fusion often is necessary when multilevel decompression is performed in myelopathic patients with severe cervical kyphosis, whether it be due to spondylosis, trauma, or previous laminectomy.[69, 110] Unlike multiple interbody grafting, long segment strut grafting is mechanically stable immediately and is not as prone to the development of late kyphosis.[110] The strut grafts typically are derived from the iliac crest, rib, or fibula.[80] Fibular grafts are stronger but incorporate slowly; typically they are reserved for patients undergoing vertebrectomy at more than three levels.[103, 108] These grafts are best seen on the lateral projection, appear-

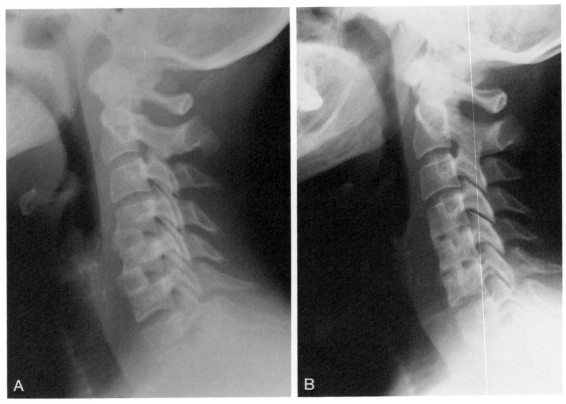

**FIGURE 18–10.** Graft collapse.
  **A** The postoperative radiograph shows Smith-Robinson grafts at C4-C5 and C5-C6.
  **B** The follow-up radiograph demonstrates loss of volume of the graft due to intrabody collapse. Loss of disc space distraction also has occurred.

ing as a rectangular strut of mature bone bridging the disc spaces and resting in notches in the intact vertebral bodies at the margins of the surgical site.[105, 108] Mechanical causes of anterior cervical graft failure can include graft fracture, collapse, resorption or frank extrusion.[76, 80] Fracture and collapse of cervical grafts are less common than in the lower spine. Autograft from osteopenic bone has little structural strength and can fracture or fragment.[76] When the graft is stronger than the vertebral endplate, it may collapse into the vertebral body, resulting in increased deformity.[80] Intravertebral collapse also is more common when the vertebral endplates have been disrupted during diskectomy or osteophyte removal (Fig. 18–10). Allograft varies in its strength, but the overall prevalence of allograft collapse appears to be higher than with autograft.[103]

Graft extrusion is a common complication, occurring in 1 to 13 per cent of patients, related to inadequate compression across the graft, failure of the graft, or failure of its interface with the adjacent vertebrae.[76, 103] This complication is seen most frequently in highly mobile spinal regions, such as the lower cervical and thoracolumbar regions. Extrusion typically is anterior or anterolateral, with resultant kyphosis (Fig. 18–11). Anterior graft extrusion in the cervical region can result in serious complications related to tracheal, esophageal, or vascular compromise.[80, 103] Posterior extrusion is rare but can produce compression of the spinal cord.

Postoperative kyphosis due to unrecognized posterior instability is a major cause of interbody graft failure and unsuccessful clinical outcome.[80, 105, 111] Posterior ligamentous incompetence is caused most frequently by trauma or postsurgical changes associated with decompressive procedures. Anterior fusion has been recommended as the optimal method of treatment of cervical burst fractures associated with neurologic deficit. Postoperative graft displacement, reangulation with loss of alignment, and progressive neurologic deficit may develop in patients with posterior ligamentous damage after an anterior operation alone.[111] Sequential or simultaneous anterior and posterior fusion may be necessary in patients with anterior deformities and posterior ligamentous instability producing neurologic deficit.[69]

It is extremely difficult to determine if successful interbody fusion for cervical spondylosis accelerates degenerative disease at adjacent disc levels owing to diminished motion at the fusion site and increased compensatory motion at adjacent levels. Progressive degenerative disease is seen in the majority of patients at long-term follow-up, typically below the fusion mass, but whether or not these changes are related to the biomechanical alterations produced by fusion is difficult to determine[112] (Fig. 18–12). Although many surgeons think that there is a risk for accelerated spondylosis after fusion, an adequate study that supports this opinion is not available. Lack of patient randomization and inability to define an adequate control group in long-term series evaluating spinal fusion make it difficult to separate surgically induced changes from the normal aging process. Gore and associates evaluated 90 patients at

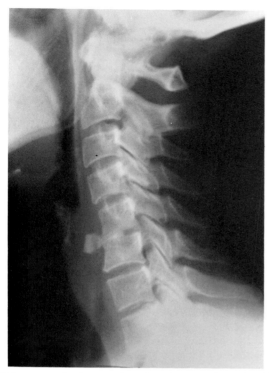

**FIGURE 18–11.** Graft extrusion. Anterior extrusion of a C5-C6 Smith-Robinson graft, loss of disc height, and mild focal kyphosis are present at the surgical level.

an average interval of 5 years after cervical fusion and found no difference in the prevalence of spondylosis between the surgical group and a nonrandomized control group.[113] These authors concluded that cervical arthrodesis does not produce significant acceleration of degenerative changes in adjacent levels.[113] At this time, the effect of fusion on adjacent levels has not been defined adequately.

Complications associated with the anterior cervical approach include esophageal injury; damage to the recurrent laryngeal, spinal accessory, phrenic, or other nerves; stellate ganglion disruption; vascular injury; thoracic duct laceration; cord damage; pneumothorax; infection; and hemorrhage.[51, 102, 103, 105, 114] Postoperative cerebrospinal fluid fistulas may be seen in patients with underlying dural erosion, dural adherence to decompression sites, or inadvertent dural laceration.[48, 115] Postoperative respiratory compromise due to tracheal compression by edema or hematoma also has been recognized as a potential cause for early postoperative morbidity and mortality.[103, 105, 116] Emery and colleagues noted the association of significant upper airway obstruction with multiple levels of cervical decompression, moderately severe underlying myopathy, and a history of heavy smoking or asthma.[116] In Emery and coworkers' study, radiographic assessment of postoperative soft tissue width did not allow prediction of those patients at risk for upper airway compromise.[116]

## SPINAL INSTRUMENTATION

The first widespread application of spinal hardware other than wiring and limited screw techniques used to achieve fusion was for the treatment of scoliosis.[2] Nonoperative treatment by casting or external bracing is uncomfortable, time consuming, and ineffective unless the deformity is flexible and residual growth potential is present.[2] Hardware was developed to allow internal correction of the scoliotic deformity and early mobilization of the patient. Its applications have since been expanded to provide rigid internal fixation for a variety of spinal disorders other than scoliosis. Spinal hardware is applied in conditions such as degenerative spondylosis, spondylolisthesis, fractures, infection, neoplasms, and congenital disorders. Rigid fixation along with bone grafting is employed to enhance the likelihood of obtaining bony fusion, to prevent pseudarthrosis, to correct deformity, and to allow early mobilization. A variety of instruments using combinations of rods, plates, pedicle screws, staples, cross-links, and hooks and wires are available currently. It must be emphasized that the purpose of instrumentation is to provide temporary, stable fixation and maintain alignment and immobilization until a solid bony spinal fusion develops.[3, 117–119] Metallic devices are unable to bear the long-term repetitive stresses to which the spine is subjected and eventually fail if a solid bone fusion is not achieved.[120] The art of selecting appropriate internal fixation devices as well as choosing the insertion techniques to be employed is extremely complex, and the biomechanical principles related to the use of these devices are complicated. Only a limited review of the various hardware systems can be presented in this chapter; the reader is referred to the excellent series of articles by Slone and coworkers that discuss the biomechanics of spinal fixation and amply illustrate the devices to be discussed.[118–121]

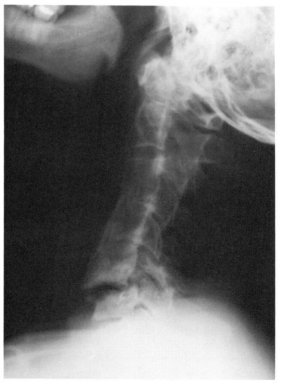

**FIGURE 18–12.** Cervical spondylosis below the level of fusion. Severe degenerative disc disease is present at the C6-C7 level. This patient has solid arthrodesis above the level of degeneration.

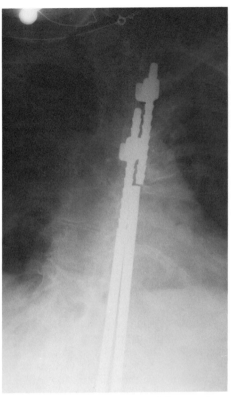

**FIGURE 18–13.** Harrington rod fracture. A fracture is seen at the junction of the fluted and straight portions of the distraction rod.

## Thoracic and Lumbar Spine

The first major spinal hardware system was developed by Harrington in the 1950s to treat children with poliomyelitis-induced neuromuscular scoliosis.[122–124] The initial design used a combination of rods and facet screws, but a ratcheted rod-hook construct was implemented early in the design of the Harrington system because of a high failure rate of the initial design.[123, 124] The system is placed posteriorly and employs distraction across the concavity of the deformity and compression along the convexity; the greater the distractive and compressive forces, the more complete the reduction.[3] The major uses for the Harrington system currently are to effect spinal fusion in the treatment of idiopathic single curve thoracic scoliosis and to provide realignment and stabilization of thoracolumbar fractures with an intact anterior longitudinal ligament.[122]

Bone grafting is used at the time of fixation as it is the bone fusion, rather than the hardware system, that is the source of long-term stability.[122] Harrington realized early in his experience that augmentation with bone graft was necessary to maintain longevity of any achieved correction in scoliotic patients.[123, 124] Although Harrington employed posterior graft alone, other surgeons have used a combination of anterior and posterior grafting to obtain solid fusion after placement of scoliosis hardware.[125, 126] Anterior grafting decreases the risk of rotational deformity (crankshaft) in skeletally immature persons.[126, 127]

The stainless steel Harrington distraction rod is 0.25 inch in diameter and is available in a variety of lengths. At the upper end of each distraction rod is a fluted section with a series of circumferential grooves designed so that the upper

hook engages on the shoulder of the groove, preventing its slippage when axial compression is applied to the hooks.[123] The superior hook generally is placed as close to the smooth portion of the rod as possible to prevent rod pull-out from the hook and fracturing at the junction of the rod and the flutes. This junction acts as a stress riser and is a major site of weakness in the system owing to an abrupt 25 per cent diminution in the cross-sectional diameter of the rod[50, 63, 128, 129] (Fig. 18–13). The lower end of the distraction rod has a narrower section (nipple) that fits through a hole in the hub of each hook.[122, 123] The Harrington compression rods come in two diameters (3 mm and 5 mm); the thinner rod is more flexible but is more likely to undergo metal fatigue and failure[50, 122, 123] (Fig. 18–14). The compression rod is fully threaded and can be employed with multiple hooks through which it is passed.[123] The use of multiple hooks across the convexity of the curve probably was the earliest form of segmental fixation. The compression rod has been said to do little to enhance the stability of the construct or improve the correction of the deformity.[2] This type of rod is used less frequently than the distraction rod of the Harrington system.

Single hooks are placed at the cranial and caudal ends of the distraction rod. The superior distraction hook is held in place with a C-shaped washer placed just distal to it. For compression rods, hexagonal nuts are used to hold the

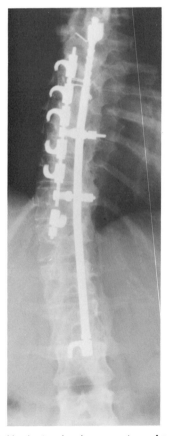

**FIGURE 18–14.** Harrington hardware system. An anteroposterior view shows a Harrington distraction rod on the left side with single upper and lower hooks. The compression rod on the right has multiple hooks and is fully threaded. Note the fracture of the compression rod above the most caudal hook. Cross-links have been placed to improve stability.

hooks in place; double nuts typically are used at the superiormost and inferiormost hooks to help maintain hook position.[123, 129] The initial hooks designed for the Harrington system were C-shaped and did not conform well to the lamina. A variety of different hook designs have since been adapted for use with the Harrington rod; these hooks may be placed into the thoracic facet, over the transverse process, or, most commonly, around the edge of the lamina.[50, 122] The Edwards ''anatomic'' hook, which has a flat contour similar to the anatomic surface of the lamina, probably is the design that is used most widely. Dislodgment of the system, which occurs in approximately 2 to 17 per cent of cases, typically is due to hook pull-out or hook-rod disengagement.[3, 50] Fractures of the rods are less common than hook dislodgment, but both complications suggest the presence of abnormal motion and pseudarthrosis[127, 130] (Fig. 18–15). Modifications in the rods or hooks (or in both), placement of multiple hooks on the distraction rod (Bobechko double upper hooks), augmentation of the rod-hook construct by sublaminar wiring (HarriLuque technique), or placement of Edwards rod sleeves between the spinous process and facets or rod linkage systems can be used to decrease the rate of dislodgment.[3, 122, 131]

The use of the Harrington system in the lower lumbar spine is associated with a higher rate of instrument failure and other complications.[122] When used in the lumbar region, contouring and a square-ended rod with square hole hooks (Moe modification) typically are employed to provide better rotational stability.[122, 129, 132] Edwards sleeves, which nestle between the spinous process and adjacent facets and help control rotation and maintain lordosis, also may be employed.[3, 131] Despite these modifications, complications related to lumbar placement develop frequently, particularly with placement below the L3 level. Problems associated with low lumbar Harrington placement include high rates of hook dislodgment, loss of lumbar lordosis (''flat-back'' deformity), abnormal gait, back pain, disability, and late dural erosion or neurologic complica-

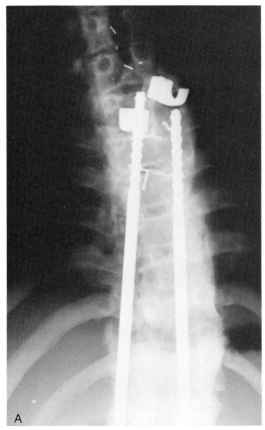

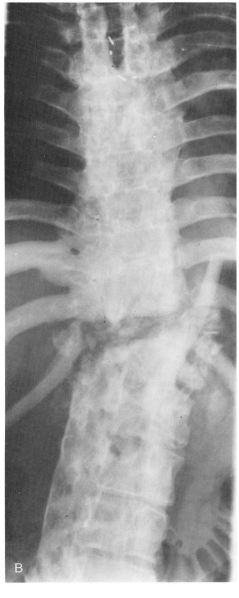

**FIGURE 18–15.** Hook pull-out.
   **A** The cranial hook has disengaged from the left Harrington distraction rod. A pseudarthrosis also is present at T11-T12 in this paraplegic patient.
   **B** The pseudarthrosis is seen to better advantage after removal of the hardware. Extensive sclerosis, subluxation, and irregularity are seen at the site of nonunion, consistent with a neuropathic spine.

tions due to migration of the caudal hook into the spinal canal.[50, 63, 126, 127, 133]

Disadvantages of the Harrington system include limited sagittal plane control, minimal derotating ability, overdistraction, a high rate of rod breakage or hook dislodgment, and a relatively high pseudarthrosis rate.[3, 50, 62, 126, 132] Application of excessive distraction stress on the hook, necessary to lock the Harrington hook, predisposes to erosion of the underlying bone, producing fractures and allowing migration of the hooks.[123, 129, 132, 133] Laminar fracture is associated with excessive operative notching, excessive distraction, osteoporosis, and low lumbar or sacral placement.[50]

Although the Harrington system was developed for scoliosis, it also has been employed widely for the reduction and maintenance of spinal alignment after traumatic injuries of the thoracic and upper lumbar regions.[60, 62, 129, 130, 134] Harrington performed the first rodding of a thoracolumbar fracture-dislocation in 1958.[122] He and other early investigators found that the major advantage of operative reduction of these injuries was the ability to start early mobilization and rehabilitation.[128, 130, 134] Since then, the Harrington hardware system has been used extensively for the management of thoracolumbar fractures. Distraction rodding is most applicable for axial load injuries, such as burst fractures producing spinal canal narrowing by means of retropulsed bone fragments. Willen and collaborators found significant improvement in midsagittal diameter and cross-sectional area of the spinal canal after Harrington instrumentation for burst fractures but noted that reduction typically was incomplete, with mean persistent postrodding narrowing of 26 per cent of the canal.[60] Compression rodding is appropriate for injuries in which posterior tensile ligamentous injury occurs but generally is not as successful owing to the limited strength of this system.[3, 50, 130] Gruca-Weiss springs were used for the same function as the compression Harrington systems, particularly in the upper thoracic region because of their strength and ease of insertion.[3, 128] This now nearly obsolete device consists of a pair of springs attached to sublaminar hooks at both ends of each spring.[3, 128] Harrington hardware is indicated primarily for use when either the anterior or the posterior longitudinal ligaments are presumed to be intact. The system is difficult to use and potentially dangerous when a grossly unstable translational or rotational injury involving all three vertebral columns is present.[50, 122, 128] Supplemental fusion at the site of fracture typically is used, along with external support.

The Harrington hardware system was not the only rod-hook construct used during the early period of spinal hardware development. Distraction across degenerative lumbar motion segments using paired fully threaded distraction rods with sublaminar hooks initially was reported by Knodt and Larrick in 1964.[135] The system was designed to distract narrowed neural foramina with short segment posterior distractive forces. The two ends of the Knodt rod are threaded in opposite directions with a central fixed nut (turnbuckle).[119] Knodt rods rarely are used today except to support vertebral body distraction in conjunction with PMMA for anterior thoracic decompression of neoplasms. The device led to significant loss of lumbar lordosis over limited segments. The slender rods also had a tendency to deform or fracture without additional support. In 1979, Jacobs designed a rod with hooks controlled by nuts and washers that allowed for hook fixation without the need for deep notches in the rod.[132] The Jacobs hooks were in an anatomic L-shaped configuration that conforms better to the lamina than the C-shaped hooks used by Harrington.[123, 132] The rod also is stronger and the hooks have a higher pull-out strength than Harrington's original design. The Jacobs system is used most appropriately for fixation of fractures at the thoracolumbar junction.[132] The bulky hooks may result in skin breakdown or discomfort when used in the upper thoracic region; hooks in the low lumbar region have a high failure rate.[132]

Traditional rod-hook systems apply concentrated vertical stresses at the superior and inferior hooks while applying only indirect corrective force to the intervening vertebral bodies. Segmental hardware systems attempt to distribute corrective forces over multiple vertebral segments. The first successful segmental spinal instrumentation system was developed by Luque in 1973 for the treatment of scoliosis.[136–138] Luque's patients included a large number of postpoliomyelitis scoliotic patients with severe osteoporosis; in this population, conventional hardware with Harrington rods resulted in a high rate of hook cut-out through the weak bone.[138] Luque hardware uses sublaminar wiring at multiple levels, combined with paired smooth rods, to apply corrective transverse forces over multiple spinal segments.[128, 136, 139] Distributing the corrective forces over multiple levels decreases bone cut-out in osteoporotic bone and provides a higher degree of stability than distraction hook and rod systems.[3, 117, 138, 140] The method of scoliosis correction is very different for the Luque segmental system than for the Harrington rod-hook system. Harrington hardware corrects by applying force in a vertical direction whereas the Luque system corrects with multiple horizontal forces.[127, 138, 141] Results from current biomechanical studies suggest that a combination of both distraction and transverse fixation forces, as is used in the HarriLuque technique, is superior to either alone.[3]

Luque rods are available in 4.8 mm or 6.3 mm diameters; the thinner rod has a tendency to break when used in patients with kyphosis or a large, rigid curve.[117, 138] Rod fracture is more likely to occur when bone arthrodesis is not accomplished and typically occurs near one end of the construct.[117] The smooth Luque rods come in various configurations, such as straight, L-shaped, box, or rectangular; in addition, there is a specialized unit rod, designed for patients requiring pelvic fixation.[138, 139] The configuration used most frequently for scoliosis is the double-L technique, with one rod's short limb directed superiorly and the other rod's short limb located inferiorly. The 90 degree bend at the end of the rod allows passage of the short limb through or under the spinous process for more stable fixation[119] (Fig. 18–16). The L shape was designed to prevent rod migration and rotation; cross-linking the two rods increases rigidity and also diminishes the risk of rod migration.[138, 139]

The unit rod for pelvic fixation is used for correction of pelvic obliquity and to help maintain upright posture in patients with truncal muscle weakness. The unit rod consists of a single rod curved back on itself to form a double rod with bilateral lateral flares at its caudal end for entry into each iliac crest.[119] Pelvic fixation of the precontoured Luque unit rods is accomplished by driving the inferior segment of rod into each ilium, a method known as the

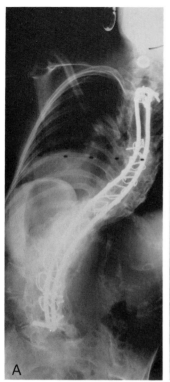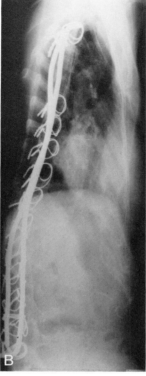

**FIGURE 18–16.** Luque L-shaped rods.
  **A** The anteroposterior view shows placement of Luque L-shaped rods for neuromuscular scoliosis. Note the short limb at one end of each rod. Multiple sublaminar wires are present.
  **B** Note the loss of normal sagittal contours on the lateral view of the spine.

Galveston technique[138] (Fig. 18–17). Ideally, 6 cm of purchase into the ilium should be obtained to optimize fixation.

The major complications of the Luque system are related to the passage of the multiple sublaminar wires. Insertion of sublaminar wires is associated with inadvertent tears of the dura even if dissection is performed carefully.[48] More importantly, the passage of sublaminar wires in scoliosis patients has been associated with a 1.8 per cent prevalence of neurologic deficit, particularly when the rod adjacent to the wire does not rest firmly on the lamina, allowing motion of the wire within the spinal canal.[50, 127, 142] When used in patients with spinal injury, sublaminar wires have been associated with neurologic injury in up to 17 per cent of cases.[50] Because of the increased risk of neurologic injury from sublaminar wire passage and the rigidity of the final correction, Luque hardware is used primarily for neuromuscular scoliosis or other problem cases.[2, 117, 127, 138]

Segmental spinal hardware with spinous process wiring offers an alternative to the sublaminar wiring technique used by Luque. Spinous process fixation is not as strong as sublaminar wiring but is safer and of adequate strength when multiple fixation points are used.[2, 141] Cut-out of the wires is common due to the thin cortical bone in the spinous process. Drummond developed a segmental spinous process fixation system that uses an 8 mm button adjacent to the spinous process.[141] The spinous process wire passes through the button (Wisconsin interspinous segmental instrumentation), providing more secure fixation and better load sharing than wires alone, thereby preventing cut-out of the wire.

Attempts to provide segmental hardware for the laminectomized spine led to the development of transpediculate screw fixation, which is not dependent on an intact posterior arch.[140] In the 1940s, screw fixation of the spine was described by various investigators who used interfacet screws to obtain fixation at the lower lumbar and lumbosacral levels.[72, 143] The short fixation screws were supplemented by bone graft, allowed for early patient mobilization, and resulted in an acceptable pseudarthrosis rate of 9.1 per cent.[143] Since that time, numerous spinal fixation systems employing screws have been developed, with the current emphasis on devices that place screws within the strong bone of the pedicles. Pedicle screw fixation systems are popular because of their strength, their ability to obtain segmental correction of deformities in all three planes, and their ability to maintain rigid segmental spinal fixation over a limited number of spinal segments, even in areas such as the lumbosacral junction that are difficult to control with other hardware systems.[2, 3, 93, 101, 119, 144] Pedicle screw fixation provides stability to all three spinal columns and allows segmental correction of lordosis, kyphosis, scoliosis, and rotation.[137, 144–146] This type of hardware system is used most frequently for immobilization in patients with painful degenerative arthritis, symptomatic spondylolisthesis, posttraumatic deformity, and severe scoliosis and for prevention or treatment of pseudarthrosis.

Currently, several different pedicle screw systems are used. These are employed predominantly in the lumbar region because of the high frequency of degenerative disease in this location, the large size of the lumbar pedicles, and the difficulty in immobilization of the low lumbar region with other systems. Less commonly, pedicle screw systems are used in the thoracolumbar or upper thoracic regions for the management of scoliosis or posttraumatic deformities. Use in the upper thoracic spine is limited by the relatively small size of the pedicles in this region,

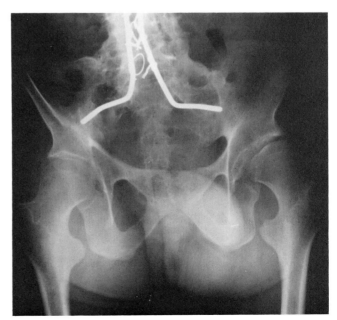

**FIGURE 18–17.** Galveston technique. The Luque unit rod with bilateral iliac bars was embedded in the iliac wings to correct pelvic obliquity. This patient with neuromuscular scoliosis also shows bilateral coxa valga deformities.

the risk of spinal cord injury, and the thinness of the overlying soft tissues, which lead to prominence of these relatively bulky devices.

Pedicle screws are available in various lengths with major screw diameters ranging from 4.5 to 7.5 mm. The screws may be cortical or cancellous and cannulated or uncannulated; pitch (distance between threads), tooth profiles, and minor diameters (which determines tooth height) also vary.[91, 121, 144, 147] Fully threaded screws of larger diameter result in the most secure fixation.[93] Preoperative CT typically can be used to measure accurately the outer cortical and inner cancellous diameters of the pedicle to select the largest acceptable screw size. Purchase of the screw tip in the anterior vertebral body cortex increases the fixation strength of the screw by 20 per cent, but routine engagement of the anterior vertebral cortex is unnecessary and increases the risk of vascular injury significantly.[91, 93, 144] The situation is different for the sacrum, where engagement of the anterior cortex increases the pull-out strength of the pedicle screw to a significant extent and is performed more often.[144] In vitro testing has shown that the sacrum, particularly the second sacral pedicle, is the weakest location for insertion.[93]

The screws connect to rods or plates either through rigid constrained linkages, as in almost all plate systems, fixators, and most of the rod systems, or through a mobile semiconstrained coupling, usually to a rod, that allows for some motion but offers more reduction capability.[91, 93, 127, 144] The early systems used plates, which are passive fixation devices, but plates are difficult to contour in both the sagittal and coronal planes and their width limits the area available for bone grafting.[131, 140] Most of the newer pedicle-screw systems use rods rather than plates to obtain rigid spinal fixation. Rigid connections between the screws and the plate or rod result in high stress concentration, which may lead to increased risk of screw loosening, hardware breakage, and stress shielding.[91, 144, 148] Loosening and subsequent fracture of the screws are more common when the sacrum is incorporated.[91, 144] One of the most important risk factors for loosening is underlying osteoporosis, which causes difficulty in obtaining purchase of the screw within the vertebral body.[93]

A pedicle screw ideally should be placed parallel to the axis of the pedicle in both the sagittal and the transverse planes (''up and in'' technique), incorporating its largest available diameter.[144, 147] ''Straight-in'' placement, as advocated by Roy-Camille, disrupts the facet joint and may result in higher rates of extraosseous screw penetration.[147, 149] Correct placement is essential to provide adequate purchase and avoid the neural structures that course alongside the pedicle. The spinal cord lies 2 to 3 mm medial to the thoracic pedicles, separated only by the dura and cerebrospinal fluid.[146, 149] The exiting nerve root passes medial and then immediately inferior to the pedicle and can be injured by incorrect screw placement. A review by the Scoliosis Research Society indicates that 3.2 per cent of patients develop neurologic compromise after placement of a pedicle screw system.[150] Injury to the dura, intervertebral disc, lateral segmental vessels, spinal nerves, lumbosacral plexus, and presacral plexus also can occur if pedicle screws are positioned incorrectly.[97, 144, 150]

The first widely used pedicle screw system employed for spinal fixation was developed by Roy-Camille and coworkers in the early 1960s.[145, 146] Initially, Roy-Camille plates were developed for fixation of the posterior cervical facets, but the hardware system rapidly evolved to encompass pedicle screw-fixation plates for the thoracic and lumbar regions. For the thoracic and thoracolumbar levels, 1 cm wide precontoured plates with reinforced holes spaced every 13 mm are used.[145, 149] Specialized plates for the lower lumbar and lumbosacral levels also are available.[145] Each screw hole is reinforced to maintain uniform strength of the plate. The reinforcements around the screws are readily apparent on the lateral view as posterior raised areas separated by clefts in the regions between the screws. The screw plate interface is not constrained rigidly, allowing micromotion in an effort to prevent screw breakage.[145]

Louis hardware is another pedicle screw-plate fixation system that can be used throughout the spine.[151] At the lumbosacral junction, the Louis system uses a butterfly-shaped single plate with two superior oval holes for the L5 pedicle screws and two obliquely oriented holes for fixation in the sacral ala.[151] Above this region, symmetric paired plates with closely spaced holes (separated by 9 mm), allowing for precise placement of the pedicle screws, are employed.[151] The sacral screws are directed obliquely 45 degrees laterally for fixation in the sacral ala, which maximizes fixation strength.[93] On most newer systems, the sacral screws are directed into the sacral promontory rather than the ala, as promontory screws have a longer depth of screw purchase and are unlikely to injure the sacroiliac joints and presacral vessels.[140] The instrument has a very low profile so it can be used for both anterior and posterior fixation.

AO dynamic compression plates (DCP) allow the screws to be angled through the holes in the plate because of their semicylindrical configuration.[94] The ability to place the screws obliquely is advantageous as it allows the screws to be oriented along the pediculate axis even if the hole in the plate is not centered directly over this structure. Up to 25 degrees of craniocaudal and 7 degrees of mediolateral angulation can be obtained.[94] The AO plates come in two widths; the wider plate has staggered holes and the narrow plate has a single row of holes spaced 16 mm apart.[94]

In the mid-1980s, plates with slots rather than holes were introduced by Steffee.[97, 131] Because slots offer considerable flexibility in the placement of the screws, the Steffee system also is known as the variable screw placement (VSP) system. The VSP system consists of bilateral 16 mm wide plates with nested slots, allowing placement of screws at various locations and angulations for fixation.[97] Washers (spacers) between the anterior surface of the plate and the screw permit level metal-to-metal contact despite screw angulation.[97] Unlike the Roy-Camille, Louis, and AO DCP systems, the VSP system does not allow any motion at the screw-plate interface, leading to increased rigidity and stress shielding.[94] Commonly available variations or alternatives to the VSP system are the Dynalok and Simmons plate-screw systems.

The use of rods, rather than plates, for pedicle screw fixation results in more active correction of deformity. Plates allow minimal correction of deformity in the sagittal plane; coronal deformity cannot be corrected but must be brought in line with the plate.[152] A variety of pedicle screw-rod systems are available commercially. The Luque segmental hardware system has been adapted to the lumbar spine, initially by transformation of the double-L rods into

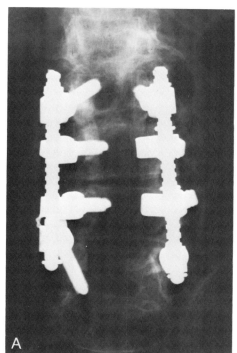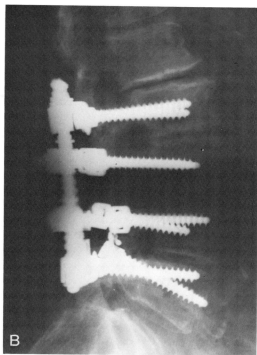

**FIGURE 18–18.** Edwards modular system.
**A** Pedicle screw fixation with the fully notched Edwards universal rods and pedicle screws.
**B** The semiconstrained pedicle connectors seen on the lateral view allow limited motion.

a semirigid screw-plate system and subsequently into a semirigid system utilizing hooks, pedicle screws, and rods instead of a plate.[139] The latest version of the Luque pedicle screw system consists of two cross-linked bars that generally are affixed to the intermediate vertebrae with pedicle screws and to the uppermost and lowermost vertebrae with sublaminar claw hooks.[139] Other systems represent modifications of skeletal external fixators adapted for internal spinal implantation. The Vermont spinal fixator consists of pedicle screws attached to both ends of a 6 mm rod via a rigid, fully constrained interface.[147] The AO internal fixator is a pedicle-screw-rod system that allows Schantz screws passed through the pedicles to be attached to threaded rods via clamps.[65]

More modular systems of pedicle-rod fixation attempt to provide flexibility in the construct to permit some motion, thereby decreasing the degree of stress shielding of the bone graft.[2] The major semiconstrained pedicle screw-rod system that has been used extensively in clinical practice is the Edwards Modular System (Fig. 18–18). This system gradually evolved from the development of Edwards rod-sleeves and an L-shaped anatomic hook in the 1980s.[131] After these early developments, numerous modifications and additions were made to the system. The current Edwards system consists of bidirectional fully ratcheted "universal" rods, anatomic hooks, screws, rod-sleeves, pedicle connectors, and cross-locks. This combination of devices allows correction of spinal deformities in almost every plane and is adaptable enough for most indications.[131] The Edwards rod lacks a discrete stress riser because the ratchets are uniformly distributed over the entire rod, resulting in rod breakage rates of less than 1 per cent.[131] The rod-sleeves also are distinctive; these polyethylene spacers contain sulfate for radiographic visualization and are used to grip the spinous process to provide translational and rota-

tional control[131] (Fig. 18–19). The Wiltse system uses a 4.75 mm serrated rod that is contoured easily and is flexible enough to limit hardware breakage and stress shielding.[152] The Puno-Winter-Bird (PWB) system is a pedicle screw-rod device that is semiconstrained, allowing some micromotion between the screw and the rod via a special coupling device.[140] The PWB rod is slender and less stiff than most other systems.

The newest development in spinal hardware is the introduction of derotational systems that can be used to apply rigid segmental fixation while also allowing for multidirection control and correction of deformity in all three planes.[3] These systems were devised initially for the correction of scoliosis, but their flexible design has expanded their use well beyond correction of scoliotic deformity. These derotational systems, represented by the Cotrel-Dubousset, Texas Scottish Rite Hospital, and Isola systems, are adaptable modular systems that can be employed for multiple indications.[3] These systems are biomechanically complex, technically demanding to insert, bulky, and expensive but they represent a major advance in spinal hardware.[2] They, along with the Edwards system, represent the first attempts at the development of a universal spinal hardware system. A truly universal system should be applicable to any region of the spine and to any pathologic spinal condition for which application of hardware is indicated.[153]

Cotrel-Dubousset (CD) hardware was developed in the early 1980s and was the first system that attempted to correct scoliotic deformities in three dimensions, unlike the uni- or bidimensional corrections of the Harrington and Luque techniques.[154] CD hardware application allows for better correction of both the coronal and the sagittal components of the deformity; the sagittal deformity was not a major consideration in prior hardware systems for scoliosis. The CD system applies mechanical correction primarily by

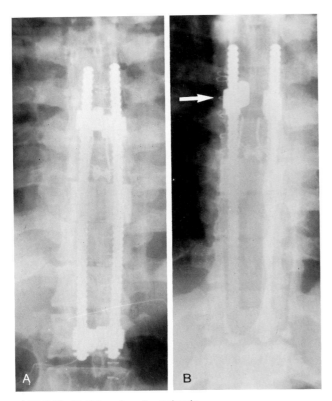

**FIGURE 18–19.** Edwards universal rods.

  **A** Anteroposterior view demonstrates paired Edwards rods with polyethylene rod sleeves abutting on the T8 spinous process. The spinous process has been wired with Drummond buttons at T7.

  **B** The upper right hook is seen to be disengaged on the follow-up examination. Note the tilting of the hook (arrow) and the development of divergence at the upper ends of the rods.

rotation of coronal deformity into the sagittal plane, thereby converting scoliotic deformity into a more physiologic kyphosis or lordosis.[2, 119, 154] The introduction of a rotational maneuver to correct spinal deformity was a major evolutionary change in the management of scoliosis.[153] The correction achieved is not as anatomic as was believed initially but still is better than can be obtained with prior hardware systems.

The CD instrument consists of a pair of 7 mm stainless steel rods that have their entire surface serrated with diamond-shaped irregularities[154] (Fig. 18–20). The rods are connected by slender threaded cross-links. Hooks or pedicle screws, or both, can be applied anywhere along the length of the rods and can face in any direction. Pedicle hooks (which have a notch between two prongs to engage the inferior pediculate cortex) and blunt-edged laminar hooks both are attached to the rod via bolting screws.[154] Pediculate fixation can be provided by blunt threaded screws that can be affixed to the same rod as the hooks or to a separate rod connected to the more superior rod with a double-beveled connector. Typically, each rod is attached to four or more laminar hooks or pedicle screws.[119] Rotational correction is accomplished by rotating the contoured rod after its insertion into the hooks placed at critical points in the spine.[2] Hooks on the same rod can be placed to act in compression or in tension. With time, the tips of the set screws may suffer wear from friction against the serrated rod, leading

to migration of the hooks or pedicle screws up or down the rod.[120]

The Texas Scottish Rite Hospital (TSRH) system has the same fundamental function as CD hardware but differs in several aspects of its design.[119, 153] It uses the same fixation principles as CD but its modifications allow for implantation and, more importantly, greater ease in removal or revision once the instrument is already in place.[153] The system has evolved from the initial development of a cross-linkage plate to a complete hardware system consisting of rods, hooks, pedicle screws, and cross-links[153] (Fig. 18–21). The differences between the CD and TSRH systems are seen in all components of the two systems. TSRH rods are roughened rather than serrated and are available in three levels of rod stiffness.[153] The cross-link is a low-profile plate with rectangular orifices for placement of bolts rather than the threaded, screwed cross-link of the CD system. The TSRH system allows for the placement of both standard (perpendicular to the rod) and variable angle pedicle screws.[119, 153] The hooks come in a wider array of configurations and sizes. CD hooks are circular; TSRH hooks are available in circular and anatomic configurations. The anatomic hooks have a more angular configuration, with a narrow shoe to provide better osseous contact and less canal compro-

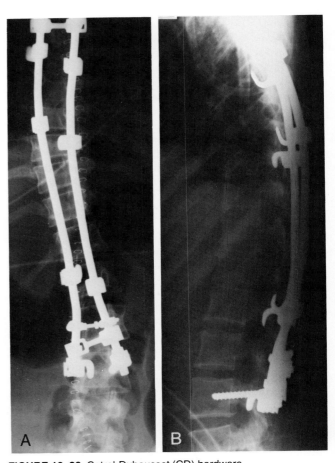

**FIGURE 18–20.** Cotrel-Dubousset (CD) hardware.

  **A** The anteroposterior view shows CD hardware placed for scoliosis correction. The serrated rods are cross-linked with both CD and TSRH devices.

  **B** The lateral view shows the C-shaped hooks and the cut set screws characteristic of CD hardware.

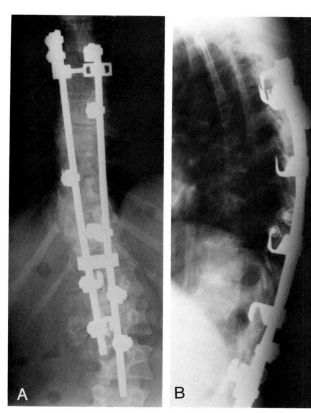

**FIGURE 18–21.** Texas Scottish Rite Hospital (TSRH) hardware.
**A** Anteroposterior view shows TSRH rods with multiple hooks and cross-links.
**B** The lateral view shows the anatomic configuration of the thoracic hooks. The uppermost vertebra is engaged by two hooks, directed toward each other in a "claw" configuration.

mise.[153] Unlike the CD system, which uses bolting screws for fixation of hooks and pedicle screws to the rods, the TSRH system employs eyebolts with large nuts for attachment.[119, 153] These eyebolts reportedly are less likely to loosen or break than the set screws on the CD system.[120] The TSRH hardware can be used to augment any existing rod system by attaching to it with its cross-link system, allowing cranial or caudal extension of any preexisting hardware.[153]

The Isola spinal implant system also is similar to the CD and TSRH devices in its function and design. The Isola system originally was devised with the intent to perfect sacral fixation.[155] It has since evolved into a modular system that is completely compatible with the VSP system developed by Steffee.[97, 155] The Isola system includes rods, plates, screws, hooks, wires, cross-links, and iliac posts (similar to Luque-Galveston unit rods).[155] The plates and pedicle screws are identical to those of the VSP system. The remainder of the hardware has some minor design differences from the TSRH system.

Compared to the vast array of posterior spinal hardware systems, relatively few anterior instrumentation systems are employed in the thoracic and lumbar regions. Anterior fixation in the thoracic and lumbar spine is used far less frequently than applications of posterior hardware, particularly since the advent of universal posterior systems that allow derotation and multiplanar correction. The anterior approach for application of hardware also is more difficult

technically and is associated with a potentially higher rate of major complications. The nonunion rate for anterior fusions typically is reported to be 10 to 50 per cent, considerably higher than with fusions accompanied by rigid posterior immobilization.[3, 63, 156] At this time, anterior thoracic and lumbar instrumentation is used primarily in patients requiring anterior decompression or in those in whom the posterior elements are deficient.[2, 3]

The first major anterior hardware system that was used extensively was reported by Dwyer in 1969. Dwyer introduced an anterior device developed for the correction of scoliosis. Placed on the convex side of the curve, the Dwyer instrument consisted of multiple staples embedded into the vertebral bodies, with vertebral body screws threaded through each staple.[119, 156, 157] A flexible braided titanium wire was passed through the screw holes and crimped and tightened, providing compression on the tensile side of the scoliotic curve. Once tightened, the device was not adjustable.[156] The Dwyer device had a high complication rate and currently is used rarely.[119, 120]

The Zielke modification of the Dwyer system replaced the cable with a thin threaded steel rod passed through slotted screw holes.[89, 119] Like the Dwyer system, the Zielke device, also known as ventral derotation spondylodesis (VDS), is applied on the convex side of the scoliotic curve and places the tensile side of the deformity under compression, allowing correction. The Zielke device, however, offered the advantage of adjustable screws, less induction of kyphosis, and fewer cases of hardware failure.[3, 156] The Zielke device permitted spinal rotation and introduced the technique of spinal derotation as a method for managing scoliosis. The Zielke device has since been supplanted by posterior hardware systems, such as Cotrel-Dubousset and TSRH rods, that perform the derotation function more safely. The TSRH system also may be employed anteriorly if necessary. Neither the Dwyer or the Zielke instruments are strong enough to be used after corpectomy or for correction of severe kyphosis.[89] Their use is limited largely to management of scoliosis in patients with grossly deficient posterior elements.

Several other anterior implantation systems were developed in the 1980s that were designed primarily for fixation after decompression of thoracolumbar fractures.[3] The Kostuik-Harrington system uses Harrington rods combined with Kostuik screws placed into the vertebral body. Two ipsilateral rods are employed in a rectangular or parallelogram fashion, improving rotational and lateral bending control in comparison to the single rod systems.[63] Cross-linking the rods provides additional stability. Typically, a distraction rod is placed anterior to a heavy compression rod, allowing correction of posttraumatic kyphosis, the most common indication for use of the Kostuik-Harrington system.[63] However, two anterior distraction rods may be used. Edwards has modified this approach through the use of universal rods and screws through which distraction can be applied initially, followed by compression to secure graft material.

In 1984, the Kaneda device was introduced for anterior vertebral stabilization; it still is one of the most widely used anterior fixation systems. It was developed primarily for fixation of thoracolumbar burst fractures, allowing decompression and fixation in one operation.[89] The Kaneda instrument incorporates both rods and plates and is inter-

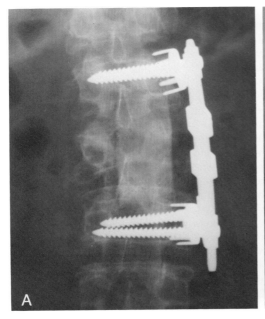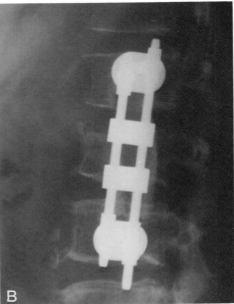

**FIGURE 18–22.** Kaneda hardware.

**A** The anteroposterior view illustrates the tetra-spiked vertebral body staple of the Kaneda system.

**B** The lateral view shows the anterior placement of the paired threaded rods. Note the large iliac strut graft placed after hemicorpectomy.

mediate between the early rod systems and newer low-profile plate systems.[89] The device consists of two tetra-spiked plates that are embedded in the vertebral body and attached to the vertebral body by screws. The two plates are connected by two 4.0 or 5.5 mm threaded rods, one anterior and one posterior, attached to the screw heads[89, 119] (Fig. 18–22). The high profile of many of these anterior instruments, particularly the obsolete Dunn device, has been associated with delayed aortic erosion and hemorrhage.[2, 51, 102] Because of the proximity of the vascular structures, current recommendations are that high-profile anterior hardware be placed on the right side or far laterally on the left to avoid wear between the metal and the pulsatile aorta.

Low-profile systems used for anterior fixation in the thoracic and lumbar regions include the contoured anterior spinal plate, AO plates, the Syracuse I plate, and the Z plate.[3, 119, 158] In general, plates provide immobilization but do not allow for significant correction of any underlying deformity. The contoured anterior spinal plate was developed by Armstrong and Chow in 1980.[158] The low-profile rectangular plate with rounded corners has a width of 2.5 cm, is available in three lengths, and has multiple perforations (arranged in three vertical rows with five holes overlying each vertebral body) through which cancellous screws are passed.[158] AO plates developed for other anatomic regions in the spine have been used to obtain anterior fixation. AO plates may be employed in either neutralization or compression modes. The Syracuse I plate, introduced by Yuan and coworkers in 1988, is a modified AO plate for spinal use that was designed to increase its resistance to rotational and translational forces.[157] The standard AO plate was modified by widening its superior and inferior margins, producing an I-configuration, removing the holes between the widened portions, and curving the plate to fit the vertebral bodies better.[157] Another device, the Z plate, allows sequential distraction and compression to help place and secure graft material.

## Cervical Spine

Posterior cervical hardware was first used by Hadra, who in 1891 described the application of silver wires wrapped around the cervical spinous processes to stabilize a fracture-dislocation.[73] Since that time, numerous techniques for posterior cervical fusion employing a combination of bone graft, wiring, or hardware application have been described. Posterior cervical hardware is used widely, primarily to obtain fusion in patients with spinal deformity and ligamentous insufficiency. Posterior cervical fusions have a relatively low complication rate[105, 159, 160]; Foley and coworkers noted a rate of 3.9 per cent, compared to 21.9 per cent after anterior surgery.[105] Inadvertent injury to the dura or spinal canal may occur but is rare. The most common complication of posterior cervical hardware is loss of fixation and recurrence of deformity.[159, 161] Hardware breakage, loosening, and pull-out typically are due to repetitive stresses applied to the fixation.

Almost all fusions at the cervico-occipital junction are performed via a posterior approach. In the lower cervical spine, both anterior and posterior hardware systems are used. Anterior approaches to the cervicocranium require either temporomandibular joint dislocation, mandibular osteotomy, transoral access with its high infection rate, or an extensive retropharyngeal dissection.[102, 103, 162] The posterior approach is easier technically and is sufficient unless an extensive anterior decompression also is necessary. Techniques using constructs of wire, bone graft, screws, plates, and PMMA all have been proposed as a means of achieving reliable fixation.[163] Most commonly, a construct consisting of both wire and onlay bone graft placed posteriorly is used at the occipitocervical and C1-C2 levels.[159, 164] In addition, more rigid hardware systems to achieve occipitocervical fusion have been developed. These include Roy-Camille plates, a modified Cotrel-Dubousset system, the Abitbol-Wiltse system, and Luque rectangle rod and wire constructs[3, 145, 159] (Fig. 18–23). Occipitocervical fusion is per-

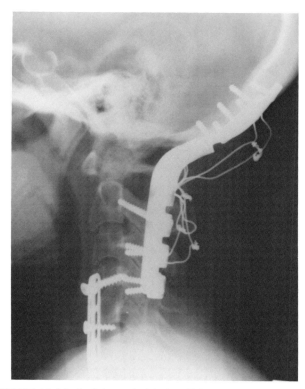

FIGURE 18–23. Occipitocervical fusion. This patient underwent occipitocervical fusion with Roy-Camille plates, bone graft, and wires for occipitocervical dislocation. Note the residual malalignment between the basion and the occiput. Also note the bulky plate reinforcement at each screw hole, characteristic of the Roy-Camille plate. An anterior cervical Caspar plate for another fracture is present in the lower cervical spine.

formed primarily for craniocervical or C1-C2 instability produced by acquired abnormalities, such as infection, inflammatory arthritis, and posttraumatic instability, or for management of unstable congenital anomalies of the occipitoatlantoaxial junction.[3, 159, 164]

Fixation at C1-C2 is employed for the treatment of a wide range of pathologic conditions that produce instability at this level. Acute trauma, nonunion of dens fractures, congenital anomalies, inflammatory arthropathies, ligamentous laxity, and degenerative disease are some of major indications for C1-C2 fusion.[163] Like cervico-occipital fusion, a combination of posterior wiring and bone graft typically is used. The Gallie fusion consists of a single midline wire passed through the C1 sublaminar space and the C2 spinous process with a single interposed iliac crest graft included in the construct.[159, 163] The Brooks fusion uses two bone grafts, one on each side, overlying the C1 and C2 laminae and compressed to them by bilaterally placed C1 and C2 sublaminar wires.[165] The Gallie fusion is safer because it avoids the passage of a C2 sublaminar wire, but the Brooks fusion offers superior stabilization, particularly during rotation.[3, 159] The McLauren fusion, the Clark technique, the Griswold method, the Meyer fusion, and numerous other methods all represent variants of these basic combined wire and bone graft fusion techniques.[105, 118, 159] C1-C2 wiring has a relatively high failure rate owing to difficulty in immobilizing this joint adequately to obtain bone fusion. Reported pseudarthrosis rates for C1-C2 fu-

sion are variable but approach 35 per cent in patients with rheumatoid arthritis.[3]

The high failure rate of C1-C2 fusion with wire has led to the development of more rigid hardware for atlantoaxial immobilization. Recently, lateral mass fixation screws passed anterosuperiorly from the lateral mass of C2 into the lateral mass of C1 have been developed. In biomechanical testing, lateral mass screws have been found to be superior to wiring techniques in resisting both anterior and posterior translation and in providing torsional and extension stability[159, 163] (Fig. 18–24). Although these screws offer superior stabilization, lateral mass screw placement is demanding technically and potentially is hazardous if the screws are not placed correctly. This technique, unlike most conventional C1-C2 fusions, allows for simultaneous decompression of the atlas and foramen magnum.[164] Fixation of type 2 odontoid fractures by screws placed via an anterior approach also has been used. Barbour and Bohler have described methods of anterior fixation of odontoid fractures using screws passed across the odontoid itself or from the lateral mass of C1 into the body of C2.[3] Anteriorly placed C1-C2 facet screws also provide a potential method of fixation but rarely are used. A variety of different screws may be employed for fixation at this level. Typical designs used include AO cannulated 3.5 or 4.0 mm screws or the Knoringer screw, which functions like the Herbert screw to provide compression across the fracture site.[118] The anterior approach for C1-C2 instrumentation for odontoid fractures is more complex technically but is being employed increasingly frequently because of the stability of fixation achieved. Currently it is used most often for fixation in patients unable to undergo rigid external immobilization who also have absence or a fracture of the posterior arch of C1, preventing posterior fusion.[3]

In the lower cervical spine, both anterior and posterior hardware systems are used to achieve immobilization. Posterior fusion is used most commonly when disruption or instability of the posterior ligamentous structures has occurred after trauma or extensive laminectomy.[105, 159–161] Other common indications include progressive deformity, pain, malignancy, inflammatory conditions, and congenital anomalies.[159, 160] Both wiring and metal hardware application, combined with bone grafting, are used widely for posterior fusion. Until recently, spinous process or facet wiring was the only method used commonly for the lower cervical region. Wiring is most effective in limiting flexion, is less effective in limiting extension, and exhibits least effectiveness in controlling rotation.[161] Wire still is the type of hardware placed most frequently in the posterior lower cervical region. Newer hardware systems, most of which are modifications of hardware developed for the lower spine, however, are being used increasingly to provide more rigid fixation. All the posterior elements, including the spinous processes, laminae, facets, and lateral masses, can be used to affix hardware.

Spinous process wiring of the lower cervical spine can be performed in a variety of ways. The original wiring technique, from which most of the current methods have evolved, is the Rogers fusion, first described in 1942.[159, 160] The Rogers fusion consists of stainless steel wire fixation of the spinous processes of adjacent vertebrae obtained by passing the wires through small transverse holes drilled at the junction of the spinous process and lamina.[160] In its

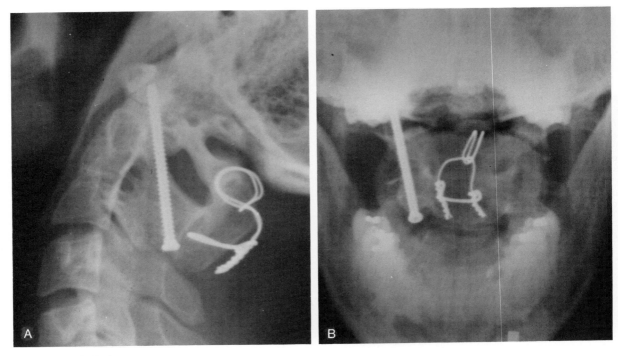

**FIGURE 18–24.** C1-C2 fusion.
  **A** Posterior midline wiring and a single interfacet screw are shown, with solid osseous fusion at C1-C2. A congenital fusion is present at C2-C3.
  **B** The anteroposterior view shows the location of the right-sided C1-C2 interfacet screw extending into the C1 lateral mass.

many modifications, wires are woven through bone grafts overlying the lamina and wrap around or pierce the bases of the spinous processes above and below the unstable level.[105] As long as the spinous processes are intact, modifications such as the Dewar procedure (which incorporates Kirschner wires), figure-of-eight wiring, and Bohlman's triple-wire technique, in conjunction with bone grafting, can be employed.[160] Songer cables, made of braided titanium or stainless steel, which have a crimped metal collar holding the ends in place, may be substituted for wire in interspinous fusions.[105]

Sublaminar or facet fusion must be performed when the spinous processes are absent or insufficient. A variety of sublaminar and facet fusion procedures are employed. The Alexander technique of sublaminar fusion consists of wiring two adjacent laminae with a stainless steel wire.[105] The Meyer technique incorporates a single wire to connect several consecutive laminae.[105] Sublaminar wiring in the cervical region, as in the remainder of the spine, places the patient at risk for neurologic injury and should be avoided in regions of stenosis or cord edema.[2] Because the lower cervical spine allows little room for error, sublaminar wiring usually is reserved for fixation at the C1 and C2 levels. Facet fusions typically are performed when the patient has had multiple laminectomies precluding a spinous process fusion (Fig. 18–25). Facet fusion originally was described in 1960 and has undergone several refinements and modifications since that time.[160, 161] Oblique wiring and wire loop techniques also are used. The Yale fusion consists of wiring each individual facet joint at the desired fusion levels.[105] Single wire techniques incorporating multiple facets may be combined with strut grafting to increase the rigidity of the fusion.[3]

Other instruments for posterior cervical fixation have been developed to provide more stability and rigid immobilization than can be achieved with wiring alone. Wiring can be combined with rods to obtain rigid segmental immobilization.[159] Other constructs employed include the AO hook-plate system developed by Magerl in 1979, the interlaminar (Halifax) clamp, first reported in 1984, and plate-screw fixation systems.[2, 118, 159, 160] The hook-plate system uses screw fixation and interlaminar clamps with hooks placed below the lower lamina and screws passed into the facet at the upper level of the fusion, supplemented by bone graft.[160] The Halifax clamp has C-shaped hooks at each end, which are connected by a screw that passes through the posterior aspect of the hooks, resisting flexion forces. The Halifax interlaminar clamp is placed unilaterally or bilaterally over the lamina and then tightened until no further flexion is possible between the two levels.[159, 160] It also may be used at the C1-C2 level, where it avoids the risk of passage of sublaminar wires.

The use of posterior cervical plates was described first by Roy-Camille and colleagues in the early 1960s.[146] The 1 cm wide plates were applied posterior to the lateral masses with screws passed into the lateral masses.[145] Two separate techniques initially were recommended for screw placement (Roy-Camille and Magerl). Screw placement with the Roy-Camille method is more likely to be in the correct anatomic zone than with the Magerl technique, with decreased risk for nerve root injury.[160] In addition, other posterior plate-screw systems, such as AO tubular and reconstruction, titanium, Haid, Harm's, and Axis posterior cervical plates, have become available.[118, 159] The use of rigid posterior cervical hardware is demanding technically and is associated with numerous complications, including injury to the

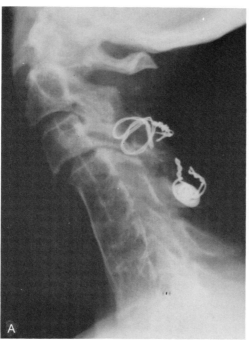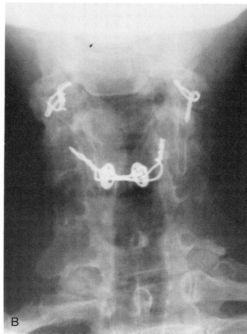

**FIGURE 18–25.** Posterior cervical fusion.

**A** The lateral view shows an anterior fusion of C4-C7. A laminectomy was performed at C2-C3. Interfacet wires are present at the C2-C3 level. Spinous process wiring at C5 with Drummond buttons also is present. The posterior bone graft from C3 to C5 is intact.

**B** The anteroposterior view shows the C2-C3 facet wiring and the C5 Drummond buttons.

vertebral arteries, nerve roots, and spinal cord.[159] Implant loosening and hardware failure also may develop.

Anterior cervical hardware developed because of the difficulty in achieving cervical fusion with anterior grafting techniques in patients with posterior cervical instability. Although traumatic instability remains an important indication for anterior instrumentation, cervical spondylosis, kyphotic deformity, spinal stenosis, and decompression of neoplasm also are frequent conditions for which anterior hardware is used. Currently, the exact indications for use of anterior hardware remain controversial. The anterior method usually is not used in single-level diskectomy; its main use is in patients undergoing multilevel decompression for spondylotic myelopathy or multilevel fusion.[3]

The first reports of anterior metallic cervical fixation appeared in the European literature in the early 1970s, when the use of AO small fragment plates, and subsequently the AO H-shaped and double-H (Orozco) plates, was described.[81, 166] The advantage noted by early investigators was the ability to perform simultaneous decompression and stabilization, obviating prolonged immobilization. Other early anterior plating systems included those developed by Roy-Camille and Louis.[3]

AO plates are affixed with screws, which should be placed solidly in the bone. Positioning of the screws within the disc space predisposes to screw pull-out, loosening, and subsequent hardware breakage.[166] The standard AO stainless steel plates require bicortical screw purchase, necessitating penetration of the posterior vertebral body cortex to achieve stable fixation.[166] The Morscher AO plate, introduced in 1986, is made of titanium and can be used with unicortical fixation of only the anterior cortex owing to the incorporation of a locking screw[81, 166] (Fig. 18–26). Initially, the Morscher screws were cannulated, contained fenestrations, and were sprayed with plasma to encourage bone ingrowth.[2, 118] The fenestrated, plasma-coated screws are no longer used, and the Morscher screw currently employed is a locking, cannulated, unicortical screw without bioactive material on its surface. The Caspar plate is a stainless steel trapezoidal plate with two rows of oval holes through which bicortical screws are placed.[118] The plate is wider at its caudal end and is slightly concave to accommodate the curvature of the vertebral bodies (Fig. 18–27). Newer plates for anterior cervical fixation, such as the Orion plate, are being introduced but experience with these constructs is limited.

## COMPLICATIONS

The failed back surgery syndrome is produced by a spectrum of disorders that are characterized by intractable postoperative pain and varying degrees of functional incapacitation. This syndrome develops in approximately 15 per cent of patients after spinal surgery.[34, 35, 167, 168] Improper patient selection and psychosocial factors probably are the single most important reasons for surgical failure. No specific anatomic lesion can be identified in a large number of patients with the failed back surgery syndrome. The most common structural lesions responsible for the failed back surgery syndrome are recurrent or persistent disc herniation, inadequate decompression of spinal stenosis, arachnoiditis, and epidural fibrosis.[34, 167, 168] Less common causes include facet instability, pseudarthrosis, nerve injury, and surgery at the wrong level.[34] Both CT and MR imaging have been used widely for evaluation of these patients. Prior to the introduction of MR imaging, plain CT or CT after intravenous enhancement with contrast agent was advocated as the most reliable method for distinguishing between the myriad conditions associated with failed surgery.[34, 169, 170] More recently, MR imaging obtained after the intravenous administration of a gadolinium contrast agent has become the procedure of choice for imaging the failed back surgery

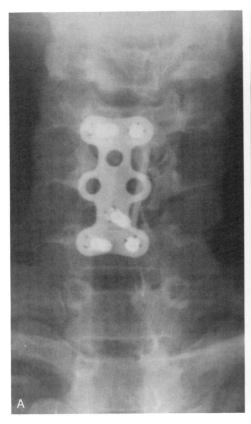

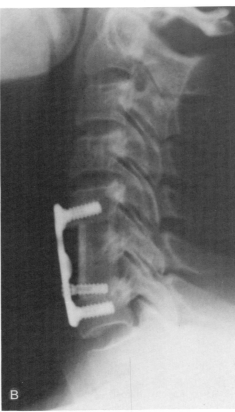

**FIGURE 18–26.** Morscher AO plate.

**A** An anteroposterior view shows a double-H configuration AO plate.

**B** The lateral view shows a corpectomy of C6 with a strut graft extending from C5 to C7. The plate is affixed with Morscher screws, which are cannulated and require purchase only in the anterior cortex.

**FIGURE 18–27.** Caspar plate.

**A** The anteroposterior view demonstrates the trapezoidal configuration of the Caspar anterior cervical plate.

**B** The screws show bicortical fixation with penetration of the posterior vertebral margin. The patient also has undergone posterior bone grafting and spinous process wiring from C3 to C6.

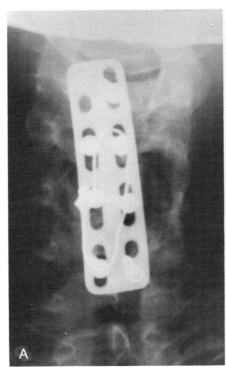

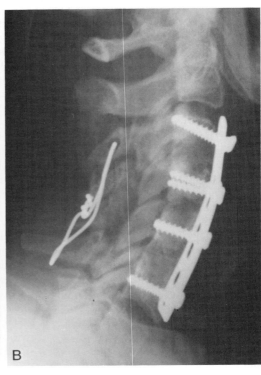

patient.[35, 167, 168, 171] The indications, roles, and imaging findings of CT and MR imaging in the postoperative spine are discussed in other chapters in this textbook (Chapters 12, 40, and 65). This chapter discusses only briefly a few of the complications that can lead to an unsuccessful surgical outcome.

## Pseudarthrosis

Pseudarthrosis or nonunion of spinal grafts is one of the major causes of failed spinal surgery.[172–174] In Frymoyer and colleagues' series, pseudarthrosis was the most common indication for repeat surgery and was associated with a significantly poorer clinical and functional result of the repeat operation.[173] Pseudarthrosis is defined as documented failure of solid osseous union 1 year after surgery.[172] The leading causes of pseudarthrosis include failed previous fusion, inadequate surgical technique, excessive motion and stresses across the fusion site, insufficient stabilization, postoperative infection, smoking, and unrecognized metabolic bone disease.[76, 103, 128, 172, 175] The lack of osseous union may result from fibrous tissue bridging the gap (fibrous nonunion) or from absence of any bridging solid tissue, allowing abnormal excessive motion.[77, 176] A fibrous nonunion may be asymptomatic, requiring no intervention if symptoms are absent.

Because there is no uniform method for diagnosing nonunion of fusion mass, considerable disparity exists regarding the pseudarthrosis rate after bone grafting. The reported prevalence of pseudarthrosis after attempted fusion ranges from 3 to 30 per cent.[172, 177] Higher rates of pseudarthrosis are encountered in patients undergoing simultaneous multilevel fusion.[108, 172, 176, 177] The rate of pseudarthosis increases substantially as additional levels are incorporated into the fusion. Cleveland and associates reported a nonunion rate of 3 per cent in single-level posterolateral lumbar fusions; the rate increased to 33 per cent when three levels were fused simultaneously.[177] The pseudarthrosis rate appears to be highest in patients operated on for nonfusion of bone graft after previous spinal fusion.[150]

The rate of nonunion for anterior cervical fusion ranges from zero to 26 per cent.[80, 108, 172] Anterior interbody fusions have a higher rate of nonunion than posterior or posterolateral fusions. Of the various posterolateral fusions employed, intertransverse fusions reportedly are less likely to undergo nonunion, with pseudarthrosis rates in the range of 7 per cent typically being reported.[33, 172] It is difficult to compare intertransverse and laminar fusion rates because the former is so much easier to assess radiographically. Long strut grafts have the highest rate of nonunion, particularly when placed for deformities and infection.[77, 80] Iliac strut grafts become incorporated more frequently and more rapidly than fibular struts, which show nonincorporation in up to 50 per cent of cases. Hardware systems are designed to immobilize the spine to enhance osseous fusion, but they are not always successful. The reported pseudarthrosis rate with rigid pedicle screw fixation varies from zero to 16 per cent.[144, 150]

Direct current electrical stimulation has been demonstrated by some studies to increase the rate of osseous spinal fusion.[172, 178] Implantable direct current stimulators have been shown by some investigators to enhance bone fusion radiographically and histologically in primary lum-

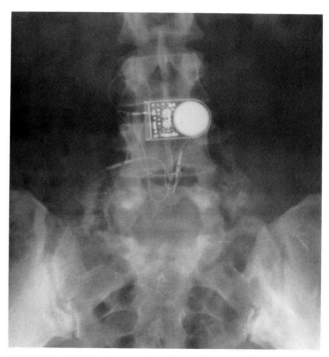

**FIGURE 18–28.** Direct current electrical stimulator. An anteroposterior view of the lumbar spine shows an extensive laminotomy defect of the caudal L5 neural arch and the upper sacrum. An electrical stimulator has been placed to enhance fusion. An intertransverse graft is present bilaterally.

bar fusions[178] (Fig. 18–28). Externally applied pulsed electromagnetic coils also are available and appear to be as effective at stimulating bone growth as implantable units. The need for routine electrical stimulation has not been established, and its role remains controversial; at this time, electrical stimulation is considered an adjunct to bone grafting in patients with established prior pseudarthrosis or those patients deemed at high risk for pseudarthrosis.[172]

Numerous imaging methods are used for the detection of pseudarthrosis; these can be divided into those that assess the morphologic structure of the grafted material and those that assess the graft functionally.[172, 179] Structural integrity is evaluated by conventional radiography and tomography, CT, and MR imaging. Distinction between frank pseudarthrosis and fibrous nonunion is difficult with these methods. Functional integrity is assessed using stress views (typically lateral flexion and extension views), dynamic fluoroscopy, stereophotogrammetric analysis, scintigraphy, and MR imaging. Of these various techniques, flexion and extension views constitute the most frequently used functional test, whereas plain films, conventional tomography, and CT scanning are used most widely for assessment of the structural integrity of spinal graft.[172, 179]

The initial diagnostic test for the evaluation of spinal fusion consists of conventional radiographs. Solid fusion results in a continuous, organized trabecular pattern across the entire grafted segment[148, 172] (Fig. 18–29). Multiple projections may be necessary to visualize the graft adequately, particularly if metal is present. Typically 6 to 9 months is required for the graft material to appear solid and continuous radiographically.[128] During the early postoperative period, pseudarthrosis is difficult to detect unless gross graft

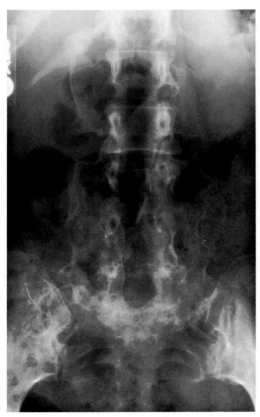

**FIGURE 18–29.** Intertransverse fusion. Solid osseous fusion with continuous trabeculae and loss of the cortical margins of the transverse processes is present at L1-L2 and at L3-L5. The L2-L3 level was not fused in this patient. Note the extensive laminectomy and foraminotomy defects.

terial. Conventional tomography has high accuracy rates for detection of pseudarthrosis; rates as high as 98 per cent have been reported.[174] The presence of hardware, particularly plate fixation systems, renders interpretation of bone fusion difficult. It has been shown that fusion tends to occur under the plate with resorption of bone graft laterally.[94] Even with conventional tomography, the region of fusion is very difficult to evaluate.

Transaxial CT scans are useful for detecting discontinuity between bone graft and the underlying vertebrae. The bone graft must be identified and followed across sequential slices to ensure that solid graft is present. Multiple slices must be integrated mentally to be certain that fragments of graft fused at one level connect to the adjacent level. CT scanning in the early postoperative period demonstrates multiple discontinuous fragments of graft; solid graft is not seen for several months after surgery. Ankylosis of the facet joints also is present as a late finding after a successful arthrodesis.[28, 34]

Failure of fusion generally is demonstrated better on re-formatted images along the course of the graft.[28, 172] Sagittal, coronal, oblique, and curved reformations all are useful in determining the continuity of bone graft material (Fig. 18–32). Direct coronal scanning of the lumbar region can be performed using a specially designed seat that places the fusion mass parallel to the CT gantry.[179] Although the direct coronal scans have superior image quality than reformations, significant improvement in diagnostic accuracy is achieved only in those patients with fusion rods, in whom exclusion of the hardware and their resultant metal streak artifacts can be achieved only by direct coronal imaging.[179] Three-dimensional CT imaging appears to be superior to

or hardware failure develops. Persistent halos or lucent areas around the graft suggest failure of incorporation and should be evaluated further with flexion-extension views. On long-term follow-up, successful arthrodesis alters the biomechanical stresses carried across the fused spinal segments. Adaptive bone remodeling, consisting primarily of focal osteoporosis of stress-shielded bone, has been demonstrated in several in vitro models[148] (Fig. 18–30). Osteoporosis in the vertebral body after successful posterior instrumentation and arthrodesis develops within 6 months of operation due to decreased motion and loading across the vertebral centrum and disc space.[148]

Conventional tomography is used widely for assessment of osseous union and detection of graft complications at sites of spinal fusion.[77, 174] Complex movement tomography, such as hypocycloidal or trispiral tomography, is necessary for optimal imaging, particularly if hardware is present. For posterolateral lumbar fusion, anteroposterior conventional tomograms alone or both anteroposterior and lateral conventional tomograms are obtained at 3 to 5 mm intervals. The anteroposterior conventional tomograms generally are more useful than the lateral projection in this region, particularly if intertransverse grafting has been performed[174] (Fig. 18–31). Lateral tomography is more useful in evaluating anterior interbody fusion, in both the cervical and the lumbar regions. The authors of this chapter often use oblique tomography if initial radiographs suggest that the oblique projection affords the best depiction of the bone graft ma-

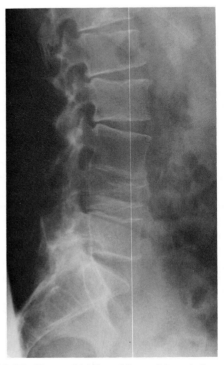

**FIGURE 18–30.** Stress shielding. After solid posterior arthrodesis from L3 to the sacrum for an L4 fracture, the lateral view demonstrates severe osteoporosis across the grafted segment due to stress shielding of the vertebral bodies.

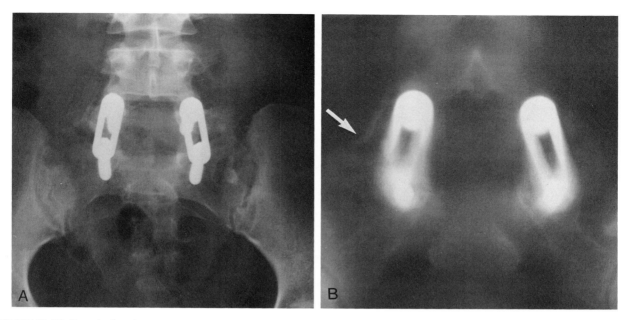

**FIGURE 18–31.** Pseudarthrosis.
**A** The anteroposterior view shows slotted Steffee plates and pedicle screws at L5 and S1. Sparse posterolateral bone graft is present.
**B** The anteroposterior conventional tomogram demonstrates bilateral failure of osseous fusion, with fragmentation of the graft (arrow).

standard reconstructions for demonstrating the extent and solidity of the fusion mass.[42]

MR imaging rarely is used to evaluate the stability or incorporation of bone graft. On the basis of the limited data now available, MR imaging does not appear to be as accurate as conventional tomography or CT scanning for evaluation of osseous fusion.[81, 180] The presence of ferromagnetic metallic wires, fixation devices, and braces limits evaluation significantly owing to the presence of metal artifacts.[35, 181–183] Most of the spinal hardware systems used are made of stainless steel, which causes marked artifacts on MR imaging because of its ferromagnetic properties. Use of biocompatible titanium hardware eliminates these artifacts and allows for undistorted imaging of the spinal canal and spinal cord adjacent to the surgical site.[181] However, wear debris from titanium may limit incorporation of this material into a fixation system.

The postoperative appearance of unincorporated graft is highly variable and depends on its initial status, amount of operative trauma, postoperative mechanics, and degree of revascularization.[81] MR imaging findings of a stable anterior vertebral body fusion include signal intensity characteristic of fat across an anteriorly grafted segment, caused by continuous marrow across the fusion site.[81, 184] Anterior graft pseudarthrosis demonstrates a gap between the native bone and the graft that is of low signal intensity on T1-weighted images and of high signal intensity on T2-weighted images.[184] MR imaging also may play a role in assessing the functional integrity of spinal grafts. In patients with a successful posterior fusion, fatty replacement of the marrow adjacent to the endplates is present, probably owing to decreased mechanical stress on the vertebrae.[180] Conversely, pseudarthrosis is associated with signal changes suggestive of edema, granulation tissue, and inflammation in the vertebral endplates at the levels of failed fusion.[180]

These alterations reflect functional changes at the vertebral body level but require at least 12 months after operation to become evident.[35]

Functional assessments of graft integrity rely on the absence of significant motion at the fusion site as the criterion for successful fusion. Segmental motion on flexion and extension views frequently is used as the standard diagnostic criterion for pseudarthrosis.[172, 177] Functional motion views are more sensitive than conventional static radiographs for identifying abnormal motion and instability.[177] Typically, lateral bending views are obtained in full flexion and extension. Cleveland and associates suggested that biplane bending views, with lateral views obtained in flexion and extension and anteroposterior views obtained with maximal lateral bending to both sides, were necessary for adequate assessment of spinal fusion.[177] Angular and translational motion can be assessed visually by obtaining tracings of comparative views, by film superimposition, or by measuring changes in intervertebral relationships using fixed anatomic landmarks.[185] Superimposing the radiographs, rather than visual inspection alone, is recommended to maximize the sensitivity of this technique.[177] Concomitant patient rotation must be avoided as the loss of superimposition of the posterior elements and change in vertebral configuration render comparison between the films extremely difficult.

Despite solid posterior fusion and intact posterior hardware, a considerable amount of movement at the disc space still may be present.[94] Anterior disc height greater than 2 mm, more than 10 degrees of angular motion, or horizontal vertebral translation greater than 3 mm have been suggested as reliable criteria for excessive movement across a fused spinal motion segment.[172] Minor degrees of intervertebral movement, the formation of an intradiscal vacuum phenomenon in extension, and the development of osteoporosis are

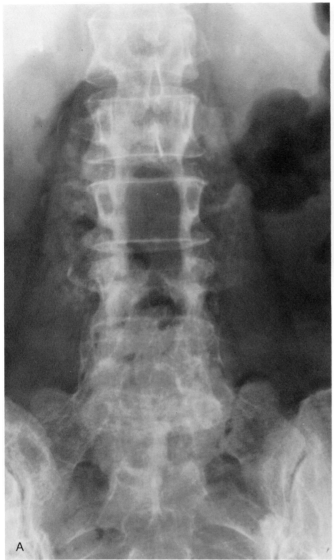

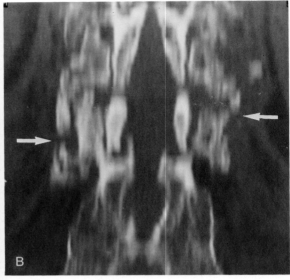

**FIGURE 18–32.** Pseudarthrosis.
**A** The anteroposterior view shows fragmented intertransverse graft bilaterally from L1 to L3. A laminectomy is present at L3 with defects in the inferior facets of L2 and L3 from decompressive foraminotomies.
**B** The curved coronal reformatted CT scan confirms discontinuity of graft material adjacent to the transverse processes (arrows).

unreliable criteria for pseudarthrosis. With successful fusion, intervertebral translations typically decrease 3 to 6 months after operation, and maximal rigidity is achieved after 1 year.[175, 177] Stereophotogrammetry is primarily a research tool for functional evaluation of spinal fusion. In this technique, small metallic spheres are implanted at the time of surgery in the posterior elements of the fused vertebrae.[175, 179] Subsequently, digitized stereoscopic radiographs of the surgical site are evaluated with the aid of computerized calibration devices for motion-induced translation in all three axes of motion.[175] Although this technique is accurate for assessing intervertebral motion, it is not used widely and probably will remain a research tool.

Despite the plethora of imaging methods available, confident diagnosis of pseudarthrosis remains a problem in a large proportion of cases.[172] Steinmann and Herkowitz have summarized the five criteria that appear most reliable in establishing nonunion. These are (1) lack of trabecular continuity; (2) collapse of graft height with a gap between the vertebral endplate and graft material; (3) shift in graft position after healing is expected to have occurred; (4) dislodgment or fracture of internal hardware after healing is expected to have occurred; and (5) unexplained pain in the area of the fusion.[172]

## Infection

Postoperative spinal infection is a very serious complication of any form of spinal surgery, occurring in approximately 1 to 3 per cent of patients.[95] Risk factors for postoperative spinal infection include advanced age, prolonged bed rest and hospitalization, obesity, diabetes, malnutrition, immunosuppression, steroid use, and infection at remote sites.[84, 95] The complexity of the operation and length of operating time also are correlated with the prevalence of infection. Laminotomy and diskectomy are associated with infection in fewer than 1 per cent of cases; spinal fusion without use of hardware carries a 1 to 5 per cent risk; fusion with hardware has an average prevalence of infection of 6 per cent or more.[1, 84, 94, 95] The most common organism implicated is *Staphylococcus aureus*, which accounts for approximately 50 per cent of all postoperative spinal infections, although infections from a variety of other causative organisms (single or multiple) may be encountered.[84, 95] Postoperative infections typically become manifest 10 to 15 days after surgery, although longer delays are not unusual.[84, 95]

Diagnostic imaging does not play a role in the detection of superficial wound infections, which are diagnosed readily clinically. Imaging does play a role in the patient with suspected deep infection, particularly when epidural or disc space infection is suspected. Disc excision creates conditions optimal for the development of infection owing to the presence of hematoma, avascular disc material, and endplate tissue in an environment with a very poor blood supply.[95] Postoperative discitis is a well-recognized complication of spinal surgery, occurring with a frequency of 0.75 to 2.8 per cent of cases.[186] The diagnosis often is delayed because the clinical presentation of pain 1 to 4 weeks after surgery is nonspecific and frequently is not associated with fever or leukocytosis, and also because of the lack of specificity of imaging methods.[95, 186]

Early conventional radiographic findings of disc space loss, osteopenia, and endplate erosion may be difficult to distinguish from some postoperative changes. With progressive infection, vertebral destruction, osseous fragmentation, and reactive sclerosis occur (Fig. 18–33). Loss of fixation and loosening of spinal hardware are seen if the infection cannot be controlled adequately with debridement, irrigation, and antibiotics. CT in the early stages of infection similarly is not reliable and scintigraphy is nonspecific, particularly in the patient operated on recently. Bone scans

using technetium-99m diphosphonate show mild to moderate increased activity within the first 3 weeks after surgery in approximately 50 per cent of patients undergoing laminectomy and diskectomy.[187] The gallium scan also becomes abnormal in 89 per cent of patients in the postoperative period.[187] Increased activity on both bone and gallium scans is related to the postoperative alterations in the bone and soft tissue and typically persists for several months; the bone scan may remain abnormal up to 1 year after operation. The normal increased activity seen on scintigraphic studies limits their usefulness in detecting postoperative spinal infection.

The MR imaging findings of postoperative discitis also show overlap with changes related to uncomplicated surgery. Boden and coworkers compared the MR imaging findings in 15 asymptomatic patients with a group of patients with documented postdiskectomy discitis.[186] The most reliable finding of postoperative infective discitis on MR images was decreased signal intensity in the vertebral marrow of both adjacent endplates in T1-weighted images with enhancement of these areas after the intravenous administration of a gadolinium contrast agent.[186] Marrow hypointensity in T1-weighted images was seen in all seven cases of infection but in only one of the asymptomatic patients.[186]

Postoperative spinal epidural empyema is a rare complication of spinal surgery, encountered in fewer than 1 per cent of patients undergoing elective surgery.[95, 188] The patient frequently has a paucity of clinical symptoms or signs to suggest the diagnosis of infection.[188] The frequent presence of an associated laminectomy allows the abscess to dissect posteriorly through the split retrospinal muscles, minimizing compression on the adjacent neural structures.[188] The CT appearance of the infected collection is very similar to a posttraumatic pseudomeningocele, although the presence of gas bubbles, loss of definition of the fat planes between the collection and the dural sac or the paraspinal muscles, and irregular enhancement of thickened walls all are suggestive of infection.[188]

## SUMMARY

Spine surgery is a rapidly evolving field, with new surgical techniques and hardware being developed continually. Familiarity with the concepts and design principles of surgical instrumentation facilitates interpretation of the placement and complications associated with use of spinal hardware. Diagnostic imaging plays an important role in determining the adequacy of surgical intervention and in detecting complications associated with spinal operations. Recent advances in CT and MR imaging have enhanced the ability to monitor both the osseous and soft tissue changes associated with spinal intervention.

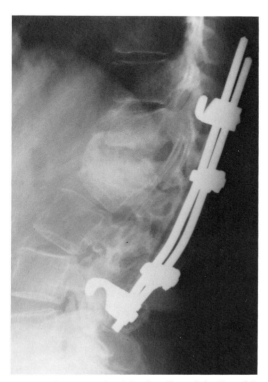

**FIGURE 18–33.** Postoperative infection. Deep infection of the L1-L2 disc and adjacent vertebrae has occurred after TSRH rodding for a burst fracture of L2. The endplates are eroded, with kyphosis and sclerosis resulting from chronic pyogenic infection.

## References

1. Garfin SR, Glover M, Booth RE, et al: Laminectomy: A review of the Pennsylvania hospital experience. J Spinal Disorders *1*:116, 1988.
2. Hu SS, Pashman RS: Spinal instrumentation: Evolution and state of the art. Invest Radiol *27*:632, 1992.
3. Cotler JM, Simpson JM, An HS: Principles, indications, and complications of spinal instrumentation: A summary chapter. *In* An HS, JM Cotler (Eds): Spinal Instrumentation. Baltimore, Williams & Wilkins, 1992, p 435.
4. El-Khoury GY, Renfrew DL: Percutaneous procedures for the diagnosis and treatment of lower back pain: Diskography, facet-joint injection, and epidural injection. AJR *157*:685, 1991.
5. Mooney V, Robertson J: The facet syndrome. Clin Orthop *115*:149, 1976.

6. Raymond J, Dumas J: Intraarticular facet block: Diagnostic test or therapeutic procedure. Radiology 151:333, 1984.
7. Fisher G: Injection therapy for herniated disks: Background and usefulness. Postgraduate Med 75:66, 1984.
8. Burton CV: Conservative management of low back pain. Postgrad Med 70:168, 1981.
9. Destouet JM, Gilula LA, Murphy WA, et al: Lumbar facet joint injection: Indication, technique, clinical correlation, and preliminary results. Radiology 145:321, 1982.
10. Ghormley RK: Low back pain. JAMA 101:1773, 1933.
11. Schellinger D, Wener L, Ragsdale BD, et al: Facet joint disorders and their role in the production of back pain and sciatica. RadioGraphics 7:923, 1987.
12. Pathria M, Sartoris DJ, Resnick D: Osteoarthritis of the facet joints: Accuracy of oblique radiographic assessment. Radiology 164:227, 1987.
13. Lilius G, Laasonen EM, Myllynen P, et al: Lumbar facet joint syndrome: a randomised clinical trial. J Bone Joint Surg [Br] 71:681, 1989.
14. Dory MA: Arthrography of the lumbar facet joints. Radiology 140:23, 1981.
15. Bjorkengren AG, Kurz LT, Resnick D, et al: Symptomatic intraspinal synovial cysts: Opacification and treatment by percutaneous injection. AJR 149:105, 1987.
16. Rothman RH, Wisneski RJ: Errors in decision making as a cause for failure of lumbar surgery. In SR Garfin (Ed): Complications of Spine Surgery. Baltimore, Williams & Wilkins, 1989, p 1.
17. Cuckler JM, Bernini PA, Wiesel SW, et al: The use of epidural steroids in the treatment of lumbar radicular pain. J Bone Joint Surg [Am] 67:63, 1985.
18. Sklar EML, Quencer RM, Green BA, et al: Complications of epidural anesthesia: MR appearance of abnormalities. Radiology 181:549, 1991.
19. Dougherty JH, Fraser RAR: Complications following intraspinal injections of steroids: Report of two cases. J Neurosurg 48:1023, 1978.
20. Kitchel SH, Brown MD: Complications of chemonucleolysis. Clin Orthop 284:63, 1992.
21. Kitchel SH, Brown MD: Complications of chemonucleolysis. In SR Garfin (Ed): Complications of Spine Surgery. Baltimore, Williams & Wilkins, 1989, p 364.
22. Cameron HU: Current concepts of the surgical treatment of low back pain. Mod Med Can 39:49, 1984.
23. Kahanovitz N: Percutaneous diskectomy. Clin Orthop 284:75, 1992.
24. Bozzao A, Gallucci M, Masciocchi C, et al: Lumbar disk herniation: MR imaging assessment of natural history in patients treated without surgery. Radiology 185:135, 1992.
25. Onik G, Maroon J, Helms C, et al: Automated percutaneous diskectomy: initial patient experience. Radiology 162:129, 1987.
26. Hijikata S: Percutaneous nucleotomy: a new concept technique and 12 years' experience. Clin Orthop 238:9, 1989.
27. Onik G, Helms CA, Ginsberg L, et al: Percutaneous lumbar diskectomy using a new aspiration probe: Porcine and cadaver model. Radiology 155:251, 1985.
28. Mall HC, Kaiser JA: The usual appearance of the postoperative lumbar spine. RadioGraphics 7:245, 1987.
29. Grabias S: The treatment of spinal stenosis. J Bone Joint Surg [Am] 62:308, 1980.
30. Wiesel SW: Neurologic complications and lumbar laminectomy: A standardized approach to the multiply operated lumbar spine. In SR Garfin (Ed): Complications of Spine Surgery. Baltimore, Williams & Wilkins, 1989, p 64.
31. Carroll SE, Wiesel SW: Neurologic complications and lumbar laminectomy: A standardized approach to the multiply-operated lumbar spine. Clin Orthop 284:14, 1992.
32. Bosacco SJ, Berman AT: Surgical management of lumbar disc disease. Radiol Clin North Am 21:377, 1983.
33. Risius B, Modic MT, Hardy Jr RW, et al: Sector computed tomographic spine scanning in the diagnosis of lumbar nerve root entrapment. Radiology 143:109, 1982.
34. Teplick JG, Haskin ME: Computed tomography of the postoperative lumbar spine. AJR 141:865, 1983.
35. Djukic S, Lang P, Morris J, et al: The postoperative spine: magnetic resonance imaging. Orthop Clin North Am 21:603,1990.
36. Herkowitz HN, Kurz LT: Degenerative lumbar spondylolisthesis with spinal stenosis. J Bone Joint Surg [Am] 73:802, 1991.
37. Katz JN, Lipson SJ, Larson MG, et al: The outcome of decompressive laminectomy for degenerative lumbar stenosis. J Bone Joint Surg [Am] 73:809, 1991.
38. Lonstein JE: Post-laminectomy kyphosis. Clin Orthop 128:93, 1977.
39. Nakai O, Ookawa A, Yamaura I: Long-term roentgenographic and functional changes in patients who were treated with wide fenestration for central lumbar stenosis. J Bone Joint Surg [Am] 73:1184, 1991.
40. Johnsson K, Willner S, Johnsson K: Postoperative instability after decompression for lumbar spinal stenosis. Spine 11:107, 1986.
41. Rothman SLG, Glenn WV, Kerber CW: Postoperative fractures of lumbar articular facets: occult cause of radiculopathy. AJR 145:779, 1985.
42. Zinreich SJ, Long DM, Davis R, et al: Three-dimensional CT imaging in postsurgical "failed back" syndrome. J Comput Assist Tomogr 14:574, 1990.
43. Hall S, Bartleson JD, Onofrio BM, et al: Lumbar spinal stenosis: Clinical features, diagnostic procedures, and results of surgical treatment in 68 patients. Ann Intern Med 103:271, 1985.
44. Delamarter RB, Bohlman HH, Dodge LD, et al: Experimental lumbar spinal stenosis. J Bone Joint Surg [Am] 72:110, 1990.
45. Deyo RA, Cherkin DC, Loeser JD, et al: Morbidity and mortality in association with operations on the lumbar spine. J Bone Joint Surg [Am] 74:536, 1992.
46. Stambough JL, Simeone FA: Vascular complications in spine surgery. In SR Garfin (Ed): Complications of Spine Surgery. Baltimore, Williams & Wilkins, 1989, p 110.
47. Horowitz SW, Azar-Kia B, Fine M: Postoperative cervical pseudomeningocele. AJNR 11:784, 1990.
48. Marshall LF: Complications of surgery for degenerative cervical and lumbar disc disease. In SR Garfin (Ed): Complications of Spine Surgery. Baltimore, Williams & Wilkins, 1989, p 75.
49. Teplick JG, Peyster RG, Teplick SK, et al: CT identification of postlaminectomy pseudomeningocele. AJR 140:1203, 1983.
50. Edwards CC, Levine AM: Complications associated with posterior instrumentation in the treatment of thoracic and lumbar injuries. In SR Garfin (Ed): Complications of Spine Surgery. Baltimore, Williams & Wilkins, 1989, p 164.
51. Stambough JL, Booth RE Jr: Complications in spine surgery as a consequence of anatomic variations. In SR Garfin (Ed): Complications of Spine Surgery. Baltimore, Williams & Wilkins, 1989, p 89.
52. Kelly JJ, Reuter KL, Waite RJ: Vascular injury complicating lumbar diskectomy: CT diagnosis. AJR 153:1233, 1989.
53. Gower DJ, Culp P, Ball M: Lateral lumbar spine roentgenograms: Potential role in complications of lumbar disc surgery. Surg Neurol 27:316, 1987.
54. Malcolm BW, Bradford DS, Winter RB, et al: Post-traumatic kyphosis: a review of forty-eight surgically treated patients. J Bone Joint Surg [Am] 63:891, 1981.
55. Court-Brown CM, Gertzbein SD: The management of burst fractures of the fifth lumbar vertebra. Spine 12:308, 1987.
56. McEvoy RD, Bradford DS: The management of burst fractures of the thoracic and lumbar spine: Experience in 53 patients. Spine 10:631, 1985.
57. Benson DR: Unstable thoracolumbar fractures, with emphasis on the burst fracture. Clin Orthop 230:14, 1988.
58. Bohlman HH: Treatment of fractures and dislocations of the thoracic and lumbar spine. J Bone Joint Surg [Am] 67:165, 1985.
59. DeWald RL: Burst fractures of the thoracic and lumbar spine. Clin Orthop 189:150, 1984.
60. Willen J, Lindahl S, Irstam L, et al: Unstable thoracolumbar fractures: A study by CT and conventional roentgenology of the reduction effect of Harrington instrumentation. Spine 9:214, 1984.
61. McAfee PC, Yuan HA, Lasda NA: The unstable burst fracture. Spine 7:365, 1982.
62. McAfee PC, Bohlman HH: Complications following Harrington instrumentation for fractures of the thoracolumbar spine. J Bone Joint Surg [Am] 67:672, 1985.
63. Kostuik JP: Anterior Kostuik-Harrington distraction systems. In HS An, JM Cotler (Eds): Spinal Instrumentation. Baltimore, Williams & Wilkins, 1992, p 359.
64. McAfee PC, Bohlman HH, Yuan HA: Anterior decompression of traumatic thoracolumbar fractures with incomplete neurological deficit using a retroperitoneal approach. J Bone Joint Surg [Am] 67:89, 1985.
65. Vazquez-Seoane P, Gertzbein SD, Yuan HA: AO internal fixator. In HS An, JM Cotler (Eds): Spinal Instrumentation. Baltimore, Williams & Wilkins, 1992, p 297.
66. Bohlman HH, Zdeblick TA: Anterior excision of herniated thoracic discs. J Bone Joint Surg [Am] 70:1038, 1988.
67. Bohlman HH, Emery SE: The pathophysiology of cervical spondylosis and myelopathy. Spine 13:843, 1988.
68. Sim FH, Svien HJ, Bickel WH, et al: Swan-neck deformity following extensive cervical laminectomy. J Bone Joint Surg [Am] 56:564, 1974.
69. McAfee PC, Bohlman HH: One-stage anterior cervical decompression and posterior stabilization with circumferential arthrodesis. J Bone Joint Surg [Am] 71:78, 1989.
70. Anderson PA, Bohlman HH: Anterior decompression and arthrodesis of the cervical spine: Long-term motor improvement. J Bone Joint Surg [Am] 74:683, 1992.
71. Bohlman HH, Anderson PA: Anterior decompression and arthrodesis of the cervical spine: Long-term motor improvement. J Bone Joint Surg [Am] 74:671, 1992.
72. Bick EM: An essay on the history of spine fusion operations. Clin Orthop 35:9, 1964.
73. Hadra BE: Wiring of the vertebrae as a means of immobilization in fracture and Pott's disease. Med Times Register 22:423, 1891. (Reprinted in Clin Orthop 112:4, 1975.)
74. Albee FH: Transplantation of a portion of the tibia into the spine for Pott's disease. JAMA 57:885, 1911.
75. Hibbs RA: An operation for progressive spinal deformities. NY Med J 93:1013, 1911.
76. Berchuck M, Garfin SR, Bauman T, Abitbol JJ: Complications of anterior intervertebral grafting. Clin Orthop 284:54, 1992.
77. Karasick D, Huettl EA, Cotler JM: Value of polydirectional tomography in the assessment of the postoperative spine after anterior decompression and vertebral body autografting. Skel Radiol 21:359, 1992.
78. Brown MD, Malinin TI, Davis PB: A roentgenographic evaluation of frozen allografts versus autografts in anterior cervical spine fusions. Clin Orthop 119:231, 1976.
79. Kurz LT, Garfin SR, Booth RE Jr: Iliac bone grafting: techniques and complications of harvesting. In SR Garfin (Ed): Complications of Spine Surgery. Baltimore, Williams & Wilkins, 1989, p 323.
80. Bauman T, Garfin SR: Complications associated with anterior grafting. In SR

Garfin (Ed): Complications of Spine Surgery. Baltimore, Williams & Wilkins, 1989, p 248.

81. Karasick D: Anterior cervical spine fusion: struts, plugs, and plates. Skel Radiol 22:85, 1993.

82. Burns BH: An operation for spondylolisthesis. Lancet 1:1233, 1933.

83. Watkins RG: Anterior lumbar interbody fusion-surgical complications. In SR Garfin (Ed): Complications of Spine Surgery. Baltimore, Williams & Wilkins, 1989, p 278.

84. Massie JB, Heller JG, Abitbol J, et al: Postoperative posterior spinal wound infections. Clin Orthop 284:99, 1992.

85. Watkins R: Anterior lumbar interbody fusion surgical complications. Clin Orthop 284:47, 1992.

86. Sartoris DJ, Gershuni DH, Akeson WH, et al: Coralline hydroxyapatite bone graft substitutes: Preliminary report of radiographic evaluation. Radiology 159:133, 1986.

87. Holmes RE, Bucholz RW, Mooney V: Porous hydroxyapatite as a bone-graft substitute in metaphyseal defects. J Bone Joint Surg [Am] 68:904, 1986.

88. McAfee PC, Bohlman HH, Ducker T, et al: Failure of stabilization of the spine with methylmethacrylate. J Bone Joint Surg [Am] 68:1145, 1986.

89. Kaneda K: Kaneda anterior spinal instrumentation for the thoracic and lumbar spine. In HS An, JM Cotler (Eds): Spinal Instrumentation. Baltimore, Williams & Wilkins, 1992, p 413.

90. Kricun R, Chovanes CE, Shoemaker EI: CT and MR appearance of cervical acrylic struts. J Comput Assist Tomogr 15:519, 1991.

91. Georgis T Jr, Rydevik B, Weinstein JN, et al: Complications of pedicle screw fixation. In SR Garfin (Ed): Complications of Spine Surgery. Baltimore, Williams & Wilkins, 1989, p 200.

92. Eismont FJ, Bohlman HH: Posterior methylmethacrylate fixation for cervical trauma. Spine 6:347, 1981.

93. Zindrick MR, Wiltse LL, Widell EH, et al: A biomechanical study of intrapeduncular screw fixations in the lumbosacral spine. Clin Orthop 203:99, 1986.

94. Sasso RC, Cotler HB, Thalgott JS: Transpedicular fixation with AO dynamic compression plates. In HS An, JM Cotler (Eds): Spinal Instrumentation. Baltimore, Williams & Wilkins, 1992, p 257.

95. Gepstein R, Eismont FJ: Postoperative spine infections. In SR Garfin (Ed): Complications of Spine Surgery. Baltimore, Williams & Wilkins, 1989, p 302.

96. Briggs H, Milligan PR: Chip fusion of the low back following exploration of the spinal canal. J Bone Joint Surg [Br] 26:125, 1944.

97. Vaccaro AR, An HS, Cotler JM: Transpedicular fixation of the spine using the variable screw placement system. In HS An, JM Cotler (Eds): Spinal Instrumentation. Baltimore, Williams & Wilkins, 1992, p 197.

98. Ray CD: The threaded fusion cage: A new method for posterior lumbar interbody fusions. Spine Surgeon 1:12, 1991.

99. Bohlman HH, Cook SS: One-stage decompression and posterolateral and interbody fusion for lumbosacral spondyloptosis through a posterior approach. J Bone Joint Surg [Am] 64:415, 1982.

100. Smith MD, Bohlman HH: Spondylolisthesis treated by a single-stage operation combining decompression with in situ posterolateral and anterior fusion. J Bone Joint Surg [Am] 72:415, 1990.

101. Hensinger RN: Spondylolysis and spondylolisthesis in children and adolescents. J Bone Joint Surg [Am] 71:1098, 1989.

102. Watkins RG: Cervical, thoracic, and lumbar complications—anterior approach. In SR Garfin (Ed): Complications of Spine Surgery. Baltimore, Williams & Wilkins, 1989, p 211.

103. An HS: Surgical exposure and fusion techniques of the spine. In HS An, JM Cotler (Eds): Spinal Instrumentation. Baltimore, Williams & Wilkins, 1992, p 1.

104. Colletta AJ, Mayer PJ: Chylothorax: An unusual complication of anterior thoracic interbody spinal fusion. Spine 7:46, 1982.

105. Foley MJ, Lee C, Calenoff L, et al: Radiologic evaluation of surgical cervical spine fusion. AJR 139:79, 1982.

106. Robinson RA, Smith GW: Anterolateral cervical disk removal and interbody fusion for cervical disk syndrome. Johns Hopkins Hosp Bull 96:223, 1955.

107. Cloward RB: The anterior approach for removal of ruptured cervical disks. J Neurosurg 15:602, 1958.

108. Whitecloud TS, LaRocca H: Fibular strut graft in reconstructive surgery of the cervical spine. Spine 1:33, 1976.

109. White AA, Jupiter J, Southwick WO, et al: An experimental study of the immediate load bearing capacity of three surgical constructions for anterior spine fusions. Clin Orthop 91:21, 1973.

110. Zdeblick TA, Bohlman HH: Cervical kyphosis and myelopathy: Treatment by anterior corpectomy and strut-grafting. J Bone Joint Surg [Am] 71:170, 1989.

111. Stauffer ES, Kelly EG: Fracture-dislocations of the cervical spine: Instability and recurrent deformity following treatment by anterior interbody fusion. J Bone Joint Surg [Am] 59:45, 1977.

112. Hunter LY, Braunstein EM, Bailey RW: Radiographic changes following anterior cervical fusion. Spine 5:399, 1980.

113. Gore DR, Gardner GM, Sepic SB, et al: Roentgenographic findings following anterior cervical fusion. Skel Radiol 15:556, 1986.

114. Fielding JW: Complications of anterior cervical disk removal and fusion. Clin Orthop 284:10, 1992.

115. Smith MD, Bolesta MJ, Leventhal M, et al: Postoperative cerebrospinal-fluid fistula associated with erosion of the dura. J Bone Joint Surg [Am] 74:270, 1992.

116. Emery SE, Smith MD, Bohlman HH: Upper-airway obstruction after multilevel cervical corpectomy for myelopathy. J Bone Joint Surg [Am] 73:544, 1991.

117. Herndon WA, Sullivan JA, Yngve DA, et al: Segmental spinal instrumentation with sublaminar wires: A critical appraisal. J Bone Joint Surg [Am] 69:851, 1987.

118. Slone RM, MacMillan M, Montgomery WJ: Spinal fixation: Part 1. Principles, basic hardware, and fixation techniques for the cervical spine. RadioGraphics 13:341, 1993.

119. Slone RM, MacMillan M, Montgomery WJ, Heare M: Spinal fixation: Part 2. Fixation techniques and hardware for the thoracic and lumbosacral spine. RadioGraphics 13:521, 1993.

120. Slone RM, MacMillan M, Montgomery WJ: Spinal fixation: Part 3. Complications of spinal instrumentation. RadioGraphics 13:797, 1993.

121. Slone RM, Heare MM, Griend RAV, et al: Orthopedic fixation devices. RadioGraphics 11:823, 1991.

122. Albert TJ, An HS, Cotler JM, et al: Harrington instrumentation and modifications. In HS An, JM Cotler (Eds): Spinal Instrumentation. Baltimore, Williams & Wilkins, 1992, p 67.

123. Harrington PR: Treatment of scoliosis: Correction and internal fixation by spine instrumentation. J Bone Joint Surg [Am] 44:591, 1962.

124. Harrington PR: The history and development of Harrington instrumentation. Clin Orthop 93:110, 1973.

125. Byrd JA, Scoles PV, Winter RB, et al: Adult idiopathic scoliosis treated by anterior and posterior spinal fusion. J Bone Joint Surg [Am] 69:843, 1987.

126. Wenger DR, Mubarak SJ, Leach J: Managing complications of posterior spinal instrumentation and fusion. Clin Orthop 284:24, 1992.

127. Wenger DR, Mubarak SJ: Managing complications of posterior spinal instrumentation and fusion. In SR Garfin (Ed): Complications of Spine Surgery. Baltimore, Williams & Wilkins, 1989, p 127.

128. Foley MJ, Calenoff L, Hendrix RW, et al: Thoracic and lumbar spine fusion: postoperative radiologic evaluation. AJR 141:373, 1983.

129. Rubenstein JD, Gertzbein S: Radiographic assessment of Harrington rod instrumentation for spine fractures. J Cana Assoc Radiol 35:159, 1984.

130. Flesch JR, Leider LL, Erickson DL, et al: Harrington instrumentation and spine fusion for unstable fractures and fracture-dislocations of the thoracic and lumbar spine. J Bone Joint Surg [Am] 59:143, 1977.

131. Edwards CC: Edwards instrumentation: a modular spinal system. In HS An, JM Cotler (Eds): Spinal Instrumentation. Baltimore, Williams & Wilkins, 1992, p 303.

132. Cerabona FP, Montesano PX: Jacobs locking hook spinal rod instrumentation. In HS An, JM Cotler (Eds): Spinal Instrumentation. Baltimore, Williams & Wilkins, 1992, p 83.

133. Hales DD, Dawson EG, Delamarter R: Late neurological complications of Harrington-rod instrumentation. J Bone Joint Surg [Am] 71:1053, 1989.

134. Dickson JH, Harrington PR, Erwin WD: Harrington instrumentation in the fractured, unstable thoracic and lumbar spine. Texas Med 69:91, 1973.

135. Knodt H, Larrick RB: Distraction fusion of the spine. Ohio State Med J 12:1140, 1964.

136. Luque ER: The anatomic basis and development of segmental spinal instrumentation. Spine 7:256, 1982.

137. Luque ER: Interpeduncular segmental fixation. Clin Orthop 203:54, 1986.

138. Thometz JG, An HS: Luque instrumentation with sublaminar wiring. In HS An, JM Cotler (Eds): Spinal Instrumentation. Baltimore, Williams & Wilkins, 1992, p 93.

139. Luque ER: Luque semirigid segmental spinal instrumentation of the lumbar spine. In HS An, JM Cotler (Eds): Spinal Instrumentation. Baltimore, Williams & Wilkins, 1992, p 219.

140. Puno RM, Byrd JA III: The Puno-Byrd (PWB) spinal system for transpedicular fixation of the lumbar spine. In HS An, JM Cotler (Eds): Spinal Instrumentation. Baltimore, Williams & Wilkins, 1992, p 281.

141. Drummond DS: Segmental spinal instrumentation with spinous process wires. In HS An, JM Cotler (Eds): Spinal Instrumentation. Baltimore, Williams & Wilkins, 1992, p 105.

142. Balderston RA: Spinal cord injury during surgery for spinal deformity. In SR Garfin (Ed): Complications of Spine Surgery. Baltimore, Williams & Wilkins, 1989, p 144.

143. King D: Internal fixation for lumbosacral fusion. J Bone Joint Surg [Am] 30:560, 1948.

144. Weinstein JN, Rydevik BL, Rauschning W: Anatomic and technical considerations of pedicle screw fixation. Clin Orthop 284:34, 1992.

145. Roy-Camille R, Mazel C, Laville C: Roy-Camille posterior screw plate fixation for cervical, thoracic, lumbar spine and sacrum. In HS An, JM Cotler (Eds): Spinal Instrumentation. Baltimore, Williams & Wilkins, 1992, p 167.

146. Roy-Camille R, Saillant G, Mazel C: Plating of thoracic, thoracolumbar, and lumbar injuries with pedicle screw plates. Orthop Clin North Am 17:147, 1986.

147. Krag MH: The Vermont spinal fixator. In HS An, JM Cotler (Eds): Spinal Instrumentation. Baltimore, Williams & Wilkins, 1992, p 237.

148. McAfee PC, Farey ID, Sutterlin CE, et al: Device-related osteoporosis with spinal instrumentation. Spine 14:919, 1989.

149. Roy-Camille R, Saillant G, Mazel C: Internal fixation of the lumbar spine with pedicle screw plating. Clin Orthop 203:7, 1986.

150. West JL III, Bradford DS, Ogilvie JW: Results of spinal arthrodesis with pedicle screw-plate fixation. J Bone Joint Surg [Am] 73:1179, 1991.

151. Louis R: Spinal internal fixation with Louis instrumentation. In HS An, JM Cotler (Eds): Spinal Instrumentation. Baltimore, Williams & Wilkins, 1992, p 183.

152. Peek RD, Wiltse LL, Hambly MF: The Wiltse system. In HS An, JM Cotler (Eds): Spinal Instrumentation. Baltimore, Williams & Wilkins, 1992, p 227.

153. Johnston CE II, Herring JA, Ashman RB: Texas Scottish Rite Hospital (TSRH) universal spinal instrumentation system. *In* HS An, JM Cotler (Eds): Spinal Instrumentation. Baltimore, Williams & Wilkins, 1992, p 127.

154. Balderston RA: Cotrel-Dubousset instrumentation. *In* HS An, JM Cotler (Eds): Spinal Instrumentation. Baltimore, Williams & Wilkins, 1992, p 113.

155. Asher MA, Strippgen WE, Heinig CF, et al: Isola spinal implant system: Principles, design, and applications. *In* HS An, JM Cotler (Eds): Spinal Instrumentation. Baltimore, Williams & Wilkins, 1992, p 325.

156. Ogilvie JW: Zielke instrumentation of the spine. *In* HS An, JM Cotler (Eds): Spinal Instrumentation. Baltimore, Williams & Wilkins, 1992, p 353.

157. Bayley JC, Yuan HA, Fredrickson BE: The Syracuse anterior I-plate. *In* HS An, JM Cotler (Eds): Spinal Instrumentation. Baltimore, Williams & Wilkins, 1992, p 397.

158. Armstrong GWD, Chow D: The contoured anterior spinal plate. *In* HS An, JM Cotler (Eds): Spinal Instrumentation. Baltimore, Williams & Wilkins, 1992, p 379.

159. An HS: Posterior instrumentation of the cervical spine. *In* HS An, JM Cotler (Eds): Spinal Instrumentation. Baltimore, Williams & Wilkins, 1992, p 33.

160. Abdu WA, Bohlman HH: Techniques of subaxial posterior cervical spine fusions: An overview. Orthopedics *15*:287, 1992.

161. Stauffer ES: Wiring techniques of the posterior cervical spine for the treatment of trauma. Orthopedics *11*:1543, 1988.

162. McAfee PC, Bohlman HH, Riley LH, et al: The anterior retropharyngeal approach to the upper part of the cervical spine. J Bone Joint Surg [Am] *69*:1371, 1987.

163. Smith MD, Kotzar G, Yoo J, et al: A biomechanical analysis of atlantoaxial stabilization methods using a bovine model: C1/C2 fixation analysis. Clin Orthop *290*:285, 1993.

164. Wertheim SB, Bohlman HH: Occipitocervical fusion: indications, technique, and long-term results in thirteen patients. J Bone Joint Surg [Am] *69*:833, 1987.

165. Southwick WO: Management of fractures of the dens (odontoid process). J Bone Joint Surg [Am] *62*:482, 1980.

166. Meyer PR Jr, Rusin JJ, Haak MH: Anterior instrumentation of the cervical spine. *In* HS An, JM Cotler (Eds): Spinal Instrumentation. Baltimore, Williams & Wilkins, 1992, p 49.

167. Ross JS, Masaryk TJ, Modic MT, et al: Lumbar spine: Postoperative assessment with surface-coil MR imaging. Radiology *164*:851, 1987.

168. Boden SD, Davis DO, Dina TS, et al: Contrast-enhanced MR imaging performed after successful lumbar disk surgery: Prospective study. Radiology *182*:59, 1992.

169. Schubiger O, Valavanis A: Postoperative lumbar CT: Technique, results and indications. AJNR *4*:595, 1983.

170. Firooznia H, Kricheff II, Rafii M, et al: Lumbar spine after surgery: Examination with intravenous contrast-enhanced CT. Radiology *163*:221, 1987.

171. Mirowitz SA, Shady KL: Gadopentetate dimeglumine–enhanced MR imaging of the postoperative lumbar spine: comparison of fat-suppressed and conventional T1-weighted images. AJR *159*:385, 1992.

172. Steinmann JC, Herkowitz HN: Pseudarthrosis of the spine. Clin Orthop *284*:80, 1992.

173. Frymoyer JW, Matteri RE, Hanley EN, et al: Failed lumbar disc surgery requiring second operation: A long-term follow-up study. Spine *3*:7, 1978.

174. Clader TJ, Dawson EG, Bassett LW: The role of tomography in the evaluation of the postoperative spinal fusion. Spine *9*:686, 1984.

175. Johnsson R, Stromqvist B, Axelsson P, et al: Influence of spinal immobilization on consolidation of posterolateral lumbosacral fusion: A roentgen stereophotogrammetric and radiographic analysis. Spine *17*:16, 1992.

176. DePalma AF, Rothman RH: The nature of pseudarthrosis. Clin Orthop *59*:113, 1968.

177. Cleveland M, Bosworth DM, Thompson FR: Pseudarthrosis in the lumbosacral spine. J Bone Joint Surg [Am] *30*:302, 1948.

178. Kahanovitz N, Arnoczky SP: The efficacy of direct current electrical stimulation to enhance canine spinal fusions. Clin Orthop *251*:295, 1990.

179. Chafetz N, Cann CE, Morris JM, et al: Pseudarthrosis following lumbar fusion: Detection by direct coronal CT scanning. Radiology *162*:803, 1987.

180. Lang P, Chafetz N, Genant HK, et al: Lumbar spinal fusion: Assessment of functional stability with magnetic resonance imaging. Spine *15*:581, 1990.

181. Mirvis SE, Geisler F, Joslyn JN, et al: Use of titanium wire in cervical spine fixation as a means to reduce MR artifacts. AJNR *9*:1229, 1988.

182. Clayman DA, Murakami ME, Vines FS: Compatibility of cervical spine braces with MR imaging: A study of nine nonferrous devices. AJNR *11*:385, 1990.

183. Lyons CJ, Betz RR, Mesgarszadeh M, et al: The effect of magnetic resonance imaging on metal spine implants. Spine *14*:670, 1989.

184. Ghazi J, Golimbu CN, Engler GL: MRI of spinal fusion pseudarthrosis. J Comput Assist Tomogr *16*:324, 1992.

185. Hanley EN, Matteri RE, Frymoyer JW: Accurate roentgenographic determination of lumbar flexion-extension. Clin Orthop *115*:145, 1976.

186. Boden SD, Davis DO, Dina TS, et al: Postoperative diskitis: Distinguishing early MR imaging findings from normal postoperative disk space changes. Radiology *184*:765, 1992.

187. Silberstein EB, Schneider HJ, Khodadad G, et al: Laminectomy: Effects on postoperative technetium and gallium scintigraphy. Radiology *151*:785, 1984.

188. Spiegelmann R, Findler G, Faibel M, et al: Postoperative spinal epidural empyema: Clinical and computed tomography features. Spine *16*:1146, 1991.

# 19

# Imaging of Joint Replacement

## Barbara N. Weissman, M.D.

The modern era of total joint replacement began in the early 1960s with the introduction of metal-to-plastic prostheses embedded in methylmethacrylate cement.[1] Changes over the years have included metal backing of the acetabular component, introduction of modular design components, the bipolar prosthesis, and the introduction of im-

proved cement fixation and additional types of fixation. With each of these modifications, the radiograph serves as the permanent record of the procedure and an important indicator of its success or failure. The expected radiographic findings after total hip replacement of various kinds and the imaging findings of the major complications of the procedure are reviewed here. Replacement of other joints is covered less extensively. The field of joint replacement surgery is recognized to be a dynamic one, and new developments in surgical technique and in imaging are likely to be forthcoming. This review attempts to provide a basis for the understanding of these developments and for the appropriate use and interpretation of imaging studies.

## TOTAL HIP REPLACEMENT

### Radiographic Technique

Radiographs are critical to following patients with total joint replacements. Unfortunately, obtaining standardized radiographs often is difficult. Methods with internal reference markers provide improved evaluation but are not readily available.[2, 3] The standard radiographic series consists of an anteroposterior view of the pelvis centered at the pubis, and an anteroposterior and frog-leg lateral view of the affected hip. Enough of the femoral shaft must be included to allow assessment of the size of the medullary canal preoperatively and of the entire femoral component and adjacent bone postoperatively. True lateral radiographs are obtained in selected cases to evaluate component position.

### Component Position

From standard radiographs, several determinations of acetabular and femoral component positions and relationships can be made.[4, 5]

#### Acetabular Inclination

Acetabular inclination indicates the tilt of the acetabular component in relation to a horizontal baseline (Fig. 19–1A). It is measured on the anteroposterior radiograph of the pelvis as the angle between lines through the medial and

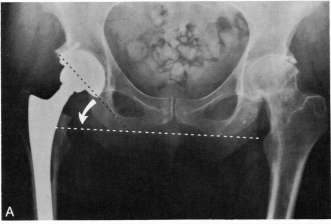

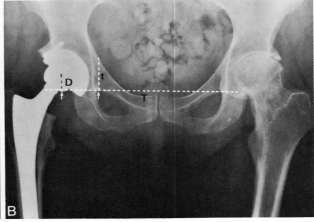

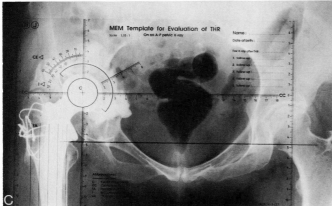

**FIGURE 19–1.** Component position.

**A** Angle of acetabular inclination. The angle between the baseline and the acetabular orifice (curved arrow) describes the tilt of the acetabular component with relation to the horizontal.

**B** Vertical and mediolateral position. The vertical position of the hip is measured as the perpendicular distance (D) from the center of the femoral head to the interteardrop line (T). The mediolateral position of the hip (between arrows) is measured as the distance along the interteardrop line from the teardrop (t) to the intersection with a perpendicular from the center of the femoral head.

**C** The ME Müller template. The template is aligned to the film with the rule (the CC line) parallel to the interteardrop line (T) and the cross is centered on the femoral head. The teardrop line can be traced onto the template. Cranial migration of the socket then can be determined on follow-up radiographs as the distance between the new interteardrop line and the original line. Medial migration of the socket is measured from point C to a perpendicular line through the teardrop.

lateral poles of the equatorial marker wire of the acetabular component and a baseline drawn along the ischial tuberosities, the teardrop shadows, or the inferior portions of the sacroiliac joints. An angle of inclination of 40 to 50 degrees has been classified as neutral, with lower measurements indicating a relatively horizontal orientation and greater measurements indicating a more vertical one. Herrlin and coworkers[6, 7] note that because this method is two-dimensional, it does not provide exact information about the angle of the acetabular component in the transverse plane. Furthermore, the tilt of the nonopaque acetabular liner of a metal-backed component cannot be appreciated on standard radiographs, although the tilt of the metal backing may be determined.

### Superoinferior Acetabular Position

Measurement of the position of the center of the hip is determined as the perpendicular distance from the center of the femoral head to a line (interteardrop line) connecting the teardrop shadows of both hips (Fig. 19–1B). When metal-backed acetabular components obscure the femoral head, the center of the cup is used as the hip center point.[8] Vertical position of the hip can be compared on serial radiographs using this method if positions are similar.

The Ranawat triangle method allows construction of a reference triangle whose position is determined from bony landmarks.[9] The superior limb of the triangle indicates the position of the subchondral bone of the acetabular roof in a

normal pelvis and may be used as a reference line for comparing component position over time.

### Mediolateral Acetabular Position

The distance along the interteardrop line from an intersection with a perpendicular line from the center of the femoral head to the teardrop allows comparison of the mediolateral position of the hip over time (Fig. 19–1B). Changes of more than 2 mm are considered significant with 10 per cent magnification. The Ranawat triangle also may be used as a reference for mediolateral prosthetic position. Kohler's line (the ilioischial line) is affected by rotation of the pelvis, making this reference of limited utility. A template designed by the Müller Foundation (ME Müller total hip replacement template, Berne, Switzerland, 1988) facilitates these measurements (Fig. 19–1C).

### Acetabular Anteversion

As emphasized by Herrlin[7] and Massin and colleagues,[8] varying concepts regarding acetabular anteversion exist. Herrlin notes true anteversion to be measured as rotation around an axis perpendicular to the transverse plane of the body. Clinically, anteversion usually is determined from the true lateral view of the hip. A parallel to the table or film edge provides the baseline in the coronal plane. The angle between a perpendicular to the baseline and the axis of the acetabular marker wire is the angle of anteversion[7] (Fig. 19–2). Frontal radiographs also allow evaluation of antever-

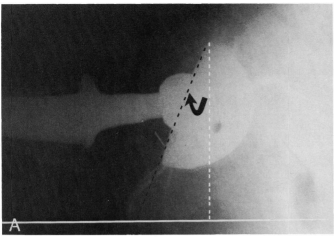
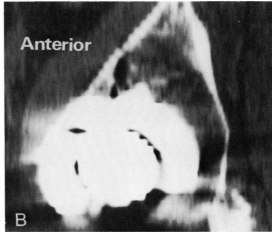

**FIGURE 19–2.** Acetabular anteversion.
  **A** The angle (curved arrow) between the axis of the acetabular marker wire and a perpendicular to the baseline (parallel to the edge of the film) is the angle of acetabular anteversion.
  **B** A reformatted CT scan shows the posterior tilt of the acetabular component in another patient.

sion. The maximal diameter of the acetabular marker ring is divided by its minimal diameter and the quotient is compared to a reference table.[10] Increasing anteversion or retroversion makes the wire appear more circular. Other methods also are available.[11, 12] CT scanning in the transaxial plane allows determination of the angle of anteversion if artifact-reducing software is available[13] (Fig. 19–2). Reformatted CT scans along the parasagittal plane allow the tilt of the acetabular component anteriorly or posteriorly to be seen directly. The correct degree of tilt is not agreed on but ranges from 0 to 25 degrees of anteversion.

### Femoral Component Position

The tip of the femoral stem should appear on the frontal radiograph to be centered in the medullary canal or to be directed medially (valgus). Femoral component anteversion may be measured on fluoroscopy in a method similar to that used for nonoperated hips. The patient undergoes fluoroscopy in the supine position. The leg is rotated under fluoroscopic visualization until the femoral neck appears longest. The angle between the vertical and the leg represents the degree of anteversion or retroversion. If the leg is rotated internally, anteversion is present.[11]

### Leg Length

Leg length is compared on the two sides by noting the distances between the proximal edge of the lesser trochanters and a baseline through the ischial tuberosity on each side.

## Component Fixation

Four major methods of component fixation to bone are used currently: press fitting, fixation with polymethylmethacrylate (PMMA) cement, bone ingrowth into porous surfaces, and hydroxyapatite coating.[14] The normal appearances and complications of each of these fixation methods are reviewed. General complications are reviewed under the discussion of cement fixation.

### Press Fitting

Press fitting of components was used primarily in the 1950s. With this type of fixation, the surgically created bed for the prosthesis is made smaller than the prosthesis itself, which then is forced into the defect.[14] In some cases, loosening occurred, and in others "stress shielding" developed when load was transferred preferentially through the prosthesis to the distal portion of the bone resulting in bone resorption in the proximal aspect of the femur and bone formation distally.

### Polymethylmethacrylate Cement Fixation

In 1961, Charnley reported the use of PMMA cement for fixation of total hip components.[1] The cement provided immediate stable fixation and functioned to distribute load more evenly to the bone. Overall, a clinical success rate of approximately 90 per cent was accomplished for cemented total hip replacements performed in the 1970s.[15] Results were disappointing, however, in younger and more active patients owing to a higher rate of prosthetic loosening.[15–17] Improvements in cementing techniques have lowered the rates of loosening on the femoral side.[18] For example, Harris and McGann[18] found aseptic loosening in only 1.7 per cent at an average of 3.3 years postoperatively. On the acetabular side, however, a nearly linear increase in acetabular loosening has been reported,[15] and improvements in cement technique are less applicable to the acetabular component. Currently, therefore, porous coated acetabular implants often are matched with cemented femoral components for older, less active patients.[19, 20] For younger patients, porous coated femoral components may be used as well.

#### Normal Appearances of Cement-Bone Interface

*Lucent Lines.* Methylmethacrylate transmits stress evenly to the underlying bone via interdigitation of the bone with the cement.[21] Indeed, pathologic examination of well-functioning femoral stems years after implantation with cement fixation has shown the host bone of the femur to have remodeled so that it was directly in contact with the cement interdigitations, usually without an intervening fibrous membrane.[22] A dense shell of bone had developed around the cement and grown into the irregular cement surface. Trabecular struts connected this inner ring of bone to the outer cortex, which was osteoporotic. The cement-bone interface was "intact and excellent throughout." On pathologic inspection of retrieved prostheses, fractures of the cement and separation of the cement from bone were seen, but the integrity of the cement-bone interface largely was intact. Radiographically this rim of new bone formation adjacent to the cement surface is not discernible.

On radiographs, thin lucent lines often are seen, however, along the cement-bone interface (Fig. 19–3). These lucent lines generally represent the end-stage of a process of necrosis and repair that results in the formation of a fibrous membrane without inflammation.[23] The appearance usually becomes stable by 2 years, with a visible radiolucent zone of 0.1 to 1.5 mm.[24] Lucent lines are distinguishable from areas of osteoporosis or residual trabecular bone by the presence of a thin line of reactive sclerosis that separates them from the adjacent bone. Without these sclerotic demarcation lines, lucent lines are difficult to evaluate and may provide a false impression of prosthetic loosening.[25]

***Standardization of Radiographic Reporting.*** Conventional nomenclature has been adapted for describing the regions of the prosthetic components (Fig. 19–4). The interface areas of the acetabulum are described as three zones after the system of DeLee and Charnley.[26] The femoral zones were divided into seven regions by Gruen and associates.[27] Additional zones may be evaluated on the lateral radiograph. Standardization of reporting of clinical and radiologic results has been attempted.[28]

**Arthrography.** Arthrography is performed most often to confirm intra-articular needle location at the time of attempted aspiration rather than specifically to identify component loosening. When the needle is introduced into the joint, every attempt should be made to obtain joint fluid. Internal rotation of the leg may be helpful. Cone and coworkers note that needle placement is an important determinant of the ability to aspirate fluid.[29] When the needle is placed on the anterior aspect of the neck of the prosthesis, fluid often cannot be obtained, whereas when the tip of the needle is placed at the medial margin of the head-neck junction, fluid usually is obtained. Instillation of nonbacteriostatic saline solution followed by reaspiration may be used when no fluid is forthcoming. Some authors suggest reaspiration of injected contrast medium, but the practice is controversial. Kim and Lachman[30] evaluated the bactericidal effects of various contrast materials on *Staphylococcus aureus*. Meglumine diatrizoate (Renografin-60, 76, or M-60) showed bactericidal or bacteriostatic effects whereas Vascoray, meglumine iothalamate (Conray), and diatrizoate sodium (Hypaque Sodium 50 per cent) did not inhibit bacterial growth. The effects were dependent on the size of the bacterial inoculum, as well as on the type and dilution of the contrast medium. Thus, it appears that if contrast material is reaspirated, it would be better not to use Renografin and to use the smallest amount of contrast medium or dilute contrast medium. Unfortunately, this may not be possible if optimal delineation of component loosening also is required. In contrast to these findings, Melson and colleagues found that arthrography with the tested contrast agents (including Renografin 76) did not interfere with subsequent bacterial cultures.[31] Interestingly, the absence of joint effusion on attempted aspiration apparently does not exclude a diagnosis of infection, as no fluid could be aspirated in

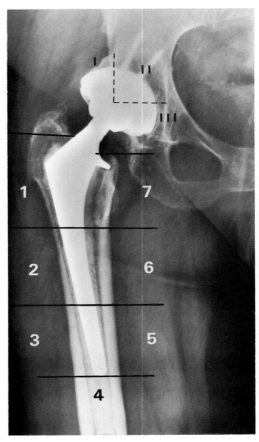

**FIGURE 19–4.** Reference zones. The zones of the acetabulum are described according to DeLee and Charnley[26] and those of the femur according to Gruen and coworkers.[27] Additional zones are added for evaluation of the lateral radiograph.

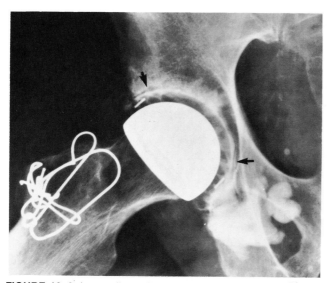

**FIGURE 19–3.** Lucent lines. A "normal" thin lucent line is present along a portion of the acetabular cement (arrows) of this surface replacement.

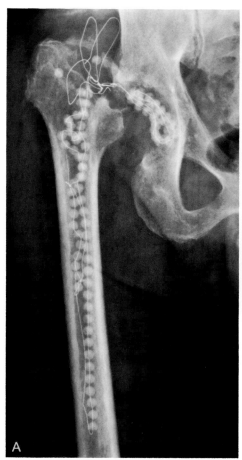

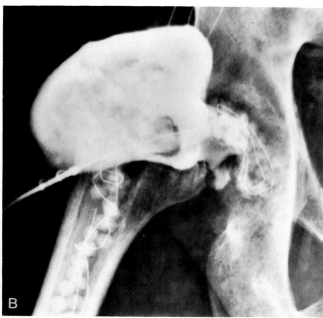

**FIGURE 19–5.** Modified Girdlestone arthroplasty.
  **A** The components of an infected total hip replacement have been removed and antibiotic methylmethacrylate beads have been inserted. The femur is subluxed superolaterally.
  **B** Joint aspiration and arthrography were performed. In this case, the needle was introduced obliquely into the acetabulum. An unusually large joint pseudocapsule has filled with contrast material.

two of six cases of infection reported by Barrack and Harris.[32–34]

After aspiration of fluid, contrast medium is injected usually until the patient has discomfort, lymphatic filling occurs, or contrast medium is seen along the cement-bone interface.[35, 36] Films taken before and after ambulation are obtained. The value of additional techniques for demonstrating component loosening is discussed later.

*Aspiration After Modified Girdlestone Arthroplasty.* After modified Girdlestone arthroplasty for removal of infected components, respiration often is used to obtain material for culture prior to reinsertion of prosthetic components (Fig. 19–5). The site of needle placement for aspiration has been described by Swan and coworkers.[37] With the patient supine, a site is chosen for needle puncture at the midpoint and slightly cephalad to a line drawn between the greater and lesser trochanters. A 20 gauge needle is directed vertically, perpendicular to this site, with the needle entrance between the resection margins of the femur and acetabulum. The needle is advanced until the posterior aspect of the acetabulum is encountered. In other instances, the depth of the pseudocapsule is uncertain and must be estimated, with aspiration attempted as the needle is withdrawn.

*Arthrographic Appearance.* Four to 5 months after surgery, a new capsule develops that is smooth and relatively small.[38] Theoretically, injected contrast material should remain confined to this space (Fig. 19–6). Capsular extensions, taking the form of bursae and cavities, were found,

however, in 43 per cent of 178 arthrograms of painful total hip replacements studied by Berquist and associates.[39] Bursae were located most frequently adjacent to the greater trochanter (32 cases), along the acetabulum (18 cases), or

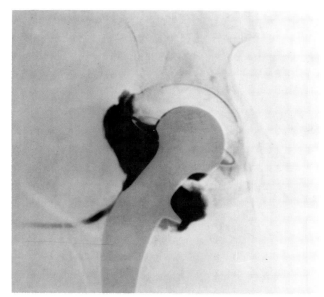

**FIGURE 19–6.** Subtraction arthrogram. No contrast material is present along the cement-bone interface about either component. The joint capsule is a little larger than usual.

**TABLE 19–1. Definitions of Prosthetic Loosening After Total Hip Arthroplasty**

| Femoral Loosening | Acetabular Loosening |
|---|---|
| *Brand* | *Brand* |
|   Any entire lucent zone ≥ 2mm, or |   Any entire lucent zone ≥ 2 mm, or |
|   Any position change ≥ 4mm, or |   Any position change ≥ 4 mm or ≥ 4 degrees |
|   Any cement fracture | |
| *Stauffer* | *Stauffer 1* |
|   Any cement-prosthesis lucent zone, or |   Any acetabular lucent zone, or |
|   Complete cement-bone lucent zone, or |   Any position change |
|   Any position change | *Stauffer 2\** |
| |   Any acetabular lucent zone, or |
| |   Any position change ≥ 4 mm or ≥ 4 degrees |
| *McBeath* | *McBeath 1* |
|   Any femoral position change |   Any position change |
| | *McBeath 2* |
| |   Any position change ≥ 4 mm or ≥ 4 degrees |
| *Cotterill* | *Cotterill 1* |
|   Any progressive lucent zone |   Any progressive lucent zone |
| *Gruen* | |
|   Any progressive lucent zone, or | |
|   Any position change, or | |
|   Any cement fracture | |
| *Harris* | |
|   Component or cement migration, or | |
|   Cement fracture, or | |
|   Development of metal-cement lucent zone | |

*Definition modified from Brand RA, Pedersen DR, Yoder SA. Clin Orthop *210*:185, 1986.

beneath the iliopsoas muscle and tendon (12 cases). Uninfected collections (bursae) usually are large and smooth-walled extensions of the capsule, whereas infected cavities typically are irregular and have synovial proliferation and a narrow, irregular communication to the joint. Recurrent dislocation is noted in one third of patients with a supra-acetabular bursa.[39] The iliopsoas bursa may become extremely enlarged,[40] appear as an inguinal mass, and compress inguinal vessels or the bladder. Greater trochanteric bursae were associated with prior revision surgery, trochanteric nonunion, prosthetic loosening, or infection or bursitis. Steinbach and colleagues note that trochanteric bursae may occur without previous trochanteric osteotomy, with trochanteric nonunion, or in association with trochanteric wires.[41] A cyst also has been reported in the rectus femoris sheath.[42]

**Bone Scan.** The expected sequence of isotope uptake around the components of a total hip replacement was evaluated by Utz and coworkers.[43] Presumably, these were cemented components, although this is not stated. In general, activity about the hip decreased over time. Nonetheless, 10 per cent of asymptomatic patients displayed increased uptake in the acetabular region for more than 3 years. By 1 year after surgery, no patient displayed more than mild radionuclide activity at the lesser trochanter or about the shaft of the prosthesis. Uptake of the radiopharmaceutical agent stabilized at the tip of the femoral stem by 10 to 12 months, but 9 per cent of patients had persistent definite uptake after 12 months. Thereafter, an increase in the uptake of the radionuclide at the tip of the femoral stem was thought to represent asymptomatic loosening. Overall the investigators concluded that "most patients will have normal bone scan approximately 1 year after surgery. Approximately 20 per cent of patients will, however, have marginally increased activity that persists for more than 1 year . . . [and] 10 per cent . . . will have a persistent definite increase in bone scan activity . . . most commonly at the greater

trochanter and prosthesis tip, which may represent remodeling or asymptomatic loosening."[43]

**Complications**

*Loosening.* Loosening is the most common cause of failure of cemented prostheses. It may be due to inadequate component fixation or to infection. Loosening rates differ in the various reported series, and comparison is made difficult by the lack of uniformity in its definition[44, 45] (Table 19–1). Improvements in cement technique have reduced loosening rates on the femoral side.[18] In contrast, acetabular loosening has been found to increase with time, and efforts at improving cement fixation have been less successful. Mechanical loosening has been reported in 41 per cent of cases.[46, 47]

*Radiographic Findings.* The radiographic findings suggesting loosening of a cemented total hip prosthesis are listed in Table 19–2.[5] They are discussed here only briefly.

CEMENT-BONE LUCENT ZONES GREATER THAN 2 MM. Cement-bone lucent zones greater than 2 mm in thickness or that are increasing in thickness suggest component loosening (Fig. 19–7). Acetabular lucent zones may be seen better if multiple views are obtained. Cain and coworkers,[48] for example, noted that additional oblique (Judet) views increased the sensitivity for detection of loosening over standard anteroposterior views and suggested that both antero-

**TABLE 19–2. Radiograph Findings Suggesting Loosening or Infection, or Both, of Cemented Total Hip Prostheses**

Cement-bone lucent zone of 2 mm or more
Widening of the cement-bone lucent zone
Migration of prosthetic components
Development or widening of metal-cement lucent zone
Cement fracture
Periosteal reaction
Motion of components demonstrable on stress views or fluoroscopy

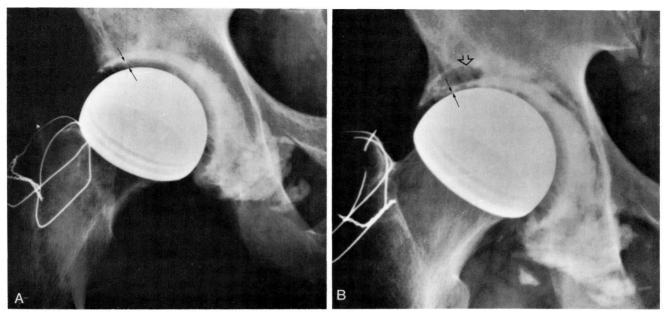

**FIGURE 19–7.** Loosening of a surface replacement with a wide cement-bone interface.

**A** A thick zone of opaque cement is noted around the acetabular component. The femoral component is cemented in place, but the interface is not visible owing to the overlying metal. The thickness of the acetabular component is shown by the arrows.

**B** Thirteen years later, the acetabular component shows wear, as evidenced by reduction in its thickness (arrows). A wide cement-bone lucent zone with adjacent sclerosis (open arrow) is seen, attesting to loosening of the acetabular component.

posterior views of the pelvis and anteroposterior views of the hip be obtained for evaluation of acetabular lucent zones.

The accuracy of the finding of a wide lucent zone for the diagnosis of loosening is thought to be greater on the femoral side than on the acetabular side.[48–52] Hodgkinson and associates[32, 33] found that the presence of a continuous lucent zone around the acetabular component indicated loosening in 94 per cent of cases. O'Neill and Harris[51] found that all acetabular sockets thought to be loose on the basis of component migration or a complete cement-bone lucent zone that measured at least 2 mm in some area proved to be loose at surgery. Many of those predicted to be well fixed, however, actually were loose. The sensitivity for acetabular loosening was only 37 per cent in this series. On the femoral side, similarly, every femoral component thought to be loose on radiographs was loose, but five components predicted on radiographs to be fixed actually were loose (sensitivity 89 per cent, specificity 100 per cent). The lucent zone visible radiographically corresponded to a synovium-like membrane that elaborated substances that resorbed bone.[53–61]

PROSTHESIS-CEMENT LUCENT LINES. Initially a thin lucent line may be present along the proximolateral aspect of the femoral component in up to 24 per cent of patients because of poor metal-cement contact in that region at the time of surgery.[24] Stable, thin lucent lines in this same region may be caused by the Mach effect.[62] The development of a lucent line, however, indicates component motion and, therefore, loosening (Fig. 19–8). This appearance of loosening is termed subsidence; it represents sinking of the femoral component inferiorly and medially. The process of subsidence was thought by Charnley to reach a point of renewed stability,[1] and, indeed, although all of these

prostheses technically are loose, many patients with such prostheses are asymptomatic.[62]

CEMENT FRACTURE. Some 1.5 per cent of cases studied by Weber and Charnley[63] demonstrated cement fracture, usually within the first year (Fig. 19–9). Other features of subsidence accompany cement fracture in most instances. Although prosthetic loosening is present, patients often are asymptomatic.

Despite the use of these well-known signs for loosening of cemented components, the criteria for loosening remain controversial. Criteria for acetabular loosening vary. Yoder and colleagues[64] defined acetabular loosening by a change in component position of greater than 4 mm or 4 degrees or by the presence of a cement-bone lucent zone of 2 mm along the entire component interface. Harris and Penenberg[46] described definite loosening as indicated by acetabular migration and impending loosening as a 2 mm continuous lucent zone. Acetabular loosening that occurs relatively early (within 10 years) is thought to be the result of deficient bone support, whereas late loosening is likely the result of component wear.[47] Migration of the acetabular component can be assessed by the methods described earlier.

Femoral component loosening has been described as definite when there is radiographic evidence of component or cement migration, as probable when a complete radiolucent zone is present, and as possible when a radiolucent line is present at the cement-bone interface involving 50 to 100 per cent of its interface.[18]

*Arthrographic Findings.* Arthrography was introduced for evaluation of total hip replacements in 1971 by Salvati and associates.[65] The appearance of injected contrast material at the bone-cement interface (Figs. 19–10 and 19–11) was considered proof of component loosening, and no

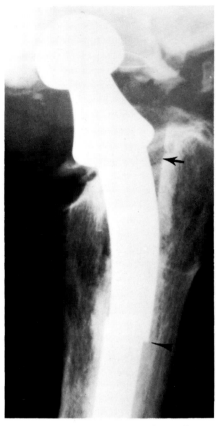

**FIGURE 19–8.** Fatigue fracture of a metal femoral stem (arrowhead) with separation at the metal-cement interface proximally (arrow).

subtraction arthrography has several advantages over photographic subtraction: it provides immediate dynamic viewing of the subtracted images, is quicker and easier, and permits the images to be manipulated.[77, 79] Walker and colleagues[78] compared photographic subtraction and digital subtraction in the assessment of 53 painful total hip replacements that subsequently required revision surgery. The digital subtraction technique improved the detection of femoral component loosening (sensitivity of photographic subtraction, 79 per cent; sensitivity of digital subtraction, 96 per cent; 100 per cent specificity for both methods). Improvement provided by the digital subtraction technique was less marked for the acetabular side of the joint. Digital subtraction images also demonstrated vascular and lymphatic opacification to advantage.

Modifications of subtraction technique include a computer processing method[74] and color subtraction.[73] Another method (K-edge digital subtraction) relies on the subtraction of two digital radiographs produced by x-ray beams above and below the K-edge of iodine.[76] This technique decreases the problem of patient motion and allows subtraction studies to be performed after exercise and in imaging planes other than the usual anteroposterior plane.

Arthrographic images obtained after the patient has walked may show evidence of component loosening not seen without ambulation. Hardy and coworkers[80] noted that the arthrographic features of loosening were more prominent after ambulation in 42 per cent of cases studied. In

false-positive cases were noted. One false-negative examination of a femoral component, however, was recorded. This initial enthusiasm was tempered by subsequent reports, particularly that of Murray and Rodrigo.[66]

Attention to the details of technique is thought to be important for improved accuracy in the diagnosis of component loosening. Underfilling of the joint, for example, may lead to failure to document loosening. This was confirmed on arthrographic studies by Hendrix and coworkers,[36] who injected relatively large volumes of contrast material into the hip until the entire cement-bone interface filled or the patient complained of pain. After injection of only 5 ml of contrast material, accuracy for the diagnosis of component loosening was 51 per cent (less than that of plain radiography), whereas the high-pressure study yielded an accuracy of 92 per cent. Tehranzadeh and associates found the arthrogram to be highly sensitive for the detection of femoral component loosening but of low sensitivity for detection of loosening of the acetabular component.[50] When the pseudocapsule is large or bursae are present that fill with the injected contrast material, attempts to opacify the cement-bone interface at arthrography may fail and lead to false-negative findings.[35]

Subtraction techniques allow the contrast medium to be differentiated from the opaque cement, making the distribution of injected contrast material easier to define.[71–79] Disadvantages to photographic subtraction include the need for strict patient immobility before and after injection, the time-consuming nature of the process, and the inability to use the technique after the patient has exercised. Digital

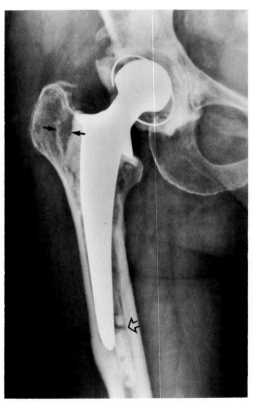

**FIGURE 19–9.** Loosening of a cemented femoral component with a cement fracture. Subsidence of the femoral stem has occurred, with settling of the stem into varus position, development of a wide cement-bone interface laterally (solid arrows), cement fracture distally (open arrow), and thickening and remodeling of the femoral cortex near the tip of the prosthesis.

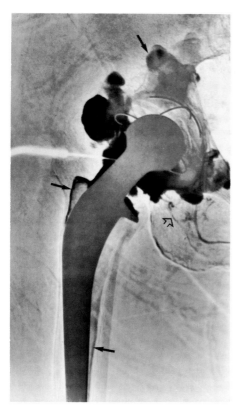

**FIGURE 19–10.** Loose cemented acetabular and femoral components shown on arthrography. The subtraction arthrogram shows the contrast medium (appearing dark) tracking along the cement about the femoral and the acetabular components (solid arrows). Faint lymphatic filling is present (open arrow).

three of 24 patients examined (12.5 per cent), the diagnosis of loosening could be made only on the postambulation films.

Reported arthrographic criteria for loosening of cemented components have varied. In 1987, Maus and associates[35] reevaluated the criteria for loosening, and their results are now in wide use (Tables 19–3 and 19–4). These authors reviewed the arthrograms of 97 hips that subsequently required surgical revision or exploration. Arthrography was performed with an attempt to generate high intra-articular pressure by injecting contrast material until lymphatic filling occurred or pain was noted. Oblique views, film subtraction, postexercise radiographs, and anesthetic injection complemented the examination. The combination of arthrographic and plain film examination allowed the diagnosis of loosening of the femoral component to be made with a sensitivity of 96 per cent and a specificity of 92 per cent. Correlation with noncontrast radiographic findings of loosening was of particular importance in cases in which the arthrogram demonstrated bursal filling, thus obviating the development of high intra-articular pressure.

On the acetabular side, revised arthrographic criteria for loosening were developed that resulted in a sensitivity of 97 per cent and a specificity of 68 per cent. This low specificity on the acetabular side is noteworthy and an important consideration when interpreting arthrograms. It seems to substantiate the findings of Murray and Rodrigo,[66] who performed arthrography in 42 asymptomatic patients with total hip replacements and found evidence of loosening of the acetabular component in 22.6 per cent. These results indicate that loosening of the acetabular component need not be symptomatic. Furthermore, these authors found

**FIGURE 19–11.** Component loosening shown on arthrography.

**A** Radiograph of revised total hip arthroplasty using a long-stem femoral component. Inadequate bone cement is present distally, with "cutting out" of the distal stem laterally (lower arrowhead). A radiolucent zone (1.5 mm) is present at the proximal bone-cement interface (upper arrowhead).

**B** Subtraction arthrogram shows contrast material along the bone-cement interface of the acetabular and femoral components (large arrows). Contrast material is observed tracking through the site of the cortical window into soft tissues (arrowhead). Lymphatic filling is noted (small arrows). (Courtesy of S. Kleiman, M.D., La Jolla, California.)

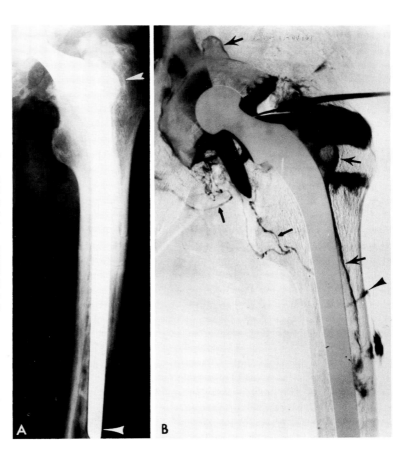

**TABLE 19–3. Arthrographic Criteria for
Acetabular Component Loosening***

Contrast material in all zones (90 per cent)†
Contrast material in zones I and II or in zones II and III
Contrast material in zones I and III with a medium or large
　pseudocapsule or bursa (57 per cent)
Contrast material more than 2 mm thick in any zone (95 per cent)
Positive signs on radiographs in a patient with a medium or large
　pseudocapsule or bursa

*From Maus TP, et al: Radiology *162*:721, 1987.
　†The number in parentheses indicates the percentage of cases with this finding that
exhibited prosthetic loosening at surgery.

loosening of the acetabular component in only seven of 12
patients who had acetabular loosening predicted arthro-
graphically. Generally, arthrography tends to produce false-
positive results for loosening of the acetabular component
and false-negative results for loosening of the femoral component.[68]

Lymphatic opacification at arthrography has been described by Coren and colleagues[81] as a nonspecific indicator
of inflammation. Dussault and coworkers[70] found lymphatic
filling in patients with prosthetic loosening and infection,
in those without such loosening or infection, and in those
with prosthetic loosening only. Bloom and associates,[82]
however, noted lymphatic opacification in 21 of 30 loose
prostheses (with or without infection) and in none of 22
prostheses that were not loose. They concluded that lymphatic opacification during arthrographic evaluation of a
total hip prosthesis was an ancillary finding of loosening
(Fig. 19–11). The sensitivity of this finding for loosening
was 70 per cent and the specificity was 100 per cent.

Anesthetic injection into a painful postoperative hip may
help to differentiate pain originating in the hip from that
related to extra-articular sources.[83] Intra-articular instillation
of an anesthetic agent most often is used as an adjunct to
arthrography. Anesthetic agents such as bupivacaine or lidocaine are injected into the joint after fluid has been aspirated for culture. Lack of pain relief is nonspecific, but
significant improvement in pain suggests an intra-articular
cause.[35] Guercio and colleagues[84] found that intra-articular
administration of an anesthetic agent reduced the pain associated with loosening of the acetabular component or
with synovitis or capsulitis but not that associated with
loosening of the femoral component. Burton and coworkers[85] found that in 95 per cent of cases, the response to
intra-articular lidocaine predicted an intra-articular cause
for the pain, amenable to revision surgery. In two cases,
patients responded to hip revision surgery despite the absence of a beneficial response to intra-articular injection of
lidocaine (8 per cent false-negative rate). Unlike the find-

**TABLE 19–4. Arthrographic Criteria for
Femoral Component Loosening***

Contrast material in prosthesis-cement interface below the
　intertrochanteric line (95 per cent)†
Contrast material in the bone-cement interface extending below the
　intertrochanteric line in regular components or to the
　midcomponent level in long-stem prostheses (98 per cent)

*From Maus TP, et al: Radiology *162*: 721, 1987.
　†Number in parentheses indicates the percentage of components that were loose at
the time of surgery.

ings of Guercio and colleagues, many of the responders had
femoral component loosening.

*Arthroscintigraphic Findings.*[85–88] Injection of isotope
(e.g. $^{99m}$Tc sulfur colloid) into the joint at the time of contrast arthrography has been advocated to improve the accuracy of detecting femoral component loosening. The acetabular component cannot be evaluated with this radionuclide
method. Femoral component loosening is detected by extension of the isotope beyond the confines of the joint
capsule, along the femoral stem. Using the combination of
arthroscintigraphy and contrast arthrography, Resnik and
associates[330] found 100 per cent sensitivity and specificity
for detection of component loosening.

Maxon and coworkers[67] used a combined isotope technique, which permitted evaluation of both the femoral and
the acetabular components. Radionuclide (100 μCi $^{111}$In-di-
ethylenetriamine pentaacetic acid) was injected intra-articularly at the time of contrast arthrography. Three hours
prior to this, 10 mCi of $^{99m}$Tc-methylene diphosphonate had
been injected intravenously. The radionuclide study proved
more specific than a contrast arthrogram (100 per cent versus 58 per cent), whereas the arthrogram was more sensitive
(100 per cent versus 64 per cent). There were five false-
positive contrast arthrograms and five false-negative radionuclide studies. The accuracy of each test was 81 per cent;
the positive predictive value was greater for the radionuclide examination, whereas the negative predictive value
was greater for the arthrographic study. Arthroscintigraphic
studies also may be helpful in delineating fistulous tracts.[87]

***Infection.*** Generally, infection or prosthetic loosening
should be considered in all cases of painful cemented hip
replacement in which extra-articular causes of pain have
been excluded. Differentiation between infection and prosthetic loosening may be difficult, but such differentiation
has important treatment implications. Clinically, pain of
sudden onset that occurs with motion suggests prosthetic
loosening, whereas pain occurring at rest or at night is more
suggestive of infection (or metastatic disease).[32–34, 89] Persistent pain after cemented total hip replacement or a history of postoperative hematoma or delayed wound healing
suggests that pain may be caused by infection.[32–34]

Diagnosis of an infected prosthesis may be made difficult
by a lack of corroborative clinical or laboratory abnormalities; for example, the temperature and leukocyte count need
not be elevated. The erythrocyte sedimentation rate normally should return to 30 mm/hour by 6 months postoperatively, and continued elevation suggests the possibility of
infection.[32–34] Evaluation of the erythrocyte sedimentation
rate in surgically proved cases of infection, however, has
shown the sensitivity of this finding to be only 60 per cent,
the specificity 65 per cent, the positive predictive value 25
per cent, and the negative predictive value 90 per cent.

Radiographic features of a rapidly developing wide cement-bone lucent zone within the first postoperative year,
endosteal scalloping, and periosteal reaction may indicate
infection.[32–34] A delay of 3 to 6 months may separate the
onset of pain and the development of these radiographic
abnormalities. Barrack and Harris[34] reviewed their cases of
revision arthroplasties and found, however, that all cases of
infection could be identified by the radiographic finding of
focal lysis, extensive nonfocal lysis, endosteal scalloping,
or periosteal reaction, or combinations of these findings.

*Aspiration Arthrography.* The prevalence of infection in

revision total hip arthroplasty is about four times as high as in primary hip replacement.[92] In many institutions, therefore, aspiration arthrography is performed in virtually all cases prior to prosthetic revision. This may not always be necessary, however. The results of aspiration arthrography need to be compared with those of scintigraphy in terms of yield and expense. The indications for joint aspiration after total hip replacement have been investigated. Tigges and associates[93] reviewed their experience with 147 hip aspirations and compared the result of aspiration culture with the findings on cultures obtained at the time of surgical revision. Of 147 cases, there were 122 true-negative, 13 true-positive, 11 false-positive, and 1 false-negative preoperative aspirations. Thus, if the preoperative aspiration was negative, the chance that the prosthesis was infected was small (negative predictive value, 99.2 per cent), whereas if it were positive, the finding was less reliable (positive predictive value, 54.2 per cent). Because of the low cost of an aspiration arthrogram it was cost effective to perform aspiration arthrography instead of more expensive nuclear medicine scans. Repeat aspiration of the hip can be done when initial results are questionable. Of clinical importance, however, the type of organism that is cultured from fluid obtained at the time of hip aspiration does not help to differentiate truly infected joints from those affected by incidental contaminants. *Staphylococcus epidermidis* is the organism recovered most commonly in both instances.

Barrack and Harris[34] reviewed 270 cases in which hip aspiration was done prior to revision surgery. They had 32 false-positive aspirations. Of six infected hips, the initial aspirations were positive in only two (four false-negative aspirations). In each infected case the patient had historic and radiographic findings that suggested the diagnosis, including focal or extensive lysis or periosteal reaction, or both. The authors, therefore, concluded that because of the high false-positive rate of joint aspirations, the high false-negative rate for infection, and the high cost of aspiration and arthrography, aspirations should be performed only in selected cases in which clinical or radiographic findings suggested that infection was present.[34] Evans and Cuckler[89] and Harris and Barrack[32, 33] have proposed algorithms for evaluation of painful total hip replacements (Fig. 19–12). Gould and colleagues[94] performed aspiration arthrograms on patients prior to revision surgery. Aspirations were negative in all cases in which the clinical suspicion of infection was low. They therefore suggested that aspiration arthrography be omitted unless there is at least some suspicion of infection. Comparison of three-phase bone scan, erythrocyte sedimentation rate, and joint aspiration for the diagnosis of infection, however, has led Levitsky and coworkers to conclude that joint aspiration is the single best test.[90] Identification of infected components is important as treatment often requires a two-stage revision.[111] Cuckler and associates[111] found that the combination of abnormal findings for erythrocyte sedimentation rate (greater than 30 mm/hour), joint aspiration, and indium scan allowed identification of all infected prostheses. If two of these studies were positive, a two-stage revision probably was necessary; if only one was positive, a repeat hip aspiration was performed.

Arthrographic features that suggest infection include an irregular contour to the joint capsule and filling of nonbursal cavities, sinus tracts, and abscesses[35, 69] (Fig. 19–13).

Infected cavities typically are more irregular than uninfected bursal collections and tend to communicate with the capsule through a narrow neck.[39] Irregular cavities were noted in 12 of 178 arthrograms in patients with symptomatic total hip prostheses studied by Berquist and associates.[39] In nine of these 12 arthrograms, the hips proved to be infected. Separate aspirations of one or more of these cavities may be necessary to establish the diagnosis, particularly if the communicating channel is narrow or opacification of these cavities after filling of the joint is slow.[41] Lymphatic filling may occur with or without infection,[35] and bursal filling is not diagnostic of infection.

*Ultrasonography.* Because of its ability to detect fluid collections, sonography may be of help in the identification of infected hip replacements.[95, 96] Fluid collections adjacent to a prosthesis may be identified and aspirated under ultrasound guidance.[96] This is particularly valuable when the fluid collection does not communicate with the joint and therefore would not have been opacified at the time of arthrography.

*Bone Scintigraphy.[97–109]* Despite initial enthusiasm for bone scanning in the evaluation of complications of total hip replacement, recent studies have indicated a more limited role for this examination.[52] For example, it has been recommended that patients with normal bone scans simply be followed, because their symptoms tend to resolve.[32, 33, 108] Tehranzadeh and colleagues[50] also believed that a normal bone scan rules out the presence of infection or loosening. Other studies have indicated that a normal bone scan does not necessarily exclude complications. Lieberman and associates[52] found falsely negative bone scans in three of 10 patients with infection, three of 44 cases of femoral component loosening, and four cases of acetabular component loosening (as documented on radiographs). Aliabadi and colleagues[106] found that even the combination of radiography and bone scintigraphy did not allow identification of all cases of prosthetic loosening. Thus, a negative bone scan does not appear to exclude either infection or loosening. Furthermore, although a positive bone scan was thought by Aliabadi and colleagues[106] and by Tehranzadeh and coworkers[50] to strongly suggest loosening or infection, other authors have noted the nonspecificity of the positive examination.[32, 33]

The pattern of uptake on bone scanning also has been of less diagnostic value than originally thought. Williamson and associates[103] found a focal pattern of uptake (uptake at the proximal and distal ends of the femoral prosthesis) to be highly suggestive of loosening, whereas diffuse uptake indicated infection (Fig. 19–14). Mountford and colleagues[104] found infection to be absent in all cases in which the bone scan demonstrated normal or focal uptake, whereas infection was present in five of six cases with diffuse uptake. In the patients evaluated by Aliabadi and colleagues,[106] however, all infected prostheses demonstrated a focal distribution of isotope and, therefore, the findings were indistinguishable from those of aseptic loosening. Of incidental note, a positive bone scan need not result from a previous hip arthrogram.[110]

*Gallium Scanning.* Gallium was first introduced for evaluation of lymphoma and later was noted to be useful in the assessment of pyogenic infection[98] and other tumors. The normal distribution of the isotope parallels the distribution of bone-seeking radionuclides and, therefore, comparison

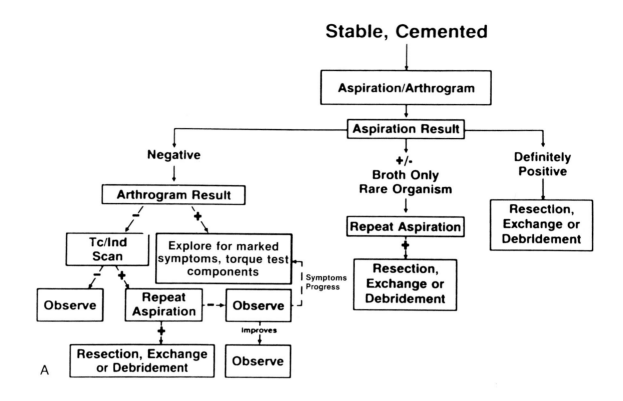

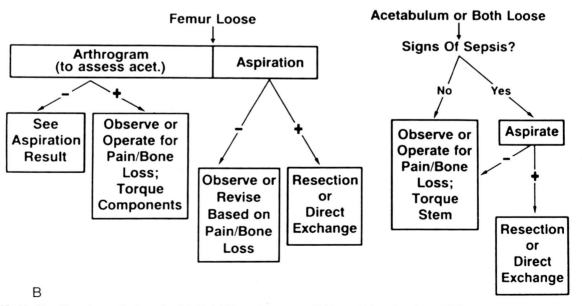

**FIGURE 19–12.** Algorithms for evaluation of painful total hip replacements. THA, total hip arthroplasty; ESR, erythrocyte sedimentation rate; CRP, C-reactive protein; WBC, white blood count; DJD, degenerative joint disease; EMG, electromyogram. (**A, B** From Harris WH, Barrack RL: Orthop Rev *22*:531, 1993. **C,** From Evans BG, Cuckler JM: Orthop Clin North Am *22*:303, 1992.)

*Illustration continued on opposite page*

The Painful THA

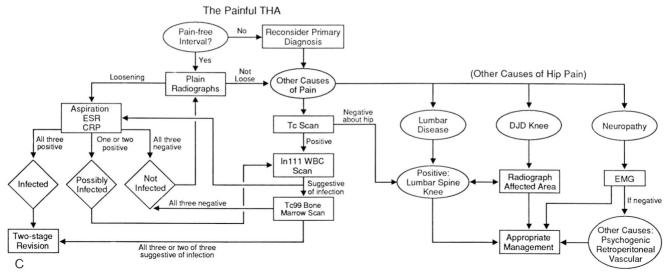

C

FIGURE 19–12 Continued

of patterns of isotope accumulation in gallium and technetium scans is necessary for correct interpretation of the gallium studies.[101] Accumulation of gallium in areas of infection depends primarily on uptake by leukocytes and by bacteria and on factors that influence tracer accumulation, such as increased regional blood flow.[98]

Although it was hoped that gallium scintigraphy would improve the accuracy for the diagnosis of prosthetic infection, the utility of this examination appears limited as judged by a low sensitivity in some series[106] and moderate specificity in others. Evaluation by Aliabadi and coworkers[106] indicated that whereas a negative gallium examination does not exclude infection, a positive one strongly suggests it.

*Indium-111 Leukocyte Scanning.*[112–122] Initial reports offered the hope that white blood cell scanning using indium-111 labeling would improve the diagnostic accuracy in cases of infection. Merkel and colleagues,[119] for example, found the accuracy of the indium-labeled leukocyte images to be 94 per cent while the combined technetium-gallium studies were only 75 per cent accurate. All patients with positive leukocyte scans were shown to have infection at the time of surgery. Changes in marrow distribution may

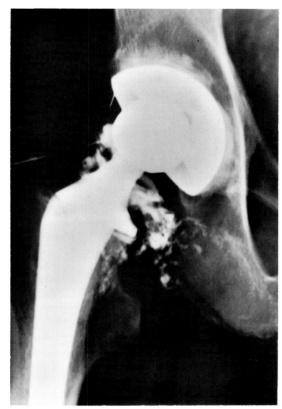

**FIGURE 19–13.** Infected total hip prosthesis. Injection of contrast agent shows filling of numerous irregular tracts extending from the joint. These tracts are virtually diagnostic of infection.

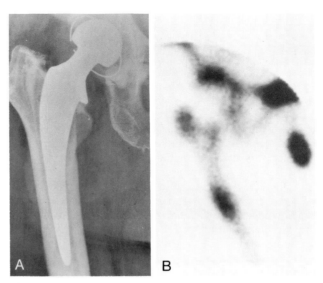

**FIGURE 19–14.** Focal uptake on bone scan.

**A** Note the radiographic evidence of loosening of the femoral component with a wide metal-cement lucent zone.

**B** The bone scan demonstrates focal isotope uptake at the proximal and distal ends of the femoral component and along the acetabular component. (From Weissman BN: Radiol Clin North Am *28*:1111, 1990.)

occur after joint replacement surgery. Whether the alterations in marrow distribution are caused by insertion of the prosthetic components or by conversion of yellow to red marrow near the prostheses is unknown.[97] Scanning with both radiocolloid (to evaluate marrow distribution) and [111]In-labeled white blood cells has been proposed as a technique to define infection even in the presence of these marrow alterations.[118, 120] A study by Seabold and coworkers[118] demonstrated improved specificity (from 59 per cent without bone marrow imaging to 92 per cent with it) of the indium scan but a decrease in its sensitivity (from 94 per cent to 88 per cent). The study of Palestro and associates[120] found a sensitivity of 100 per cent, specificity of 97 per cent, and accuracy of 98 per cent for the combined radionuclide examination.

[111]In-labeled leukocyte scanning is relatively time-consuming and expensive.[115] Other disadvantages include the potential for iatrogenic errors in administration (and the small attendant risk of human immunodeficiency virus infection).[102, 121] In addition, Zilkens and associates[109] found positive [111]In-labeled leukocyte scans in a high percentage of patients with loose, but not infected, total hip prostheses. Wellman and colleagues[86] noted inability to differentiate between cellulitis and an infected prosthesis with [111]In-labeled leukocyte scanning. An increased uptake of [111]In-labeled leukocytes may occur in acute osteomyelitis, acute exacerbation of chronic osteomyelitis, septic arthritis, rheumatoid arthritis, abscesses, fractures, recent surgical wounds and procedures, heterotopic bone formation, osteosarcoma, Paget's disease, eosinophilic granuloma, and pigmented villonodular synovitis.[123, 124] The sensitivity of the examination decreases as the chronicity of the infection increases.[86, 117] The combination of bone and [111]In-labeled leukocyte scanning improves the specificity of the indium examination but decreases its sensitivity.[121, 124] Furthermore, sensitivity for demonstrating infections involving the central skeleton is reduced in comparison to those of peripheral regions.[102] After review of the status of [111]In-labeled leukocyte imaging for osteomyelitis, Alazraki concluded that although the indium-leukocyte study is the best test available, in view of the multiple problems attached to indium-leukocyte imaging other radionuclide studies that could serve as alternatives for imaging of infection should be sought.[102]

[99m]Tc-HMPAO (hexamethylpropylene-amine oxime) also has been introduced as a method for labeling leukocytes. Its advantages over [111]In-labeled leukocyte examinations include lower radiation exposure, improved image resolution, and same day imaging.[115, 125] Labeled white cell scans are best for detecting infections with a granulocytic rather than a lymphocytic response. This is especially true when pure granulocyte preparations, rather than mixed white blood cells, are used.[125] Tc-HMPAO produces a more pure granulocyte marker and may be less sensitive to the presence of chronic infections. Roddie and coworkers[115] found excellent sensitivity (100 per cent) and specificity (93 per cent) for the detection of osteomyelitis, septic arthritis, or infected prostheses. Glithero and associates,[125] however, found reduced sensitivity for the detection of insidious infection using either [111]In-oxine labeled or [99m]Tc-HMPAO labeled white cell scans. Only three of eight total hip replacements evaluated by indium oxine were identified as infected. Five other infected hips were imaged with

HMPAO and no evidence of infection was detected in any of these five hips. The results for total knee prostheses were better with all five infected knees predicted by the Tc-HMPAO scans. No false-positive results were reported. The disappointing sensitivity of these scanning methods was thought to be attributed to the chronicity of the infection; the average interval from the time of surgery to that of imaging was significantly shorter in cases of true-positive scans than in those of false-negative scans.

*Other Radionuclide Studies.* Other isotopes have been used for the detection of infection, including infected joint replacements. [99m]Tc nanocolloid leaks into the extracellular space in areas of inflammation and has been used to study orthopedic infection and septic loosening of joint replacements.[116] The same specificity (93 per cent) and a slightly greater sensitivity (87 per cent) have been found for the nanocolloid examinations than for [111]In-labeled leukocyte scintigraphy.

Monoclonal antibodies also have been used to evaluate infection. Sciuk and colleagues[121] used monoclonal mouse antibodies directed against a granulocyte surface antigen labeled with technetium-99m or iodine-123 with the advantage over labeled leukocyte scans of ready availability and ease of preparation. A sensitivity of 89 per cent, specificity of 84 per cent, and accuracy of 86 per cent were noted when these scans were interpreted in conjunction with the bone scan. Nonspecific deposition of leukocytes in hematoma, contusion, or noninfected sites of inflammation may produce diagnostic difficulty.[126] In addition, false-negative results may accompany chronic infection. Oyen and colleagues[127] used [111]In-labeled nonspecific human immunoglobulin G scanning to evaluate infection. In an evaluation of 31 total hip replacements, seven true-positive, 21 truenegative, two false-positive, and one false-negative case were reported. False-positive studies were attributed to other inflammatory processes.

***Aggressive Granulomatous Disease (Cement Disease).*** Harris and coworkers[128] first described extensive localized areas of bone resorption around the femoral stems in four patients with cemented total hip replacements. The components were only slightly loose at the time of revision surgery. Histologic examination showed sheets of macrophages, birefringent intracellular and extracellular material, foreign body giant cells, and the absence of acute or chronic inflammatory cells. The birefringent material was believed to be more consistent with PMMA cement than with polyethylene. Santavirta and associates[129] described these lesions as distinct histologically (as well as radiographically) from the usual findings associated with prosthetic loosening, although this point is controversial. Subsequently, Jasty and colleagues[331] noted the same response adjacent to wellfixed hip components. Abundant PMMA cement particles were present, and the possibility of micromotion producing shedding of particles was discussed. Santavirta and associates noted that the immunohistologic finding of multinucleated giant cells and monocyte macrophages supported a foreign body reaction.[129] The condition became known as "cement disease," and its elimination was believed to be possible only with the elimination of cement.[130] Prosthetic fixation without cement has not alleviated the problem, however. The condition has been reported in association with wear of both the methylmethacrylate and polyethylene components,[131] with and without prosthetic loosening, with or without cement fixation,[132–135] with polyethylene particles alone,[138] and without either cement or polyethylene.[136] Maguire and coworkers[131] postulated that either PMMA cement or polyethylene could incite a giant cell response if the size, surface areas, and rate of particle production were suitable. Boynton and colleagues[137] studied the membranes around various loose prostheses that had been inserted with and without polyethylene and with and without cement, and these investigators found the presence of giant cells to be related predominantly to the presence of polyethylene wear debris.

Several authors have suggested a relationship between benign fibrous membranes around components or active membranes associated with component loosening and these focal areas of bone destruction.[137] Boynton and colleagues[137] postulated that a combination of biologic and mechanical events apparently occurs and leads to a threshold level of particulate matter, which causes a transformation of the macrophages in a relatively benign membrane into an active bone-resorbing unit. These authors believed that polyethylene debris is responsible for the threshold levels being exceeded.[137] Schmalzried and coworkers[132] found that despite the differing radiographic appearances (i.e., diffuse linear lucent zones or focal lytic lesions), the bone resorption was related to macrophages laden with polyethylene debris. These authors suggested that joint fluid (and therefore particles) can penetrate extensively around even a well-fixed component (in the "effective joint space"). Often this penetration is greater in extent than is apparent on arthrography. The difference between localized bone lesions and linear cement-bone lucent zones may be related to the distribution and concentration of particulate material. Debris-activated macrophages and giant cells release prostagandin E2, interleukin-1, and osteoclast activating factors that destroy bone, eventuating in focal granulomatous lesions or, more often, in a more slowly developing membrane with eventual prosthetic loosening in a small proportion of these cases.[139] A recent study of the relationship of cement failure and prosthetic loosening has demonstrated that particles of PMMA cement (1 to 12 mm in size) are engulfed by macrophages, whereas larger particles are not. Tissue culture has shown that phagocytosis of these particles leads to an increased production of tumor necrosis factor (a cytokine) by macrophages, which then may lead to bone resorption and loosening of the prosthesis. Thus, mechanical failure of the cement mantle may lead to the production of small particles (1 to 12 $\mu$m) that are phagocytized by macrophages. This causes cell death and release of bone-resorbing mediators, including tumor necrosis factor, leading to bone resorption at the cement-bone interface. Whether the implant loosens first, allowing wear debris to enter the effective joint space, or whether the wear debris causes the initial loosening, is controversial.[133, 140] Transport of polyethylene debris to local lymph nodes has been reported.[141]

Osteolytic lesions appear on radiographs as well-defined focal areas of bone resorption that do not conform to the shape of the prosthesis[142–144] (Fig. 19–15). They occur most often near the tip of the femoral component or along its medial border.[142] Scott and associates[142] found five cases of focal bone resorption in 79 cemented prostheses followed

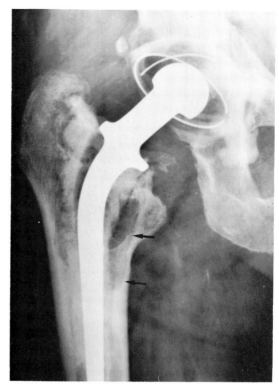

**FIGURE 19–15.** Aggressive granulomatous disease. Loosening of the cemented femoral stem is present, as shown by wide metal-cement lucent zones. Well-defined focal areas of bone destruction (arrows) indicate aggressive granulomatous disease. (From Weissman BN: Radiol Clin North Am *28*:1111, 1990.)

for at least 10 years. Santavirta and coworkers[61] noted such bone resorption in 5 per cent of patients undergoing revision for prosthetic loosening; loosening appeared to precede the lytic lesions by 11 to 48 months in all cases.

*Acetabular Wear.* Most currently used prostheses consist of a combination of metal and high density polyethylene. The polyethylene liner is thought to wear at a rate of 0.2 mm/year.[145] This rate may be accelerated in young, active men.[146] The average rate of wear may lead to the production of several hundred million to several billion wear particles per year.[139] Because particulate debris from polyethylene wear may produce bone resorption and loosening, research has been directed toward finding improved prosthetic surfaces. Creation of ceramic femoral heads matched with polyethylene acetabular components is one attempt to decrease prosthetic wear[147, 148] (Fig. 19–16). Investigations of the metal used in the creation of the femoral head that articulates with the polyethylene acetabular component[149] and of the ideal femoral head size[150] are being undertaken to determine which prosthetic components minimize wear.

The decrease in thickness of the acetabular polyethylene component that is seen on radiographs is thought to reflect a combination of abrasive wear, creep, and plastic deformation.[149] Usually, however, the change in the thickness of the polyethylene is taken as an indicator of wear[149] and, therefore, as an indicator of the production of wear debris. Gross wear of the acetabular liner is indicated by the development of an eccentric position of the femoral head within the acetabular component (Figs. 19–7 and 19–17). More

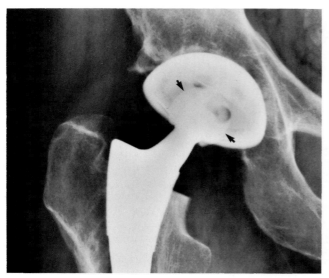

**FIGURE 19–16.** Ceramic femoral head. A ceramic femoral head (arrows) was used in an attempt to decrease acetabular wear.

subtle degrees of wear require careful measurements. Initially, Charnley and Halley[151] used radiographic measurements to assess wear and reported that wear in a 9 to 10 year period averaged 1.3 mm/year. Their measurement technique later was questioned.[152] Subsequent measurements using a revised technique indicated prosthetic wear to average 0.15 mm/year. The rate of wear was noted to decrease with time.[145] Griffith and coworkers[146] discussed several positioning variables that affected measurement results. Some studies have compared radiographically determined wear with direct measurements of the thickness of the acetabular components. The technique utilized by Livermore and coworkers[150] incorporated early and late radiographic measurements, corrected for magnification. Comparison with actual specimens demonstrated a mean

discrepancy of 0.075 mm (range, 0 to 0.4 mm).[150] Thus, radiographic measurement seems an accurate tool for assessing polyethylene wear.

*Prosthetic Dislocation.* Radiographs are essential for confirming prosthetic dislocation, defining any underlying cause, and disclosing any complications or conditions that interfere with reduction. Generally, the diagnosis of prosthetic dislocation is readily apparent. Such dislocation occurs in 0.3 to 5.8 per cent of total hip or bipolar prostheses[152] and occurs most often in the immediate postoperative period. When prosthetic dislocation occurs more than 3 months after surgery, underlying component malposition should be suspected.[11] Fackler and Poss[11] found 44 patients with prosthetic dislocation to have component malposition (defined as acetabular or femoral component retroversion or acetabular anteversion of more than 25 degrees), whereas only 6 per cent of patients without prosthetic dislocation showed similar findings. Detachment of the greater trochanter (displacement of fragments of cement or wire into the joint[154]) and component dissociation should be sought on radiographs.

*Dissociation of Prosthetic Components.* Charnley's initial design for total hip prostheses consisted of a high density polyethylene acetabular component matched with a one-piece femoral head-stem component.[1] Modifications to that design have included metal backing of the acetabular component (introduced in the 1970s to allow replacement of the acetabular liner for wear), screws to stabilize the metal backed components, modular femoral head and neck-stem components, attachable collars, distal and proximal sleeves, and porous coated surface.[154] At each of the modular interfaces, complications may occur. Examples include metal debris from screw fretting, corrosion at the head-neck taper when different metals are used, dissociation of the femoral head from the neck,[156, 158, 159] cracking of polyethylene liners at their superior surface, and separation and inferior rotation of the acetabular liner. Quale and associates[160] reported three hip replacements in which the acetab-

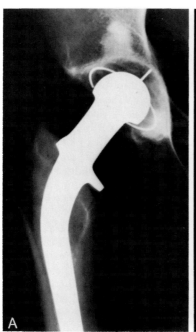 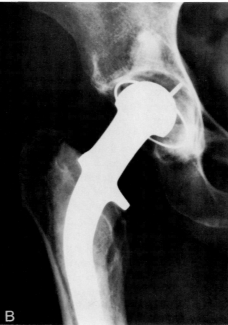

**FIGURE 19–17.** Acetabular wear.

**A** This frontal radiograph was obtained shortly after total hip replacement.

**B** An examination 13 years later shows the shift in the position of the femoral head within the acetabulum, attesting to the acetabular wear that has occurred.

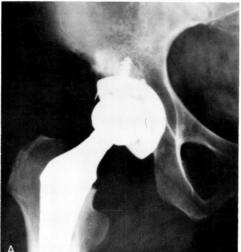
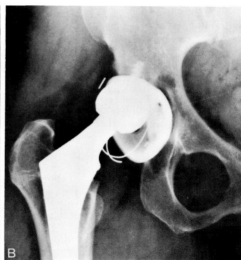

**FIGURE 19–18.** Acetabular disruption.

**A** The frontal radiograph shows no loosening of the bone ingrowth acetabular component. The marker wires of the acetabular liner are visible.

**B** Follow-up radiograph shows displacement of the bone ingrowth acetabular component from the bone and displacement of the acetabular liner (as shown by the marker wire).

ular liner separated from the metal backing and rotated inferiorly, allowing the metal femoral head (chrome-cobalt) to articulate with and erode the metal (titanium) backing of the acetabulum (Fig. 19–18). Radiographs (including magnification or soft tissue techniques, conventional tomography, or phosphor plate images) showed the rotated polyethylene liner reliably as a crescentic lucent zone in the joint. The femoral head was noted to be displaced laterally. Metal deposition in the joint produced an opaque curvilinear dense shadow corresponding to the shape of the joint capsule. Predisposing causes for this disruption include prior dislocation,[155] certain design features of the prosthesis, and a vertical position of the acetabular component.[154] Correct diagnosis requires close scrutiny of postreduction radiographs for lucent areas that may represent a displaced liner and for eccentric position of the femoral head in the acetabular shell as well as for dense lines indicating metal debris. In some cases of liner displacement, the femoral head will appear more deeply seated within the acetabular shell.

***Heterotopic Bone Formation.*** The cause of heterotopic bone formation after total hip replacement is unknown. Its prevalence ranges from 5 to 90 per cent,[161] and this frequency is thought to be increased in men with osteoarthrosis,[161] hypertrophic osteoarthrosis, prior heterotopic ossification or contralateral ossification,[164] ankylosing spondylitis,[163] diffuse idiopathic-skeletal hyperostosis,[164] posttraumatic arthritis, prior surgery, or extensive operative trauma[165] and in those who undergo various surgical techniques.[167] An increased frequency and severity of heterotopic bone formation have been noted in patients undergoing bone ingrowth femoral fixation in comparison to those in whom the femoral component had been inserted with cement fixation.[161] It has been postulated that escape of femoral bone marrow elements and particulate bone debris is greater when an uncemented rather than a cemented component is used.[161] The origin of the cells responsible for the formation of heterotopic ossification likewise is uncertain. Thomas[164] notes that pluripotential mesenchymal cells from the perivascular tissues may differentiate into osteoblastic cells, which form the heterotopic bone. Because this differentiation occurs within 16 hours after surgery,[164] preventive strategies must be implemented preoperatively or shortly postoperatively.

Radiographically, the ossification usually is visible by 2 to 4 weeks after surgery.[5, 161] The classification by Brooker and associates is a convenient method for grading the quantity of bone formed[166] (Table 19–5). Although easy to use, this classification does not allow for differences in component size and placement, which could influence the spacing between areas of ossification.[167] Maloney and colleagues[161] suggest adding a modifier to Brooker grades III and IV to indicate the functional impact of the ossification (A indicating no functional limitation and B indicating limitation).

A minority of patients (10 per cent or fewer) with heterotopic ossification demonstrate symptoms of limited motion, pain, or both.[168] Heterotopic bone formation may be prevented by nonsteroidal anti-inflammatory medication or radiation therapy. Such medication has been shown to prevent the formation of heterotopic ossification but also to inhibit bone formation about porous coated components.[164, 169] Similarly, the risk of development of heterotopic ossification is reduced to less than 10 per cent after such radiation therapy.[167] Because irradiation also interferes with bone ingrowth, the regions of the porous coating are shielded from the primary radiation beam.[164, 169] The trochanteric osteotomy site likewise is shielded. Complications of prophylactic irradiation in these cases include malpositioning of the radiation shields so that the periarticular region is erroneously shielded or the bone ingrowth areas are irradiated. No radiation-induced sarcomas have been reported with the treatment schedules utilized.

***Tumors.***[170–174] On rare occasions, malignant tumors have been associated with total hip replacements. Brien and coworkers[171] noted that 11 malignant tumors arising near a

**TABLE 19–5. Grading of Heterotopic Ossification About the Hip***

| | |
|---|---|
| Class I | Islands of bone within the soft tissues |
| Class II | Bone about the pelvis or proximal end of the femur leaving at least 1 cm between apposing bony surfaces |
| Class III | Bone about the pelvis or proximal end of the femur reducing the space between apposing bone surfaces to less than 1 cm |
| Class IV | Apparent bony ankylosis |

*From Brooker AF, et al: J Bone Joint Surg [Am] 55:1629, 1973.

hip prostheses had been reported prior to 1990, and additional tumors have been reported with other types of orthopedic hardware. Tumors have occurred in both bone and soft tissue and included osteosarcomas, fibrosarcomas, malignant fibrous histiocytomas, high grade sarcomas, epithelioid sarcomas, and synovial sarcomas. Radiographically, these tumors must be differentiated from pseudotumors associated with foreign body reactions to debris. Malignant lesions in the presence of total joint replacement are of particular concern because of the possible carcinogenic effect of metals, polyethylene, or methylmethacrylate. The use of bone ingrowth components, with their large surface areas in contact with tissues, is of additional concern and offers opportunity for close scrutiny.

### Bone Ingrowth (Porous Coated, Biologic) Fixation[175–195]

Cementless fixation was developed in the 1970s[14] in response to the reported high prevalence of aseptic loosening of cemented components. The goals of surgery with porous coated implants are to provide a durable arthroplasty with a lasting satisfactory clinical result, to avoid cement, and to maintain bone stock.[15] Initial use of porous coating of implants with ceramics and polymers largely has been replaced by the use of porous metallic coatings applied to solid metal components[178] (Fig. 19–19). With these techniques it is hoped that bone will grow into the porous surface. Retrieval studies, however, have shown that bone ingrowth is limited and occurs more often into the femoral (rather than the acetabular) component in the hip and into the femoral more than the tibial component in total knee replacements[183] (Fig. 19–20). In a review, Haddad and associates[178] concluded that a combination of limited ingrowth of bone and extensive ingrowth of fibrous tissue is adequate for fixation.

Newer models of femoral components, with proximal areas for bone ingrowth, have replaced the early designs in which bone ingrowth surfaces covered all or nearly all of

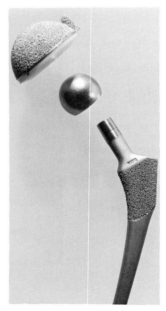

**FIGURE 19–19.** Bone ingrowth components. A polyethylene acetabular component is covered with a metallic cap. Note the irregular coated portions of the acetabular and femoral components. The femoral head component is interchangeable, allowing some adjustment in the length of the femoral component.

the length of the prosthesis. The advantages of coating only the proximal regions include the smaller surface area for corrosion and metal release, the decreased likelihood of distal stem fixation with proximal loosening leading to stem fracture, and easier implant removal should it be required.[190]

Bone ingrowth around porous coated prostheses depends on the presence of certain prosthetic design characteristics, close apposition of the host bone to the porous surface, and initial stabilization of the components by means of press fitting or use of additional fixation, such as screws or

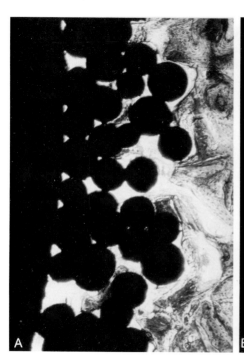
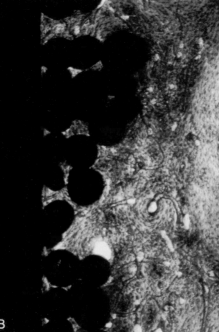

**FIGURE 19–20.** Bone ingrowth around a porous coated implant.
**A** Photomicrograph 6.5 months after surgery shows osteocytes deep within the surface porosity (20x). (From Bobyn JD, Engh CA: Orthopedics 7:1410, 1984.)
**B** Photomicrograph 3 years after surgery shows excellent bone ingrowth between the pores and filling in of spaces to the depth of the implant surface. (From Engh CA, Bobyn JD: Biological Fixation in Total Hip Arthroplasty. Thorofare, NJ, Slack Inc, 1985.)

pegs.[178, 184] Bone ingrowth should occur by 4[181] to 6 weeks[187] after surgery, and patients often are kept on incomplete weight-bearing until 6 weeks after surgery. Comparison of cemented and cementless prostheses, with mean follow-up periods of approximately 4 years, showed a higher function score in the uncemented group,[196] although equivalent pain relief was noted.

Engh and colleagues indicate two assessments that must be made when evaluating porous coated prostheses: evaluation of the presence or absence of ''osseointegration'' (bonding of the prosthesis directly to the bone without a fibrous layer), and evaluation of prosthetic ''stability'' (the absence of visible motion between the implant and the bone under load such as may be applied in the operating room).[184] When osseointegration is present, the component is always stable.

Stabilization of bone ingrowth components may occur as a result of either bone or fibrous tissue ingrowth. Bone ingrowth is considered ideal. Even at surgery, it may be impossible, however, to differentiate between a stable prosthesis resulting from bone or fibrous fixation. Evaluation of the stability of porous coated prostheses depends heavily on radiographic interpretation. Three categories of biologic fixation and stability were described by Engh and Massin[192] on the basis of appearances on an initial radiograph and one obtained 2 years later. An optimal appearance is one showing fixation by bone ingrowth; a suboptimal but stable appearance is caused by development of delayed stabilization by fibrous tissue; and in an unstable fixation, neither bone nor dense fibrous tissue develops about the prosthesis within the first year. Stabilization by bone ingrowth is indicated by the absence of reactive lines around the porous part of the implant and the presence of new bone filling the area between the endosteal surface and the porous portion of the implant[184] (Fig. 19–21). When stabilization by fibrous tissue occurs, it is evident on radiographs obtained 1 year after surgery by the presence of thin sclerotic lines (demarcation lines) paralleling the porous surface of the implant and separated from it by a thin lucent zone. Stabilization of the prosthesis may be assessed in these cases only by further follow-up. Engh and Massin[192] believed that if this interface remains unchanged and no change has occurred in the position of the prosthesis by 2 years after surgery, the component probably is held firm by strong fibrous tissue ingrowth and bone formation beneath the collar and at the stem tip. Conversely, if further migration of the prosthesis occurs, the prosthesis is unstable. Using these signs a score could be developed that reflects prosthetic fixation and stability (Table 19–6).

Several radiographic signs should be assessed when evaluating a bone ingrowth component. These include (1) the signs of bone or fibrous tissue ingrowth (spot welding and demarcation lines); (2) signs of stability or motion; and (3) signs of remodeling occurring as a result of changing stress (rounding, bone resorption or corticocancellization of the medial femoral cortex, hypertrophy of endosteal cancellous bone at the margin of the bone ingrowth surface, and cortical hypertrophy near the distal aspect of the stem). As indicated earlier, thin lucent zones with adjacent thin sclerotic lines (demarcation lines) may appear along the porous coated portion of the prosthesis. Progression of lucent zones in either width or length has been noted to occur even in asymptomatic persons.[187] Callaghan and coworkers[175] found

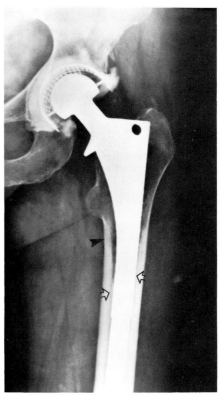

**FIGURE 19–21.** Stable porous coated femoral stem with bone ingrowth. At the time of a 4.5 year follow-up radiographic examination, new bone fills the gap from the cortex to the end of the bone ingrowth area (arrows). Loss of bone has occurred proximally with thinning of the cortices, bone loss from the medial femoral cortex, and loss of density of the cortex medially (arrowhead), termed corticocancellization.

progression of the lucent zone with its accompanying thin sclerotic rim in 41 per cent of asymptomatic persons. Acetabular lucent zones are uncommon but are seen most often along zone 3, where they have been observed in 18[186] to 52

**TABLE 19–6. Radiographic Signs of Bone Ingrowth Fixation and Stability***

| | Major Signs | Minor Signs |
|---|---|---|
| Osteointegration | No reactive line along porous surface | |
| | Endosteal bone bridging gap to porous surface (''spot welds'') | |
| Absence of osteo-integration | Extensive reactive lines along porous surface (½ of zones) | Absence of spot welds |
| Implant instability | Progressive implant migration | Reactive lines about the smooth stem |
| | | Widening of canal |
| | | Pedestal formation plus reactive lines |
| | | Late progressive bead shedding |
| | | Widening of lucent zone or divergence of lucent zone |
| | | Calcar hypertrophy |

*After Engh CA, et al: Clin Orthop 257:107, 1990.

per cent[175, 188] in various series. Longer follow-up is necessary to understand completely the significance of these thin but increasing lucent zones.

When bone ingrowth occurs along the porous surface no interposed lucent line is seen between the host bone and the beaded surface. Correlation of radiographic features of bone ingrowth around acetabular components with findings on postmortem histologic examination has shown that the radiographs overestimated the occurrence of bone apposition and underestimated the presence of gap areas.[177] Bone ingrowth averaged about one third of the available surface and well-organized fibrous tissue occupied most of the remaining surface of these well-functioning components.

**Radiographic Findings of Stability or Motion.** Evidence of bone ingrowth or the absence of signs of loosening indicates stability of the prosthetic components. Even in well-fixed prostheses, however, relative motion may occur between the prosthesis and the bone owing to differences in the stiffness of these materials and bone. Thus, for a given load, the deformation of the prosthesis is less than that of the cortical bone distal to the prosthesis, resulting in relative motion between the two.[186] This motion is indicated by a thin lucent line along the smooth portion of the stem of the prosthesis. A high frequency of radiolucent lines (bordered by thin sclerotic lines) along the smooth uncoated portion of bone ingrowth prostheses and at the proximal portion of the femoral component laterally in the region of the greater trochanter has been noted (Fig. 19–22).

Design changes in components may make the distal part of the prosthesis less rigid and, therefore, decrease the relative motion. Use of components made of titanium alloy, which has a lower modulus of elasticity than cobalt alloy, may be helpful in this regard. Splitting of the distal end of

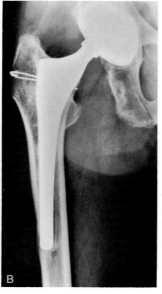

**FIGURE 19–22.** Lucent lines, probable prosthetic loosening.

**A** The bone ingrowth femoral component is in varus position. A thin lucent region is present along the smooth portion of the stem, but no lucent zones are present at the bone ingrowth area.

**B** Three years later, subsidence of the femoral stem has occurred with increased varus alignment of the stem and development of a proximal zone of lucency between the prosthesis and the greater trochanter. No lucent regions are present at the medial bone ingrowth surface.

the stem makes it more flexible. Too much flexibility, however, may lead to weakening of the stem or high bone-implant shear stresses that predispose to prosthetic loosening.[190]

Engh and colleagues[184] graded the stability of the distal stem by comparing findings on initial and final radiographs. Instability was considered to be present when the initial films showed the distal tip of the prosthesis to fill the medullary canal completely and comparable final radiographs showed that the stem no longer contacted the endosteal surface. Stability of the stem was present when the stem continued to fill the canal, no reactive lines developed, and no settling of the component occurred. When the component did not fill the canal initially and no changes occurred on follow-up, the stem was considered stable. If less of the canal was filled or reactive lines developed at the stem tip, the stem was considered unstable.

*Prosthetic Migration.* Acetabular migration is measured with minimal difficulty using constructed baselines, the Ranawat triangle, or a template as described earlier. Change in femoral component position over time may be more difficult to determine. Engh and coworkers[177] defined prosthetic migration as a change in the distance between the lateral shoulder of the prosthesis and the superior tip of the greater trochanter of 2 mm or more. Callaghan and associates[175] measured vertical subsidence as a decrease of 5 mm or more between the superomedial extent of the porous coating and the top of the lesser trochanter. Vertical subsidence of the femoral stem of more than 5 mm was found in 14 per cent of porous coated anatomic (PCA) prostheses followed for a mean of 3 years.[179] Vertical settling tended to be greater when less of the canal was filled by the prosthesis. Kattapuram and colleagues[185] measured settling from the superomedial edge of the porous coating of the PCA prosthesis to the most proximal aspect of the medial femoral cortex.[185] This radiographic finding proved to be the major indicator of clinical outcome; greater degrees of subsidence were associated with a poorer clinical result, particularly if the subsidence increased after the first year. Subsidence of more than 10 mm or that continuing after the first year are poor prognostic indicators.

*Bead Loss.* The significance of displacement of beads into the adjacent soft tissues depends on its chronology. Engh and Massin[192] noted displacement of surface beads in 4 per cent of 343 anatomic medullary locking (AML) prostheses. In five of 13 cases this finding was present on the initial radiograph and did not progress on subsequent radiographs. Presumably, in these cases, the beads were displaced during insertion of the components. In all of these patients, a stable fixation occurred, either by early bone ingrowth or by delayed fibrous fixation. Progressive displacement of beads occurred in five cases; two had unstable femoral components and three showed delayed fibrous stabilization. Thus, progressive displacement of beads suggests an unstable component (Fig. 19–23). The finding is not uncommon, having been noted around 28 per cent of femoral and 18 per cent of acetabular components in one 2 year series.[175] Kattapuram and coworkers[185] found displaced beads around four of five failed prostheses, but also about stable prostheses.[185]

*Cortical Thickening.* Focal thickening of the femoral cortex may be generated by a number of mechanisms. It may reflect poor fixation of the prosthesis proximally and

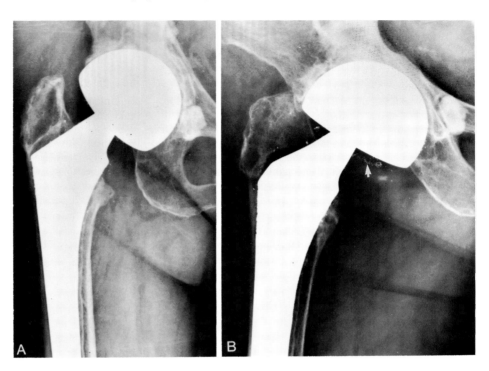

**FIGURE 19–23.** Loosening of bone ingrowth femoral component with migration and bead displacement.

**A** Bone ingrowth bipolar prosthesis was inserted during a revision of a previously loose prosthesis. Three years later, settling of the femoral component is seen with widening of the lucent zone at the junction of the prosthesis and the bone. The wide lucent zone along the bone ingrowth surface and extending along the smooth portion of the stem as well as the increased numbers of displaced beads attest to prosthetic loosening.

**B** One year later, further evidence of loosening of the femoral component and displacement of a large number of beads into the joint (arrow) are seen.

medially, with varus migration of the prosthesis. Loosening with mediolateral toggle produces a windshield-wiper effect, resulting in thickening of the cortex both medially and laterally, generally accompanied by other evidence of prosthetic loosening. Cortical thickening also may occur in fixed femoral components as a result of the relative bending of the bone in relation to the stiffer femoral stem.[187]

*Canal Filling.* The size of the femoral stem in relation to the femoral shaft has prognostic implications. Engh and Massin[192] found this to be the most important factor contributing to bone ingrowth fixation: When the canal was filled by the prosthesis, stable bone ingrowth fixation was likely at the time of follow-up examination. Unfortunately, canal filling also is more likely to be accompanied by proximal bone resorption (stress shielding).[190] Callaghan and coworkers[175] considered that an excellent fit of the femoral stem was present if the frontal radiograph showed the stem to be in contact with the cortical bone in at least one area both medially and laterally, and the lateral radiograph showed the surface of the component to be within 2 mm of the anterior cortex at the proximal and distal ends of the prosthesis and the posterior cortex at the site of the posterior bow of the component. Engh and Bobyn[190] defined canal filling as contact of the implant with the medial and lateral endosteal cortex at the same level within the isthmus.

*Stress Shielding.* Stress shielding refers to the loss of bone that occurs adjacent to a prostheses when stress is diverted from the area. The finding is related to the stiffness of the prosthesis (it is greater with chrome-cobalt prostheses than with titanium-alloy components) and with the type and location of fixation. Stress will travel through the stiffest portion of a system if there is good interface contact.[181] Thus, if the prosthesis is bonded to the bone, the stress will enter one end of the prosthesis and exit through the other end, diverting stress from the surrounding bone. The presence of stress shielding, therefore, indicates that bone in-

growth has occurred.[192] Factors that contribute to more severe degrees of stress shielding include large stem size (greater than or equal to 13.5 mm), two thirds or full porous coating of the stem, filling of the canal by the stem, radiographic appearance of bone ingrowth, and patient age of 50 years or older.[190]

Bone loss caused by stress shielding is manifested on radiographs as intracortical tunneling (corticocancellization), rounding or bone resorption in the medial aspect of the femoral neck, and "periosteal atrophy,"[184] usually most prominent in the medial femoral cortex. Engh and Massin[192] found stress shielding in 14 per cent of patients with AML femoral stems 5 years after implantation. Callaghan and associates[175] found 66 per cent of patients to exhibit loss of proximal femoral density and 70 per cent to reveal rounding of the calcar on 2 year follow-up examinations. Wixson and colleagues[20] found rounding of the femoral neck in 67 per cent of patients, resorption of the femoral neck in 20 per cent, and corticocancellization in 70 per cent. Differentiation of bone loss caused by stress shielding from that caused by other factors, including particles produced by wear debris, depends on its time of appearance. Bone resorption as a consequence of wear debris and granuloma formation occurs late and often is progressive, whereas stress shielding occurs within the first year after surgery and stabilizes by the second postoperative year.[190]

*Bone Pedestal.* The "pedestal" refers to a shelf of new bone that develops at the tip of the femoral stem as a response to increased load in the area. It may be associated with stable or unstable components. When the components are stable, no new radiolucent zones or reactive lines at the tip of the stem are present.

*Enlargement of Diameter of Medullary Canal.* Remodeling changes occur in the diaphysis of a bone after insertion of a femoral component. Enlargement of the diameter of the shaft as well as of the intramedullary canal occurs.

The canal enlargement is greater in patients with unstable bone ingrowth stems.[192]

**Scintigraphic Findings.**[193–195] As might be expected from the remodeling that occurs in association with bone ingrowth components, uptake of isotope may be detected on bone scans, even in asymptomatic subjects. Quantitative assessment of bone scans in asymptomatic patients with AML bone ingrowth prostheses has shown that the ratio of radionuclide accumulation about the stem to that in the normal contralateral femur or in the sacroiliac joint is stable 1 year or more after surgery. The pattern of isotope uptake may differ, however, depending on the design of the component.[193] Radionuclide uptake was seen on delayed bone scan images in all bone ingrowth cases studied by Oswald and coworkers.[194] The amount of uptake about the medial segment of the tip of the prosthesis tended to remain stable or decrease over time and to be less than or equal to radionuclide uptake on the lateral side of the tip. Increased uptake about the femoral component occurred frequently on [111]In-labeled leukocyte scans during the first 24 months.[194] In most cases, this uptake was less than or equal to that on bone scans and remained stable or decreased during the 6 to 24 month period of study. Data derived from this study indicated that complications should be expected when

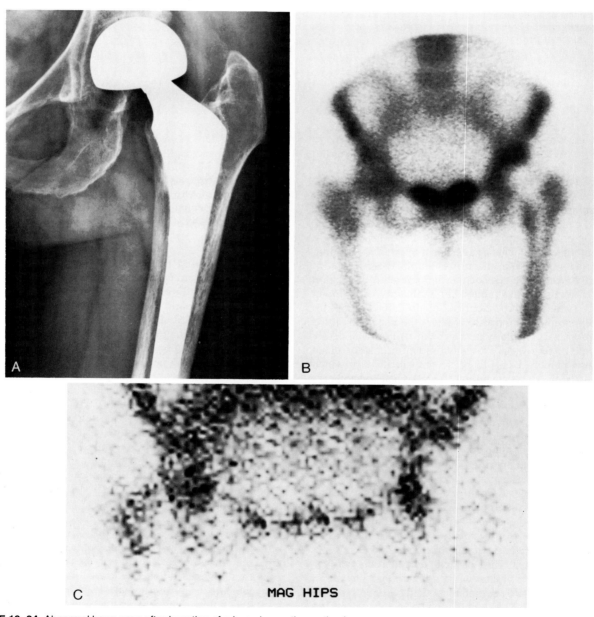

**FIGURE 19–24.** Abnormal bone scan after insertion of a bone ingrowth prosthesis.

**A** Radiograph shows mild settling of the femoral component of the bipolar prosthesis. Sclerotic areas are seen adjacent to the bone ingrowth area. Sclerosis of the superior portion of the acetabulum is present. Clinically, pain and a question of infection were present.

**B** Bone scan demonstrates increased uptake, particularly about the tip and trochanteric region of the femoral component, suggesting loosening. Increased uptake also is noted along the acetabulum.

**C** The [111]In-labeled leukocyte scan shows mild increased uptake in the acetabulum consistent with inflammation. At surgery, no loosening of the femoral stem was found.

either the uptake of the radionuclide in the flow phase of a three phase bone scan was increased or focal blood-pool activity was present; when such uptake in the medial aspect of the tip of the prosthesis was greater than that in lateral aspect or increased with time (3 to 24 months); or when such uptake in the prosthetic tip was greater than that in the iliac crest (Fig. 19–24). Infection should be suspected when radionuclide uptake on an [111]In-labeled leukocyte scan was greater than that in the iliac crest, occurred in a pattern other than a focal or diffuse linear one, or increased on serial scans obtained 6 months or more after surgery.[195]

**Arthrographic and Arthroscintigraphic Findings.**[197, 198] Incomplete ingrowth of bone around the porous surface of a bone ingrowth prosthesis may create channels that allow contrast material or isotope to collect, leading to an erroneous diagnosis of prosthetic loosening of a bone ingrowth component on arthrography or arthroscintigraphy.[198] Harris and associates[199] described such a case, in which a large amount of contrast material was seen around the bone ingrowth component, with filling of draining veins, but rigid fixation was found at the time of surgery. In fact, both false-positive and false-negative studies have been identified. Harris and Barrack[32, 332] have studied the utility of arthrography in assessing painful uncemented hip prostheses. Arthrograms of 24 uncemented femoral stems were reviewed. False-positive examinations for loosening occurred in four cases and false-negative examinations in six cases (sensitivity, 57 per cent; specificity, 60 per cent; accuracy, 58 per cent). Swan and coworkers[197] performed standard arthrography with radiopaque contrast material and nuclear arthrography in 12 patients with painful bone ingrowth prostheses who subsequently underwent additional surgery. Three hours prior to standard arthrography, [99m]Tc-methylene diphosphonate was administered intravenously. The intra-articular injection of contrast material was supplemented by intra-articular injection of 0.1 mCi of [111]In-labeled chloride in saline solution. The joint then was exercised passively. Only the femoral component was assessed. With regard to prosthetic loosening, contrast arthrography yielded a sensitivity of 50 per cent and a specificity of 100 per cent. Nuclear arthrography yielded a sensitivity of 70 per cent and a specificity of 100 per cent. Simultaneous analysis of results of both studies revealed improved sensitivity to 90 per cent while 100 per cent specificity was maintained for the diagnosis of femoral loosening. Additional studies evaluating the roles of contrast and radionuclide arthrography for assessment of uncemented prosthetic components are necessary.

### Additional Findings

***Thigh Pain.*** Thigh pain rarely is observed after cemented arthroplasties, but it is not uncommon after uncemented total hip replacement. In one report, thigh pain was observed in 25 per cent of patients with uncemented femoral components and none of a similar group of patients with cemented components followed for at least 2 years.[19] Bands and associates[179] found thigh pain to occur in 43 per cent of patients after PCA prostheses, at some time in the postoperative course. Early in the postoperative course, this pain may result from micromotion of the prosthetic components; the pain may diminish as prosthetic fixation occurs.[179] Continued thigh pain after the first postoperative year suggests that stable prosthetic fixation has not been achieved. Hedley and colleagues[188] found thigh pain in 30 per cent of patients

at 6 months after surgery, in 8 per cent at 1 year after surgery, and in 4 per cent at 2 years after surgery. No correlation has been found between the presence of thigh pain and the extent of radiolucent regions at the bone-prosthesis interface, the fit of the femoral stem,[179] the amount of filling of the canal by the prosthesis, the formation of endosteal new bone, or the presence of cortical hypertrophy near the distal stem. Varus position of the femoral stem may predispose to thigh pain, however.[186]

***Fracture.*** For bone ingrowth to occur, the prosthesis must be stable within the bone at the time of surgery. On the acetabular side, this stability may be maintained by screws or pegs, whereas on the femoral side it is maintained by the press fit of the component into the femur. Because of this tight fit and the relatively large femoral components that are used to maximize contact of the prosthesis with the femoral cortex, femoral fracture may occur. The postoperative radiograph must include visualization of the bone past the tip of the component to allow for proper assessment of this complication.

***Focal Bone Loss and Prosthetic Loosening.*** As discussed earlier, focal bone resorption, first described in cemented prostheses, has been described subsequently in uncemented components, including those in which bone ingrowth has occurred (Fig. 19–25). In 1990, Maloney and collaborators described focal osteolysis adjacent to stable uncemented components.[176] This finding was seen in about 3 per cent of patients and generally occurred at least 3 years after insertion of the prosthesis. Histologic specimens from two cases revealed aggregates of macrophages with partic-

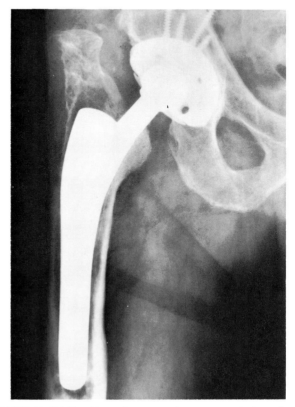

**FIGURE 19–25.** Focal bone loss around an uncemented prosthesis. Loosening of the press fit femoral stem with marked subsidence and a focal expansile area of lucency at the tip of the prosthesis are seen.

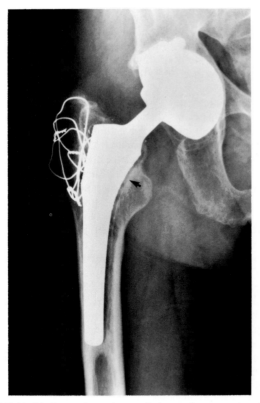

**FIGURE 19–26.** Loose bone ingrowth femoral component. A wide zone of lucency is seen along the area of bone ingrowth (arrow) as well as along the smooth portion of the femoral stem. Several beads are noted in the soft tissues.

ulate polyethylene and metallic debris. Follow-up examinations in 154 patients with uncemented Harris-Galante porous coated implants for 20 to 77 months disclosed endosteal cortical erosion in 20 (13 per cent).[135] Osteolytic lesions were noted on radiographs at 12 to 66 months. The lesions most often involved the femur adjacent to the distal, smooth portion of the femoral stem. As with cemented components, the lytic lesions usually increase in size with time.

Osteolysis has been noted at the rim of bone ingrowth acetabular components.[177] Engh and coworkers[177] found evidence of osteolysis about the acetabular components in almost 20 per cent of patients more than 8 years after operation but in fewer than 5 per cent of those followed for less than 5 years.

Pathologic examination has shown that, as with cemented components, membranes are formed along the surfaces of bone ingrowth components (Fig. 19–26). In loose bone ingrowth components, these interface membranes are composed largely of well-vascularized, loosely organized connective tissue with large active fibroblasts and islands of woven bone.[57] Macrophages containing hemosiderin and metal also are noted and metal debris is found within mast cells. Such cells are significant as they may be involved in chronic inflammation and in pathologic bone resorption.

***Release of Metal Particles.***[201–206] Metal debris may result from loosening and fretting of sintered particles, wear of titanium modular heads, or corrosion or abrasion of the femoral component that is in contact with bone.[135] Debris is more common with titanium components, particularly

when they are used for the articular surface.[203–205] The role of metal debris in loosening and osteolysis is less certain than are the roles of PMMA cement or polyethylene.[134] There is concern, however, regarding possible effects of metal released from the prosthetic components. Elevated concentrations of metal have been found in the blood and urine of patients with prostheses. Jacobs and coworkers[201] noted serum concentrations of titanium in patients with loose titanium-alloy hip prostheses to be approximately double those of control subjects. Sensitivity to metal also has been suggested as a cause of prosthetic loosening.[108]

### Bipolar Prostheses

Bipolar hip prostheses were introduced as alternatives to hemiarthroplasty (e.g., Moore and Thompson prostheses). Theoretically, the increased motion at the articulation between the acetabular component and the femoral head allows less motion at the prosthesis-acetabular articulation and thus decreases acetabular wear.[208, 209] Other theoretical advantages of bipolar prostheses include a lower frequency of prosthetic dislocation and the ability to revise the acetabular component to a total hip replacement if the need arises. Some studies, however, have shown progressive, decreased motion at the inner bearing of the prosthesis.[209]

Complications of bipolar prostheses include fracture of the ipsilateral femur,[210] component fracture and separation, abnormal wear of the acetabulum, and wear of the acetabular liner[209] (Figs. 19–27 and 19–28). Deformation of the acetabular liner may occur, owing to static or dynamic

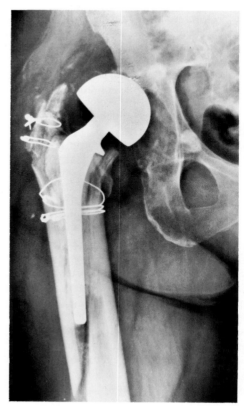

**FIGURE 19–27.** Subluxation of bipolar prosthesis and femoral fracture. The bipolar acetabular component is displaced superolaterally to the acetabulum. Bone loss has occurred from the superolateral portion of the acetabulum and residual cement is present from prior total hip replacement. A femoral fracture has occurred.

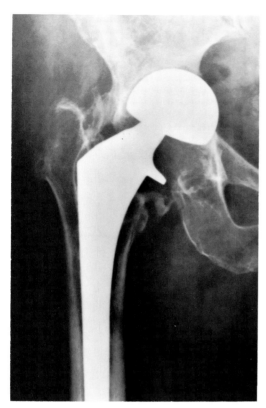

**FIGURE 19–28.** Bipolar prosthesis with acetabular protrusion. The bipolar prosthesis has migrated superomedially.

loading or absorption of moisture. Stress on the superolateral aspect of the acetabular component leads to wear of the acetabular liner and tilt of the acetabular shell into a varus position. Incavo and associates[209] reported three patients in whom wear of the polyethylene liner led to contact between the medial acetabular rim and the medial femoral component, producing a groove in its surface. This groove was visible only on radiographs obtained after acetabular revision.

The "unipolar" prosthesis has replaced the bipolar prosthesis in some cases. The unipolar prosthesis functions as a hemiarthroplasty but has modular components to allow adjustment of neck length (Fig. 19–29).

### Hydroxyapatite Coated Prostheses[211–215]

Hydroxyapatite coating of prostheses allows chemical bonds to form with the adjacent bone[211] and promotes bone apposition. The coating, which is not visible radiographically, is plasma sprayed onto the proximal portion of the femoral component. Acetabular components also may be prepared in a similar fashion. The hydroxyapatite surface is nontoxic and resorbs slowly over time.[212]

Hydroxyapatite coating allows direct bone apposition without interposition of a fibrous membrane[213] and, therefore, radiographs can be expected to show bone in direct apposition to the prosthetic surface without an intervening lucent line. Follow-up evaluation 2 years or longer after hydroxyapatite coated prostheses have been inserted have shown areas of new bone formation adjacent to the junction of the coated and uncoated segments of the prostheses.[211, 212] A thin lucent region often parallels the uncoated portion of

the stem, owing to differences in stiffness of the implant and the bone, with resultant micromotion. Mild subsidence of the prosthesis may occur. Resorption of the calcar, presumably due to stress shielding, occurred in almost half of the cases evaluated by D'Antonio and colleagues.[212] Cortical thickening of the femur occurs most often in zones 3 and 5. Remodeling generally occurs within the first postoperative year (Fig. 19–30).

## TOTAL KNEE REPLACEMENT

Total knee replacement is used to alleviate pain and disability not responsive to medical management, particularly in cases of rheumatoid arthritis and osteoarthritis (especially in older patients).[216] Osteotomy often is used in preference to total joint replacement in patients with osteoarthritis who are less than 60 years of age, manual laborers, athletes, or grossly overweight.

The term "total knee replacement" refers either to resurfacing of the femorotibial compartments or to resurfacing of the femorotibial and patellofemoral compartments. Three categories of total knee prostheses are described, according to the degree of stability (or constraint to knee motion) that they provide.[217] Nonconstrained components provide no inherent stability and allow considerable motion. The stability of the prostheses is dependent on intact or reconstructed soft tissue. The older resurfacing types of prostheses, such as the geometric and polycentric prostheses, are examples of nonconstrained prostheses. Constrained prostheses provide inherent stability so that the cruciate or collateral ligaments of the knee need not be intact. These components limit the motion of the joint. Older hinge prostheses (e.g., Guepar hinge, Walldius hinge) are of this type. Unfortunately, these older constrained prostheses were complicated by high rates of loosening and infection.[218] Newer con-

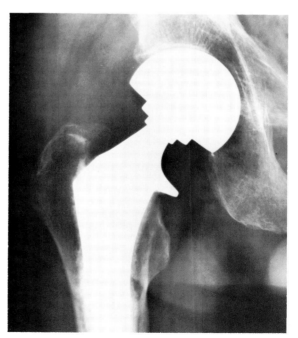

**FIGURE 19–29.** Unipolar prosthesis. The modular femoral and acetabular components are linked and function as a hemiarthroplasty. Motion occurs only between the native acetabulum and the prosthesis.

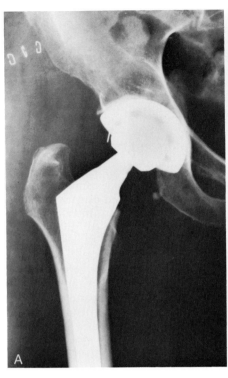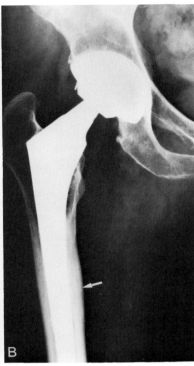

**FIGURE 19–30.** Hydroxyapatite-coated prosthesis.

**A** Initial examination. The hydroxyapatite coating is not visible.

**B** Several years later, remodeling has occurred with bone thickening distally (arrow) and resorption proximally. (Courtesy of A. Newberg, Boston, Massachusetts.)

strained prostheses have been developed that have metal-to-polyethylene articulations and allow some gliding and rotatory motion (e.g., the Kinematic rotating hinge, the constrained posterior stabilized prosthesis)[218] (Fig. 19–31). Most prostheses are semiconstrained. These include a group of cruciate sparing prostheses (e.g., the duopatellar, Kinematic, Press Fit Condylar Knee) in which a posterior cutout allows the intact posterior cruciate ligament to remain in position, and a group of cruciate sacrificing prostheses (e.g., total condylar prosthesis) (Fig. 19–32).

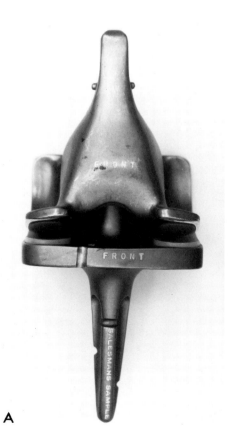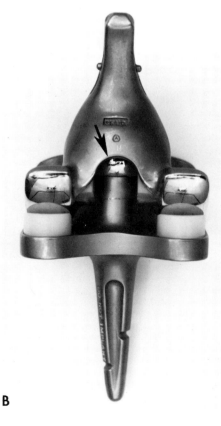

**FIGURE 19–31.** Constrained total knee prosthesis. Spherocentric prosthesis (Howmedica Inc). Anterior **(A)** and posterior **(B)** views. Polyethylene pads are present on the tibial component for articulation with the metallic femoral component. Full constraint is provided by central ball-and-socket articulation (arrow).

**A**                          **B**

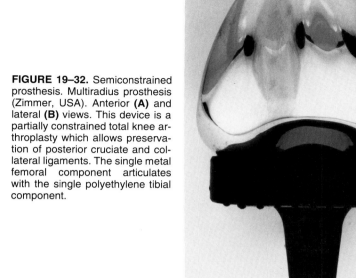
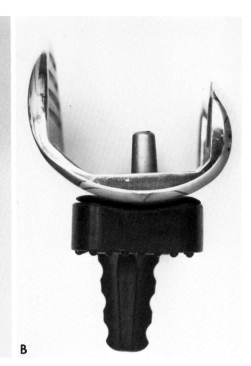

**FIGURE 19–32.** Semiconstrained prosthesis. Multiradius prosthesis (Zimmer, USA). Anterior **(A)** and lateral **(B)** views. This device is a partially constrained total knee arthroplasty which allows preservation of posterior cruciate and collateral ligaments. The single metal femoral component articulates with the single polyethylene tibial component.

Unicompartmental prostheses (unicondylar prostheses) resurface both the femoral and tibial sides of a damaged compartment (Fig. 19–33). Unicompartmental prostheses are used only in cases of osteoarthritis in which damage is limited to a single compartment and the ligaments are intact. Because inflammatory disorders (e.g., rheumatoid arthritis) typically involve all three compartments of the knee,

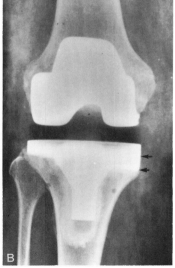

**FIGURE 19–33.** Loose unicondylar prosthesis.
**A** Radiography of the knee (obtained with the patient erect) shows a unicondylar replacement with overall varus alignment of the knee. Settling of the tibial component has occurred into the tibia, and a 1 mm cement-bone lucent zone is visible beneath the tibial component cement. Probable wear of the tibial articular surface is present.
**B** Revision with the insertion of a total knee prosthesis has led to restoration of normal valgus alignment. A metal wedge that is thicker medially (thickness shown by the arrows) has been inserted beneath the medial aspect of the tibial tray to help fill the area of bone loss.

unicondylar prostheses are not used for these conditions. Hemiarthroplasty involves resurfacing one side of the joint and rarely is used.

Total knee arthroplasty is an exacting operation, requiring attention to the detail of component positioning and the balance of soft tissue structures. The final tibiofemoral angulation of the knee should be 7 to 9 degrees of valgus.[216] This angulation should recreate the normal mechanical axis of the leg (determined by constructing a line from the center of the femoral head through the center of the knee and the center of the ankle). Bone defects remaining after the femoral and tibial resections are made are filled with cement, graft, custom prostheses, or wedges. Fixation with cement or bone ingrowth has been utilized. Windsor and Insall[216] recommend routine resurfacing of the patella when practical, but this issue is debated.[219, 222, 223] Patients with rheumatoid arthritis who have involvement of the knee usually undergo patellar resurfacing to decrease the rate of recurrent inflammation associated with retained cartilage.

## Postoperative Appearance

Anteroposterior views of the knee taken in supine and standing positions, along with lateral and tangential patellar views, are obtained routinely for follow-up of patients with total knee replacements. Standing views of the entire leg are useful for preoperative planning and to document component position postoperatively. Fluoroscopy has been suggested to view the cement-bone interface in profile, but it generally is not used. As reproducible radiographs are ideal for following patients over time, standardized positioning has been attempted. Siu and coworkers,[222] for example, used a frame apparatus. The radiographs are digitized and corrected for parallax, and a number of angular measurements are generated by computer. Because these techniques require a specialized apparatus, they do not appear to be generally applicable.

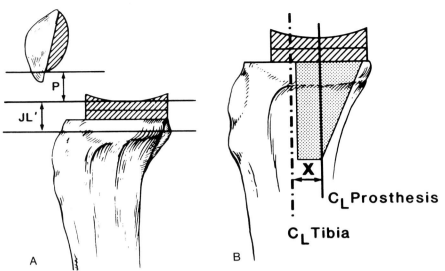

**FIGURE 19–34.** Measurement of the joint line height, patellar height, and central position of the tibial component.

**A** The distance from the tibial tubercle to the articular surface on the lateral radiograph represents the height of the joint line (JL). The height of the patella (P) is measured from the joint line to the patellar component.

**B** The relationship of the center of the tibial component and the center line of the tibia can be compared. (From Figgie HE, et al: J Bone Joint Surg [Am] *68*:1035, 1986.)

In the normal situation, anteroposterior views show femorotibial alignment of 7 to 9 degrees of valgus. If standing views of the knee are obtained, the center of the knee should lie on the mechanical axis of the leg. Such restoration of normal alignment results in lower stresses at the implant-bone interface. The tibial component should be perpendicular in relation to the tibial shaft or up to 2 degrees of varus alignment.[224] The distance of the edge of the tibial component to the tibial margins as well as the presence and thickness of any cement-bone and prosthesis-bone lucent regions should be evaluated. Varus position of the tibial component refers to relative tilting of the component medially. Lee and coworkers[224] found radiolucent lines to be related to medial shift of the tibial component by more than 4 mm or placement of the tibial component in more than 2 degrees of varus angulation. When intramedullary, rather than extramedullary, alignment systems are used for positioning the components, the tract from the apparatus may be visible on immediate postoperative radiographs.

On the lateral view, evaluation often includes assessment of the distance of the tibial component from the anterior and posterior tibial margins, the tilt of the tibial and femoral components in relation to the respective shafts of the tibia and femur, the distance of the center of the tibial component to the center of the tibia, and the height of the joint line[225] (Fig. 19–34). These parameters can be compared on pre- and postoperative studies. The level of the joint line can be measured on the lateral radiograph as the distance from the tibial tubercle to the lowest portion of the tibial prosthetic articular surface, or the tip of the fibula can be used as the reference point.[226] Figgie and associates[225] found that, postoperatively, the highest functional knee scores were associated with a posterior position of the tibial component with relation to the center line of the tibia, maintenance of the inferior pole of the patellar implant proximal to the joint line, and minimum change in the joint line. A range of measurements was associated with good or excellent knee scores (the "neutral" range): anteroposterior tibial component position greater than or equal to zero, a change in the joint line of 8 mm or less, and a patellar height of 10 to 30 mm.[225]

The position of the patellar component is judged on lateral and tangential patellar views. On the lateral view, the height of the patellar component is measured as the perpendicular distance from the joint line to the inferior edge of the patellar articular surface.[227] The suggested range for patellar height is 10 to 30 mm.[225] On the tangential patellar view, the prosthesis should contact the femoral component symmetrically. Other measurements have been described by Gomes and coworkers.[227]

A normal area of bone rarefaction occurs in the anterior portion of the femur, beneath the femoral component, in about two thirds of cases after total knee arthroplasty.[228] This represents bone loss in response to stress shielding and is not evidence of prosthetic loosening (Fig. 19–35). Such

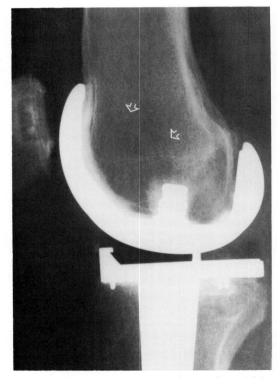

**FIGURE 19–35.** Stress changes in the femur after total knee replacement. A poorly defined area of osteopenia without a sclerotic margin is noted in the anterior aspect of the femur (arrows).

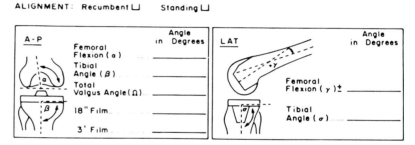

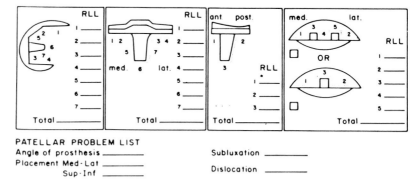

**FIGURE 19–36.** A standardized reporting system for knee arthroplasties. (From Ewald FC: Clin Orthop *248*:9, 1989.)

bone loss may be differentiated from significant lucent lines by the absence of an accompanying line of bone sclerosis (demarcation line).

The width and location of lucent lines should be noted. Wright and associates[226] reviewed radiographs obtained 5 to 9 years after insertion of a cruciate ligament sparing prosthesis (Kinematic total knee). They found nonprogressive lucent zones measuring less than 1 mm wide in 40 per cent of tibial components and 30 per cent of femoral components. A standardized recording system for this radiographic feature has been proposed by the Knee Society[229] (Fig. 19–36). The final score of each component is the sum of the thickness of each radiolucent line in each zone, measured in millimeters.

## Clinical Results

The clinical results of total knee replacement are good. Long-term follow-up assessments by Buechel and Pappas,[230] for example, have shown that more than 90 per cent of cemented prostheses remained in situ and were associated with satisfactory (better than poor) knee scores more than 10 years after surgery. Uncemented prostheses followed for 6 years showed almost uniform success. Lee and colleagues[224] found that 95 per cent of posterior cruciate condylar prostheses followed for at least 7 years were associated with excellent results, and Wright and coworkers[226] found 90 per cent of cases followed for 5 to 9 years to be associated with good or excellent results. Rand and Ilstrup[231] evaluated 9200 total knee arthroplasties and found four independent variables that, when present, led to a 97 per cent probability that the implant would be in place at the time of a 10 year follow-up examination. These factors were primary total joint replacement, a diagnosis of rheumatoid arthritis, an age of 60 years or more, and the use of

a condylar prosthesis with a metal-backed tibial component. Five year results have shown comparable survival rates of prostheses fixed with or without cement.[231]

## Complications

### Patellar Complications

The need for revision surgery after total knee arthroplasty relates most commonly to patellar complications.[226] Stress fracture of the patella, loosening of the patellar component, and dislocation or subluxation of the patellar component are the most common problems encountered. Prostheses with a more constrained patellofemoral joint appear to have a higher frequency of patellar component loosening.

Patellar stress fractures are reported in up to 21 per cent of cases.[232] These fractures often are detected as incidental findings on radiographs (Fig. 19–37). The prevalence of patellar stress fractures has increased in the elderly and as more sophisticated prostheses are used. According to Brick and Scott,[232] fracture fixation is indicated if a fracture is displaced more than 2 cm, if a significant extensor lag is present causing instability, or if the component is displaced. Goldberg and coworkers[233] concluded that fractures not accompanied by patellar dislocation, component loosening, or complete disruption of the extensor mechanism may be treated nonsurgically. Although lateral release was thought to predispose to patellar fracture, comparison of patients with and without lateral release has shown patellar fractures to be more frequent in those without this procedure.

Loosening of the patellar component, as in loosening of other components, may be asymptomatic. Osteonecrosis of the patella is thought to predispose to both loosening and stress fracture.

Patellar malposition is readily recognizable on radio-

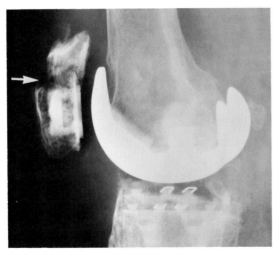

**FIGURE 19–37.** Patellar fracture. A transverse fracture has occurred at the bone-prosthesis interface. (From Weissman BN: In CB Sledge, et al (Eds): Arthritis Surgery. Philadelphia, W.B. Saunders Co, 1994.)

graphic examination. Some 24 symptomatic patellar subluxations or dislocations occurred in 2887 total knee replacements evaluated by Brick and Scott.[232] Patellar subluxation is caused by imbalance of soft tissue, component malposition, malalignment, hemarthrosis, and trauma.

Initially, polyethylene patellar components were used without metal backing. Newer components were designed with metal backing in an attempt to transmit load more uniformly to bone, to decrease the tendency of the polyethylene to deform, and to add a porous surface for bone

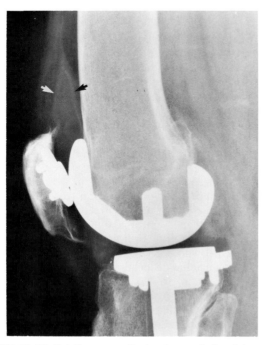

**FIGURE 19–38.** Patellar wear with development of metal synovitis. A white outline (arrows) of the suprapatellar pouch (the "metal line" sign) developed in this patient during the follow-up period. This finding is a strong indicator of metal synovitis. In this case, abnormal tilt of the patellar component is seen, suggesting patellar wear as the source of the metal.

ingrowth.[234] Despite apparent success with metal backing of tibial[236] and acetabular components, the metal backing of the patellar component requires a thinner polyethylene surface and ultimately may result in polyethylene wear. Bayley and Scott[237] found cracking of the polyethylene over the sharp edge of the metal backing laterally in 16 of 25 cases of failure of the patellar component.[237] Wearing or splitting of the polyethylene, or its displacement from the metal backing,[238] allows the metal of the femoral component to rub against the metal backing of the patellar component, resulting in the production of metal debris and synovitis. Such synovitis may be associated with black discoloration of aspirated joint fluid in some patients.[239]

Radiographic examination usually allows a preoperative diagnosis of patellar component disruption. Thinning or displacement of the polyethylene articular surface usually is visible on radiographs.[235] Fatigue fractures of the junction of the fixation pegs and metal backing, separation of the porous coating from the underlying metal, and displacement of the metal backing with fracture at the peg-plate junction also have been documented radiographically.[235] The metal synovitis often is visible radiographically, usually as a line of increased opacity outlining the distended joint (the "metal line" sign) or as a diffuse opaqueness of the joint fluid[240] (Fig. 19–38). These complications have resulted in the elimination of metal backing in newer patellar components.

### Joint Instability

Joint instability may be a complication of total knee replacement when soft tissue constraints remain inadequate (Fig. 19–39).

### Prosthetic Loosening

Tibial component loosening generally is considered to be the most frequent cause for complete revision of a total knee replacement.[224] Wright and coworkers,[226] however, noted no cases of femoral or tibial loosening. Insall[333] found loosening in 1.8 per cent of total condylar prostheses. The incidence of prosthetic loosening, therefore, seems to be less than that occurring after total hip replacement. The tibial component is involved most often and the loosening develops most frequently at the cement-bone interface. A wide (2 mm or more) or enlarging lucent zone, collapse of subjacent trabecular bone, fragmentation of underlying cement, changes in component position, development of a metal-cement lucent region, and change in the angulation of the knee on weight-bearing radiographs are indications of loosening of cemented components[5] (Figs. 19–40 and 19–41). In addition, continued shedding of beads from the surface of bone ingrowth components after the first 3 to 6 months postoperatively suggests prosthetic loosening.[241]

Bone scanning often shows mildly to moderately increased isotope activity for years after total knee replacement.[242] A normal scan is good evidence that no loosening or infection is present.

Arthrography may confirm loosening of components by showing contrast agent insinuation within the cement-bone interface (Fig. 19–42). Generally, radiopaque contrast material is used, which is injected until the suprapatellar pouch is full. Anteroposterior, oblique, and lateral radiographs are obtained after exercise of the knee and walking, with and without traction placed on the extremity.

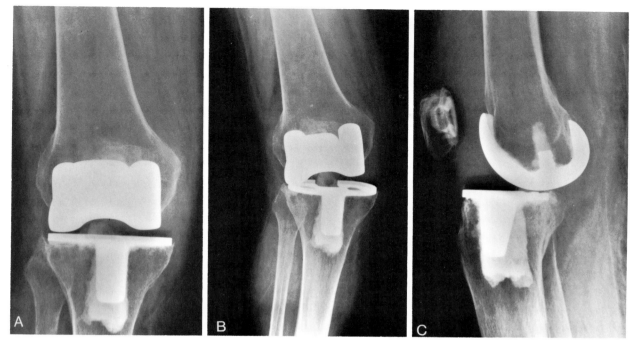

**FIGURE 19–39.** Joint instability.
  **A** Supine examination shows a semiconstrained prosthesis in place with valgus alignment of the knee.
  **B** The degree of valgus angulation is markedly increased on the standing view.
  **C** The lateral view demonstrates anterior tibial subluxation, the result of soft tissue imbalance.

### Prosthetic Wear[240, 243–254]

Deposition of metal in the joint after total knee replacement may be caused by wear of a metal-to-metal hinge or of polyethylene articular surfaces, allowing the metal of the femoral component to articulate against the metal backing of the tibial component or the metal backing of the patellar component. In the series of cases of metal synovitis reported by Weissman and colleagues,[240] two cases resulted from hinge wear, 10 from wear of metal-backed patellar components, and six from wear of the tibial prosthetic sur-

face. The consequent shedding of metal into the joint may be visible as a curvilinear radiodense line outlining the joint capsule (the ''metal line'' sign) or as diffuse opacity of the joint fluid (Fig. 19–43). Titanium is particularly prone to such wear. Breen and Stoker[243] reported three patients with titanium alloy megaprostheses inserted in the knee after tumor resection who developed large fluid-filled cysts along the anterior aspects of the tibial components and problems with extensor function.

The problem of component wear has received considerable attention.[244–247] Wear debris consisting of polyethylene,

**FIGURE 19–40.** Tibial component loosening.
  **A** The initial standing radiograph shows the knee in slight varus alignment. The tibial component is small, compared with the width of the tibial plateau.
  **B** Standing radiograph seven years later documents shift of the tibial component position, with sinking of its medial aspect, metal-cement lucent areas laterally and at the tibial stem, increased varus alignment, and thinning of the medial polyethylene liner consistent with wear.

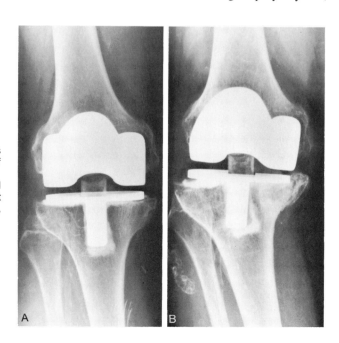

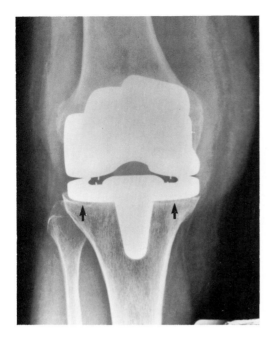

**FIGURE 19–41.** Loosening of bone ingrowth tibial component. A 1 to 2 mm lucent line is noted beneath the tibial tray (arrows) with a thinner lucent zone around the tibial stem.

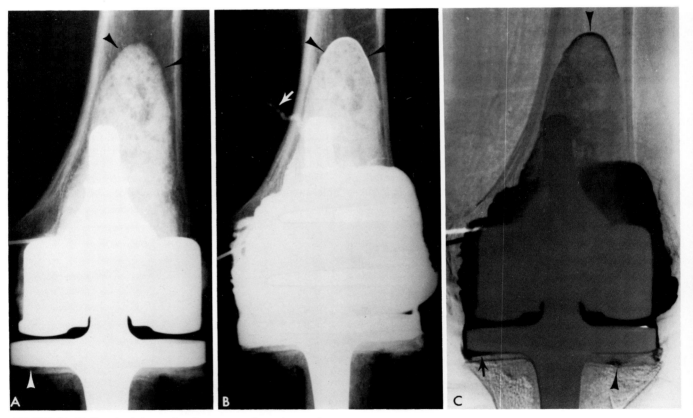

**FIGURE 19–42.** Prosthetic loosening demonstrated at arthrography.
   **A** Radiograph of spherocentric total knee arthroplasty. Narrow (1 mm) radiolucent zones are noted at the bone-cement interface of the femoral component and the metal-cement interface of the tibial component (arrowheads).
   **B** Arthrogram shows contrast material entering the bone-cement interface of the femoral component (arrowheads) and lymphatic filling (white arrow). Contrast material entering the metal-cement interface along the tibial component is appreciated more easily in the subtraction radiograph **(C).**
   **C** Subtraction arthrogram demonstrates contrast material entering the metal-cement interface of the tibial component (arrow) as well as the bone-cement interface of both components (arrowheads).

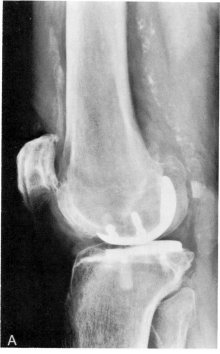
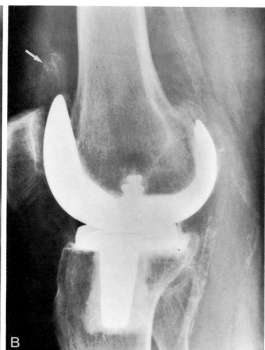

**FIGURE 19–43.** Metal synovitis.

**A** Lateral radiograph of a patient with a medial unicondylar prosthesis shows a dense white line in the suprapatellar pouch, indicating metal synovitis ("metal line" sign). The finding resulted from wear of the tibial component.

**B** In another patient who currently was asymptomatic, a radiograph shows a white line outlining the suprapatellar pouch (arrow), indicative of metal synovitis.

metal, or both, may result in the formation of a hypertrophic synovium-like membrane capable of producing substances that induce bone resorption. This membrane appears to be responsible for osteolysis (that may be marked) around even uninfected, stable uncemented total knee components, and it appears to be similar or identical in type to the membrane that occurs around loose prostheses[252] (Fig. 19–44). The process is analogous to that in the hip. The size of the particles released and their number appear to influence the tissue response. Smaller particles are associated with a histiocytic response and bone loss, whereas larger particles are associated with a giant cell response.[249]

Several cases of osteolysis around uncemented knee prostheses have been reported.[248, 249, 253] In a review of 174 consecutive bone ingrowth total knee arthroplasties by Peters and coworkers,[249] 16 per cent of implants demonstrated osteolysis, most often seen in the medial tibial metaphysis, and progressing around the tibial base plate and along the

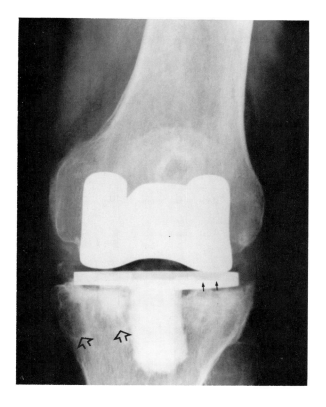

**FIGURE 19–44.** Histiocytic response. This patient had metal synovitis at surgery with wear of the lateral tibial tray (solid arrows) due to instability. A wide metal-cement lucent zone and multiple well-defined lucent areas (open arrows) have developed at the cement-bone interface.

medial fixation screw. A large volume of small particles was found in all patients with osteolysis. In other cases, femoral lysis has been massive. Radiographic documentation of early tibial component wear may be possible by paying careful attention to diminution of joint space on standing views or to a change in the mechanical axis of the knee on such radiographs.[245] The process of stereophotogrammetry may be useful for this assessment.

Attempts to improve the polyethylene articular surface by the addition of carbon fiber reinforcement apparently have been unsuccessful.[251] Carbon fibers and polyethylene have been reported in external iliac lymph nodes of a patient with a well-functioning knee prosthesis without apparent loosening.[250] No synovitis was apparent in the knee. Radiographs obtained 9 years after insertion of the prosthesis showed thinning of the polyethylene, especially of the patellar component, but no prosthetic loosening was apparent.

In summary, in the knee as in the hip, bone cement is not necessary for a foreign body membrane to form or for osteolysis to occur. This condition (termed ''cementless disease'') may be attributable to polyethylene wear and deposition of metal particles.

### Infection

Infection is the most frequent reason for failure of a total knee prosthesis[236] (Figs. 16–45 to 16–47). The prevalence of infection after total knee arthroplasty ranges from 1.1 to 12.4 per cent.[255] Evaluation of more than 4000 total knee arthroplasties implanted from 1973 to 1987 revealed 67 with infection (1.6 per cent) and demonstrated an increased risk of infection in those patients with rheumatoid arthritis, skin ulcerations, and prior knee surgery.[256] Although infections may occur early in the postoperative course, their appearance may be delayed for several years, particularly in rheumatoid arthritis patients.

The utility of various radionuclide methods for the diagnosis of infection after total knee replacement has indicated that combined leukocyte-labeled and sulfur colloid scans offer the highest accuracy (95 per cent).[257–260]

## TOTAL SHOULDER REPLACEMENT[262–283]

Total shoulder prostheses theoretically should restore normal anatomic relationships and provide functional stability. The earliest prostheses were constrained designs, however, in which the glenoid and humeral components were linked about a fixed center of rotation. These prostheses provided stability, prevented upward migration of the humeral component, and could be used in patients with severe defects in the rotator cuff; examples were the Stanmore, Michael Reese, and Gristina prostheses. Nonconstrained prostheses have no physical connection between the glenoid and humeral components and require intact soft tissues for stability (e.g., the Neer II prosthesis). Semiconstrained components incorporate a superior extension to the glenoid component in an attempt to limit upward subluxation of the humerus (e.g., the McNab-English prosthesis). As in the hip, a bipolar arthroplasty has been developed for the shoulder. The bipolar cup articulates with both the acromion and the glenoid. As the name indicates, motion occurs at two levels, between the humeral head and the glenoid cup and between the cup and the bony glenoid.

### Complications

Review of total shoulder replacement has shown loosening of the glenoid component and component instability to

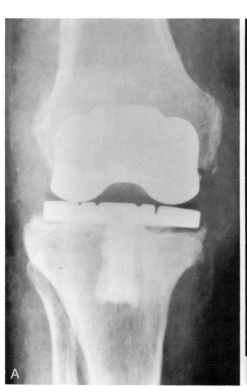
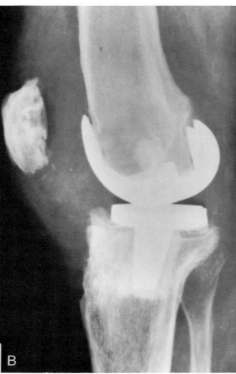

**FIGURE 19–45.** Infected total knee replacement. Frontal **(A)** and lateral **(B)** views show marked intra-articular soft tissue swelling. Tibial component loosening and periosteal reaction along the femur are seen. (**A** From Weissman BN: In CB Sledge, et al (Eds): Arthritis Surgery. Philadelphia, WB Saunders Co, 1994.)

**FIGURE 19–46.** Infected total knee replacement.

**A** Radiograph shows no evidence of prosthetic loosening, bone destruction, or periosteal reaction to suggest infection.

**B** Bone scan indicates increased uptake around the tibial component and the patella.

**C** The ¹¹¹In-labeled leukocyte scan reveals increased uptake within the joint, indicative of articular infection or inflammation.

(**A** From Weissman BN: Radiol Clin North Am *28*:1111, 1990.)

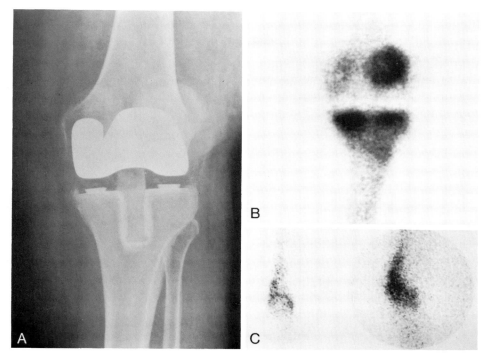

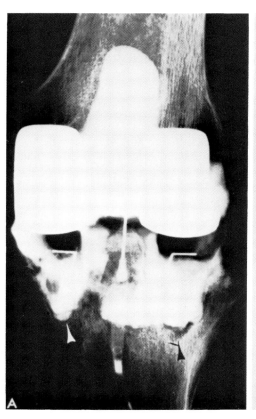

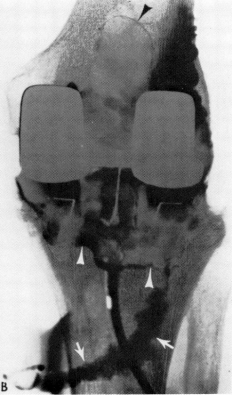

**FIGURE 19–47.** Infected total knee replacement demonstrated with arthrography.

**A** Preliminary anteroposterior radiograph with needle in place (geometric total knee arthroplasty, patella removed). A wide radiolucent zone (2.5 mm) is present around the bone-cement interface of the tibial component (arrowheads).

**B** Anteroposterior subtraction arthrogram shows contrast material tracking along the bone-cement interface of both components (arrowheads). A sinus tract is demonstrated extending from the base of the tibial component to the skin (arrows).

be the complications that most often require revision.[277] Reported glenoid loosening rates have varied from 2.7 per cent for unconstrained total shoulder replacements for non–rheumatoid arthritis patients to 10.4 per cent for constrained total shoulder replacements in rheumatoid arthritis patients. Instability was most frequent in the non–rheumatoid arthritis patients with a constrained prosthesis (10.2 per cent). Superior subluxation of the humeral head occurs quite often, particularly in patients with rheumatoid arthritis with nonconstrained prostheses (9 per cent), but it may not result in poor clinical outcome.[277]

### Radiographic Findings

The posterior oblique radiograph with the humerus in external rotation is the single most informative postoperative radiograph[262, 266] (Fig. 19–48). An additional internal rotation view of the shoulder usually is added to complete the routine examination.

The author's experience is largely with the Neer unconstrained prosthesis. The humeral component is positioned in 30 to 35 degrees of retroversion, and when the humerus is rotated externally and the patient is turned into the posterior oblique position, both components are seen in profile. The posterior oblique view of this prosthesis also generally shows the inferior edge of the humeral component and the inferior edge of the glenoid component to be aligned. The superior margin of the prosthetic head should be higher than the greater tuberosity. The glenoid component orientation on the frontal projection may be assessed by measuring the facing angle (the angle between the long axis of the glenoid component and the medial border of the scapula). When the glenoid component is tilted downward (closed angle) the possibility of upward subluxation of the humerus is thought to be reduced.

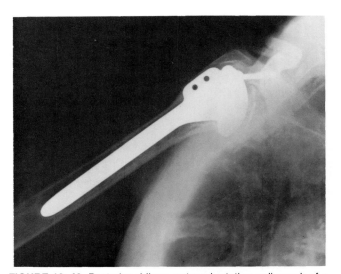

**FIGURE 19–48.** Posterior oblique, external rotation radiograph of a Neer total shoulder replacement. This view allows the components to be seen in profile. The humeral component is uncemented (press fit). The nonmetal-backed glenoid component is cemented; the marker wire beneath the articular surface is evidenced by wide metal-bone and cement-bone lucent zones. A screw is present in the coracoid process consequent to coracoid osteotomy. (Reprinted with permission from Aliabadi P, Weissman BN: In RJ Friedman (Ed): Arthroplasty of the Shoulder. New York, Thieme, 1994. Copyright, Thieme Medical Publishers, Inc.)

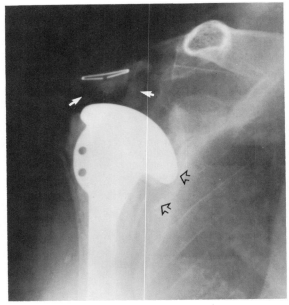

**FIGURE 19–49.** Glenoid component displacement. The external rotation view shows the glenoid component (solid arrows) displaced from the glenoid fossa (open arrows). (Reprinted with permission from Aliabadi P, Weissman BN: In RJ Friedman (Ed): Arthroplasty of the Shoulder. New York, Thieme, 1994. Copyright, Thieme Medical Publishers, Inc.)

Retroversion of the humeral component may be measured directly on radiographs (the method of Mukherjee-Sivaya[263]) or may be determined geometrically from anteroposterior views of the humerus obtained with the forearm in 35 degrees of internal rotation.[274] Retroversion may be determined either by using a formula, by comparison with a standard table, or by approximation, subtracting 40 degrees from the measured angle between a perpendicular to the humeral head ellipse and a perpendicular to the axis of the humeral shaft. In most circumstances, the result of such estimation is within 5 degrees of the actual figure.

Lucent zones delineated by thin lines of sclerosis occur more often along the glenoid components of total shoulder prostheses than along the humeral components. Cement-bone lucent zones greater than 2 mm wide raise the suspicion of component loosening (Fig. 19–48). The glenoid component may become completely dislodged from the underlying bone and lie free within the joint (Fig. 19–49). Bone ingrowth components produce changes in the adjacent bone in accordance with transmitted stress. McElwain and English[270] studied 13 bone ingrowth semiconstrained total shoulder prostheses and found resorption of the proximal humeral cortex in nine patients, cancellous new bone formation in seven, and proximal humeral remodeling in five.

Subluxation or dislocation may occur early or late in the postoperative course. Moeckel and associates[284] classified instability occurring after unconstrained total shoulder replacement as superior, inferior, anterior, and posterior. Superior instability is most common and is documented by the high position of the humerus in relation to the glenoid (Fig. 19–50). Usually this appearance indicates deficiency of the rotator cuff, but component malposition, such as upward tilting of the glenoid component or relative lengthening of the humerus, may cause or exacerbate this instability.[284] Boyd and colleagues[268] indicated the condition to be present when the humeral head was proximal to the

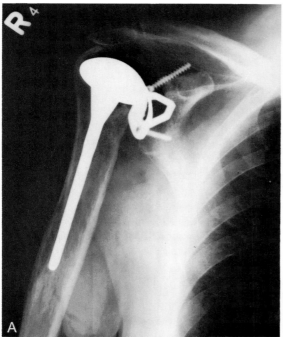

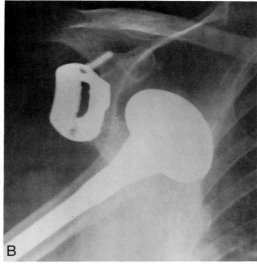

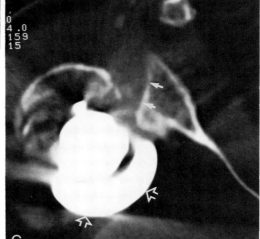

**FIGURE 19–50.** Subluxation after total shoulder arthroplasty. Findings in 3 different patients.
   **A** Upward subluxation of the humeral head in relation to the glenoid has occurred.
   **B** Medial dislocation of the humeral component is observed. Additional views confirmed the *anterior* position of the humeral head.
   **C** *Posterior* dislocation of a humeral hemiarthroplasty (open arrows) with relation to the glenoid (arrows).
   (Reprinted with permission from Aliabadi P, Weissman BN: In RJ Friedman (Ed): Arthroplasty of the Shoulder. New York, Thieme, 1994. Copyright, Thieme Medical Publishers, Inc.)

center of rotation of the glenoid. A summary of postoperative complications indicates that instability occurs most often after constrained prosthetic replacement and least often after hemiarthroplasty.[277]

Inferior subluxation is caused most frequently by residual shortening of the humerus, usually as a consequence of a humeral fracture. Weakness of the deltoid muscle also may result in inferior humeral subluxation. Anterior humeral subluxation or dislocation may result from soft tissue imbalance or component malposition. Exaggerated humeral or glenoid anteversion predisposes to this complication. Posterior subluxation or dislocation of the humeral component also relates to soft tissue imbalance and alteration in articular anatomy. Glenoid or humeral component retroversion may lead to this complication. Inadequate correction for posterior bone loss from the glenoid predisposes to retroversion of the glenoid component. It is helpful, therefore, to evaluate the status of the glenoid region preoperatively with radiographs and CT scanning, if necessary.

Aliabadi and Weissman[262] defined loosening of cemented components as the presence of a cement-bone lucent zone of 2 mm or more along the entire interface or any lucent zone developing at the prosthesis-cement interface. As with prostheses in other joints, these findings may not be associated with symptoms. Loosening also is indicated by a change in component position over time. Subsidence of an uncemented humeral component has been noted in 5 per cent of press fit Neer humeral components.[269] Displacement of the glenoid component may result in the component's lying free within the joint. Careful inspection of the relationships of the glenoid component to the adjacent scapula is warranted at the time of each radiographic follow-up examination to avoid overlooking such displacement.

The features of bone ingrowth total shoulder prostheses have not been evaluated completely. It is likely that loosening of a bone ingrowth prosthesis is present when a lucent zone 2 mm or wider is present between the irregular surface of the prosthesis and the bone, particularly if this zone increases in size over time. In the hip, and presumably in the shoulder, lucent zones that remain unchanged after 2 years suggest the formation of a stable fibrous tissue interface. Progressive or marked subsidence of components, progressive shedding of beads, and changes in component position indicate loosening (Fig. 19–51).

Infection is a less common complication than joint instability or prosthetic loosening. A literature review indicates

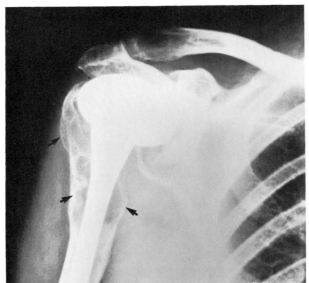

**FIGURE 19–51.** Loosening of glenoid component with histiocytic response due to glenoid wear. An internal rotation view of the humerus in a young homemaker shows well-defined areas of lucency (arrows) about the humeral component. The glenoid component has become worn.

that this complication has occurred in 1.0 per cent of non-constrained total shoulder arthroplasties in patients with rheumatoid arthritis and in 2.4 per cent of constrained total shoulder prostheses in subjects without rheumatoid arthritis.[277] Poorly marginated areas of bone destruction, periosteal reaction, and wide lucent zones at the bone-cement or prosthesis-bone interface (especially if the accompanying sclerotic demarcation zone is absent) suggest infection. Infection also may be present without radiographic abnormalities.

Component disruption, including dissociation of a snap fit glenoid liner, dissociation of modular heads, and component fracture, has been reported.[275] Intraoperative fractures have been noted in 2.5 per cent of nonconstrained total shoulder replacements in rheumatoid arthritis patients.[277] Postoperative fractures occurred in 2.4 per cent of 127 constrained total shoulder replacements in patients without rheumatoid arthritis. These fractures may occur distal to the tip of the humeral component, underscoring the need to include this region on all postoperative radiographs.

## TOTAL ELBOW REPLACEMENT[285–292]

Total elbow arthroplasty is performed primarily in patients with rheumatoid arthritis in whom pain is uncontrolled by medical management.[285] Initially developed prostheses were of the hinge type, popularized in the early 1970s. As with all constrained devices, prosthetic loosening was responsible for the greatest number of failures. Semiconstrained hinge prostheses in which a loose metal-to-plastic bearing was present between the components produced a less constrained device (e.g., triaxial prosthesis) with consequent lower loosening rates. Nonconstrained resurfacing prostheses (e.g., capitellocondylar prosthesis) have no linkage between the components. Loosening rates are lower than with constrained prostheses, but dislocation may occur if the para-articular soft tissues are inadequate.

Lateral radiographs of the capitellocondylar prosthesis should show the stem of the ulnar component to roughly parallel the proximal anterior ulnar cortex (Fig. 19–52). The humeral stem should parallel the humeral shaft, and the center of rotation should be in line with the anterior humeral cortex.[290] On the anteroposterior view, the articular surface should be located centrally in relation to the distal end of the humerus. The capitellar portion of the prosthesis articulates with soft tissue or with a radial head component

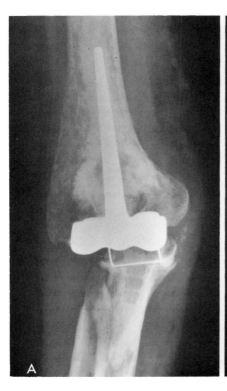
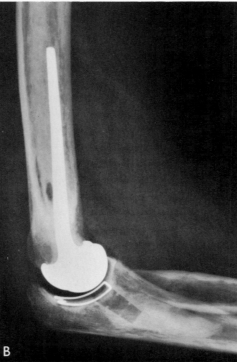

**FIGURE 19–52.** Unconstrained capitellocondylar prosthesis. The capitellar portion of the prosthesis articulates with the soft tissues in this case. Both components are cemented. (From Weissman BN: In CB Sledge, et al (Eds): Arthritis Surgery. Philadelphia, WB Saunders Co, 1994.)

composed of silicone rubber. Cement should extend past the tips of the humeral and ulnar stems. Briggs and Smith[287] described a set of two anteroposterior radiographs that may be used to determine the axial rotation of the prosthetic components. As with other joints, careful assessment of the cement-bone interface should be done at the time of each follow-up study. A standardized form for following components is available.[286]

Ewald and coworkers[288] found improvement in pain, functional status, and range of motion (with the exception of extension) in patients who underwent capitellocondylar elbow replacement. Similarly, Morrey and Adams[289] reported pain relief in 91 per cent of patients after insertion of semiconstrained modified Conrad prostheses.

Complications of total elbow replacement include prosthetic loosening or dislocation, infection, and fracture (Fig. 19–53). The nonconstrained prostheses may dislocate, as was found in 6 per cent of capitellocondylar prostheses reviewed by Ruth and Wilde[286] and in 3.5 per cent of such prostheses studied by Ewald and colleagues.[288] Lateral translation of the components may be seen on radiographs but is not considered a clinical problem.[288] Prosthetic loosening is thought to be less frequent in nonconstrained prostheses than in constrained designs, but revision was necessary in 1.5 per cent of cases in the series of 202 nonconstrained prostheses studied by Ewald and colleagues.[288] Infection rates are relatively high (1.5 to 8 per cent).[286, 288, 292]

## TOTAL ANKLE REPLACEMENT[293–304]

Total ankle replacement is used to provide a painless, stable, and functional ankle joint capable of allowing the patient to perform normal activities of daily living.[293] The operation is reserved most often for patients with rheumatoid arthritis who have polyarticular involvement[295, 296, 301] (Fig. 19–54). Older or debilitated patients with posttraumatic arthritis also may be candidates for the procedure,[297]

but in younger, more active patients, ankle fusion usually is the procedure of choice. Unfortunately, the success of this procedure has not been as great as that of total hip replacement. Long-term follow-up has shown high rates of loosening (e.g., 90 per cent at 10 years for a constrained prosthesis[303]) and limited pain relief, leading Jensen and Kroner[304] to conclude that the overall results of ankle joint replacement are so poor that it should be indicated in only a few carefully selected cases.

Prostheses may be constrained (allowing primarily flexion and extension—e.g., Oregon, Mayo, Buchholz, TPR prostheses); unconstrained, allowing motion in multiple planes (e.g., Waugh, Smith prostheses); or semiconstrained, permitting flexion and extension and some multiaxial rotation.[298] The components are placed with the tibial component perpendicular to the long axis of the tibia and with the talar component parallel both to the long axis of the talus and to the plane of the resected surface of the tibia with the foot in neutral position.[298] Complications of total ankle replacement are primarily loosening and infection.[297]

### Radiographic Findings

Radiographic assessment includes evaluation of the following features[294] (Fig. 19–55).

#### Center of Rotation

The curve of the superior surface of the talus is identified on the lateral view, and the center of rotation is determined using a template of concentric circles. The preoperative and postoperative centers of rotation then can be compared.

#### Migration of Components

Migration of the talar component was noted in 14 of 15 cases studied by Unger and coworkers.[294] Measurements for anteroposterior displacement of the talus are calculated as the perpendicular distance from the center of rotation to the tibial midshaft axis. Inferior migration of the talar compo-

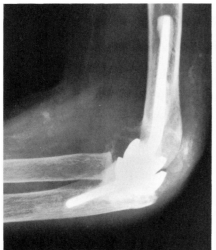
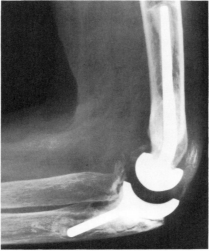
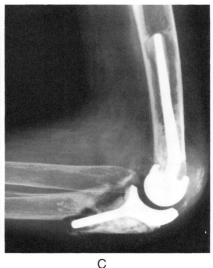

|   A   |   B   |   C   |

**FIGURE 19–53.** Loose capitellocondylar prosthesis with fracture.
 **A** A metal-backed capitellocondylar prosthesis has been inserted.
 **B** Follow-up examination 1.5 years later shows widening of the cement-bone interface of the ulnar component, indicating loosening.
 **C** Follow-up examination almost three years after **A** shows a fracture through the area of loosening. Revision with a more constrained prosthesis was performed.

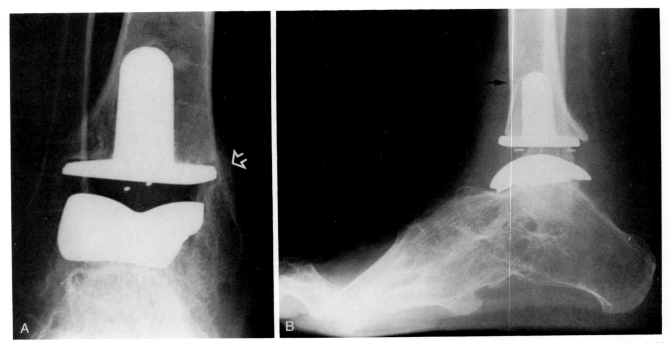

**FIGURE 19–54.** Total ankle replacement. Anteroposterior **(A)** and lateral **(B)** views of the ankle in a patient with severe rheumatoid arthritis and extensive hindfoot and midfoot fusion show a bone ingrowth total ankle replacement. The disruption in the anterior tibial cortex (solid arrow) is a surgical defect. Periosteal reaction is present at the site of a medial malleolar fracture (open arrow).

nent (subsidence) is measured by noting changes in the perpendicular distance from the center of rotation to the calcaneal baseline. The angulation of the talar component is measured as the angle between the talar component and a perpendicular from the calcaneal baseline.

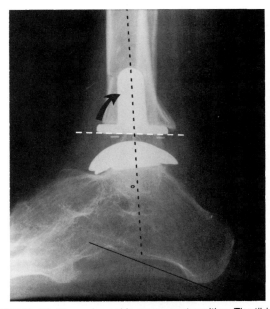

**FIGURE 19–55.** Measuring ankle component position. The tibial axis (blacked dashed line), tibial component axis (white dashed line), and angle between them (arrow) are indicated. The calcaneal baseline (solid line) and approximate center of rotation of the prosthesis (circle) are indicated. These reference points are used for documenting changes in component position. (After Unger AS, et al: Foot Ankle *8*:173, 1988. Copyright American Orthopaedic Society, Inc.)

Tibial migration in the anteroposterior direction may be measured as the change in distance from the anterior and posterior margins of the tibial component to the respective edges of the tibia on the lateral projection. Changes in angulation of the tibial component are measured with relation to a perpendicular to the midtibial axis line on anteroposterior views. Settling of the tibia in relation to the tibial component (vertical subluxation of the prosthesis) may occur, although quantification of this finding has proved difficult.

### Radiolucent Areas

Radiolucent areas are most common along the tibial component. In one series, at the time of follow-up examinations that averaged 5.6 years after surgery, cement-bone lucent regions were present about 14 of 15 tibial components, and tibial component tilting occurred in 12 of these cases.[294]

### Motion of Components on Stress Views

Component loosening may be documented at fluoroscopy or on stress views by changes in component position with relation to the adjacent bone. Such changes were seen in four of 18 arthroplasties that were followed for an average of only 36 months[299] and in 10 per cent of total ankle replacement that were followed for an average of only 14.7 months.[301]

### Miscellaneous Findings

Other abnormalities include intraoperative fracture of the medial or lateral malleolus (not to be confused with the anterior tibial defect that may be produced during surgical exposure using an anterior approach), impingement of the lateral malleolus on the talus, and recurrence of deformity.[300]

## SILICONE RUBBER PROSTHESES[305–329]

Silicone rubber elastomer prostheses have been used for replacement of the metacarpophalangeal and interphalangeal joints,[309, 322, 323] the radiocarpal articulation,[307, 308, 320] the carpal bones (especially the scaphoid, lunate, and trapezium),[319, 326, 327] the ulnar styloid, the radial head, the disc of the temporomandibular joint, and the first metatarsophalangeal joint[328] (Figs. 19–56 to 19–58).

### Radiographic Findings

Silicone rubber prostheses are only slightly denser than soft tissue on radiographs, making the components difficult to identify. The Swanson metacarpophalangeal joint prosthesis allows joint motion to occur, because of both the hinge action of the central portion of the prosthesis and the pistoning of the prosthetic stems within the bone. At the metacarpophalangeal joints, the rectangular central hinge portion of the prosthesis should be parallel to the resection margins of the metacarpal bones in posteroanterior radiographs.[5] The anterior concavity of the hinge portion of the prosthesis can be seen on the lateral view. A thin sclerotic rim usually develops along the intramedullary stems of the prosthesis, making it more apparent.

### Complications

Results of long-term follow-up have emphasized the complications associated with these prostheses, particularly fracture and silicone-induced synovitis. Other complications include infection (about 1 per cent), implant dislocation (less than 1 per cent), and recurrent deformity. Infec-

tion is suggested on radiographs by the development of osteoporosis, bone destruction, periosteal reaction, and soft tissue swelling. Because these prostheses function largely as spacers, a joint capsule develops around them that may provide stability, even when prosthetic fractures occur.

### Fractures of Prostheses

Fractures of silicone rubber prostheses are quite frequent in some locations. More than half of wrist prostheses in one series were fractured.[307] Twenty-six per cent of Swanson metacarpophalangeal joint prostheses were noted to be fractured in another series.[322] Fracture of metacarpophalangeal joint components is suggested if recurrence of joint deformity, shortening of the digit, change in the position of the digit, or disruption of the component occurs.[313]

### Silicone Synovitis

Silicone synovitis represents the response to the shedding of silicone particles from prostheses that are damaged by shear and compressive forces.[312] The complication appears more frequent after carpal prostheses than after metacarpophalangeal, proximal interphalangeal, and radiocarpal joint replacements,[312] perhaps, in part, owing to the lower compressive forces that occur in the joints of the fingers. Carter and associates[321] found radiographic evidence of silicone synovitis in 75 per cent of scaphoid implants, 55 per cent of lunate implants, and 75 per cent of scapholunate implants. A study of Swanson wrist prostheses by Fatti and coworkers[308] showed that whereas no cases of silicone synovitis were seen in the first review of patients followed more than 2.5 years, reexamination at an average of 5.6 years after surgery showed presumed silicone synovitis in 10 of 35 wrists. Jolly and associates[307] noted a 30 per cent

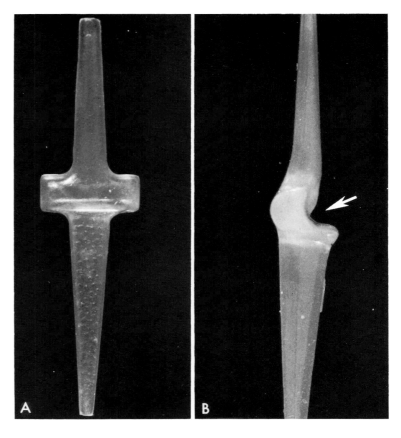

**FIGURE 19–56.** Swanson metacarpophalangeal joint prosthesis. **A** Dorsal aspect. **B** Lateral aspect. The metacarpal stem is longer. A concavity on the volar aspect allows flexion (arrow).

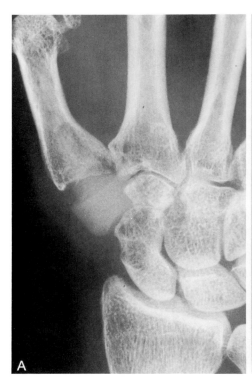

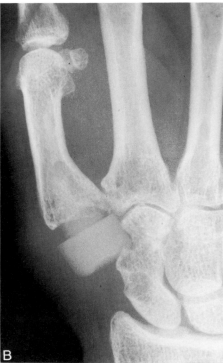

**FIGURE 19–57.** Subluxation of a trapezium prosthesis.

**A** Initial postoperative radiograph after removal of the trapezium and its replacement with a silicone spacer implanted into the base of the first metacarpal bone.

**B** Follow-up radiograph 4 months later shows subluxation of the prosthesis relative to the scaphoid.

**FIGURE 19–58.** Fracture of silicone rubber prosthesis: Silicone metacarpophalangeal joint implants. A fracture of the second metacarpophalangeal joint prosthesis is manifested by subluxation (arrow). A fracture of the third metacarpophalangeal joint prosthesis shows narrowing of the joint space with extrusion of silicone fragments (arrowheads). The remaining implants appear intact.

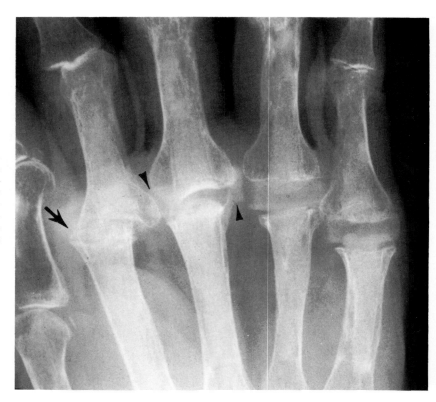

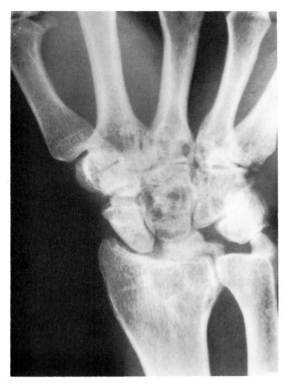

**FIGURE 19–59.** Silicone synovitis. A lunate prosthesis is in place but is thinned. Well-defined lucent lesions are present in the carpal bones and the distal end of the radius owing to the giant cell reaction to silicone particles. The cartilage spaces are mildly narrow. The bone density is preserved. (From Weissman BN: Radiol Clin North Am 28:1111, 1990.)

prevalence of silicone synovitis in patients followed at least 44 months. Clinically, painful synovitis occurs months or years after an otherwise uneventful course. Some patients remain asymptomatic despite typical radiographic changes of the condition. It is postulated that fibrillation of the prosthesis occurs, leading to shedding of silicone elastomer particles that become embedded in the synovium with resulting synovial hypertrophy, chronic inflammatory and giant cell infiltration of the synovial membrane, invasion of adjacent bones, and eventual collapse or fracture.[318] Pathologic examination reveals intracellular and extracellular silicone particles that are refractile under polarized light,[312] are not birefringent, and range in size from 6 to 100 μm in diameter.[324] Transport of these particles to regional lymph nodes may produce nodal enlargement that may be striking enough to suggest malignancy.[310, 311, 315, 329] Silicone particles also have been found in bone marrow sites that are remote from the implant.[324]

The radiographic appearance of silicone synovitis is typical (Fig. 19–59). Deformity or fracture of the prosthesis may be visible but is not always apparent. Well-defined subchondral lucent defects and erosions (often with thin sclerotic margins),[316, 317] preservation of the cartilage spaces, and soft tissue swelling are typical features.[314, 317] Osteoporosis is not a prominent finding, usually allowing differentiation of this condition from infection. Left untreated, the lesions tend to enlarge. Radiographic diagnosis usually is not difficult, but differential diagnostic possibilities include pigmented villonodular synovitis, amyloidosis, and tuberculous or fungal infection. MR imaging theoretically may play a role in the diagnosis of this condition; these prostheses and their particles are low in signal intensity on T1-weighted and T2-weighted images (Fig. 19–60).

## SUMMARY

As advances and improvements are made in joint replacement technology and surgical technique, imaging remains an important means of monitoring the patient's postoperative progress and identifying complications. Radiographs provide a permanent record of the procedure and can document success or failure of the operation. This chapter presents the information required for accurate interpretation of radiographs after various fixation devices and cement materials have been used. It also reviews expected findings, both normal and abnormal, of total hip replace-

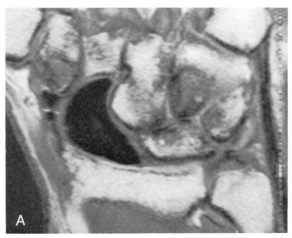
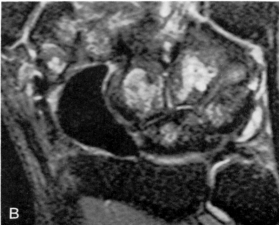

**FIGURE 19–60.** Silicone synovitis. A silastic implant was used to replace a fractured scaphoid bone.
**A** A coronal T1-weighted (TRITE, 733/20) spin echo MR image shows the signal void of the scaphoid implant. Note regions of low signal intensity in multiple carpal bones, corresponding to fluid within cystic lesions. The lunate-capitate joint space is narrowed.
**B** A coronal short tau inversion recovery (STIR) MR image (TRITE, 2000/30; inversion time, 140 msec) reveals the implant of low signal intensity and carpal cysts and joint fluid of high signal intensity. Small particles of silastic are evident in the radial aspect of the wrist.
(**A, B,** Courtesy of S. Eilenberg, M.D., San Diego, California.)

ment as well as replacements of the knee, shoulder, elbow, and ankle. Complications of each operation are discussed, as are the relative sensitivity and specificity of various imaging methods.

Some of the information presented in this chapter has been presented in Weissman BN: Radiographic evaluation of total joint replacement. In: Textbook of Rheumatology, Kelley WN, Harris ED, Ruddy S, Sledge CB (eds.), 4th Edition, Volume 2, 1993, pp. 1881–1934 and Weissman BN: Current topics in the radiology of joint replacement surgery. Radiol Clin North Am *18*:1111, 1990.

The author recognizes with gratitude the illustrations contributed by Dr. Thomas G. Goergen and the Musculoskeletal Radiology Group of the Brigham and Women's Hospital (Drs. Piran Aliabadi, Nancy D. Baker, J. Leland Sosman, and Carl S. Winalski) and the secretarial help of Mrs. Roberta Otis. Sincere thanks to Dr. John Wright of the Department of Orthopedics for reviewing this manuscript.

## References

1. Charnley J: Arthroplasty of the hip. A new operation. Lancet *1*:1129, 1961.
2. Mulroy RD Jr, Sedlacek RC, O'Connor DO, et al: Technique to detect migration of femoral components of total hip replacements on conventional radiographs. J Arthroplasty 6(Suppl)¹–S4, 1991.
3. Baldursson H, Hansson LI, Olsson TH, et al: Maturation of acetabuler socket after bone hip replacement determined with roentgen stereophotogrammetry. Acta Orthop Scand *51*:535, 1980.
4. Weissman BN: Current topics in the radiology of joint replacement surgery. Radiol Clin North Am 28:1111, 1990.
5. Weissman BN: Radiographic evaluation of total joint replacement. *In* WN Kelley, et al: (Eds): Textbook of Rheumatology. (4th Ed.) Philadelphia, WB Saunders Co, 1993, p 1881.
6. Herrlin K, Selvik G, Pettersson H: Space orientation of total hip prosthesis. A method for three-dimensional determination. Acta Radiol Diagn 27:618, 1986.
7. Herrlin K: Radiology of the total hip prosthesis. Prosthetic position, orientation, design, component interaction and dislocation. University Hospital Lund, Sweden (Thesis) 1988.
8. Massin P, Schmidt L, Engh CA: Evaluation of cementless acetabular component migration. An experimental study. J Arthroplasty 4:245, 1989.
9. Ranawat CS, Dorr LD, Inglis AE: Total hip arthroplasty in protrusio acetabuli of rheumatoid arthritis. J Bone Joint Surg [Am] 62:1059, 1980.
10. McLaren RH: Prosthetic hip angulation. Radiology 107:705, 1973.
11. Fackler CD, Poss R: Dislocation in total hip arthroplasties. Clin Orthop 151:169, 1980.
12. Ghelman B: Radiographic localization of the acetabular component of a hip prosthesis. Radiology 130:540, 1979.
13. Mian SW, Truchly G, Pflum FA: Computed tomography measurement of acetabular cup anteversion and retroversion in total hip arthroplasty. Clin Orthop 276:206, 1992.
14. Szivek JA: Bioceramic coatings for artificial joint fixation. Invest Radiol 27:553, 1992.
15. Mehloff MA, Sledge CB: Comparison of cemented and cementless hip and knee replacements. Arthritis Rheum 33:293, 1990.
16. Halley DK, Charnley J: Results of low friction arthroplasty in patients 30 years of age or younger. Clin Orthop 112:180, 1975.
17. Callaghan JJ: Results of primary total hip arthroplasty in young patients. J Bone Joint Surg [Am] 75:1728, 1993.
18. Harris WH, McGann WA: Loosening of the femoral component after use of the medullary-plug cementing technique. Follow-up note with a minimum five-year follow-up. J Bone Joint Surg [Am] 6:1064, 1986.
19. Maloney WJ, Harris WH: Comparison of a hybrid with an uncemented total hip replacement. J Bone Joint Surg [Am] 72:1349, 1990.
20. Wixson RL, Stulberg SD, Mehlhoff M: Total hip replacement with cemented, uncemented, and hybrid prostheses. J Bone Joint Surg [Am] 73:257, 1991.
21. Freitag TA, Cannon SL: Fracture characteristics of acrylic bone cements. I. Fracture toughness. J Biomed Mater Res 10:805, 1976.
22. Jasty M, Malone WH, Bragdon CR, et al: Histomorphological studies of the long-term skeletal responses to well fixed cemented femoral components. J Bone Joint Surg [Am] 72:1220, 1990.
23. Willert H-G, Ludwig J, Semlitsch M: Reaction of bone to methacrylate after hip arthroplasty. A long-term gross, light microscopic, and scanning electron microscopic study. J Bone Joint Surg [Am] 56:1368, 1974.
24. Beckenbaugh RD, Ilstrup DM: Total hip arthroplasty. A review of 333 cases with long follow-up. J Bone Joint Surg [Am] 60:306, 1978.
25. Kwong LM, Jasty M, Mulroy RD: The histology of the radiolucent line. J Bone Joint Surg [Br] 74:67, 1992.
26. DeLee JG, Charnley J: Radiological demarcation of cemented sockets in total hip replacement. Clin Orthop 121:20, 1976.
27. Gruen MS, McNeice GM, Amstutz HC: "Modes of failure" of cemented stem-type femoral components. Clin Orthop 141:17, 1979.
28. Johnston RC, Fitzgerald RH, Harris WH, et al: Clinical and radiographic evaluation of total hip replacement. J Bone Joint Surg [Am] 72:161, 1990.
29. Cone RO, Yaru N, Resnick D, et al: Intracapsular pressure monitoring during arthrographic evaluation of painful hip prostheses. AJR 141:885, 1983.
30. Kim KS, Lachman R: In vitro effects of iodinated contrast media on the growth of staphylococci. Invest Radiol 17:305, 1982.
31. Melson GL, McDaniel RC, Southern PM, et al: *In vitro* effects of iodinated arthrographic contrast media on bacterial growth. Radiology 112:593, 1974.
32. Harris WH, Barrack RL: Developments in diagnosis of the painful total hip replacement. Orthop Rev 22:439, 1993.
33. Harris WH, Barrack RL: Contemporary algorithms for evaluation of the painful total hip replacement. Orthop Rev 22:531, 1993.
34. Barrack RL, Harris WH: The value of aspiration of the hip joint before revision total hip arthroplasty. J Bone Joint Surg [Am] 75:66, 1993.
35. Maus TP, Berquist TH, Bender CE, et al: Arthrographic study of painful total hip arthroplasty: Refined criteria. Radiology 162:721, 1987.
36. Hendrix RW, Wixson RL, Rana NA, et al: Arthrography after total hip arthroplasty: A modified technique used in the diagnosis of pain. Radiology 148:647, 1983.
37. Swan JS, Braunstein EM, Capello W: Aspiration of the hip in patients treated with Girdlestone arthroplasty. AJR 156:545, 1991.
38. Gelman MI: Arthrography in total hip prosthesis complications. AJR 126:743, 1976.
39. Berquist TH, Bender CE, Maus TP, et al: Pseudobursae: A useful finding in patients with painful hip arthroplasty. AJR 148:103, 1987.
40. Matsumoto K, Hukuda S, Nishioka J, et al: Iliopsoas bursal distention caused by acetabular loosening after total hip arthroplasty. Clin Orthop 279:144, 1992.
41. Steinbach LS, Schneider R, Goldman AB, et al: Bursae and abscess cavities communicating with the hip. Radiology 156:303, 1985.
42. Fritz P, Mariette X, Clerc D, et al: Rectus femoris sheath: A new localization of hip synovial cyst. J Rheumatol 16:1575, 1989.
43. Utz JA, Lull RJ, Galvin EG: Asymptomatic total hip prosthesis: Natural history determined using Tc-99m MDP bone scans. Radiology 161:509, 1986.
44. Brand RA, Pedersen DR, Yoder SA: How definition of "loosening" affects the incidence of loose total hip reconstructions. Clin Orthop 210:185, 1986.
45. Mjöberg B, Brismar J, Hansson LI, et al: Definition of endoprosthetic loosening. Comparison of arthrography, scintigraphy and roentgen stereophotogrammetry in prosthetic hips. Acta Orthop Scand 56:469, 1985.
46. Harris WH, Penenberg BL: Further follow-up on socket fixation using a metal-backed acetabular component for total hip replacement: A minimum ten-year follow-up study. J Bone Joint Surg [Am] 69:1140, 1987.
47. Garcia-Cimbrelo E, Munuera L: Early and late loosening of the acetabular cup after low-friction arthroplasty. J Bone Joint Surg [Am] 74:1119, 1992.
48. Cain TM, Fon GT, Brumby S, et al: Plain film and arthrographic findings in painful total hip arthroplasties with surgical correlation. Australas Radiol 34:211, 1990.
49. Gelman ME, Coleman RE, Stevens PM, et al: Radiography, radionuclide imaging, and arthrography in the evaluation of total hip and knee replacement. Radiology 128:677, 1978.
50. Tehranzadeh J, Gubernick I, Blaha D: Prospective study of sequential technetium-99m phosphate and gallium imaging in painful hip prostheses (comparison of diagnostic modalities). Clin Nucl Med 13:229, 1988.
51. O'Neill DA, Harris WH: Failed total hip replacement: Assessment by plain radiographs, arthrograms, and aspiration of the hip joint. J Bone Joint Surg [Am] 66:540, 1984.
52. Lieberman JR, Huo MH, Schneider R, et al: Evaluation of painful hip arthroplasties. J Bone Joint Surg [Br] 75:475, 1993.
53. Goldring SR, Schiller AL, Roelke M, et al: The synovial-like membrane at the bone-cement interface in loose total hip replacements and its proposed role in bone lysis. J Bone Joint Surg [Am] 65:575, 1983.
54. Goldring, Jasty MJ, Roelke MS, et al: Formation of a synovial-like membrane at the bone-cement interface. Arthritis Rheum 29:836, 1986.
55. Spector M, Shortkroff S, Hsu H-P, et al: Tissue changes around loose prostheses. A canine model to investigate the effects of an antiinflammatory. Clin Orthop 261:140, 1990.
56. Johanson NA, Bullough PG, Wilson PD, et al: The microscopic anatomy of the bone-cement interface in failed total hip arthroplasties. Clin Orthop 218:123, 1987.
57. Lennox DW, Schofield BH, McDonald DF, et al: A histologic comparison of aseptic loosening of cemented, press-fit and biologic ingrowth prostheses. Clin Orthop 225:171, 1987.
58. Ohlin A, Johnell O, Lerner UH: The pathogenesis of loosening of total hip arthroplasties. Clin Orthop 253:287, 1990.
59. Horowitz SM, Doty SB, Lane JM, et al: Studies of the mechanism by which the mechanical failure of polymethylmethacrylate leads to bone resorption. J Bone Joint Surg [Am] 75:802, 1993.
60. Jiranek WA, Machado M, Jasty M, et al: Production of cytokines around loosened cemented acetabular components. J Bone Joint Surg [Am] 75:863, 1993.
61. Santavirta S, Sorsa T, Konttinen YT, et al: Role of mesenchymal collagenase in the loosening of total hip prosthesis. Clin Orthop 290:206, 1993.

62. DeSmet AA, Kramer D, Martel W: The metal-cement interface in total hip prostheses. AJR *129*:279, 1977.

63. Weber FA, Charnley J: A radiological study of fractures of acrylic cement in relation to the stem of a femoral head prosthesis. J Bone Joint Surg [Br] *57*:297, 1975.

64. Yoder SA, Brand RA, Pendersen DR, et al: Total hip acetabular component position affects component loosening rates. Clin Orthop *220*:79, 1988.

65. Salvati EA, Freiberger RH, Wilson PD: Arthrography for complications of total hip replacement: A review of thirty-one arthrograms. J Bone Joint Surg [Am] *53*:701, 1971.

66. Murray WR, Rodrigo JJ: Arthrography for the assessment of pain after total hip replacement. J Bone Joint Surg [Am] *57*:1060, 1975.

67. Maxon HR, Schneider HJ, Hopson CN, et al: A comparative study of indium-111 DTPA radionuclide and iothalamate meglumine roentgenographic arthrography in the evaluation of painful total hip arthroplasty. Clin Orthop *245*:156, 1989.

68. Phillips WC, Kattapuram SV: Prosthetic hip replacements: Plain films and arthrography for component loosening. AJR *138*:677, 1982.

69. Brown CS, Knickerbocker WJ: Radiologic studies in the investigation of the causes of total hip replacement failure. J Can Assoc Radiol *24*:245, 1973.

70. Dussault RG, Goldman AB, Ghelman B: Radiologic diagnosis of loosening and infection in hip prostheses. J Can Assoc Radiol *28*:119, 1977.

71. Anderson LS, Staple TW: Arthrography of total hip replacement using subtraction technique. Radiology *109*:470, 1973.

72. Firooznia H, Baruch H, Seliger G, et al: The value of subtraction in hip arthrography after total hip replacement. Bull Hosp Joint Dis *35*:36, 1974.

73. Drinker H, Turner RH, Mckenzie JD, et al: Color subtraction arthrography in the diagnosis of component loosening in hip arthroplasty. Orthopedics *1*:224, 1978.

74. Bassett LW, Loftus AA, Mankovich NJ: Computer-processed subtraction arthrography. Radiology *157*:821, 1985.

75. Salvati EA, Ghelman B, McLaren T, et al: Subtraction technique in arthrography for loosening of total hip replacement fixed with radiopaque cement. Clin Orthop *101*:105, 1974.

76. Kelcz F, Peppler WW, Mistretta CA, et al: K-edge digital subtraction arthrography of the painful hip prosthesis: A feasibility study. AJR *155*:1053, 1990.

77. van der Lande BAE, van Helmond EPM, Scholten ET, et al: Digital subtraction arthrography of hip joint prostheses. Diagn Imaging *55*:228, 1986.

78. Walker CW, FitzRandolph RL, Collins DN, et al: Arthrography of painful hips following arthroplasty: Digital versus plain film subtraction. Skel Radiol *20*:403, 1991.

79. Resnick D, Kerr R, André M, et al: Digital arthrography in the evaluation of painful joint prostheses. Invest Radiol *19*:432, 1984.

80. Hardy DC, Reinus WR, Totty WG: Arthrography after total hip arthroplasty: Utility of postambulation radiographs. Skel Radiol *17*:20, 1988.

81. Coren GS, Curtis J, Dalinka M: Lymphatic visualization during hip arthrography. Radiology *115*:621, 1975.

82. Bloom RA, Gheorghiu D, Krausz Y: Lymphatic opacification in the prosthetic hip. Skel Radiol *20*:43, 1991.

83. Daum WJ: Use of local anesthetic with the hip arthrogram as a diagnostic aid. Orthop Rev *27*:123, 1988.

84. Guercio N, Orsini G, Broggi S, et al: Arthrography of the prosthesetized painful hip: The importance of imaging and functional testing. Ital J Orthop Traumatol *16*:93, 1990.

85. Burton DS, Propst-Proctor SL, Schurman DJ: Anesthetic hip arthrography in the diagnosis of postoperative hip pathology. Contemp Orthop *7*:17, 1988.

86. Wellman HN, Schauwecker DS, Capello WN: Evaluation of metallic osseous implants with nuclear medicine. Semin Nucl Med *28*:126, 1988.

87. Jain CU, Yang DC, Patel DM, et al: Cutaneous fistula communicating with the hip in a patient with a painful total hip prosthesis demonstrated by radionuclide arthrography. Clin Nucl Med *11*:820, 1988.

88. Abdel-Dayem HM, Bardowala YM, Papademitrio T, et al: Loose hip prosthesis appearance in radionuclide arthrography. Clin Nucl Med *11*:713, 1986.

89. Evans BG, Cuckler JM: Evaluation of the painful total hip arthroplasty. Orthop Clin North Am *22*:303, 1992.

90. Levitsky KA, Hozack WJ, Balderston RA, et al: Evaluation of the painful prosthetic joint. J Arthroplasty *6*:237, 1991.

91. Bergstrom B, Lidgren L, Lindberg L: Radiographic abnormalities caused by postoperative infection following total hip replacement. Clin Orthop *99*:95, 1974.

92. Dupont JA: Significance of operative cultures in total hip arthroplasty. Clin Orthop *211*:122, 1986.

93. Tigges S, Stiles RG, Meli RJ, et al: Hip aspiration: A cost-effective and accurate method of evaluating the potentially infected hip prosthesis. Radiology *189*:485, 1993.

94. Gould ES, Potter HG, Bober SE: Role of routine percutaneous hip aspirations prior to prosthesis revision. Skel Radiol *19*:427, 1990.

95. Foldes K, Gaal M, Balint P, et al: Ultrasonography after hip arthroplasty. Skel Radiol *21*:297, 1992.

96. Graif M, Schwartz E, Strauss S, et al: Occult infection of hip prosthesis: Sonographic evaluation. J Am Geriatr Soc *39*:203, 1991.

97. Rosenthall L: Radionuclide investigation of osteomyelitis. Curr Opin Radiol *4*:62, 1992.

98. Kirchner PT, Simon MA: Radioisotopic evaluation of skeletal disease. J Bone Joint Surg [Am] *63*:673, 1981.

99. Horoszowski H, Ganel A, Kamhin M, et al: Sequential use of technetium 99m MDP and gallium 67 citrate imaging in the evaluation of painful total hip replacement. Br J Radiol *53*:1169, 1980.

100. Williams F, McCall IW, Park WM, et al: Gallium-67 scanning in the painful total hip replacement. Clin Radiol *32*:431, 1981.

101. Rosenthall L, Lisbona R, Hernandez M, et al: $^{99m}$Tc-PP and $^{67}$Ga imaging following insertion of orthopedic devices. Radiology *133*:717, 1979.

102. Alazraki NP: Diagnosing prosthetic joint infection. J Nucl Med *31*:1955, 1990.

103. Williamson BRJ, McLaughlin RE, Wang G-J, et al: Radionuclide bone imaging as a means of differentiating loosening and infection in patients with painful total hip prosthesis. Radiology *133*:723, 1979.

104. Mountford PJ, Coakley AJ: Role of technetium-99m phosphonate bone and indium-111 leukocyte scanning for detecting the infected hip prosthesis. J Nucl Med *30*:562, 1989.

105. Weiss PE, Mall JC, Hoffer PB, et al: $^{99m}$Tc-methylene diphosphonate bone imaging in the evaluation of total hip prostheses. Radiology *133*:727, 1979.

106. Aliabadi P, Tumeh SS, Weissman BN, et al: Cemented total hip prosthesis: Radiographic and scintigraphic evaluation. Radiology *173*:203, 1989.

107. Chafetz N, Hattner RS, Ruarke WC, et al: Multinuclide digital subtraction imaging in symptomatic prosthetic joints. AJR *144*:1255, 1985.

108. Reing CM, Richin PF, Kenmore PI: Differential bone-scanning in the evaluation of a painful total joint replacement. J Bone Joint Surg [Am] *61*:933, 1979.

109. Zilkens KW, Wicke A, Zilkens J, et al: Nuclear imaging in loosening of hip-joint endoprostheses. Arch Orthop Trauma Surg *107*:288, 1988.

110. Traughber PD, Manaster BJ, Murphy K, et al: Negative bone scans of joints after aspiration or arthrography: Experimental studies. AJR *146*:87, 1986.

111. Cuckler JM, Stark AM, Alavi A, et al: Diagnosis and management of the infected total joint arthroplasty. Orthop Clin North Am *22*:523, 1991.

112. Magnuson JE, Brown ML, Hauser MF, et al: In-111-labeled leukocyte scintigraphy in suspected orthopedic prosthesis infection: Comparison with other imaging modalities. Radiology *168*:235, 1988.

113. Mountford PJ, Hall FM, Wells CP, et al: $^{99}$Tc$^m$-MDP, $^{67}$Ga-citrate and $^{111}$In-leukocytes for detecting prosthetic hip infection. Nucl Med Commun *7*:113, 1986.

114. Gómez-Luzuriaga MA, Galán V, Villar JM: Scintigraphy with Tc, Ga and In in painful total hip prostheses. Int Orthop (SICOT) *12*:163, 1988.

115. Roddie ME, Peters AM, Osman S, et al: Osteomyelitis. Nucl Med Commun *9*:713, 1988.

116. Streule K, De Schrijver M, Fridrich R: $^{99}$Tc$^m$-labelled HSA-nanocolloid versus $^{111}$In oxine-labelled granulocytes in detecting skeletal septic process. Nucl Med Commun *9*:59, 1988.

117. McAfee JG, Samin A: In-111 labeled leukocytes: A review of problems in image interpretation. Radiology *155*:221, 1985.

118. Seabold JE, Nepola JV, Marsh JL, et al: Postoperative bone marrow alterations: Potential pitfalls in the diagnosis of osteomyelitis with In-111-labeled leukocyte scintigraphy. Radiology *180*:741, 1991.

119. Merkel KD, Brown LM, Dewanjee MK, et al: Comparison of indium-labeled-leukocyte imaging with sequential technetium-gallium scanning in the diagnosis of low-grade musculoskeletal sepsis. J Bone Joint Surg [Am] *67*:465, 1985.

120. Palestro CJ, Kim CK, Swyer AJ, et al: Total-hip arthroplasty: Periprosthetic indium-111-labeled leukocyte activity and complementary technetium-99m-sulfur colloid imaging in suspected infection. J Nucl Med *31*:1950, 1990.

121. Sciuk J, Puskas C, Greitemann B, et al: White blood cell scintigraphy with monoclonal antibodies in the study of the infected endoprosthesis. Eur J Nucl Med *19*:497, 1992.

122. Oyen WG, van Horn JR, Claessens RAMJ, et al: Diagnosing prosthetic joint infection. J Nucl Med *32*:2195, 1991.

123. Johnson JA, Christie MJ, Sandler MP, et al: Detection of occult infection following total joint arthroplasty using sequential technetium-99m HDP bone scintigraphy and indium-111 WBC imaging. J Nucl Med *29*:1347, 1988.

124. Wukich DK, Abreu SH, Callaghan JJ, et al: Diagnosis of infection by preoperative scintigraphy with indium-labeled white blood cells. J Bone Joint Surg [Am] *69*:1353, 1987.

125. Glithero PR, Grigori P, Harding LK, et al: White cell scans and infected joint replacements. J Bone Joint Surg [Br] *75*:371, 1993.

126. Reuland P, Winker KH, Heuchert T, et al: Detection of infection in postoperative orthopedic patients with technetium-99m-labeled monoclonal antibodies against granulocytes. J Nucl Med *32*:2209, 1991.

127. Oyen WG, van Horn JR, Claessens RAMJ, et al: Diagnosis of bone, joint, and joint prosthesis infections with In-111-labeled nonspecific human immunoglobulin G scintigraphy. Radiology *182*:195, 1992.

128. Harris WH, Schiller AL, Scholler JM, et al: Extensive localized bone resorption in the femur following total hip replacement. J Bone Joint Surg [Am] *58*:612, 1976.

129. Santavirta S, Konttinen YT, Bergroth C, et al: Aggressive granulomatous lesions associated with hip arthroplasty. J Bone Joint Surg *72*:252, 1990.

130. Jones LC, Hungerford DS: Cement disease. Clin Orthop *225*:192, 1987.

131. Maguire JK, Coscia MF, Lynch MH: Foreign body reaction to polymeric debris following total hip arthroplasty. Clin Orthop *216*:213, 1987.

132. Schmalzried TP, Jasty M, Harris WH: Periprosthetic bone loss in total hip arthroplasty. J Bone Joint Surg [Am] *74*:849, 1992.

133. Hodge WA, Collier JP, Supernant BA, et al: Failure of a well-fixed bone-ingrown titanium hip prosthesis. Orthop Rev *22*:719, 1993.

134. Maloney WJ, Peters P, Engh CA, et al: Severe osteolysis of the pelvis in association with acetabular replacement without cement. J Bone Joint Surg [Am] *75*:1627, 1993.

135. Tanzer M, Maloney WJ, Jasty M, et al: The progression of femoral cortical

osteolysis in association with total hip arthroplasty without cement. J Bone Joint Surg [Am] 74:404, 1992.

136. Borssén B, Kärrholm J, Snorrason F: Osteolysis after ceramic-on-ceramic hip arthroplasty. Acta Orthop Scand 62:73, 1991.

137. Boynton E, Waddel JP, Morton J, et al: Aseptic loosening in total hip implants: The role of polyethylene wear debris. Can J Surg 34:599, 1991.

138. Howie DW, Vernon-Roberts B, Oakeshott R, et al: A rat model of resorption of bone at the cement-bone interface in the presence of polyethylene wear particles. J Bone Joint Surg [Am] 70:257, 1988.

139. Bobyn JD: Polyethylene wear debris. Quill on scalpel (Editorial). Can J Surg 34:530, 1991.

140. Franzé H, Mjöberg B: Wear and loosening of the hip prosthesis. Acta Orthop Scand 61:499, 1990.

141. Gray MH, Talbert ML, Talbert WM, et al: Changes seen in lymph nodes draining the sites of large joint prostheses. Am J Surg Pathol 13:1050, 1989.

142. Scott WW, Riley LH, Dorfman HD: Focal lytic lesions associated with femoral stem loosening in total hip prosthesis. AJR 144:977, 1985.

143. Chew FS, Lev MH: Polyethylene osteolysis. AJR 159:1254, 1992.

144. Reinus WR, Gilula LA, Kyriakos M, et al: Histiocytic reaction to hip arthroplasty. Radiology 155:315, 1985.

145. Charnley J, Halley DK: Rate of wear in total hip replacement. Clin Orthop 112:170, 1975.

146. Griffith MJ, Seidenstein MK, Williams D: Socket wear in Charnley low friction arthroplasty of the hip. Clin Orthop 137:37, 1978.

147. Mahoney OM, Dimon JH: Unsatisfactory results with a ceramic total hip prosthesis. J Bone Joint Surg [Am] 72:663, 1990.

148. Winter M, Griss P, Scheller G, et al: Ten-to-14-year results of a ceramic hip prosthesis. Clin Orthop 282:73, 1992.

149. Bankston AB, Faris PM, Keating EM, et al: Polyethylene wear in total hip arthroplasty in patient-matched groups. J Arthroplasty 8:315, 1933.

150. Livermore J, Ilstrup D, Morrey B: Effect of femoral head size on wear of the polyethylene acetabular component. J Bone Joint Surg [Am] 72:518, 1990.

151. Charnley J, Cupic A: The nine and ten year results of the low-friction arthroplasty on the hip. Clin Orthop 95:9, 1973.

152. Clark IC, Black K, Rennie C, et al: Can wear in total hip arthroplasties be assessed from radiographs? Clin Orthop 121:126, 1976.

153. Mullins MF, Sutton RN, Lodwick GS: Complications of total hip replacement. A roentgen evaluation. AJR 121:545, 1974.

154. Collier JP, Major MB, Jensen RE, et al: Mechanisms of failure of modular prostheses. Clin Orthop 285:129, 1992.

155. Kitziger JK, Delee JC, Evans JA: Disassembly of a modular acetabular component of a total hip-replacement arthroplasty. J Bone Joint Surg [Am] 72:621, 1990.

156. Pellicci PM, Haas SB: Disassembly of a modular femoral component during closed reduction of the dislocated femoral component. J Bone Joint Surg [Am] 72:619, 1990.

157. Brien WW, Salvati EA, Wright TM, et al: Dissociation of acetabular components after total hip arthroplasty. J Bone Joint Surg [Am] 72:2548, 1990.

158. Woolson ST, Pottorff GT: Disassembly of the modular femoral prosthesis after dislocation of the femoral component. J Bone Joint Surg [Am] 72:624, 1990.

159. Barrack RL, Burke DW, Cook SD, et al: Complications related to modularity of total hip components. J Bone Joint Surg [Br] 75:688, 1993.

160. Quale JS, Murphey MD, Huntrakoon M, et al: Titanium-induced arthropathy associated with polyethylene-metal separation after total joint replacement. Radiology 182:855, 1992.

161. Maloney WJ, Krushell RJ, Jasty M, et al: Incidence of heterotopic ossification after total hip replacement: Effect of the type of fixation of the femoral component. J Bone Joint Surg [Am] 73:191, 1991.

162. Sumner DR, Tuerner TM, Pierson RH, et al: Effects of radiation on fixation of non-cemented porous-coated implants in a canine model. J Bone Joint Surg [Am] 72:1527, 1990.

163. Wilde AH, Collins RH, Mackenzie AH: Reankylosis of the hip joint in ankylosing spondylitis after total hip replacement. Arthritis Rheum 15:493, 1972.

164. Thomas BJ: Heterotopic bone formation. In CA Harlan (Ed): Hip Arthroplasty. New York, Churchill Livingstone, 1991, p 405.

165. Seegenschmiedt MH, Goldmann AR, Martus P, et al: Prophylactic radiation therapy for prevention of heterotopic ossification after hip arthroplasty: Results in 141 high-risk hips. Radiology 188:257, 1993.

166. Brooker AF, Bowerman JW, Robinson RA, et al: Ectopic ossification following total hip replacement. J Bone Joint Surg [Am] 55:1629, 1973.

167. Velasco AD, Allan DB, Wroblewski BM: Psoas tenotomy and heterotopic ossification after Charnley low-friction arthroplasty. Clin Orthop 291:193, 1993.

168. Schmidt SA, Kjaersgaard-Andersen P, Pedersen NW, et al: The use of indomethacin to prevent the formation of heterostopic bone after total hip replacement. J Bone Joint Surg [Am] 70:834, 1988.

169. Konski AA, Pellegrini VD: Postoperative irradiation for prevention of heterotopic bone after total hip arthroplasty. Int J Radiol Oncol Biol Phys 19:809, 1990.

170. Martin A, Bauer TW, Manley MT, et al: Osteosarcoma at the site of total hip replacement. J Bone Joint Surg [Am] 70:1561, 1988.

171. Brien WW, Salvati EA, Healey JH, et al: Osteogenic sarcoma arising in the area of a total hip replacement. J Bone Joint Surg [Am] 72:1097, 1990.

172. Lamovec J, Zidar A, Cucek-Plenicar M: Synovial sarcoma associated with total hip replacement. J Bone Joint Surg [Am] 70:1558, 1988.

173. Svensson O, Mathiesen EB, Reinholt FP, et al: Formation of a fulminant soft-tissue pseudotumor after uncemented hip arthroplasty. J Bone Joint Surg [Am] 70:1238, 1998.

174. Ryu RKN, Bovill EG, Skinner HB, et al: Soft tissue sarcoma associated with aluminum oxide ceramic total hip arthroplasty. Clin Orthop 216:207, 1987.

175. Callaghan JJ, Dysart SH, Savory CG: The uncemented porous-coated anatomic total hip prosthesis. J Bone Joint Surg [Am] 70:337, 1988.

176. Maloney J, Jasty M, Harris WH, et al: Endosteal erosion in association with stable uncemented femoral components. J Bone Joint Surg [Am] 72:1025, 1990.

177. Engh CA, Zeittl-Schaffer KF, Kukita Y, et al: Histological and radiographic assessment of well functioning porous-coated acetabular components. J Bone Joint Surg [Am] 75:814, 1993.

178. Haddad RJ, Cood SD, Thomas KA: Biological fixation of porous-coated implants. J Bone Joint Surg [Am] 69A:1459, 1987.

179. Bands R, Pelker RR, Shine J, et al: The noncemented porous-coated hip prosthesis. Clin Orthop 269:209, 1991.

180. Sielewicz M, Scholz J, Hanslik L: A five year follow-up of 605 cases of the MCCL (metal-cancellous cementless Lubeck) total hip prosthesis. Ital J Orthop Traumatol 15:433, 1989.

181. Cameron HU: Six-year results with a microporous-coated metal hip prosthesis. Clin Orthop 208:81, 1986.

182. Boyes C: Norwich cementless total hip replacement. Radiography Today 56:17, 1990.

183. Barbos MP: Bone ingrowth into madreporic prostheses. J Bone Joint Surg [Am] 70:85, 1988.

184. Engh CA, Massin P, Suthers KE: Roentgenographic assessment of the biologic fixation of porous-surfaced femoral components. Clin Orthop 257:107, 1990.

185. Kattapuram SV, Lodwick GS, Chandler H, et al: Porous-coated anatomic total hip prostheses: Radiographic analysis and clinical correlation. Radiology 174:861, 1990.

186. Dodge BM, Fitzrandolph R, Collins DN: Noncemented porous-coated anatomic total hip arthroplasty. Clin Orthop 269:16, 1991.

187. Kaplan PA, Montesi SA, Jardon OM, et al: Bone in-growth hip prostheses in asymptomatic patients: Radiographic features. Radiology 169:221, 1988.

188. Hedley AK, Gruen TA, Ruoff DP: Revision of failed total hip arthroplasties with uncemented porous-coated anatomic components. Clin Orthop 235:75, 1988.

189. Schmalzried TP, Finerman GAM: Osteolysis in aseptic failure. In Fitzgerald R (Ed): Non-cemented Total Hip Arthroplasty. New York, Raven Press, 1988, p 303.

190. Engh CA, Bobyn JD: The influence of stem size and extent of porous coating on femoral bone resorption after primary cementless hip arthroplasty. Clin Orthop 231:7, 1988.

191. Perner HS, Voth E, Reith HG, et al: Cementless implantation of Zweymueller-Endler total endoprostheses of the hip. Clinical, radiological and scintigraphic follow-up for 2 years. Nucl Med 25:55, 1986.

192. Engh CA, Massin P: Cementless total hip arthroplasty using the anatomic medullary locking stem. Clin Orthop 249:141, 1989.

193. Rosenthall L, Ghazal ME, Brooks CE: Quantitative analysis of radiophosphate uptakes in asymptomatic porous-coated hip endoprostheses. J Nucl Med 32:1391, 1991.

194. Oswald SG, Van Nostrand D, Savory CG, et al: Three-phase bone scan and indium white blood cell scintigraphy following porous coated hip arthroplasty: A prospective study of the prosthetic tip. J Nucl Med 30:1321, 1989.

195. Oswald SG, Van Nostrand D: Atlas of normal bone scan and [111]In white blood cell findings in porous-coated hip prostheses. In Abreu SH, van Nostrand D, Zeissman HH (Eds): Selected Atlases of Bone Scintigraphy. New York, Springer-Verlag, 1992.

196. Hozack WJ, Rothman RH, Booth RE, et al: Cemented versus cementless total hip arthroplasty. A comparative study of equivalent patient populations. Clin Orthop 289:161, 1993.

197. Swan JS, Braunstein EM, Wellman HN, et al: Contrast and nuclear arthrography in loosening of the uncemented hip prosthesis. Skel Radiol 20:15, 1991.

198. Oswald SG, Herzwurm PJ: False-positive radionuclide arthroscintigraphy with a porous-coated total hip prosthesis. Clin Nucl Med 16:815, 1991.

199. Harris WH, Mulroy RD, Maloney WJ, et al: Intraoperative measurement of rotational stability of femoral components of total hip arthroplasty. Clin Orthop 266:119, 1991.

200. Hedley AK: The Hip. Proceedings of the 14th Open Scientific Meeting, St. Louis, CV Mosby, 1987, pp 225–250.

201. Jacobs JJ, Skipor AK, Black P, et al: Release and excretion of metal in patients who have a total hip-replacement component made of titanium-base alloy. J Bone Joint Surg [Am] 73:1475, 1991.

202. Lalor PA, Gray AB, Wright S: Contact sensitivity to titanium in a hip prosthesis? Contact Dermatitis 23:193, 1990.

203. Salvati EA, Betts F, Doty SB: Particulate metallic debris in cemented total hip arthroplasty. Clin Orthop 293:160, 1993.

204. Cameron HU: Failure of a titanium endoprosthesis—a case report. Can J Surg 34:625, 1991.

205. Spector M: Biomaterial failure. Orthop Clin North Am 23:211, 1992.

206. Haynes DR, Rogers SD, Hay S, et al: The differences in toxicity and release of bone-resorbing mediators induced by titanium and cobalt-chromium alloy wear particles. J Bone Joint Surg [Am] 75:825, 1993.

207. Maloney WJ, Smith RL, Castro F, et al: Fibroblast response to metallic debris in vitro. J Bone Joint Surg [Am] 75:835, 1993.

208. Lockie K, Binns M, Fisher J, et al: Assessment of the deformation of the

Bateman bipolar hip prosthesis inner bearing due to moisture absorption and creep. Injury 23:116, 1992.

209. Incavo SJ, Ninomiya J, Howe JG, et al: Failure of the polyethylene liner leading to notching of the femoral component in bipolar prostheses. Orthop Rev 22:728, 1993.

210. Overgaard S, Jensen TT, Bonde G, et al: The uncemented bipolar hemiarthroplasty for displaced femoral neck fractures. Acta Orthop Scand 62:115, 1991.

211. Geesink RGT: Experimental and clinical experience with hydroxyapatite-coated hip implants. Orthopedics 12:1239, 1989.

212. D'Antonio JA, Capello WN, Crothers OD, et al: Early clinical experience with hydroxyapatite-coated femoral implants. J Bone Joint Surg [Am] 74:995, 1992.

213. Soballe K, Gotfredsen K, Brockstedt-Rasmussen, et al: Histologic analysis of a retrieved hydroxyapatite-coated femoral prosthesis. Clin Orthop 272:255, 1991.

214. Abrahams TG, Crothers OD: Radiographic analysis of an investigational hydroxyapatite-coated total hip replacement. Invest Radiol 27:779, 1992.

215. Bauer TW, Geesink RCT, Zimmerman R, et al: Hydroxyapatite-coated femoral stems. J Bone Joint Surg [Am] 73:1439, 1991.

216. Windsor RE, Insall JN: Surgery of the knee. In CB Sledge, et al (Eds): Arthritis Surgery. Philadelphia, WB Saunders, 1994, p 794.

217. Peterson LFA: Current status of total knee arthroplasty. Arch Surg 112:1099, 1977.

218. Scuderi GR, Insall JN, Windsor RE, et al: Survivorship of cemented knee replacements. J Bone Joint Surg [Br] 71:798, 1989.

219. Rand JA: Patellar resurfacing in total knee arthroplasty. Clin Orthop 260:110, 1990.

220. Picetti GD, McGann WA, Welch RB: The patellofemoral joint after total knee arthroplasty without patellar resurfacing. J Bone Joint Surg [Am] 72:1379, 1990.

221. Enis JE, Gardner R, Robledo MA, et al: Comparison of patellar resurfacing versus nonresurfacing in bilateral total knee arthroplasty. Clin Orthop 260:38, 1990.

222. Siu D, Cooke TDV, Broekhoven LD, et al: A standardized technique for lower limb radiography: Practice, applications, and error analysis. Invest Radiol 26:71, 1991.

223. Abraham W, Buchanan JR, Daubert H, et al: Should the patella be resurfaced in total knee arthroplasty? Clin Orthop 236:128, 1986.

224. Lee JG, Keating EM, Ritter MA, et al: Review of the all-polyethylene tibial component in total knee arthroplasty. Clin Orthop 260:87, 1990.

225. Figgie HE III, Goldberg VM, Hieple KG: The influence of tibial-patellofemoral location on function of the knee in patients with the posterior stabilized condylar knee prosthesis. J Bone Joint Surg [Am] 68A:1035, 1986.

226. Wright J, Ewald FC, Walker PS: Total arthroplasty with the kinematic prosthesis. J Bone Joint Surg [Am] 72:1003, 1990.

227. Gomes LSM, Bechtold JE, Gustilo RB: Patellar prosthesis positioning in total knee arthroplasty. Clin Orthop 236:72, 1998.

228. Mintzer CM, Robertson DD, Rackemann S, et al: Bone loss in the distal anterior femur after total knee arthroplasty. Clin Orthop 260:135, 1990.

229. Ewald FC: The Knee Society total knee arthroplasty. Roentgenographic evaluation and scoring system. Clin Orthop 248:9, 1989.

230. Buechel FF, Pappas MJ: Long-term survivorship analysis of cruciate-sparing versus cruciate-sacrificing knee prostheses using meniscal bearings. Clin Orthop 260:162, 1990.

231. Rand JA, Ilstrup DM: Survivorship analysis of total knee arthroplasty. J Bone Joint Surg 73:397, 1991.

232. Brick GW, Scott RD: The patellofemoral component of total knee arthroplasty. Clin Orthop 231:163, 1988.

233. Goldberg VM, Figgie HE III, Inglis AE, et al: Patellar fracture type and prognosis in condylar total knee arthroplasty. Clin Orthop 236:115, 1988.

234. Ritter MA, Campbell ED: Postoperative patellar complications with or without lateral release during total knee arthroplasty. Clin Orthop 219:163, 1987.

235. Piraino D, Richmond B, Freed H, et al: Total knee replacement: Radiologic findings in failure of porous-coated metal-backed patellar component. AJR 155:555, 1990.

236. Rand JA: Comparison of metal-backed and all-polyethylene tibial components in cruciate condylar total knee arthroplasty. J Arthroplasty 8:307, 1993.

237. Bayley JC, Scott RD: Further observations on metal-backed patellar component failure. Clin Orthop 236:82, 1988.

238. Lombardi AV, Engh GA, Volz RG, et al: Fracture/dissociation of the polyethylene in metal-backed patellar components in total knee arthroplasty. J Bone Joint Surg [Am] 70:675, 1988.

239. Bayley JC, Scott RD, Ewald FC, et al: Failure of the metal-backed patellar component after total knee replacement. J Bone Joint Surg [Am] 70:668, 1988.

240. Weissman BN, Scott RD, Brick GW, et al: Radiographic detection of metal-induced synovitis as a complication of arthroplasty of the knee. J Bone Joint Surg [Am] 73:1002, 1991.

241. Dodd CAF, Hungerford MD, Karckow KA: Total knee arthroplasty fixation. Comparison of the early results of paired cemented versus uncemented porous coated anatomic knee prostheses. Clin Orthop 260:66, 1990.

242. Schneider R, Hood RW, Ranawat CS: Radiologic evaluation of knee arthroplasty. Orthop Clin North Am 13:225, 1982.

243. Breen DJ, Stoker DJ: Titanium lines: A manifestation of metallosis and tissue response to titanium alloy megaprostheses at the knee. Clin Radiol 47:274, 1993.

244. Plante-Bordeneuve P, Freeman MAR: Tibial high-density polyethylene wear in conforming tibiofemoral prostheses. J Bone Joint Surg [Br] 75:630, 1993.

245. Goodman S, Lidgren L: Polyethylene wear in knee arthroplasty. Acta Orthop Scand 63:358, 1992.

246. Lindstrand A, Stenström A: Polyethylene wear of the PCA unicompartmental knee. Acta Orthop Scand 63:260, 1992.

247. Blunn GW, Joshi AT, Lilley PA, et al: Polyethylene wear in unicondylar knee prostheses. 106 retrieved Marmor, PCA, and St Georg tibial components compared. Acta Orthop Scand 63:247, 1992.

248. Gross TP, Lennox DW: Osteolytic cyst-like area associated with polyethylene and metallic debris after total knee replacement with an uncemented vitallium prosthesis. J Bone Joint Surg 74:1096, 1992.

249. Peters PC, Engh GA, Dwyer KA, et al: Osteolysis after total knee arthroplasty without cement. J Bone Joint Surg [Am] 74:864, 1992.

250. Bauer TW, Saltarelli M, McMahon JT, et al: Regional dissemination of wear debris from a total knee prosthesis. J Bone Joint Surg [Am] 75:106, 1993.

251. Wright TM, Rimnac CM, Faris PM, et al: Analysis of surface damage in retrieved carbon fiber–reinforced and plain polyethylene tibial components from posterior stabilized total knee replacements. J Bone Joint Surg [Am] 70:1312, 1988.

252. Berry DJ, Wold LE, Rand JA: Extensive osteolysis around an aseptic, stable, uncemented total knee replacement. Clin Orthop 293:204, 1993.

253. Kilgus DJ, Funahashi TT, Campbell PA: Massive femoral osteolysis and early disintegration of a polyethylene-bearing surface of a total knee replacement. J Bone Joint Surg [Am] 74:770, 1992.

254. Rhoads DD, Noble PC, Reuben JD, et al: The effect of femoral component position on patellar tracking after total knee arthroplasty. Clin Orthop 260:43, 1990.

255. Schoiff SC, Morrey BF: Treatment of infection after total knee arthroplasty by debridement with retention of the components. J Bone Joint Surg [Am] 72:1383, 1990.

256. Wilson MG, Kelley K, Thornhill TS: Infection as a complication of total knee-replacement arthroplasty. J Bone Joint Surg [Am] 72:878, 1990.

257. Minoves M, Garcia JR, Mane S, et al: Infected knee prosthesis: Visualization of the fistulous tract by Tc-99m HMPAO leukocyte scintigraphy. Clin Nuc Med 17:593, 1992.

258. Hunter JC, Hattner RS, Murray WR, et al: Loosening of the total knee arthroplasty: Detection by radionuclide bone scanning. AJR 135:131, 1980.

259. Schneider R, Soundry M: Radiographic and scintigraphic evaluation of total knee arthroplasty. Clin Orthop 205:108, 1986.

260. Rosenthall L, Lepanto L, Raymond F: Radiophosphate uptake in asymptomatic knee arthroplasty. J Nucl Med 29:1546, 1987.

261. Palestro CJ, Swyer AJ, Kim CK, et al: Infected knee prosthesis: Diagnosis with In-111 leukocyte, Tc-99m sulfur colloid, and Tc-99m MDP imaging. Radiology 179:645, 1991.

262. Aliabadi P, Weissman BN: Radiology of total shoulder arthroplasty. In RJ Friedman (Ed): Arthroplasty of the Shoulder. New York, Thieme, 1994, p 53.

263. Saha AK: Dynamic stability of the glenohumeral joint. Acta Orthop Scand 42:491, 1971.

264. Neer CS, Watson KC, Stanton FJ: Recent experience in total shoulder replacement. J Bone Joint Surg [Am] 64:319, 1982.

265. Cofield RH: Total shoulder arthroplasty with Neer prosthesis. J Bone Joint Surg [Am] 66:899, 1984.

266. Aliabadi P, Weissman BN, Thornhill T, et al: Evaluation of a nonconstrained total shoulder prosthesis. AJR 151:1169, 1988.

267. Amstutz HC, Sew Hoy AL, Clarke IC: UCLA anatomic total shoulder arthroplasty. Clin Orthop 155:7, 1981.

268. Boyd AD, Aliabadi P, Thronhill TS: Postoperative proximal migration in total shoulder arthroplasty. Incidence and significance. J Arthroplasty 6:31, 1991.

269. Gristina AG, Roman RL, Kammire GC, et al: Total shoulder replacement. Orthop Clin North Am 18:445, 1987.

270. McElwain JP, English E: The early results of porous-coated total shoulder arthroplasty. Clin Orthop 218:217, 1987.

271. Post M, Jablon M: Constrained total shoulder arthroplasty. Long-term follow-up observations. Clin Orthop 173:109, 1983.

272. Sledge CB, Kozinn SC, Thronhill TS, et al: Total shoulder arthroplasty in rheumatoid arthritis. Rheumatology 12:95, 1989.

273. Ovesen J, Nielsen S: Prosthesis position in shoulder arthroplasty. Acta Orthop Scand 56:330, 1985.

274. Frich LH, Moller BN: Retroversion of the humeral prosthesis in shoulder arthroplasty. Measurements of angle from standard radiographs. J Arthroplasty 4:277, 1989.

275. Driessnack RP, Ferlic DC, Wiedel JD: Dissociation of the glenoid component in the Macnab/English total shoulder arthroplasty. J Arthroplasty 5:15, 1990.

276. Groh GI, Rockwood CA Jr.: Surgical anatomy and technique. In RJ Friedman (Ed): Arthroplasty of the Shoulder. New York, Thieme, 1994, p 80.

277. Silliman JF, Hawkins RJ: Complications following shoulder arthroplasty. In J Friedman (Ed): Arthroplasty of the Shoulder. New York, Thieme, 1994, p 242.

278. Brukhead WZ: Cementless shoulder arthroplasty. In J Friedman (Ed): Arthroplasty of the Shoulder. New York, Thieme, 1994, p 281.

279. Cofield RH: Unconstrained total shoulder prostheses. Clin Orthop 173:97, 1983.

280. Post M, Haskell SS, Jablon M: Total shoulder replacement with a constrained prosthesis. J Bone Joint Surg [Am] 62:327, 1980.

281. Coughlin MJ, Morris JM, West WF: The semiconstrained total shoulder arthroplasty. J Bone Joint Surg [Am] 61:574, 1979.

282. Frich LH, Moller BN, Sneppen O: Shoulder arthroplasty with the Neer Mark-II prosthesis. Arch Orthop Trauma Surg 107:110, 1998.

283. Thornhill TS, Karr MJ, Averill RM, et al: Total shoulder arthroplasty: The Brigham experience. Orthop Trans 7:497, 1983.

284. Moeckel BH, Warren RF, Dines DM, et al: The unstable shoulder arthroplasty. *In* RJ Friedman (Ed): Arthroplasty of the Shoulder. New York, Thieme, 1994, p 254.

285. Weiss AA, Berman AT, O'Brien J: What are the current indications for total elbow arthroplasty? Report of a case using allograft for TEA. Orthopedics 16:237, 1993.

286. Ruth JT, Wilde AH: Capitellocondylar total elbow replacement. J Bone Joint Surg [Am] 74:95, 1992.

287. Briggs PJ, Smith SR: Radiographic assessment of component orientation in elbow arthroplasty. Acta Orthop Scand 64:212, 1993.

288. Ewald FC, Simmons ED, Sullivan JA, et al: Capitellocondylar total elbow replacement in rheumatoid arthritis. J Bone Joint Surg [Am] 75:498, 1993.

289. Morrey BF, Adams RA: Semiconstrained arthroplasty for the treatment of rheumatoid arthritis of the elbow. J Bone Joint Surg [Am] 74:479, 1992.

290. Weissman BN: Prosthetic replacement of the elbow. Semin Roentgenol 21:66, 1986.

291. Pritchard RW: Total elbow joint arthroplasty in patients with rheumatoid arthritis. Semin Arthritis Rheum 21:24, 1991.

292. Wolfe SW, Figgie MP, Inglis AE, et al: Management of infection about total elbow prostheses. J Bone Joint Surg [Am] 72:198, 1990.

293. Spaulding JM, Megesi RG, Figgie HE, et al: Total ankle arthroplasty. AORN J 48:201, 1988.

294. Unger AS, Inglis AE, Mow CS, et al: Total ankle arthroplasty in rheumatoid arthritis: A long-term follow-up study. Foot Ankle 8:173, 1988.

295. Takakura Y, Tanaka Y, Sugimoto K, et al: Ankle arthroplasty: A comparative study of cemented metal and uncemented ceramic prostheses. Clin Orthop 252:209, 1990.

296. Newton SE: An artificial ankle joint. Clin Orthop 142:141, 1979.

297. McGuire MR, Kyle RF, Gustilo RB, et al: Comparative analysis of ankle arthroplasty versus ankle arthrodesis. Clin Orthop 226:174, 1988.

298. Scholz KC: Total ankle arthroplasty using biological fixation components compared to ankle arthrodesis. Orthopedics 10:125, 1987.

299. Herberts P, Goldie IF, Korner L, et al: Endoprosthetic arthroplasty of the ankle joint. Acta Orthop Scand 53:687, 1982.

300. Dini AA, Bassett FH: Evaluation of the early result of Smith total ankle replacement. Clin Orthop 146:228, 1980.

301. Demottaz JD, Mazur JM, Thomas WH: Clinical study of total ankle replacement with gait analysis. J Bone Joint Surg [Am] 61:976, 1979.

302. Saltzman CL, Johnson KA: Surgery of the ankle and foot. *In* CB Sledge (Ed): Arthritis Surgery. Philadelphia, WB Saunders 1993, p 828.

303. Wynn AH, Wilde AH: Long-term follow-up of the Conaxial (Beck-Steffee) total ankle arthroplasty. Foot Ankle 13:303, 1992.

304. Jensen NC, Kroner K: Total ankle joint replacement: A clinical follow-up. Orthopedics 15:236, 1992.

305. Smahel J, Meyer V: Structure of capsules around silicone implants in hand surgery. Hand 15:47, 1983.

306. Lagier R: Case report 719. Skel Radiol 21:137, 1992.

307. Jolly SL, Ferlic DC, Clayton ML, et al: Swanson silicone arthroplasty of the wrist in rheumatoid arthritis: A long-term follow-up. J Hand Surg [Am] 17:142, 1992.

308. Fatti JF, Palmer AK, Greensky S, et al: Long-term results of Swanson interpositional wrist arthroplasty. Part II. J Hand Surg [Am] 16:432, 1991.

309. Swanson AB, de Groot Swanson G: Flexible implant resection arthroplasty: A method for reconstruction of small joints in the extremities. AADS Instructional Course Lectures 27:27, 1978.

310. Kircher T: Silicone lymphadenopathy: A complication of silicone elastomer finger joint prostheses. Hum Pathol 11:240, 1908.

311. Sammarco GJ, Tabatowski K: Silicone lymphadenopathy associated with failed prosthesis of the hallux: A case report and literature review. Foot Ankle 13:273, 1992.

312. Atkinson RE, Smith RJ: Silicone synovitis following silicone implant arthroplasty. Hand Clin 2:291, 1986.

313. Ferlic DC, Clayton ML, Holloway M: Complications of silicone implant surgery in the metacarpophalangeal joint. J Bone Joint Surg [Am] 57:991, 1975.

314. Bansal M, Goldman AB, Bullough PG, et al: Case report 706. Skel Radiol 21:49, 1992.

315. Groff GD, Schned AR, Taylor TH: Silicone-induced adenopathy eight years after metacarpophalangeal arthroplasty. Arthritis Rheum 24:1578, 1981.

316. Rosenthal DI, Rosenberg AE, Schiller AL, et al: Destructive arthritis due to silicone: A foreign-body reaction. Radiology 149:69, 1983.

317. Schneider HJ, Weiss MA, Stern PJ: Silicone-induced erosive arthritis: Radiologic features in seven cases. AJR 148:923, 1987.

318. Smith RJ, Atkinson RE, Jupiter JB: Silicone synovitis of the wrist. J Hand Surg [Am] 10:47, 1985.

319. Pellegrini VD, Burton RI: Surgical management of basal joint arthritis of the thumb. Part I. Long-term results of silicone implant arthroplasty. J Hand Surg [Am] 11:309, 1986.

320. Comstock CP, Louis DS, Eckenrode JF: Silicone wrist implant: Long-term follow-up study. J Hand Surg [Am] 31:201, 1988.

321. Carter PR, Benton LJ, Dysert PA: Silicone rubber carpal implants: A study of the incidence of late osseous complications. J Hand Surg [Am] 11:639, 1986.

322. Beckenbaugh RD, Dobyns JH, Linscheid RL, et al: Review and analysis of silicone-rubber metacarpophalangeal implants. J Bone Joint Surg [Am] 58:483, 1976.

323. Bieber EJ, Weiland AJ, Volenec-Dowling S: Silicone-rubber implant arthroplasty of the metacarpophalangeal joints for rheumatoid arthritis. J Bone Joint Surg [Am] 68:206, 1986.

324. Gordon M, Bullough PG: Synovial and osseous inflammation in failed silicone-rubber prostheses. J Bone Joint Surg [Am] 64:574, 1982.

325. Westesson P-L, Eriksson L, Lindström C: Destructive lesions of the mandibular condyle following diskectomy with temporary silicone implant. Oral Surg 63:143, 1987.

326. Hofammann DY, Ferlic DC, Clayton ML: Arthroplasty of the basal joint of the thumb using a silicone prosthesis. J Bone Joint Surg [Am] 69:993, 1987.

327. Swanson AB, de Groot Swanson G, Maupin BK, et al: Failed carpal bone arthroplasty: Causes and treatment. J Hand Surg [Am] 14:417, 1989.

328. Broughton NS, Doran A, Meggitt BF: Silastic ball spacer arthroplasty in the management of hallux valgus and hallux rigidus. Foot Ankle 10:61, 1989.

329. Christie AJ, Weinberger KA, Dietrich M: Silicone lymphadenopathy and synovitis: Complications of silicone elastomer finger joint prostheses. JAMA 237:1463, 1977.

330. Resnick CS, Fratkin MJ, Cardea JA: Arthroscintigraphic evaluation of the painful total hip prosthesis. Clin Nucl Med 11:242, 1986.

331. Jasty MJ, Floyd WE III, Schiller AL, et al: Localized osteolysis in stable, nonseptic total hip replacement. J Bone Joint Surg [Am] 68:912, 1986.

332. Barrack RL, Tanzer M, Kattapuram SV, et al: The value of contrast arthrography in assessing loosening of symptomatic uncemented total hip components. Skeletal Radiol 23:37, 1994.

333. Insall JN: Presidential address to the Knee Society. Choices and compromises in total knee arthroplasty. Clin Orthop 226:43, 1988.

# INDEX

▼

Note: Page numbers in *italics* refer to illustrations; page numbers followed by (t) refer to tables.

Rugby, injuries in, 3230
Rugger-jersey spine, in hyperparathyroidism, 2021, 2030, 2035
in primary oxalosis, 1690, *1692*
in renal osteodystrophy, *1473*, 1904, *1905*, 2036, *2039–2040*, 4010, *4012*
Running, fatigue fractures in, 2580, 2583
femoral stress fracture in, 2590
fibular stress fracture in, 2589, *2593*
injuries in, 3230
joint loads in, 793
meniscal degeneration in, 3254
tarsal navicular stress fracture in, 2588–2589, *2592*
tibial stress fracture in, 2590
Rupture(s). See specific structures, e.g., *Achilles tendon.*
Rush pin, 492, *492*

**S**

Saber shin, in acquired syphilis, 2499
in congenital syphilis, 2493, 2495, *2496, 2497*
in rickets, 1894
in yaws, 2499
Sac, synovial, *306*
Saccular recess, dilation of, *98*
Sacral nerve root, disruption of, sacral fracture and, 2804
Sacralization, of fifth lumbar vertebra, 717
Sacrococcygeal agenesis, 4287–4288, *4289*
maternal diabetes mellitus and, 2088
Sacrococcygeal joint, 717
chordoma of, 3848, *3849*, 3852, *3852*
obliteration of, 717
Sacrococcygeal ligaments, 717
*Sacrocystis lindemanni*, 2537(t)
Sacroiliac joint(s), 717–718, *718, 719*. See also *Ilium; Pelvis; Sacrum.*
abnormalities of, differential diagnosis of, 957–958, 958t
distribution of, 1062t
in paralysis, 3375
pelvic sepsis and, in paralysis, 3375
accessory, degenerative disease of, 1319–1320
age-related changes of, 1313, *1314*
alkaptonuria of, 1679, *1679*, 1780
ankylosing spondylitis of, *859*, 957–958, 958(t), 988t, 1011–1012, *1011, 1018–1021*
computed tomography of, 1057, *1060*
differential diagnosis of, 1064–1065, 1064(t), *1065*
distribution of, *1779*, 1780
juvenile-onset, *974*, 988(t)
ossification in, *854*
scintigraphy of, 1055, 1057, *1058–1059*
ankylosis of, in ankylosing spondylitis, *854*, 988(t), 1013, *1018, 1020*
in juvenile chronic arthritis, 988t
in myositis ossificans progressiva, 4128
in rheumatoid arthritis, 988t
arthritis of, tuberculous, *2481, 2482*
arthrography of, 399, *399*
bony ankylosis of, 718
in Paget's disease, *1954*
Brucella infection of, 2457
calcium pyrophosphate dihydrate crystal deposition disease of, 1601, *1601*
conventional tomography of, 111
cryptococcosis of, 2506
degenerative joint disease of, 1064–1065
differential diagnosis of, 1319, 1319(t)
distribution of, *1779*, 1780
diastasis of, *2565*

Sacroiliac joint(s) *(Continued)*
in pregnancy, 2096
symphysis pubis subluxation and, 2636
disease distribution in, *1779*, 1779–1780
eburnation of. See also *Osteitis condensans ilii.*
in ankylosing spondylitis, *1020*
enthesopathy of, in ankylosing spondylitis, *1017*
erosion of, in ankylosing spondylitis, 988(t), 1013, *1018, 1020, 1021*
in juvenile chronic arthritis, 988t
in multicentric reticulohistiocytosis, 2207, *2212*
in rheumatoid arthritis, 988t
fibrous capsule of, 717
fracture of, 2807–2808
radiation and, 3292, *3293*
gout of, 1064–1065, 1064t, 1536, *1536, 1779, 1780*
immobilization of, 1780
in adolescents, 50, *50*
in ankylosing spondylitis, *1017, 1020*
in Behçet's syndrome, 1780
in Crohn's disease, 1127, *1128*, 1129
in diffuse idiopathic skeletal hyperostosis, 1465, 1471, *1473*
in familial Mediterranean fever, 1151, *1151*, 1152t, 1152(t), 1780
in Gaucher's disease, 2198
in hyperparathyroidism, 1064, 1064t, 1065, *1779*, 1780, 2021, *2022*
in inflammatory bowel disease, *1779*, 1780
in juvenile chronic arthritis, 988t
in multicentric reticulohistiocytosis, 2207, *2212*
in osteitis condensans ilii, 1064, 1064(t), 1065, 2089, *2090*, 2091t. See also *Osteitis condensans ilii.*
in Paget's disease, *1954*
in paralysis, 1065, 3378, 3380, *3380*
vs. ankylosing spondylitis, 3378, 3380, *3380*
in poliomyelitis, *3366*
in polymyalgia rheumatica, 1238
in pregnancy, 2089
in Reiter's syndrome, 1064, 1065, *1065*, 1105, *1105*, 1112–1117, *1113, 1116, 1779*, 1780
in SAPHO syndrome, 4450, *4450*
in sickle cell anemia, 2111, *2113*
in sternocostoclavicular hyperostosis, 4456
in systemic lupus erythematosus, 1179, 1183, *1183*
in traumatic paraplegia, 3378
in ulcerative colitis, 1123–1124, *1123–1125*
in Whipple's disease, 1131, *1133*
in X-linked hypophosphatemia, 1908, *1908*
infection of, 1064–1065, 1064(t), *1779*, 1780, 2436, 2439–2441. See also *Sacroiliitis.*
clinical manifestations of, 2439
computed tomography in, 2440–2441, *2441, 2442*
decubitus ulcer and, 2439, *2439*
differential diagnosis of, 2441, *2444*
drug abuse and, *2392*, 2440, 2441
magnetic resonance imaging in, 2441, *2442, 2443*
radiographic-pathologic correlation in, 2439–2440, *2440*
routes of, 2436, 2439, *2439*
vs. Reiter's syndrome, *2444*
joint space narrowing of, in neuromuscular disorders, 3378
in paralysis, *3380*
in rheumatoid arthritis, 924, *925*

Sacroiliac joint(s) *(Continued)*
in traumatic paraplegia, 3378
juvenile chronic arthritis of, *1779*, 1780
mechanical stress on, osteitis condensans ilii from, 2089
mobility of, 25
movement of, 718
multicentric reticulohistiocytosis of, 2207, *2212*
non-Hodgkin's lymphoma of, *2265*
obliteration of, simulation of, 50, *50*
ochronotic arthropathy of, 1683
ossification of, in ankylosing spondylitis, 1013, *1018, 1019*
osteoarthritis of, 1064–1065, 1064t, 1313–1320, *1314–1320*, 1319(t). See also *Osteoarthritis, sacroiliac joint.*
osteomyelitis of, gallium-67 imaging in, 443, *444*
intravenous drug abuse and, *2440*
scintigraphy in, 443, *444*
osteonecrosis of, radiation therapy and, 3292, *3292*
osteophytes of, in diffuse idiopathic skeletal hyperostosis, *1473*
osteosarcoma of, *3670*
osteosclerosis of, in ankylosing spondylitis, 1013, *1020, 1021*
in Gaucher's disease, 2198
in polymyalgia rheumatica, 1238
in sickle cell anemia, 2111, *2113*
pain in, in ankylosing spondylitis, 1010
plain film radiography of, 25, *26, 27*
anteroposterior, 25, *26*
craniocaudal, 25, *27*
in adolescents, 50, *50*
oblique, 25, *26*
plasmacytoma of, *2168*
POEMS syndrome of, 2172
preauricular sulci of, 50, *51*
psoriatic arthritis of, 1064, 1065, *1065*, 1077, *1077*, 1082, *1088–1089*
distribution of, *1779*, 1780
scintigraphy of, *1093*
psoriatic spondylitis of, 1064, 1064t
radiation therapy of, 3292, *3292*
radiography of, 718
relapsing polychondritis of, 1152(t), 1153, *1155*, 1780
rheumatoid arthritis of, 924, *925*, 957–958, 958(t), 988t, 1064, 1064(t), 1065
distribution of, *1779*, 1780
radiography of, 924, *925*
scintigraphy in, 462
sarcoidosis of, 4344
septic arthritis of, *153*
intravenous drug abuse and, *2440*
stress changes at, in poliomyelitis, *3366*
subchondral bone condensation in, 1313
subchondral resorption of, in hyperparathyroidism, 2021, *2022*
subluxation of, 2804, *2805*, 2807, *2810*
in acetabular fracture, *2811*
widening of, radiation therapy and, 3292, *3292*
Sacroiliac ligaments, 718, *720*
ankylosis of, *859*
calcification of, in X-linked hypophosphatemia, 1908, *1908*
in pelvic fracture, *2803*
interosseous, 717–718
ossification of, in diffuse idiopathic skeletal hyperostosis, *1474*
ventral, 717, *719*
Sacroiliitis, after intestinal bypass surgery, 1121t, 1134–1135, *1135*
circumscribed, 1319, *1320*

ISBN 0-7216-5067-8

T